COMMUNITY HEALTH NURSING
Caring in Action, 2nd Edition

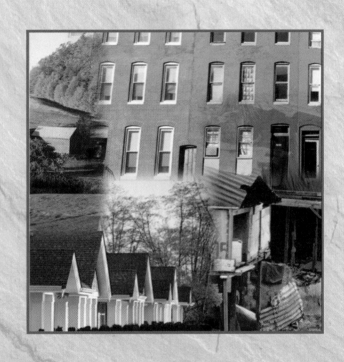

About the
ONLINE COMPANION™

Delmar Learning offers a series of Online Companions.™ Through the Delmar site on the World Wide Web, the Online Companions™ let readers access online companions that update the information in the books.

To access the *Community Health Nursing, 2E* site simply point your browser to:

http://www.DelmarNursing.com

COMMUNITY HEALTH NURSING
Caring in Action, 2nd Edition

Janice E. Hitchcock, DNSc, RN
Professor Emeritus
Department of Nursing
Sonoma State University
Rohnert Park, California

Phyllis E. Schubert, DNSc, RN, MA
Nurse Educator (retired)
California State University System
Fresno and Rohnert Park, California
Nurse Therapist, Private Practice
Carmichael, California

Sue A. Thomas, EdD, RN
Professor Emeritus
Department of Nursing
Sonoma State University
Rohnert Park, California

THOMSON
™
DELMAR LEARNING

Australia Canada Mexico Singapore Spain United Kingdom United States

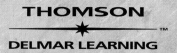

THOMSON
DELMAR LEARNING

Community Health Nursing: Caring in Action, 2e
by Janice E. Hitchcock, Phyllis E. Schubert, and Sue A. Thomas

Health Care Publishing Director:
William Brottmiller

Executive Editor
Cathy L. Esperti

Acquisitions Editor:
Matthew Filimonov

Developmental Editor:
Marah Bellegarde

Editorial Assistant:
Patricia Osborn

Executive Marketing Manager:
Dawn F. Gerrain

Channel Manager:
Jennifer McAvey

Project Editor:
Mary Ellen Cox

Production Coordinator:
Anne Sherman

Art/Design Coordinator:
Robert Plante

Technology Project Manager:
Laurie Davis

Technology Project Specialist:
Victoria Moore

Production Assistant:
Sherry McGaughan

For permission to use material from this text or product, contact us by
Tel   (800) 730-2214
Fax   (800) 730-2215
www.thomsonrights.com

Library of Congress Cataloging-in-Publication Data
Community health nursing: caring in action / [edited by] Janice Hitchcock, Phyllis E. Schubert, Sue A. Thomas.—2nd ed.
    p. ; cm.
  Includes bibliographical references and index.
  ISBN 0-7668-3497-2 (alk. paper)
  1. Community health nursing. 2. Public health nursing. I. Hitchcock, Janice E. II. Schubert, Phyllis E. III. Thomas, Sue A.
  [DNLM: 1. Community Health Nursing. 2. Public Health Nursing. WY 106 C734289 2003]
RT98.H58 2003
610.73'43—dc21   2001053866

NOTICE TO THE READER

Publisher does not warrant or guarantee any of the products described herein or perform any independent analysis in connection with any of the product information contained herein. Publisher does not assume, and expressly disclaims, any obligation to obtain and include information other than that provided to it by the manufacturer.

The reader is expressly warned to consider and adopt all safety precautions that might be indicated by the activities described herein and to avoid all potential hazards. By following the instructions contained herein, the reader willingly assumes all risks in connection with such instructions.

The publisher makes no representations or warranties of any kind, including but not limited to, the warranties of fitness for particular purpose or merchantability, nor are any such representations implied with respect to the material set forth herein, and the publisher takes no responsibility with respect to such material. The publisher shall not be liable for any special, consequential, or exemplary damages resulting, in whole or in part, from the readers' use of, or reliance upon, this material.

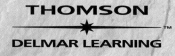

THOMSON
DELMAR LEARNING

Australia Canada Mexico Singapore Spain United Kingdom United States

Dedication

To all my friends and colleagues:
You have enriched my life beyond words. To the
memory of my family: You were always my strongest
supporters. To my students: I have learned so much
from you throughout the years.
Janice Hitchcock

To all community health nursing students, to all
nurses who work in community health settings, and
to all nurses who apply these principles. In other
words, to all nurses committed to excellence and
caring in nursing practice everywhere.
Phyllis Schubert

To my family, friends, and colleagues for their
continued support and encouragement throughout
the completion of this second edition. Your love and
caring has been very important. To my former
students and all other nurses who care!
Special thanks to the memory of my parents and
other family members who were committed to giving
back to their communities. They were highly
respected leaders and truly cared.
Sue Thomas

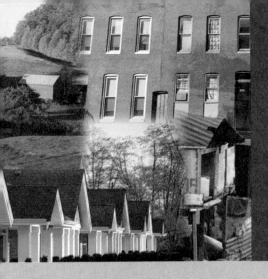

BRIEF CONTENTS

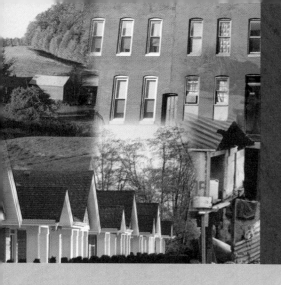

CONTENTS

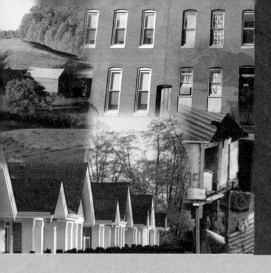

PREFACE

*C*ommunity Health Nursing: Caring in Action, second edition, now in full color, is a concise yet comprehensive text designed for nursing students and practicing nurses to provide a foundation in community health nursing practice. This new edition prepares nurses to take advantage of the opportunities and challenges present when working in the community and the ever-changing health care system.

Throughout history, community health nurses have been an integral part of health promotion and disease prevention activities as well as health care reform. With the evolving health care system and challenges that clients face in the community, the importance and necessity of community health nurses continues. There is growing awareness of the importance of strategies to promote health and prevent disease at global and national levels. More and more, there is an increasing need for nurses to care for clients in the community and provide them with services designed to promote, protect, and preserve their health. The importance of addressing aggregate needs through program planning in partnership with the community has emerged as a major strategy to improve the health of the community. With the increased complexity of health care, client advocacy is imperative.

With these issues and countless others encountered in today's world, the goals of this text are to provide a broad-based perspective of the many dimensions of public health and community health nursing.

CONCEPTUAL FRAMEWORKS

Community Health Nursing: Caring in Action, second edition, was written and designed with the reader in mind. The text builds on knowledge and skills common to all nurses, including nursing process, nursing theory, communication process, human development, and nursing care of individuals. It provides opportunities for the reader to critically apply the knowledge presented and to learn how to seek answers to questions that arise. The conceptual approach to this text is based on the following:

- *International perspectives* are interwoven as nursing is challenged to meet the health care needs of people, both nationally and internationally. It is no longer possible in today's world to look only at regional health concerns. A sense of global connectedness is necessary. The text includes contributors from Canada and Australia, countries with well-recognized public and community health systems, to enhance an international perspective.

- *Caring frameworks* are used as a basis for practice. We believe that nursing and nursing education must focus on building caring environments to promote health and healing. Caring requires a partnership between students and faculty and with clients as well as other health care professionals. It requires respect for the student's ability to think and practice and respect for the client's right to make health decisions coupled with their capacity to make appropriate decisions when given adequate health-related information.

- *Community and family concepts* are stressed throughout to prepare the student to work in the community with the family as a unit, not just with individuals within the family. Population-focused practice as well as multidimensional family dynamics and family aspects are emphasized throughout the text.

- *Integrative health practices* including healing modalities, energetic healing, visualization, and imagery are incorporated. The concept of mutual connectedness provides a framework for examining the nature of healing processes and outcomes.

- *Healthy People 2010 objectives* are fully integrated throughout the text.

ORGANIZATION

Unit I introduces the student to the practice of community health nursing as a population-focused specialty, with a presentation of caring as central to practice and an overview of caring models. The historical perspective is discussed with an emphasis on health and healing within a public health context.

Unit II highlights the many dimensions of the current health status and health care delivery system, including economic issues, in the United States and internationally. The imperative for examining health status and health care systems from a global perspective is explored.

Unit III provides the foundations of community health nursing. Philosophical, ethical, cultural, spiritual, and environmental perspectives are explored as well as the many dimensions of caring communication, defined as teaching/learning and counseling/communication. Issues in health promotion health protection and disease prevention are explored. A new chapter on integrative health care practices has been included.

Unit IV focuses on caring for populations with an emphasis on the application of the nursing process at the community level. Aggregate populations are examined along with an exploration of population-focused practice and epidemiology as a public health science. Community assessment, program planning, implementation, and evaluation are discussed in detail. Politics of health care and public policy are explained and explored. A new chapter on quality management has been added. The roles of the community health nurse take many forms, and these roles are examined and explained as well as practice specialties in community health nursing.

Unit V emphasizes caring for individuals and families in the community. Community health nurses work with families in their homes, schools, and other settings. The many aspects of the home visit are delineated and discussed. The growth and development of individuals from infancy through old age are examined. Because nurses work with individuals in all phases of the life cycle, they are expected to understand what is considered normal and recognize deviations from this pattern. Risk factors at each stage of development are emphasized. The multidimensional nature of families is explored through a discussion of frameworks for assessing families and family environments and an exploration of family functioning. The relationship of these matters to the health of the family is explored.

Unit VI deals with issues regarding the care of vulnerable populations, that is, those populations that are at high risk for health problems. Problems such as communicable disease, chronic illness, developmental disorders, mental health problems, family and community violence, substance abuse, homelessness, and rural health issues are discussed. A new chapter has been added on poverty. These are all major health problems with which community health nurses deal on a regular basis. Communicable disease, chronic disease and illness, and developmental disorders have long been the focus of community health nursing. Mental health, substance abuse, family violence, poverty, and homelessness are community health problems that the community health nurse must also address because of the magnitude in the community. We have added a section on terrorism to the Family and Community Violence chapter. It's impact on the health of a community and what part the public

health can play in dealing with its effects are discussed. Rural health needs continue to challenge the resources of community health nurses.

SPECIAL FEATURES

There are numerous special features in *Community Health Nursing: Caring in Action* designed to stimulate critical thinking and self-exploration and to encourage readers to synthesize and apply critical knowledge presented in the text.

Making the Connection boxes, a new feature, open each chapter offering linkages between the information given in a specific chapter and related textual information as discussed in other chapters.

Reflective Thinking boxes encourage readers to examine their own personal views on given topics in order to identify their own thoughts and feelings and to understand the varying viewpoints they may encounter in clients and co-workers. These boxes are designed to encourage reflection on an issue from a personal context, to raise awareness, and to stimulate critical thinking and active problem solving.

Decision Making boxes encourage the reader to develop sensitivity to ethical and moral issues. The boxes guide the reader to think critically in community health nursing practice and be active in problem-solving and decision-making processes.

Research Focus boxes feature a discussion of current research and the implications of the research on nursing practice.

Perspectives offer community health insights from the perspective of nursing students, faculty, practicing nurses, and clients. This true-life feature allows the reader to see the types of issues, experiences, and people encountered while practicing in the community.

Out of the Box, another new feature that can be found in the chapters, describes a project or a program that is on the cutting edge of community health nursing. It provides the student with examples of how creative thinking and teamwork can make positive differences in the world.

Community Health Nursing View features real-world scenarios to assist the reader in making the connection between theory and practice more easily. This feature offers critical thinking questions that provide opportunities for the reader to assess and act within the nursing environment while reinforcing knowledge of the nursing process in assessing, diagnosing, identifying outcomes, planning care, performing interventions, and evaluating the outcomes of the care.

PEDAGOGICAL FEATURES

Community Health Nursing: Caring in Action, second edition, also includes many pedagogical features that promote learning and accessibility of information.

Illustrations highlight the theories and concepts of community health nursing, and the **photographs** give insight to the many persons, places, and things that make up our local communities and the world.

Competencies open each chapter and introduce the main areas targeted for mastery in each chapter, providing a checkpoint for study.

Key Terms are boldfaced and defined in the text the first time they are used. You will also find a key term listing at the beginning of each chapter that can be used to study and check comprehension.

References at the end of the text document the theoretical basis of each chapter, and provide resources for continued study.

Web Resources found at the end of the text present web sites that contain related information pertinent to the chapter. Note: URL's change frequently. The URL's listed were current as of press date.

Glossary at the end of the book defines all key terms used in the text and serves as a comprehensive resource for study and review.

Index facilitates comprehensive access to material.

CHANGES IN THE NEW EDITION

The most visible change in this new edition is the addition of *full color* to the text. The use of full color makes the identification of the pedagogical and special features easy and the illustration come alive and provides the student with a visually appealing experience.

Three new chapters have been added: *Chapter 12, Integrative Health Care Perspectives* discusses the increasing use of integrative therapies, an overview of the thought traditions and perspectives of health care, nursing theory, and the use of integrative therapies in community health nursing and its implications for practice. *Chapter 17, Quality Management* explores the concept of quality, the historical development of the meaning of quality in health care, the use of evaluative models in quality management, and the implications it has in community health nursing. *Chapter 32, Poverty* recognizes the proliferation of poverty and its impact on health care. Dimensions of poverty are explored as well as how the community health nurse can make a significant impact on the health of the poor.

We have strived to make the content more succinct and remove redundancy found in the last edition by adding the *Making the Connection* boxes, rearranging chapter order, and making content less wordy and more clear to the reader. Chapter order has been revised in Units II and IV to improve flow of content. Nutrition content has been integrated throughout the text instead of in one chapter to stress that nutrition difficulties are affected by many variables.

Other changes or additions include:

- Discussion of terrorism and its effects
- *Healthy People 2000* goals and objectives achievement and the inclusion of *Healthy People 2010*

- Incorporation of more community/public health nursing examples
- An explanation of community-based and community-oriented nursing
- Cultural competence and its importance in community health nursing
- Introduction to concepts of social capital and capacity building
- Inclusion of block and forensic nursing
- Telemedicine and telehealth
- More information on migrant health and disaster nursing
- New theories and models, including holographic theory, the ASTDN public health nursing model, and the Donebadian model
- A *free* CD-ROM at the back of the book that contains Flashcard software that reviews concepts on a chapter-by-chapter basis
- The Hitchcock home page (http://www.delmarnursing.com/olcs/hitchcock), which contains chapter objectives, PowerPoint notes, and web links

EXTENSIVE TEACHING/LEARNING PACKAGE

The complete supplement package was developed to achieve two goals:

1. To assist students in learning the essential information needed to promote their understanding of community health nursing practice
2. To assist instructors in planning and implementing their programs for the most efficient use of time and other resources

Student Tutorial CD-ROM

A *free* student tutorial CD-ROM is packaged with each text. It is a computerized flashcard program designed to help users learn and retain large amounts of information quickly and easily. This CD-ROM contains terms and definitions in a question-and-answer format to aid in overall understanding of community health nursing. This unique program provides a fun, self-paced environment for anyone learning or brushing up on nursing concepts. User-defined preferences control how information is present—in what order, pause length between question, and more. FLASH! displays the question with the answer automatically or manually. System requirements are 100 MHz Pentium, 24 MB RAM, Microsoft Windows 95 or newer, AVGA 24-bit color display, and 8 MB disk space.

On-line Companion

Delmar offers a series of on-line companions. Through the Delmar site on the World Wide Web, the Hitchcock, Schubert, Thomas on-line companion allows users of

Community Health Nursing; Caring in Action, second edition, to access a wealth of information designed to enhance the book:

- Student resources such as Power Notes (an on-line PowerPoint presentation that supplements the text's coverage); chapter objectives that students may access anyplace, anytime; and web links to find supporting or related materials to chapter content and community assessment tools.

- Instructor resources including downloadable supplements and weblinks. See Instructor's Web Site information later on in the preface for more detailed description.

To access the site for *Community Health Nursing: Caring in Action,* second edition, simply point your browser to http://www.delmarnursing.com/olcs/hitchcock.

Community Health Nursing Case Study CD-ROM

Order number: 0-7668-3499-9.

A compilation of 20 case studies with critical thinking questions provides the student with real-life scenarios to apply community nursing principles they have learned. Topics include HIV testing, TB, herbal supplement use, well-water problems, and how they affect individuals and communities both locally and globally.

Handbook of Community Health Nursing: Tools and Resources

By Daryle Wane.

Order number: 1-4018-1273-2.

This must-have reference contains a compilation of community health assessment tools that a nurse would use when evaluating family and community health. Content includes resource data, assessment tools, screening tools, teaching tools, and intervention strategies.

Community Health and Wellness Needs Assessment: A Step-by-Step Guide

By Deena Nardi and Josy Petr.

Order number: 0-7668-3498-0.

This step-by-step guide provides the essential concepts of how to conduct a community health and wellness assessment and can be later used as a resource following graduation and transition into practice. Content is based on the Ontario Needs Impact Based Model, *Healthy People 2010* goals, and the WHO definition of health. Each chapter includes learning objectives, definitions of key terms, examples to illustrate how to conduct a community needs assessment, and examples of assessment and analysis of specific data addressing *Healthy People 2010*

goals. Community assessment tools can be found at www.delmarnursing.com/olcs/hitchcock.

ELECTRONIC INSTRUCTOR'S RESOURCE KIT

Order number: 1-4018-1279-1.

A must-have for all instructors, this comprehensive CD-ROM resource includes:

Instructor's Manual

- **Key Terms** list the key terms for each chapter alphabetically, with corresponding definitions.

- **Instructional Strategies** center on the competencies presented in each chapter and include three to five questions for the instructors to pose to students to pique their interest. These strategies also include possible answers.

- **Case Study/Theory Application** feature includes community health scenarios that allow the student to apply theory and offer the instructors helpful hints to stimulate discussion, individual exercises, group exercises, and Internet activities to reinforce the theory applications.

- **Suggested Answers** correspond to the decision-making type questions presented in the Community Nursing View feature.

Computerized Testbank

A computerized testbank contains modifiable multiple-choice questions and answers. The user can also add their own questions or let the software create tests in less than 5 minutes. Instructors can print out quizzes and tests in a variety of layouts. Innovative electronic take-home testing (put test on disk) and Internet-based testing capabilities are perfect for distance learning. Additionally, the software allows the user to include video and audio in the electronic tests.

PowerPoint

A vital resource for instructors, this PowerPoint presentation parallels the content found in the book, serving as a foundation on which instructors may customize their own unique presentations.

INSTRUCTOR'S WEB SITE

Found at http://www.delmarnursing.com/olcs/hitchcock, content includes the *Instructor's Manual* and the *PowerPoint presentation* found on the CD-ROM as well as web links for more related chapter information.

ABOUT THE AUTHORS

Janice E. Hitchcock received her diploma in nursing from New England Deaconess Hospital, Boston, Massachusetts. She obtained her baccalaureate degree from Simmons College, Boston, Massachusetts, her master's degree in psychiatric–mental health nursing/community health nursing, and her doctorate in nursing science from the University of California, San Francisco. Dr. Hitchcock is a licensed Marriage, Family and Child Counselor (MFCC) and, while continuing to teach, she also maintained a private practice in individual, couple, and family therapy for 15 years. She is currently Professor Emeritus in the Department of Nursing at Sonoma State University, Rohnert Park, California.

Dr. Hitchcock has worked in and taught psychiatric–mental health nursing and community health nursing for more than four decades. She also taught communication theory, human sexuality, and family theory. She was a founding faculty member of the Second Step nursing program at Sonoma State University in 1972. This program was the first of its kind to be accredited by the National League for Nursing. More recently, she helped to initiate a basic baccalaureate program at the same university.

Since the early 1980s until retirement she taught a general education course in human sexuality that was well received by students from all disciplines and continues to be an important part of the university curriculum. She has a special interest in gay health care and has worked with master's degree students in the nursing department and throughout the country who have replicated her doctoral research in which she developed a basic social process called "Personal Risking." This process evolved from a grounded theory analysis of interviews with lesbians in the San Francisco Bay area regarding their decision-making process of self-disclosure of their sexual orientation to health providers.

Dr. Hitchcock has a number of publications to her credit and is a member of several professional organizations, including the American Nurses Association, American Association of Sex Educators, Counselors, and Therapists, American Association of Marriage and Family Therapists, and the Society for the Scientific Study of Sex.

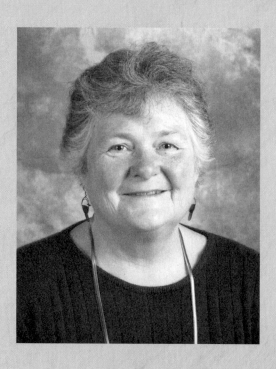

Phyllis E. Schubert received her basic nursing education in a diploma program at Los Angeles County General Hospital in California. She earned a baccalaureate degree in nursing, a master's degree in community health nursing with a school nursing focus, and a second master's degree in counseling from California State University, Fresno. She earned a doctor of nursing science degree in community health nursing with a focus in holistic nursing practice from the University of California, San Francisco.

Dr. Schubert's career in nursing has spanned the field of nursing and has included medical-surgical nursing, long-term care, school nursing in elementary and secondary schools in programs for migrant and learning disabled children, and inpatient psychiatric evaluation and care of children. She has served on nursing faculties while teaching community health nursing, nursing theory, communication skills, and holistic nursing approaches at California State University, Fresno, and Sonoma State University in Rohnert Park, California. Since retiring from the California State University System, she cofounded Nursing Therapeutics Institute in Cotati, California, an organization dedicated to the practice, education, and research of holistic nursing therapies and approaches; she has also provided health promotion and healing therapies for clients in private holistic nursing practice settings.

She has been practicing and teaching Therapeutic Touch (TT) for over 20 years and is recognized as a qualified teacher of TT by the Nurse Healers—Professional Associates, Inc. and is thus a member of the Therapeutic Touch Teachers Cooperative. She is certified by Jin Shin Jyutsu, Inc. of Scottsdale, Arizona, to practice Jin Shin Jyutsu (JSJ) and to teach JSJ self-help classes; and is certified by the Academy for Guided Imagery of Mill Valley, California, to practice Interactive Guided Imagery. She currently holds membership in the American Nurses Association/California, Nurse Healers—Professional Associates, Inc., the International Association of Interactive Imagery, the National Alliance for the Mentally Ill (NAMI), and the National Health Ministries Association. She is especially interested in the area of spiritual health, the role of the parish nurse, and developments within the field of parish nursing.

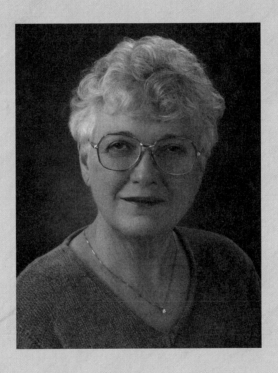

Sue A. Thomas received her baccalaureate degree in nursing at the University of California, San Francisco, attending both the University of California, Berkeley, and the University of California, San Francisco. Her master's degree in community health nursing, with a focus on administration and supervision, was obtained from Boston University School of Nursing. A Doctor of Education in Organization and Leadership was received from the University of San Francisco.

Dr. Thomas's professional career in nursing has included a variety of experiences both in the United States and in Australia. Her clinical practice in San Francisco included medical-surgical nursing, public health nursing in San Francisco's multicultural communities, school nursing within the context of public health nursing, and supervision of staff in public health nursing. She is a Professor Emeritus of nursing at Sonoma State University, Rohnert Park, California. She was responsible for coordinating the community health nursing program at Sonoma State University, teaching both community health nursing theory and clinical courses. Dr. Thomas was a founding faculty member of the Second Step nursing program at Sonoma State University in 1972, the first of its type in the nation. She also taught graduate courses in leadership and management as well as graduate and undergraduate research and served as Graduate Coordinator. Prior to teaching at Sonoma State University, Dr. Thomas also taught community health nursing theory and practice at San Francisco State University.

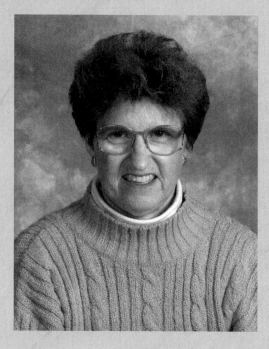

One of Dr. Thomas's major interests is international health and international nursing. She has also taught in Australia, primarily in the Melbourne area, at La Trobe University School of Nursing. She was a Visiting Fellow at the Royal Melbourne Institute of Technology School of Nursing (formerly Phillip Institute of Technology) in Melbourne. In addition, she served as nursing consultant in a variety of capacities, one of which was Curriculum Consultant at Deakin University (formerly Victoria College). In addition to teaching and consulting in Australia, Dr. Thomas was the International Coordinator of the 1992 International Caring Conference held in Melbourne, Australia—cosponsored by the International Association for Human Caring (IAHC) and the Royal College of Nursing Australia, with nurses from 14 countries represented. She was one of the charter members of the IAHC, having served for a number of years in the 1990s on the board and as a board officer. Dr. Thomas is currently on the Board of Directors of the IAHC and member of the Editorial Review Board for the *International Journal for Human Caring*.

In addition, Dr. Thomas has participated as a coinvestigator in a collaborative research team since the early 1990s, having completed state and cross-national studies focused on care delivery patterns, published in refereed journals. The cross-national study was presented at the Sigma Theta Tau, Int. International Research Congress in Utrecht, Netherlands, July 1998. Since 1998, Dr. Thomas was the principal investigator of a national study focused on care delivery regulations, also published in a refereed journal.

Dr. Thomas is also especially interested in the delivery of care to vulnerable populations, the emerging field of parish nursing, and the study of caring worldwide. She currently serves on the Advisory Council for a Nursing Center designed to meet the needs of the homeless and near homeless in an Interfaith Council Agency in the North-Bay region in California. Dr. Thomas is currently a member of the American Public Health Association, Sigma Theta Tau, Int., and the International Association for Human Caring.

ACKNOWLEDGMENTS

This text, now in it's second edition, is one that continues to highlight the essence of caring in action at local, national, and international levels. Community/public health nurses have a rich history of caring for the communities they serve in order to improve the public's health.

The authors wish to acknowledge those who have been a part of the creation of this second edition of our text. Their efforts to enrich this text are examples of caring in action. These contributors have worked diligently to share their expert knowledge and scholarship. Their endeavors reflect the future of nursing and an enthusiasm and pride in the profession—a commitment to excellence.

Students and colleagues have greatly enriched the book through generous contributions of their own clinical and personal experiences. These offerings have significantly helped to make the chapters come alive and give life to the theories and concepts presented in the text. We would like to thank Dr. Barbara Place from Melbourne, Australia, for her ongoing support of our efforts to increase the international focus in this text. She was consistently available to share her valuable ideas regarding this second edition.

The staff at Delmar have been consistently encouraging and supportive. They always came through with ideas and resources when they were needed. Marah Bellegarde, developmental editor, and Matt Filimonov, acquisitions editor, have been most helpful in responding to our questions and concerns, thereby assisting us in the completion of this project. We would like to thank Mary Ellen Cox, Anne Sherman, Bob Plante, Laurie Davis, Victoria Moore, and Sherry McGaughan, members of the production and technology staff, for their invaluable efforts.

We also want to thank all our reviewers, whose comments were helpful and who provided us with different perspectives which added considerably to the final outcome of the text.

Finally, we apologize if we have missed anyone. It was not intentional. We have valued everyone who has contributed to this project.

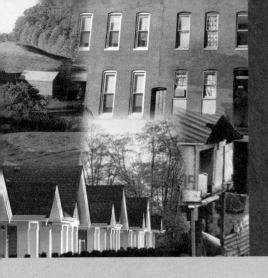

CONTRIBUTORS

David Becker, MS, RN, CS
Associate Professor of Nursing
Roxbury Community College
Boston, MA
Clinical Nurse Specialist
Community Clinical Services
McLean Hospital
Belmont, MA
Chapter 29: Mental Health and Illness

Anne L. Biggins, RN, RM, BN, MPHC
Coordinator, Quality Improvement Program for Far North
Queensland
Catholic Diocese Aged Care Services
Adelaide, Australia
Chapter 13: Population-Focused Practice

Patricia Biteman, RN, MSN
Lecturer
Humboldt State University
Arcata, CA
Chapter 34: Rural Health

Claire Budgen, RN, BSN, MSN, PhD
Professor
Okanagan University College
Kelowna, British Columbia, Canada
Adjunct Professor
University of British Columbia
Vancouver, British Columbia, Canada
Chapter 16: Program Planning, Implementation, and
Evaluation

Doris Callaghan, BScN, MSc
Associate Professor
Okanagan University College
Kelowna, British Columbia, Canada
Chapter 27: Chronic Illness

Gail Cameron, RN, BSN, MN
Professor
Okanagan University College
Kelowna, British Columbia, Canada
Chapter 16: Program Planning, Implementation, and
Evaluation

Nancy Kiernan Case, PhD, RN
Director of Clinical Support Programs
Exemplar Lutheran Medical Center
Wheat Ridge, CO
Chapter 7: Philosophical and Ethical Perspectives

Greg Crow, EdD, RN
Professor of Nursing
Sonoma State University
Rohnert Park, CA
Chapter 6: Health Care Economics

Rebekah Jo Damazo, RN, MSN
Professor of Nursing
California State University, Chico
Chico, CA
Chapter 26: Communicable Diseases

Jenny Donovan, RN, RM, MCHN, BN, MSC
Stream Coordinator, Child Adolescent and Family Health
Nursing
Senior Lecturer
School of Nursing and Midwifery
Flinders University
Adelaide, Australia
Chapter 13: Population-Focused Practice

Linda G. Dumas, PhD, RN, ANP
Associate Professor and Chairperson
Department of Community and Family Nursing
University of Massachusetts
Boston, MA
Chapter 31: Substance Abuse

Mary Beatrice Hennessey Wohn, RN, MSN
Instructor
College of Nursing
University of Massachusetts
Boston, MA
Chapter 31: Substance Abuse
Chapter 33: Homelessness

Deborah Klaas, RN, PhD
Associate Professor
Sonoma State University
Rohnert Park, CA
Chapter 23: Care of Young, Middle, and Older Adults
Chapter 28: Developmental Disorders

Carol Ann Lockhart, PhD, RN, FAAN
President
C. Lockhart Associates
Tempe, AZ
Chapter 4: Health Care Delivery in the United States

Barbara Mandleco, RN, PhD
Associate Dean of Research and Scholarship
Brigham Young University
Provo, UT
Chapter 22: Care of Infants, Children, and Adolescents

Cynthia Conger O'Neill, PhD, RN
Assistant Professor of Clinical Nursing
The University of Texas at Austin
Austin, TX
Chapter 18: Power, Politics, and Public Policy

Lindsey K. Phillips, RN, MS
Quality Assurance/Utilization Review Systems Consultant
Huckleberry Youth Programs
San Francisco, CA
Chapter 14: Epidemiology

Michelle Porter, RN, MSN, FNP
Family Practice with Jay Zaslow and Lana Nguyen
Sonoma County, CA
Sonoma County Public Health: Juvenile Health
Sonoma County, CA
Chapter 30: Family and Community Violence

June Hart Romeo, PhD, RN, NP-C
Director, Center for Poverty Studies
Cleveland State University
Cleveland, OH
Chapter 32: Poverty

Aida Sahud, DrPH, MSN, RN
Public Health Nurse (District Nurse), City of Berkeley
Berkeley, CA
Chapter 15: Assessing the Community

Diane Stafanson, RN, MSN, NP(c)
Associate Professor (Retired)
Holy Names College
Oakland, CA
Women's Health Care Nurse Practitioner
Oakland, CA
Chapter 19: Varied Roles of Community Health Nursing
Chapter 20: Practice Specialties in Community Health Nursing

Marshelle Thobaben, RN, C, MS, APNP, FNP, PHN
Professor of Nursing
Humboldt State University
Arcata, CA
Chapter 34: Rural Health

Eileen M. Willis, BEd, MEd
Senior Lecturer
School of Nursing and Midwifery
Flinders University
Adelaide, Australia
Chapter 13: Population-Focused Practice

Janice Young, RN, MS
Tuberculosis Nurse Consultant
California Department of Health Services
TB Control Branch
Berkeley, CA
Chapter 14: Epidemiology

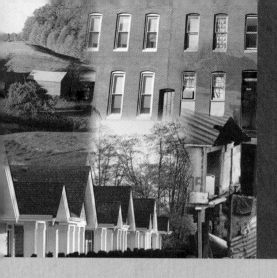

REVIEWERS

Joan Baldwin, DNSc, RN
Professor, Brigham Young University
College of Nursing
Provo, UT

Anne Dollins, CNM, PhD, MPH, MSN
Assistant Professor, Department of Nursing
Director, BSN Program
Assistant Dean, College of Professional Studies and
Education
Northern Kentucky University
Highland Heights, KY

Margaret L. Hopkins, MS, RN
Assistant Professor, Nursing Education Program
Elmira College
Elmira, NY

Patricia Leary, MEd
Professor
Ferris State University
Big Rapids, MI

Nancy Rudner Lugo, DrPH, MSN
Maitland, FL

Mary Ann Madewell, DNS, RNC
Assistant Professor of Clinical Nursing
College of Nursing
University of Cincinnati
Cincinnati, OH

Shirley Mason, EdD, RN
University of North Carolina
School of Nursing, Chapel Hill
Chapel Hill, NC

Marylyn Morris McEwen, MS, RN, CNS
Associate Specialist Interdisciplinary
School of Nursing
University of Arizona
Tucson, AZ

Deana Molinari, RN, MSN, Doctoral Candidate
School of Nursing
Brigham Young University
Provo, UT

Donald Morisky, ScD, MSPH, ScM
Professor and Vice Chair
Department of Community Health Sciences
University of California
Los Angeles, CA

Virginia Nehring, PhD, RN
Associate Professor
College of Nursing and Health
Wright State University
Dayton, OH

Karen Plotkin, RN, MS, CS, PhD(c)
University of Massachusetts at Amherst
Amherst, MA

Rebecca W. Robinson, RN, PhD
Associate Professor
West Texas A&M University
Amarillo, TX

Rachel E. Spector, PhD, RN, CTN, FAAN
Associate Professor
School of Nursing
Boston College
Chestnut Hill, MA

Carol Voght, DrPH, RN
Director of Health Service Management Program
Nursing Faculty Member
Cabarrus College of Health Sciences
Concord, NC

HOW TO USE THIS TEXT

Subject matter is presented in an innovative, interesting, and engaging manner throughout the text. The following suggests how you can use the features of this text to gain competence and confidence in community health nursing.

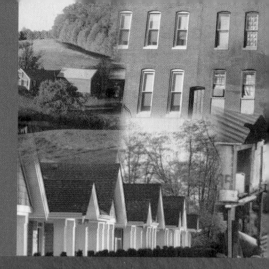

COMPETENCIES

Upon completion of this chapter, the reader should be able to:

- Recount the history of communicable diseases and identify efforts throughout history to control these diseases.
- Recognize the importance of a global perspective on communicable disease control.
- Identify modes of transmission for communicable diseases.
- Explain the difference between acquired, natural, and active immunity.

Competencies

Read the chapter competencies before reading the chapter content to set the stage for learning. Return to the competencies when the chapter study is complete to see which entries you can respond to by saying, "Yes, I can do that."

Making the Connection

Refer to these boxes before beginning a chapter to tie content between information given in a specific chapter and related information discussed in other chapters.

MAKING THE CONNECTION

Chapter 1 Caring in Community Health Nursing

Chapter 8 Cultural and Spiritual Perspectives

Chapter 10 Caring Communication and Client Teaching/Learning

Chapter 11 Health Promotion and Disease Prevention Perspectives

KEY TERMS

amended	incrementalism
author	killed
coalition	lobby
collective	policy
health care policy	political action/political activism
healthy public policy	
house of origin	

Key Terms

After reading the chapter, go back and review this list to test your comprehension of the key terms.

Reflective Thinking

This feature can help you to develop or enhance sensitivity to ethical and moral issues. You may choose to read through each one and explore issues before reading the chapter. Upon reading through the chapter, readdress each Reflective Thinking and evaluate your original thoughts. If you choose to read them as you go through the chapter, perhaps write your thoughts down, to look at them later.

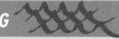

REFLECTIVE THINKING

Assessing the Problem

You are visiting Mrs. Sayer, a 70-year-old woman with severe emphysema, and her husband. Mrs. Sayer is continuously on oxygen. On her table, you notice an ashtray holding several half-smoked cigarettes.

- What is your first reaction to this observation?
- What issues of your own must you address before approaching the client regarding this observation?
- How would you develop your teaching goal? Why?
- How would you include Mr. Sayer in your teaching?

DECISION MAKING

The Age to Retire

Imagine you are a community health nurse working with the family of a frail 85-year-old woman. She lives with her daughter and her husband. The son-in-law is 68 years old, has a chronic heart problem, and receives a disability stipend. The daughter is 62 years old and has been employed as a bookkeeper at a fruit cannery for many years. She states she has not been feeling well and is finding it difficult to work all day and come home to care for her mother, who is needing more and more help. She says she would like to retire so she could stay at home with her mother but is afraid there will not be enough income to keep their home and maintain their lifestyle.

- What factors must be considered in her decision?
- How can you assist her in making this decision?

Decision Making

This feature allows you to assess and act within the community health nursing environment by offering the opportunity for you to think critically and problem solve as well as allowing you to develop sensitivity to ethical and moral issues. You may choose to read through each one and explore the situation before reading the chapter. Then as you read through the chapter, readdress each Decision Making and reevaluate your original thoughts. If you choose to read them as you go through the chapter, perhaps write your thoughts down, then go back and look at them at a later date.

Out
of the Box

Foundations Enhancing Health in Young Adulthood

Community health nurses are actively and courageously paving the way for healthy young adulthood by providing diligent, effective and creative care to teens. While adolescent behaviors are often addressed in the media, when it comes to seeking health care, they are a silent and neglected cohort, despite vast physical/mental changes, concerns, and risks. An example of nurse-led care for adolescents began in 1990 in Flagstaff, Arizona. During a youth town hall meeting, several area teens expressed desires for free, confidential health care services, particularly related to the issues of sexuality, pregnancy, violence, and substance abuse. Initially the county Department of Health Services and a Behavioral Health Center collaborated to start the Teen Wellness Clinic in which pregnancy testing and counseling were provided. The services quickly expanded to provide primary health care services for youth ages 13–19 years. Care provided by a community health nurse, two family nurse practitioners, and a behavioral health specialist now includes physical, behavioral, mental health, and social needs. All services are free and confidential, except in the case of physical illness not related to sexual activity. In this situation, parents must be contacted for consent to treat.

Seventy-five percent of client visits involved pregnancy issues when the clinic first started. Now, 10 years later, data show just 50% of visits address reproduction and pregnancy, sexually transmitted diseases (STDs), and other physical problems while 50% of the

visits address behavioral and mental health issues. Based on the success of the Teen Wellness Clinic, in 2000 funding was received to focus more on the needs of adolescent males. This clinic has been a primary factor in decreasing the teen pregnancy rate in the county and in fact has become the medical home for many at-risk, disenfranchised adolescents who would otherwise not be served or served minimally.

The clinic is open two afternoons a week from 2 P.M. until 6 P.M. on a first-come, first-served, walk-in basis. Despite the fact that clients are growing in numbers (nearly 150 are seen in a month), no teen is ever turned away. They may have to return for examinations but will always have at least the opportunity to talk with the community health nurse manager, the nurse practitioner, or the behavioral health specialist. The clinic focuses on assessment of physical and psychological issues as well as works in collaboration with other local health care agencies for appropriate referrals as necessary. The community health nurse manager is responsible for referral and follow-up for the teens seen in the clinic by the nurse practitioner and the behavioral health specialist. This community health nurse is also responsible for accountability to the various funding agencies. The Teen Wellness Clinic in Flagstaff, Arizona, is a model for an effective nurse-run community intervention that maximizes the potential for experiencing a healthy young adulthood by serving adolescents, particularly those at risk. ■

—*Kathy Ingelse, FNP, MS*
Teen Wellness Clinic

Out of the Box

As you read these stories of innovative community health programs, think about how each relates to your community. Is it something that may work in your community? Why or why not? How could it be tailored for your community? Consider the problem or challenge for which the program was designed. Brainstorm ideas with fellow students on programs you could develop that would address the same problem or challenge.

Research Focus

Emphasize the importance of clinical research in nursing by linking findings to practice. This useful learning tool focuses attention on current issues and trends in nursing, stresses the significance of evidence-based practice, and illustrates the correct way to write an abstract for a research project.

RESEARCH FOCUS

Depression and Stress in Street Youth

Study Problem/Purpose

This study explored the depression levels and coping methods of 27 youths living on the streets in Canada. Results were compared with a control group of an equal number of nonrunaway peers. The study was conducted to increase understanding of the effects of homelessness on youth in order to guide professionals to develop more effective interventions.

Methods

A questionnaire consisting of six sections (demographics, depression, self-esteem, coping methods, family background, and stress) was administered to random samples of street youths and housed high school students. Depression, self-esteem, and life stress were evaluated using standardized scales. Evaluation of the other factors is discussed.

Findings

The street youths had a significantly higher mean level of depression with the most commonly cited reasons:

money, shelter, food, family stress, and separation from friends. Street youths had a significantly higher current stress level than the nonrunaway group and reported even higher stress when living at home. The street youths generally employed less positive coping mechanisms and were more apt to engage in drug and alcohol use and self-harm. The author cautions regarding the interpretation of coping mechanisms because some of those considered maladaptive might actual serve an adaptive purpose for a child living on the street.

Implications

The article points out the necessity to evaluate homeless youths for depression, levels of stress, and danger of self-harm. Care must be taken to explore the youths' total situation when examining coping mechanisms. By first understanding the purpose of the coping mechanism, the youths might be helped to develop less harmful techniques.

Source: Ayerst, S. L. (1999). Depression and stress in street youth. Adolescence, 34 (135), 567–575.

KEY CONCEPTS

◆ The healthy family has certain identifiable characteristics that reflect its multidimensional nature. It is important to keep in mind that each family is unique and addresses these dimensions in its own way.

◆ Five major family functions are important in the nurse's work with families: the affective, socialization, economic, reproductive, and health care functions.

◆ Family process comprises several interacting dimensions that facilitate the development of family life. The major structural components are role, communication, values, power, decision making, and coping. Each of these is multifaceted.

◆ The resiliency model of family stress, adjustment, and adaptation emphasizes family adaptation and enumerates family types and levels of vulnerability. This model helps nurses deal with families in crisis.

Key Concepts

Review these main points of the chapter and use them for a beginning point of study and review.

COMMUNITY NURSING VIEW

Eiswari Osler is a divorced, 57-year-old woman. Her two daughters are grown, live in distant cities, are busy with families of their own, and call their mother approximately once a month. Eiswari works in a very busy accounting office, shouldering heavy responsibilities and working long hours. She is also active in several community organizations, filling her time with activities.

Eiswari attended a community nursing clinic for a routine physical because one of her friends worked there as a nurse. She completed a computerized health risk appraisal and was interviewed by the nurse, who took a thorough health history. The nurse identified and recorded the following lifestyle factors that placed Eiswari at risk for certain health conditions.

Physical: Walks one block each morning from her car to the office. She has a very full schedule and has not planned for further exercise. She says she enjoys these brief walks and enjoyed swimming when she was younger.

Psychological: Feels intense pressure from being in a middle-management position at work. States she feels angry a lot but tries not to lash out, and she does not have a good way to express her anger. States she has been thinking about joining a support group for women in management positions.

Sociological/physical: Has four or five female friends who exchange phone calls and meet her for lunch from time to time. Attends many social events associated with work and her community-organization activities. Tends to eat fatty, salted foods with others at work and at social events because these snack foods are always available. Smokes one pack per day and drinks scotch and water after work and at social events. Takes Valium three or four times a day for stress.

Spiritual: States she has not identified her life meaning or purpose. She simply wants to save enough money for her older years so that she will not be a burden to her children.

Environmental: Lives in the inner city and states she is concerned about traffic and safety in the streets. She carries a beeper that makes a loud noise in her purse in case of attack.

Nursing Considerations

Assessment

◆ You find that her physical examination is essentially negative. What, if any, tests (other than physical) might be indicated in her assessment?

Diagnosis

◆ Based on the information you have, what nursing diagnoses might you identify?

◆ What risk factors are inherent in Eiswari's situation?

◆ For what diseases and/or conditions would you expect her to be at risk?

Outcome Identification

◆ What are the client's goals for health behavior change?

◆ How can you help her set realistic goals?

◆ What are signs of accomplishment? Discouragement?

◆ How can you encourage and support her progress?

Planning/Interventions

◆ What strategies would you use for building a therapeutic relationship with Eiswari?

◆ How might you initiate development of a treatment plan and a contract with her?

◆ What is she choosing to work on?

◆ Does she wish to change any of her health behaviors?

◆ How will you introduce your concerns, or will you introduce them? (Refer to Chapter 10 for the mutual problem-solving process nursing checklist and follow the suggestions there.)

◆ What specific nursing therapies could you use?

◆ How would you use teaching? Counseling? Deep relaxation or guided imagery? Touch therapies?

◆ Where would you start with an educational program?

◆ What medical or community health programs might be appropriate referrals for Eiswari?

Evaluation

◆ What indicators might help you determine whether the plan is working for Eiswari?

◆ How will you know whether the plan is successful?

Community Nursing View

Community Nursing Views help you make the connection between theory and practice more easily. After you have finished the chapter, read the story presented. Then answer the critical thinking questions. Discuss your answers with fellow students. If your answers differ, consider why they differ. After hearing an explanation of an answer that differs from your own, consider whether you agree or disagree and why.

Perspectives...

INSIGHTS OF A COMMUNITY HEALTH NURSE

I work for a public health department, providing care to people who have communicable diseases. This work has given me a lot of field experience teaching people about bacteria and "bugs." Sometimes, my teaching falls on deaf ears. The population we serve is culturally diverse: Vietnamese, Laotian, Cambodian, Eretrian, Filipino, Korean, Japanese, and Spanish-speaking. I am bilingual in Spanish and English, so much of the teaching I do is with the Spanish-speaking community.

Our staff of public health aides reflects a smattering of our client population, and they are superhelpful to we Caucasian nurses regarding the culturally sensitive issues of our clients. Even so, my interventions are not always heeded, and I get disappointed. I tell myself not to have expectations—to go with the flow—but it is easy to assume that people will act how I think they should ... and when they do not, I get really disappointed. Other times, I think the people are a certain way—so I think they live in a certain kind of house, and it ends up different than what I expected. So I am often surprised because I have expectations, and things are often different than what I think they will be. I will give you a couple of examples.

A Vietnamese public health aide helped us to understand why a young Chinese woman refused to have blood drawn around the time of the Chinese New Year. He explained that it is a bad omen to take blood out of the body at any time, but especially at the New Year.

We could, then, understand why—no matter how easy we made it for this educated Chinese student—she did not follow through with our instructions. One nurse was able to use a lot of coaxing to get her to do her blood test.

Another time, I was doing follow-up on an active TB case who was Hispanic. I went to a lumbermill where the contact was the only woman who worked in the mill, a middle-aged Caucasian woman who does cleanup. She wore a hard hat, flannel jeans, work pants, and boots, and even after washing her hands, they looked dirty. The dirt was embedded in her skin. When she came to clinic appointments, she dressed the same, except without the hard hat. Her 12-year-old daughter (who could not stop talking) was also a contact. The girl was given a PPD test at the clinic and came back three days later to have it read. When the repeat PPD was done three months later there were transportation problems. I ended up taking the mom home from the clinic so I could read the girl's skin test. My expectation (I cannot get away from them) was that they would live in some sort of shack or very low-income apartment or cottage. As I pulled up to this large, modern, ranch home, I was surprised. The home was very much one you would find in any middle-class suburb. The furnishings were simple and plain.

—Anonymous

Perspectives

These musings from the student or professional nurse are intended to provide a snapshot of actual practice. They are included as a reality check as you read through the text content. It may be helpful for you to keep a running journal of your own experiences—did a certain experience affect you in some way? Journal writing is a wonderful way to begin to examine your own responses and provide other aspiring nurses the wisdom of your experiences.

NURSING AND CARING IN THE COMMUNITY

This unit introduces the student to the practice and history of community health nursing and the importance of the concepts of caring, collaboration, and partnership as they pertain to nursing, specifically community health nursing.

IN THIS UNIT

MAKING THE CONNECTION

Caring is the foundation stone of respect for human dignity and worth upon which everything else should be built. . . . When all else fails, as it eventually must in the lives of all of us, a society that gives a priority to caring . . . is worthy of praise.

—*Callahan, 1990, p. 149*

COMPETENCIES

Upon completion of this chapter, the reader should be able to:

- Identify the major goal of community health nursing practice.
- Discuss the definitions of community health and public health nursing.
- Describe the focus of community health nursing practice.
- Discuss caring as the context for nursing practice.
- Describe the concept of caring in specific relation to community health nursing.
- Discuss the meaning of caring in nursing.
- Consider the importance of establishing caring partnerships with individuals, families, and groups.
- Define *health, health promotion, health protection, healing,* and *disease/injury prevention.*
- Define public health and its focus.

KEY TERMS

aggregate	health balance
caring	health potential
community	health promotion
community-based nursing	health protection
community health	holism
community health nursing	model
community-oriented nursing practice	moral obligation
compassion	partnership
determinants of health	population-focused practice
disease and injury prevention	primary prevention
downstream thinking	public health
ecological system	public health nursing
empowerment	risk
epistemologic	secondary prevention
healing	social justice
health	tertiary prevention
	upstream thinking
	wellness

Community health nurses have a rich tradition of providing care to individuals, families, and communities. They are committed to social justice, health promotion, health protection, disease prevention, and the facilitation of healing. The major goal of community health nursing is the preservation and improvement of the health of populations and communities worldwide. To accomplish this goal, community health nurses practice in the neighborhoods and homes of individuals and families in the United States as well as in other nations. Community health nurses are keenly aware of the special application of human caring to their practice.

Community health nurses are leaders in improving the quality of health care for individuals, families, and communities. They have the knowledge and skills to work in geographically and culturally diverse settings, from large cities to isolated rural areas. Community health nurses work with many families and groups within their communities and in a variety of community health agencies, from state and national health departments to community-based neighborhood groups. The services they provide range from examining infants in a clinic setting to providing case management services to frail elders in the home. Community health nurses also carry out epidemiologic investigations and participate in health policy analysis and decision making. They are in a position to contribute to the development of community-based systems that address the current and projected health needs of populations.

This book focuses on the unique contributions that community health nurses make to improving the health of our communities and on the nature of the knowledge that these nurses must have in order to practice in the community. An emphasis on caring in this book demonstrates the authors' belief that caring is a vital force for human growth, fulfillment, promotion of health, and survival. In this opening chapter, which serves as an introduction to subsequent chapters, community health nursing is viewed within the context of caring for the health of individuals, families, and populations. This approach requires a discussion of the concept of caring and its significance to community health nursing. To illustrate the caring mission of community health nursing practice, this chapter also explores the concepts of health, public health, social justice, health promotion, health protection, disease/injury prevention, and healing.

DEFINITION AND FOCUS OF COMMUNITY HEALTH/PUBLIC HEALTH NURSING

The focus of community health/public health nursing is the health of populations. **Health** is defined as a state of well-being resulting from harmonious interaction of body, mind, spirit, and the environment. **Community health** is achieved by meeting the collective needs of the community and society by identifying problems and supporting community participation in the process. Community health nursing's scope of concern and commitment is to the entire population as distinguished from a designated individual or family focus. Community health

✴ DECISION MAKING

Community Awareness

◆ What existing health problems are you aware of in your community?

◆ If you were a community health nurse, what activities might you propose to decrease the health problems in your community?

◆ What activities are currently taking place in your community to address identified health problems?

nurses work with individuals and families within the context of the larger community. The goals of care are health promotion, health protection, the prevention of disease and injury, and healing. Health promotion activities and prevention efforts may be directed at the total population or at individuals and families within that population **aggregate,** or subgroup. Because the focus is the community, nurses must be prepared to promote the health of the community through health promotion activities and prevention efforts that address the health problems of populations.

Considerable discussion and debate have centered on the definition and focus of public health nursing and community health nursing practice. Public health nursing has certain characteristics and is viewed as a specialized field of practice within the broad arena of community health nursing (Williams, 2000). This view is consistent with those recommendations developed at a Consensus Conference on the Essentials of Public Health Nursing Practice and Education, sponsored by the U.S. Department of Health and Human Services, Division of Nursing in 1985.

Freeman (1963) provides a classic definition of **public health nursing:**

Public health nursing may be defined as a field of professional practice in nursing and in public health in which technical nursing, interpersonal, analytical, and organizational skills are applied to problems of health as they affect the community. These skills are applied in concert with those of other persons engaged in health care and through comprehensive nursing care of families and other groups and through measures for evaluation or control of threats to health, for health education of the public, and for mobilization of the public for health action. (p. 34)

The American Public Health Association (APHA) Ad Hoc Committee on Public Health Nursing (1981) put forth the following definition of public health nursing in the delivery of health care:

Public health nursing synthesizes the body of knowledge from the public health sciences and profes-

sional nursing theories for the purpose of improving the health of the entire community. This goal lies at the heart of primary prevention and health promotion and is the foundation for public health nursing practice. . . . Identifying subgroups (aggregates) within the population which are at high risk of illness, disability, or premature death, and directing resources toward these groups, is the most effective approach for accomplishing the goal of [public health nursing]. (p. 10)

The most current update of the definition of public health nursing by the APHA, Public Health Nursing Section was formulated in 1996:

Public health nursing is the practice of promoting and protecting the health of populations using knowledge from nursing, social, and public health sciences. . . . The primary focus of public health nursing is to promote health and prevent disease for entire population groups. Public health nurses work with other providers of care to plan, develop, and support systems and programs in the community to prevent problems and provide access to care. (pp. 1, 2)

The practice of public health nursing is a systematic process by which:

1. The health and health care needs of a population are assessed in order to identify those who would benefit from health promotion or who are at risk of illness, injury, disability, or premature death.

2. A plan for intervention is developed in partnership with the community to meet identified needs that takes into account resource availability, the various activities that contribute to health, and the prevention of illness, injury, disability, and premature death.

3. The plan is implemented in an effective, efficient, and equitable manner.

4. Evaluations are conducted to determine the outcomes on the health status of individuals and the population.

5. The results of the process are used to influence and direct the current delivery of care, use of health resources, and policy development and research at local, regional, state, and national levels in order to promote health and prevent disease (APHA, Public Health Nursing Section, 1996).

As can be seen, the 1996 definition of public health nursing reaffirms the 1981 definition.

Williams (2000) proposes one of the major factors that should distinguish public health nursing from other areas of specialization in nursing is practice that is community oriented and population focused, noting that a population focus is historically consistent with public health philosophy. **Community-oriented nursing prac-**

tice refers to the provision of health care through a focus on the assessment of major health and environmental problems, health surveillance, and monitoring of population health status in order to promote, protect, and maintain health and prevent disease/injury.

Community health nursing is another term that has been used, a term developed to apply to those nurses who practice in the community in contrast to institutional settings (such as school nurses, occupational nurses, nurses in clinic centers, parish nurses, and others). Since the 1980s the terms *public health nursing* and *community health nursing* have been used in the United States to describe population-focused community-oriented practice. As mentioned previously, however, public health nursing can be viewed as a specialized field of practice within the broad arena of community health nursing. Public health nurses work primarily in the public sector.

In 1980, the American Nurses Association (ANA) defined **community health nursing** as follows:

Community health nursing is a synthesis of nursing practice and public health practice applied to promoting and preserving the health of populations. The practice is general and comprehensive. It is not limited to a particular age group or diagnosis and is continuing, not episodic. The dominant responsibility is to the population as a whole; nursing directed to individuals, families, or groups contributes to the health of the total population. Health promotion, health maintenance, health education and management, as well as coordination and continuity of care are utilized in a holistic approach to the management of the health care of individuals, families, and groups in a community. (p. 2)

The Task Force on Community Health Nursing Education, Association of Community Health Nursing Educators (ACHNE) (1990), described the term *community health nursing,* stating:

Community health nursing is the synthesis of nursing theory and public health theory applied to promoting and preserving the health of populations. The focus of community health nursing practice is the community as a whole, with nursing care of individuals, families, and groups being provided within the context of promoting and preserving the health of the community. (p. 1)

Community health nursing will be used in this textbook as a broad-based term that includes the various specialty fields of practice: public health nursing, school nursing, occupational health nursing, parish nursing, and others. Recently, discussion has occurred regarding the emergence of a term in nursing—**community-based nursing.** In 1998, a statement on the Scope of Public Health Practice was developed by the Quad Council of

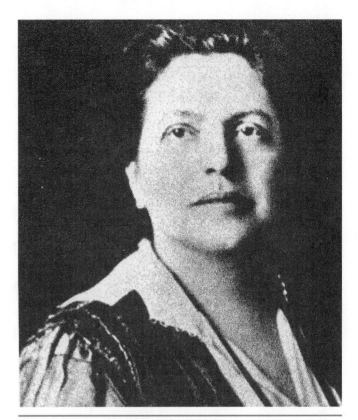

Lillian Wald. Photo courtesy of American Nurses Association.

the American Nurses Association in order to clarify the difference between community-based nursing and public health/community health nursing (Williams, 2000). Community-based nursing is referred to as that practice in nursing which focuses on the provision of personal care to individuals and families in the community. In contrast, public health and community health nursing generalists and specialists focus on the population as a whole.

Early public health nursing pioneers demonstrated the distinction between the definitions. In the late 1800s, Lillian Wald, at Henry Street Settlement House, New York City, and Mary Brewster, New York City Visiting Nurse Service, not only focused on the importance of working with individuals and families in the community but also recognized the need to become social activists. They worked toward the improvement of health education and health standards in their communities. Both Wald and Brewster recognized the need to bring nursing services into the homes of those who were experiencing poor health and who were living under unhealthy conditions in the community. Their vision extended beyond caring for families during illness to include a reform agenda aimed at effecting public policy to improve the unhealthy conditions in their city. Early public health nurses led many of the policy revolutions that helped bring family planning, workplace safety, and maternal child health services to populations in need (Salmon, 1993).

RESEARCH FOCUS

Preparing Currently Employed Public Health Nurses for Changes in the Health System

Study Problem/Purpose

Changes taking place in health services require additional skills in assessment, policy development, and assurance. In order to provide both public health practice at the community level and population-focused individual health care services, public health nurses need further preparation. The purpose of this study was to describe a core public health nursing curriculum, part of a larger project designed to identify the skills needed by public health nurses in the current and future public health system.

Methods

Two focus groups of key informants representing state and local public health nursing practice, public health nursing education, federal agencies, organizations interested in public health and nursing education, and academia outlined key content for a continuing education curriculum for current public health nurses. Material was synthesized from multiple sources.

The first focus group was comprised of 25 informants selected on the basis of elected and appointed positions, publication history, and peer recommendation. The participants in the second group included rep-

resentatives from the first group, with additional participants who were state nursing directors, each of whom was accompanied by one staff public health nurse.

Findings

The skills and knowledge identified as most needed were those required for data analysis/statistics, epidemiology and its application, health status measurement and organizational change, how people connect to organizations, skills to bring about organizational change, conducting population-based interventions, coalition building, environmental health, developing interdisciplinary teams and policy development, program evaluation, and quality improvement.

Implications

It is essential that collaboration takes place between public health nursing practice and education. Partnerships also with other public health agencies will be necessary in order for public health nurses to develop the required skills necessary to enhance their ability to address public health infrastructure needs.

Source: Gebbie, K. M., & Hwang, I. (2000). Preparing currently employed public health nurses for changes in the health system. American Journal of Public Health, 90 (5), 716–721.

Wald (1971) and her colleagues utilized direct clinical nursing practice in the home combined with collective political activities as their two major approaches to improve the health of the **community,** a group of people sharing common interests, needs, resources, and environment. Although these early public health nurses worked closely with individuals and families within communities, they realized that the social and environmental **determinants of health** (factors that influence the risk for health outcomes, such as pollution, poverty, and child labor) required collective action aimed at improving the social and environmental conditions. The need to affirm direct clinical practice and social activism as the two approaches applied in community health nursing practice is just as pertinent today. Interesting parallels exist between the late-20th-century and early-21st-century dilemmas and those confronted by Wald and her public health nurse associates over 100 years ago. Now, as then, frightening diseases, alienation of the poor, a problematic economic climate, and unmet health care needs of populations at great risk constitute serious

health care issues. In the last two decades, many U.S. cities had epidemics that challenged the belief that such occurrences in industrialized nations were a thing of the past, conditions such as human immunodeficiency virus (HIV), asthma, and tuberculosis. Those at the margins of society—the homeless, the incarcerated in prisons, those living in extreme poverty—experience rates of poor health many times higher than other members of the population (Freudenberg, 2000). This is clearly a moment in time when nurses can provide assistance in meeting societal needs for community-based health care.

Population-Focused Practice

It is important to understand that population-focused practice is central to community health nursing; this perspective is different from that of nursing practice focused primarily on providing services to individuals and families. Population-focused practice is discussed in greater detail in Chapter 13, but an introduction is in order here.

REFLECTIVE THINKING

Social Mission of Nursing

- What does social activism mean to you?
- What feelings arise for you when you consider the level of poverty in your community? What does poverty mean to you?
- What do you think are the unmet needs in your neighborhood?

Population-focused practice, as differentiated from individual practice, is based on the notion that an understanding of the population's health is critical. A population's problems and strengths (assets) are defined (diagnoses) and solutions (interventions) are proposed, in contrast to diagnoses and interventions at the individual client level. The population focus is consistent with public health philosophy and is a fundamental principle that distinguishes community health nursing from the other nursing specialties.

A population focus requires thinking upstream, looking beyond the individual. McKinlay (1979) challenged health professionals to focus more on **upstream thinking,** "where real problems lie" (p. 9). Upstream strategies focus on identifying and modifying economic, political, and environmental variables that are contributing factors to poor health worldwide. For example, a population focus would require consideration of those who may need particular services but who either have not entered the health care system or do not have access to an acceptable, compassionate service system (e.g., homeless or near-homeless elderly persons with untreated hypertension, diabetes, or foot infections; nonimmunized children). **Downstream thinking** refers to a microscopic focus characterized primarily by short-term, individual-based interventions. Out of the Box tells the story of a successful population-focused practice.

Out
of the Box

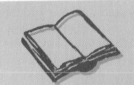

In 1991, a committee was formed by a group of professional women committed to eliminating elder homelessness in Boston. The committee, called the Committee to End Elder Homelessness (CEEH), continues to exist to this day. The original and continuing Board President is Anna Bissonnette, RN, MS, a community health nurse and faculty member at Boston University School of Medicine. Bissonnette was also a founder of CEEH. Her vision, leadership, and activism in advocating for the rights of elders helped increase public awareness of the problem of elder homelessness. She has worked to reach out to elders at risk and to create housing and health service options for homeless individuals. The CEEH conducted a comprehensive survey to determine the extent of elder homelessness, worked to create a shared-living home for formerly homeless women in Jamaica Plain, sponsored apartments for homeless men and women, and developed an extensive outreach program to assist the homeless. In 1996, CEEH launched a second project: the renovation of a former warehouse into 40 apartments for homeless elderly men and women who are coping with mental and/or physical health problems. The project was completed in 1997. Health services are provided within this South Boston facility, creating a model assisted-living program. In 2000, a third housing project in Brookline, Massachusetts, was completed. Because of the ingenuity, compassion, and commitment with which Anna Bissonnette and her committee have worked to meet the health care needs of people in their community, Bissonnette received the Robert Wood Johnson Leadership Award in 1994, the Massachusetts Gerontology Louis Lowy Award and the Massachusetts Health Council Award in 1998, in addition to being recognized by the mayor of Boston for her advocacy for justice for the elderly homeless.

Since 2000, the outstanding leadership and activism of Anna Bissonnette and her committee continues, demonstrating their ongoing commitment to improve the health of the homeless elderly. A fourth residence opened in the fall of 2001 in Roxbury, Massachusetts. This residence is the first of its kind in Massachusetts, an assisted-living facility targeting homeless and frail elders. The very poorest of frail elders will have access to this service-enriched senior housing. This project of the CEEH is yet another example of how caring action can truly make a difference! ■

INTRODUCTION TO CARING IN COMMUNITY HEALTH NURSING

Caring is defined as those assistive, enabling, supportive, or facilitative behaviors toward or for another individual or group to promote health, prevent disease, injury, and facilitate healing. Historically, community health nurses have worked to establish caring **partnerships** with families and communities. As such, they focus on developing relationships with those they serve, basing their services on the **empowerment** (enabling others to acquire the knowledge and skills needed for informed decision making and affording others the authority to make decisions that affect them) of others and on fostering mutual respect and cooperation. The nurse's facilitation of a humane and healing environment is central to community nursing practice.

Community health nurses manifest their caring perspective through their work with individuals, families, and groups as well as through their participation in formulating public policy. Many community health nurses work with marginalized populations—the poor or disenfranchised. Consistent with the definition of caring, they work to develop trusting relationships with the families and communities in order to promote health, prevent disease, and facilitate healing. Community health nurses are thus essential instruments of caring and can assist in transforming the present and future health care system by demonstrating actions that are courageous, competent, compassionate, and creative at local, state, national, and international levels. As Roach (1991) suggests:

> The nursing profession, by its very nature and mandate, has the great privilege of standing in the health care world with a tradition of . . . caring. Its power for moving the world toward a more humane resolution of the crises it now experiences is both formidable and reassuring. (p. 8)

Nurses offer important means of assessing the health of populations and the impact of environmental hazards on that health, establishing open lines of communication within the community and conveying information about health standards and **risks.** As trusted health professionals, nurses are frequently able to enter and move within communities in ways not possible for others. The community health nurse knows ways to reach out to people, facilitate growth in the direction of wholeness and health, and encourage the development of trust.

Meaning of Caring for Community Health Nurses

The concept of caring is central to community health nursing practice. It is a constructive concept, that is, one that affirms those qualities that foster health and facilitate healing. Caring provides both the context and energy for nurses to work in diverse communities ranging from isolated rural areas to the crowded cities.

Caring is a dynamic state of consciousness (Gaut, 1993) where nurses' thoughts, feelings, and actions determine how deeply they care about the communities they serve, the nature of their work with individuals, families, and groups as well as their participation in public policy making and change. The power of caring enables community health nurses to awaken those energies that illuminate and enable their participation in social transformation. As community health nurses become engaged in creating new possibilities for the health care system worldwide, social transformation becomes a reality.

To meet the health needs of the population, the community health nurse brings a sensitivity to the many individuals and groups in the community, with respect for their cultural lifeways and patterns, spiritual needs, values, health beliefs, and methods of managing their unique problems. The practice of community nursing is diverse and adaptable to different age and socioeconomic groups as well as cultural and ethnic groups in a variety of settings. Within the context of this diverse nursing practice, the nurse has the opportunity and responsibility to foster health by providing a caring presence in the company of human vulnerability and suffering. At the population level, the community health nurse would demonstrate caring by, for example, examining the prevalence of hypertension among different age, racial, gender, and socioeconomic groups, identifying those subpopulations with the highest rates of untreated hypertension, and determining those programs that could reduce the prevalence of untreated hypertension.

An increasing number of nurses worldwide are recognizing the power of caring in relation to their work with individuals, families, and communities. Caring en-

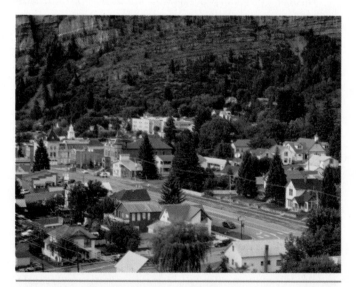

Community health nurses provide care to people in a variety of settings.

ables nurses to identify problems, recognize possible solutions, and implement those solutions (Benner & Wrubel, 1989) within the context of a healing environment. **Holism** is the belief that living beings are interacting wholes who are more than the mere sum of their parts. A caring, holistic practice perspective "enlarges the notion of the human from a duality of mind and body, to one that respects the simultaneous and continuous interaction of person, environment and health" (Gaut, 1993a, p. 167). As such, human beings are viewed in the context of the **ecological system** (the interrelationship between living things and their environment)—as part and parcel of a whole. Health and healing, together with the concept of wholeness, are integrated in family and community life.

Believing that caring is central to nursing practice, nurse scholars have studied dimensions of caring in different contexts. An increasing number of nurses from countries around the world are interested in studying care and caring from philosophical, **epistemologic** (pertaining to the nature and foundation of knowledge), economic, administrative, educational, and practice perspectives. Human caring is viewed as one of the most essential characteristics that assist people to maintain health, recover from illness, and die with dignity. As Roach (1991) succinctly states, "Caring is the expression of our humanity, and it is essential to our development and fulfillment as human beings" (p. 8).

The earliest studies of caring in nursing trace back to the early 1960s and the Gadsups of New Guinea, when Leininger (1977) identified various perceptions of caring, such as protection, nurturance, and surveillance. On the basis of her early work, Leininger (1977) went on to describe the phenomenon of care and caring as an essential human need, necessary for health, well-being, human development, and survival. In subsequent work, Leininger further explored the concept of caring from a combined anthropological and nursing perspective, with the cultural meaning of human caring being the focus of concern. Leininger's important discoveries related to the concept of caring laid the foundation for other researchers to follow.

The concept of caring continues to receive increased attention and emphasis in health care and nursing. In addition, caring has been recognized as an important concept to many other disciplines, as reflected in the various meanings of human caring described by those in the sociobehavioral sciences, anthropology, fine arts, psychoneuroimmunology, philosophy and ethics, and theology (Lakomy, 1993). Lakomy points out that "the meanings of caring have suggested both diversity and a universal theme" (1993, p. 181). An understanding of caring in a variety of contexts is therefore imperative for community health nursing. The systematic study of caring; the development of theoretical models of caring; the significance of caring in relation to individual, family, and community outcomes; and the examination of car-

ing from health policy perspectives and in comparative contexts are of major importance. A recent international conference in June 2001, for example, sponsored by the International Association for Human Caring and the University of Stirling in Scotland highlighted the importance of exploring the phenomenon of caring approaches to the study of caring across disciplines. The conference focused on "creating communities of caring—global initiatives." Nurses from Australia, Canada, the Netherlands, New Zealand, the United Kingdom, Germany, Japan, Sweden, Taiwan, and the United States participated in the conference, attesting to the importance of caring in nursing.

The implications of caring for community health nurses are clear. A caring perspective requires the community health nurse to approach individuals, families, and groups from a holistic viewpoint, where principles of wholeness, harmony, and healing speak strongly to the nature of health.

Definitions of Caring

Caring has been defined in a number of different ways. A review of the various definitions suggests a diversity in the conceptualization of caring. Each of the definitions is important for community health nurses to examine because each has implications for practice. Leininger (1991) defines caring as "those actions and activities directed toward assisting, supporting, or enabling another individual or group with evident or anticipated needs to ameliorate or improve a human condition or lifeway" (p. 4) or to face death. Larson (1986) defines caring as the intentional attitudes and actions that convey emotional concern and physical care and that promote a sense of safeness and security in another.

Other definitions of caring emphasize that caring is a motivation to protect the welfare of another person or to assist that person to grow and actualize the self (Gaylin, 1976; Mayeroff, 1971).

Fry (1993) states that human caring "is a moral concept when caring is directed toward human needs and is perceived as a duty to respond to need" (p. 176). Watson (1985, 1988) characterizes caring as the moral ideal of nursing; a commitment, an intention. Caring has also been conceptualized as the human mode of being (Roach, 1991). As the human mode of being, caring is not unique to nursing but, rather, is unique in nursing as the concept

> which subsumes all the attributes descriptive of nursing as a human, helping discipline. Nursing is no more or no less than the professionalization of the human capacity to care through the acquisition and application of the knowledge, attitudes, and skills appropriate to nursing's prescribed roles. (p. 9)

FIGURE 1-1 Dimensions of Caring

Compassion

Competence

Confidence

Conscience

Commitment

Roach (1991) proposed that caring involves five different expressons.

REFLECTIVE THINKING

The Meaning of Caring

- What does caring mean to you?
- What are some examples of a nurse who demonstrates caring behaviors with families and populations?
- How might you feel if you thought a nurse was uncaring?

Roach proposes a helpful categorization of the concept of caring, stating that caring involves a number of different expressions. She identified these expressions as the five C's: compassion, competence, confidence, conscience, and commitment (see Figure 1-1). These dimensions of caring have significance for community health nurses as these nurses develop partnerships with individuals, families, communities, and health team members.

Boykin and Schoenhofer (1993) describe caring as "the intentional and authentic presence of the nurse with another who is recognized as person living caring and growing in caring" (p. 25). The nurse-client relationship is viewed as egalitarian and a shared lived experience.

Caring provides the central focus for community nursing practice. Community health nurses work with vulnerable populations—the wounded and those who are suffering. Because the community health nurse enters into the lives of people in their homes, in schools, in clinics, and in other settings, it is essential that nurses develop a philosophical and ethical framework to guide and evaluate their nursing practice. Understanding the meaning of caring is central to developing effective relationships and to promoting health and **wellness** (a group's progression to a higher level of functioning) within the context of community health nursing practice.

Ray (1999) clearly points out that the future of caring in our challenging health care environment is social, transcultural, and "communal moral caring" (p. 10). Ray further states:

It is a commitment to a communitarian agenda—to a new reflective and ethical imagination that upholds and enhances the dignity of clients, health care professionals, and all citizens. It is a call to act now to advance a compassionate and just health care system for all, regardless of cultural identity, health status, personal income, or political persuasion. It is a time when nurses must take a more profound leadership role in health and social policy development. (p. 10)

Caring Themes and Models

Just as no consensus exists regarding the definition of caring, the concept itself can be viewed through different lenses. Caring is understood in a context. In other words, various behaviors may be experienced as caring, depending on the needs and values of the individual, family, or group. As Snyder, Brandt, and Tseng (2000) note, "No one definition of caring emerges. What is clear—is that caring is a multidimensional phenomenon which involves physical, mental, emotional, and spiritual aspects and is a critical component of patient care provided by nurses" (p. 37).

An examination of the concept of caring by Morse, Bottorff, Neander, and Solberg (1991) resulted in the identification of five epistemological perspectives, based on their content analysis of 35 definitions of caring. These perspectives included caring as a human trait, caring as a moral imperative or ideal, caring as an affect, caring as an interpersonal relationship, and caring as a therapeutic nursing intervention. Community health nurses must learn to identify the meanings that the various conceptual categories have for them. Nurses must also learn to identify the meaning of caring from the perspectives of the individuals, families, and communities they serve.

Fry (1991, 1993) developed a helpful description of the models of human caring that emphasizes the various attributes of the concept. A **model** provides a frame of reference for members of a discipline to guide their thinking about observations and interpretations (Fawcett, 1995). A conceptual model refers to ideas about individuals, groups, situations, and events of interest. Models are based on the concepts considered to be relevant. The first and most widely used model of caring is the cultural model developed from anthropological and sociological studies of caring behaviors in various cultural groups. The cultural model relates caring to cultural beliefs, practices, and human survival (Leininger, 1984). It is discussed in greater detail in Chapter 8.

A feminist model of caring relates human caring to the perspective of feminine moral development (Gilligan, 1977) and identifies caring as an attitude that can be learned and nurtured through education (Noddings, 1984). Noddings described caring as an attitude that expresses our earliest memories of being "cared for." The feminist model has received a great deal of attention in nursing.

Another model, described as a humanistic model of caring, relates human caring to a **moral obligation** or duty (Pellegrino, 1985). Pellegrino believes that caring as a professional duty is an obligation to promote the good of someone—to promote the welfare and well-being of the client.

Humanistic models of caring have been developed by a number of nurse scholars (Gadow, 1980, 1985; Gaut, 1981, 1989; Ray, 1981, 1987; Roach, 1989; Watson, 1985). These authors characterize caring as an intention, a will, a commitment, and an ideal. Caring is viewed as a way of being that is supported by a philosophy of moral commitment directed toward preserving humanity and protecting human dignity.

Fry (1991) proposed an obligation model of caring, which emphasizes compassion, doing good for others, and competence. The purpose of caring is directed toward the good of the individual. Fry (1993) also proposed a covenant-oriented model of caring, which emphasizes the presence of fidelity in relationships. Fidelity between persons flows from the covenant made between persons when they exist in particular relationships with each other: teacher and student, nurse and client, mother and child. Nurse caring, as proposed in this model, embodies **compassion:** doing for others, respect for persons, and the protection of human dignity.

Thus different conceptual approaches have been developed in the attempt to understand the phenomenon of human caring. Each of the models of caring is important because it indicates that caring encompasses different dimensions in a variety of contexts. In community health nursing, caring is more than an ideal, a commitment, or a sentiment; it is a science, an art, an action, and definitely not an exercise in passivity. Caring is a moral obligation that requires nurses to manifest those acts and processes directed toward meeting expressed or anticipated human needs in ways that are perceived as competent, compassionate, supportive, and growth enhancing.

CONTEXT FOR COMMUNITY HEALTH NURSING

The major goal of community health nursing is the preservation of the health of populations through a focus on health promotion, health protection, and health maintenance. In order to accomplish this goal, the community health nurse is oriented toward health and the identification of populations at risk. For the purpose of illustrating the caring mission of community health nursing as a population-focused practice, the concepts of health, public health, social justice, health promotion, health protection, disease/injury prevention, and healing are explored.

Health

The term *health* has been defined in a number of different ways and is an evolving concept. The World Health Organization (WHO) (1974) formulated a classic definition of health as "a state of complete physical, mental, and social well-being and not merely the absence of disease or infirmity" (p. 1). This definition of health introduced the area of social well-being, thereby linking health and social life and health and social policy. The WHO definition thus called attention to the multidimensional nature of health. The WHO views health within the social context. Health is not only a personal responsibility but is influenced by the physical and social environments.

Pickett and Hanlon (1990) describe health as being on a continuum and emphasize the absence of disability. They state that "a disease or injury is any phenomenon that may lead to impairment" (p. 5). Kickbusch (1989) suggests that we need to reexamine our understanding of health itself in view of both the changing lifestyles of our societies and the new, more inner directed values emerging in industrialized countries. Value orientations today view human beings in the context of the ecological system, with the individual a part of a whole. In this context, the health of an individual is related not only to the physical self but also to the mind and spirit. Kickbusch (1989) states, "Health is integrated in family and community life, is dependent on the physical as much as on the socioeconomic environment. It is constituted through the interaction of human biology and personal behavior and is created within a totality of culture and biosphere" (p. 48). Further discussion of environmental factors will be discussed in Chapters 3 and 9.

Health is therefore viewed as a necessary element in improving peoples' lives; however, Rodriquez-Garcia and Akhter (2000) suggest that health alone, separate from social, economic, and political developments and social justice, cannot improve the human condition or promote human development. Health issues must therefore be placed in the arena of public concern.

Health, as Pender (1996) points out, is increasingly recognized as a concept that is not only multidimensional but applicable to individuals and population aggregates as well. Health is a dynamic process inherent in the life experience of families and communities.

Over the course of time, views on health and illness have diverged significantly and in various systems of sociocultural values. Differences can be noticed among subcultures, smaller communities, and individuals. Thus, health is a complex phenomenon that is given form and meaning according to how it is perceived (Nijuis, 1989). It is, therefore, imperative that the community health nurse examine the ways individuals, families, and communities define health.

Public Health

Many attempts have been made to define the term *public health,* and, clearly, the definitions have changed over time. Early definitions focused on the sanitary measures utilized against nuisances and health hazards (Pickett & Hanlon, 1990). With the bacteriologic and immunologic discoveries of the late 19th and early 20th centuries and the development of techniques for the application of these discoveries, the concept of disease prevention was added. Public health then came to be viewed as an integration of sanitation and medical sciences. Today, public health is also regarded as a social science.

One of the best known and most widely accepted definitions of public health was the one formulated by Winslow in 1920 (Hanlon & Pickett, 1984):

Public Health is the science and art of (1) preventing disease, (2) prolonging life, and (3) promoting health and efficiency through organized community effort for

a. the sanitation of the environment

b. the control of communicable infections

c. the education of the individual in personal hygiene

d. the organization of medical and nursing services for the early diagnosis and preventive treatment of disease

e. the development of social machinery to ensure everyone a standard of living adequate for the maintenance of health, so organizing these benefits enables every citizen to realize his birthright of health and longevity. (p. 4)

A more recent definition of public health was published in the 1988 Institute of Medicine (IOM) Report, which addressed the future of public health. In that report, **public health** was defined as "organized community efforts aimed at the prevention of disease and promotion of health" (IOM, 1988, p. 41). Public health was also described as "what we, as a society, do collectively to assure the conditions in which people can be healthy" (IOM, 1988, p. 41).

In its 1988 report, the IOM indicated that the mission of public health could be addressed by both private and public groups as well as by individuals but that the government had a specific function: ensuring that the vital elements are in place and that the mission is adequately addressed (IOM, 1988). In order to clarify the govern-

ment's role, the report refers to the public health core functions at all levels of government: (1) assessment of the population and monitoring of the population's health status and disseminating that information; (2) policy development, which refers to developing policies that use scientific knowledge in decision making for the purpose of promoting the health of the population; and (3) assurance, which refers to the role of public health in making sure that basic, communitywide health services are available and accessible as well as ensuring that a competent public health staff is available. The purpose of public health in the United States is to prevent epidemics and the spread of disease, protect against environmental hazards, prevent injuries, promote and encourage healthy behaviors, respond to disasters and assist communities in their recovery, and ensure the quality and accessibility of health services (Public Health Functions Steering Committee, 1994).

Organized public health efforts a century ago were developed in the political arena of social reform. Many of the public health pioneers were social policy reformers. They were pioneers in relation to promoting an understanding of the relationship between health, work, labor, housing, and sanitation from the perspectives of various disciplines and political alignments (Kickbusch, 1989). Various sectors of the community worked together to bring about the major changes in the health of populations at the turn of the century. Much of this early innovation was introduced by local authorities at the city level. The early public health efforts were linked to social policy, environmental health, and housing policy. These efforts were viewed as an expression of societal progress.

Over the past 100 years, the focus of public health has changed. Kickbusch (1989) contends that public health has become medicalized, with a primary focus on large-scale, disease-based interventions. These interventions focused primarily on the organization of medical services rather than on systems that promote health and prevent illness. The link to social policy had become less obvious. Measures such as health promotion, prevention, environmental protection, and social interventions became less important in a system focused on disease and disease intervention.

Since the late 1980s, however, the WHO (1989) recognized the need to reaffirm the basic tenets of the "old public health," to create a renaissance of public health thinking and action. Public health is once again based on a "social and ecological understanding of health" (WHO, 1989, p. 44) with public health in a stage "where it aims to move from planning for sick factors to truly planning for health. That implies setting goals for policy action and not just goals to alter individual and family behavior" (pp. 46–47). In 1978 WHO (1989) articulated the goal that, by the year 2000, all people in all countries should have a level of health that will enable them to work productively and to participate actively in the social life of the community in which they live. This WHO initiative

REFLECTIVE THINKING

The Meaning of Health

- What does the term *health* mean to you?
- How would you describe the health of your community?
- What health-promotion activities that might transform the health of your community would you support?

became known as Health for All by 2000 and will be discussed further in Chapter 2.

In 1998, the WHO reaffirmed the Health for All process and endorsed the new World Health Declaration and new global health policy—"Health For All in the 21st Century" (WHO, 1998a). This new policy builds on past achievements and guides actions and policy for health at international, national, regional, and local levels. It also identifies global priorities and targets for the first 20 years of this century (WHO, 1998b). In the United States, Healthy People 2010 is an example of a national response to the WHO global health policy. Further discussion of these global and national policies will be discussed in subsequent chapters.

In 1989, Kickbusch, from the WHO, pointed out that the link between political action, social reform, and public health efforts—characteristic of the earlier public health approach—had to be reestablished. Public health efforts also had to be linked to societal planning and to a notion of social change (Kickbusch, 1989). Since 1989, action has taken place at local, state, national, and international levels to improve the health of cities and communities. Interest in world health has grown as well as interest in ways to improve it. As just stated previously, in 1998 for example, the WHO discussed strategies for achieving the goals of Health for All (HFA) and the identification of global priorities and 10 global targets for the first 20 years of the 21st century. In Chapters 2 and 5, these actions, strategies, and targets are discussed in greater detail. Community health nurses have a very significant role to play in terms of planning for the transformative process that must occur.

Public Health Essential Services

As previously mentioned, the IOM in 1988 published a report which identified the public health core functions at all governmental levels: assessment, policy development, and assurance. Public health nurses are thus expected to incorporate the core public health functions within the

framework of their practice. This means that public health nurses require additional skills in population assessment, policy development, and assurance to provide necessary population-based services at community, family, and individual levels (Gebbie & Hwang, 2000).

In 1994, the Public Health Service Functions Steering Committee (1994) identified essential public health services that address the core functions discussed previously:

1. Monitor health status to identify community health problems.
2. Diagnose and investigate health problems and health hazards in the community.
3. Inform, educate, and empower people about health issues.
4. Mobilize community partnerships to identify and solve problems.
5. Develop policies and plans that support individual and community health efforts.
6. Enforce laws and regulations that protect health and ensure safety.
7. Link people to needed personal health services and assure the provision of health care when otherwise unavailable.
8. Assure a competent public health and personal health care work force.
9. Evaluate effectiveness, accessibility, and quality of personal and population-based health services.
10. Research new insights and innovative solutions to health problems.

It is critical that public health nurses be prepared to develop skills in these areas since they are expected to provide many of these services throughout the United States.

Social Justice

Social justice is the mission of public health. With its focus on the protection and preservation of the health of the population, public health has an egalitarian tradition. **Social justice** is that form of justice that entitles all persons to basic provisions such as adequate income and health protection. In the event that persons are not able to provide for their basic necessities, collective action is taken to make such necessities available. In public health, therefore, collective action addresses a health ethic that focuses on health and the identification of populations at risk in order to promote and preserve health. Thus, public health policy addresses not only lifestyle changes but also social and environmental factors that impinge on health. It should be pointed out here that, in the United States, the predominant model of justice is the *market justice* model, a model that assigns entitlement based on that which has been gained through primarily individual efforts.

As Rodriquez-Garcia and Akhter (2000) so clearly point out, however, the values that are basic to public health are the values of human rights. Thus, "when social justice is compromised, human suffering escalates— We must foster a social consciousness among decision makers, in both the private and public sectors. We must educate health professionals about the universal principles and values that prescribe social justice and adherence to human rights" (p. 694).

Ensuring social justice for all people is essential to prevent human suffering and advance human development. As Ray (1999) suggests, there is a need to "cultivate a reflective, social, and moral conscience as the foundation to the creation of authentic community, and subsequently, health care reform for health security is necessary" (p. 10).

Health Promotion and Health Protection

I believe promotion of health is far more important than the care of the sick. I believe there is more to be gained by helping every man learn how to be healthy than by preparing the most skilled therapists for service to those in crises. (Henderson, 1993, p. 40)

The concepts of health promotion, health protection, and disease/injury prevention are crucial ones in relation to understanding the mission of public health and, thus, community health nursing. The ideas for health promotion and disease prevention continue to evolve, in addition to increasing access to and improving the quality of health care, reducing risk behavior, and improving social conditions (Freudenberg, 2000).

Health promotion can be defined as those activities related to individual lifestyle and choices and designed to improve or maintain health. Noack (1987) emphasizes that health promotion comprises those efforts directed toward the protection, maintenance, and improvement of **health potential** (the ability to cope with environmental changes) and, hence, **health balance** (the state of well-being resulting from the harmonious interaction of body, mind, spirit, and the environment). Thus, there is an individual as well as a community component to health promotion. The individual component seeks to improve health potential through immunizations, adequate nutrition, education, counseling, exercise, and social support. The community component aims to improve the health of the community through multisectoral, holistic, political, legislative, and administrative efforts. The community's health is sustained through the maintenance or establishment of health services, healthy working environments, information networks, and self-help programs.

Probably the most widely cited definition of health promotion can be found in the Ottawa Charter for Health Promotion (1987):

DECISION MAKING

Health Promotion

◆ What activities or programs in your community emphasize health promotion?

◆ How might you find out about such activities?

◆ Do any of the "health programs" in your community benefit you or your family? If so, how? If not, how might you assist in developing a program of benefit to you? To others in your community?

Health promotion is the process of enabling people to increase control over, and to improve, their health. To reach a state of complete physical, mental, and social well-being, an individual or group must be able to identify and to realize aspirations, to satisfy needs, and to change or cope with the environment. Health is, therefore, seen as a resource for everyday life, not the objective of living. Health is a positive concept emphasizing social and personal resources, as well as physical capabilities. Therefore, health promotion is not just the responsibility of the health sector, but goes beyond healthy lifestyles to well-being. (p. iii)

This Ottawa definition of health promotion reflects an integration of community and personal efforts by a focus on enabling individuals or groups, through social action, to improve their health. The WHO (1989) Regional Office for Europe considers health promotion as the process of enabling individuals and communities to increase their control over the determinants of health and thus improve their health. Health promotion is viewed as a unifying concept for those who recognize the need for change in the ways and conditions of living in order to promote health. As noted by the WHO, Regional Office for Europe (1984):

Health promotion best enhances health through integrated action at different levels on factors influencing health—economic, environmental, social, and personal. Given these basic principles, an almost unlimited list of issues for health promotion could be generated: food policy, housing, smoking, coping skills, social networks. (p. 3)

Since the First International Conference on Health Promotion held in Ottawa, Canada, in 1986, which resulted in the previously mentioned Ottawa Charter for Health Promotion, there have been five global conferences on health promotion. The last conference was held in June 2000 in Mexico City, organized jointly by the WHO, the Pan American Health Organization, and the

FIGURE 1-2 Examples of Three Levels of Prevention

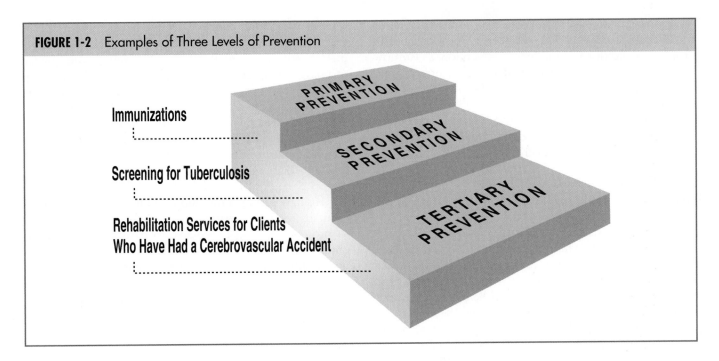

Immunizations

Screening for Tuberculosis

Rehabilitation Services for Clients
Who Have Had a Cerebrovascular Accident

Ministry of Health in Mexico (Ippolito-Shepherd & Cerqueria, 2000). These conferences attest to the recognition of the importance of health promotion efforts at national and international levels. The global priorities and strategies will be discussed in Chapter 5.

As consensus on the meaning of health promotion evolves, social action to strengthen members of society will surface as a central tenet. Health promotion can act as a mediating strategy between people and their environments, combining personal choice with social responsibility. As a principle, health promotion involves the whole population in the context of their everyday life. Thus, health promotion involves close cooperation between all sectors of the community—including government—to ensure that the total environment is conducive to health.

Health promotion includes strategies [U.S. Department of Health and Human Services (USDHHS), 1991] related to individual and family lifestyles coupled with personal choices made in a social context that significantly influence overall health. Examples include increased physical activity, improved nutrition, decreased tobacco use, decreased use of alcohol and other drugs, family planning with the goal of fewer teen pregnancies and unwanted pregnancies, reduced family violence, improved mental health, and the development of educational and community-based programs in schools and workplaces.

Two important public health tenets clearly underlie the concept of health promotion: a multisectoral approach and community involvement. If health promotion best enhances health through integrated action, and if health emerges from the influence of a variety of factors, then close cooperation among different sectors of the community is needed. With health promotion becoming more prominent on the health agenda, care must be taken to reach out to those populations most in need. In the United States, those who have historically been neglected in relation to health matters are the poor, racial and ethnic minority groups, and elders. Health promotion activities in the workplace and in schools and other neighborhood sites are ways to reach out to all people.

Health protection refers to activities designed to actively prevent illness, detect illness early, thwart disease processes, or maintain functioning within the constraints of illness (Pender, 1996). Health protection includes environmental or regulatory strategies that confer protection on large population groups specific to occupational health and safety, environmental health, food and drug safety, oral health, and unintentional injuries (USDHHS, 1991).

Disease and Injury Prevention

Prevention is another major concept central to public health and the caring mission of community health nursing. **Disease and injury prevention** refers to those activities designed to protect persons from disease and injuries and their consequences. In order to understand the concept of prevention, Leavell and Clark (1958) proposed the classic definition delineating three levels of prevention. These levels are defined and examples are provided in Figure 1-2.

Primary prevention—activities designed to prevent a problem or disease before it occurs

Secondary prevention—activities related to early diagnosis and treatment, including screening for diseases

Tertiary prevention—activities designed to treat a disease state or injury and to prevent it from further progressing

Disease and injury prevention is not synonymous with health promotion. The relationship between health promotion and disease and injury prevention, as Breslow (1990) suggests, may be viewed more accurately as a continuum ranging from "extreme infirmity to bounding health" (p. 13). A person's degree of health may be found somewhere on the continuum. Health promotion focuses on facilitating the maintenance of a person's current position on the continuum relative to age, with movement toward the positive end. Disease and injury prevention, however, focuses on preventing specific diseases and injuries that carry one to the negative end of the health spectrum.

Many industrialized nations have reached a point at which health, rather than merely the control of disease, is on the agenda of health care priorities. Although diseases must continue to be confronted, coupled with ways to minimize them, a focus on health is necessary. Community health nurses as well as other health professionals have a special role in health promotion, health protection, and disease and injury prevention: to delineate the prospects for preserving life and extending health for most persons, to determine the barriers to achieving health potential, and to advocate the social and personal actions necessary to meet these ends.

Healing

Healing has emerged as an important concept to nursing and public health. Healing enhances, promotes, and preserves the individual, family, or group. The term *healing* is derived from the word *hale,* meaning "whole." Thus, the literal meaning of healing is "becoming whole."

Healing refers to wholeness and balance. Implicit in this concept is a recognition of the unity of life and an emphasis on the harmony between persons and their environment. **Healing** is therefore defined as the restoration of health, harmony, and well-being to the body, mind, spirit, and environment.

An important concept related to healing is presence. Being present is a major principle central to healing (Engebretson, 2000). Presence refers to the quality of being open, receptive, available to the experience of another person or persons through a reciprocal interpersonal interaction (Patterson & Zderad, 1976). Presence refers to the creation of a space for healing. Presence has been identified by Gaut (1992) as a principal component of human caring. Caring presence therefore is a critical concept for nursing practice (Dossey, 1997; Gaut, 1992; Snyder & Lindquist, 1998).

Human caring transactions with persons and communities requiring health care services have the capacity to promote healing processes, to ease suffering. When community health nurses work with families and groups within the context of a caring environment, the potential for self-healing arises. The recognition of the healing power within individuals, families, and communities, and the use of that power to promote health and well-being, is a central mission of community health nursing.

REFLECTIVE THINKING

Community Involvement

- Do you know of nurses in your community who demonstrate an interest in the health of the populations who live there? If so, how are those nurses involved in health care?
- How would you assess your own involvement in your community? What role do you think you could play in the future?

Perspectives...

INSIGHTS OF A COMMUNITY HEALTH NURSE

Reflections

We ponder and reflect
listening
to the sounds of our own voices.
Coming together
to reach out to others,
Aspiring to care
in ways that are our own.

We open ourselves
learning about others
Learning about living, loving,
dying.
We are enriched, touched,
by those
who have taught us
so much.

We learn once again
to share our own light
experience our own energy.
Soaring
like a bird in flight
Seeking
new ways of being
and becoming.

—Sue A. Thomas, November 1990

CARING FOR POPULATIONS: POPULATION-FOCUSED PRACTICE

As was the case over 100 years ago, nurses today are in a position to participate in transforming our health care systems. Community health nurses can participate by contributing to the development of a unifying structure for the delivery of comprehensive, quality health care—a system focused not only on disease control and prevention but on health promotion as well. The Pew Health Professions Commission commented on the failure of health services to manage a person's safe passage through the health care system so that health is enhanced, illness prevention is incorporated, and death is dignified (Shugars, O'Neil, & Bader, 1991). Broad-based case management and coordination of care are services needed to facilitate "safe passage."

With a focus on providing care to populations, community health nurses are able to participate in coordinating health care services. Further, they possess a practice knowledge indispensable in a quality health care system: practice in providing case management as well as health education services to vulnerable populations; skill in coordinating care and developing trusting relationships through the establishment of caring partnerships with members of the community; and knowledge of the personal, environmental, political, social, spiritual, and cultural dimensions of health.

Community health nurses work in a variety of settings in the community, including homes, clinics, schools, workplaces, and organizations. They are also involved as members of health-planning agencies and councils, and they serve their communities as elected political officials. Community health nurses are concerned about the needs of those who do not receive health care services as well as the enhancement of health for those who do have access to the health care system. They are skilled in providing services to populations at high risk for illness, aging populations, homeless persons, children and adults with chronic illnesses

COMMUNITY NURSING VIEW

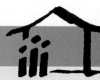

Heather Voss was an RN-BSN student at Sonoma State University who recognized the need for a nursing center in Marin County, California—a center designed to provide free nursing health care services to the homeless and near-homeless population. This center would become a program in an interfaith council agency serving the homeless and near-homeless population. Heather believed that in order to enhance health promotion, disease and injury prevention, and healing in a very vulnerable population, nursing services should be based on the philosophy of caring practice—respect, compassion, competence, and dignity. Her vision became a reality in 1995 with the opening of a nursing center staffed by nurses and nurse practitioners. Heather subsequently became a nurse practitioner and program director of the nursing center. The center is a part of an agency that serves the homeless and near-homeless population primarily and provides basic health services, health screening and referral, and case management. It continues today as a well-recognized community service, one that provides professional, compassionate health services.

Nursing Considerations

Assessment

◆ What did Heather observe that may have precipitated her action to create a nursing center?

Diagnosis

◆ Lack of adequate housing is an obvious issue for the homeless population.

◆ Identify other possible problems faced by the homeless and formulate a nursing diagnosis for each.

Outcome Identification

◆ What outcomes would be expected for the populations served?

Planning/Interventions

◆ Provide a plan for reaching the vulnerable population to be served by the center.

◆ How would the services offered be publicized?

◆ What interventions would be offered?

Evaluation

◆ What would indicate that the center succeeded in its initial goal to enhance health promotion, disease prevention, and healing?

◆ How might client satisfaction be determined?

and disabilities, persons struggling with alcohol and chemical dependencies, families trying to cope with violence in their homes and neighborhoods, and persons confronting the return of acute or chronic communicable diseases (Zerwekh, 1993).

As Gebbie and Hwang (2000) indicate, community health nurses must use a population-focused approach to practice. Although individuals and organizations may be responsible for subpopulations in the community (e.g., a health department responsible for a teen-parent program), population-focused practice addresses the larger community. Inherent in such an approach is examination of the health needs and assets of the population and of the nature of the health care resources designed to meet those needs. The community is viewed as a whole, and questions are raised about its overall health and those factors contributing to that health. A population focus in community health nursing uses a scientific approach based on assessment of the community or population. This assessment is used for participation in policy development and evaluation purposes to assure that essential community-oriented health services are available.

In planning and providing care to populations, community health nurses are interested in the phenomena of human care, caring, and healing. The perspective of the nurse is a holistic vision of the community's health. In order to promote individual, family, and community health, a holistic approach requires partnerships among many different sectors in the community. Partnerships based on the principles of empowerment, cooperation, and negotiation facilitate the creation of an environment where transformation can occur.

An increasing number of nurses are awakening to the possibilities of caring—caring about families, organizations, communities, nations, and the biosphere. As these nurses reaffirm caring as a concept with central importance in the study and practice of nursing, the possibilities of transformation become a reality where community health nurses fulfill their obligations in human caring through effective population-focused nursing practice.

KEY CONCEPTS

◆ The focus of community health/public health nursing is caring for the health of populations.

◆ The preservation and improvement of health of populations give direction to community health nursing practice.

◆ The development of knowledge and skills in performing the public health core functions is critical for community/public health nurses.

◆ The ANA and APHA definitions of community health nursing emphasize the synthesis of nursing and public health knowledge as a foundation for the scope of practice.

◆ The concept of caring is of central importance in community health nursing.

◆ A caring perspective requires the community nurse to approach individuals, families, and groups from a holistic view.

◆ The creation of caring partnerships with individuals, families, and communities is basic to community health nursing practice.

◆ The concepts of social justice, health, public health, health promotion, health protection, disease and injury prevention, and facilitation of healing are central to community health nursing.

◆ Principles of wholeness, harmony, and healing are important in understanding the nature of health.

◆ Community health nurses work in a variety of community settings, as well as serve as members of agency boards, planning teams, and councils.

RESOURCES

Agency for Health Care Research and Quality: http://www.ahcpr.gov
American Public Health Association: http://www.apha.org
Centers for Disease Control and Prevention:
    Health Alert Network: http://www.phppo.cdc.gov/han
    Mortality and Weekly Report: http://www.cdc.gov/mmwr
International Association for Human Caring: http://www.humancaring.org
National Institutes of Health: http://www.nih.gov
U.S. Department of Health and Human Services, Office of Disease Prevention and Health Promotion, Healthy People: http://www.health.gov/healthypeople
World Health Organization: http://www.who.org

Chapter

2

HISTORICAL DEVELOPMENT
OF COMMUNITY HEALTH NURSING

Sue A. Thomas, EdD, RN

MAKING THE CONNECTION

No occupation can be intelligently followed or correctly understood unless it is, at least to some extent, illumined by the light of history interpreted from the human standpoint.

—Dock & Stewart, 1938, p. 3

COMPETENCIES

Upon completion of this chapter, the reader should be able to:

- Examine community health nursing from a historical perspective.
- Describe the development of major public health events in Europe and the United States.
- Examine the central elements of two major international initiatives for community health.
- Describe the contributions of the early public health nursing leaders who played a central role in the development of nursing practice in the community.
- Identify the major contributions of early public health leaders.
- Discuss the evolution of major organizations relative to public health and community health nursing.
- Describe the ways how World War I and World War II influenced the development of community health nursing.
- Discuss the impact of the Health for all and Healthy Cities projects on community health nursing.

KEY TERMS

epidemic	primary health care
incidence	sustainable
pandemic	development
prevalence	vital statistics

To understand the nature of community health nursing and the factors influencing its development, one must examine the historical context. This chapter describes early practices that formed a foundation for the organizations and methods we now term *community health and public health nursing.*

Community health nursing, as discussed in Chapter 1, was introduced as a term in 1980 by the American Nurses Association to broadly identify those nurses whose focus of practice is the community. *Public health nursing* is a term that was introduced earlier in the history of nursing. Public health nursing is viewed as a specialty area in community health nursing, as are school nursing, hospice and home health nursing, occupational health nursing, and an emerging area of practice called parish nursing. In this view, public health nursing takes place within a public agency funded by governmental sources

REFLECTIVE THINKING

Nursing History

- What does the study of nursing history mean to you in relation to understanding nursing as a profession?
- What historical information do you think is important for nurses to examine?
- How would you describe your introduction to nursing history in previous academic endeavors?

to protect the public health, such as in a county or state health department.

This chapter further traces the evolution of modern practices. Donahue (1991) succinctly summarized the meaning of historical knowledge to nursing when she stated that history enables one to speculate and reflect, throwing light on the origins of persistent problems and issues and thus providing a basis for analysis. This analysis may provide insight into possible resolutions. As Keeling and Ramos (1995) also emphasized, in order to fully understand their heritage, nurses must study nursing history.

A review of nursing history also expands the knowledge base of nurses and promotes understanding of the social and intellectual origins of the profession (Booth, 1989; Donahue, 1991; Friedman, 1990). Community health nursing has developed from social pressures that exist in new as well as familiar forms. As Keeling and Ramos (1995) pointed out, current practice and health care dilemmas "are not easily understood nor challenges addressed in the absence of such insight" (p. 31).

Public health and community health nurses in the United States have historically focused on improving the health of the community. Since the late 1890s, when public health nursing emerged as a specialty in the United States, there has been a focus on prevention of disease and disability, the control of infectious diseases, an emphasis on environmental conditions such as sanitation, health education, and provision of care for the sick in their homes. Community and public health nurses have placed a major emphasis on improving the health status of vulnerable populations, working within the context of multidisciplinary practice.

HISTORICAL BACKGROUND OF PUBLIC HEALTH EFFORTS

This section provides a broad overview of the historical and political influences on public health activities, thereby laying the foundation for the sections on public health nursing and community health nursing. Although this information is discussed separately with regard to European and American history, the accompanying tables interlace events of all geographic areas in order to show their temporal relationships.

International Background

Early historical evidence suggests that personal as well as community hygiene and health care were practiced during the pre–Christian era. Many primitive tribes developed practices such as the removal of the dead and the burial of excreta, along with rules against fouling tribal quarters (Hanlon, 1964). Whether these practices were based more on superstition than on concerns surrounding sanitation is unknown. What can be surmised is that many primitive people recognized the existence of disease and engaged in various activities to drive away the evil spirits of disease (Hanlon & Pickett, 1984).

Table 2-1 lists some early activities that reflect an interest in public health. Early Greek civilization, for example, emphasized personal cleanliness, exercise, and nutrition—health promotion activities still encouraged today (Hanlon, 1964). Around 1500 B.C., the Hebrews were practicing public health measures, such as protection of food and water supplies as well as specific disease control (Anderson et al., 1978).

The Middle Ages

When the Christian era began, a change in philosophy toward community health and personal health began to emerge. The early Christian church, representing the thinking of the time, believed that Roman and Grecian life patterns, as discussed previously and in Table 2-1, focused on the body rather than the soul. The resulting philosophical shift to emphasizing neglect of the body for the purposes of enhancing the spiritual self led to a number of health problems (Kelly, 1981).

Because of the decline in community and personal prevention efforts during the Middle Ages, **epidemics** (disease rates beyond the usual frequency) of terrifying **pandemic** (worldwide epidemic) proportions occurred. Bubonic plague, for example, appeared in China, Egypt, India, Armenia, Europe, and other locations. The total mortality from bubonic plague is estimated to have been more than 60 million. In France, only one-tenth of the population is said to have survived. Over time, other diseases such as syphilis, diphtheria, streptococcal infections, dysenteries, and typhoid also took their toll (Pickett & Hanlon, 1990).

Early Christianity did, however, emphasize personal responsibility for the care of others and organized care of the sick to help meet the needs of society (Brainard, 1985). The sick, poor, and needy were cared for in hospitals, asylums, and almshouses.

The Renaissance

In Europe, after a depressing period associated with a focus on disease as punishment for sin, the concept of human dignity began to resurface. Intellectual inquiry and the search for scientific truth emerged. The Renaissance (A.D. 1500–1700) also led to awareness of society's responsibility for the health and welfare of its citizens. Of particular interest to community health nursing was the growing interest in care of the ill and aged in their homes. Founding of the Sisters of Charity in France set the stage for the emergence of visiting nurse services. (The work of these sisters and of St. Vincent de Paul is discussed further in the section on establishment of community and public health nursing practice.) See Table 2-2 for a list of events and actions that occurred during the Renaissance (including Colonial American events, to be discussed later).

The Industrial Revolution

The Industrial Revolution of the 1700s had a major influence on the health of the community. Industrialization and rapid urbanization throughout Europe resulted in higher infant mortality, poor working conditions, occupational diseases, overcrowding in poor urban areas, and populations vulnerable to epidemic infectious diseases (Ashton, 1992). The emphasis on industry and production overshadowed many of the gains made during the Renaissance. Similar conditions were taking place in the late 1700s in the United States.

The 18th and 19th Centuries in Europe

During the 18th and 19th centuries, the growth of populations in Europe led to greater emphasis on sanitation and

TABLE 2-1   Pre-Christian Era Events Related to Public Regulation of Health Practices

ERA	EVENT
ca. 3000 B.C.	Sewage disposal system developed in Egypt (Hanlon, 1964).
ca. 2000 B.C.	Code of Hammurabi specifies health practices and regulates physician conduct in ancient Babylonia (Anderson, Morton, & Greene, 1978).
ca. 1500 B.C.	Hebrews' Mosaic law specifies personal and community responsibilities for maternal and child health, communicable disease control, sewage disposal, etc. (Anderson et al., 1978).
498 B.C.	In Rome, office created to supervise health concerns such as garbage removal and sewage systems (Winslow, 1923).

vital statistics (the systematic use of data from registration of life events such as birth, deaths, and marriages to track health and social needs). There was a high **incidence** (frequency of new cases in a specified population) and **prevalence** (number of existing cases) of infectious diseases such as smallpox, cholera, and tuberculosis. The poor were living in "appalling, unsanitary conditions, crowded into slums" (Ashton, 1992, p. 1), where they were vulnerable to epidemic infectious disease.

In response to growing public awareness of existing sanitary and social problems, Great Britain enacted the first sanitation legislation in 1837. During this period, death rates were high in cities such as Liverpool, where more than half of the children of working-class families died before age five. The average age at death was 22 years for tradespeople, 36 years for gentry, and 16 years for laborers (Pickett & Hanlon, 1990).

In the 1840s public health, as it is known today, began with Edwin Chadwick in Great Britain. In 1842 Chadwick became known for his significant "Report on an Inquiry into the Sanitary Conditions of the Labouring Population of Great Britain." One result of this report was the establishment in 1848 of a General Board of Health in England (Hanlon & Pickett, 1984). Improvements soon followed with the enactment of legislation concerning factory management, child welfare, care of the aged and the mentally ill, education, and other social reform measures. Chadwick's answers to the appalling conditions of the poor—sewers, housing improvements, and water supply—had more to do with urban planning than with health services as we know them today.

Historical Development in America

On the North American continent, public health problems were recognized quite early by the colonists, who set the stage for later development. Table 2-2 lists some

17th-century European and Colonial American health-related events.

Colonial America

As early as 1639, a mandate by the Massachusetts Bay Colony required official reporting of vital statistics. Similar laws were enacted by the Plymouth Colony (Chadwick, 1937). Very little further progress of a public health nature occurred prior to the American Revolution, although temporary boards of health were established in response to particular epidemic health problems such as yellow fever, smallpox, typhoid fever, and typhus. The first permanent board of health was established in 1780.

With the development of the Marine Hospital in 1798 came the provision of health care to sick and disabled merchant seamen. The hospital concept was of particular significance because it was the beginning of what later came to be known as the U.S. Public Health Service (Hanlon, 1964). A public health committee formed in New York City at about the same time focused on sanitation and other health-related measures. The term *public health* has since been used to refer to government-run health services, which now constitute only one segment of the broader concept of community health.

The 18th and 19th Centuries in America

As can be inferred from Table 2-3, few major health-related events occurred in the 18th century. Although the United States expanded considerably during the first half of the 19th century, public health activities did not advance. Epidemics of smallpox, yellow fever, and other infectious diseases crossed the land. In Massachusetts, the tuberculosis death rate exceeded 300 per 100,000 population in 1850; during the same time period, infant mortality was estimated at approximately 200 per 1000 live births (Hanlon, 1964). As the United States grew, the number of cities increased, and the poor, as in Europe, crowded into substandard housing with unsanitary conditions, thereby creating the environment for illnesses to flourish (Rosen, 1958).

In response to the problems that emerged during the late 1700s and that continued into the 1800s, some larger cities, such as New York and Philadelphia, established city health departments. These city departments—along with the first state board of health, established in 1869—set the stage for the four levels of official public health action, now including national and international agencies.

Lemuel Shattuck, public health pioneer, issued a Census of Boston, which revealed startling statistics about the high infant and maternal death rates. Shattuck's 1850 report of the Sanitary Commission of Massachusetts has been viewed as one of the most remarkable reports in U.S. history, and one well ahead of its time (Hanlon, 1964). The report included a discussion of present and future public health needs of Massachusetts as well as of the nation. The report provided information related to

TABLE 2-2	Health-Related Events of the 17th Century
YEAR(S)	**EVENT**
1601	Elizabethan Poor Law enacted in England addresses care for the aged and disabled.
1600s	St. Vincent de Paul founds order of Sisters of Charity in France to care for the sick and poor at home.
1639	Massachusetts and Plymouth colonies mandate reporting of births and deaths (Chadwick, 1937).
1647	Massachusetts passes legislation prohibiting pollution of Boston Harbor.
1669	First visiting nurses sponsored by St. Vincent de Paul in France.

TABLE 2-3   Events of the 18th and 19th Centuries That Influenced Public Health and Community Health Nursing

YEAR(S)	EVENT
1701	Massachusetts enacts laws regarding isolation of smallpox victims and ship quarantine.
1780	First permanent local board of health organized in Petersbury, Virginia [Public Health Service (PHS), 1958].
1789–1799	Boards of health established in Philadelphia, New York, Baltimore, and Boston (PHS, 1958).
1798	U.S. Congress creates Marine Hospital.
1812	Irish Sisters of Charity founded in London, initiating home visiting by nuns.
1837	Great Britain enacts first sanitation legislation.
1839	American Statistical Society founded by Shattuck.
1842	Chadwick's Inquiry into the Sanitary Conditions of the Labouring Population of Great Britain published (Pickett & Hanlon, 1990).
1844	Healthy Towns associations formed in London in response to threats posed by urbanization and industrialization and to enact legislation to improve public health (Finer, 1952).
1848	Public Health Act passed in Parliament in London, unifying the organization of public health efforts.
	General Board of Health for England established to deal with child welfare, care of mentally ill and disabled, and other social actions.
1850	Shattuck's Report of the Sanitary Commission of Massachusetts published.
1854	Nightingale begins her involvement in the Crimean War, addressing environmental and health care issues.
1859	Rathbone promotes establishment of district nursing in Liverpool, England.
1869	First state board of health established in Massachusetts.
1870	Second state board of health established in California.
1872	American Public Health Association founded.
1875	Ward-Richardson shares vision of "Hygeia: A City of Health in England" to encourage passage of Public Health Act in Great Britain, which included prevention measures and occupational health and safety (Cassedy, 1962).
1876	Pasteur and Koch usher in the mechanistic biomedical paradigm, with its emphasis on identification and treatment of germ-related causes of disease (Duhl & Hancock, 1988).
1877	First home visiting nurses employed by a volunteer agency in the United States.
1879	Ethical and Cultural Society of New York employs four nurses in dispensaries.
1882	American Red Cross founded by Clara Barton to supply nurses for service during World War I.
1885–1886	Visiting Nurse associations established in Buffalo and Philadelphia.
1892	School nursing established in London.
1893	Henry Street Settlement founded by Lillian Wald.
	Dock, Robb, and Nutting organize the American Society of Superintendents of Training Schools for Nurses in the United States and Canada.
1895	Vermont Marble Company employs first occupational health nurse.
1896	First rural nursing service in United States started by Ellen M. Wood in Westchester County, New York.
1898	Los Angeles becomes the first city to hire a nurse in an official health department.

environmental, food, drug, and infectious disease patterns and recommended keeping vital statistics records. Although Shattuck's visionary report called for these and many other reforms that seem modern even today, it "remained almost unnoticed by the community or by the profession for many years, and its recommendations were ignored" (Hanlon, 1964, p. 50).

Not until 1869, 19 years later, was the first state board of health established in Massachusetts, as earlier recommended by Shattuck. This state health department, under Henry Bowditch's leadership, focused on public and professional education related to hygiene, housing, communicable diseases, and living conditions of the poor, among other issues. By the end of the 19th century, 18 other states had established state health departments; in the early part of the 20th century, the remaining states followed suit.

With the increased focus on the public's health toward the end of the 19th century, people became more concerned about the plight of the poor, and, as a result, greater emphasis was placed on the abolition of child labor, improved housing, and maternal and child health. Many voluntary organizations were founded, including the Red Cross, the American Society for the Control of Cancer, and the National Tuberculosis Association. The American Public Health Association (APHA), founded in 1872, became the formal organization for public health

professionals (Fee, 1991). Formation of the APHA represented a significant advance in public health expansion. Its early meetings focused on aspects of sanitation, transmission and control of diseases, longevity, hygiene, and other subjects (Hanlon & Pickett, 1984). The APHA today remains a major organization in the United States, serving its members and the public with information and advocacy for improvement of health in communities throughout the nation.

The 20th Century

Soon after the turn of the century, the U.S. Public Health Service (USPHS) was created. This federal service actually began in 1902, with the Public Health and Marine Hospital Service. Renamed the U.S. Public Health Service in 1912, it grew rapidly as U.S. society became increasingly complex and experienced several wars and economic depressions (Hanlon & Pickett, 1984).

The chief officer of the USPHS became the Surgeon General, with the passage of federal legislation mandating federal involvement in health promotion. In the early years of the 20th century, health needs of special population groups began to be recognized, leading to development of federal programs related to maternal and child health, sexually transmitted diseases, mental illness, and other health concerns. Today, the USPHS is the most important federal health agency. Table 2-4 lists 20th-century events that influenced community health nursing.

REFLECTIVE THINKING

Public Health Achievements

- Think about one modern-day public health problem. What progress has been made in addressing the problem since recorded history?
- How do some of the public health problems documented from earlier centuries compare with those of today?

TABLE 2-4 Events of the 20th Century That Influenced Public and Community Health Nursing

YEAR(S)	EVENT
1902	Lina Rogers, on loan from Henry Street Settlement House, starts school of nursing in New York.
1904	Los Angeles becomes the first city in the United States to hire school nurses.
1909	Metropolitan Life Insurance Company offers visiting nurse services to policyholders in New York (first national system of insurance coverage for home-based care).
	First White House Conference for Children held.
1910	Mary Adelaide Nutting starts first postgraduate course in public health nursing at Teacher's College, Columbia University, New York.
1911	Metropolitan Life Insurance Company initiates visiting nurse services throughout the United States.
1912	U.S. Children's Bureau and U.S. Public Health Service created.
	American Red Cross Town and Country Nursing Service established.
	National Organization for Public Health Nursing (NOPHN) formed, with Lillian Wald as first president.
1920	U.S. legislation giving women the right to vote passes.
1921	Shepherd-Towner Act passes, authorizing grants to states to provide care to at-risk maternal aggregates.
1922	Harlem Committee of New York Tuberculosis and Health Association established, based on Mabel Staupers' community assessment.
1923	Goldmark Report published, recommending that nursing education be offered in institutions of higher learning.
1925	Frontier Nursing Service started by Mary Breckinridge in Kentucky.

(continues)

YEAR(S)	EVENT
1930	National Institutes of Health created in the United States.
1934	Mabel Staupers appointed as first nurse executive of National Association of Colored Graduate Nurses.
	Pearl McIver becomes the first public health nurse hired by the U.S. Public Health Service.
1935	Social Security Act passes in U.S. Congress, establishing Old Age, Survivors, and Disability Insurance (OASDI) program.
1951	National organizations in the United States recommend that college-based nursing programs include content in public health.
1952	NOHPN absorbed into the National League for Nursing (NLN).
1953	U.S. Department of Health, Education, and Welfare created.
1963	NLN requires baccalaureate nursing programs to include public health nursing content and practice in the curriculum, as recommended in 1951.
1964	Economic Opportunity Act passes, providing funds for neighborhood health centers, Head Start, and other community programs.
1966	Comprehensive Health Planning and Public Health Services Act passes.
	Social Security Act amended to include Medicare program.
1967	U.S. Congress passes Medicaid provision of Social Security Act to provide care for the poor.
1974	LaLonde Report ("A New Perspective on the Health of Canadians") published in Canada.
	National Health Planning and Resources Development Act passes in United States as an attempt to create systematic health care planning.
1976	McKeown's statistical analysis of infectious disease mortality in England and Wales published.
1978	International Conference on Primary Health held, resulting in the World Health Organization (WHO) initiative known as the Alma Ata declaration on Primary Health Care.
1981	Global Strategy for Health for All by the Year 2000 agreement adopted by member nations of WHO.
1983	Prospective payment system [diagnosis-related groups (DRGs)] instituted under Medicare.
1985, 1991	WHO Regional Office for Europe publishes Targets for Health for All reports.
1986	Ottawa Charter for Health Promotion developed at the First International Conference on Health Promotion, held in Canada.
	1990 Health Objectives for the Nation published.
	Healthy Cities Project created, WHO European Office.
	Development of Healthy Cities Projects begins throughout the world, continues through the 1990s.
1988	Health for All Australians report developed in response to WHO's Health for All initiative.
1989	New Zealand Health Goals and Targets for the Year 2000 report published.
1990s	Health care systems in Western and developing nations undergo restructuring.
1990	U.S. Healthy People 2000 Objectives published.
1986–1993	Healthy Cities Projects developed throughout the world.
1993	First International Healthy Cities and Communities Conference held in San Francisco.
1996	U.S. Healthy People 2000, Midcourse Review and 1995 Revisions published.
1999	World Health Report, 1999, published by WHO.
	Public Health Nursing Quad Council through the American Nurses Association develops a new scope and standards of public health nursing document, identifying the differences between community-oriented and community-based nursing practice.
2000	U.S. Healthy People 2010 published.
	WHO's (2000) *World Health Report 2000-Health Systems: Improving performance* published.

INTERNATIONAL INITIATIVES IN PUBLIC HEALTH

The study of international initiatives in public health during the 20th century provides the background necessary to understand public health projections for this century. Particularly from the 1930s through the early 1970s, public policy on health in Great Britain and many other countries, including the United States, was dominated by a treatment orientation, with the implicit assumption that "magic bullets could be provided by the pharmaceutical industry for all conditions" (Ashton, 1992, p. 3).

By the early 1970s, however, the therapeutic approach was being challenged. Most countries, including developing countries, were experiencing a crisis in health care costs. Many had adopted the Western pattern of building large hospitals that incorporated highly trained professionals. Such facilities took up the bulk of the health care budget, leaving little funding for rural areas or for primary care. From the problems associated with this development, the two concepts of primary health care and emphasis on community development began to surface (Ashton, 1992).

In Great Britain, McKeown's (1976) statistical analysis demonstrated that most of the decline in infectious disease mortality in England and Wales between 1840 and 1970 occurred before medical therapeutic intervention. This analysis resulted in a revived interest in public health and prevention efforts. McKeown concluded that a number of factors contributed to improved health outcomes in Great Britain. These were:

- Limitation of family size
- Increase in food supplies
- A healthier physical environment
- Specific preventive and therapeutic measures

A review of international literature specific to public health refers to McKeown's work as a benchmark for what has become known as the New Public Health. This approach seeks a synthesis of the environmental and personal preventive and the therapeutic eras in public health history. It focuses on public policy as well as personal behavior and lifestyle (Ashton, 1992).

The LaLonde Report, "A New Perspective on the Health of Canadians," published in Canada in 1974 and discussed in Chapter 5, has been viewed as a restatement of earlier public health reports on sanitary conditions among laboring populations. The LaLonde Report has been applied at different levels in various nations and continues to shape public policy this century.

Declaration of Alma Ata

Since the LaLonde Report, the World Health Organization (WHO) has generated several initiatives. At the International Conference on Primary Health Care, held in 1978 at Alma Ata, participants from 143 countries identified primary health care as the best possible way to attain health for all by the year 2000. The Alma Ata Declaration, referred to as Health for All by the Year 2000, resulted in countries throughout the world taking action to create national initiatives focused on implementing primary care measures to improve the health of their people. Health itself was described as a basic human right and world-wide social goal (Basch, 1990). The Health for All initiative continues to provide directions for this century, with health placed at the core of the global development agenda (Brundtland, 1999).

Primary health care emphasizes the preventive rather than the curative end of the health care continuum. This approach to care focuses on equity, community participation, accessibility of services, and the importance of the environment in relation to the health of individuals and communities (Lamont & Lees, 1994). The Alma Ata primary health care focus, by its very nature, requires a coordinated, intersectoral approach. It is transdisciplinary, broad in nature, and a more integrated approach to the health and social well-being of the community.

The central elements of both WHO initiatives, the Alma Ata Declaration and the Healthy Cities Project (discussed below), are a focus on the poor and disenfranchised; the need to reorient the focus of medical and health systems away from hospital care and toward primary health care; the importance of a consumer focus in health care; and the creation of partnerships between public, private, and voluntary sectors. The concept of health promotion embedded in these initiatives reaffirms the importance of public policy and environmental action as well as personal lifestyle. Health promotion is discussed further in Chapters 5 and 11.

Health for All Initiative

The WHO policy of Health for All by the Year 2000 resulted in the setting of goals and targets to improve the public's health worldwide. Two years after Health for All was adopted by WHO in 1981, the U.S. Surgeon General's Report on Health Promotion and Disease Prevention was developed, subsequently resulting in the publication of the Healthy People 2000 objectives in 1990 [U.S. Department of Health and Human Services (USDHHS), 1990]. The WHO's European Regional Office published the first set of Targets for Health for All in 1985 (WHO, 1985). This report was updated in 1991 on the basis of broad representation from the various European member states (WHO, 1991). In 1988, Australia published its first national goals and targets for population health for the year 2000 and beyond (Health Targets and Implementation Committee, 1988). In 1989, the New Zealand Health Charter was developed, making area health boards accountable to the New Zealand government for achieving objectives in order to justify their budgets. With the change in government in 1990, however, New Zealand abandoned these goals and targets (Green, 1996).

The Australian and U.S. approaches, in contrast to the New Zealand model, provided opportunities for states and communities to decide whether to adopt or adapt the national health objectives in their own policies and plans. These approaches have been effective ones. In the United States an interstate initiative was put in place to translate the national objectives to meet various state needs and priorities. This interstate network resulted in consensus-building efforts, effective consultation procedures, and coalition building activities that continue in the implementation of the Healthy People 2010 initiative. Community partnerships are viewed as critical in improving the health of communities.

Healthy People 2010 builds on the intitatives pursued over the past 20 years. It presents a nationwide health promotion and disease prevention agenda, designed to achieve two main goals: (1) increase quality and years of healthy life and (2) eliminate health disparities among segments of the population. These two goals will be monitored in 28 focus areas through 467 objectives. Each objective has a target for specific improvements to be achieved by 2010 (USDHHS, 2000).

As can be seen, the WHO initiative Health for All by the Year 2000 resulted in the creation of a momentum among nations that embodies the spirit of partnership, collaboration, and consensus building. It is anticipated that through the process of working together, we can continue to build healthier cities and communities worldwide this century.

Healthy Cities and Communities

The Healthy Cities initiative was started in 1986 by the European office of the WHO. A proposal that included four to six cities was developed. This project was thought by many world cities and towns to be a useful vehicle for translating the WHO Health for All by the Year 2000 strategy and the 30 European Targets for Health for All into local programs.

In 1993, the first International Healthy Cities and Communities Conference was held in San Francisco, California. Participants from around the world gathered to discuss various activities related to the creation of the Healthy Cities Project and actions to improve the health of those in their communities. The conference was very successful, providing the opportunity for participants to share their experiences with each other—participants from countries such as Australia and countries in Asia, South America, Europe, and North America.

The WHO initiatives indicate recognition of the need to reduce fragmentation of services—to work toward creating seamless, integrated health care systems that focus on consumer needs. The challenge today is whether the global initiatives of the 1990s can be as effective as the national initiatives established in Britain in the 1840s. As Ashton (1992) pointed out, "It is imperative that broad-

---

✳ DECISION MAKING

Creating Community Partnerships

◆ Building partnerships among organizations in the community reflects an effort to improve the nature of health care delivery and, ultimately, the health of the community. Through collaboration, health care problems and issues can be and are being addressed in a more comprehensive way. Creating partnerships between providers and consumers is another endeavor to enhance care delivery.

◆ What types of activities have occurred in your community in relation to creating partnerships for health care delivery?

◆ What do you think about the idea of creating partnerships among organizations to enhance health care delivery? What about partnerships between providers and consumers? What does consumer-focused care mean to you?

◆ How might you participate in the process?

---

based professional, public, and political coalitions be built to tackle the problems which confront us" (pp. 10–11).

Duhl (1992), one of the primary leaders of the WHO Healthy Cities Project, suggests that if living areas contain diverse groups, cultures, values, and goals, as they do in cities throughout the world, then "a new means must emerge for dealing with health" (p. 17). The values built into the Health Promotion, Healthy Public Policy, and Healthy Cities initiatives are such a response. The Healthy Cities/Communities model respects diversity, encourages participation, and calls for equity, asking that providers and consumers sit together, explore perceptions of health needs, investigate various visions, and create responsive systems.

In 2001, the focus on the development of healthy communities continues. For example, the vision for U.S. Healthy People 2010 is "healthy people in healthy communities." Addressing the challenge of health improvement is viewed as a shared responsibility that will continue to be based on community partnerships, comprised of government leaders (state, local, and national), policymakers, health care professionals, business executives, educators, community leaders, and the public (USDHHS, 2000).

An example that highlights the emphasis on creating healthy communities was an international conference in nursing, held in Scotland in June 2001, titled "Creating Communities of Caring—Global Initiatives." The conference was an international collaborative effort between the International Association for Human Caring and the University of Stirling in Scotland. It is important to note that caring was highlighted as a central focus for community building.

EVOLUTION OF COMMUNITY HEALTH NURSING— CARING AND HEALING PRACTICE

Caring and Healing in Community Health Nursing

Over the past century, community health nurses have demonstrated courage and commitment in providing care to people in their communities. In the United States as well other countries, community health and public health nursing can trace its origins to those first nurses who provided care to poor people in their homes, neighborhoods, workplaces, schools, and clinics. In Great Britain, Australia, Canada, the United States, and other nations, these nurses were frequently the only providers of care to underprivileged individuals and families. They also visited families in outlying areas, traveling by many different modes of transportation. Among early community health nurses, caring for the people included raising needed funds for services and political support. In this way, community health nurses fulfilled social as well as professional roles.

In San Francisco in November 1993, the APHA recognized the outstanding contributions of public health nurses to improving the health of their communities. That year, public health nurses in the United States celebrated a century of caring—caring for communities, aggregates, and families. Across the nation, nurses came together to honor their founders—leaders such as Lillian Wald, Mary Brewster, Margaret Sanger, and Lavinia Dock. Public health nursing in the United States began with those nurses, who provided nursing services to needy families in their homes.

The first public health nurses were caring women with compassion for the communities they served. They recognized the overwhelming health problems in the late 1800s and committed themselves to providing care to families in homes, their workplaces, schools, neighborhoods, and clinics, reaching out to care for those in their communities (APHA, 1993).

Public health nurses have served people of all ages and have practiced in a variety of settings, focusing on health promotion, disease prevention, treatment, and rehabilitation in their efforts to address health needs (Freeman, 1964). The early public health nurses were able to mobilize community resources in creating enlightened models for care—models that are still relevant today. Many of the early nursing leaders were involved in the social issues of their time, including women's suffrage, public health, and child labor laws (Donahue, 1991), as discussed in subsequent sections.

The Legacy of Florence Nightingale—The Evolution of Modern Nursing

Nursing is an art; . . . it requires as exclusive a devotion, as hard a preparation as any painter's or sculptor's work; for what is having to do with dead canvas or cold marble, compared with having to do with the living body; the temple of God's spirit? (Nightingale, 1867, p. 149)

Florence Nightingale, the woman credited with establishing modern nursing, was born in 1820 to an established English family. She was well educated and concerned about hygiene and health (Goodnow, 1933). In her youth, Nightingale longed to be a nurse; however, nursing was not yet a recognized field of study. Further, being a nurse was viewed as less than socially desirable; therefore "respectable" people did not do the work.

Not until she was 31 years of age did Nightingale enter nurse's training under the direction of Pastor Fliedner at Kaiserwerth Hospital on the Rhine in Germany. Nightingale also studied the organization of the Sisters of Charity in Paris as well as nursing systems in Austria, France, Germany, and Italy (Dock & Stewart, 1925).

In 1854, Nightingale responded to the Crimean War at Scutari in Turkey, where she became a pioneer in improving conditions for wounded soldiers. When Nightingale arrived at Scutari, she found that the hospital, built for 1700 patients, actually held 3000 to 4000 wounded men. The men were lying naked, and there were no beds, no blankets, no laundry, and no eating areas (Goodnow, 1933).

Nightingale not only made major reforms in hospital operations within a few months; she also recognized the importance of keeping statistical information about the death rates of soldiers in the Crimean hospital, comparing these rates with the death rates in hospitals in Manchester and in or near London.

Because of Nightingale's meticulous attention to maintaining statistical records, she was able to clearly demonstrate that, by the end of the Crimean War, her reforms had resulted in lower death rates of soldiers. Nightingale also

REFLECTIVE THINKING

The Legacy of Florence Nightingale

- What do you think were Florence Nightingale's most important contributions?
- What were some of her contributions that have relevance for today?

established community services and activities for soldiers, such as rest-and-recreation facilities. In addition, care for families was organized (Dock & Stewart, 1925).

Florence Nightingale demonstrated, in an exemplary way, that public health principles are central to health care services. One of her greatest contributions was in relation to sanitation reform. As noted by Cohen (1984) and Grier and Grier (1978), Nightingale was concerned about the environmental determinants associated with health and disease. She also demonstrated the value of utilizing statistics to describe population factors, statistics that could be used for political advocacy on behalf of the population aggregate. The development and application of statistical procedures continued after her return to London in 1856, at the close of the Crimean War.

Florence Nightingale was a visionary, and she left a rich legacy to those of us in the latter part of the 20th century and beyond. Styles (1992), in her commentary for a commemorative edition of Florence Nightingale's *Notes on Nursing,* describes Nightingale as

> our enduring symbol. . . . She represents many of the values we continue to hold dear. The origins of many of today's nursing movements can be traced to the Nightingale legacy. She was preaching vehemently about the environment, the community (or district), sanitation, hygiene, healthy living, and preserving the vitality of patients more than a century before primary health care was elevated to the rank of worldwide gospel at Alma Ata. (pp. 72–75)

Nightingale was influential in the reformation of hospitals and in promoting public health policies for the British Sanitary System (Kalisch & Kalisch, 1982). She was the first nurse to exert political pressure on government,

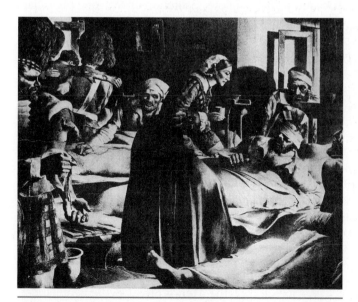

Florence Nightingale in the Crimea. Photo courtesy of Pfizer Consumer Group, Pfizer, Inc.

taking social action at a time when nursing was not a recognized or highly valued endeavor.

Establishment of Community Health Nursing and Public Health Practice

Community health nursing began in 1669 with the first visiting nurses, who were sponsored by St. Vincent de Paul in Paris. St. Vincent de Paul organized the Sisterhood of the Dames de Charité, introducing the principles of visiting nursing and social welfare. He focused on helping people to help themselves. The work of the sisterhood emphasized the belief that home visiting required not just kindness and intuition but also sound knowledge of scientific principles (Maynard, 1939). The voluntary association of friendly visitors established by St. Francis de Paul to care for the sick and poor in their homes represents another early form of visiting nursing (Dolan, 1978).

Other early forerunners of community health nursing were the first two nursing orders in Great Britain. Mary Aikenhead (Sister Mary Augustine), who started the Irish Sisters of Charity in Dublin in 1812, developed a nursing model whereby the nuns visited the sick in their homes. The community health nursing movement owes its further development to William Rathbone of Liverpool, England, a Quaker who in 1859 became impressed by the skilled care his wife received during a fatal illness. As Gardner (1919) states, "It is to Mr. Rathbone that we owe the first definitely formulated district nursing association" (p. 14). A philanthropist, Rathbone promoted the establishment of district nursing, or visiting nursing service, for the sick poor of Liverpool. Rathbone believed that if nursing care could help his wife, who had the money to purchase services, those who were sick and poor might benefit from the needed services even more.

Rathbone employed Mary Robinson, the first nurse to visit the sick poor in their homes. She was not only to provide therapeutic nursing care for the sick but also to instruct the patients and their families in the care of the sick, the maintenance of hygienic practices in the home, and those things that contributed to healthful living. The service provided was so effective that Rathbone decided to establish a permanent district nursing service in Liverpool (McNeil, 1967). Liverpool was organized into 18 districts, each of which would have a nurse and a social worker to meet the needs of its communities.

In order to obtain qualified nurses who would be able to do this difficult work, Rathbone asked for assistance from Florence Nightingale, who helped him establish a training school for visiting nurses in affiliation with the Roy Infirmary of Liverpool. From the beginning, Nightingale referred to the graduates of the visiting nursing program as "health visitors." The model was very successful and eventually expanded to the national level under voluntary agencies (Rosen, 1958).

Community Health Nursing in the United States

In the United States, as in Great Britain, community health nursing developed from district and home visiting, with the first nurses employed in 1877 by the Women's Branch of the New York City Mission, a voluntary agency (Waters, 1912). Frances Root, a graduate nurse, was the first salaried U.S. nurse to provide nursing care to the sick poor in their homes. In 1878, the Ethical Culture Society of New York employed four nurses in dispensaries to serve in an ambulatory care role in the community. These nurses worked under the supervision of a physician, incorporating health teaching as well as illness care in their practice (Brainard, 1985).

Within the next few years, the idea spread, with nursing associations, later called visiting nursing associations, established initially in Buffalo and Boston in 1885 and in Philadelphia in 1886. These associations relied on support from lay contributions and on small service charges. The Boston Instructive Visiting Nurse Association emphasized the community health nursing education role as well as care of the sick, ushering in the beginning of the health promotion focus that now characterizes community health nursing. By 1890, visiting nurse services were organized in 21 U.S. cities (Novak, 1988).

Visiting nursing in the United States, as in Great Britain, was begun by people who were concerned about the conditions in which the poor lived. Then, as now, many of the most serious public health problems were in poverty-stricken communities, with hunger, family violence, homelessness, crime, youth alienation, deterioration of the physical environment, and unemployment clearly evident.

Contributions of Lillian Wald and Others

In 1893, Lillian Wald and Mary Brewster cofounded the first organized public health nursing agency, or settlement house, in New York City. They rented an apartment in lower Manhattan, beginning what came to be known as the Henry Street Settlement, eventually the New York Visiting Nurse Association. Mary Brewster and Lillian Wald were able to obtain funds from philanthropists in order to offer care to needy persons. It was Wald, a nurse, who coined the title *public health nurse*. Wald used the word *public* so that all people would know that this type of service was available to them (Haupt, 1953). Wald claimed that she selected the title public health nurse to emphasize the community value of the nurse, whose service attitudes were built on an understanding of the social and economic problems associated with illness and disease.

Wald and Brewster developed a model based on the premise that nurses should be available to anyone who needed them, without the intervention of a doctor, thereby highlighting nursing as an independent profession. Wald's settlement house was different from the

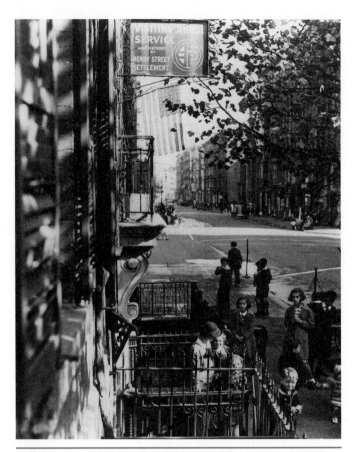

Nurses at the Henry Street Settlement in New York City. Photo courtesy of the Visiting Nurse Service of New York.

other visiting nursing services of that time, the latter associated with sectarian organizations or dispensaries. Wald believed that the nursing agency should not be associated with a religious institution or with one physician. Further, she believed that nurses should live in the neighborhood where they provided services in order to more fully understand the needs of the families they served. Both Wald and Brewster lived in the area of the Henry Street Settlement.

Like Nightingale, Lillian Wald and Mary Brewster were wealthy young women and trained nurses who traveled a different path than did many other women in their social class. They were very concerned about the care of the poor, who faced overwhelming physical, social, emotional, and economic problems. The Henry Street Settlement went beyond the individual efforts of community health nurses of earlier times. Lillian Wald had a vision that public health nurses would be available to those in need in homes, in workplaces, in schools, on street corners, in clinics—anywhere that people in need lived, worked, played, and died.

As director of the Henry Street Settlement House, Wald is legendary not only for her nursing accomplishments but also for her dedication to social reform. Wald and Brewster's collective vision focused not only on

REFLECTIVE THINKING

Visions of Nursing Leaders

- It is important to examine the visions of early nursing leaders and to consider how these visions might be relevant today.
- What relevance do the visions of the early community health nursing leaders hold today?
- How do you think our public health problems today compare with those of Lillian Wald's period?
- What problems do you see in your own community? How should they be handled? By whom?

investment because doing so could reduce mortality and would limit the benefits paid by the company. Wald and Frankel recommended that Metropolitan Life hire visiting nurses to care for policyholders during illness. The two principles underlying the insurance coverage for nursing services were that the company would utilize existing public health nursing services rather than employing their own, if at all possible, and that services would be available to anyone, with payment based on the ability to pay. Both of these principles continue today in health agencies in the United States.

Metropolitan Life Insurance Company began providing nursing services on an experimental, three-month basis in June 1909. Nurses from the Henry Street Settlement visited sick Metropolitan Life policyholders referred by agents in one section of the city. Results were compared with those for similar policyholders in another section of the city who did not receive nurse visits. The three-month experiment was such a success that the Metropolitan Life directors authorized an extension of the program to cover policyholders throughout the city (Hamilton, 1989), resulting in the first national system of insurance coverage for home-based care.

By 1911, Metropolitan Life started offering nursing services throughout the United States. Wherever possible, Metropolitan Life contracted with visiting nurse associations to provide care; when this was not possible, the insurance company employed its own nurses to provide care. By 1916, the services of a visiting nurse were available to 90% of the insurance company's 10.5 million policyholders in 2000 Canadian and U.S. cities. By 1925, Metropolitan Life reported that 240,000 lives had been saved, translating to an estimated savings of $43 million for the company (Hamilton, 1989).

For many years, Metropolitan Life Insurance Company financed approximately one-third of the budgets of most visiting nurse associations. After 44 successful years, the Metropolitan project ended in 1953. The shift from voluntary responsibility for health care to professional community organizations was one of the major reasons for the change. The Metropolitan project, however, demonstrated how nursing and a business endeavor could work together to accomplish their goals, contributed to the establishment of a cost-accounting system for visiting nurse associations that is still in use today, demonstrated that nursing services could reduce deaths from infectious diseases, and educated nurses in relation to marketing services and recruitment (Haupt, 1953).

School Nursing

The health of mothers and children was yet another concern of Lillian Wald and other social activists of her time. The nurses from Henry Street Settlement and other service programs identified children who had been excluded from school because of illness. (The preceding perspective box, which contains an excerpt from Lillian Wald's notes, highlights the conditions in which some children were living.)

By 1902, the health conditions of school children in New York City, for example, were of major concern. Many students had diseases such as pediculosis, trachoma, ringworm, scabies, and impetigo. Fifteen to 20 children in each school were being sent home daily. This high level of school absence due to the childhood illnesses convinced Wald to contact Dr. Lederle, Commissioner of Health in New York City, whom she convinced to try a school nursing experiment (Buhler-Wilkerson, 1985).

Lina Rogers, a public health nurse from Henry Street Settlement, was loaned to the New York City Health Department to work in a school (Dock & Stewart, 1925). Subsequently, other nurses from Henry Street Settlement were assigned to three other New York City schools in a pilot project. This project was so successful that school nurses were hired on a widespread basis. These nurses provided health teaching to students and their families, treated minor infections, and performed physical assessments.

The concept of school nursing soon spread to other parts of the United States. Los Angeles became the first city to hire nurses in schools (Gardner, 1952). School nursing began with an emphasis on preventing the spread of communicable diseases and treating other problems associated with school-age children. By the 1930s, however, school nursing also incorporated a focus on health promotion activities such as casefinding, integrating healthy lifestyle concepts in the curriculum, and maintaining a safe and healthy physical school environment (Igoe, 1980).

Rural Nursing

In cities and towns, public health nursing was developing rapidly; in rural areas, however, progress was slower. The first rural nursing service was established by Ellen Morris Wood in Westchester County, New York, in 1896. In 1906, a nursing service for both the well-to-do and the poor was started in Salisbury, Connecticut.

In addition to her work in the city, Lillian Wald was also concerned about providing health services to those in rural areas. In 1912, she asked her wealthy friend Jacob Shiff to donate money to the American Red Cross so that it could establish a rural nursing service. She was successful in her actions, convincing the American Red Cross to direct its attention to creating a new department, the Town and Country Nursing Service. The service extended community health nursing services to rural areas (Brainard, 1985). The purpose of the service was to provide rural areas and small towns with public health nurses and to supervise the work of these nurses. The Town and Country Nursing Service later became known as the Bureau of Public Health Nursing.

Another very important development in the expansion of rural nursing and community health outreach programs was the work of a nurse named Mary Breckinridge. Born in 1881 into a prominent American family, Mary Breckinridge in her early years traveled to many parts of the world—Russia, France, Switzerland, and the British Isles. After the death of her two children, she devoted herself to the service of others, particularly children (Frontier Nursing Service, 1999).

Breckinridge played a vital role in community health by founding the Frontier Nursing Service (FNS) of Kentucky. She was committed to promoting the health care of disadvantaged women and children and used part of the money left to her by her grandmother to start the FNS (Browne, 1966).

The first health center organized by Breckinridge was established in a five-room cabin in Leslie County, Kentucky in 1925. At that time Leslie County was one of the poorest and most inaccessible areas in the United States. Breckinridge chose the Kentucky mountains because of their inaccessibility. She introduced the first nurse midwives in the country. Riding their horses up into the mountains and across streams in blizzards, fog, or floods, the FNS brought health care to families throughout the area.

By 1930, six outpost nursing centers had been built. Through fund-raising efforts, Breckinridge was able to provide leadership in establishing medical, surgical, and dental clinics and 24-hour nursing and midwifery services, serving nearly 10,000 people over 700 square miles. Until her death in 1965, Mary Breckinridge was the driving force behind the FNS (FNS, 1999).

The FNS continues today, playing a vital role in the delivery of community health nursing services. Through the Frontier School of Midwifery and Family Nursing, hundreds of nurses have been prepared to serve their respective communities. Today the FNS is organized as a parent holding company for Mary Breckinridge Health Care. The services include a home health agency, two outpost clinics, one primary health care clinic in the hospital, and the Frontier School of Midwifery and Family Nursing, the largest nurse midwifery program in the United States (FNS, 1999).

Occupational Health Nursing

Occupational health nursing is another area of focus in community health nursing. Margaret Sanger, PHN, was instrumental in addressing the health problems of factory workers (women, in particular) in the lower East Side of Manhattan. In addition, Vermont's Governor Proctor hired nurses to address the health needs of those living in villages associated with the Vermont Marble Company (Novak, 1988). By 1897 the Employees Benefit Association of John Wanamaker's department store in New York City had hired nurses to provide services to employees in their homes. These nurses soon expanded their role to include disease and injury prevention and first aid in the workplace. From 1910 to 1919, the number of firms employing nurses grew from 66 to 871 (Brainard, 1985).

Equality in Nursing and Services to Special-Population Groups

In the early 1900s, injustices in the U.S. health care system were apparent, particularly in relation to community health services for African Americans and the poor. Mabel K. Staupers recognized these injustices and devoted her life to improving community health services for African Americans in Philadelphia and Harlem (Mosley, 1995). She is recognized as a renowned nursing leader who clearly demonstrated caring in practice.

When Staupers was 13, her family moved to Harlem from the British West Indies. After completing her high school education, she decided to become a nurse. In 1914, segregation in schools of nursing limited African American women's choices to Chicago, New York, and Washington, D.C. Mabel attended and in 1917 graduated from the Training School for Nurses at Freedman's Hospital in Washington, D.C. (Mosley, 1995).

Like many African American nurses at that time, Staupers, after receiving her nursing diploma, was employed primarily to care for patients of her own race in hospitals and in private-duty nursing. Staupers worked as a nurse in the District of Columbia area until 1920, when she returned to New York City and noted the living and health

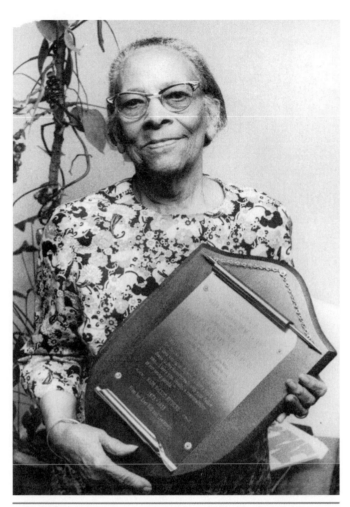

Mabel K. Staupers. Photo courtesy of Foundation of the New York State Nurses Association, Guilderland, NY.

Tuberculosis and Health Association was established in 1922 (Osofsky, 1966).

According to Osofsky (1966), the major efforts of the Harlem Committee focused on eradicating tuberculosis. The committee, however, did not view its role as being limited to this cause and subsequently organized health clinics to provide services ranging from social hygiene and nutrition to prenatal care. Serving as the executive secretary of the committee for 12 years, Staupers attracted public attention and was commended for her work. She organized health education activities provided in churches, schools, and other organizations. She also helped organize free prenatal dental care for expectant mothers who were registered with the Visiting Nurse Association, free dental service for children in schools, neighborhood health education programs in Harlem, a health-examination service, nutrition classes for children, a free diagnostic clinic for those unable to pay, and a health information program (Kiernan, 1952). Eventually, the various services developed by Staupers became a part of the Central Harlem Health Center.

In addition to her outstanding leadership in community health characterized by her efforts to establish community-based outreach health care services in Harlem, Staupers was also an activist in the struggle for equality in the professionalization of African American nurses, who sought the opportunity to work in a variety of agencies. In 1934, Staupers was appointed the first nurse executive of the National Association of Colored Graduate Nurses (NACGN); in 1949, she was elected president. Staupers was a very active executive director and president, significantly influencing the professional process for African American nurses in relation to job placement, promotion, educational opportunities, and curriculum improvements in African American

conditions in the African American community. In Harlem alone, many African American women were dying from childbirth complications. The mortality rate from tuberculosis among African Americans of all ages was three to four times that of the general population of New York City. In fact, tuberculosis was Harlem's major killer (Harding, 1926).

Health services in the Harlem community were very limited (Mosley, 1995). Staupers joined two physicians, Louis T. Wright and James L. Wilson, in opening the Booker T. Washington Sanitorium, the first African American–owned and African American–managed hospital in Harlem. She served as director of nurses there, helping to relieve the suffering among the people in the community.

Staupers later left the sanatorium. After working for a time in Philadelphia as a director of nurses, Staupers returned to New York, where she was hired to work with the New York Tuberculosis and Health Association. She conducted a survey of Harlem's community health needs, and, as a result, the Harlem Committee of the New York

REFLECTIVE THINKING

Social Activism in Nursing

- One of the issues in nursing and health care has been equality for special-population groups. What do you think about Mabel Staupers' contributions?
- When you think about a nurse as a social activist, what does this mean to you? What comes to mind?
- Do you think that social activism should be a major role of the community health nurse? Why? Why not?

schools of nursing. Within the American Nurses Association, the National League for Nursing Education, and the National Organization for Public Health Nursing, Staupers also made significant inroads in increasing awareness of the problems encountered by African American nurses (Mosley, 1995).

NURSING ORGANIZATIONS AND NURSING EDUCATION

Beginning in the late 19th century in the United States and Canada, the value of organized efforts among nurses was recognized. In 1893, Isabel Hampton Robb led the effort to create the American Society of Superintendents of Training Schools of Nursing in the United States and Canada. This society, which later became known as the National League for Nursing (NLN) (Goldwater & Zusy, 1990; Kelly, 1991), established training standards and promoted collaborative relationships among nurses. In 1895, the Nurses Association Alumnae of the United States and Canada was formed, later becoming the American Nurses Association (ANA). The purposes of this organization were to strengthen nursing organizations, promote ethical standards, and improve nursing education (Lancaster, 1996).

By 1911, efforts were being made to standardize nursing services outside the hospital. A joint committee was organized with representatives from the ANA and the American Society of Superintendents of Training Schools. Lillian Wald served as chairperson. The committee recommended the formation of a new organization to meet the needs of community health nurses. After considerable discussion with representatives of such organizations as city and state boards of health and education, visiting nurse associations, tuberculosis leagues, hospitals, dispensaries, day nurseries, settlements, and churches and other charitable organizations, the National Organization of Public Health Nursing (NOPHN) was formed. This was the first national nursing organization to have a paid staff and a designated headquarters (Fagin, 1978).

Following the development of the NOPHN, public health nursing expanded to meet societal needs. Allen (1991) points out the ways whereby the development of district nursing, and later public health nursing, fostered the concepts inherent in holistic nursing. To public health nursing, nursing meant caring for the whole person, family, friends, neighbors, and the community in relation to health and illness needs. As Allen comments:

> The ideas of wholeness implicit in the public health nursing movement were important in providing its direction, significant in the notion that it was a type of nursing set apart and above other specialties, and crucial to the movement of nursing education into the universities and nursing's recognition as a profession. (p. 75)

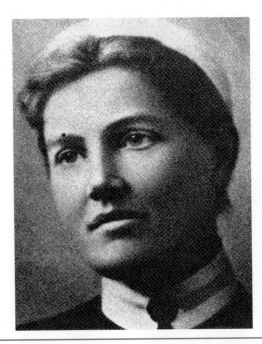

Isabel Hampton Robb. Photo courtesy of American Nurses Association.

It became apparent that public health nursing called for special educational preparation. Traditionally, all nurses were prepared in apprentice-type programs in hospitals. The curriculum was determined by hospital needs and under the direction of physicians. The focus of study was individual illness oriented and did not adequately prepare the nurse to provide services in a community setting. Public health nurses in the community functioned more independently, performed casefinding and health teaching, made referrals, and viewed their domain as the community—serving individuals, families, and population aggregates from a holistic perspective.

With the recognition that community health nurses needed additional preparation beyond the hospital-based curriculum, nursing leaders in the United States, after considerable debate, decided that all nurses needed some community health training. Basic undergraduate courses began to include community health in the curriculum, with Boston offering the first undergraduate community health nursing course (Lancaster, 1996).

As community health nursing grew and the broad scope of community health nursing became more apparent, the need for postgraduate work in community nursing also became apparent. In 1910, Mary Adelaide Nutting started the first postgraduate community health nursing course at Teacher's College in conjunction with the Henry Street Settlement (Deloughery, 1977). Because of community health nursing's concerns with social and educational problems, many of the early university-based public health nursing programs were offered through teacher's colleges or university departments of social work in sociology. By 1921, 15 colleges and universities in the United States offered courses in public health nursing, meeting the standards set forth by the NOPHN (Jensen, 1959).

In 1923, a landmark study called the Report of the Committee for Study of Nursing Education was published. This study, which began in 1919, came to be known as the Goldmark Report. Under the auspices of the Rockefeller Foundation, the Committee for the Study of Public Health Nursing Education began with a focus on public health nursing education. The following year, however, the focus expanded to nursing education in general. The report findings affected not only public health nursing but all of nursing as well. The report recommended that nursing education take place in institutions of higher learning. Subsequently, Yale University School of Nursing and the Frances Payne Bolton School of Nursing at Case Western Reserve University opened in 1923. Community health nursing content was included in both programs (Tinkham & Voorhies, 1977).

In addition to the offering of community health nursing content at institutions of higher learning, a change in the employment of public health nurses occurred in the 1920s. Prior to this time, most public health nursing services were provided by voluntary agencies such as the American Red Cross and other organizations. During the 1920s, however, official governmental agencies such as local and state health departments began to incorporate public health nursing services (Tinkham & Voorhies, 1977).

Schools of nursing expanded throughout the United States during the 1920s. Collegiate programs in nursing increasingly included content in public health, with the first basic collegiate program in nursing accredited in 1944. That program included adequate preparation in community health so that graduates did not have to take additional courses to practice public health nursing (National Organization of Public Health Nursing, 1944). Beginning in 1963, the NLN required baccalaureate nursing programs to include public health nursing content and practice in order to be considered for accreditation.

THE INFLUENCE OF THE WAR YEARS ON COMMUNITY HEALTH NURSING

Both World War I and World War II affected the development of public health programs and of community health nursing. This section illustrates the particular ways that many aspects of community health nursing and life in general changed because of these wars.

World War I and After

By the time World War I began in 1917, the role of the community health nurse was well established. The onset of World War I, however, required thousands of nurses to work for the war effort, leaving very few to provide

services in the public health setting. The American Red Cross helped maintain community health nursing by establishing a roster of nurses who could be asked to supply health care services. These services focused on educational programs for the community as well as the control of communicable diseases (Roberts, 1954).

During World War I, a nurse was loaned to the USPHS from the NOPHN to establish a community health nursing program for military outposts. This program resulted in the first community health service to become a part of the federal government (Gardner, 1919).

After World War I, many changes occurred that affected community health nursing, such as economic prosperity and the use of the automobile. The automobile enabled nurses to reach rural areas and to provide services to those in areas that were less accessible. Public health services expanded throughout the nation. Many federally funded relief projects utilized nurses, resulting in the recognition that federally employed nurses were needed to provide consultation to the states. Public health, as noted by Smillie (1952), became a subject of nationwide interest and importance. By 1920, 28 states had statewide public health nursing programs; 5 of these states included divisions of public health nursing within their state health departments (Roberts, 1954).

One of the major events that also occurred after World War I was the Great Depression. By the early 1930s, the effects of the Depression were clearly evident. Salaries decreased, unemployment was rising, and public health nursing services had to be reduced. Because public health nursing had formulated its objectives, however, and had developed a sound basis for organization, it was able to withstand the Depression. The need for services increased, and public health nursing was able to respond (Tinkham & Voorhies, 1977). The results of the Depression required that the federal government assume more responsibility for the general welfare of the people, largely because there was a growing realization that the good of the people was central to the government's mission (Tinkham & Voorhies, 1977).

In 1934, Pearl McIver, a well-qualified public health nurse, became the first nurse employed by the USPHS to provide consultant services to the states for nurses working in federal relief projects. Prior to 1936, as noted by Lancaster (1996), "only a few states had budgeted community health nursing positions" (p. 13). By 1936, however, all states were allocating budget funds for some type of public health nursing consultant position.

In 1930, the National Institutes of Health (NIH) was created, providing federal support for health care research in the United States. After the Great Depression of the 1930s, the federal government expanded health and social welfare programs. The first of these initiatives was the Social Security Act in 1935, which addressed the financial needs of elders through the Old

Age, Survivors, and Disability Insurance (OASDI) program. In 1966, the Social Security Act was amended to create the Medicare program, which provides health care insurance for older Americans. In 1967, Medicaid was passed to provide health insurance for low-income Americans.

World War II and After

After World War II began in 1941, many nurses joined the Army and Navy Nurse Corps. In response to the increased need for nurses, the National Nursing Council, comprising six national nursing organizations, assisted by the U.S. Department of Education, asked for and received $1 million to increase nursing education facilities. The USPHS administered these nursing education funds.

World War II, like World War I and the Great Depression, had a major effect on community health nursing. Specifically, the war resulted in an expansion of community health nursing practice and health care delivery. The prosperous postwar economy affected community health nursing practice. Furthermore, even greater numbers of community health nurses found it possible to see far more people due to the increased use of the automobile.

A particularly important effect of World War II on community health nursing had to do with returning veterans. During the war, approximately 15 million U.S. servicemen were exposed to quality health care, some of them for the first time. Further, wartime service called attention to the poor health of many young and middle-aged males. The high-quality, broader scope of care received by veterans during the war led them to expect the same on the home front. Local health departments thus soon found themselves besieged not only by a burgeoning group of clients who expected high-quality services but also by a sudden increase in accidents, emotional problems, alcoholism, and other health problems not previously considered to be a part of their responsibility (Roberts & Heinrich, 1985).

When the war was over in 1945, President Harry Truman presented to Congress the following proposals for a health care system (Kalisch & Kalisch, 1982):

1. Prepayment of medical costs with compulsory insurance and general revenues
2. Protection from loss of wages as a result of sickness
3. Expansion of services related to the public's health, including maternal and child health services
4. Governmental aid to medical schools for research
5. Increased construction of hospitals, clinics, and medical institutions (p. 21)

National health insurance was proposed; however, charges of socialism from the American Medical Association ended the debate about national coverage in 1949 and 1950 (Kalisch & Kalisch, 1995). But increased

---

> ### REFLECTIVE THINKING
>
> #### Community Health Nursing Contributions
>
> - What characteristics do you think community health nurses must have in order to be effective in the health care arena?
> - How do you think nurses might participate in improving the health of their communities?

---

demand for services led to an increase in funding for specific health problems such as venereal disease, cancer, tuberculosis, and mental illness. Increased demand also led to new arrangements for financing health care and a subsequent expansion of the health insurance industry (Ginzberg, 1985).

Local health departments also increased significantly in the United States. By 1955, 72% of all counties in the continental United States had full-time local public health services, with public health nurses composing a large proportion of the staffing. During the 1950s, interest increased in nurse midwifery, equality and advancement of African American nurses in public health, cost analysis studies, and improved coordination of organized nursing (Roberts & Heinrich, 1985).

Ruth Freeman, a well-known public health nursing educator, consultant, author, and leader in nursing, contributed significantly to the practice of public health nursing in the United States in the 1940s, 1950s, and beyond. She greatly influenced public health nurses and physicians through her contributions as director of nursing at the American Red Cross and consultant to the National Security Board in Washington, D.C. (1946–1950).

In addition, Ruth Freeman served as Professor of Public Health Administration and coordinator of the nursing program at John Hopkins University, School of Hygiene and Public Health from 1950 to 1971. She was the author of many publications, including two community health/public health nursing texts which became widely used as major texts in nursing programs. Ruth Freeman was appointed to many national positions—as a member of the 1958 White House Conference on Children and Youth and as consultant to the WHO and Pan American Health Organization (Bullough, Church, & Stern, 1988).

The 1960s brought a revolution in health care in the United States that affected public health and public health nursing. The Economic Opportunity Act provided funds for neighborhood health centers, Head Start, and many other community programs designed to improve the health of the community. Programs for maternal and child health, mental health, mental retardation, and pub-

RESEARCH FOCUS

The Caring Connection in Nursing: A Concept Analysis

Study Problem/Purpose

The concept of connection has been used in the nursing literature in the context of a caring relationship in nursing; however, the concept needs further description. Because caring is viewed as the essence of nursing, it is important to examine the concept of connection within the caring context. The purpose of this study was to conduct a concept analysis in order to explicate the concept of "connection" in relation to the caring literature in nursing.

Methods

The process of concept analysis was used, incorporating the methods of Walker and Avant (1995) and Rodgers (1989). Publications for the proceedings of the Caring Conferences for the International Association for Human Caring over the past two decades were the primary sources of information and CINAHL was used to search the nursing literature for the key word *connection* under the subject of caring.

Findings

The concept analysis of connection was identified as a dynamic concept that has different meanings depending on whether the term is used as a verb or a noun. Connection was viewed as an outcome, a consequence of the process of connecting. Establishing a meaningful connection with the client was one of five conceptualizations found in the nursing literature. Critical attributes, the process attributes (those related to connecting) included (1) effective communication skills (being present, empowering, attending, listening) and (2) intentionality (involves choice or the decision by the nurse to engage in the nurse–client relationship; includes copresence, depth in the relationship, and transcendence).

As an outcome, connections included synchrony, rhythm, harmony, and unity. Connection enables healing.

Implications

The concept of connection is one that can be most important in nursing education and practice, a concept that is central to the caring mission of nursing. The moments of connection make a difference in the lives of individuals and families, moments that can be ones of healing and transcendence. The concept of connection in nursing is embedded in the caring literature. The special moments shared with clients can be ones of harmony, healing, and diminishing of vulnerability, thereby fostering opportunities to enhance healing. Establishing connections with clients should be modeled by experienced nurses and nourished in beginning nurses. The caring connection in nursing is needed.

Source: Wilder, M. H. (1997). The caring connection in nursing: A concept analysis. International Journal for Human Caring 1(1), 18–24.

---

lic health training also saw increases in funding. New programs funded care for elders and the poor. As Lancaster (1995) notes, however, the revised act did not include coverage for preventive health care, and home health care was reimbursed only when ordered by a physician. Funding for home health services, however, resulted in the rapid expansion of home health agencies, including for-profit agencies. At the same time, however, there was a decline in many health promotion and disease prevention activities because of limited funding. Today, home health care is one of the major growth areas in the health care industry.

In 1965, the nurse practitioner movement began at the University of Colorado, with the development of the first pediatric nurse practitioner program. This program prepared nurses to provide comprehensive well-child care in ambulatory settings (Ford & Silver, 1967). This development set the stage for nursing's role expansion into providing primary health care to select populations. The early public health movement was the forerunner of today's primary care movement (Fagin, 1978). Public health nurses were the first nurse practitioners, and although many remained in public health, others left to work in a variety of clinical arenas. In public health agencies, nurse practitioners have continued to play an important role in providing primary health care to individuals and families in inner cities, rural areas, and other underserved areas.

In the 1970s, community health nurses played important roles in the hospice movement, the birthing center initiative, drug and substance abuse programs, day care for elders and those with disabilities, and rehabilitation services in long-term care (Roberts & Heinrich, 1985). Prevention once again was viewed as critical at the federal level, and cost effectiveness emerged as a new concern for health care. Because nurses were viewed as cost-effective providers of primary care, the way was cleared for community nursing to expand into new areas.

In this new economic climate, nurses in other specialty areas of nursing, including medical-surgical, maternal and child health, and psychiatric, began to work with individuals and families outside the hospital setting (Ruth & Partridge, 1978). Public health nurses had been the first to promote the idea that nursing could best meet the total health needs of people, and their focus continued to include aggregates as well as individuals and families in the community.

The Influences of the 1980s, 1990s, and After

The 1980s ushered in a period of change throughout the world. The Healthy Cities concept linked the Health Care for All initiative to an implementation model that is being utilized today as a model for change and development in community health.

In the United States, cost effectiveness of health care became a major concern. Health promotion and disease prevention programs were assigned lower priority as funding was shifted to meet increased costs of hospital care and technological medical procedures. In 1983, a prospective payment system for hospital care based on diagnosis related groups (DRGs) was instituted under Medicare. Ambulatory services and home health care grew rapidly. The number of nurses in home health care, however, increased. Other community outreach centers were developed, such as community nursing centers and linkages with schools. People were more often expected to assume caregiving roles for family members and for themselves. Health education, a major role of public health nursing since Lillian Wald's time, became more important. Self-care became more of a focus in health care approaches.

In the latter part of the 1980s, funding for public health declined. As a result, fewer public health nurses were employed in official agencies. The reduced public support, financing, and impact of public health services was clearly identified in the landmark publication for the Institute of Medicine (IOM, 1988), *The Future of Public Health*. The IOMs' report was a call for action to improve public health funding and services in order to address the mission of public health nationally.

The IOM report and the Health for All initiative coupled with the Healthy Cities/Communities movement reemphasized the importance of public health. In addition, WHO highlighted the concept of **sustainable development,** a relatively new concept that focuses on justice and opportunities for all people throughout the world, not just a privileged few. Sustainable development is a "process in which economic, fiscal, commercial, energy, agricultural, and industrial policies are conceived so as to achieve development that is economically, socially, and environmentally sustainable" (Pan American Association, World Health Association Document, 2001, p. 4). Further discussion of sustainable development will be included in Chapters 5 and 9. As WHO so clearly pointed out, among the essential public health functions the health sector must address in relation to sustainable development are monitoring, measuring, and championing the safety of the physical and social environments, ensuring that all development is evaluated in terms of its environmental and social impact on the population's health, in particular those who are the most vulnerable and unprotected. Strategies for improving the public's health has once again emerged as a major national and international effort.

Caring for our most vulnerable populations has long been the tradition of public health nursing, when our early public health nursing leaders such as Lillian Wald and others highlighted the importance of the impact of physical and social environmental factors on population health. In 1993, as discussed previously in this chapter, public health nursing celebrated "A Century of Caring," recognizing the caring of community health nurses over the century—caring that encompassed courage, commitment, compassion, and respect for the populations served. Reaching out to assist people who were the most vulnerable, those who were underserved, and those with major health problems comprised public health nurses' caring for the health of people in need (USPHS, 1993). Caring for our most vulnerable populations and working to promote sustainable development within the community will continue to be critical roles for public/community health nurses in the future.

The 1990s brought restructuring of the health care systems in the United States and other Western nations, a process that continues today. Increasingly, nursing care is delivered in community settings, with greater emphasis being placed on primary health care, case management, long-term care management, and the care of the acutely ill in their homes and in other ambulatory settings.

At the National and International Case Management Conference in Melbourne, Australia, in July 1995, participants from Australia, Great Britain, and the United States talked about practice issues, ideas, and concerns related to health care practice and the need for case management. Various case management models were discussed, whether the setting was long-term care, ambulatory care, acute care, or home care. A focus on consumer needs and on a more community-responsive system that encourages consumer decision making was stressed. Nursing was identified as central to the process of working together with other disciplines in ensuring that consumers receive comprehensive care in a seamless system. Health providers and consumers alike recognize that the health care system is difficult to negotiate and that consumers clearly need assistance in moving through the system. Community health nurses have played and continue to play an important role in this process.

COMMUNITY NURSING VIEW

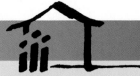

A public health nurse is working in a neighborhood of ethnically diverse, low-income people. The nurse makes home visits to various clients, including 75-year-old Emanuel, who receives assistance from an in-home support service program. Emanuel lives alone in an apartment and has a history of alcohol abuse, which has been successfully treated. He attends Alcoholics Anonymous. He has a variety of medical problems that require long-term care management services. The nurse has been visiting Emanuel in his home for the past month.

During the nurse's most recent home visit, Joan, a neighbor from next door, makes a visit to Emanuel's home. Before the nurse leaves, Joan asks the nurse to take her blood pressure. Joan complains that she has been having headaches and blurred vision for the past two days, is worried about her blood pressure, and will soon be evicted from her apartment with nowhere to go. Joan states that she lives alone, has a car, and may be forced to stay in a storage room. Joan says that she understands that public health nurses help people in need of services. When asked about access to health care, Joan states that she receives medical care from a nonprofit health maintenance organization (HMO) in the same town but that she has neither seen nor called her doctor yet. "I have been so busy and so stressed. I know I should have gone or at least called. I thought that you could help me when Emanuel told me you would be visiting today." This is the first time that the nurse has met Joan.

Nursing Considerations

Assessment

◆ What additional data are needed to assess Joan's situation?

◆ How would a knowledge of community health nursing history affect assessment in this situation?

Diagnosis

◆ On the basis of the information given, what diagnosis would be made?

Outcome identification

◆ What outcome would be expected for Joan?

Planning/Interventions

◆ How might the issue of impending homelessness be addressed?

◆ How might the public health nurse respond to this situation?

◆ What actions might be taken?

Evaluation

◆ What would indicate that the plan and intervention were successful?

It is projected that consumers in the future will play an even more important role as informed participants in making decisions about their own care. In addition, ambulatory, primary health care systems are expected to assume an increasingly significant place in health care. These projections apply not only in the United States but also in Australia, Canada, Great Britain, and other Western nations.

In many developing nations however, serious imbalances exist in terms of human and physical resources, technology, and pharmaceuticals. In addition, many have too few qualified health personnel. In the world's poorest countries, particularly sub-Saharan Africa, most people, particularly the poor, have to pay for health care out-of-pocket, often when they are sick and most in need of it. They have less access than better-off groups to subsidized services, because the better-off groups are likely to be members of job-based prepayment schemes (WHO, 2000). One of the outcomes related to this financial issue is health inequities—a higher proportion of preventable deaths and disabilities occur in our developing, low-income nations. This problem

is a major concern of WHO. Further discussion regarding the problem is included in Chapter 4. Because of WHO's concern, it is anticipated that policymakers will work to improve primary health care services for the poor.

Two major reasons for the reconfiguration of health care delivery systems are cost containment and elimination of health disparities among segments of the population who are at higher risk. Community health nurses, as well as other nurses, are in a prime position to assist in the paradigm shift. Nurses must take leadership roles in emphasizing the need for humanistic care and practice, rather than focusing primarily on the principles of economic rationalism. Community health nurses must collaborate with other health professionals and consumers in order to develop comprehensive advocacy programs that will promote and protect the health of people. Working together to promote health for all remains a challenge for the future. Developing partnerships to reduce health disparities and improve health system performance is a most important worldwide agenda where nurses must play a major role.

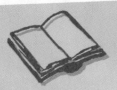

Out
of the Box

Developing innovative partnerships that will work to improve the public's health worldwide is critical. It is of utmost importance that community health nurses are knowledgeable about these partnerships, given the history of the population focus of the practice and the increased emphasis on global perspectives in health care.

A new global health commission, the Commission on Macroeconomics and Health, was launched in January 2000 by the WHO Director-General Gro Harlem Brundtland. The purpose of this commission is to examine the way improvements in health can be used to reduce poverty. Issues such as debt relief, trade negotiation, the acquired immunodeficiency syndrome (AIDS) crisis, essential drug availability, and spiraling health care costs have made it clear that health has a central place in the world economy.

A series of studies will have been conducted by the end of 2001, studies that focus on how health interventions can enhance economic growth and reduce inequity in developing countries. Prior to the beginning of 2002, a final report will be produced.

This new global health commission includes representatives from World Bank, the International Monetary Fund, the United Nations Development Program, and the Economic Commission on Africa. The commission will assess and provide information on:

1. *The nature and magnitude of economic outcomes as they relate to health investments*
2. *The economics of incentives for research and the development of vaccines and drugs that primarily affect those populations who are poor*
3. *The mobilization of resources necessary to provide effective and equitable services that deal with major disease problems that affect the poor*
4. *Costs and cost-effective mechanisms that address the major diseases of the poor*

The strengths of this international commission are that it is based on the partnership model and that it focuses on the study of the linkages between poverty and health—a major global public health concern. ■

A basic principle of community health nursing, then, is to understand the concerns of the people they serve. The community health nurse sees where people work, play, worship, live, study, and die. Community health nurses work with groups, families, and individual clients as well as function in multidisciplinary teams and programs. They participate in identifying the strengths of the communities they serve as well as in defining and addressing health problems. They have worked and continue to work with people in their own environments.

Community health nurses have fostered the caring, healing, and health model of nursing, a model that is once again coming to the forefront. In the early days, community health nurses worked to create community models of caring. Today, community health nurses must participate with other disciplines and with consumers in creating healthier caring communities, with health viewed in its broadest sense, from a holistic perspective.

KEY CONCEPTS

- ◆ To understand the nature of community health nursing and future developments, one must examine the historical context of early public health and community health nursing efforts.

- ◆ A number of factors influenced the development of public health and community health nursing: early Christianity, the Industrial Revolution, heightened public awareness of community problems, two major wars, a major economic depression, and social action on the part of community health nursing leaders.

- ◆ The Health for All and Healthy Cities/Communities initiatives are rooted in a spirit of partnership, collaboration, and consensus building.

- ◆ The mission of public health nursing has historically been twofold: personal advocacy and social activism.

- ◆ Since their inception, the roles of community health nurses have been multifaceted, complex, and challenging.

- ◆ Public health and community health nursing organizations matured as a result of both the vision of the nurses themselves and evolving community needs.

- ◆ The years during and after the two world wars brought expansion of health care concepts as well as new roles for public health and community health nurses.

- ◆ An intersectoral approach to planning and implementing health care for all is basic to public health philosophy.

RESOURCES

American Public Health Association: www.apha.org
American Association for the History of Nursing: www.aahn.org
Center for the Study of Nursing History: www.nursing.upenn.edu/history
Frontier Nursing Service: www.frontiernursing.org
Institute of Medicine: www.iom.org
Johns Hopkins University Center for Communication Programs: www.jhuccp.org
Pan American Health Organization: www.paho.org
US Department of Health and Human Services, Office of Disease Prevention and Health Promotion: www.health.gov
World Health Organization: www.who.org

II

HEALTH CARE: NATIONAL AND INTERNATIONAL PERSPECTIVES

T*his unit highlights the dimensions of health care systems around the world. This will serve as a basis of comparison with the U.S. health care delivery system. Also included is information on the steps being taken to change the current U.S. health care delivery system and the economic aspects that affect it.*

IN THIS UNIT

Chapter

3

NATIONAL AND INTERNATIONAL HEALTH PERSPECTIVES

Sue A. Thomas, EdD, RN

No health system can be sustained if it acts at cross-purposes with its core. We must create a milieu where caring and healing connections make it possible to address health as the first priority of the system. . . . We must join together with communities in a mutually beneficial effort to produce sustainable health at both personal and collective levels.

—*Tim Porter-O'Grady (1995)*

COMPETENCIES

Upon completion of this chapter, the reader should be able to:

- Discuss population health from national and international perspectives.
- Identify the determinants of population health, including the changes that have occurred in health professional perspectives.
- Identify the changes in the measurement of global health status from a public health perspective.
- Identify selected health problems from a population-based approach.
- Compare and contrast selected population changes with an international focus.
- Explain the community health nursing role in relation to caring for the health of communities from a national and international perspective.
- Discuss the implications for change in global health planning efforts.

KEY TERMS

disability-adjusted life
   year (DALY)

global burden of
   disease (GBD)

Community health nurses provide care to clients in various communities throughout the world. The community health nurse functions within the multidisciplinary care model, a model that contributes to the comprehensive care of communities. When effective, the comprehensive holistic model exemplifies the collective spirit, the creation of caring communities in which human beings are respected, nurtured, and celebrated.

In order to function effectively in communities, community health nurses must examine the health of communities from national and international perspectives. Community health nurses must have knowledge of the various health problems that exist within the populations. Population characteristics need to be addressed in order to gain an understanding of changing population needs. It is also important to examine those factors that contribute to the health of populations, such as environmental and social determinants, as well as organizational efforts that are related to health status assessment, prevention, and control.

The purpose of this chapter is to examine the health of populations from national and international perspectives. Population health and selected characteristics will be discussed, in addition to those determinants that have an impact on health. The chapter will conclude with a

discussion of the community health nursing role and community efforts to address community health.

POPULATION HEALTH

There are a variety of ways to describe the health of a population. There are different ways in which health and illness are defined and many different ways that people have thought about the relationship between the two.

In this chapter, a review of general and infant mortality estimates and life expectancy will provide a background for examining health progress. In addition, current thinking about approaches to measuring health status will be discussed. An initial examination of historical trends will demonstrate how the patterns of disease and life expectancy have changed dramatically over the course of this century.

Historical Perspectives

Since the 18th century, there has been a major shift in the health of populations, particularly in industrialized nations, and a significant decline in the death rate during the past 200 years (Lee & Estes, 1994). This decline reflects the decrease in the incidence of infectious diseases in industrialized nations that once claimed the lives of individuals in their early years. As McKeown (1978) pointed out, "over 90% of the reduction was due to a decrease of deaths from infectious diseases" (p. 6).

For example, in the 1800s, respiratory tuberculosis was the single largest cause of death (McKeown, 1978). There were remarkable changes in the course of the disease, however, as evidenced by the decline in British tuberculosis death rates from approximately 450 deaths per 100,000 people in 1810 to 180 per 100,000 in 1890 (Dubos & Dubos, 1952). This significant improvement could be linked to the sanitary reform movement, a reaction to the adverse impact of the Industrial Revolution. Even though the growth of industries brought about many benefits, the movement of workers and their families into cities not equipped to handle such influx resulted in very poor living conditions for many (Rosenberg, 1962).

In various cities throughout the world, pigs, dogs, and goats roamed the streets, serving as garbage disposal agents. In some cities, people had to get water from a pump in the street. Rooms were small, poorly lit and poorly ventilated, and often overcrowded. Infectious diseases such as tuberculosis, measles, diphtheria, and typhoid fever flourished. The inner city poor suffered the most; however, other social classes were also affected (Fee, 1987).

The development of the sulfonamides in the 1930s, penicillin in the 1940s, and broad-spectrum antibiotics in the 1940s and early 1950s played an important role in the declines in mortality from some of the infectious diseases;

however, as the late British physician McKeown noted, "the role of individual medical care in preventing sickness and premature death is secondary to that of other influences" (p. 12, as cited in Lee & Estes, 1994). McKeown argued that medical science and service are not the primary determinants of health; rather, environment and personal behavior play a significant role. Improved nutrition; a safer, cleaner environment; a change to fewer children in families; and changes in other personal health habits were more significant. The determinants of health will be explored further later in this chapter.

Today, the leading causes of death in many of the industrialized nations such as the United States are chronic diseases: for example, heart disease, cancer, and strokes. In industrialized nations, chronic diseases will remain the major causes of death in the future. In developing countries, however, infectious diseases will remain the leading causes of death. An infectious disease crisis of global proportions is threatening gains in health and life expectancy. Infectious diseases are now identified as the world's major killer of children and young adults [World Health Association (WHO), 1999b]. As the economies of the developing nations improve, however, noncommunicable diseases are projected to account for an increasing share of disease burden.

In the United States over the past 25 years, significant improvements have been made in reducing the mortality from heart disease and stroke: Death rates for heart disease and stroke have declined by 49% and 58%, respectively. Much of this success has been attributed to a dual strategy that includes a high-risk and population approach. Improved high blood pressure control and high blood cholesterol control have been identified as the principal initiatives [U.S. Department of Health and Human Services (USDHHS), 2000b]. In *Healthy People 2010*, major health disparities and gaps were shown to exist among population groups and geographic regions, with a disproportionate burden of death and disability in minority and low-income groups and those with the least education (USDHHS, 2000b).

Even though there has been a significant improvement in the mortality associated with certain chronic diseases in industrialized nations, the level of disability and handicap associated with chronic illness has increased. Many of the chronic illnesses are long term in nature, posing different types of problems in the community. More than 500 million people experience special needs related to disabilities. Up to 10% of the global population lives with disabilities that can cause difficulties in daily activities. An estimated 80% of the world's disabled people live in developing nations [American Public Health Association (APHA), 2000a].

Chronic disability conditions in the United States caused major activity limitations for 10.6% of the population in 1993, an increase from 9.4% in 1988. Over 21% of the population, or more than 54 million people, in the United States have some level of disability. As the population ages in the coming years, those people with dis-

abilities will rise. Clients with disabilities tend to report more pain, anxiety, days of depression, and sleeplessness and fewer days of vitality than those without activity limitations. Many people with disabilities lack access to medical care and other health services. Chronic disability was identified as a target area in the *Health People 2010* objectives, with a recognition of the need for health promotion of people with disabilities, prevention of secondary conditions, and elimination of disparities between people with and those without disabilities in the United States (USDHHS, 2000). Chronic disability conditions in the United States and worldwide lead to physical, emotional, social, and economic costs to individuals, families, and nations.

The next two decades will see major changes in the health needs of all the world's populations. By the year 2020, noncommunicable diseases are expected to account for seven out of every 10 deaths in the developing nations of the world, compared with less than half in the latter part of the 20th century. These changes are expected because of the rapid aging of the populations in the developing countries worldwide. As the population ages, the major health problems become those of adults rather than children. The rapidity of change will present significant challenges to health care systems and will result in difficult decisions about the allocation of scarce resources (Murray & Lopez, 1996).

In the early decades of the 21st century, therefore, it will be necessary to confront the challenges of a double burden of disease: first, the emerging epidemics of noncommunicable diseases and injuries, which are becoming more prevalent in both industrialized and developing nations, and, second, the continued problems of infectious diseases, malnutrition, and childbirth complications, which more disproportionately affect those who live in poverty. Reducing the burden of the inequality that exists among the world's disadvantaged populations, in comparison to those who are not poverty stricken, is a priority in international health (WHO, 1999a).

REFLECTIVE THINKING

Chronicity and Health Promotion

- What do you think can be done at national and international levels to deal with problems associated with chronicity?
- How might you participate at the community level to assist in health promotion and disease prevention activities to decrease the incidence of chronic diseases?

Determinants of Health

As mentioned previously in this text, in order for nurses to promote health in individuals, families, and groups, they must view health from a population perspective as well as from a focus on individuals and families. It is important to examine the determinants of health in populations.

The health of a population is influenced by various factors: biology, lifestyle, environment, and the health care system. Determinants of health include not only health behaviors of clients and the influence of their family history but also social and environmental determinants. The different determinants of health have a profound effect on the health of individuals and communities. An evaluation of the determinants is a critical part of working with clients to improve health and well-being (USDHHS, 2000b).

An examination of the distribution of mortality and morbidity between social groups is necessary, as is an examination of the environmental determinants that affect health. As noted by Blane (1995), there is a definite consistency in the distribution of mortality and morbidity between social groups. The more advantaged groups, whether identified in terms of income, education, social class, or ethnicity, tend to have better health than the other members of society. The distribution is graded, not bipolar (advantaged versus others), so that a change in the level of advantage or disadvantage is associated with a change in health patterns, as measured by mortality and morbidity.

For most people, their cultural heritage, social roles, and economic situation have a profound influence on health behaviors and health outcomes. Blane (1995) states:

This social patterning of health is important for a number of reasons. The size of the gap between the mortality rates of the most and least advantaged groups gives some indication of the potential for improvement in a nation's health. Identification of the groups who are at greatest risk of poor health can inform sound governance of medical services. . . . Understanding the causes of social variations in health should lead to intervention strategies which can reduce them. (p. 903)

The economic situation of people has a major influence on health outcomes. Poverty in all its forms was identified as the greatest challenge to the international community (Annan, Johnston, Kohler, & Wolfensohn, 2000). Around the world, one person in five lives on less than $1 a day—and one in seven suffers chronic hunger. In many developing countries, poverty is a major contributor to the risk of death and inhibits mental and physical development. South Asia has the greatest numbers of poor; however, the proportion of poor people is highest in sub-Saharan Africa. Even though there are currently major international efforts to reduce poverty by 2015,

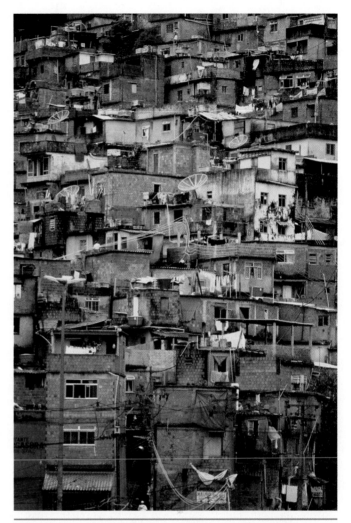

Poverty is a global concern. This photo is of a low-income area in Brazil where having adequate housing and food is a daily concern. Courtesy of Photodisc.

approximately 900 million people will still be left in extreme poverty (United Nations et al., 2000b).

As clearly pointed out by Nijhius (1989), health is a complex phenomenon that is given form and meaning by the way it is perceived, but it is also definitely linked within the social context of living. The social environment has a profound effect on health, at the individual, family, and community levels. The quality of the social environment is a major determinant of health (USDHHS, 2000b).

The environment is also critical in promoting the health of the population. Throughout history, citizens and leaders have made changes to improve their communities (Duhl & Drake, 1995). Whether making water available, removing sewage, or reducing the exposure to physical hazards at work sites, the ultimate goal has been to improve the quality of life. The physical environment can promote good health, for example, by providing clean, safe places for people to work, exercise, and play. As Duhl and Drake (1995) have stated, "Before the scientific age of medicine, there was always an awareness of the interconnectedness of health and the environment" (p. 105).

When Florence Nightingale returned from the Crimean War in 1860, she focused her energies on the health implications of broader issues. In the United States, Lillian Wald, Mary Brewster, and Lavinia Dock, among others, also recognized the linkage between health, the environment, and social determinants. They too focused on broader social and environmental issues related to health, as noted in Chapter 2.

Although morbidity and mortality are affected by many interrelated factors, with the advent of the Industrial Age in the 18th century, a new intervention model emerged. A linear, rational, and reductionist model replaced the holistic perspective, which viewed health issues in a broader context. The new model suggested that successful intervention came from finding a causative agent associated with the problem and then removing it (Duhl & Drake, 1995).

The reductionist model views the body as a machine that can be examined in terms of its parts, separate from the psychological, social, spiritual, and environmental aspects of illness. By focusing on the individual, this approach causes health professionals to ignore the complex interrelated web of relationships in a community and the interdependence of individual health and the social, ecological systems of which we are all a part.

As has been previously claimed, the medical model, with its focus on the individual, has resulted in life span improvement, a decrease in illness, and improvement in the well-being of people. McKeown, however, explained with statistical detail, as noted by Kickbusch (1989), those factors that brought about the significant changes in the health of the population at the beginning of the 20th century. These factors were improved living conditions and better nutrition, in other words, changes in the standard of living.

Environmental Challenges—Global Perspectives

As discussed in Chapters 1 and 9, the environment is a major determinant of population health. The health of the biosphere significantly impacts human health. Global atmospheric change, ecotoxicity, and the depletion of natural resources pose serious environmentally based threats this century. An estimated 25% of preventable illnesses can be attributed to poor environmental quality worldwide. Air pollution alone contributes to premature deaths and billions of dollars in health-related costs annually—air pollutants such as ozone (outdoor) and environmental tobacco smoke (indoor) (USDHHS, 2000b).

Poor air quality contributes to respiratory illnesses such as asthma, cardiovascular disease, and cancer. A major concern worldwide is the increase in asthma cases. Environmental triggers in both indoor and outdoor air contribute to asthma's development and severity. In the

United States alone, there is a rapidly growing asthma epidemic, whose victims are projected to more than double by 2020 with 1 in 14 Americans affected unless the rates are decreased. In 2010 the projected number of persons in the United States with asthma will be over 20 million, and by 2020 it is projected to be over 25 million, approaching 30 million (Pew Environmental Health Commission, 2000).

Global atmospheric change has the potential to affect population health in a number of ways. The depletion of the ozone layer and the associated increase in ultraviolet radiation reaching the earth pose serious problems, e.g., increased rates of cataracts and skin cancer, with possible immune system interference. Acid rain continues to be a serious problem because of its effects on ecosystems and association with respiratory diseases. Global warming is another major change with the potential to result in agricultural disruption, which could result in malnutrition, famine, and an increase in tropical infectious diseases transmitted by insects (Hancock & Garrett, 1995).

Ecotoxicity, the effect of toxic chemical pollutants, also threatens health. The effects of air and water pollution, including pollution caused by seepage of toxic chemicals stored in the ground, have received a great deal of attention. Effects including detrimental genetic, hormonal, immunologic, and psychologic consequences may pose serious problems (Hancock & Garrett, 1995). Environmental toxification is a health threat that requires immediate attention and action.

Depletion of natural resources also has an impact on health, both directly and indirectly. The shrinking of pasturelands through desertification and erosion and the decline of harvestable terrestrial, marine, and freshwater species can lead to malnutrition and famine. Ground and surface water pollution threaten not only safe drinking water supplies but agricultural production as well. The development of safe and sustainable alternatives to dwindling fossil fuel resources is necessary to prevent energy supply problems, including heating of homes, transportation of agricultural products, and provision of basic services. As Hancock and Garrett (1995) point out:

> What is needed is a system of economic development that avoids harming the health of the ecosystem of which we are part and the global life support system upon which we depend for our health and survival. This will require a shift in the industrialized world toward a more environmentally sustainable form of economic development in the context of a consumer society. (p. 940)

Achieving and maintaining health in this century will require broad-based actions that address environmental health as well as the other major determinants of health at national and international levels. Policies and strategies have emerged to deal with these global challenges, strategies such as healthy public policy, sustainable development, and investment in health through intersectoral collaboration. Because of the global concerns about our environment and the loss of environmental resources such as tropical forests, active partnerships are emerging in order to promote sustainable development. The World Bank, International Monetary Fund, Organization for Economic Co-Operation and Development, and the United Nations, for example, worked together in a partnership endeavor and formulated a goal to implement national strategies for sustainable development by 2005 (United Nations et al., 2000b). Through unsustainable harvesting and degradation that occurred in the early 1990s, about 17 million hectares of tropical forests were cleared annually. Lost forests can no longer conserve soil and water resources, mitigate climate change, sustain biodiversity, or protect natural and cultural heritage.

The growth in the development and application of the strategies associated with sustainable development and healthy public policy is occurring. They have the potential to continue to bring about changes in the 21st century, whereby people and communities can take part in defining and achieving progress in population health. The future of our health in the 21st century "involves much more than the future of medical care, since the major factors affecting health are environmental, social, and economic ones" (Hancock & Garrett, 1995, p. 935).

Measuring Health Status

Measuring the health status of a population, a nation, or the world is a systematic approach that is a major responsibility of public health and other health-related organizations. Monitoring and evaluating the health status are essential for purposes of evidence-based public health policymaking. It is essential therefore that community health nurses understand the processes and methods used to measure health status.

Health status can be measured by birth and death rates, life expectancy, morbidity from specific diseases, risk factors, quality of life, use of health care services, accessibility to health services, health insurance coverage, and other factors. More recently, greater emphasis has been placed on also monitoring behaviors, environmental factors, and health systems (USDHHS, 2000b). Traditionally, mortality and life expectancy have been important indicators of population health. However, morbidity and health-related quality of life in addition to mortality are now viewed as critical indicators also (Melse, Essink-Bot, Kramers, & Hoeymans, 2000). Chapter 14 focuses on the study of those basic public health measures used to assess health status.

A new approach for measuring health status, called the **global burden of disease (GBD),** was developed by Murray and Lopez (1996). This approach was reported in their landmark publication, *The Global Burden of Disease and Injury Series,* published in 1996. The publication was the result of a major study that involved a five-year effort—a collaborative effort of the WHO, the World Bank, and the Harvard School of Public Health. This effort included projections of disease and injury to 2020. The method quantifies not only the number of deaths but also the impact of premature death and disability on a population. These indicators are then combined into a single unit of measurement of the global burden of disease. The GBD study reported the first estimates of mortality and disability that could be related to certain risk factors for disease, such as tobacco, alcohol, unsafe sex, and sanitation (Murray & Lopez, 1996). The use of the GBD approach is expanding worldwide, and many countries have completed or are undertaking national burden of disease assessments. In addition, WHO publishes burden of disease results and promotes its development and application. A major revision of the GBD for the year 2000 has been launched (Murray & Lopez, 2000). It is currently being developed.

The GBD has three aims (Murray & Lopez, 1996):

1. To include nonfatal conditions, as well as mortality data, in assessments of health status. In many countries, the statistics on the health status of populations are limited, and the number of deaths from specific causes each year are difficult to obtain; thus only estimates can be made. Traditionally, mortality data have been widely used as indicators of health status; however, even in countries where the data are available, such as industrialized nations, they fail to identify the impact of nonfatal outcomes of disease and injury, such as blindness, dementia, or severe respiratory diseases on population health.

2. To produce "objective, independent, and demographically plausible assessments of the burdens of particular conditions and diseases" (p. 6).

3. To measure disease and injury burden in ways that can allow comparisons of the relative cost effectiveness of different interventions, in terms of cost per unit of disease burden averted, e.g., the treatment of long-term care for schizophrenia versus ischemic heart disease. Rational allocation of scarce resources requires this comparison.

The single measure of disease burden for the GBD is called the **disability-adjusted life year (DALY),** an internationally standardized measure. The DALY expresses years of life lost to premature death and years lived with a disability of specified severity and duration. One DALY is therefore one lost year of healthy life. In this measure, a premature death is defined as "one that occurs before the age to which the dying person could have expected to survive if [he or she] were a member of a standardized model population with a life expectancy at birth equal to that of the world's longest-surviving population, Japan" (Murray & Lopez, 1996, p. 7).

The DALY is a measure that makes comparisons between health losses due to mortality and morbidity and health losses attributable to different diseases. As Melse et al (2000) point out, "Burden of disease calculations in DALYs may . . . help in setting priorities among diseases and disorders for policy-making, interventions, and research" (p. 1241).

The inclusion of information about the GBD in this chapter is important for community health nurses to begin to understand because of the implications this landmark measurement has on examining the health status of nations. The reporting of health outcomes from a global perspective, using a different public health measure, is a true challenge for the future.

Life Expectancy

Life expectancy is one of the measures that is used to assess health status. Life expectancy is the "average number of years people born in a given year are expected to live based on a set of age-specific death rates (USDHHS, 2000b, p. 8). Global average life expectancy at birth in 1955 was 48 years, in 1995 it was 65 years, and in 2025 it is estimated that life expectancy will be 73 years. By the year 2025, WHO expects that no country will have a life expectancy of less than 50 years (WHO, 1998).

Differences in life expectancy between countries, however, suggest a major need for improvement. More than 50 million people live in countries with a life expectancy of less than 45 years. Over 5 billion people in 120 countries in 1998 had a life expectancy of more than 60 years. At least 18 countries with populations of 1 million or more may have life expectancies greater than the United States for both men and women (USDHHS, 2000b).

Risk Factor Surveillance to Promote Global Health

Surveillance is a major focus of public health. A global health perspective requires a worldwide system to monitor risk factors in different population groups, identify emerging health problems that are critical at the international or regional level, and develop effective prevention strategies to deal with the problems (Morabia, 2000). Surveillance of risk factors is needed to track outcomes of chronic disease, for example, hypertension and lifestyles associated with cardiovascular disease. Surveillance is also needed to track other risk factors, such as those associated with infectious diseases, injuries and accidents, and mental illness and mental disorders.

Worldwide surveillance programs, however, are in their infancy. A variety of methods have been used since the 1960s, primarily national surveys that are conducted in various countries. A variety of other strategies have been used in Europe. Morabia (2000) suggests that a centralized Internet database may be the most accessible and efficient way to combine collected data from different countries. An attempt to provide reports of current epidemic outbreaks was established by WHO in April 2000. A global outbreaks alert and response network was developed. Those that are considered to have potential international importance are included in a weekly e-mail service distributed to global surveillance partners and public health professionals worldwide.

It is clear that international and regional cooperation and collaboration are needed in a system of worldwide risk factor surveillance, thus providing an opportunity to benefit from public health researchers around the world. Those regions that lack surveillance infrastructure and resources could be assisted by shared expertise and by coordinated fund-raising efforts for core functions such as database maintenance (Morabia, 2000).

GLOBAL MORTALITY ESTIMATES

Worldwide, one death in every three in 1990 was from the category Group I in the GBD—communicable, maternal, perinatal, and nutritional conditions. Most all of these deaths were in the developing regions. One death in 10 was from Group III causes (injuries) in the GBD, and just over half were from Group II causes (noncommunicable diseases) (Murray & Lopez, 1996). Table 3-1 offers a listing of the different types of categories used in the Global Burden of Disease and Injury Series.

The developing regions of the world were estimated to have 47.4% of deaths attributable to noncommunicable diseases and maternal, perinatal, and nutritional conditions and 10.7% to injuries. In the industrialized regions of the world, 86.2% of deaths were due to noncommunicable diseases, with 7.6% due to injuries and 6.1% due to communicable, maternal, perinatal, and nutritional conditions. Only in India and sub-Saharan Africa did communicable diseases and maternal, perinatal, and nutritional conditions dominate as the major categories for deaths, accounting for 51% and 65% of deaths, respec-

TABLE 3-1 Global Burden of Disease and Injury Series Categories

GROUP I	GROUP II	GROUP III
Communicable diseases	Noncommunicable diseases	Injuries
Maternal conditions		
Perinatal conditions		
Nutritional conditions		

Source: Adapted from Summary: The Global Burden of Disease, Global Burden of Disease and Injury Series, *by C. J. Murray and A. D. Lopez, 1996, Cambridge, MA: Harvard School of Public Health on Behalf of the World Health Organization and the World Bank, Harvard University Press.*

tively. In Latin America and the Caribbean, there were almost twice as many deaths from noncommunicable disease as from those reported in the communicable disease category; whereas in China there were four and a half times as many deaths from noncommunicable diseases as from the communicable disease category (Murray & Lopez, 1996).

In the recent WHO World Health Report (1998), communicable diseases in Group I will continue to dominate in developing countries as the major cause of death. As the economies of the developing nations improve, however, noncommunicable diseases from Group II will become more prevalent. As noted in the report, this increase "will be due largely to the adoption of 'western' lifestyles and their accompanying risk factors—smoking, high-fat diet, obesity, and lack of exercise" (WHO, 1998, p. 3).

Leading Causes of Death Worldwide

In 1990, just over 50 million people died worldwide, with ischemic heart disease (IHD) causing more deaths than any other disease or injury (Murray & Lopez, 1996). Only 2.7 million of the 6.3 million who died of IHD were in the industrialized nations, thus pointing to the need for

RESEARCH FOCUS

Socioeconomic Inequalities in Mortality among Women and Men: An International Study

Study Problem/Purpose

Socioeconomic inequalities in mortality have been studied in countries around the world. Inequalities in mortality have been documented; however, many of the studies have been confined to men, partly because the most frequently used socioeconomic classification is based on occupation and thus can be less easily applied to women. Women who are not in paid employment cannot be classified based on their own occupational class; thus, they would be left out of the study. Because of the problem associated with the use of occupation as a socioeconomic indicator for women, educational level was selected as a more adequate indicator.

The purpose of the study was to examine differences in total and cause specific mortality by educational level among women compared to men in seven countries: the United States, Finland, Norway, Sweden, Italy, the Czech Republic, Hungary, and Estonia.

Methods

National data were obtained for the period ca. 1980–1990 using national longitudinal studies, national census, and national unlinked cross-sectional studies. Poisson regression analysis was used to calculate age-adjusted ratios comparing a broad lower educational group with a broad upper educational group. Causes of death were coded using the *International Classification of Diseases*, 9th revision.

Findings

This international study found that socioeconomic inequalities in total mortality was smaller among women than among men. It also showed that sex differences in the size of the inequality varied significantly between countries, from almost none in Norway to the highest in the Czech Republic. In terms of mortality, higher mortality rates among lower educated women were found for most causes of death, but not for neoplasms. Relative inequalities in mortality were generally larger among men than among women. The only cause of death for which inequalities were larger among women than men was cardiovascular disease. Neoplasms and cardiovascular disease accounted for a large majority of all deaths, in both men and women, but neoplasms had a larger share in total female mortality than in total male mortality.

Implications

The interaction of gender with educational level in terms of the effect of socioeconomic status on mortality appears to provide important clues for understanding reasons that contribute to socioeconomic inequalities in mortality. Further study of the interaction between gender, socioeconomic factors, and mortality may provide additional knowledge regarding important clues to the explanation of inequalities in health among women and men.

Source: Mackenbach, J. P., Kunst, A. E., Groenhof, F., Borgan, J., Costa, G., Faggiano, F., Jozan, P., Leinsalu, M., Mortikainen, P., Rychtarikova, J., & Valkonen, T. (1999). *Socioeconomic inequalities in mortality among women and among men: An international study*. American Journal of Public Health, 89(12), 1800–1813.

greater recognition of the changing mortality patterns in the developing nations.

In 1997, there was a global total of 52.2 million deaths, with 15.3 due to circulatory diseases. In 1997, 17.3 million deaths worldwide were due to infectious and parasitic diseases, and 3.6 million were due to perinatal conditions. An estimate of 1.8 million adults died of AIDS in 1997 (WHO, 1998). In 1998, there was a worldwide threat of 53.9 million deaths from all causes, with 31% due to cardiovascular disease, 25% due to infectious diseases, 13% due to cancers, and 11% due to injuries. Respiratory and digestive deaths accounted for 9%, maternal deaths 5%, and other causes 6% (WHO, 1999b). An examination of the mortality patterns worldwide is necessary to examine in order to plan effective responses to deal with the problems.

Maternal and Women's Health

Maternal and women's health issues are critical to examine from a global perspective. Ninety-nine percent of maternal deaths occur in developing countries, most of them preventable. Infections, blood loss, and unsafe abortion account for most of the deaths (United Nations et al., 2000b). An estimate of 514,000 women died during pregnancy and childbirth in 1995 and many millions more suffered with treatment. Maternal mortality varies widely among the regions of the world—low in Latin America, but very high in Africa. In many of the poor African countries, one mother dies from pregnancy complications and delivery per every 100 live births (United Nations et al., 2000b).

Although the rate of maternal deaths in developing nations can be reduced through access to services and treatment of pregnancy complications, major efforts are needed to reduce maternal mortality in the developing regions. The goal of the World Bank and the United Nations is to reduce maternal rates by three-quarters by 2015. In order to reduce the maternal mortality, the necessary services include family planning, basic maternity care, skilled birth attendants, neonatal care, and the pre-vention and treatment of unsafe abortions as well as complications of pregnancy and delivery (United Nations et al., 2000b). These services are often unavailable, inaccessible, and unaffordable to women in the developing nations, particularly in Africa (Anderson, 1996). Africa now has the largest percentage of its population living in poverty, with Nigeria accounting for nearly a quarter of sub-Saharan Africa (United Nations et al., 2000b).

In order to deal with the problems of maternal mortality, a global initiative was started by WHO and UNICEF to reform the services received by women and children in developing countries (Heiby, 1998). These organizations called for government initiatives to address maternal mortality. Since then, the World Bank, the International Monetary Fund, the Organization for Economic Co-Operation and Development, and the United Nations have also highlighted the importance of reducing maternal mortality, investing more in health systems to improve the quality and coverage of delivery services and providing prenatal/postnatal care to the poor, particularly those in the developing nations. These four organizations called for government actions to reduce maternal mortality, to assist those who are the most vulnerable throughout the world. Through their work as partners in the global effort, anti-poverty strategies are being implemented with governments to improve maternal mortality and other key social indicators (United Nations et al., 2000b).

Health of Infants and Small Children

The significance of infant mortality as an indicator of a nation's health status and well-being has been well documented in the social and biomedical research literature. Since the early part of the 20th century in the United States, for example, significant progress was made in infant survival through improved sanitation and socioeconomic conditions, success against infectious diseases, improved nutrition and access to prenatal care, and the use of technology in neonatal intensive care units (Rice, 1994).

The overall mortality rates have improved significantly over the last century. In the United States, much of this improvement can be attributed to the progressive child welfare movement inspired by Lillian Wald and other women of that time. Infant mortality was defined as a social problem, with multiple causes. The poverty paradigm was used by these socially conscious women, who collected empirical evidence, built community consensus, and harnessed political will to deal with the child welfare problem. Through the effectiveness of the child welfare movement—the reduction of poverty and the amelioration of the effects of poverty on the poor—the improvement of individual health occurred. The provision of safe milk supplies, improved housing and elimination of environmental hazards, elimination of exploitive child labor practices, as well as an increase in parenting education all provided a powerful means for public health action.

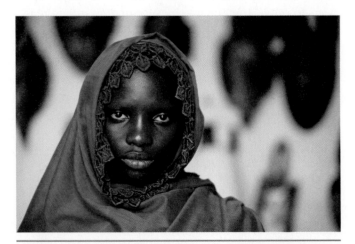

Maternal mortality rates are very high in Africa.

Although the infant mortality rate in the United States has declined steadily since 1933, it has been consistently higher than that found in many industrialized countries (Singh & Yu, 1995). The rate of decline in the United States has not equaled that of other industrialized countries. In 1960, the United States ranked 12th internationally in infant mortality. In 1988, the United States ranked 23rd in the world (MacDorman & Rosenberg, 1993). By 1991, compared with other industrialized nations, the United States ranked 24th in infant mortality (USDHHS, 1996).

Even though the infant mortality rate in the United States has significantly declined over the past four decades, the infant mortality rate among African Americans remains more than double that for whites. In addition, Native Americans and Alaska Natives have an infant mortality rate almost double that for whites (USDHHS, 2000b).

In 1995, the infant mortality rate per 1000 live births worldwide was 59 compared with 148 in 1955. It is projected to be 29 in 2025. The under-5-years of age mortality rates per 1000 live births for 1955 was 210, 78 for 1995, and projected to be 37 in 2025. Significant progress has been made in reducing under-5 mortality since 1955, and it is projected to continue. Overall, there were about 10 million under-5 deaths in 1997 compared with 21 million in 1995 (WHO, 1998).

Using the statistical reporting regions by WHO, in 1998 the infant mortality rate per 1000 live births in Africa was 91; in Southeast Asia (including India), 68; and in the Western Hemisphere as a whole, 39. In Europe, which includes the nations of the former Soviet Union, the rate was 21 and in the United States it was 7 (WHO, 1999b).

By 2025, it is projected that globally there will be approximately 5 million deaths among children under 5—97% of them in developing countries, with most of them due to infectious diseases such as pneumonia and diarrhea combined with nutritional deficiencies (Group I-GBD). There are approximately 24 million low-birthweight babies born every year, with many likely to die early (WHO, 1998).

Malnutrition of infants and young children is currently one of the most severe global public health problems. Malnutrition continues to contribute to nearly half of the 10.5 million deaths per year among preschool children worldwide. In January 2001, the executive board of WHO adopted a resolution calling for protection, promotion, and support of breastfeeding and complementary practices in addition to improving the nutrition of women of reproductive age worldwide, especially during and after pregnancy (WHO, 2001a).

Health of Older Children and Adolescents

According to the WHO (1998) World Health Report, one of the major 21st-century problems confronting children will be the continuing spread of HIV/AIDS. In 1997,

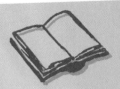

Out of the Box

Reducing infant mortality and low-birthweight infants is a major public health concern. In order to address this concern, collaborative efforts are needed to address this problem. The project discussed here is an example of an innovative effort at the local level. This effective innovative project is the Prenatal Advantage Black Infant Health Project in San Mateo County Health Services, California.

The purpose of this project is to reduce the infant mortality, low birthweight, and sudden infant death syndrome (SIDS) rates in the African American community. The program includes pregnant and parenting African American women and their families, in particular those at risk of delivering a low-birthweight infant.

In order to fulfill the purpose, a variety of comprehensive services are provided: prenatal outreach, coordination of health, social services, public health nursing services, parent education classes, social support and empowerment classes, childbirth education and labor/delivery tour, case management support for young fathers, and AIDS outreach and education. Services are provided to the African American women up to 24 months following delivery as well as parenting support for young fathers. Public health nurses play a major role in this project.

In order to encourage community awareness, support and advocacy for healthy African American infants, a Black Infant Health Advisory Group works to facilitate community mobilization and collaborative efforts. The advisory group collaborates with other programs, such as the Prenatal to Three Program, Adolescent Family Life Project, March of Dimes, Mid-Coastal California Perinatal Outreach Project, and others. The Prenatal to Three initiative is another collaborative team in San Mateo County which includes public health nurses. ∎

590,000 children 15 years of age became infected with HIV. This disease alone could reverse some of the major gains made in child health over the last 50 years. Other factors in the coming years will pose major risks in the transition from childhood to adulthood—such things as violence, delinquency, drug use, alcohol abuse, motor accidents, and sexual hazards such as HIV. Those most likely to be most at risk are children growing up in poor urban environments (WHO, 1998).

It is projected that the number of young women aged 15–19 will increase from 251 million in 1995 to 307 million in 2025. In 1995, young women aged 15–19 years delivered 17 million infants. Because of projected population increase, it is expected that the number of infants will decrease only to 16 million in 2025. Pregnancy and childbirth in the adolescent years pose higher risks for both mother and infant (WHO, 1998).

Tobacco is another major problem that is taking its toll on children worldwide. One in five children in developing countries smokes, according to the new WHO (2000a) survey published in the *WHO Bulletin*. In the 12 countries surveyed—Barbados, China, Costa Rica, Fiji, Jordan, Poland, Russia, South Africa, Sri Lanka, Ukraine, Venezuela, and Zimbabwe—nearly 25% of the children who smoked began before age 10 and more than two-thirds wanted to quit. It is estimated that the number of smoking-related deaths worldwide, across age groups, will rise to 10 million per year by 2030, with 70% of the deaths occurring in developing countries. Thus, smoking patterns among children are critical and contribute to the global epidemic of tobacco-related death and disease.

HEALTH TRENDS AND PATTERNS

The Emergence and Reemergence of Infectious Diseases

Since 1986, a reemergence of concern about infectious diseases has occurred. As suggested by Khabbaz, Peters, and Berkelman from the U.S. National Center for Infectious Diseases, Centers for Disease Control and Prevention (CDC, 1995), "The claim of victory over infectious diseases made by prominent U.S. public health officials during the past two decades has unfortunately proven to be false" (p. 10). Infectious diseases continue to remain the cause of significant morbidity and mortality worldwide. In addition, emerging and reemerging infections continue to present themselves as problems. As reported by WHO (1999a), an infectious disease crisis of global proportions threatens hard-won gains in health and life expectancy. Infectious diseases account for more than 13 million deaths a year—one in two deaths in developing countries. Most deaths from infectious diseases occur in developing countries, the countries with the least money to spend on health care, with about one-third of the population—1.3 billion people—living on income of less than $1 a day (WHO, 1999a). Infectious diseases are not just a developing country problem, however. The crisis has the potential to threaten industrialized nations as well. The significant increase in travel has meant that disease can now be transmitted from one continent to another in short periods of time. Increasingly, infectious diseases are moving across borders between nations. For example, over 12,000 cases of

malaria were reported among European travelers in 1999 (WHO, 2000). In addition, the arsenal of drugs now available to treat infectious diseases is depleted due to increased resistance of microbes to antimicrobial drugs. Many of the complex factors involved in disease emergence and reemergence are present, including the significant increase in population movements over the past 10 years. In 1996, as many as 50 million people—1% of the global population—were uprooted from their homes, making them especially vulnerable to infectious disease. Other factors include the growth of densely populated urban areas with unsafe water, poor sanitation, and widespread poverty (WHO, 1999a). Changes in land use, growth in international trade and biological products, socioeconomic instability, and political unrest also contribute to the infectious disease emergence.

There are three major infectious diseases that are threatening the health of populations worldwide: tuberculosis, HIV/AIDS, and malaria. Collectively, they cause over 300 million illnesses and more than 5 million deaths each year (WHO, 2000c).

As Wilson (1995) stated:

> Only a small fraction of the microbes that exist on the earth have been identified and characterized. As we probe the recesses of the earth we will continue to uncover microbial life as yet unknown. It is folly to think we have already discovered all existing microbes with pathogenic potential for humans. In addition, microbes mutate, recombine, and undergo genetic shift and drift. Because of their short generation time, microbes have the capacity for rapid adaptation through genetic change. Bacteria are enormously versatile, and have great metabolic diversity. (p. 93)

Wilson (1995) further pointed out that epidemiologic approaches will facilitate the detection and characterization of microbes, techniques such as constructing evolutionary trees, with the molecular mapping of the location and spread of a certain strain in different parts of the world. The focus on emerging diseases must integrate knowledge and skills from many disciplines in the social, biological, and physical sciences, because it is evident that the causes of various diseases and their prevention are multifactorial.

Tuberculosis

One of the major infectious diseases to reemerge in industrialized countries is tuberculosis (TBc). In developing nations, however, TBc has historically been a major infection that contributes to mortality (WHO Fact Sheet, 2000b). Worldwide, respiratory tuberculosis was the single largest cause of death in the mid-19th century, with mortality from the disease declining after 1938, when it was first registered in England and Wales as a cause of death (McKeown, 1978).

Tuberculosis and its control are related to social and economic determinants. During the Industrial Revolution, as noted by Friedan (1994), crowding and other factors contributed to the increase in the number of TBc cases. During the 20th century, TBc rates fell steadily in most industrialized countries, except during periods of social stress such as war, with higher rates occurring among immigrants from countries with high prevalence rates (Dubos & Dubos, 1952).

With the discovery of anti-TBc medications and the development of early detection and follow-up programs, the decline in TBc rates was noted, bringing about the possibility of eliminating TBc from the United States, for example (CDC, 1988). Because TBc declined in the United States in the 1970s and 1980s, many of the follow-up programs established for its control, often carried out by public health nurses in local health departments, were disbanded (Brodney & Dobkin, 1991). In 1980, many people incorrectly assumed that TBc in the United States had been controlled; therefore, the effective programs were no longer needed. Fueled by poverty, homelessness, and AIDS, as well as erosion of the public health infrastructure, the reemergence of TBc occurred (Hamburg, 1995). Since the early 1990s, however, in response to the increased incidence of TBc, federal, state, and local efforts have reestablished effective TBc control programs.

The decline in the number of TBc cases reported annually in the United States during 1992–1995 (14.5%) has been attributed to a variety of factors: (1) improved laboratory methods to allow for prompt identification of *Mycobacterium tuberculosis,* (2) broader use of drug susceptibility testing, (3) increased use of preventive therapy in high-risk groups, (4) decreased transmission of the bacillus in congregated settings (e.g., correctional facilities and hospitals) through adherence to infection control guidelines, (5) improved follow-up of persons with TBc initially reported to the health department, and (6) increased federal resources for state and local TBc control efforts. Various activities demonstrated the recognition in the United States that TBc, as a serious infectious disease, required continued and ongoing program efforts.

The national decreases in TBc morbidity in the United States can continue if efforts to promptly identify, treat, and follow those persons with TBc are sustained. In addition, TBc skin tests among high-risk persons, such as the homeless and near homeless, will enable the identification of those who could potentially benefit from preventive chemotherapy.

Worldwide, tuberculosis results in 2.9 million deaths each year (WHO, 1998). An estimate of 8 million people acquire TBc each year. Over 1.5 million cases per year occur in sub-Sahara Africa, and the rate is rising significantly as a result of the HIV/AIDS epidemic. Nearly 3 million TBc cases occur per year in southeast Asia and over a quarter of a million TBc cases per year in Eastern Europe. In Eastern Europe, TBc deaths are increasing after almost 40 years of decline. As can be seen, the biggest burden of TBc is in southeast Asia (WHO, 2000b).

The global epidemic of TBc is growing. It is estimated by WHO (2000b) that, between 2000 and 2020, nearly 1 billion people will be newly infected, 200 million will get sick, and 35 million will die from TBc if control measures are not further developed. The breakdown in health services, the spread of HIV/AIDS, and the emergence of multidrug-resistant TBc are factors contributing to the rise in TBc. Because of WHO's concern about the rising incidence of TBc worldwide, in 1993 WHO declared TBc to be a global emergency. Since that time WHO and its international partners have formed the DOTS-Plus Working Group, which is working to determine the best possible strategy to manage multidrug-resistant TBc, which is rising in some countries, particularly the former Soviet Union. The WHO strategy for detection and cure of TBc includes five elements: political commitment, microscopy services, drug supplies, surveillance and monitoring systems, and the use of efficacious regimens with direct observation of treatment. By the end of 1998, the WHO strategy for TBc detection and control was adopted by 22 of the high-burden countries, which had 80% of the estimated cases of TBc (WHO, 2000b).

Acquired Immunodeficiency Syndrome

Another major occurrence specific to infectious diseases is the emergence of AIDS, which has become a leading cause of death worldwide. A record 2.6 million people throughout the world died of AIDS in 1999, while an estimated 5.6 million children and adults became newly infected with HIV (APHA, 2000b).

Since the AIDS epidemic began in the 1980s, 50 million people worldwide have been infected with HIV, while more than 16 million have died (APHA, 2000b). The challenges the global epidemic poses to families, societies, governments, and science continue. In the United States, nearly 700,000 cases of AIDS have been reported since the epidemic began. The latest estimates suggest that 800,000–900,000 people in the United States currently are infected with HIV, with about one-half of all new HIV infections among those who are under 25 years (USDHHS, 2000a). More than 400,000 lives have been taken prematurely in the United States since the AIDS crisis began (USDHHS, 2000b).

Despite the steady advances in prevention science and in treatments to improve survival among AIDS-infected persons, HIV remains a major public health threat in the United States (Fleming, Wortley, Karon, DeCork, & Janssen, 2000). Even though a 42% decline in death rates occurred between 1996 and 1997, followed by a 20% decline between 1997 and 1998, the total number of people who need care for HIV is increasing (USDHHS, 2000a). Also, although significant declines in the number of AIDS cases and deaths have occurred since 1996 among men and women, all racial/ethnic groups, and all behavioral risk categories, the rates of decline have not been uniform. Proportionate declines in AIDS incidence and deaths have been smaller among African Americans than whites and among women than men. It was estimated in the early 1990s that 13 million people were infected worldwide (World Bank, 1993). As was predicted, HIV disease continues to rise. In 1997, there were 2.3 million global deaths from HIV/AIDS (WHO, 1998). By 2020 it is projected that HIV could rank as high as tenth as a leading cause of global disease burden (see Table 3-2).

As noted by the CDC, HIV disease has a devastating impact on those who are already marginalized members of society. Growing numbers of HIV infection and AIDS cases occur among poor residents of inner cities. AIDS afflicts many people enduring social problems in the United States and other nations—poverty, drug use, prostitution, and discrimination, as well as limited access to health care. As pointed out by the National Commission on AIDS (CDC, 1993), the association of poverty, homelessness, and disease is dramatized by the impact of the HIV epidemic on those who are disenfranchised, those in inner cities who are living at the margins of society. Without permanent addresses or steady incomes, the homeless and many of America's poor often are precluded from all but the most basic health care.

Global projections for HIV demonstrate that the death toll from AIDS may be even greater than expected in the future. In sub-Saharan Africa, for example, death rates from HIV/AIDS are expected to peak around 2005, with approximately 800,000 deaths per year. In India, death rates are expected to peak around 2010, at approximately half a million a year. During the year 2006, HIV deaths are anticipated to peak worldwide, with an estimate of 1.7 million deaths that year. It must be understood, however, that these projections are estimates only (Murray & Lopez, 1996).

Malaria

Malaria is an infectious disease that has been singled out by WHO for concerted global action. It was described in the WHO report (1999a) as an exemplar of an "unfinished agenda" of infectious diseases. In addition to suffering and death, malaria penalizes the poor communities, perpetuating poverty through work loss and increased social instability. In Africa, for example, the gross domestic product would be up to $100 billion greater if malaria had been eliminated (WHO Fact Sheet, 2000c).

Between 300 and 500 million cases of malaria occur worldwide each year. There is an estimate of one million malaria deaths each year. The countries where malaria is endemic include some of the most poverty stricken in the world. Most of the deaths occur in sub-Saharan Africa. In 1997, 165 malaria deaths per 100,000 population occurred in sub-Saharan Africa, in comparison to 18 per 100,000 worldwide. The disease affects children primarily in Africa, accounting for one in four of all childhood deaths in that country (WHO, 1999a).

A resurgence of malaria has occurred primarily because of a number of factors: civil conflict and human migration, climatic and environmental changes, deteriorating health systems, and increasing resistance to antimalarial drugs and increasing resistance to insecticides. Addressing

TABLE 3-2 Twelve Leading Causes of Global Burden of Disease and Injury

1990	2020
Pneumonia	Ischemic heart disease
Diarrheal disease	Depression
Perinatal conditions	Road traffic accidents
Unipolar major depression	Cerebrovascular disease
Cerebrovascular disease	Lower respiratory infections
Tuberculosis	Tuberculosis
Measles	War
Road traffic accidents	Diarrheal diseases
Congenital anomalies	HIV
Malaria	Perinatal conditions
Chronic obstructive pulmonary disease	Violence

Source: Adapted from Summary: The Global Burden of Disease, Global Burden of Disease and Injury Series, *by C. J. Murray and A. D. Lopez, 1996, Cambridge, MA: Harvard School of Public Health on Behalf of the World Health Organization and the World Bank, Harvard University Press.*

REFLECTIVE THINKING

Infectious Diseases

- What contributions do you think you could make in the prevention of infectious diseases such as tuberculosis or AIDS?
- Why is it important to have a global understanding of the distribution and emergence of infectious diseases?
- What infectious diseases are prevalent in your community? Why would it be important to know the incidence and prevalence of these diseases?

the problem of malaria is thus a major battle in the war against poverty. To deal with the problem, WHO has been working with international organizations, governments, academic institutions, the private sector, and nongovernmental organizations to promote the development of tools to control malaria and assist in strengthening health systems to prevent and treat malaria. The new initiative was launched in 1998 in partnership with the United Nations (UN) Children's Fund, the UN Development Program, and the World Bank (WHO, 1999a).

Understanding and coping with infectious disease emergence require a global perspective, geographically and conceptually. The globalization of infectious diseases is of concern because an outbreak in one nation may potentially affect others. The need for international cooperation on epidemic alert and response is critical today because of the global public health threat of emerging infectious disease agents, drug-resistant infectious agents, and epidemics. As WHO points out, however, there is a window of opportunity to deal with diseases such as malaria, TBc, HIV, and diarrheal diseases through prevention and treatment strategies now available that can be provided to developing nations who experience most deaths from infectious diseases. In April 2000 a global outbreak alert and response network was established by WHO, referred to earlier in this chapter. Reports of current epidemic outbreaks received by WHO that are of international importance are communicated to public health officials and global surveillance partners via e-mail on a weekly basis (WHO, 2001a).

Another major action taken by WHO was the recent opening of a new WHO office in Lyon, France, in February 2001. This new office is a part of the WHO Department of Disease, Surveillance, and Response. The major mission of the new office is to improve the capacity of developing countries to contain epidemics of emerging communicable diseases, including drug-resistant infection. The Lyon WHO office will assist in the training of specialists worldwide who work to control epidemics, thus preparing them to effectively and rapidly detect the major epidemic and emerging diseases. The WHO office in Lyon will also assist in setting up a network of national laboratories in developing nations (WHO, 2001d).

Injuries and Accidents

Although injuries are another major cause of morbidity and mortality worldwide, many countries lack adequate data to routinely monitor these conditions. Injuries have not received the attention given to conditions of comparable or lesser public health importance (Murray & Lopez, 1996). Injuries, however, are important to examine, both fatal and nonfatal, as emphasized in *The Global Burden of Disease and Injury Series* (see Table 3-2).

Deaths from injuries (unintentional injuries) are among the most frequently recorded causes of death in populations for which mortality data are available and reasonably complete. Because of the availability of data, most injury research focuses on fatalities. As mentioned in *Healthy People 2010: Understanding and Improving Health* (USDHHS, 2000b), unintentionally fatal injuries include motor vehicle accidents, poisonings, drownings, falls, residential fires, and firearms primarily. More than 400 Americans die each day due primarily to these injuries, with motor vehicle crashes being the most common cause of serious injury. In 1998, there were 15.6 deaths per 100,000 persons from motor vehicle crashes, with nearly 40% of traffic fatalities in 1997 being alcohol related. Thus the reduction of injuries and deaths due to unintentional injuries was identified as one of the major target objectives for 2010 in the United States.

Worldwide, in 1990, approximately 5 million people died of injuries of all types; two-thirds of them were men, with most of the deaths being concentrated among young adults. Road traffic accidents, suicide, war, fire, and violence all were included within the 10 leading causes of death. Among adults aged 15–44 worldwide, road traffic accidents were the leading cause of death for men, fifth for women. Suicide was second only to TBc as a cause of death for women between age 15 and 44. In China, in 1990, more than 180,000 women killed themselves. In sub-Saharan Africa, the leading cause of fatal injuries was war (Murray & Lopez, 1996). One of the significant health challenges of noncommunicable health problems includes unintentional and intentional injuries (WHO, 1999b). These injuries accounted for 15% of the global disease burden in 1990, posing a large and neglected health problem in regions of the world.

The global burden of injury in 1990 was highest in the formerly socialist economies of Europe, with almost 19% of all burden attributed to injury causes. China had the second highest injury burden; Latin America and the Caribbean third highest and sub-Saharan Africa fourth (Murray & Lopez, 1996). In almost all regions of the world, except the Middle East crescent, unintentional injuries were a much bigger source of ill health in 1990 than injuries that were intentional, such as war and violence.

The challenge remains for health professionals to routinely inquire and counsel clients about their activities at home and in automobiles. Primary care providers can help to prevent injuries. In addition, there needs to be a greater emphasis on surveillance of injury morbidity, disability, and costs in order to identify risk factors and to evaluate injury prevention programs. Community health nurses have a very important role to play in the prevention efforts.

Chronic Diseases and Disability

As discussed earlier in this chapter, chronic diseases and disabilities pose serious problems for both developing and industrialized nations now and in the future. In addition to the challenges of infectious diseases and injuries discussed previously, chronic or noncommunicable diseases are becoming more prevalent in both developing and industrialized nations. Chronic diseases are expected to increase worldwide as the population ages, augmented by the large numbers of people in developing regions who are now exposed to tobacco. The prevention and treatment of chronic diseases worldwide pose major challenges in the future.

In 1990, the three leading causes of global disease burden were pneumonia, diarrheal diseases, and perinatal conditions, in descending order. Projected to take their place by 2020 are ischemic heart disease, depression, and road traffic accidents. Table 3-2 lists the top 12 leading causes of global disease burden from 1990 as compared with estimates for 2020. In a WHO (1999b) report, lung cancer was identified as a major health challenge for the future also—among cancers, the most significant cause of disease burden, with the major contributor to lung cancer being smoking.

Tobacco, Obesity, and Alcohol

Tobacco is the number one contributor to premature death and disability worldwide. Tobacco is expected to increase its share to just under 9% of the total global burden of disease in 2020, compared with just under 6% for ischemic heart disease, the leading projected disease. In 1990, the level of 2.6% of all disease burden worldwide was attributed to tobacco use. As Murray and Lopez (1996) stated, "This is a global emergency that many governments have yet to confront" (p. 38).

WHO (1999b) reported that the death toll from smoking may have been seriously underestimated. As many as one in two long-term smokers die from their habit throughout the world. By the year 2030 (10 years after the GBD study), if current trends continue, tobacco will kill 10 million people a year—over 70% of them in developing countries. Because of this global emergency, WHO called for a worldwide ban on all tobacco advertising and promotion, for sustained tax increases on cigarettes, for wider access to tobacco substitutes, and for the formation of tobacco control coalitions. While calling for these actions in 1999, WHO also noted that effective tobacco controls did exist, and where these have been used, governments were effective in reducing the increase in tobacco use.

In the United States, cigarette smoking is the single most preventable cause of disease and death. It results in more deaths per year than AIDS, alcohol, cocaine, heroin, homicide, suicide, motor vehicle crashes, and fires combined (USDHHS, 2000b). Tobacco-related deaths number more than 430,000 per year among U.S. adults. A major concern is the increase in the percentage of adolescents who were cigarette smokers in 1999 compared to 1998. In 1999, 35% smoked in comparison to 24% in 1998. Adolescent rates of smoking increased in the 1990s among white, African American, and Hispanic high school students after years of declining rates in the 1970s and 1980s. Although this increase in smoking has occurred, the number of cigarettes smoked per person in the United States overall is on the decline, falling some 42% between 1980 and 1999 (Worldwatch Institute, 2000). The commitment to tobacco control in the United States is therefore critical and its use has been included as a target objective in *Healthy People 2010*.

Obesity is the second major contributor to premature death and disability worldwide, following tobacco. Because of the increasing worldwide concern about this problem, it is critical that community health nurses focus on this problem also. At the end of the year 2000, Worldwatch Institute, a nonprofit Washington public policy research organization dedicated to informing policymakers and the public about emerging global problems and trends, issued an alert. This alert pointed out that obesity is reaching epidemic proportions, affecting a growing number of people in both industrialized and developing countries (Worldwatch Institute, 2000). Obesity and overweight are major contributors to the increased incidence of heart disease, stroke, breast cancer, colon cancer, arthritis, adult-onset diabetes, sleep disturbances, and problems breathing (USDHHS, 2000b).

In the United States, the CDC estimates that 300,000 Americans now die each year from obesity-related diseases. For the first time in history, the number of overweight people, which has climbed to 1.1 billion worldwide, rivals the number of undernourished and underweight people. In the United States, 61% of all adults are estimated to be overweight or obese; in Russia, the figure is 54%; in the United Kingdom 51%; and in Germany 50%. Overweight and obesity are increasing rapidly in the developing nations also. In

Brazil and Columbia, for example, 35% and 41% of the population respectively are overweight. Not only are more people worldwide overweight than ever before, but the rates are increasing (Worldwatch Institute, 2000).

There is a challenge worldwide to increase the emphasis on making nutritional well-being a priority, to fund health programs that are designed to improve nutrition and physical activity, and to place greater governmental educational efforts on nutrition issues. Taking action to reduce the prevalence of obesity is a must, and it is a target objective in *Healthy People 2010.*

Alcohol is the third major factor that contributes to the disease burden worldwide. In 1990 alcohol contributed to approximately 3.5% of the total disease burden throughout the world (Murray & Lopez, 1996). Alcohol causes the heaviest burden in men in the industrialized regions of the world. Alcohol is the leading cause of disability for men in the industrialized nations and the fourth leading cause of disability in developing nations (WHO, 1999b).

In the United States, alcohol abuse alone is associated with motor vehicle crashes, homicides, suicides, and drowning—the leading causes of death among youth. In addition, long-term drinking can lead to heart disease, cancer, alcohol-related liver disease, and pancreatitis (USDHHS, 2000b). Alcohol and illicit drug use in the United States are associated with many of the most serious problems, including violence, injury, and HIV infection. In 1995, the annual economic costs from alcohol abuse in the United States were estimated to be $167 billion (USDHHS, 2000b). Because of the nation's concern about alcohol and illicit drug use, one of the target objectives in *Healthy People 2010* addresses this problem.

Mental Illness and Mental Disorders

The burdens of mental illness, such as depression, alcohol dependence, and schizophrenia, for example, have been seriously underestimated by health status measures that do not take into account disability. Psychiatric conditions account for almost 11% of the disease burden worldwide (Murray & Lopez, 1996). Of the 10 leading causes of disability worldwide in 1990, measured in years lived with the disability, 5 were psychotic conditions: unipolar depression, alcohol use, bipolar affective disorder (manic depression), schizophrenia, and obsessive-compulsive disorder. The predominance of these conditions was not restricted to wealthy countries, although the burden is highest in the industrialized nations, such as the United States and Great Britain.

Since 1990, the incidence of mental illness and mental disorders worldwide has been increasing, thus causing extensive disability in both industrialized and developing nations. Major depression ranked fifth in the 10 leading causes of global disease burden in 1998. After major depression, the most important causes of neu-

ropsychiatric burden are alcohol dependence, bipolar affective disorders, and schizophrenia. In high-income countries, dementias are the third leading cause of neuropsychiatric burden (Brundtland, 2000).

It is clear that a higher priority must be given to mental health worldwide. As Brundtland (2000) so clearly states, "mental health depends on some measure of social justice; and mental illness given its scale, must be treated at the primary level where possible" (p. 411).

World Mental Health Perspectives

The past 50 years have seen significant improvements in the general level of physical public health in countries worldwide. Life expectancy has increased, infant mortality rates are reduced, and many of the common infectious diseases are less of a threat, although they still require concerted and ongoing surveillance, identification, treatment, and follow-up (Heggenhougen, 1995). Yet as Heggenhougen (1995) stated, "Public health, in terms of mental and behavioral problems, including human rights abuses and social pathologies, is appalling throughout the world, requiring immediate attention and a new perspective" (p. 267).

The burden of psychiatric conditions has been seriously underestimated. Unipolar depression was the leading cause of disability worldwide in 1990, with an estimated 50.8 million people affected, constituting 10.7% of the total percentage of the leading causes of disability in the world (Murray & Lopez, 1996). As estimated by the World Bank in 1993, neuropsychiatric disorders in adults in developing countries contributed 12% to the global distribution. It was projected that by the year 2000, the number of cases of schizophrenia in developing countries would increase by 45% from the 1985 rate, to 24.4 million. Mental retardation and epilepsy rates were more than three times higher in developing nations than in industrialized countries. Seventy-five percent of the elderly with dementia were projected to live in developing nations (approximately 80 million) by the year 2025 (World Bank, 1993).

As reported by Brundtland (2000), Director General of WHO, 5 of the 10 leading causes of disability worldwide (major depression, schizophrenia, bipolar disorders, alcohol use, and obsessive-compulsive disorders) are mental problems. These problems are as relevant in developing nations as in wealthy nations and are projected to increase significantly in the coming years.

A major study conducted by the WHO International Consortium in Psychiatric Epidemiology (2000a) examined data from 30,000 people in seven countries—Brazil, Canada, Germany, Mexico, the Netherlands, Turkey, and the United States. The purpose of the study was to examine cross-national comparative studies of the prevalences and correlates of mental disorders. The investigators found that 48% of those studied in the

United States experienced at least one mental disorder in their lifetime, compared to 40% in the Netherlands, 38% in Germany, 37% in Canada, 36% in Brazil, 20% in Mexico, and 12% in Turkey. An examination of the data showed that mental disorders were most often chronic. (Mental disorders were classified as anxiety disorders, mood disorders, or substance-use disorders.) All three classes of the disorders were positively related to people with low income and below-average education or who were unemployed or unmarried. Delays in seeking treatment were widespread among early-onset cases and only a minority of the people with prevailing disorders received any treatment. The WHO International Consortium in Psychiatric Epidemiology (2000a) stated, "Mental disorders are among the most burdensome of all classes of disease because of their high prevalence and chronicity, early age onset, and resulting serious impairment. There is a need for demonstration projects of early outreach and intervention programmes for people with early-onset mental disorders, as well as quality assurance programmes to look into the widespread problem of inadequate treatment" (p. 413).

In the United States, as reported in the 1996 *Healthy People 2000* document (USDHHS, 2000b), an estimated 41.1 million adults have had a mental disorder at some time in their lives. An estimated 7.5 million children suffered from mental and emotional disturbances, such as autism, attention-deficit disorder, and depression. In the United States, major depression accounted for more bed days than any impairment except for cardiovascular disease. In the *Healthy People 2010* report (USDHHS, 2000b), approximately 20% of the U.S. population is affected by mental illness during a given year. Depression is the most common disorder of all mental illnesses, with more than 19 million adults in the United States suffering from depression. Major depression is the leading cause of disability and the cause of more than two-thirds of the suicides per year. In 1997, only 23% of adults diagnosed with depression sought treatment. The misunderstanding of mental illness and the associated stigmatization prevent many people with depression from seeking professional assistance.

Heggenhougen (1995) suggests that a new paradigm for understanding the processes contributing to the health of communities and societies is needed. The concern must be for human suffering in all of its various forms: social maladies, such as violence and mental and behavioral pathologies; human rights abuses; and the basic concern for physical health. Public health lies at the intersection of these various forms. Heggenhougen's suggestion is as relevant today as it was in 1995.

Although there are major mental and social health problems worldwide, major efforts to deal with the problems have emerged. New pharmaceutical agents have enabled the effective treatment of many of the most severe mental illnesses. Community-based, integrated programs that focus on families have been shown to have great potential for improving lives (Heggenhougen, 1995). Creative public health initiatives focused on violence, abuse of women, and substance abuse are emerging in communities. New public health models have been introduced, including epidemiologic models for research and risk evaluation, with research focused on addressing the social and cultural context of particular behaviors. There is greater recognition of local strengths and resources, with community assets identified and reinforced. Because of its concern about mental health, WHO launched a Mental Health 2001 year-long campaign focused on mental health, which culminated in a World Health Report 2001 on mental health. This report includes topics such as the prevalence of mental disorders, organization and financing of programs, prevention strategies, and projections for the future (WHO, 2001b). World Health Day 2001 is another WHO action effort, and its focus is mental health. The aim is to raise awareness about barriers to treatment and also about solutions to deal with mental and brain disorders.

Higher priority must be given to mental health, however. Providing resources—human and material—for relevant programs and policies must be included. As Heggenhougen (1995) states, "Mental health represents one of the great frontiers in the improvement of the human condition—mental health must be placed on the international agenda" (p. 269).

Millions of people today suffer from mental health problems—many characterized by undue suffering and premature death. We must rise to the challenge posed by mental health problems worldwide. Community health nurses are in a vital position to participate in prevention strategies, community action, and collaborative efforts at local, national, and international levels.

Violence

Violence is one of the major public health problems that has received a greater public health emphasis, as discussed in Chapter 30. The public health focus on violence has helped to redefine the problem in measurable terms. One of the current definitions of violence is "the threatened or actual use of physical force or power against another person, against oneself, or against a group or community, that either results in or has a high likelihood of resulting in injury, death, or deprivation" (Mercy, Rosenberg, Powell, Broome, & Roper, as cited in Foege, Rosenberg, & Mercy, 1995, p. 2). The injuries may be psychological or physical. Violence includes suicide or attempted suicide, as well as interpersonal violence such as domestic and child abuse, rape, elder abuse, or assaults (Rosenberg & Fenley, 1990).

Violence has contributed to the rates of premature mortality worldwide. Violence can also be interrupted with interventions to break the cycle. The search for solutions must focus on the social and economic factors that contribute to violence as well as individual factors (Foege et al., 1995).

Receiving attention is the connection between violence involving individuals or families and violence involving cultures, societies, and nations. Violence is a global problem, with interpersonal violence, ethnic violence, and national conflict being interrelated (Foege et al., 1995).

Violence must be considered a major public health problem because of the toll it takes on society. In the United States, for example, injuries from violence resulted in the loss of over 149,000 lives in 1991 and resulted in the loss of more years of potential life than heart disease, cancer, and stroke together (National Center for Health Statistics, 1992). In comparison with other industrialized countries, the United States experienced the highest homicide rates among males 15–24 years of age from 1988 to 1991 (WHO, 1991). In 1998, the homicide rate in the United States fell to its lowest level in three decades—6.5 homicides per 100,000 persons. In 1997, 32,436 individuals died from firearm injuries, and of these, 42% were homicide victims. In 1997, homicide was the third leading cause of death for children aged 5–14 years (USDHHS, 2000b).

According to Foege et al. (1995), violence in the United States among young people is an epidemic out of control. Violence is a major problem of concern to public health; however, it is a problem of concern to other branches of government and other countries as well. Public health focuses on primary prevention and thus views the prevention of violence as critical. The public health and community health nursing approach to violence focuses on ways to break the cycle of violence, whatever the form, and stops a pattern that so often begins in infancy and childhood and carries over into young adulthood, middle age, and older age. The public health approach focuses on the bridging of many different disciplines, different parts of government, and outreach to the public and private sectors as well as to community residents themselves.

Community health nurses are in vital positions to participate in collaborative multidisciplinary, community-based coalitions to work on developing multiple complementary activities that can assist in preventing violence effectively. The challenge is a major one that will require compassion and courage to assist those in need.

An examination of world health data at the end of the 20th century clearly indicated the major differences in world health. Monitoring risk factors in different populations and identifying emerging health problems in both industrialized and developing nations worldwide are critical. Such indicators point to the need for global collaboration to assist in dealing with the inequalities in health status. The findings pose definite challenges to public policy formation and health initiatives in this century.

POPULATION CHARACTERISTICS— PROJECTED CHANGES

Population growth and changes have a significant impact on social and economic conditions. Population changes also have an influence on health and well-being and rank among the major determinants of health care needs.

Changes in Population Age Structures

One of the major changes in the population in many countries throughout the world, in both developing and industrialized nations, has been significant shifts in population age structures. These shifts have been characterized, to a great extent, by a decline in fertility, declining mortality levels at older ages, and growth of the elderly populations (United Nations Population Division, 2001, p. 14). These shifts are projected to result in important consequences and implications for various countries. It is necessary, therefore, to have an understanding of these changes and their projected results. It is also necessary to examine the contributing factors that influence the population age structure.

In the following discussion, global changes in the age structure are reviewed. It is important to mention that the major source of population estimates is the population census. Census data, as well as survey data, on age distribution in a number of developing countries may be significantly biased by misreporting of ages and age-selective undernumeration. Results of the analysis should therefore be viewed with these factors in mind.

The population of the world will be presented initially, with long-range projections to the year 2050. These projections, presented by the United Nations in 2001, are based on possible scenarios of future levels of fertility and mortality, both central demographic determinants affecting population age structures. The projections are in no way to be viewed as a prevision of the future population trends in the world.

The population of the world reached 6.1 billion in mid-2000 and is currently growing at an annual rate of 1.2%, or 77 million people per year (United Nations Population Division, 2001, p. v). Six countries account for half of this annual growth: India, China, Pakistan, Nigeria, Bangladesh, and Indonesia. By 2050, the world population is estimated to be between 7.9 billion (low estimate) and 10.9 billion (high estimate), with the medium estimated at 9.3 billion (United Nations Population Division, 2001).

The population growth of the industrialized regions is anticipated to change little during the next 50 years, primarily because fertility levels are expected to remain low. In contrast, the population of the developing regions is projected to rise steadily from 4.9 in 2000 to 8.2 billion in 2050 (medium estimate), based on the assumption that there will be continuing declines in fertility. Particularly rapid growth is expected among the group of 48 countries identified as among the poorest and least developed, with their population expected to increase from 658 million in 2000 to 1.8 billion by 2050 (United Nations Population Division, 2001).

There are expected to be major changes in the age structure of the world's population. Globally, the world population will have aged significantly by 2050. Over the next 50 years, the proportion of children is projected to decrease by a third, reaching 21% in 2050, in contrast to the proportion of older persons. The number of persons age 60 years and over will more than triple, with a projected increase from 606 million in 2000 to nearly 2 billion by 2050. One of the most dramatic changes is the increase in the number of those aged 80 and over, from 69 million in 2000 to 379 million in 2050, more than a fivefold increase (United Nations Population Division, 2001).

By 2050, 19 countries are expected to have at least 10% of their population aged 80 years or over: Austria, Belgium, Channel Islands, Finland, France, Germany, Greece, Hong Kong (SAR of China), Italy, Japan, Macao, the Netherlands, Norway, Singapore, Slovenia, Spain, Sweden, Switzerland, and the United Kingdom. In addition, six countries are projected to have more than 10 million people age 80 years or over: China (99 million), India (48 million), the United States (30 million), Japan (17 million), Brazil (10 million), and Indonesia (10 million). These six countries combined will account for 57% of all the oldest people in the world (United Nations Population Division, 2001). These changes will have major implications for health care professionals in the years to come.

In addition, the number of older, disabled persons will also increase as the population ages. If the rates of disability among the elderly continue to rise (as has occurred in industrialized countries), the number of disabled persons will be enormous. The anticipated continued aging of populations will result in the need for substantially reorganized health services.

The demographic transition, with its changing age of death and the existence of large numbers of people affected with chronic degenerative diseases and disabilities, is therefore very important for planning health services and education of health professionals.

Population Growth and Urbanization

Another major change in the population in many countries is the rapid growth of the world's population who will live in cities. By 2030 it is estimated that the urban population will reach 4.9 billion—60% of the world's population (United Nations Population Division, 2000). A major portion of the population is projected to be in the cities of developing countries, whose population will double to nearly 4 billion by 2030, as reported in an important previous edition by Johns Hopkins University, Population Information Program (2001).

REFLECTIVE THINKING

Population Increases

- What impact do you think the changing population age structures will have on health care service needs?
- What recommendations do you have in relation to dealing with the projected population increases in older adults?
- How might you participate in community-based initiatives that focus on health promotion activities for older adults?

An increasing number of people in the developing world live in "megacities," or cities of at least 10 million people. In 1975 only five cities throughout the world had 10 million or more people—Tokyo, New York, Shanghai, Mexico City, and Sao Paulo. As can be seen, three of these cities were in developing countries. The number of cities with 10 million or more people is projected to increase to 23 by 2015, and all but 4 of them will be in developing countries. In 2015, the largest cities in the world, with 20 million people in each city, will be Tokyo, Bombay, Lagos, Dhaka, and Sao Paulo (United Nations Population Division, 2000).

Given the rapid growth in cities throughout the world, particularly in developing countries, natural resources are under increasing pressure, threatening public health and development. Such things as water shortages together with poor sanitation, degradation of arable land for food production, air and water pollution, increased pressure on half of all coastal ecosystems by high population densities and urban development, and global warming, which is due largely to burning fossil fuels, pose major global challenges for the future.

This rapid growth of populations in cities therefore presents a number of global public health challenges on natural resources. It is clearly evident that without practicing sustainable development, we will face the possibility of a deteriorating environment and ecological threats (Johns Hopkins University, Population Information Program, 2000). Taking steps toward sustainability must be implemented now and in the future in order to preserve the public's health. These include the efficient use of energy, protecting freshwater sources, preserving arable land and increasing food production, recycling, managing coastal zones and fisheries to protect the coasts from pollution, protecting biodiversity, and adopting an international agreement to reduce the burning of fossil fuels, which contribute to global warming.

Another important promising strategy for improving health and slowing population growth is meeting the family planning needs of city residents (Brockherhoff, 2000). Programs can improve services to reach the urban poor, including recent migrants, who live in areas that have often not been well served. Since the 1960s, family planning programs have played a key role in slowing population growth in developing countries (Upadhuay & Robey, 1999). Slowing population growth would assist in improving living standards in order to buy time for sustainable, environmentally friendly policies to take effect (Brockherhoff, 2000).

Community health nurses at all levels—local, state, national, and international—can work together to promote sustainable development in their respective areas as well as the improvement of family planning services to reach the urban poor. Developing knowledge about sustainable development strategies worldwide is the first step in the process. Strategies that address sustainability through legislative action, community partnerships, and development of international agreements on climate change (global warming) are examples of caring in action!

COMMUNITY HEALTH NURSING ROLE

A focus on global population health, changing population characteristics, and factors that contribute to population health is necessary in community health nursing. Community health nurses have excellent opportunities to participate in communitywide health care and will have even more in the future. Community health nurses have the ability to integrate concepts of health and disease, individual and aggregate approaches, public health and nursing, and health promotion and disease prevention. Nurses can demonstrate understanding of the relationships between the personal and environmental factors that affect health and thus are able to intervene at individual, family, and community levels.

Community health nurses can play a vital role in building partnerships with communities that assist in addressing the current and projected health needs. Participating in partnerships with other health care professionals and members of the community—local, state, national, and international—will assist in the creation of healthier communities.

The International Healthy Cities/Communities movement, referred to in Chapter 1, focuses on mobilizing local resources and political, professional, and community members to improve the health of the community. It is a public health approach that examines the many interrelated factors that influence the health of a community. In order to participate in this movement and in the process of population health improvement, community health nurses must function in multidisciplinary teams, working with community residents and leaders and participating together in changing health care delivery systems.

Community health nurses can participate in policy making at local, state, national, and international levels to improve access to basic and preventive care, taking the

Perspectives...

INSIGHTS OF A PROFESSOR EMERITUS

It is critically important for community health nurses, and other nurses as well, to develop a knowledge of global health problems and issues. We live in a global society, and it is no longer sufficient for nurses to focus only on the population health needs in their respective countries. Nurses are in a vital position to assist in shaping public policy at national and international levels.

Having had the opportunity to participate in a variety of international professional activities—consulting, teaching, coordinating an international conference, presenting at research colloquia, and participating in conducting cross-national research—I have been provided with a rich tapestry of knowledge about nursing and health care issues in other countries. It is evident that a global knowledge of health concerns and needs, as well knowledge of nursing's role in building caring, healthy communities, is imperative for our profession now and in this century. Faculty members have a major responsibility to expand their focus on population health to include global perspectives. It is also an imperative to expand our knowledge in cultural care, on the cultural strategies that groups and communities use for negotiating our various health care systems. Listening to the perceptions of nurses, health care providers, and consumers from other countries share their knowledge with us is critical.

We are interconnected as nations; we do not exist in isolation. As nurses, we must become knowledgeable about global health problems and issues, cultural negotiation strategies, and the role that we can play in shaping healthy public policy at local, state, national, and international levels. It is through our global interconnectedness with nurses in other countries that we can work together to promote health throughout the world. As Ramos (1997) so clearly states, "If the world is to be a healthier place, we cannot limit our caring to the interface with patients. There are huge steps to be taken in unifying health care professionals to design . . . care delivery systems that bring health to the people of the world. . . . If we care about the world we live in, if we translate our caring into a larger effort, we can make a difference" (p. 16).

Let us move forward with courage, commitment, compassion, excitement, and confidence that we, as nurses, can participate, personally and collectively, in building healthier communities worldwide.

—Sue A. Thomas, EdD, RN

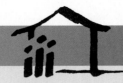

COMMUNITY NURSING VIEW

A community health nurse is working in a community with a large population of at-risk and high-risk child-bearing and childrearing Hispanic women, many of whom sought prenatal care late in their pregnancies. The infant mortality rate is higher in this community than in others surrounding it. Goals for this community are to reduce barriers to prenatal care and provide care that is culturally relevant. The community health nurse is asked to serve as project director of a new program designed to reduce barriers to early prenatal care.

Nursing Considerations

Assessment

◆ What should the community health nurse include in the needs assessment process?

◆ What data should be collected regarding barriers to prenatal care? Who should collect the data?

◆ What factors need to be considered specific to data collection?

Diagnosis

◆ Who should be involved in the formulation of community health diagnoses?

Outcome Identification

◆ What outcomes could be formulated specific to the prenatal care issue?

◆ What is the benefit to the community? To the mothers?

Planning/Interventions

◆ Who should be involved in the planning with regard to the where, when, who, and how of program development?

◆ What factors should be considered when planning the program?

◆ What methods might be used to reduce barriers to prenatal care for the Hispanic women?

Evaluation

◆ What indicators would suggest that the program has been effective?

◆ What might be suggested as the next course of action if the program is determined to be unsuccessful? Successful?

initiative to work with community residents, leaders, and other health professionals to usher in the necessary changes. The nurse must place greater emphasis on participating in policy development aimed at quality-of-life issues, based on the caring concepts of mutual respect, trust, compassion, and courage. The community health nurse educates the public about population health problems and issues and elicits their perspectives about their own community's health and population needs. The community health nurse is in a position to influence health outcomes and policy changes. The nurse can talk to policymakers about identified health needs and populations at risk and can serve on committees that address population health improvement strategies, such as educational programs, outreach services, and legislative action, among others. The nurse can also assist in identifying priorities and strategic planning for local, national, and international action as well as participate in program evaluation research.

Participating with community leaders and citizens to establish a balanced approach to health improvement is another role for the nurse. Population health improvement efforts must balance an emphasis on personal responsibility with the social, structural, and environmental dimensions of health. Community health nurses are in pivotal positions to assist in this effort.

Because community health problems and issues transcend international borders, an international focus in community health nursing is also needed. Knowledge of the importance of the *Global Burden of Disease Study* can provide the nurse with a much needed picture of global projections for the future as well as knowledge of the more current public health measures used to assess the health status of nations. International cooperation is required to deal with the challenges for the future. Basic to international collaborative efforts is the need for health care professionals to be culturally informed and cognizant of cultural differences.

Although disease, disability, injury, birth, death, and aging are universal, there are cultural differences in ways of defining health and illness, different systems for preventing and treating deviations from health, and different ways of coping with developmental and situational events (Dreher, 1996). Because of these differences, health care in the future will call for culturally informed health professionals. As countries become even more interconnected, nurses as healers will be challenged to discover cultural meanings of health events, health beliefs, practices, and behaviors. Working with nurses and colleagues from both developing and industrialized nations will require cultural knowledge and sensitivity to culturally diverse ways of being. Appreciating cultural diversity will enhance nursing's contribution to building healthier communities.

The focus on healthy public policy, sustainable development, and the concept of investing in health are important concepts in building healthier communities. Building healthy communities is a public health approach that encompasses the recognition that health and well-being are interconnected with social, cultural, physical, economic, environmental, and other factors and that community participation and collaboration are necessary to improve health and the quality of life.

The growing worldwide movement for healthy cities and communities, which was initiated by WHO in the 1980s, could result in improved public health systems in the 21st century, ones that will be just as effective in improving health as their counterparts were in the 19th century. Community health nurses have the potential to play a vital role in the creation of healthier communities, as did nursing leaders such as Florence Nightingale, Lillian Wald, Mary Brewster, and Lavinia Dock, among others, over a century ago. Community health nurses are in a position to participate in the debates regarding changing priorities for public health in the decades ahead.

KEY CONCEPTS

- It is essential that community health nurses have a knowledge of population health problems from both national and international perspectives in order to function effectively in the global community as well as in their own community.

- Population health assessments must include knowledge not only of global mortality patterns but also of disease patterns, disabilities, and injuries in populations.

- Chronic diseases and disabilities are expected to increase as the population ages.

- The crusade against infectious disease must continue because of emergence and reemergence of infectious diseases worldwide.

- Mental illnesses and mental disorders are increasing worldwide, thus requiring concerted global action to deal with the problem.

- There needs to be greater emphasis on surveillance of injury morbidity, disability, and costs in order to identify risk factors and to evaluate injury prevention programs.

- It is of vital importance to examine changing perspectives related to understanding the determinants of health.

- The global burden of disease (GBD) quantifies not only the number of deaths but also the impact of premature death and disability on a population.

- Changing global population growth patterns have a major impact on the nature of health care service needs.

- Knowledge of the importance of sustainable development is critical.

- Knowledge of cultural factors is critical in the building of healthy communities.

- Community health nurses are in a vital position to contribute to the creation of community partnerships for the purpose of enhancing community health at local, state, national, and international levels.

✳ DECISION MAKING

Culturally Congruent Care

- A community health nurse is working in a multicultural urban neighborhood with families representing different racial and ethnic groups from different countries of origin. One of the major goals of the community health nurse is to provide services that are culturally congruent. Nursing interventions that are culturally relevant and sensitive to client and community needs decrease the possibility of conflict arising from cultural misunderstanding.

- What assessment domains should be included in order to understand the health needs of the selected populations in the neighborhood?

- What pertinent cultural factors should be included in a community nursing assessment?

- Why is cultural information important in the care of all clients?

RESOURCES

American Public Health Association: www.apha.org
Global Health Council: www.globalhealth.org
International Institute for Sustainable Development: www.iisd.org
Johns Hopkins University, School of Public Health, Center for Communication Programs: www.jhuccp.org
Pan American Health Organization: www.paho.org
Pew Environmental Health Commission: www.pewenviro-health.jhsph.edu
U.S. Department of Health and Human Services, Centers for Disease Control and Prevention: www.cdc.gov
World Federation of Public Health Associations: www.wfpha.org
World Health Organization: www.who.int
Worldwatch Institute: www.worldwatch.org

HEALTH CARE DELIVERY IN THE UNITED STATES

Carol A. Lockhart, PhD, RN, FAAN

MAKING THE CONNECTION

Many Americans are critical about our health care system. But not nearly as many are knowledgeable about it. Maybe I should call it our health scare system, or our health care non-system. Unfortunately, there is no system in the way Americans scramble for health care.

—Koop, 1991, p. 302

COMPETENCIES

Upon completion of this chapter, the reader should be able to:

- Describe how health services are planned and organized in the United States.
- Discuss the influence of the U.S. political culture on the health care system.
- Identify the role of health insurance and public health in providing access to health care services.
- Examine the incentives relating to managed care.
- Identify the types of health service organizations that deliver care.
- Describe the responsibilities of public health organizations at national, state, and local levels.
- Discuss the focus of community nursing organizations and centers and their potential role in health service delivery.
- Discuss the influences on the consumer's choice of health services.
- Describe the paradigm shift that is beginning in health care.
- Describe the focus of community health nursing under the new paradigm.
- Identify trends that will shape public health and health care in the next decade.

KEY TERMS

allopathic	managed care
complementary health care services	managed competition
	osteopathy
fee-for-service (FFS)	paradigm
homeopathy	preexisting condition
indemnity insurance	

Public health organizations and the community health nurses working within them are committed to caring for the populations, families, and individuals that make up a community. Most nations, particularly the industrialized nations, have an organized national health system whose goal is to deliver the full range of available care to its citizens. Through such a system, the government defines and sets national health goals that are supported by modifying the national system. Although the goals are not always achieved, there exists a national direction and plan for the health care offered to the citizens of the given country.

This, however, is not true of the United States. Whereas we do deliver sophisticated and technologically advanced health care services and, in many senses, the best individualized care in the world, we do not have a national system for delivering that care or for ensuring our population's health and well-being. A system provides "a set or arrangement of things so related or connected as to form a unity or organic whole" (*Webster's New World College Dictionary*, 1999, p. 1453). In the United States, health care is treated as a private business rather than a publicly produced good or service that should be available in some coordinated way to all citizens as part of citizenship. A wide range of services are offered through individual private practitioners, organizations, and programs. Although services are sometimes coordinated between the various providers, this is usually not the case, and there exists no specific responsibility for doing so.

The federal government of the United States does, however, attempt to influence the nature and direction of the health of the nation. In 1980, the U.S. Department of Health and Human Services (USDHHS) issued a report, *Healthy People: The Surgeon General's Report on Health Promotion and Disease Prevention*. It set goals that sought to reduce mortality among infants, children, adolescents and young adults, and adults. It also sought to increase independence among older adults. In 1990, USDHHS issued *Healthy People 2000: National Health Promotion and Disease Prevention Objectives* with three broad goals: (1) to increase the span of healthy life for Americans, (2) to reduce health disparities among Americans, and (3) to achieve access to preventive services for all Americans. There were 300 national objectives in 22 priority areas set in conjunction with other government agencies, voluntary and professional organizations, businesses, and individuals.

The latest effort to guide the nation toward improved health is *Healthy People 2010 Objectives: Understanding and Improving Health* (USDHHS, 2000), which presents 26 areas for improvement and a full list of objectives for each area. Two broad goals guide the objectives: (1) to increase quality and years of healthy life and (2) to eliminate health disparities in health status, health risks, and use of preventive interventions among population groups. Objectives focus on promoting healthy behaviors, healthy and safe communities, improving systems for personal and public health, and prevention and reduction of diseases and disorders. (You can request a copy of the full report from the U.S. Government Printing Office by asking for stock number 017-001-00543-6.)

In the 20 years between the 1980 Surgeon General's report and *Healthy People 2010*, health professionals and the public have become more aware of and receptive to the idea of setting national health objectives. This latest publication is helping to shape health initiatives planned in the USDHHS, state health departments, managed-care organizations, and private care settings across the country. In particular, it has made the differences in health status for various populations clearly visible and helped initiate some of the broadest, coordinated efforts ever to occur in this country that are aimed at improving health status indicators and reducing the risks of disease and disorders.

Multiple private groups, associations, and like bodies, such as the National Academy of Science's Institute of Medicine (IOM), also provide overall public policy direction through publication of reports such as *The Future of Public Health* (IOM, 1988) and *Healthy Communities: New Partnerships for the Future of Public Health* (IOM, 1996). The 1988 report set forth a vision for public health and identified the mission and substance of governmental public health agencies. During preparation of the 1996 report, the IOM committee preparing the report noted that many of the problems and issues noted in 1988 remained true, even though progress was being made on the recommendations for improvement. What was seen as needed was not a revision of the future of public health but an enhancement to the report which would address the relationship between public health agencies and the public's health and managed care plus the role of the public health agency in the community. A subsequent report in 1997 by the IOM, *Improving Health in the Community: A Role for Performance Monitoring,* continued the focus on enhancing efforts at improving the public's health. Accomplishing the suggested goals, however, is difficult because no nationally organized delivery system or responsible party is charged with achieving them, and there is no way to require private providers to work toward them. Still, knowing and agreeing upon a target is helping to drive plans for change.

This seemingly impossible and improbable situation constitutes the subject of this chapter. Community health nurses deal with whole communities, not just with single individuals, practitioners, or institutions. To be able to understand and assist a community to achieve or maintain a certain health status, community health nurses must know how health care is financed, organized, and delivered in the United States, including the strengths U.S. health care offers and the gaps or failures that limit it. This chapter, then, explores the ways that health care services are organized and delivered and the impact that this has on populations and on community health nursing practice.

HEALTH CARE IN THE UNITED STATES

Health care in the United States is provided by a wide range of people and encompasses both the organized health care services and the informal health care (attention and protection) offered by individuals, families, and friends. Self-care and the care offered to children, loved ones, and friends on a daily basis actually constitute the bulk of the health care provided in this country.

Organized health care services, including public health, are the organized delivery components of health care wherein services are offered by individual practitioners, organizations, and institutions to the client or consumer of the services. Increasingly, the dominant, Western **allopathic** (practices derived from scientific models and technology) medical model of health care is being challenged to acknowledge and incorporate alternative modes of care such as **osteopathy** (a system of medical practice based on the theory that diseases are due chiefly to a loss of structural integrity), **homeopathy** [a system of medical practice that treats certain diseases by the administration of small doses of a remedy (drugs) that would, in healthy persons, produce symptoms of the disease being treated], and **complementary health care services** such as those offered by Eastern medicine, traditional healers, and folk medicine. Complementary health care services are those not used in general medical practice and have not been tested by scientific study in the United States. These services are used by clients in addition to their mainstream medical care. In acknowledgment of this trend, the National Institutes of Health, the health research arm of the federal government, created an Office of Alternative Medicine in 1991. Further discussion of alternative/complementary care practices is included in Chapter 12.

Regardless of the health care model, payment to the provider of services may come wholly or in part from the individual, the employer, government tax revenue, or voluntary organizations that choose to support specific services as part of a charitable mission. These four types of payors finance the delivery of health care services in the United States (see Figure 4-1). Although the bulk of the money spent in the system goes to allopathic health care services, it is estimated that many billions of dollars are spent on alternative medicine, with the vast majority of this money coming from the individual's own pocket (Eisenberg et al, 1993). Slightly over 3% of the expenditures on health care in 1998 went for "other personal health care," or services outside hospital, physician, dental, home health, and other services which are considered part of allopathic delivery of care (Levit et al., 2000). (See Chapter 6 for a more in-depth discussion of health economics.)

The Political Foundation of Health Care

No look at U.S. health care can be undertaken without first understanding the political context within which the delivery system developed. Elazar (1966) describes the political culture of this country as being one of (1) individualism; (2) civil liberties; (3) equality (of process, not

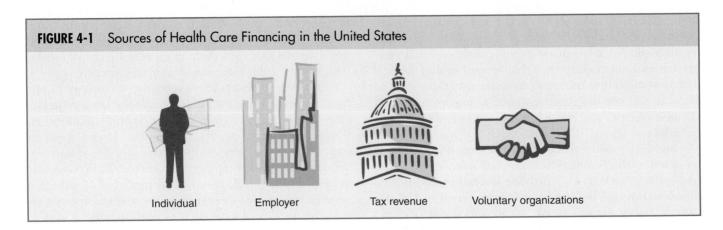

FIGURE 4-1 Sources of Health Care Financing in the United States

Individual   Employer   Tax revenue   Voluntary organizations

outcomes); (4) popular sovereignty and representative democracy; (5) belief in private property, capitalism, and the free market; (6) rationality, which is reflected in self-interest and competition; (7) a Protestant work ethic; and (8) separation of church and state. Our country is a federation of states whose citizens have chosen to decentralize power throughout federal, state, county, and local governments. Nowhere in our nation do we look to a central authority or body to dictate the lives of our citizens. Centralized control is against every belief and structure we have created as a nation.

Not surprisingly, then, the United States has consistently supported a health delivery approach that allows as much individual and state/local government control as possible. We have supported health care as a private business not only because we are a capitalist nation but also because this approach fits with the beliefs we hold about ourselves as individuals and about the role of government.

In the United States, government's role in our lives is generally expected to be limited rather than enhanced by public policy decisions. Even when government's role is expanded, new programs are designed to fit with and build on existing law and on our independent and business-centered market approach to health care. Incremental or gradual change rather than wholesale modification characterizes our political process. Proposals that seek to enlarge government—even generally positive federal and public health programs—are often criticized by legislators and individuals as being too intrusive and contrary to the political philosophy of the country. In the political environment of the 1980s, 1990s, and into the 21st century federal programs changed to reduce the requirements that states must meet to qualify for program funding under both Republican and Democratic administrations. Block grants (lump sums of money) or other approaches are allowing states to set their own rules and regulations to a significant degree. Welfare reform and Medicaid (health care for the poor) reforms that allow use of managed care are two examples of this reform trend.

Payors have financed the creation of a health system rich in resources. We have used those resources to de-

REFLECTIVE THINKING

Political Structure

- Describe the political culture of your state. How has it shaped access to health and welfare services?
- What efforts are underway, or have already taken place, to reform health or welfare in your state?
- As a citizen and a community health nurse, how can you be involved in the political life of your community?

velop medical research and technology that place us at the forefront of medical care and quality worldwide but that do not necessarily ensure optimal health status outcomes for our people. We use billions of dollars each year to provide wonderful physical structures, machines and instruments, new pharmaceuticals, and well-prepared health professionals. We expect our science and technology to fix most things, including poor health and disease. But whether a person has access to all these riches and enjoys their benefits depend in great part on whether that person has insurance and where that person lives.

The Insured

Nearly all health services in the United States are financed through private insurance purchased by an employer or through public insurance paid for with tax revenues from local, state, or federal taxes. A much more limited number of services are offered to the public as part of general public health programs or by charitable organizations. (See Chapter 6 for a detailed discussion of health insurance.)

Private insurance is offered by employers, usually with the employee paying some share of the premium cost. The federal Medicare and Medicaid programs represent the bulk of publicly financed insurance. Under Medicare, a person is eligible by virtue of age or disability. With Medicaid, a shared federal-state program, the means, or income, of a person determines whether they are eligible according to that state's eligibility criteria.

Health insurance began in the 1930s as a plan to pay hospitals fees for services provided to clients. That plan (the third party) became Blue Cross. A short time later, a Blue Shield plan was developed to pay physicians fees (Williams & Torrens, 1999). Other insurance approaches grew out of these initial efforts.

Indemnity insurance plans (which pay a cash benefit to the insured) have largely used **fee-for-service (FFS)** payment approaches, wherein fees are paid for a single episode of care, mostly acute episodes of care. As a payment system, insurance is not responsible for the health care delivery system that provides the care and coordinates its various components to ensure a person either stays well or is returned to maximum attainable health status. By adopting a fee-for-service payment approach, providers of care had the opportunity to increase the number of single services they delivered in order to increase the number of fees received (income or profit). The more fees paid, the greater the revenue generated for the provider (physician, hospital, etc.) and the greater the cost to the insurance company and the private or public payor (individual, company, or government) purchasing the insurance. Utilization of health service increased under these conditions, as did the dollars spent to provide the services. This is the genesis of much of the concern regarding rising health service costs in the last quarter of this century, because the federal insurance schemes (Medicare, Medicaid, and CHAMPUS) and employer insurance traditionally used fee-for-service as their primary payment approach.

The rising cost of health care and the fragmentation and inefficiency of the existing health care delivery structure have prompted the largest payors for health care services (both employers and government) to question whether the current system deserves their support. Increasingly, they are turning to managed care in the hope that it will provide the quality and quantity of care needed to ensure people's health and well-being.

Managed care refers to a variety of organizational arrangements. Managed care, however, seeks to provide, coordinate, and manage the services offered to the client, all within one financing and delivery system. In other words, the financing, payment, and delivery components are all linked within the managed-care plan and thus should be able to decrease episodes of fragmented care and unnecessary utilization while improving care cost efficiency and effectiveness.

The Uninsured and the Underinsured

In a given year, somewhere between 80% and 85% of the population has access to insurance in one form or an-

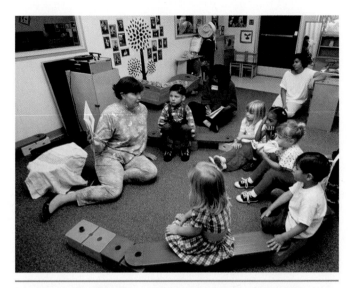

In order for this day care worker to have health care insurance, she must pay the entire cost herself. Unfortunately, her wage is not adequate to cover this expense along with her other living expenses. Consequently, she does without insurance.

other. Some people, however, may lose their insurance for short or long periods for a variety of reasons, including (1) being unable to pay the premium; (2) having a **preexisting condition** (health problem that was diagnosed or treated or that existed prior to issuance of an insurance policy) that an insurer either refuses to cover (thereby making the person uninsurable) or delays covering for fear that the insuree will need care and cost money; (3) becoming ineligible for Medicaid or some other government-related program; (4) changing jobs or going to work for a company that does not offer insurance, such as is often the case in farming, housekeeping, and other job situations where people are employed in low-wage jobs; or (5) going to work for an employer who passes most of the cost of insurance on to the employee, an expense that the employee cannot afford. In other words, an uninsured person may be almost anyone, and in 1999, the uninsured accounted for 17.5% of the population (Employee Benefit Research Institute, 2000).

Those who are unemployed or self-employed or work in small businesses often have difficulty buying health insurance because they lack the purchasing and bargaining power of large organizations. Many uninsured persons either have made too much money in the previous year to qualify for a public program or do not make enough money to feel that they can afford to purchase insurance on their own; and many of those who do purchase insurance are financially limited to buying policies that offer little in the way of services, in effect rendering insurees underinsured.

Yet another segment of the uninsured are employed by employers who do contribute to the cost of insurance, but these individuals are healthy and do not believe they

REFLECTIVE THINKING

Uninsured/Underinsured Families

Many families in the United States are either underinsured or uninsured. This is a major problem for the families and for the community health nurses who provide services to them.

- What do you think should be done to deal with this problem in our country? What are the issues?
- How might you assist families to obtain the care they need?

will need care. They therefore choose not to use any of their income to buy health insurance. Young adults often fall into this category of the uninsured.

A number of health reform efforts at both federal and state levels have repeatedly attempted to extend coverage to the uninsured and uninsurable. In the absence of some mandatory national or state programs, millions will at some time in their lives find themselves without health insurance coverage and therefore limited in the health care they can hope to receive.

Employer payors are using their purchasing power by banding together in business coalitions, alliances, and various affiliated groups to purchase care directly from networks of providers instead of insurance companies and managed-care plans. Rather than having to take the price offered by an insurance company or plan, these large groups negotiate premium rates on their own. In some cases, these groups control the health care purchasing for so many people that they can, to a significant

degree, set the price they are willing to pay. As networks, the managed-care plans and insurance companies compete with each other to enroll employer, Medicaid, and Medicare clients. The effort by purchasers to introduce competition into a health care market that is seen as having little real competition is termed **managed competition.** The hope is that such competition will force insurers and providers to lower their prices in order to capture more business and gain access to more people able to pay for health care coverage.

The impact of these changes is that caregivers and institutions must shift from seeking to provide as many services as possible under a fee-for-service payment approach to keeping the client well and providing fewer services so as to protect their best interests in an atmosphere of prepayment and negotiated contracts. In a fee-for-service system, the concern is that a client might receive too many or unnecessary services; in a prepaid system, the concern is that too few services might be given in order to save the provider and the managed-care plan money. Table 4-1 compares the potential consequences of fee-for-service and managed-care approaches.

Whether it is fee-for-service or managed care in a private or public insurance scheme, equalizing access, cost, and quality remains an elusive goal within the health care system. Figure 4-2 shows a triangle with the points identified as access, quality, and cost. Each reform in the health care system attempts to improve one or the other points. But with each change, the other points are pushed out of alignment, and the perfect triangle is destroyed. Indemnity insurance, Medicaid, and Medicare sought to increase access and quality but in the end increased costs because of the increase in the number and price of services delivered. Managed care tried to control costs, but its critics suggest a significant portion of the energy in managed-care organizations has gone to managing costs, rather than quality, or access to care. The result is that approaches to the financing and delivery of health

TABLE 4-1   Possible Outcomes of Fee-for-Service and Managed-Care Capitation Payment Approaches

FEE-FOR-SERVICE	MANAGED CARE USING CAPITATION
Increased services	Decreased services
Single service	Continuum of services
Episodic care	Prevention/wellness care
Emphasis on specialty care	Emphasis on primary care/case management
Shift of costs to other payors	Cost management within premium
Independent providers	Integrated providers
Limited peer review	Extensive peer review
Little or no financial risk	Managed-care plan and providers placed at financial risk

Note: It is important to remember that these are potential consequences of the different payment approaches; the likelihood and severity of these consequences (harm to the patient) depend on the philosophy and perspective of the individual and groups providing the care.

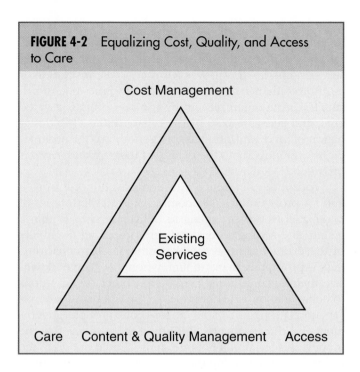

FIGURE 4-2 Equalizing Cost, Quality, and Access to Care

Cost Management

Existing Services

Care   Content & Quality Management   Access

For the majority of employed insured individuals and families, the impact of rationing efforts is minimal or, at least, acceptable. These insurees pay a small portion of their health care costs—a portion that is within their financial means—and the insurance pays for most, if not all, of the costs associated with the services they require. For the uninsured and underinsured and for many persons covered by Medicare and Medicaid, sharing in the cost of care may be a much greater burden depending on the size of their share. Those who find the financial burden too great may forgo necessary care because of associated costs.

The proportion of the nation's income and expenditures that goes toward buying health care has steadily climbed over the years. At the same time, other things such as housing, food, and education continue to demand our dollars. Resources available to fund the health care system, thus, are not unlimited. This dictates judicious use of resources and services on the part of community health nurses and others who seek to ensure that the national population has access to needed services to ensure an acceptable health status.

care remain uncertain, with different ones being tried and discarded and pieces of each taken on to the next approach. What is evolving is a hybrid of fee-for-service and managed-care features that, so far, presents no clear picture of what the healthy delivery and payment system will look like by 2010.

What is even less clear is how public health will be integrated into any revised system. Public health services and prevention approaches have been, and continue to be, poorly integrated into insurance and managed-care systems. Efforts to link approaches to care that can improve the health status for whole populations are and will remain a focus of public health agencies and community health nurses. It is they who will have to lead others in efforts to meet *Healthy People 2010* objectives and other communitywide and national efforts to improve the health of America.

Those persons without insurance, those denied insurance because of their health status, and those with inadequate insurance or with public or private insurance that purposely restricts access to certain care, to timely care, or to quantities of care are faced with rationing of the health services. Rationing is not new in the United States. For years the uninsured have been denied health services or have received limited services only. Although rationing in one form or another has always existed in the U.S. health care system, not until the last 15–20 years has it been purposely used to help control ever-increasing health care costs. At one time, the ability to charge some payors higher prices left room for providers to offer services for free or at reduced cost to select clients. This practice of shifting the cost of care from one payor to another is becoming increasingly limited under current payment and delivery schemes such as managed care.

COORDINATION AND INTEGRATION OF HEALTH CARE SERVICES

The organizations and individuals who offer health care services are usually independent providers. Physicians, hospitals, nursing homes, rehabilitation programs, and others provide care within the scope of their services and often leave clients to find and manage the other services they might need.

The local delivery system the client must turn to has also been left to its own devices in determining, planning, and designing the services that are to be made available within a community. "Hospitals can open or close according to community resources, preference, and the dictates of an open market for hospital services. Also, physicians are free to establish their practice where they choose" (De Law, Greenberg, & Kinchen, 1992, p. 151). Nothing has changed in the last 10 years. To the extent planning is done in this country, it is done largely in response to budgetary decisions and is based on the amount of funds available in private businesses or public coffers.

Community health planning, which sought to direct the location and size of facilities and equipment, was popular during the 1970s and early 1980s. In the years since, popularity has diminished largely because the political climate at national and state levels shifted away from a regulatory approach and toward deregulation under Presidents Reagan and Bush. It has continued to do so under a Republican-controlled Congress and a national conservative trend. There are no health-planning requirements at the federal level, and states require health planning to varying degrees. Construction of hospitals and nursing homes as well as purchase of some large-capital investments such as magnetic resonance imaging machines may be reviewed in some states. Even so, most buildings and equipment are eventually purchased and developed as an organization or individual wishes, as long as that organization or individual has the required funds.

Governmental and charitable programs are frequently left to fill the gaps created when private providers do not, or will not, offer a service in a particular locale. In many cases, the areas left unserved are inner cities or small rural communities, where income levels may mean that residents do not have the insurance or resources to buy health care. To fill this gap in available care, the government develops or encourages development of a geographically well positioned range of services to afford individuals access to acceptable and desirable care. In many such programs, community health nurses are key providers, such as in community health and mental health centers. Uncertain and often dwindling funding makes the future of such programs precarious, however.

Until recently, almost all health care was controlled by locally owned organizations or hospitals that had little or no relationship with each other. Now, health services may actually be part of larger, private health plans, alliances, and corporations with national, state, and local offices, facilities, or programs. Where facilities are located (or purchased) is increasingly dictated by the ways that the national organizations plan to compete for clients. Many smaller and locally owned organizations cannot compete or survive in this kind of environment and are being bought by or are merging with larger systems. For the community health nurse, a work setting that was once a locally owned and run visiting nursing service or home health agency may thus now be part of a larger statewide or national organization.

OWNERSHIP OF HEALTH DELIVERY ORGANIZATIONS

Health services are delivered to the insured and uninsured alike by private and public entities. Private ownership can be divided into two categories: (1) not-for-profit, voluntary, or charitable entities and (2) for-profit, investor-owned entities. Public or governmental ownership rests with government bodies at the federal, state, and local levels, where tax dollars are used directly to purchase care or deliver services. (The structure of government-owned public health organizations is discussed in greater detail later in this chapter.)

Private physicians' offices and those of nurse practitioners and other health professionals, hospitals of all types, nursing homes, managed-care organizations, clinics, freestanding surgical centers, psychiatric facilities, and all other entities or groups that provide services may fall within the definition of private for-profit or not-for-profit ownership.

Historically, private not-for-profit voluntary health care institutions were developed by religious and charitable organizations that received tax-free status in return for the good they provided the community. The behavior and charitable mission of these groups dictated their services, and any profit was returned to the institution or group to enhance or expand services. In the case of private for-profit organizations, by contrast, profit is a stated goal, and taxes are paid by the organizations. The designation of an organization as for-profit or not-for-profit indicates nothing about the quality of the care and services provided.

Today, the difference between private not-for-profit and for-profit entities is becoming blurred. Both types of organizations are struggling to deliver services within a health care setting where costs are outpacing the ability of these organizations to absorb them. Cost consciousness is prompting many to limit whom they serve, downsize their organizations, merge with other organizations to achieve economies of scale, sell, or close. When not-for-profit groups are sold to for-profit groups, government and the courts are supporting the position that the money accrued under tax-free status should not go to the for-profit entity making the purchase. Instead, the "profits" are to be used to create foundations that will continue to have a community/charitable goal. Such foundations may represent a significant source of money for local health care programs in coming years.

In order to understand the incentives, issues, and disputes that arise surrounding both defining the services to be delivered and paying for those services, it is important to know who owns a health care business. Figure 4-3 displays the types of private health care institutions and organizations from which individuals receive their care. The private health care services delivery sector and the businesses that support it—such as pharmaceutical companies and medical equipment and supply companies—constitute what many refer to as the "health care industry." The word *industry* has been applied to health care in recent years because it describes the nature of the business attitude and processes that now dominate health care.

For some, this "industry" approach fostered by a for-profit system is the antithesis of what they espouse for health care. "Faith-based" organizations are, in many cases, trying to revive and enhance the original voluntary and charitable nature of not-for-profit care. The repeated failure of the health care system to reach segments of society with the services and support necessary to allow them to improve their lives and their health status is prompting religiously affiliated groups to develop innovative approaches to the delivery of health promotion, disease prevention, and treatment services. These approaches allow churches, synagogues, and mosques to serve their own members or multiple congregations and the broader community. Nurses in such roles are often referred to as "parish nurses." For those individuals receiving these services, they offer a context within which they can accept and learn how to manage their own health for a better future.

FIGURE 4-3 Types of Private Ownership in the Health Care Service Delivery System

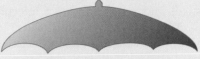

NOT-FOR-PROFIT (Voluntary/Charitable)	**FOR-PROFIT (Investor Owned)**
Sectarian or religiously affiliated	Individually owned
Community-based groups	Partnerships
Fraternal organizations (e.g., Shriners, Kiwanis)	Limited liability companies
Business and industry (e.g., Kaiser-Permanente Plan)	Corporations
Unions	
Disease-specific groups (e.g., Cancer Society)	
Foundations (e.g., Pew, Robert Wood Johnson)	
Professional associations	
Some insurance companies (e.g., some Blue Cross/Blue Shields)	

HEALTH SERVICE ORGANIZATIONS

Health service organizations (HSOs) are formed to deliver care, with the number and variety of organizations created influenced by both the ways we choose to finance and pay for that care and the technology available. Payors are influencing those choices by asking that the dollars spent result in more than just a tally of the number of services provided. They are asking that the services actually produce outcomes of value to the client and that plans and providers be able to report on outcomes for the populations to which they provide care—a positive step toward improved health status.

Along with outcomes, purchasers of care are asking for evidence-based medicine. Providers of care at all levels, physicians, nurses, and allied health care givers are being asked to provide the evidence, or research that proves that the care they offer is the most appropriate and will result in the best outcome for their patients. In many cases the evidence does not exist. The next decade will see significant efforts put toward developing that evidence in all areas of health care. To some extent, public health may be ahead of other areas simply because it has had to justify itself so consistently in all settings. The use of immunizations, maternal and child health care services, disease tracking, and other public health activities consistently provide evidence to support the need for and benefit of such services. Proving its importance to the public and other disciplines is nothing new for public health.

Following is a brief discussion of some of the most common types of health service organizations, including public health organizations. The inclusion of public health in this discussion is intentional, because as simply one component of the U.S. organized health care system, public health must be examined within the context of that system. It should be further noted that the following discussion can by no means be considered exhaustive, because new health service organizations and groupings of services are constantly being created.

The Public Health System

Even though we might wish it were so, the public health system is not one of the major components of the health system in the United States in terms of funding. Money for government public health activities comprised only 3.6% of the expenditures on health in 1998, or slightly over $36 billion out of expenditures of over $1 trillion (Levit, et al., 2000). This is actually up from 1.5% in 1990.

Ellencweig and Yoshpe (1984) suggest that public health services are intended to protect the community against the hazards of group living. This is a simple statement, but it encompasses the goal that community public health nurses work toward and that public health has always sought to do for populations.

REFLECTIVE THINKING

Impact of Different Types of Health Care Systems

- What are the strengths and weaknesses of a privately owned, business-oriented health care system?
- What impact does a private system of care have on health and wellness?
- What role do you think government should play in the health care system?

During the latter half of the 19th century, communicable diseases were spurred by unsafe drinking water and food and by poor sanitation. People died of acute gastrointestinal and respiratory tract infections such as pneumonia. Tuberculosis was one of the few diseases with which people lived long enough to have the disease be considered chronic. Public health efforts designed to improve sanitation and food handling reduced the number of people affected by communicable diseases or eliminated many such diseases (Dieckmann, 2000).

By the early 1900s, attention had shifted from general public health issues affecting whole communities to single acute episodes of illness experienced by individuals. Developing technologies, medications, and health insurance helped encourage this shift in focus from public health to acute illness.

At the public level, services and programs respond to broad community needs that are not usually addressed by privately owned and more narrowly defined service providers. While privately owned entities do indeed provide research and education, these efforts do not always coincide with all the perceived needs of the public. Consequently, government (primarily at the federal level) funds extensive research and education believed to be in the interest of national goals for health and safety. Public health and welfare are further protected by the public (governmental) sector through regulation, licensing, and monitoring of select health services, health professionals, and health programs (primarily at the state and local levels). When the private sector is involved, it is most often as a contractor to government or as a grant recipient implementing programs planned by government or by private foundations.

The IOM's report *The Future of Public Health* defines the mission of public health "as fulfilling society's interest in assuring conditions in which people can be healthy" (1988, p. 7). To do this, public health agencies at different levels of government provide the epidemiological and community assessment necessary to define health need; develop and modify the policies, laws, and programs required to respond to that need; and work to ensure that the programs are implemented in a manner so as to have the desired effect. This process is not simple, because actions are carried out largely within the political arena and in a setting where government budgets dictate much of that which can or cannot be done. Furthermore, elected officials most often think in terms of immediately fulfilling campaign promises, rather than in planting the seeds of positive impact 10 or 15 years hence when a preventive public health program they earlier supported might finally demonstrate success.

Federal, state, and local levels of government may provide any or all of the following: direct services, research, education, development/planning, and regulation of health care services. Table 4-2 indicates the range of health-related services offered by state and local governmental bodies. The majority of public health–related ser-

TABLE 4-2 Examples of State and Local Public Programs and Services

DIRECT/CONTRACTED SERVICES

Public health and primary care services

Mental health hospitals and services

City/county/university hospitals and medical schools

Nursing home care

Hospital districts or authorities

Animal control

POLICY DEVELOPMENT/PLANNING

Monitoring, data collection, analysis—epidemiological assessment

Development/implementation of health laws and regulation

REGULATION

Licensing of health care facilities (hospitals, nursing homes, etc.)

Licensing of health care agencies (home health, hospice, ambulances, etc.)

Licensing of health care professionals

Licensing of restaurants and food handlers

Regulation of environment (water, sewer, sanitation, air)

EDUCATION/RESEARCH

Health education, promotion, and disease prevention

Training/educational programs

Research (often as part of data gathering)

vices provided are under state or local direction because the Constitution grants the states the power and responsibility to protect the public health. Core public health functions carried out by state and local governments, as suggested by the Association of State and Territorial Health Officials (1994), are related to the following: (1) monitoring the health of the population and developing policies to promote healthy behavior and health; (2) mobilizing and training specialists to investigate, prevent, and control epidemics, disease, and disasters; (3) organizing communities for action; and (4) protecting the public by monitoring and regulating medical services, the environment, the workplace, housing, food, and water.

Funds may be appropriated by any level of government for use in any of the activities carried out by a public health agency. Most often, however, we hear about the distribution of federal monies to the states, which may use the monies themselves or may in turn distribute the monies to local governments. The grants or allocations

FIGURE 4-4 U.S. Department of Health and Human Services Organizational Chart

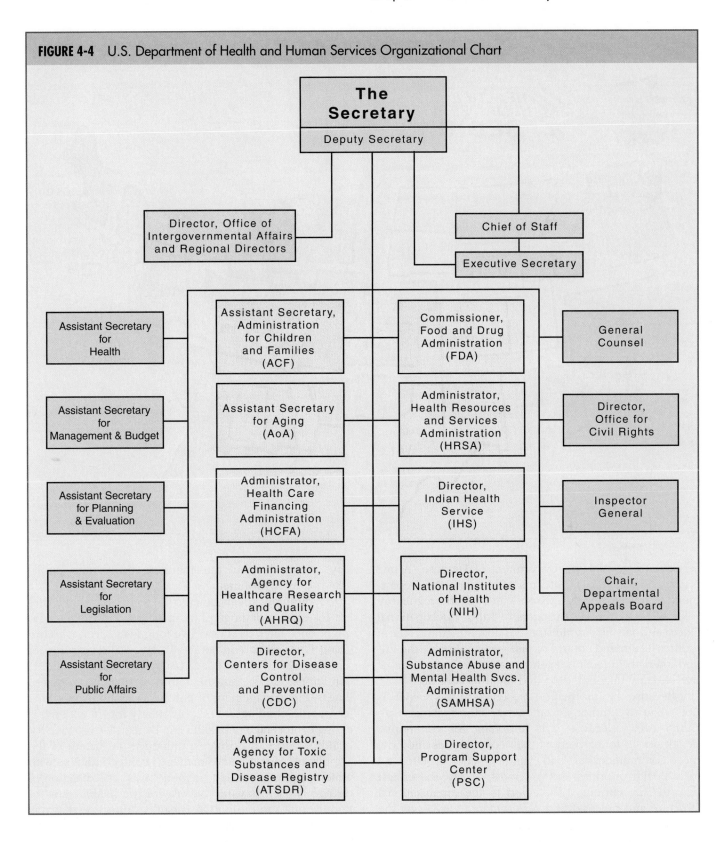

may be in lump sums (block grants, which have broad guidelines and allow the receiving group wide latitude in defining how grant money is used) or tied to an activity or service for which requirements are specified in detail.

Figure 4-4 lists the specific departments and agencies of the USDHHS. In addition, Figure 4-5 displays the 10 regions into which the USDHHS has divided the nation to allow it to focus its work with the states located in each region.

While the USDHHS encompasses most of the agencies responsible for health at the federal level, other departments do have a health role, such as (1) the direct

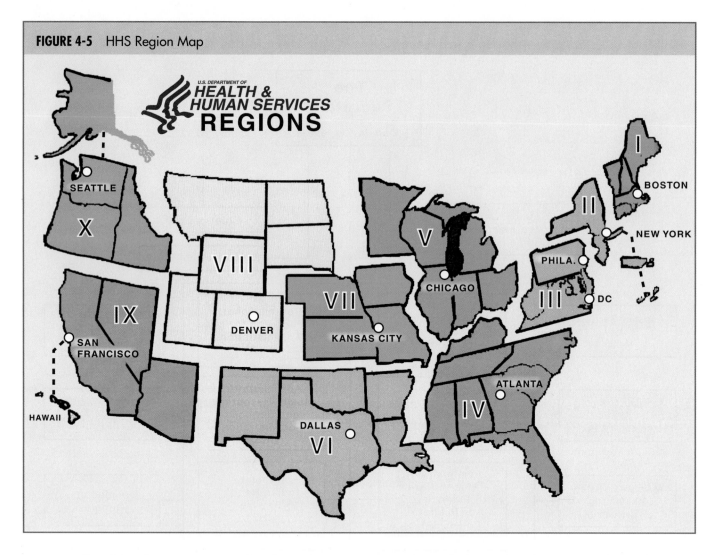

FIGURE 4-5 HHS Region Map

services offered by the Department of Defense (Army, Navy, and Air Force), Veterans Affairs, and the Department of Justice (federal prisons) and (2) the regulatory roles filled by the Departments of Labor (Occupational Safety and Health Administration) and Agriculture (farm worker health and control of disease in animals), the Environmental Protection Agency, and the Department of the Treasury (alcohol, drug and firearms control).

Because the information presented in this section is not exhaustive and organizational structures change with nearly every election, it is important for community health nurses to learn about their communities and how those communities relate to changing national, state, and local health priorities and programs. Today, the easiest way to stay current with regard to the organizational structure and function of a government entity is via the Internet. All of the agencies that are part of the USDHHS may be reached by logging onto the web at www.hhs.gov. The links from the site can take you to the White House and numerous other sites of interest. Each provides a wealth of information by posting reports, news briefs, and updates about current activities. Use the web to search for the information you want and need to

stay informed about the changing health and public health care environment.

Continuing advancements in technology and care are fostering a demographic transition. Individuals who might once have died now live long lives, even with ongoing illnesses or conditions. Today, acute episodes of illness may in fact be exacerbations of existing chronic conditions. Rather than treatment of single episodes of illness, the management of chronic conditions over time for people of all ages, and particularly for the elderly, is taking center stage in health care. Demand is growing for health services to positively influence the health of the population served and to manage health conditions with which people live on an ongoing basis. The direction of change is back toward concern for the health status of populations and the public's health, a direction that was missing in the U.S. health care delivery system in the latter half of the 20th century. Public health is and will continue to be in competition for its share of available health care funding. Its often unseen importance to the community and the individual makes it difficult to gain support for increasing public health–related services and dollars. As more of these services are presumed to be part of the scope of services offered in managed-care settings, cooperation between public health agencies and private bodies will be increasingly necessary to ensure that the needs of the population are addressed.

Significant efforts are underway across the country to revitalize and enhance the public health infrastructure that supports the core functions of public health. A renewed interest in defining how public health monitoring, education, and services can articulate with private and managed-care services has prompted initiatives by private foundations, medical societies, and government at the local, state, and federal levels. *Healthy People 2010* and the IOM reports are helping drive some of these initiatives. But overall, there is greater interest in public health because of the reality that many of the problems and issues facing the nation in the next decade can only be dealt with at a community level.

Primary Health Care Systems

Primary health care as an organizational movement officially began at the 30th World Health Organization (WHO) Assembly in 1977 with the adoption of a resolution identifying the goal of health attainment that would enable citizens of the world to live socially and economically productive lives. As a WHO member nation, the United States endorsed primary health care as a way to achieve the goal of Health for All by the Year 2000.

Primary health care has been defined as essential care made universally accessible and available to individuals and families within a community, with an emphasis on disease prevention, health promotion, community involvement, multisectoral cooperation, and a cost that the community and country can afford (WHO, 1978). The primary health care system includes a comprehensive range of services such as public health, prevention, diagnostic, therapeutic, and rehabilitative services. Primary health care services are community focused with an emphasis on health promotion and preventive services rather than the acute medical care services offered in a hospital. Primary health care services include health education, nutrition, maternal-child health care, family planning, immunization, prevention and control of locally endemic diseases, treatment of commonly occurring diseases and injuries, provision of essential medications, and safe water and basic sanitation. Primary health care is part of ambulatory care, public health, acute, long-term health and mental health care settings.

The scope of primary care means it is the largest component of health care provided in the nation. Many primary care services are not identified as separate items in the tally of how health care dollars are used. By adding together some of those that are listed, however, we get a sense of the magnitude of the dollars spent on primary care in the United States. If we include things like physician services, dental services, other professional services, prescription drugs, vision products, other personal health care, and government public health activities, we see that roughly $435 billion goes toward primary care. Right behind primary care in expenditures is hospital care, at nearly $383 billion (Levit et al., 2000).

Hospitals

Today's hospital care is focused largely on secondary and tertiary care or the acute care required for both simple and complex problems (specialty care) requiring 30 or fewer days of medical, surgical, and nursing care or emergency services. Hospitals have been a part of society for thousands of years as houses for the ill, poor, and dying. Not until the latter half of the 19th century, however, did improvements in technology allow for the beginnings of safe and effective organization and delivery of services. Discoveries and advances in antisepsis, asepsis, inhalation procedures, and anesthesia made it possible for invasive surgery to be planned and effective as opposed to being the last of a number of poor options for saving a life. Developments in radiography, blood typing, and clinical laboratories plus increased understanding of clinical care and client responses allowed hospitals to offer improved medical and surgical interventions (Shi & Singh, 2000).

The work of Florence Nightingale in British hospitals also brought improvements and understanding in the areas of sanitation and the organization and operation of hospitals (Kopf, 1991). Nightingale's use of fundamental public health and epidemiological principals provided direction for the development of all health care services, and her efforts at training nurses to work in the hospital helped increase the use of organized hospital services and laid the basis for today's hospital nursing practice.

Most hospitals were created as private, not-for-profit corporations responding to community need and the needs of the poor. Every community wants a hospital of its own. In recent years, however, hospitals (particularly small hospitals) have begun to close as falling occupancy rates, controls on length of hospital stays, movement of care to the community, and mergers reduce the need and competition for hospital beds. If clients do not require intensive medical or nursing care, they are discharged to recover at home.

Psychiatric hospitals differ from acute-care hospitals, both in the type of care they provide and in ownership. Most were created as public facilities where the mentally ill were warehoused and often committed involuntarily. Not until after World War II, when technological advances prompted by the war led to the development of psychoactive drugs, were the mentally ill given new hope for control over and recovery from their conditions. In response to the changes facilitated by medication and treatment advances, the 1963 Community Mental Health Center Act sought to foster the movement of mental health clients from psychiatric hospitals to community-based centers where they could be treated outside an institutional setting. This shift, combined with further advances in the development of medications and treatments, fostered the expectation that clients could and should be treated more appropriately in the community. The resources necessary to adequately implement such an approach, however, have never been forthcoming, leaving many mental health clients with inadequate treatment and community supports such as housing.

Insurance coverage for mental health services has been limited. Private insurance pays more readily for physical care than for mental health care and, typically, provides only limited coverage for psychiatric problems. Thus, public funding may be the only recourse for a mental health client, but, often, this funding is also limited. Insurance parity, or equality of treatment and payment for physical and mental health services, has been enacted into law in some states, but it is still a goal to be achieved nationally in the 21st century.

Ambulatory Surgery

Technology has helped reduce the amount of time clients must remain in the hospital. For years, select surgeries have been performed with the client being admitted and discharged from the hospital on the same day. Only since the early 1970s, however, have large numbers of surgeries been performed on an outpatient (rather than as a hospital inpatient) basis (Morgan, 1986). Hospitals, freestanding surgical centers, and physicians' offices today offer surgery to the ambulatory patient.

By not admitting clients for overnight care, the use of costly hospital facilities, 24-hour nursing care, and ancillary services such as food and laundry is avoided. Clients spend the day and return to their homes to heal.

The interest in reducing both hospital costs and the cost of health care in general has contributed to the rise in same-day surgery. Short-acting anesthetics, new surgical procedures, and technology that allows for very small incisions that heal quickly have all contributed to the growth of outpatient surgical procedures. In some cases, insurance will pay for certain surgeries only if they are performed on an outpatient basis.

Long-Term Care Facilities and Home- and Community-Based Care

Long-term care refers to the range of services that people with functional impairments require to be maintained "in safety and dignity, and to pursue the most meaningful lives that their disabilities permit" (Fogel, Brock, Goldscheider, & Royall, 1994, p. 1). The need for long-

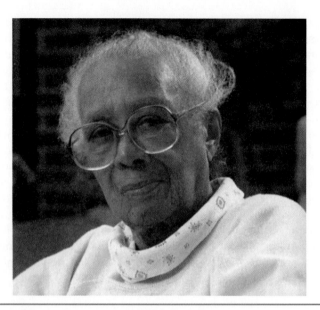

The growing number of elders with chronic health conditions increases the need for home and community-based services and quality of long-term care facilities.

term care arises when individuals can no longer maintain themselves without assistance or supervision because of mental, physical, or social impairment and because the environments within which they live cannot or will not offer them the support they need.

The United States and other industrialized nations are facing growing populations of elderly individuals. Health care and technology have allowed individuals to live longer lives with chronic conditions that may impair their health or functioning without causing death. Growing numbers of elders require assistance and care to maintain themselves in (1) their homes, with family members, nurses, and others providing intermittent care and support; (2) residential housing, where they can live in some variation of congregate housing and receive limited amounts of support from people employed to assist those living there; (3) community day care settings, where families can leave elders during work hours and then return to take their elderly family members home in the evening; and (4) nursing homes, where various levels of care are offered according to the clients' needs.

Nursing Homes

Nursing homes are probably the best known long-term care facilities. They grew out of the community almshouses, or poorhouses, and, later, the privately owned "boarding houses" sponsored by churches and those caring for the wealthy aged. Social Security legislation passed in 1935 included an Old Age Assistance (OAA) program, which paid for residents of private facilities meeting minimal requirements set by the federal government, thereby encouraging small, private, for-profit boarding houses to increase in number in response to the private-market financial incentive (Rakich, Longest, & Darr, 1992). The law specified coverage for private facilities only, primarily because the private sector had the most effective lobbying efforts.

By 1950, nursing homes were licensed in every state (American Nursing Home Association, 1993). Whereas Medicare provides limited funding for skilled nursing care services, Medicaid pays for many of the nursing home beds in use in this country. The federal Medicare program specifies the requirements that must be met by nursing home facilities, but the states perform the compliance reviews and provide state licensing. Stryker (1988) notes that the model for nursing home care is based on a hospital medical disease model rather than on a model focusing on quality of life. This focus limits the social supports available to nursing home clients. In some cases, clients who need only social supports could more appropriately remain at home. Some funding exists for such support services but, where offered, the services are bound by regulation and constraints that limit the total availability of services.

Costs for nursing home care accounted for 8.6% of the spending for personal health care in 1998 (Levit et al., 2000). Nursing home costs constitute the fourth largest expense behind those for hospitals, physician services, and pharmaceuticals. Nursing home care will have significant budget implications as the number of elderly persons increases in this century. Alternatives to nursing homes will become more important to elected leaders as the number of elders requiring assistance increases—and as those same elders use the power of their votes to have their demands met.

Home Health Care

Home care services are provided by home health agencies, visiting nursing services, some public health agencies, and private companies. Lillian Wald is credited with establishing the first continuing program in the United States, with the creation of the Visiting Nursing Service of New York City in 1893 (Mundinger, 1983). Wald's vision significantly shaped the character and content of community public health nursing.

Home health care is usually thought of in terms of the definition used by the Medicare program, which covers physician care, skilled nursing services, physical therapy, occupational and speech therapy, social work services, and home health aide services. Skilled nursing care is defined as intermittent, part-time services delivered by a nurse in the residence of a home-bound client.

In 1960, home health care was so rarely used that it was not included in the calculations of national health care expenditures. By 1980, home health care accounted for $1.3 billion, growing to $9.8 billion in 1991 and $29.3 billion in 1998 (Letsch, 1993; Levit et al., 2000). Budget constraints placed on home health in the late 1990s have slowed the growth of home health services, but it is doubtful this will or can continue, given the growing number of elderly and people with chronic disease. It is expected that expenditures for home health care and other long-term care services will increase as the number of elders continues to surge with the aging of the post–World War II baby boomers.

Hospice

The modern version of hospice was developed in the 1960s in England by Cicely Saunders, MD (Manning, 1984). It spread to the United States, where independent, community-based programs using volunteers trained to deal with death and dying provided care to clients and their families.

Hospice programs focus on palliative care and comfort for the client who is expected to die within the near future. Support is offered to the client and family during and after the death of the ill family member. Today, volunteers and an interdisciplinary team of health professionals and chaplains work to provide a wide range of physical and emotional supports to clients and families.

REFLECTIVE THINKING

Encouraging Public Health Concepts

- How might interest in public health issues be improved?
- What roles do you think community health nurses could fill in health service organizations and managed-care organizations?
- What can you do to foster public health and preventive health concepts in your work setting?

Ambulatory Care

Ambulatory care is care delivered in an office or other setting at the time and place of the client's choosing. Once the care is provided, the client returns to home or work. Ambulatory care constitutes much of the primary care offered in this country and, often, the first point of contact for the client with the health care system.

Physicians' offices, emergency rooms, and outpatient clinics of acute-care hospitals, urgent-care centers, and freestanding clinics and centers offer ambulatory/primary care. Walk-in diagnostic imaging centers and mobile mammography examinations are examples of the growing variety in types of ambulatory settings and services.

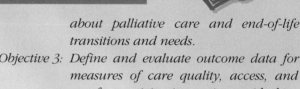

Out of the Box

Phoenix-based Hospice of the Valley (HOV) is one of the four largest hospices in the nation with a long history of caring for dying patients. What that experience has revealed is that patients with serious chronic illnesses need assistance long before they are eligible for hospice care during what is expected to be the last six months of their life. To respond to that need, HOV applied for and received a three-year grant (1999–2001) to be one of 21 Robert Wood Johnson (RWJ) Promoting Excellence in End-of-Life Care Project participants. The demonstration project, Phoenix-Care, which continues to operate through private donations and funding, provides palliative coordinated care to people who are not "clearly terminal" and therefore not eligible for hospice care. The project provides home-based services to seriously chronically ill individuals who are at risk of death from their advanced disease state but who are not yet eligible for or are unwilling to participate in a hospice program. PhoenixCare nurse case managers visit the home to provide both the palliative services usually associated with hospice care and the coordination and disease management associated with care for people with chronic illnesses.

Although discussions were occurring nationally about the need for palliative care in a prehospice home setting, little had been done to do so, since there are few insurance companies that will pay for such care. PhoenixCare and several other of the participants in the RWJ Project sought to define a program that might provide such positive patient outcomes that payers would cover the cost of care.

PhoenixCare has four key objectives:

Objective 1: Refine, structure, and implement differing levels of in-home care.

Objective 2: Educate participating patients/families, clinicians, and personnel from health plans, hospitals, and provider groups about palliative care and end-of-life transitions and needs.

Objective 3: Define and evaluate outcome data for measures of care quality, access, and cost for participating patients with three diagnoses (metastatic cancer, congestive heart failure, and chronic obstructive pulmonary disease).

Objective 4: Assess care quality, access, and cost components in order to develop a delivery and payment model which supports varying levels of palliative care as a benefit within a single health plan.

The PhoenixCare demonstration assesses whether there is improved quality of care and access to care for patients when compared to a control group not receiving PhoenixCare services. Differences in utilization of services, perceived quality of care, and cost are examined. The PhoenixCare model was implemented with patients referred from managed-care plans, the predominant insurers in the Phoenix metropolitan area. Data and information are used to assess the potential for a delivery and payment model for prehospice care within managed health care systems and to provide a better understanding of programs such as PhoenixCare.

The PhoenixCare model is now part of a new demonstration called Medicaring. Based on the PhoenixCare research design, educational tools, and clinical experience of the Project, HOV applied for and was awarded one of 15 slots for a Coordinated Care Demonstration Project by the Centers for Medicare and Medicaid Systems. It is the only hospice-based project to participate in the four-year (2001–2005) national demonstration exploring how to improve care for chronically ill Medicare beneficiaries. It is one more step toward finding payment sources for home-based palliative and coordinated care. ■

As is the case with ambulatory surgery, ambulatory care settings offer increasingly sophisticated and complex treatments to clients who simply stop in for care and then go on their way. Emergency rooms are frequently used to provide ambulatory care. The cost of the care, however, is far more expensive than if it was delivered in a physician's office or clinic. In order to shift clients whose cases are not true emergencies to the less expensive clinic setting, some hospitals are establishing ambulatory clinics in conjunction with their emergency rooms. Insurance companies discourage the use of the emergency room as an ambulatory care site. Most, in fact, reduce the amount they will contribute and require a greater out-of-pocket payment by the client than if the client had been seen in another ambulatory care site.

Community Nursing Organizations/ Community Nursing Centers

Community nursing organizations (CNOs) or centers (CNCs) also offer ambulatory/primary care services. A CNO can be a single setting where clients visit but, more often, encompasses a wide range of services offered by nurses in a variety of practice arrangements and settings in the community. Both CNOs and CNCs offer nurse-managed services to clients across the continuum of care in the home, community, hospital, or nursing home setting (Aydellotte et al., 1987; Riesch, 1990; Sharp, 1992). They usually offer both illness management services (comparable to a medical acute-care model) and nursing care and coordination. Advanced-practice nurses offer the acute care to clients and bill insurance companies if possible (Safriet, 1992). Community health and other nurses offer nursing care, coordination, and education. The majority of the care provided by advanced-practice, community health, and other nurses is not reimbursable under insurance; thus, other payment sources such as grants and direct contracts with employers, city and state governments, and others must replace the unavailable insurance revenue (Lockhart, 1994).

Although the CNO has a difficult time as an independent financial entity, the model for care is being adopted by groups of providers who want to use the approach to market coordinated care to the public. Advanced-practice, community health, and other nurses are serving as the first contacts and managers of care for various institutions, employers, and insurance companies. They are expected to do so in increasing numbers as payors demand coordinated care for insured individuals. Although CNCs began to expand in the early 1960s, the American Nurses Association (Aydellotte et al., 1987) and Glass (1989) suggest their origins lie in the public health nursing centers, nurse settlements, and rural nursing services of 100 years ago.

ASSESSING TRENDS AND INFLUENCES ON HEALTH SERVICES DELIVERY

As has already been discussed, multiple influences affect the health care system and the ways it operates. Figure 4-6 presents one model (Lockhart, 1992) for analyzing those trends and influences as they affect the choices and purchases made by consumers and their providers. This model highlights the structures that shape a consumer's choice of services within the health care delivery system. It also can be used to analyze the trends and influences on local, state, or national approaches to care and can

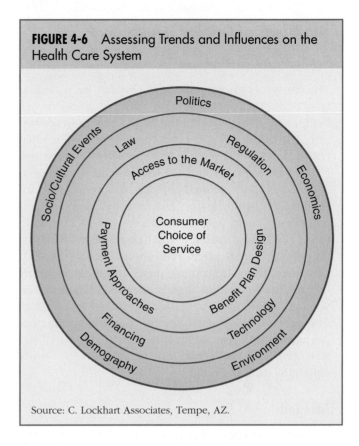

FIGURE 4-6 Assessing Trends and Influences on the Health Care System

Source: C. Lockhart Associates, Tempe, AZ.

help community health nurses identify areas where they or others can seek to intervene as advocates for clients.

The outer circle of the figure identifies the overall influences of sociocultural, political, economic, demographic, and environmental events. The cultural diversity of our nation, increases or decreases in the population, and/or the ages of population members all change the type and number of services needed and wanted. In 1997 women represented 46% of the work force and will reach parity with men in the next century. They will require specific services, particularly those relating to children (Judy & D'Amico, 1997). Social issues such as drug use, homicide, and other crimes also influence the types and number of services required to respond to the population's needs and demands.

Whereas at one point in time we could chart our country's economic future by how well the economy and production were managed, today our economic future is linked to the global economy and thus surges or declines along with the economies of other countries throughout the world. Turns in the economy affect the wealth of individuals and the nation and, thereby, the money both are willing to commit to health services.

Politically, our nation changes its focus as leaders change and espouse what are called conservative or liberal agendas. It is increasingly difficult to define exactly what those terms mean; however, it is true that whoever holds political power sets the agenda for establishing laws and regulations and determining the availability of

Attributes of Quality Health Care

Study Problem/Purpose

The consumer's perception of quality has been studied less often than professionally defined measures of health care quality within the health care delivery setting. The purposes of this study were (1) to define what consumers identify as the attributes of health care and nursing care quality and (2) to examine the relationship of consumer-defined perspectives on quality to indicators of health status and selected demographic variables. Quality has most often been looked at in terms of the information useful to consumers in choosing among health plans, rather than looking at what consumers want from those plans and their providers of care. Recent studies suggest there is a link between what people expect and their perceived satisfaction. The general expectations for care and the specific expectations for a visit are linked to the final sense of satisfaction with the actual care received. This study sought to examine both.

Methods

The study used an exploratory design in which 239 consumers were recruited from waiting rooms of clinics (n = 122, or 51%) and in neighborhoods in door-to-door visits (n = 117, or 49%) of a large metropolitan area in the midwestern United States. Both urban and suburban populations were included. Participants completed a survey developed by the study investigators [Quality Health Care Questionnaire (QHCQ)] where participants rated the importance of 27 attributes of health care and nursing care quality. Factor analysis resulted in identifying six factors that accounted for 64% of the variance, including medical care, teaching by the nurse, provider competence, choice of provider, nurse-patient interaction, and convenience of appointments. Participants also completed the SF-36 Health Survey, a 36-item instrument widely used by researchers to measure health status in eight general areas: social and physical functioning, bodily pain, general health, vitality, and role limitations due to physical health problems, emotional problems, and mental health.

Findings

A total of 149 women and 87 men participated in the study ranging in age from 18 to 92 years. Most had insurance, with 140 having private insurance through an employer, 68 having Medicare, 39 covered as veterans, and 18 having Medicaid.

The findings suggest that the most important indicators of quality health care to these consumers are (1) whether they get better and (2) whether they have the opportunity to be cared for by physicians who are well informed and have up-to-date knowledge. Similarly, the most important indicators of quality nursing care to these consumers are (1) being cared for by nurses who are well informed and possess up-to-date knowledge and (2) being able to communicate with the nurse. The study found that spending enough time with the nurse and not feeling rushed during the visit were important indicators of quality, as was having a nurse teach about the illness, medications, treatments, and staying healthy. Consumers wanted to be able to call a nurse with questions. There were some differences in perceptions according to race, age, years of education, income, and health status. Teaching by the nurse was more important for consumers with reported poorer health status and chronic illness and less education and income and among African Americans.

Implications

This study adds to the body of literature on efforts to understand the consumer's perceptions of quality health and nursing care. It helps to guide practitioners by highlighting those actions important to consumers and, in this case, suggests that the health education and teaching carried out by nurses are important components of perceived quality to consumers. The importance that consumers place on teaching by the nurse was emphasized, particularly among people with less education, low income levels, and chronic illness.

Although important, the study and the study specific survey need to be replicated under more closely controlled conditions to see if the findings are valid and reliable. The number of participants seems adequate for this study, but the manner of selection (door to door and being approached in a clinic) may have introduced bias as to who would be willing to participate. The study participants themselves varied widely in sociodemographic and health-related data and, because of the limited sample size, may not be truly representative of their populations. Since this is one of the few studies attempting this research, it is an important addition to the literature and, even with its limitations, lays a good basis for further research in the area.

Source: Oermann, M. H., & Templin, T. (2000). Important attributes of quality health care: Consumer perspectives. *Journal of Nursing Scholarship, 32,2.*

education and services for such things as birth control, abortion, and acquired immunodeficiency syndrome (AIDS).

The environment in which all this transpires is more healthy or less healthy depending on the attitudes and beliefs of the politicians and society within which we live and, thereby, the efforts undertaken to ensure clean air, safe drinking water, soils free of contaminants, and other factors that create not only a safe but a pleasant environment. The ways that those safeguards affect the viability of industry and business influence whether certain rules and regulations are enacted. The ultimate cost to the health of the population is often weighed against the cost of the loss of jobs.

The laws, regulations, technology, and financing depicted in the second outermost circle in Figure 4-6 are all affected by the influences in the outermost circle, just discussed. Although the political influences on laws and regulations may be the most obvious, the choices and trade-offs made in response to the political, economic, social, demographic, and environmental factors in the outermost circle affect all the variables in the second outermost circle. The results shape our country's financial well-being and, therefore, the number of dollars believed available to provide health care to our population.

Financing for health care insurance is done primarily through the employment setting for the working population and through government for the elderly and specific populations. Those who provide the financing and the amounts available ultimately define which health and public health services are offered and the ways they are offered, particularly with regard to health technology (see Figure 4-7). The passage or failure of laws, regulations, and policies that (1) make it easy or difficult to bring new technology to market and (2) allow for or restrict payment for that technology dictates the technology that will be developed and used.

In Figure 4-6, the third and last set of influences on consumer choice—payment approaches, benefit plan design, and access to the market—are all specific to the ability to offer and purchase a service in the health care market.

Who has access to the market in order to provide services is dictated by both who is licensed to care for clients and who is eligible to be reimbursed for the care provided. Nurse access to the market is limited sometimes by law but most often by a program, plan, or insurance policy that excludes nurses from the definition of a provider, limits the services for which nurses will be paid, or pays an amount different from (usually less than) that paid to other providers offering the same service. In addition, the design of the benefit plan determines the type of services eligible for payment under the plan. If a service or provider, including a public health provider, is not listed as one of those eligible for payment or coverage, the client and provider must decide whether to pursue the service at the client's own expense.

All the items listed in the circles of influence act on each other and on the consumer. Finally, the consumer's personal choices, listed in the center of the circle of influences in Figure 4-6, are shaped by considerations such as the following:

- What is the quality of the service?
- How much of it will I need (quantity)?
- How much does it cost (price)? Can I afford to share in the cost or to pay for it completely on my own?
- Where is it offered (location)? Is it convenient to my home? Can I get there from where I live?
- Can I afford the time? Does it require time away from work? Loss of pay?
- What are my preferences for care? Do I simply like a certain physician or nurse?

When buying health care, the strength of these last influences may vary because individuals may not have enough information to make a choice or may have so little responsibility for the cost of the service that they simply go where their physician or plan suggests. This is in part the reason that health care really does not resemble a normal market for goods and services. Even so, consumer choices are influenced by these factors, and as health care continues to change, one of the changes will be demand for greater involvement of clients in the choices and uses of the services offered them.

Trends Shaping the Future of Public Health

A number of the trends changing and molding the health care of the future have already been discussed as part of the description of the health care delivery system. Areas

---

FIGURE 4-7 Technological Methods

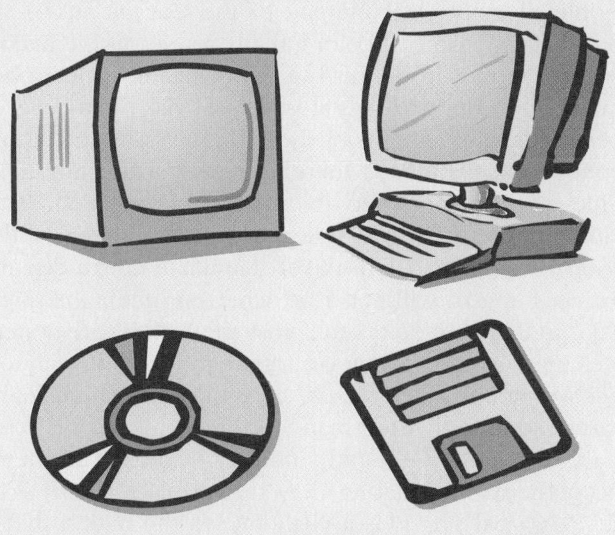

What are your thoughts regarding the delivery of care through these technological methods? What about the quality of care? What sort of care could be offered through these methods?

✳ DECISION MAKING

Importance of Healthy Lifestyles

Healthy People 2010 identifies improved quality and years of life as a goal. For most people, the single most important thing they could do to improve their health status and ensure healthy years of life would be to change their lifestyle choices on a daily basis. Making the decision to institute changes in lifestyle is difficult and one many people fail to make.

As a community/public health nurse, living by example is one way to help influence those you care for in your work setting to make positive decisions about their lifestyle. Your own involvement with regular exercise, a balanced diet, maintaining proper weight, low or moderate use of alcohol, and no use of tobacco and illegal drugs speaks louder than any lectures you might provide. Beyond that, however, how can you incorporate positive messages about lifestyle choices in your daily practice with clients? When people have long-established negative habits, how can you help them understand the impact those choices are having on their health and future? For many with complex and complicated lives, particularly those in poverty, how do you approach them about lifestyle choices when they may be more worried about just surviving another day, not years? Deciding to "live" a healthy life sounds good, but how do you make it meaningful in the variety of settings in which you encounter clients and among the various populations you serve?

that will continue to shape that future were highlighted in the previous section on assessing health care trends and influences. This section identifies selected trends and issues that public health will be required to address in the next decade if it is to ensure the health of the populations within our society.

The first goal of *Healthy People 2010* is to "increase quality and years of healthy life." Our nation's changing demographics will dictate much of that focus for public health in the 21st century. The nation's population is growing and aging, and with that growth and age will come increased demand for primary health care and public health services, particularly since for many people the longer years of life they are living are not healthy ones.

The aging of the population has taken center stage in most discussions of the future because of the sheer in-

crease in numbers that will be experienced because of the aging of the post–World War II baby-boom generation. Our total population is often displayed as a "pyramid." Vast numbers of young are portrayed at the bottom, with decreasing numbers depicted in each successive age group going up the pyramid, until at the top relatively few older people are shown as still alive.

This pyramid, however, is beginning to look like a box, with the numbers of individuals at each age group nearly equal to every other. It is not until after the age of 70 years that there is a notable decline in the number of elderly compared to other groups, with the most significant drop in numbers not occurring until after 80 years of age (see Figure 4-8). Even though the absolute numbers of elderly are increasing at a faster rate than those in the other age groups, it does not mean that the numbers in those age groups are declining. Populations of all ages, sex, and racial/ethnic mix will need increased efforts at health promotion and disease prevention throughout the life span if we are to improve or even maintain the current health status achieved to date.

The focus of health care is shifting to chronic disease and diseases that result from poor lifestyle choices. Too often, the decline and disabilities that can accompany such diseases are the only picture people have of their future if they are diagnosed with such illnesses. Helping people to change and control their environments and educating people about how to prevent or lessen the impact of such diseases will necessarily be significant components of community health nursing. Without that focus, longer lives will be seen as a burden rather than a gift. The availability of community-based support from nurses and others prepared to provide the range of services needed will be significant determinants of what futures they experience.

By 2010, one-third of the nation's people will be people of color (U.S. Bureau of the Census, 2000). In some states people of color already represent the majority of the population. This is a public health concern because when the health status, health risks, and use of preventive interventions by these populations and ethnic groups are examined, there is a disparity with their achievements compared to the total population. This finding prompted the adoption of the second goal of the *Healthy People 2010* objectives: Eliminate health disparities. Such a goal will never be achieved unless there is a major initiative undertaken across the health care system to change the factors that contribute to health disparities. This will not be an easy task, since these disparities have existed so long that too many of the people themselves, health care providers and "industry," and governments accept them as inevitable. They are not. The *Healthy People 2010* goal provides a challenge to the nation that it must, in all fairness to its citizens, seek to meet. Community health nurses are at the forefront of the battle that will need to be waged to change the status quo. We have

FIGURE 4-8 Projected Resident Population of the United States as of July 1, 2025

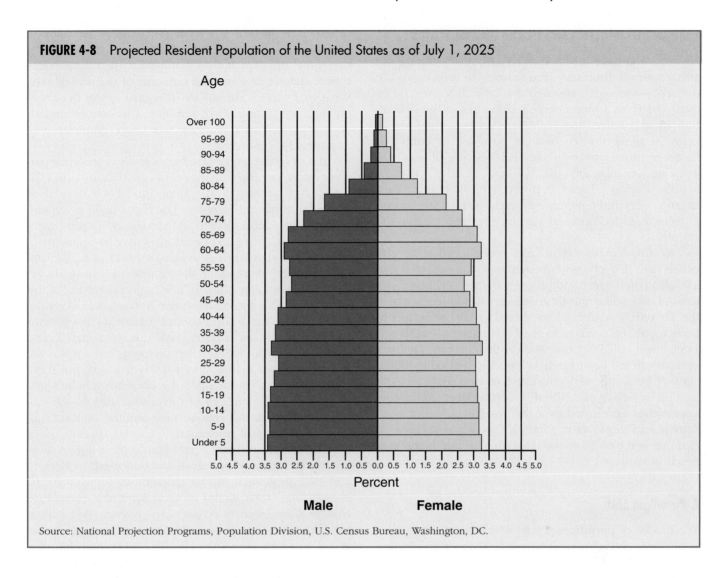

Source: National Projection Programs, Population Division, U.S. Census Bureau, Washington, DC.

far too few nurses who are from the wealth of racial and ethnic backgrounds that make up this vibrant country of ours. Community health nurses must reach out to all communities, and be part of those communities, whatever the racial/ethnic mix or age mix.

Violence and crime within families, communities, and between and within nations is an ever greater burden on society. The threats of biological terrorism and natural or man-made disasters are ones for which most local and state public health agencies are ill prepared. Detecting, tracking, and treating such planned or unplanned events are beyond the capabilities of the public health infrastructure currently operating. Efforts are underway to improve the capabilities of communities to deal with violence to individuals and populations, but the work has only begun. Significantly more funding and personnel will be needed if the system is to deal effectively with any of these threats. Again, *Healthy People 2010* has identified objectives which seek to improve systems for personal and public health. One set of objectives speaks specifically to improving the

public health infrastructure by improving the training and competencies of public health workers, monitoring capabilities, and epidemiology and laboratory services. All will be needed if we are to deal with the threats posed.

Whether it be in urban or rural settings, growing numbers of people, houses, consumer goods, cars, and waste will stress our fragile environment and its ability to respond and repair itself. Clean water will be an ever more serious issue throughout the nation, not just in arid parts of the country, but in those that have depleted groundwater or polluted their streams, lakes, and groundwater. Assuring access to reliable sources of power will challenge assumptions about how water, wind, oil, and nuclear energy are used, or misused. Public health agencies and personnel and communities should be in the forefront of the debates about how to use and protect the environment and natural resources. *Healthy People 2010* identifies objectives to promote healthy and safe communities, a difficult and important task in an increasingly dense society.

REFORMING HEALTH CARE IN THE UNITED STATES

National and state health care reform efforts during the 1990s spurred the health care industry to respond to the threat of government-imposed change with actions the industry believes address perceived failures in the system. Individual practices and institutions are becoming part of larger systems through outright purchase or contracts. Large organizations with national systems of care are evolving, organizations that will seek to offer outcome-specific, evidence-based, cost-effective, and efficient care to employers and government purchasers for use by employees and Medicaid and Medicare enrollees across the country.

As this consolidation and reorganization of the health care delivery system continues, it is expected that a relatively few large and privately owned organized systems of care will control the delivery of health services in the United States. Employer-based coverage will continue to be the primary method of financing health services, even in light of questions to the contrary. Delivery options offered to privately or publicly funded individuals will be a mix of fee-for-service, managed-care, utilization review, precertification procedures, and other approaches developed over the last 20 years. But, consumers and employer payors will have a real say in what that mix will look like, even though its shape is still very much in shadow.

A Paradigm Shift

The model, or **paradigm,** under which health care is currently delivered is undergoing a shift. The various changes previously discussed as being underway do not constitute a true paradigm shift, however. In a paradigm shift, as described first by Thomas Kuhn (1986), the underlying beliefs about a thing are shaken and changed forever.

To date, the primary change in health care has been a movement of the payment system away from fee-for-service and toward some level of managed care and prepayment. Now it is shifting back again. New on the horizon is the expectation that a price paid for services should deliver an expected outcome of defined quality. What that quality should be in regard to the design of the delivery system is not yet clear. Discussions regarding the definition of quality will likely continue well into the 21st century.

But even these changes do not really represent a paradigm shift, because the model of care that underlies the delivery of services is the same model we have used throughout the 20th century. The focus is on acute episodes of care provided to individuals by single practitioners. Thus, although practitioners may be operating in a newly linked or larger system, to a great extent, the care and the delivery are much the same as they have always been. The paradigm shift, then, is largely rhetorical at this point. Health for the client is often a stated but poorly defined goal of the insurance and managed-care systems being created. Cost controls, new quality demands, and compliance with payment requirements have made the system different than it was a few years ago, but these things have not yet changed the underlying beliefs, expectations, and practices of those operating in the system. A true shift will require time and the education of both providers and consumers.

Health care reform, a paradigm shift, is a goal nursing has consistently embraced and endorsed. In 1993, to add to a growing national momentum for change, 62 nursing organizations put forward *Nursing's Agenda for Health Care Reform* (American Nurses Association [ANA], 1993). This document supports efforts to ensure access to a core of essential health care services for all at an affordable cost. Health care would be restructured to focus on consumers and to work toward wellness and care rather than illness and cure. The ANA's *Nursing's Vision for Primary Health Care in the 21st Century* (Marion, 1996) continued the thrust toward a change in the paradigm for health care by advocating for a shift from acute sickness care to community-based primary care and an enhanced public health system.

This agenda and others like it have been put forward by groups and individuals who want to see a true paradigm shift within the health care system. That shift is about changing the purpose for which the system is created and then designing the delivery system, services, payment, and financing to ensure that health and well-being are attainable for the population served. This is a far greater change than simply modifying payment or even restructuring the delivery system; it requires that we ask anew which services are needed (whether or not they are currently covered by insurance) and how best to deliver them to ensure healthy populations.

Answering questions about those things needed to keep people healthy requires consideration of more than just acute medical care. It requires examining the human ecosystem with regard to the ways it influences

---

REFLECTIVE THINKING

Nursing Influence

- At what points do you believe you could influence health care choices and access to care in the model illustrated in Figure 4-6 and discussed in this section?
- What would you do if an insurer refused to pay for an examination or care for yourself? Your child? Your spouse? Your parent? A friend? Your client?

health and determining that which must be done to support or change those influences in a given individual, family, or community. It also requires consideration of the ways that consumer choices are, or might conceivably be, influenced to support health. Instead of reacting, a reformed health care system should consider how to proactively influence positive health and lifestyle choices through the design of the system and the services offered.

Designing a proactive, positive health system requires leadership by people who understand clients and the full range of care and services they might need. Nurses, and particularly community health nurses, understand the human ecosystem and the holistic nature of health care and services. In addition, community health nurses understand how to meet the needs of populations. Community health nurses should thus play a primary role in defining the new paradigm in health care. Membership on local, state, and national governmental and private health planning boards and committees can afford community health nurses the opportunity to speak to the character of the care and services needed in a responsive health care system operating under a new paradigm. Three key concepts in that new paradigm are discussed next.

Consumer Sovereignty and Responsibility

Consumer sovereignty is a major paradigm shift from traditional values that view professional autonomy above other consumer values. Consumer sovereignty, as used here, suggests that clients have the power, authority, and responsibility to be involved in their health care and services. Personal health care involves the daily choices and actions taken to ensure ongoing health. Health care services are used to prevent disease, promote health, and treat illness. Consumers' choices may be limited by some rationing method, but within the scope of the choices available, the consumer should have a say about what is or is not done.

The Center for Biomedical Ethics of the University of Minnesota conducted an interdisciplinary research project that examined the values framework of the U.S. health care system (Priester, 1992). An assessment of the current values of professionals and the public alike placed professional autonomy above all other values, including client autonomy, consumer sovereignty, client advocacy, access to care, and quality of care.

The concept of consumer sovereignty is contradictory to the way our current health care system operates but is consistent with our political and cultural philosophy. Consumers have surrendered control of their health to health professionals. In no other areas of their lives do Americans do this. A true paradigm shift demands that consumers exercise control over their health status.

Women will be significant players within any redefined system, because they are the primary purchasers and managers of health care for their families and themselves. Community health nurses must therefore help educate women to be informed and assertive consumers empowered to make choices and able to manage the health status of themselves and their families.

Population projections suggest that the United States will become even more culturally diverse in the next century. Community health nurses must be comfortable with and become part of the cultures and races represented throughout the nation. Diversity will be a reality, and community health nurses themselves must both reflect that diversity and allow it to shape the type and manner of services they provide to clients.

Wellness and Care

This text proposes wellness and care (as opposed to illness and cure) as the preferred model for health services. This still-evolving paradigm is one that nursing can support and advance.

Biotechnology developments and genetic research currently underway will ultimately provide the information necessary to predict who will become ill and develop certain diseases and conditions. Such predictions will be able to be made long before we learn how to change the genes that cause the related problems, however. Research by physicians, nurses, and others will help define ways that clients can maintain wellness. It will also identify the personal care and health services needed by individuals in order to prevent crossing from wellness into illness states requiring cure. This paradigm, again, is different from the one that currently exists. This paradigm presumes people can be taught and assisted in their efforts to remain well and that this approach will work to a significant degree. Rather than meaning that people will not have chronic and other health problems, this paradigm presumes that enough support and education

---

REFLECTIVE THINKING

The Wellness and Care Paradigm

- What changes might you expect to see in the health care delivery system under a wellness and care paradigm?
- What must community health nurses do to prepare to function under such a model?
- What can you and other community health nurses do to foster the adoption of such a model?

Perspectives... ✳

INSIGHTS OF A PROFESSOR EMERITUS

The U.S. health care system is undergoing change. In the United States, cost, access, and quality are major issues that are being addressed in a number of different ways. One of the major changes, the shift from acute to community-based care, has resulted in the expansion of nursing services in the community. A greater emphasis is placed on developing community partnerships and population-focused practice. Rather than seeing clients apart from their environment, clients are viewed within the context of community in order to ensure that all aspects of health are considered. In addition to the previously mentioned changes, there is also a focus on multidisciplinary care that emphasizes care from a variety of different professionals working in a coordinated system around client needs.

The various changes in the U.S. health care system are having a significant impact on community health nursing and the role of faculty in teaching students to prepare for practice. In the early development of nursing, people were cared for in their homes. Hospitals were developed to assist in the care of the homeless and poor. Today, and in the future, a vast majority of health care services will continue to be provided in the home, in schools, in community-based centers, in faith communities, and in other settings. As the population ages, there will be an even greater need for long-term

care management services for clients in their homes, as well as home health services following hospital discharge. There will also be a need for improved coordination of care services for young families—child bearing and child-rearing. Vulnerable population groups such as the homeless and near homeless will require creative, innovative partnerships in communities to address their health care needs. Community health nursing faculty have a major role to play in preparing students for these changes.

I think that community health nurses have a vital role to play in building caring communities—communities where partnerships are fostered, where multidisciplinary and community members work together to identify client health care needs and services to meet those needs provided at a cost that the community can afford. Delivering caring, compassionate ser-vices to families in the midst of change is an imperative. Exploring the meaning of caring within the context of community and discussing the need to develop a seamless health care system where partnerships among institutions and agencies will ultimately enhance health and healing are important for students. Opportunities for students to participate in such efforts must be provided.

—Sue A. Thomas, EdD, RN

will be provided to clients to help them make the choices and take the actions necessary to limit any health risks. This, then, is a proactive approach to keeping people well, rather than a retrospective effort at curing that which has already gone wrong. Again, community health nurses must be at the forefront of change.

The advances made will also raise significant ethical issues. Individuals will need to learn to manage the courses of their own health and plan their lives in light of the knowledge that they carry genes that may negatively affect their health. Because the outcomes will dictate the approaches to well-being for the client populations they serve, community health nurses must be in the forefront of the ethical debates that will arise.

The education and care community health nurses offer will increasingly be provided with the help of electronic media, computers, video, and other technology, facilitating provision of care across communities and into rural and isolated areas. Clinical practice guidelines and general care guidelines being developed by the Agency for Health Care Research and Quality, professional asso-

ciations, insurance companies, and managed-care plans will seek to identify the most likely range of services, education, and actions needed to achieve a positive health outcome. Guidelines and outcomes definition will of necessity require the input of professionals and consumers alike. Community health nurses should seek to participate in guideline development at all levels to ensure that public health and care concerns are addressed.

Care in the Community

As previously stated, care is moving from institutions to the community. Hospitals and institutional settings are increasingly used for only limited periods of time when clients are acutely ill, with clients being discharged home for most of their recovery. In response, some nurses are moving to the community to serve the clients. Still others are working to provide care to a defined population across the continuum of settings serving the clients. Community health nurses must take on leadership and management roles in such programs and must help define how community nursing

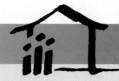

COMMUNITY NURSING VIEW

A public health nurse is working in a county with a significant number of homeless and near-homeless persons. In the county, an Interfaith Council agency serves this population and is known for its compassion and outreach to them. The agency provides counseling, clothing, assistance with job placement, and a day service center where the homeless can take showers, use phones, etc. The nurse has visited the program site and identified the need for developing a nursing center there, a nursing center that would provide basic health screening and follow-up, treatment of minor conditions, case management, and client advocacy. Many of the clients who use the agency programs have indicated that they would definitely like to have a nursing center available to them. Many of them have indicated that they feel "safe," "respected," and "treated with dignity" at the Interfaith agency.

Nursing Considerations

Assessment

◆ What information would you need from the agency director and staff to assist in deciding whether to initiate the development of a nursing center?

◆ What questions would you ask to obtain the information?

Diagnosis

◆ Identify several nursing diagnoses that may pertain to the health needs of the homeless population.

◆ Which of the listed diagnoses could be addressed by having a nursing center in the community?

Outcome Identification

◆ What outcomes would indicate that the nursing center had achieved its objectives?

Planning/Interventions

◆ Who would need to be involved in the planning process?

◆ What services could be offered?

◆ Would outside financing be needed? If so, when could it be obtained?

Evaluation

◆ What process could be used to determine the type of outcome measurements that would provide the evaluation data needed?

---

organizations and other nurse-managed services can provide significant components of the prevention, primary care, community-based services and client-centered care required in the new paradigm. The community health nurse will need to work with government and managed-care plans to monitor and assess both the health status of the populations served and the impact of the service provided on the entire community within which the community health nurse works. What we do as practitioners will influence the ultimate shape of both.

KEY CONCEPTS

◆ Health services in the United States are, to a great extent, privately planned and organized, with little local, state, or national governmental input.

◆ Since 1980, the U.S. Department of Health and Human Services has set goals for improving the nation's health. The latest, *Healthy People 2010,* has two overarching goals: (1) to increase quality

and years of healthy life and (2) to eliminate health disparities among population groups.

◆ The public health system receives only a very small portion of the dollars spent on health care in America. Efforts at revitalizing and enhancing the public health infrastructure that supports the core functions of public health are needed to allow the nation to address many of the health problems facing it.

◆ The U.S. political culture fosters individualism and entrepreneurial efforts in the economy and in all sectors of society, including health care.

◆ Privately or publicly provided health insurance is the primary vehicle through which people gain access to health services. In the absence of insurance, individuals must pay out of their own pockets or face going without services except in emergencies.

◆ A wide range of health service organizations exist, with new configurations being created in response to changes in financing and delivery demands.

◆ Community nursing organizations/centers offer ambulatory care and community nursing services focusing on primary care and prevention.

◆ The consumer's choice of health services is affected by political, economic, social/cultural, demographic, and environmental factors and a wide range of approaches and practices that derive from these factors.

◆ A true shift in the underlying beliefs about health care would require that the health of the client be defined as the goal for the delivery of health services.

◆ Wellness and care, consumer sovereignty, and community-based care are concepts that would characterize a health care system operating under a new paradigm.

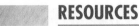 **RESOURCES**

Agency for Healthcare Quality and Research (AHQR): www.ahcpr.gov

American Medical Association: www.ama-assn.org

American Nurses Association: www.ana.org

Centers for Disease Control and Prevention: www.cdc.gov

Commonwealth Fund: www.cmwf.org

Employee Benefits Research Institute: www.ebri.org

Families USA: www.familiesusa.org

General Consumer Information Sites: www.drkoop.com; www.healthcentral.com; www.webmd.com

National Academy of Sciences, Institute of Medicine: www.nas.edu/nas/nashom

Robert Wood Johnson Foundation: www.rwjf.org

Social Science Gateway: www.sosig.ac.UK

U.S. Bureau of the Census: www.census.gov

Chapter

5

HEALTH CARE SYSTEMS IN THE WORLD

Sue A. Thomas, EdD, RN

MAKING THE CONNECTION

Today and everyday, the lives of vast numbers of people lie in the hands of health systems. From the safe delivery of a healthy baby to the care with dignity of the frail elderly, health systems have a vital and continuing responsibility to people throughout the life span. They are crucial to the healthy development of individuals, families, and societies everywhere.

—World Health Organization, 2000, xi

COMPETENCIES

Upon completion of this chapter, the reader should be able to:

- Discuss the major international health and health promotion efforts from a global perspective.
- Discuss the role of primary health care in promoting the health of nations.
- Identify the major national and international health initiatives that affect public health.
- Describe major international health organizations and their contributions to promoting health.
- Discuss the nature of health system performance and improvement from an international perspective.
- Discuss selected health care system trends in the United Kingdom, Australia, Canada, and Russia.
- Discuss cross-sectoral and cross-national collaboration as emerging strategies for the future.
- Discuss nursing's contribution to cross-sectoral collaboration efforts.

KEY TERMS

intergovernmental organizations

International Council of Nurses (ICN)

official international health organizations

Pan-American Health Organization (PAHO)

philanthropic foundations

private organizations

private voluntary organizations

Sigma Theta Tau, International (STT)

United Nations Children's Emergency Fund (UNICEF)

World Bank

World Health Organization (WHO)

Because of the recognition of the global connectedness among nations and the increasing concern for international health and health care, community health nurses need to understand the organizational issues in health care delivery systems from an international perspective. Exploring the nature of the changes that are occurring in health care delivery can assist in the analysis of various approaches to international health care.

As Dreher (1997) states:

It is clear that worldwide health cannot be achieved by a single nation. Indeed, even the health of a single nation cannot be achieved only through the ef-

forts of that nation. Damage to the rain forest in Brazil affects the atmosphere that the whole world breathes, wars in Eastern Europe impact countless other nations, a virus originating in Africa has pandemic implications and television violence from the U.S. is broadcast throughout the world. Health is a dynamic and worldwide relationship between human societies and their environments. Like it or not, we live in a global society, and health is a global responsibility. (p. 5)

This chapter provides a discussion of international health initiatives that have particular relevance for community health nursing. It also discusses the major international health organizations, including those in nursing. Changing perspectives in health care delivery systems are described, with a focus on selected health care systems. Last, implications for the future are explored.

INTERNATIONAL HEALTH AND HEALTH PROMOTION

As discussed in earlier chapters, the World Health Organization (WHO) initiative Health for All by the Year 2000 (HFA 2000) resulted in significant growth of interest in world health and how best to achieve it. This interest is reflected in the recognition of the need to better understand health care issues and concerns on a global level.

All countries of the world have health problems and concerns. There is a difference in the nature of the problems and how to deal with them, however. Some countries experience higher infant and child mortality rates than others, as discussed in Chapter 3. Some countries have higher rates of certain infectious diseases, differences in environmental health hazards, chronic diseases, lifestyles, and mental health problems, among others. Examining the major problems and concerns of the world's health is of critical importance to community health nurses. One of the major ways WHO proposes to deal with various health problems and concerns is through a greater emphasis on health promotion and disease prevention efforts as well as improvement in health system performance.

As Murray (2000), Director of WHO's Global Program on Evidence for Health policy, noted very clearly, even though significant progress over the past decades has been achieved in the health of populations, virtually all countries are underutilizing the various resources that are available. This underutilization thus results in large numbers of preventable deaths and disabilities, suffering, injustice, inequality, and denial of an individual's basic rights to health and well-being.

Health Promotion

Health promotion is central to the work of community health nurses, as well as all health professionals, whether in Australia, Canada, Russia, Finland, Brazil, the United Kingdom, the United States, or other countries. The emphasis on health promotion is an expanding one in nursing and health care generally, as discussed in Chapters 1 and 11.

Health promotion reflects a shift in focus toward care in community settings and an increased emphasis on the public's health. At the international level, health promotion efforts are enhanced through the process of countries working together for the purpose of sharing knowledge, resources, and skills to promote world health. An integrated approach reflects the important position that health promotion increasingly occupies in nursing and in all of the various health care activities in many countries throughout the world. It is an approach that focuses on the premise that the basic conditions and resources for health are peace, shelter, food, income, education, a stable ecosystem, sustainable resources, social justice, and equity (WHO, 1986). The integrated approach is based on the WHO health promotion initiatives, which acknowledge the global nature of many of today's health problems and the importance of the environment and ecological sustainability in promoting world health.

Health promotion is central to the whole view of health and caring, not marginal to mainstream care (Pike & Forster, 1995). It is a major challenge for this century. Health promotion is not a new concept; however, it has historically been viewed primarily as the province of public health in Western industrialized nations. The crisis in health care costs together with the demographic changes, changing patterns of health and disease, and the recognition that prevention can reduce costs and illness have led to a far greater emphasis on community health and on health promotion.

Health promotion in this chapter and book is viewed within the context of Ottawa's Charter for Health Promotion and the WHO targets for Health for All (WHO, 1993; Messias, 2001). The Ottawa Charter has become influential in promoting health and assisting the process to make it operational. This charter integrated the concept of healthy public policy with the need for personal and individual involvement in health promotion. The charter was based on principles of social justice, equity, and the achievement of Health for All by the Year 2000 (Pike, 1995). The Ottawa strategy emphasizes both individual and community dimensions of health promotion, with the recognition that the two need to work together. It clearly points out that both the individual context and a public/community approach are vital to health promotion.

WHO recognized the significance of the Ottawa Charter and through the Healthy Cities/Communities movement has developed a far greater emphasis on public health and environmental issues. WHO shifted from a major focus on individual and lifestyle behaviors to a far greater emphasis on public health and the environment, thus attempting to create and maintain a better balance between lifestyle, the environment, and health service issues. In addition, in 2000 WHO conducted its first ever analysis of the world's health systems from all of the 191 WHO member states. Thus, the performance of the health systems that serve people around the world is also viewed as critical to health and well-being. As Brundtland (2001) clearly points out, the defining purpose of health systems is to improve and protect health.

The Role of Primary Health Care

Primary health care in international health is associated with the global conference held at Alma Ata in 1978, the conference that promoted the initiative Health for All by the Year 2000 (WHO, 1978). Primary health care (PHC), defined broadly at Alma Ata, emphasized universal health care access to all individuals and families, encouraged participation by community members in all aspects of health care planning and implementation, and promoted the delivery of care that would be "scientifically sound, technically effective, socially relevant and acceptable" (WHO, 1978, p. 2).

A major initiative produced in 1974, which had an influence at Alma Ata, was the LaLonde report, called "A New Perspective on the Health of Canadians." This report stimulated discussion regarding the need for a new perspective on the health of the Canadian population. As the Canadian Minister of National Health and Welfare, LaLonde recommended a more comprehensive approach to health care. LaLonde identified the major determinants of health as human biology, environment, lifestyle, and health care. Ashton and Seymour (1988) argued that this report was a major turning point in international policy with the reaffirmation of earlier public health strategies that focused on a broader approach to health rather than only a personal approach.

Thus, a major shift in perspective that emerged from the LaLonde report, the Alma Ata conference, and the Healthy Cities/Communities movement, referred to initially in Chapter 1, was the shift from an individual focus to one of community participation. The incorporation of a public health approach to primary health care placed

---

REFLECTIVE THINKING

Health System Performance

- What do you think makes a good health system?
- What do you think makes a system fair?
- How do we know whether a health system in any given country is performing as well as it could? How do you think health system performance should be measured?

the emphasis in principle on the community and its participation, self-reliance, and self-determination. Adoption of this interpretation of primary health care is identified as one area for action in Health for All in the 21st Century (WHO, 1999).

The involvement of community members as participants in planning for health is viewed as a critical ingredient for effective public health practice for this century. The commitment to shared values and common goals enables the group to deal with complex problems and issues more effectively than individuals alone. Thus, community health nurses are in a vital position to participate as leaders in the process.

Katz and Kreuter (1997) suggest that the justification for making community participation an essential aspect for public health practice can be summarized as follows:

- Nonmedical factors, such as social conditions and community values, have a major influence on health status.
- Planners and policymakers must actively involve the public in the development of solutions to health problems because medical interventions alone are not sufficient to result in health status improvements.
- Policy development requires the active involvement of people who are affected by public health programs.

MAJOR INTERNATIONAL ORGANIZATIONS

There are a variety of organizations concerned with international health. Because nursing is a global discipline and health is a global concern, nurses must be knowledgeable about international health organizations that work to improve the world's health.

Types of International Health Organizations

International health organizations can be classified as private voluntary agencies, philanthropic foundations, private organizations, and official (governmental, intergovernmental) agencies as well as professional and technical organizations (Basch, 1990). **Private voluntary organizations** include both religious and secular groups that provide different health care assistance programs. Many of the religious institutions, such as the Maryknoll Missionaries from the Catholic Church, conduct health service projects worldwide. Secular groups, such as the International Council of Voluntary Agencies, assist in coordination activities. Other examples are Project HOPE and CARE.

Philanthropic foundations are those that use funds from private endowments to provide grants for health-related projects. Examples of the philanthropic

organizations involved in health care globally include the Rockefeller Foundation, the W. K. Kellogg Foundation, and the Hewlett Foundation. The program goals and projects vary. **Private organizations** such as pharmaceutical companies provide financial and technical assistance for health care, employment, and access to health care.

Official international health organizations are those agencies throughout the world that participate in collaborative arrangements via official governmental structures. Bilateral arrangements may occur between countries through various governmental organizations. Many of these arrangements are made between two countries with the focus on a single project. **Intergovernmental organizations** also exist. These organizations deal with health concerns on an ongoing basis and collaborate with governments, private foundations, and other efforts to improve health. Professional and technical organizations address specific professional as well as scientific goals and participate in the sharing of knowledge. An example is the International Council of Nurses.

The major intergovernmental organization that deals with health concerns at the international level is the **World Health Organization (WHO).** WHO was created in 1946 through the efforts of the League of Nations, which became the United Nations (UN). WHO was the outcome of a variety of global activities begun in the mid-1880s, directed by various countries to control cholera (Basch, 1990). The UN Charter resulted in formation of a special health agency that could deal with global health problems. The central office for WHO is in Geneva, Switzerland, with six regional offices in Copenhagen, Alexandria, Brazzaville, Manila, New Delhi, and Washington, D.C. In 2001, WHO opened a new office in Lyon, France, to assist developing countries detect and contain epidemics and emerging communicable diseases (WHO, 2001a). The World Health Assembly, which meets yearly in May, is the policy formation arena for WHO. The scope of WHO's responsibilities is comprehensive and consists of many major functions, with over 100 subfunctions. The objective of WHO is the attainment by all peoples of the highest possible level of health. It is responsible for monitoring global disease incidence and prevalence and for setting international health standards specific to sanitation, laboratory procedures, pharmaceutical manufacturing, and biological products. It also monitors environmental pollution and sponsors a variety of programs with emphasis on training medical personnel, health services development, primary health care, and disease control programs. WHO, in cooperation with other specialized agencies, promotes the improvement of nutrition, housing, sanitation, recreation, economic or working conditions, and other aspects of environmental hygiene. Another major function is the promotion of activities in the field of mental health.

At the World Health Assembly in Geneva in 1999, for example, WHO unveiled its vision for global health for the next decade. It recommended a new direction to increase healthy life expectancy for all while ensuring improvement for the world's poorest people. Placing health at the core of the global development agenda was highlighted by WHO Director General Harlem Brundtland (WHO, 1999).

Three other international organizations are also well known for their health-related efforts: the World Bank, the United Nations Children's Fund, and the Pan-American Health Organization. The **World Bank** is an organization that places its major emphasis on assisting countries where economic development is needed. It provides financial assistance to governments and foundations to develop projects that address the health of those countries where economic development is limited. The bank assists with projects that focus on economic growth, affordable housing, safe and usable water, and sanitation systems, among others.

The **United Nations Children's Emergency Fund (UNICEF)** was formed after World War II to assist the children who lived in European war countries. Since that time, however, UNICEF expanded its focus worldwide. Health projects have been developed throughout the world to control leprosy, tuberculosis, yaws, and other diseases. Maternal and child health programs are other global efforts supported by UNICEF.

The **Pan-American Health Organization (PAHO),** founded in 1902, was developed to assist countries of the Western Hemisphere. It focuses its efforts on the Americas, all of the countries of the Western Hemisphere, particularly those in Latin America. PAHO works with all countries of the Americas to improve health and raise the living standards of the people. Two of its major functions are to identify public health hazards and to distribute public health data that include epidemiological informa-

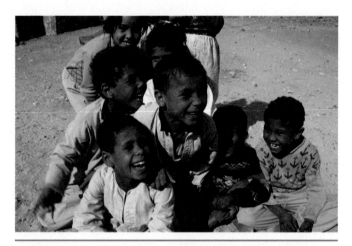

UNICEF has initiated maternal and child health programs and health projects that have controlled the spread of various diseases. Courtesy of Photodisc.

tion, information about the health systems within the countries, and various environmental issues. The PAHO supports public health research efforts and professional education. The national profiles it creates provide significant assistance to health-planning efforts.

Major concerns of the PAHO are the spread of AIDS and the health needs of the most vulnerable populations in the Americas. To address these concerns, PAHO works with both governmental and nongovernmental organizations. For example, a new strategic plan to prevent and control AIDS in the Caribbean was launched by PAHO in February 2001 in agreement with other organizations such as the U.S. Agency for International Development, the Canadian International Development Agency, and the Commission of the European Community, among others. The reason for the focus on the Caribbean is that 9 of the 12 countries with the highest infection rates in the Americas are in the Caribbean basin (PAHO, 2001).

Another organization that addresses international health is the Global Health Council (GHC). The GHC is a 29-year-old membership organization composed of professionals in the health care field, nongovernmental and governmental organizations, academic institutions, foundations and corporations. The council is dedicated to improving health worldwide.

The mission of the organization is to mobilize effective action by advocating for needed health care policies and resources, building alliances among the various membership groups in order to improve health, and communicating ideas, knowledge, and best practices in the health care arena.

The GHC is a U.S.-based nonprofit organization created initially to identify priority world health problems and report them to the U.S. public, Congress, international and domestic government agencies, academic institutions, and the broader global health community. The

✳ DECISION MAKING

International Health Care

Select a country or area of the world outside the United States that interests you.

◆ How might you find out about the status of health care in that country, its major health problems, and which international health organizations are involved with health care delivery in that country?

◆ What types of questions would you need to ask in order to determine the role of primary health care in that country and the role of the community health nurse?

priorities of the council highlight the major contributors to the global health burden of ill health such as child health, HIV/AIDS, reproductive and maternal health, infectious diseases, and emerging global health threats.

The council works to build alliances and communicate knowledge of global health issues and actions through annual conferences, forums, and two on-line publications: Global HealthLink and AIDSLink. In addition, another powerful tool is the council's web site (www.globalhealth.org), which is used to communicate ideas and best practices, conference and forum events, advocacy actions such as the introduction of the Global Health Act of 2000, and examples of alliance building.

Major International Nursing Organizations

In nursing, two major international organizations need to be discussed: the International Council of Nurses and Sigma Theta Tau, International. The **International Council of Nurses (ICN)** represents a federation of national nurses associations, representing nurses in more than 120 countries.

The ICN was the first international organization for professional women in history and is the only organization that represents the nursing profession worldwide. The ICN is the primary organization for the advancement of international nursing. The mission of ICN is to represent nursing worldwide, advancing the profession and influencing health policy. ICN works to ensure quality nursing care for all, sound health policies globally, the advancement of nursing knowledge, the presence worldwide of a respected nursing profession, and a competent and satisfied nursing workforce (ICN, 2001).

ICN is headquartered in Geneva, Switzerland, and serves as an advocate for healthy communities and sustainable development. It works to identify health needs of populations at risk together with nursing and other health-related organizations. ICN's vision is a healthy world where access to health is a basic human right. It works with governments and international organizations to attain a level of health that will assist populations in living a socially and economically productive life (ICN, 2000).

Sigma Theta Tau, International (STT) is the international honor society of nursing. It was founded in 1922 at the Indiana University Training School for Nurses. In 1997, STT celebrated its seventy-fifth anniversary, with more than 200,000 members worldwide who live and work in 73 nations. There are 356 chapters located at colleges and universities in Australia, Canada, Puerto Rico, South Korea, Taiwan, and the United States. It is the second largest nursing organization in the United States and one of the five largest in the world.

The purpose of STT is to recognize, encourage, and support nursing excellence in clinical practice, education, research, and leadership. The organization is dedicated to improving the health of people worldwide through increasing the scientific base of nursing practice.

HEALTH CARE SYSTEMS: CHANGING PERSPECTIVES

It is important that nurses recognize the significance of global sharing of knowledge about the provision of health services in different countries. Because nursing is a global enterprise and is committed to improving the health of citizens worldwide, a discussion of various health systems is included in this chapter. As Dreher (1997) points out, most of the major changes in disease prevention and control came not from medicine, as it is currently understood and practiced, but from public health practice, in which nurses have the primary responsibility for promoting healthy lifestyles, providing health education, and improving sanitation and hygiene. Thus, a focus on global knowledge related to health care systems is critical because nurses can work together throughout the world to enhance care and caring in changing political climates.

As the world's people become more interdependent, it is imperative that nurses be prepared to deal with international health and that international health be integrated into the nursing curriculum. Wright, Godue, Manfredi, and Korniewicz (1998) conducted a study that focused on how nursing education and associated activities prepared nurses to develop a knowledge of international health. This study is particularly significant because it was the first known study that focused on the extent and nature of international health activities among U.S. schools of nursing and from schools in Latin America and the Caribbean. See the accompanying Research Focus for further exploration.

Health care systems in countries throughout the world vary in relation to their philosophies, structures, and functions. Several basic elements, however, are addressed in all the various systems (Basch, 1990): (1) the type of coverage a citizen or consumer could anticipate, (2) who can utilize the system, (3) the providers and the types of care they provide, (4) location of the health care

---

✳ DECISION MAKING

Global Levels of Health Care

It is most important that nurses develop knowledge of international health and those activities that contribute to the health of people worldwide. You have been asked to participate in a discussion focused on international health.

♦ What information do you think you would need to discuss international health issues? From what sources might you obtain information regarding the major international health problems?

♦ How do you think nurses should be prepared to think and act at both local and global levels?

RESEARCH FOCUS

Nursing Education and International Health in the United States, Latin America, and the Caribbean

Study Problem/Purpose

There is little research about the preparation and activities of nurses to assist them in dealing with international health and little information about the extent of international health activities in U.S. schools of nursing. The purpose of this study was to identify international health activities in schools of nursing in the United States, Latin America, and the Caribbean.

Methods

A descriptive study design with a 16-item survey questionnaire was used to obtain information from a random sample of 100 U.S. university schools of nursing and 15 schools with known international activities (10 from the United States and 5 from Latin America and the Caribbean). Responses were received from 59 of the U.S. randomly sampled schools and from 8 of those known to have international activities. All 5 schools from Latin America and the Caribbean responded.

Findings

International health as a topic was found in one-third of the U.S. schools of nursing, but international health was not integrated with other subjects. Of the U.S. respondents, 54 (84%) expressed interest in the field of international health. All 5 of the Latin American and Caribbean schools of nursing confirmed the PAHO's indications of international health activities. International health activities were usually individual initiatives with limited institutional support.

Implications

This study indicates a growing interest in international health among schools of nursing. However, the schools have contributed in a limited way to the development of the international health field. The study reveals a definite need for schools of nursing to include a nursing curriculum with international health, an interdisciplinary approach to the international health curriculum, and a vision of international health as a leadership responsibility for nurses.

Source: Wright, M. M., Godue, C., Manfredi, M., & Korniewicz, D. (1998). Nursing education and international health in the United States, Latin America, and the Caribbean. Image: Journal of Nursing Scholarship, 30(1), 31–36.

---

services and nature of the facilities, and (5) who has the influence or power to determine access and availability. There is currently one additional major element that many are experiencing: rapidity of change. System changes are occurring throughout the world. The context of change and changes in government policy in various countries are occurring in all elements of services and in all types of services, including services for the elderly, child health and welfare, mental health, alcohol and drug services, and disability services.

Health Systems: A Global Perspective

Health System Performance

In 2000, a major report titled *The World Health Report 2000: Health Systems: Improving Performance* was published by WHO. This significant report focused on the first ever analysis of the systems conducted by WHO, referred to previously in this chapter. As WHO noted in the report, "better health is unquestionably the primary goal of a health system" (p. 21). A second goal of health systems is fairness in providing financial contribution for those whose health care can be catastrophically costly, and the third goal is responsiveness to expectations of the population, reflecting the importance of respect for dignity, autonomy, and confidentiality of information. Progress toward goal attainment depends on how well health care systems carry out four vital functions: service provision, resource generation, financing, and stewardship.

Thus, WHO engaged in the major effort of assessing health system performance to determine how far health systems in the member states are achieving these goals for which they should be accountable and how efficiently resources are used. In order to provide an evidence base to assist policymakers to improve health system performance, WHO focused on five performance indicators to measure health systems in the 191 member states (WHO, 2000). WHO's assessment system included:

1. Overall level of population health
2. Health inequalities (or disparities) within the population
3. Overall level of health system responsiveness (a combination of patient satisfaction and how well the system acts)

4. Distribution of responsiveness within the population (how well people of different socioeconomic levels perceive that they are served by the health system)

5. Distribution of the health system's financial burden within the population (who pays the costs)

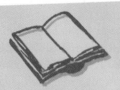

Out of the Box

There is a major need to bring life-saving medicine and necessary care to the most vulnerable populations in the world. Many poor in developing countries die each year from infectious diseases because they do not have access to medicines. Because of this problem, a campaign was launched in 2000, the Access to Essential Medicines Campaign.

Working to bring medicines to needy countries is a campaign initiated by Medecins Sans Frontieres (also known as Doctors Without Borders or MSF). MSF, a private nonprofit organization, was founded in 1971 by a group of French physicians who believed that all people have the right to health care and that the needs of these people cross national borders. It is an international network with sections in 18 countries. On a yearly basis, more than 2000 volunteer nurses, physicians, and other medical professionals, water/sanitation engineers, and administrators work with 15,000 locally hired staff to provide health care assistance in more than 80 countries.

Among the core activities of the current Access to Essential Medicines Campaign is an effort to influence world trade negotiations so that life-saving medications are not treated like other consumer goods. Since 2000, MSF has worked to prioritize access to affordable medicines in planning the use of international health funds. A number of strategies have been proposed to ensure the availability of lowest cost medicines and other health-related goods. Among the strategies are:

Encouraging generic competition
Creating an information database on drug prices and quality as well as client status
Encouraging purchase of medicines from lowest cost suppliers, including generic companies

Through its Medicines Campaign, MSF is confronting the problems faced by those in the developing world who need access to affordable, effective treatments for infectious diseases. ■

For each performance indicator, WHO used existing sources or newly generated data to calculate measures of attainment for those countries where information was available. WHO's Christopher Murray and Julio Frenk were the primary persons who formulated the framework for the report. The development of new analytical methods and summary indicators, new international data collection efforts, and empirical analysis for the report involved over 50 persons, the majority from the WHO Global Programme on Evidence for Health Policy. Demography, cause of death, burden of disease, life expectancy, disability-adjusted life expectancy (DALE), health inequalities, fairness of financial contribution, health system preferences, national health accounts and profiles, performance analysis, and basic economic data were all used for performance assessment purposes.

The findings from WHO's assessment of the world's health systems revealed that the U.S. health system spends a higher portion of its gross domestic product (GDP) than any other country but ranks 37 out of 191 countries according to its performance. The United Kingdom, which spends 6% of its GDP on health services, ranks 18th. The WHO study, using the five performance indicators, reported that France provides the best overall health care, followed by Italy, Spain, Oman, Austria, and Japan. Most of the countries that were ranked the lowest are in sub-Saharan Africa where life expectancies are low. Because of the HIV/AIDS epidemic, healthy life expectancy for infants born in 2000 in the sub-Saharan region has dropped to 40 years or less.

In Europe, health systems in Mediterranean countries such as France, Italy, and Spain were rated higher than others in the continent. Norway was rated the highest Scandinavian nation, at 11th. In the Latin American nations, Columbia, Chile, Costa Rica, and Cuba were rated highest—22nd, 23rd, 36th, and 39th in the world, respectively.

In the Pacific region, Australia ranked 32nd overall, while New Zealand was 41st. In the Middle East and North Africa, many countries ranked highly: Oman was in 8th place overall, Saudi Arabia 26th, United Arab Emirates 27th, and Morocco, 29th.

Performance Measures

Overall Level of Health

The measure WHO used to assess overall population health was the DALE. The DALE is a measurement estimated from three kinds of information: "the fraction of the population surviving to each age, calculated from birth and death rates; the prevalence of each type of disability at each age; and the weight assigned to each type of disability, which may or may not vary with age. Survival at each age is adjusted downward by the sum of all the disability effects" (WHO, 2000, p. 28).

DALE was estimated to equal or exceed 70 years in 24 countries and 60 years in over half of the 191 member countries of WHO. In 32 countries, however, DALE was estimated to be less than 40 years. In many of these countries, major epidemics of HIV/AIDS were contributing factors, among other causes.

Distribution of Health in Populations

Health inequalities in populations are also a health system concern. A health system has the responsibility to try to reduce inequalities by prioritizing actions to improve the health of those who experience poor health wherever the inequalities are caused by conditions amenable to interventions.

Child and adult mortality data were used by WHO in their health system performance assessment in a small number of countries—six in particular—because for most countries it was possible only to use child mortality data. The highest ranking countries that have fewer health inequalities based on mortality data are primarily European, high-income countries. Except for Afghanistan and Pakistan, all the countries that ranked lowest on child health equality were in sub-Saharan Africa, where child mortality remains high. WHO plans to use adult mortality data in the future when it is available.

The country where health is most equally distributed is in Japan, with considerably more inequality in Mexico and the United States. Australia and Norway both show more symmetric distributions.

Responsiveness

Responsiveness refers to how the system performs relative to meeting a population's expectations of how it should be treated. A key informant survey consisting of 1791 interviews in 35 countries was used resulting in scores (from 0 to 10) on seven different elements of responsiveness related to respect for persons (e.g., respect for dignity, autonomy) and client orientation (prompt attention, quality of amenities, access to social support networks, and choice of provider).

Respondents were asked to rank the seven elements in order of their importance. Respect for persons and client orientation were rated as equally important overall. The three elements of respect for persons were also rated as equally important. However, the four elements of client orientation resulted in different rankings— therefore unequal weights. Prompt attention (immediate attention in emergencies and reasonable waiting times for nonemergencies) received the highest rating, followed by the quality of amenities (e.g., cleanliness, space), access to social support networks for those receiving care (families and friends), and choice of provider (freedom to select which individuals or organization delivers one's care).

In almost every country where key informants were surveyed, the poor were identified as the main disadvantaged group. They were considered to be treated with less respect, to have less choice of providers, and to be offered amenities of poorer quality than the nonpoor. Rural populations were viewed to be treated worse

than urban populations, suffering from less prompt attention, less choice of providers, and lower quality of amenities. Those who were viewed as receiving worse treatment than others in the population were women, children or adolescents, and indigenous or tribal groups (WHO, 2000).

Distribution of Financing

This indicator refers to fair financing in health systems, which means that the risks each household faces due to the costs of the health system are distributed according to ability to pay, not to the risk of illness. A fairly financed system ensures financial protection for everyone. The WHO report (2000) suggested that countries spending less than around $60 per person per year on health result in their populations being unable to access health services from an adequate performing system.

Families that spend 50% or more of their nonfood expenditure on health are likely to be impoverished as a result. Household surveys conducted by WHO showed that in Brazil, Bulgaria, Jamaica, Kyrgyzstan, Mexico, Nepal, Nicaragua, Paraguay, Peru, the Russian Federation, Vietnam, and Zambia more than 1% of all households had to spend half or more of their full monthly capacity to pay on health. In the WHO report of 2000, great inequality characterized China, Nepal, and Vietnam, in which nearly all health spending is out of pocket.

Health Sector Reform

The emergence of health sector reform as a major international public health issue suggests that there is a widespread recognition of health sector problems and the need for solutions. Berman (1996) suggested that health sector reform may be defined as "sustained, purposeful, and fundamental change in the policies, programs, and institutions providing health care services" (p. 34). *Sustained change* refers to an effort over time—a process. It does not mean a single action. *Purposeful change* requires goals and implies that outcomes can be evaluated. *Fundamental change* differentiates the nature of health sector reform, with the inclusion of programs, institutions, and policies, from a specific programmatic change.

Health sector reform is needed in order to meet the current diverse health needs of populations and to incorporate rapid technological change. The goal of health sector reform is to provide health care that is affordable and manageable for future generations—to create systems that will be driven not by market forces alone but also by public policy and government.

Countries with different social and economic conditions are considering or developing programs to meet future needs. In the higher income countries, a variety of concerns have resulted in reform efforts: (1) the rapid increase in health care costs, (2) consumer dissatisfaction with access to and the quality of their health care, and (3) major disparities in access to health care for certain population groups. These factors are important in the examination of reform efforts in such countries as the United Kingdom, Sweden, and the Netherlands. In 1994 reform efforts were the major motivational factors for the unsuccessful health reform proposals in the United States.

In the formerly socialist countries, such as the former Soviet Union, Eastern Europe, Vietnam, and China, because of the major political and economic changes, government-financed and government-operated health care services can no longer rely on adequate government support. There are current efforts to find new ways to satisfy the health care need. Many of these countries are struggling, however, with the issues of providing care to their populations, particularly those who are poor and vulnerable.

Middle-income and poorer countries have different pressures for reform. Countries such as Mexico, Colombia, and Thailand are experiencing shifts in disease patterns from high rates of infectious and communicable diseases to high rates of chronic diseases while, at the same time, trying to deal with the poor population groups who suffer from the conditions found in the poorest countries. In the poorest countries such as those in sub-Saharan Africa they too are trying to deal with the HIV/AIDS epidemic that is occurring, particularly among the poor.

In addition to the concern about the high rates of infectious and communicable diseases as well as high rates of chronic diseases, there is an increased emphasis on the predicted worldwide rise in mental and neurological disorders—primarily unipolar depression, schizophrenia, bipolar and obsessive-compulsive disorders, as well as alcohol use (WHO, 2001b). Based on data gathered from 181 countries by Project ATLAS, a WHO project, it was found that 78 countries (43%) have no mental health policy, 37 (23%) have no legislation on mental health, 69 (38%) have no community care facilities, and in 73 (41%) the treatment of severe mental disorders is not available in primary health care systems (WHO, 2001b). These findings point to the major need for health sector reform action worldwide. They are a wake-up call for the world.

In many of the poorer countries such as those in Latin America and sub-Saharan Africa, declining incomes and public revenues have resulted in reduction in government health care expenditures. The most basic health care services have become more limited as a result.

As Berman (1996) stated:

Although there is no single formula for health sector reform among such diverse countries, there are common themes. These include social solidarity in redistributing resources from the wealthier to the poorer and from the healthier to the sicker groups; increased use of regulated market-like forces to encourage efficiency and quality; focus of resources on more cost effective services; and increased recognition and wise use of pluralism in government and private participation in the health sector. (p. 36)

Brundtland (2000), Director General of WHO, clearly stated:

Whatever standard we apply, it is evident that health systems in some countries perform well, while others perform poorly. This is not due just to differences in income or expenditure: we know that performance can vary markedly, even in countries with very similar levels of health spending. . . .

Performance assessment . . . invites reflection on the forces that shape performance and the actions that can improve it. (pp. vii–viii)

Countries have developed many different types of health care systems; however, the current predominant theme is performance assessment and health system improvement. Even though nursing varies from country to country and nurses' roles are diverse given the nature of the different health care systems, nursing is in a position to make a difference during this period of change. We need to assist each other through global sharing of knowledge, participating in healthy public policy development, and caring about one another with respect for our various cultures.

Selected Health Care Systems

United Kingdom

The United Kingdom (UK) uses a government health system, the National Health Service (NHS). It began in 1946 for the purpose of providing everyone with health services and is supported by individual and corporate taxation. Services are administered through a system of health authorities. The services provided by the health authorities include general medicine, disability, surgery, and rehabilitation. Services are made available through private physicians, hospitals, nurses and allied health professionals, clinics, health outreach programs such as hospice, boroughs, district nursing, and environmental health services.

The British health care system still provides the majority of health care services, but it has undergone many changes. The changes have been particularly rapid since the mid-1980s, primarily in relation to the delivery process. The NHS is changing so that it not only focuses on treating people when they are ill but also works in partnership with others to improve health through health system improvement: better planning, increasing fairness, and reducing health inequalities. In the White Paper, The New NHS, the government in the United Kingdom formulated a vision for a national health service that provides equal access to high-quality treatment everywhere and services that are faster and more convenient [United Kingdom Department of Health (UKDOH), 2000].

One of the major pressures to change health services has been to contain costs, and this has resulted in the movement toward a more businesslike climate. The NHS is the largest item of central government expenditure after social security and is Europe's largest organization (UKDOH, 2000). Therefore, there is a greater emphasis on providing efficient and effective services. As a result, disease prevention and health promotion activities are receiving increased funding. Decision makers and health care providers are recognizing that it makes sense to try to curtail spending on high-technology hospital treatment (curative in nature) by preventing any need for it, and they are acknowledging the burden of preventable diseases. The shift of the balance of funding toward a greater emphasis on prevention and health promotion is also consistent with the WHO strategy and the focus on primary health care (Pike, 1995).

The shift in funding has resulted in the orientation toward a community basis for the delivery of care. This community focus is occurring in the health sector and in social work and social care. Large institutions such as those that housed people with mental health problems, institutions for those with learning disabilities, large homes for older adults, and many of the larger hospitals that were a legacy from the last century are disappearing. Smaller units in the community are thought to be more appropriate. Larger institutions are often viewed as too expensive to manage. Community care is viewed as a more appropriate model because many of the conditions today are amenable to a caring approach rather than a primary focus on curing actions.

A number of conditions are bringing about the changes in the British health system plans for the future. The rise in the incidence of chronic diseases, degenerative conditions, and disability, along with the increase in the number of older adults in the population, has resulted in the recognition of the need for changes in health delivery. Mental health problems concerned with depression, stress, and substance abuse are also issues that require a community care focus. Thus, particular groups such as older adults, people with disabilities and long-term illnesses, and mental health service users are viewed as distinct groups, ensuring that the NHS is meeting their needs by developing a systematic approach to caring for them. The emphasis on quality of care and health system performance in order to expand best practice is a major focus of the new NHS (UKDOH, 2000).

Most people suffering from chronic diseases and disability are cared for in the community, not in institutions or hospitals. Thus, there is greater recognition in the United Kingdom than there is in the United States that health problems need to be prevented. Health promotion is viewed as a most important way to deal with current and future health problems.

Australia

Australia also uses a government system, a system of national health insurance for basic health care services—acute, subacute, and home care—for all persons in the population. Medicare, Australia's system of national health insurance, was instituted in 1984. Australia's health care system has three levels within the public sphere: Commonwealth, state, and local. In general, the Commonwealth (federal) government is responsible for the funding of health services. The states and territories have the primary responsibility for the direct provision of health services, and the health responsibility of the local government, which varies from state to state or territory, lies primarily with environmental control measures and a range of community-based and home care services.

Australia also has a private sector which is involved at all levels in funding (insurance and out-of-pocket personal payments) and in the provision of services (general practice, medical specialists, diagnostics, hospitals, and aged care). Individuals purchase private insurance to supplement services provided through Medicare. Health care funding, however, is dominated by the public sector, which accounts for 69.1% of all funding (Bloom, 2000).

Australian governments have historically held the view that private markets will not ensure that those who are economically or socially disadvantaged will have adequate access to high-quality affordable care. Public finance of essential basic health care services is thus justified to alleviate poverty, including the poverty that might result from having to pay unexpected large health care bills. Thus, financial fairness has been one of the underpinnings of the Australian health care system (Podger & Hagan, 2000).

Changes in government policy and in the role and structure of Australian families, the aging of the population, and the recognition of the need to control health care costs all began in the 1980s. Given these changes, significant shifts have occurred in the Australian health care system also. In Australia, as in the United States, there has been a major shift away from acute-care institutions to home-based care in all service sectors, including services for the aging, child welfare, mental health, alcohol and drug abuse, and disability services (Zamurs, 1995). Thus, community-based care plays a major role in the health care system.

Community-based care in Australia now involves diverse providers and requires coordination of services. The major changes in the acute-care system, based on technological changes, improved clinical practice, and further development of care management and nursing services at home, have reduced the length of stay in hospitals. Because of this shift, improving the linkages between the hospital and community-based services has been increasingly emphasized in order to continue improvements in care management through effective discharge planning.

One of the results of earlier hospital discharges, coupled with the changing demographics and the resultant increase in the proportion of people with chronic health conditions, is the ever-increasing demand on family caregivers; these patterns are also identified in the United

States. Complex care demands related to the increased acuity of family members being cared for at home have resulted in difficulty for the health and well-being of caregivers, particularly those without supportive families or community networks to share responsibilities (Zamurs, 1995).

In Australia, there is a great emphasis on shifting resources to the primary and continuing care system, because it is anticipated that the greatest demand and need will be for community-based services. With the shift to community-based services, health promotion and well-being receive greater emphasis.

The health services in Australia, similar to those in the United Kingdom and the United States, are operated in a climate influenced by privatization, economic considerations, and the culture of consumerism. There is a great emphasis on the need for efficient and effective services.

One of the health and community service provisions is the national health insurance system, called Medicare, referred to earlier. The national health insurance system is popular with consumers, "playing a central role in making Australia a just society" (Duckett, 1995, p. 15). The five principles underpinning Medicare are universality, access, equity, efficiency, and simplicity (Commonwealth Department of Health, Housing, and Community Services, 1992). All residents are eligible for benefits, which include access to free inpatient and outpatient treatment in public hospitals and private medical services. Medicare covers all Australians for medical services outside hospitals (at 85% of the fee schedule set by Medicare) and for the cost of hospital treatment (Bloom, 2000). Individuals who wish to use the services of a private medical practitioner of their choice will receive a benefit of 85% of the schedule fees (Commonwealth Department of Human Services and Health, 1995). Medicare has historically been very strongly supported by the Australian people. Because of this support, even though Medicare was an issue in the late 1990s, the government focused on incremental changes to the existing system rather than devising new systems to solve existing problems (Somjen, 2000).

Although the national health insurance system is viewed as a strength, it has problems, such as lengthy hospital waiting lists, limited access to costly new technology, gaps in service provisions for people with chronic conditions, and difficulty in navigating the complexity of an array of programs and services. Because of the identified problems, changing community expectations, the changing care environment, and pressures on government to control costs, reform was viewed as necessary (Duckett, 1995).

The Council of Australian Governments (COAG) in 1994 identified reforms of health and community services that it viewed as necessary for the future (Duckett, 1995). The COAG approach to dealing with the identified problems was to conceptualize "streams of care as the basis for change." Three major categories of care were identified:

1. General care—Refers to primary health care, home and community care services, and selected outpatient services considered episodic in nature.

2. Acute care—Refers to care in day surgery centers and acute-care hospitals. Viewed as all activities directly related to the services provided prior to the acute intervention, the acute-care service itself, and any postacute services directly related to the specific acute episode.

3. Coordinated care—Refers particularly to care and support that are long term and complex. Coordinated care services, provided by a care coordinator, are believed to be particularly important for persons with chronic diseases—the frail elderly, disabled, those with long-term psychiatric problems, and those with long-term rehabilitation problems. Such care coordination has been identified as one way to prevent other health problems from arising and to address them early when they do, thus reducing the need for hospitalization or institutionalization. Nurses, particularly community health nurses, can play a vital role in this effort.

Australia, as evidenced in other industrialized countries, has a government which plays a large part in financing and regulating the health system. The Australian government has played a major role in funding the provision of health services because of the interplay of several factors. These factors include the belief that unregulated markets for health care do not work as efficiently and social concerns about the equitable distribution of health care. Health is valued because it is fundamental to the definition of how one lives. During the late 1990s, however, Australia, evident in other countries as well, was either planning or implementing reforms in order to control costs, improve access, and maintain the quality of health care (Somjen, 2000).

Canada

The Canadian health care system is also based on a national health insurance program. It is a predominantly publicly financed, privately delivered system that is known as "Medicare." The system provides access to universal, comprehensive coverage for medically necessary hospital care and inpatient and outpatient physician services—the dominant features of the system. Health care in Canada is financed primarily through taxation—provincial and federal personal and corporate incomes taxes.

The management and delivery of health services are the responsibility of the individual provinces or territories. The Canada Health Act specifies the criteria that provincial health plans must meet in order for a province to qualify for the full federal transfer of payments (Health System and Policy Division, Health Canada, 1999).

Canada's health care system relies primarily on primary care physicians, who account for approximately 51% of all active physicians in the country. They are usually the initial contact in the system and control access to most specialists and other services. Canada does not have a system of "socialized medicine," with physicians employed by the government. Most doctors are private practitioners (Health System and Policy Division, Health Canada, 1999).

In addition to insured hospitals and physician services, provinces and territories also provide some public coverage for other services that are not included in the national health insurance framework for certain population groups (e.g., seniors, children, welfare recipients). These supplemental benefits often include such therapies as dental and vision care, prescription drugs, and assistive equipment. Although the provinces/territories do provide some additional benefits, supplementary health services are primarily privately financed. Individuals and families may acquire private insurance or benefit from an employer-based group insurance plan to help pay for expenses associated with supplementary health services.

Federal legislation to institute national health insurance was enacted in 1957 and has evolved into its present form. Prior to the late 1940s, private medicine dominated health care in Canada, with access to care based on ability to pay. Currently Canada's health system is based on five principles that are specified in the Canada Health Act of 1984 (Health System and Policy Division, Health Canada, 1999; Ross Kerr, 1997):

1. Universality—Extending coverage to the entire population rather than to selected groups

2. Comprehensiveness—Coverage of all medically necessary services

3. Accessibility—Reasonable access to health care services

4. Portability—Coverage required for residents of one province when they move to another province and require services

5. Public administration—Nonprofit operation by an organization fiscally responsible to the provincial government

In 1998, total expenditures in Canada were $82.5 billion, or $2694 per capita. Health expenditures accounted for 9.3% of GDP in 1998, down from the 1992 peak level of 10.1%. Public sector funding represents approximately 68.7% of total health expenditures, with the remaining 31.3% privately financed out of pocket or through employer-sponsored benefits or supplementary insurance (Health System and Policy Division, Health Canada, 1999).

In the 1980s and 1990s the rising costs of health care, specifically hospital and physician services, served as a major impetus for change in the Canadian system. The aging of the population, increasing rates of health care utilization, and rising costs raised issues that are being debated regarding payment for health services. These debates have given impetus to health system changes (Ross Kerr, 1997) that place greater emphasis on community-based care.

With the movement toward community-based care, major restructuring efforts are occurring in Canada. With the intent to increase the efficiency of service delivery and yet maintain quality of care, critical issues are being discussed in Canada, as in other countries. In addition to the increased emphasis on health promotion and cost efficiency, there is a greater recognition of the various determinants of health discussed in the landmark LaLonde report, determinants such as income, education, and the environment. Health is being viewed more broadly than as being merely the absence of illness, and new approaches are being examined in relation to the meaning of health (Ross Kerr, 1997).

By adopting a determinant of health framework which recognizes the broader determinants of health and shifting the emphasis of the health care system from institutionally based delivery models to integrated community-based models which place increased emphasis on health promotion and disease prevention, the federal and provincial governments are responding to the need for system changes (Health System and Policy Division, Health Canada, 1999). Moving to a community-based model emphasizing disease prevention, health promotion, and multidisciplinary collaboration is viewed as holding the greatest potential for improving health (Ross Kerr, 1997).

Because of the changes occurring in Canada, providing accessible primary and community-based health care and linkages between hospitals and community services are challenges for the future. Although it is recognized that there are limits to the nature and amount of care that can be provided, measures need to be taken to ensure that universal availability and access to needed services are provided in a publicly funded, nonprofit, affordable system. Canadians regard health care as a right, and they value their health system because it exemplifies the shared values of the Canadian society—equity, fairness, compassion, and respect for the fundamental dignity of all. Adherence to the principles of the Canada Health Act will remain an important characteristic of their health care system (Health System and Policy Division, Health Canada, 1999).

Russia

Health care in Russia is also in the midst of major changes. A discussion of health care must be viewed within the context of the political changes that occurred in Russia since 1991 and the significant changes that have occurred in nursing in that country. The Independent Republic of the Russian Federation, a reality since December 25, 1991, and its constitution set forth a health care system free of charge to all citizens (Smith, 1997).

Before 1991, health care was delivered by a centrally ordered, hierarchical system (Curtis, Petukhova, & Taket, 1995). Clients did not pay for care directly, and health care professionals were considered state employees. Health care concerns were given a lower priority than other governmental endeavors such as industrial and military activities. The GDP for health care spending was approximately 2.4% (Curtis et al., 1995). Because of this lower priority rating, chronic underfunding and rationing occurred. Long waits for service and medicinal supply shortages were prevalent.

Since 1991, Russia has struggled to enact social reforms and a market-driven economy. Russia is a nation trying to overcome its history of oppression and human rights violations, as is evident in its new national charter. With this effort, problems have arisen. Inflation, poverty, crime, and concerns about the infrastructure are having a major impact on the people. The crumbling infrastructure and political changes are posing very serious problems for the health care system in Russia (Smith, 1997). Health care funding is not a priority of the government.

Hospitals are finding it difficult to operate, with shortages of food, supplies, and medicines in many areas. Each hospital has two parts; one part is designated for people without money or insurance. Their care is free, but they receive no or few medications and limited attention. The other part of the hospital is reserved for clients who pay for their care. These clients receive medications and more attention from staff. In addition, they are better fed because of their ability to pay for their care. Some hospitals provide little or no food on the free side because of severe funding shortages. Family members are expected to bring food, but clients who have no family have a very serious problem (Smith, 1997).

Because nursing constitutes a major portion of the health professional work force, it is important to describe the historical context and the changes that have taken place in nursing in Russia. Historically, nursing was and still remains a physician-dominated, task-oriented profession. The status and income of nursing are low. Nurses' wages have been just above the poverty line (Perfiljeva, 1997). The working conditions are poor, and nurses are required to increase the workload, which has resulted in work that is very demanding. As Perfiljeva states, "Most of them hold down two jobs to make ends meet" (p. 8).

Since 1991, however, physician dominance has been fading. Through the vision of Perfiljeva, who is the Dean of the School of Nursing at the Moscow Medical Academy, the academy initiated the first master's program in nursing in the country (Smith, 1997). In very difficult circumstances, progress has been made in nursing education in Russia, with curricula focused on both hospital nursing and community nursing at the baccalaureate level as well.

Perfiljeva (1997) comments:

It is recognized in the country that effectiveness, efficiency, and humanity—the cornerstones of a high quality service—depend to a large extent on the work of nurses. As the national debt rises and economic pressures continue to affect health care budgets, providing the most efficient and cost effective care is vital. Nurses can potentially save hospitals a great deal of money by working daily with patients in the community to prevent serious illnesses, or prevent people going into the hospital in the first place. (p. 8)

Thus health promotion and disease prevention efforts will become a major role for nurses in the future. Perfiljeva also states, "We are very proud of our nursing students—They are the change agents in the health care delivery system and particularly, in their health care settings" (p. 9).

IMPLICATIONS FOR THE FUTURE

Many nations are engaged in health system improvements that imply substantial changes in policies, programs, and institutions providing health care services. These changes require health professionals to reexamine their present and future roles. Given the nature of these changes, it is increasingly recognized that to improve the health of the community, address health problems, and respond to economic and performance pressures, interdisciplinary, cross-cultural collaboration is necessary. Collaboration within and between countries can provide powerful strategies for dealing with current and future health care delivery problems.

Because of the health inequalities that exist globally, there is a need for continued emphasis on the Health for All policy and framework originally proposed in Alma Ata in 1978 (Messias, 2001). The need for a continued global response to health inequalities is critical. Despite significant progress in improving the health of the world's population, as indicated by improved life expectancy, declining infant mortality rates, improved access to safe drinking water and sanitation, and increased immunization coverage, health inequalities continue to exist, particularly in the poorest nations (Brundtland, 2000; WHO, 1999). Health for all thus continues to be a call for equity and social justice—a global issue that must be dealt with by health systems around the world.

Health professionals are working in a rapidly changing world environment. These changes present a valuable opportunity to engage in collaborative endeavors for the purpose of learning from each other and taking a proactive approach to dealing with current and future health care environments. These collaborative efforts can enhance not only the health of the individuals and populations that health professionals serve but also their own

Perspectives... ✳

INSIGHTS OF A PROFESSOR EMERITUS

Developing a knowledge of international perspectives about health and health care systems is an imperative for nursing today and in the future. The importance of sharing knowledge about the world's health problems and the nature of the health care delivery systems cannot be underestimated. We live in a global society, and as nurses we have knowledge to share, knowledge of the commonalities and differences in nursing and health care worldwide. We can assist each other, as colleagues and friends, in health promotion and disease prevention efforts. We must work together as nurses and with other health professionals to build healthy, caring communities.

One of the challenges for nursing in this century is to incorporate into nursing curricula a much greater emphasis on global health perspectives. As a faculty member who had the opportunity to teach and consult in a country outside the United States since the 1980s and to participate in the development of an international association in nursing, I have found that there is a growing interest in international health in nursing. There is a need, however, to encourage the study of international health in schools of nursing and to conduct research that reflects cross-national collaborative efforts. Providing opportuni-

ties for faculty and students to learn more about international health and international health issues in nursing will require formal commitments by schools and their universities to develop partnerships, student exchange programs, and faculty projects with universities in other countries. If we truly believe that we live in a global society, then we must expand our knowledge of global health and participate in international health efforts.

As community health nurses, with our understanding of the global public health and primary health care initiatives, we have a broad perspective of health care that incorporates a tradition in the international health field. We can assist others in this challenge for the future, developing knowledge about health and disease patterns throughout the world, coupled with the recognition of the cultural significance of health, disease, and illness. Throughout our journey of global sharing, our exchanges will need to be culturally sensitive, modified, and negotiated. As nurses we must view ourselves as part of the global community in which problems, resources, and opportunities for community action efforts are shared.

—Sue A. Thomas

effectiveness and influence. By working together, health professionals can be active participants in advancing the goal of health for all the world's people.

Cross-sectoral and cross-national partnerships provide the opportunity to bring together a broad range of health professionals, community leaders, and health organizations. International cooperation through international organizations, universities, and consulting firms has assisted national leaders to develop health sector information that can and does assist in health improvement efforts. Continued exchange and transfer of knowledge, technology, and experience between and within countries will assist in dealing with problems in financing, organizing, and managing health care systems.

As cross-sectoral collaboration within countries and cross-national collaborative efforts expand, it will be critical that community health nurses, as well as all nurses, develop knowledge and competencies in intersectoral and interdisciplinary collaboration as well as knowledge of the major global health care system issues. Collaboration enhances each health sector's stature and sphere of

influence (Lasker and the Committee on Medicine and Public Health, 1997). It requires competencies in negotiation, communication, and community development; a population focus; the ability to use information systems; and the ability to use culturally congruent care strategies to improve health care.

The collaborative paradigm was a framework used by leaders in public health and medicine in the 19th century when they worked together on health boards and sanitary reforms. Lillian Wald, the founder of public health nursing in the United States, demonstrated the value of collaborative efforts toward the beginning of the 20th century, as did Lavinia Dock and Mary Brewster, among others. Today, such a framework enhances the ability of community health nurses and other health professionals to achieve the powerful synergies of cross-sectoral collaboration.

Nurses face the challenge of embracing a global perspective and the Health for All framework. To bring global perspectives to their practices, nurses must be willing to take leadership in reorienting local and national

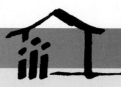

COMMUNITY NURSING VIEW

A community health nurse working in a city has been asked to be on a steering committee to identify and implement the process for assessing the health of the city using the WHO Healthy Cities model. The ultimate purpose of the community assessment project is to provide a document that will assist in building a healthier city through the formulation of community health diagnoses and proposed interventions. The community itself is multicultural, with varying socioeconomic levels represented. The community health nurse is well known for his or her knowledge of the community as well as knowledge of the community assessment process. The community health nurse previously served on several other citywide committees whose purposes were to address special target population needs, such as high rates of family violence and of older adults with chronic disabling conditions, many of whom were identified as poor.

Nursing Considerations

Assessment

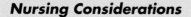

- What steps should be taken to begin the assessment process?
- Who should be involved in the community assessment process?

- What kind of structure, organization, and funding will be necessary?
- What data will be needed? From what sources?

Diagnosis

- Who should participate in formulating the diagnoses? In setting priorities?
- What process would you recommend specific to the analysis?

Outcome Identification

- What outcome indicators would you use to evaluate the assessment?

Planning/Interventions

- Who should participate in planning the interventions?
- What methods would you recommend?
- How should the priority problems and proposed interventions be determined?

Evaluation

- Who should participate in the evaluation process?
- What methods would you suggest? Why?

---

health care systems toward the principles of primary health care and health for all (McElmurry & Keeney, 1999). Community health nurses have a vital role in this endeavor at local, national, and international levels. Given the nature of our global burden of disease and the economic and social disparities manifest in poverty, the major public health challenge of this century will be to reduce these disparities (Brundtland, 2000; WHO, 1999).

As we think about the future, it is important to emphasize that what each of us does contributes to tomorrow. Salmon (1998) so clearly states, "What is good about today reflects what we have done in the past. So, too, will the future be a mirror of what each of us cares about, is committed to, knows and does" (p. 3).

Working together to improve the health of our communities, nationally and internationally, is an example of caring in action. As Roach (1995) concluded, "Caring is the human mode of being" (p. 9). Thus, caring actions are critical, actions that include respect for others and compassion for those whose health care and life are compromised. Empowering community members, nurses, and

other health professionals through interdisciplinary cross-national collaborative efforts will provide opportunities to demonstrate caring in action. Caring represents an ongoing commitment to work together to help meet the health care needs of the people throughout the world.

KEY CONCEPTS

- Health for all of the world's people is an international goal and is promoted by the major world health organizations.
- Primary health care and health for all are the key strategies for promoting the health of the world's populations.
- The major international health organizations that are involved in world health include (1) private voluntary agencies, (2) philanthropic foundations, (3) private organizations, (4) official (governmental

and intergovernmental) agencies, and
(5) professional and technical organizations.

◆ Health system improvement has emerged as a major international public health issue with the recognition of health sector problems that need to be addressed.

◆ Cross-sectoral collaboration within countries is a framework that offers health professionals powerful strategies for dealing with current and future health care problems and challenges.

◆ Cross-national collaboration provides opportunities for health professionals to assist others in their endeavors to improve the health of their communities.

◆ Community health nurses, as well as other nurses, must develop a knowledge of global health and health care system issues.

RESOURCES

UNITED STATES

American Public Health Association: http://www.apha.org
Sigma Theta Tau, International: http://www.nursingsociety.org

AUSTRALIA

Australian Institute for Health and Welfare:
    http://www.aihw.gov.au

Public Health Association of Australia, Inc.:
    http://www.pha.org.au

UNITED KINGDOM

Department of Health, United Kingdom:
    http://www.doh.gov.uk

CANADA

Canadian Society for International Health: http://esih.org
Health Canada: http://www.hc-sc.gc.ca

EUROPE

European Public Health Alliance: http://www.epha.org
European Union: http://europa.eu.int

GLOBAL

Global Health Council: http://www.globalhealth.org
International Council of Nurses: http://www.icn.org
Pan American Health Organization: http://www.paho.org
United Nations: http://www.unsystem.org
United Nations Children's Fund: http://www.unicef.org
World Bank: http://worldbank.org
World Federation of Public Health Associations:
    http://www.apha.org/wfpha
World Health Organization: http://www.who.int

Chapter

6

HEALTH CARE ECONOMICS

Gregory L. Crow, EdD, RN

MAKING THE CONNECTION

We live in a universe of creative emergence.

—Wilber, 1996, p. 25

COMPETENCIES

Upon completion of this chapter, the reader should be able to:

- Describe the U.S. health care system, including the way it functions.
- Define general and health care economic terms.
- Discuss the federal, state, and local governmental roles in health care.
- Identify the mechanisms by which health care costs are controlled.
- Compare and contrast the European health care financing model with that of the United States.
- Describe the ways that emerging health care financing trends shape health care in the United States.
- Apply the concept of caring to health care economics.

KEY TERMS

capitation	managed competition
case management	market system
client cost sharing	Medicaid
copayment	Medicare Part A
diagnosis-related groups (DRGs)	Medicare Part B
economic policy	microeconomics
economics	out-of-pocket expenses
fee-for-service	preferred-provider organization (PPO)
finance controls	rationing
financing	regulatory finance controls
gross domestic product (GDP)	reimbursement
health maintenance organizations (HMOs)	reimbursement controls
inflation	third-party payor
macroeconomics	usual and customary reimbursement
managed care	utilization controls
managed-care organization	

With the advent of managed care in the United States in the last decades of the 20th century, a new and often uneasy relationship emerged between payers, providers, and consumers of health care. Prior to managed care, the payers of health care sent payments in the form of premiums to health care insurers who then paid the provider, be they physician, hospital, home health agency, nursing home, or pharmacy. Under this old system the provider decided how much care a client would receive and where they would receive it.

Under managed care, payers (employers, insurers, and government) took a very active role in managing every aspect of the client's care. This active role monitored the decisions providers made about how much health care a client would receive and where they would receive their care (acute-care hospital, home care, ambulatory care or long-term care facility). Perhaps the most revolutionary aspect of managed care was that the provider shared the financial risks involved in providing all aspects of care and the payer established up front the amount a provider would be reimbursed for services rendered.

The new reimbursement scheme forced all providers to examine the processes and practices they used to deliver client care. Suddenly, economics and financing of health care took center stage, causing unprecedented change in all aspects of the U.S. health care system. The old paradigm of pay as you go and quality at any cost was no more—the new paradigm of balancing cost with quality had arrived.

Evidence that cost and quality are playing a coequal role in health care delivery in managed care is emerging. The *New York Times* and other national magazines such as *Time* and *Newsweek* have documented this trend. The *New York Times* (July 2, 2001, p. C1) reported that managed-care organizations are implementing new reimbursement policies that reward providers for the quality of their care as well as controlling the costs. In the recent past, almost all managed-care organizations rewarded providers based on their ability to keep health care costs down. Each bill was scrutinized to make sure providers were not ordering more high-priced tests and procedures.

This movement toward rewarding quality is a plus for consumers because providers will now have incentives to improve client care rather than just cutting costs. Employers are also hailing the trend as they believe it will benefit them as employee absences will decrease (*New York Times,* July 2, 2001, p. C1).

However, there could be a downside to this trend. Because nothing is free, the cost of quality bonuses will be passed on to the employer and to their employees in the form of higher premiums. This coupled with a decline in the U.S. economy and the resulting layoffs in almost all industries and service sectors might backfire, driving health care costs so high that we will again find ourselves in the midst of a managed-care movement where controlling costs is a major thrust.

For most of the 20th century, the economics and financing of health care were the exclusive domain of management. In nursing schools, students were often told that their role in the health care system was to take care of the client and to let someone else worry about the money. Moreover, they were told that the cost of care should pay no role in where, when, and how health care was provided. Hospitals would often keep clients in the hospital until the weekend so that the family would be there to take care of them, and nurses routinely sent clients home with supplies to tide them over until they could purchase their own supplies. The journey to the new reality of managed care has not been an easy one to say the least.

To understand and flourish in the new paradigm require that all providers and employers gain knowledge and understanding of health care economics and share in the development of strategies to cut costs. The accountability for the economic viability of all health care organizations has become more decentralized, placing both managers and staff in an awkward alliance. To say that the clinical staff did not greet this new shared accountability with open arms is an understatement. Moreover, to say that managers were eager to share power and control over the allocation of increasingly meager and finite resources is also an understatement. This situation often led to a disconnect between management and staff as caring, the core of nursing, appeared to be displaced in favor of economics. This phenomenon led many nurses and consumers to the conclusion that the organizations in which they practiced and received care had placed quality and caring second to economics (Crow, 2001).

This chapter is meant to provide the reader with an overview of health care economics. For the foreseeable future economics will play a significant role in all aspects of health care. You might ask: Why is this important when all I want to do is provide quality care to my community?

Knowledge of health care economics is essential if nurses are to play an ever-increasing role in the viability of the community health agencies in which they practice and ensure that quality and caring are at least considered as equal components in the design of care. To be active and influential stakeholders in the economic decisions that impact client care, nurses must understand and speak the language of economics and finance. Think about it—a conversation between two or more community health nurses about the care of a client in the community is accurate, productive, and efficient because they speak the same language and do not have to rely on someone to interpret the conversation. As long as language hinders their abilities to be active and influential in the allocation of resources, nurses will continue to be the recipients of the economic policies and decisions of others, which has for far too long been the case.

Policymakers, employers, health care providers, insurance companies, and consumers are searching for ways to enhance, provide, and control allocations of finite health care resources. Figure 6-1 illustrates the sources and the targets of the U.S. health care dollar in 1999 (Health Care Financing Administration, Office of the Actuary [HCFA OA], 2001a). As can be seen, governmental (Medicare, Medicaid) and other private programs accounted for $0.46 of every dollar spent; private health insurance, out-of-pocket payments, and other private sources accounted for the remainder ($0.54). The targets of this spending demonstrate that most health care dollars continue to be spent on acute hospital care ($0.03). Other spending (includes dentist, durable medical equipment, over-the-counter drugs, public health, research, and construction) accounted for $0.26; physician services consumed $0.20 of each dollar, with nursing home care, prescription drugs, and program administration accounting for the remainder ($0.21). Figure 6-2 demonstrates that from 1960 to 2000, national health care expenditures rose from $26.7 billion to $1,299.5 billion. At the same time, out-of-pocket nonreimbursable expenses rose from $12.9 billion nationally to $194.5 billion (HCFA, OA, 2000b).

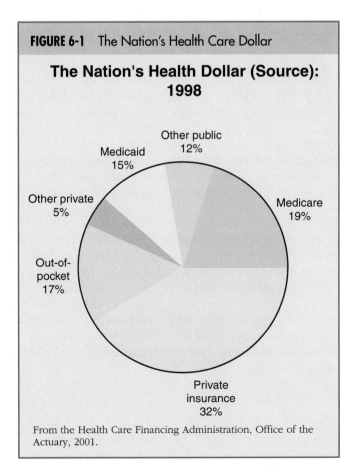

FIGURE 6-1 The Nation's Health Care Dollar

The Nation's Health Dollar (Source): 1998

- Other public 12%
- Medicaid 15%
- Other private 5%
- Out-of-pocket 17%
- Medicare 19%
- Private insurance 32%

From the Health Care Financing Administration, Office of the Actuary, 2001.

FIGURE 6-2 The Nation's Health Care Dollar (Spending)

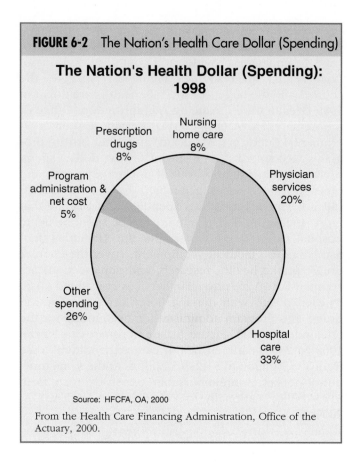

The Nation's Health Dollar (Spending): 1998

Source: HFCFA, OA, 2000

From the Health Care Financing Administration, Office of the Actuary, 2000.

ECONOMICS

The first step in wisdom is "getting things by their right names" (Wilson, 1998, p. 13). Because economics plays such a vital role in health care, community health nurses must increase their knowledge and awareness of those forces that shape health care financing in the United States. Specifically, the nurse must understand a number of terms in order to understand the economics of health care.

Economics is the science concerned with the ways that society allocates scarce resources commonly known as goods and services (Finkler & Kovner, 2000). Economics addresses the supply and demand on the part of an environment for a product or service. Examples of economic health care environments are individual consumers, insurance companies, employers, and state and federal governments. Resources include inputs such as labor, capital, and technology. Resources are considered scarce when society demands more resources and goods than are generally available. Economics viewed from a market perspective is divided into macroeconomics and microeconomics.

Macroeconomics

Macroeconomics is one of two major economic theories. The prefix *macro* means "large," indicating that **macroeconomics** is the study of the market system on a large scale. Macroeconomics focuses on the aggregate performance of all markets in a market system and on the choices made by that large system in an economy (Finkler & Kovner, 2000). In health care, one macroeconomic market is the entire U.S. health care system, including the way that it performs in terms of profit, loss, and efficiency.

Microeconomics

Microeconomics is the second major economic theory. The prefix *micro* means "small," indicating that **microeconomics** is the study of the market system on a small scale. Microeconomics focuses on the individual markets that make up the market system and on the choices made by small economic units such as individual consumers and individual firms (Finkler & Kovner, 2000). One example of a microeconomic system is the individual consumer or small-business owner and the ways that these markets interact and influence each other in the provision of health services. Macroeconomics and microeconomics are both influenced by economic policy formulated at federal, state, and local levels.

The state microeconomic system can influence the federal macroeconomic system because the number of state enrollees in health care plans, partially funded by federal programs, can rise or fall depending on state law or policy. As the number of state enrollees rises or falls, the amount of funds transferred from federal macroeconomic programs to state microeconomic programs will fluctuate. Vice versa, the federal macroeconomic system can influence the state microeconomic system by limiting the total amount of dollars available for funding or by establishing federal laws that influence how states spend health care dollars.

Economic Policy

Economic policy is a course of action intended to influence or control the behavior of an economy. Economic policy is typically implemented and administered by the government (Wessels, 1993). The U.S. federal, state, and local governments are attempting to develop economic policies to control health care costs (Heshmat, 2001). It should be noted, however, that the U.S. health care system, or market, has not reacted to health care economic policy in the manner that other markets have typically responded to governmental policy decisions. Typically, as a commodity becomes scarce, the price increases, and, conversely, as the market becomes flooded with a commodity, the price goes down. Regardless of health care policy, supply, or demand, however, the United States has experienced a consistent increase in costs associated with health care.

Federal, state, and local governments have traditionally attempted to control health care costs via economic policy, financing, and reimbursement. **Financing** is the amount of dollars that flow from payors to an insurance plan, either private or governmental. **Reimbursement** is the flow of dollars from the insurance companies to providers or hospitals. The flow of dollars within health care is focused on a market, whether that market be local, state, or federal.

Market System

A **market system** is a mechanism by which society allocates scarce resources (Finkler & Kovner, 2000). In the United States, several types of market systems allocate scarce health care resources. The federal government allocates resources via programs such as Medicare, Medicaid, and the U.S. Public Health Service. At the state level, public health service and community district hospitals represent the primary sources in the market system. On the private side of the health care market system are profit and not-for-profit health maintenance organizations, private hospitals, insurance companies, and group or individual medical practices (Mechanic, 1994). The way that a market system operates in terms of efficiency or waste affects the gross domestic product of the country in question. The **gross domestic product (GDP)** is all the goods and services produced for domestic use by a nation in one year and represents a microeconomic theoretical base. It also constitutes a way of comparing one nation with another in terms of economic function. In comparative studies, the collective health care expenditures of each of a number of nations are often each expressed as a percentage of the GDP (Duffy, 1993). One factor that influences the GDP is the theory of supply and demand for a product or service. The GDP does not take into account any products produced by another nation and transported to the United States for consumption. Therefore the GDP is concerned only with goods and services produced and consumed within the borders of the United States in a one-year period (see Table 6-1).

Inflation

Inflation, a rise in the general level of prices, is a term generally associated with macroeconomic theory (Finkler & Kovner, 2000). Inflation is closely related to the concepts of supply and demand discussed earlier. A frus-

trating aspect of inflation and its relation to health care in the United States is that our costs appear to inflate whether or not there is ample supply or decreased demand. In fact, during the Kennedy and Johnson administrations, as the supply of health care increased, the cost increased as well. Currently, the federal government is attempting to control the cost of health care by decreasing the supply and controlling how health care dollars are spent. While inflation has not proceeded at the rate it did in the 1970s and 1980s, it nonetheless is still increasing. Federal and state governments and consumers are turning to managed care and managed competition as means to control the inflationary tendencies of health care costs.

HEALTH CARE ECONOMIC TERMS

The following discussion highlights health care economic terms with which the nurse should become familiar.

Capitation

Capitation is a dollar amount established to cover the cost of health care services delivered to a person for a specific length of time, usually one year. The term usually refers to a negotiated, per-capita (per-person) rate to be paid periodically by a managed-care organization to a health care provider. The provider is then responsible for delivering or arranging for the delivery of all health services required by the covered person under the conditions of the provider contract. Capitation may also refer to the amount paid to a managed-care organization by the HCFA on behalf of Medicare or Medicaid recipients or by a state (HCFA, 1998a).

Case Management

Case management is the process whereby all health-related matters of a case are managed by a physician or nurse. Nurse and physician case managers coordinate designated components of health care, such as appropriate referral to consultants, specialists, hospitals, and services. Case management is intended to ensure continuity of services and accessibility and to negate the provision

TABLE 6-1 Health Care Expenditures as Percentage of GDP, 1960–2000						
	1960	**1970**	**1980**	**1990**	**1995**	**2000**
Percentage of Gross Domestic Product	5.1	7.0	8.8	12.0	13.4	13.2

From Health Care Financing Administration, Office of the Actuary, National Health Expenditures Aggregate: 1960–2000 *[On-line].*
Available: http://www.hcfa.gov/stats/nhe-oact/tables/nhegdp00.csv.

of fragmented services and redundant care and the misutilization of facilities and resources. It also attempts to match the appropriate intensity of services with the client's needs over time (HCFA, 1998b).

Copayment and Out-of-Pocket Expenses

Copayment is a cost-sharing arrangement whereby the person who is insured pays a specified charge (e.g., $10.00 for an office visit). The person is usually responsible for payment at the time that the service is rendered (HCFA, 1998a).

Out-of-pocket expenses are expenses not covered by a health care plan and, thus, borne by the individual (see Table 6-2) (HCFA, 1998a).

Diagnosis-Related Groups (DRGs)

Diagnosis-related groups refer to a prospective cost reimbursement classification system for inpatient services based on diagnosis, age, sex, and presence of complications. It is used as a means of both identifying costs for providing services associated with given diagnoses and reimbursing hospitals and selecting other providers for services rendered. The amount of payment is predetermined (HCFA, 1998b).

Fee for Service

Fee for service is a payment system whereby nurses, physicians, hospitals, and other providers are paid a specific amount for each service performed as it is rendered and identified by a claim for payment. Because costs of providing care vary depending on geographic location, fees also vary depending on region of the United States (HCFA, 1998b). For instance, the cost to build and operate a hospital in downtown San Francisco is more than in rural California. In general, the costs of property, labor, and supplies are higher in cities as opposed to rural settings.

Managed Care

Heshmat (2001) defines **managed care** as the external monitoring and comanaging of an ongoing provider-client relationship to ensure that the provider delivers

only appropriate care. Staines (1993) notes that if all acute health care services were delivered through managed-care systems, national health care expenditures might be decreased by as much as 10%. Managed care is seen as a means to control cost while also maintaining quality and access to appropriate care. Managed care is also a mechanism for introducing competition into the health care market and, thereby, for making the health care market respond in the expected fashion to the supply and demand cycle.

A **managed-care organization** is an entity that integrates financing and management and the delivery of health care services to an enrolled population. Managed-care organizations provide, offer, or arrange for coverage of designated health services needed by members for a fixed, prepaid amount (HCFA, 1998a).

A **preferred-provider organization (PPO)** is a health care delivery system that contracts with providers of medical care to provide services at discounted fees to members. Members may seek care from nonparticipating providers but are generally penalized financially for doing so, via loss of discounts and higher copays and deductibles (HCFA, 1998b).

Health maintenance organizations (HMOs) are a type of insurance. An HMO contracts with and enrolls individuals and groups to provide comprehensive health care services on a prepaid basis. These agencies can be profit or nonprofit. Health maintenance organizations emphasize preventive health services, and most provide inpatient and outpatient services (HCFA, 1998a). For a further discussion of HMOs, see Chapter 4.

Managed Competition

Enthoven (1993) defines **managed competition** as "a purchasing strategy to obtain maximum value for employers and consumers" (p. 28). The theoretical foundation of managed competition is microeconomics, which rewards those suppliers who do the most efficient job of providing health care services that improve quality, cut costs, and satisfy consumers. The goal of managed care and managed competition is to limit expensive care that is unnecessary without interfering with appropriate treatment (Heshmat, 2001). Both managed care and managed competition are seen as potential strategies for third-

TABLE 6-2 National Health Care Expenditures and Out-of-Pocket Costs, 1960–2000						
	1960	**1970**	**1980**	**1990**	**1995**	**2000**
National expenditures	26.7	73.1	245.8	696.0	990.2	1,299.5
Out-of-pocket	12.9	25.1	55.3	137.3	146.5	194.5

From Health Care Financing Administration, Office of the Actuary, 2000, National Health Expenditures Aggregate: 1960–2000. *[On-line]. Available: http://www.hcfa.gov/stats/nhe-oact/tables/nhe00.csv.*

party payors to control both the financial and reimbursement costs of the health care market.

Third-Party Payor

Third-party payors for health care services vary and are determined by one's health care coverage. *Third party* refers to an entity other than the provider or the consumer that is responsible for total or partial payment of health care costs (Levit, Olin, & Letsch, 1992). Whether the third party pays all or a portion depends on the type of coverage. If the consumer is required to make partial payment, that payment is commonly referred to as a copay. For elderly persons, the third-party payor is Medicare; for the poor, it is Medicaid; and for the insured, it is the insurance company. The prevalence of third-party payors decreases the role that price plays in determining the supply and demand of health care services. Because the bill is sent directly from the provider to the payor, effectively bypassing the consumer, the consumer is unaware of the cost. Remember, the cost of a product is determined by the price that the consumer is willing to pay for that product. If consumers are not aware of the costs of their care, there is little incentive for providers to control those costs.

Medicare

Medicare Part A, or the Hospital Insurance (HI) program, helps pay for hospital, home health, skilled nursing facility, and hospice care for the aged and disabled. Part A is financed primarily by payroll taxes paid by workers and employers. The taxes paid each year are used mainly to pay benefits for current beneficiaries. Income not currently needed to pay benefits and related expenses is held in the HI trust fund and invested in U.S. Treasury securities. At age 65, people are automatically enrolled in Part A regardless of whether they are retired. A person and his or her spouse who have paid into the Social Security system via employment for 40 quarters or more are eligible for Social Security. People who have paid into the Social Security system for fewer than 40 quarters can enroll in Part A by paying a monthly premium. People who are totally and permanently disabled and are under age 65 may enroll in Part A after having received Social Security disability benefits for 24 months. People with chronic renal disease requiring dialysis or a transplant are also eligible for Part A after a 24-month waiting period.

A qualified hospital stay is one that meets the following criteria:

1. A doctor prescribes inpatient hospital care for an illness or injury.

2. The illness or injury requires care that can be provided only in a hospital.

3. The hospital participates in the Medicare program.

4. The hospital's utilization review committee agrees with the need for hospitalization.

A qualified nursing facility care stay must meet the following criteria to be reimbursed by Medicare Part A:

1. The enrollee requires skilled nursing or rehabilitation services that can be provided only in a skilled nursing facility.

2. The enrollee was in a hospital for 3 days in a row, not counting the day of discharge, before entering the skilled nursing facility.

3. The enrollee is admitted to a facility within a short period of time (generally 30 days) after leaving the hospital.

4. The condition for which the enrollee is receiving skilled nursing facility care was treated in the hospital or arose while the person was receiving care in the hospital.

5. A medical professional certifies that daily skilled nursing or rehabilitation care is necessary.

Medicare Part A qualified home health care must meet the following criteria:

1. The enrollee requires intermittent skilled nursing care, physical therapy, or speech-language therapy.

2. The enrollee is confined to home.

3. A physician determines that the enrollee needs home health care and sets up a plan for the person to receive care at home.

4. The home health agency providing the care participates in Medicare.

Medicare Part A also covers hospice care if the enrollee meets the following criteria:

1. The enrollee's physician and the hospice's physician certify that the enrollee is terminally ill.

2. The enrollee chooses to receive hospice care instead of the standard Medicare benefits for the illness.

3. The care is provided by a Medicare participating hospice program.

See Table 6-3 for a summary of Medicare Part A benefits.

Medicare Part B, or the Supplementary Medical Insurance (SMI) program, pays for physician, outpatient hospital, and other services for the aged and disabled. Part B is financed primarily by transfers from the general fund (tax revenues) of the U.S. Treasury (approximately 75%) and by monthly premiums paid by beneficiaries. Income not currently needed to pay benefits and related

TABLE 6-3   Medicare A and B Summary of Benefits

MEDICARE PART A

Who Is Eligible

A person is eligible for Medicare Part A if the person or his or her spouse worked for at least 10 years in Medicare-covered employment and the person is 65 years of age and a citizen or permanent resident of the United States.

Benefits

Inpatient hospitalization	Days 1–60: Medicare Part A pays except for the $812 deductible.	Days 61–90: Medicare Part A pays except for $203/day.	Days 91–150: Medicare Part A pays except for $406/day. (*Note:* Beyond 150 days with lifetime reserve days used, Medicare Part A pays nothing.)
Skilled nursing facility	Days 1–20: Medicare Part A pays the full cost of services.	Days 21–100: Medicare Part A pays all but $101.50/day.	After 100 days, Medicare Part A does not pay for services.
Home health care	All services covered if enrollee meets the Medicare Part A criteria for home health care.	Medicare Part A pays the full cost of some medical supplies if billed through the home health agency.	Medicare Part A pays 20% of approved durable medical equipment such as wheel-chairs, hospital beds, oxygen supplies, and walkers.
Hospice care	Patient must elect to take the Medicare Part A hospice care instead of the standard Medicare inpatient hospital benefits. The patient's physician must certify that the person suffers from a terminal illness.	Medicare pays the entire bill for hospice service.	There is a copay of $5 for each drug prescription.

MEDICARE PART B

Who Is Eligible

All Medicare Part A enrollees who elect to pay the monthly Part B premium of $54.00 are eligible.

Benefits

Medical expenses	Medicare Part B pays a portion of the bill for all medically necessary services.	Medically necessary services are physician care, physical and occupational therapy, medical equipment, diagnostic tests, and speech therapy.	Medicare pays 80% of approved amount after the enrollee pays the $100 annual deductible.
Preventive care	Medicare Part B will pay for services no matter where the enrollee receives them (inpatient or outpatient).	Medicare Part B pays for screening pap smears, breast prostheses following mastectomy, screening mammograms, artificial limbs, and eyes.	
Outpatient medications	Medicare Part B does not cover medications.		

*From Centers for Medicare & Medicaid Services. (2002). Medicare and you. **Baltimore, MD: author. Retrieved from http://www.medicare.gov.***

expenses is held in the SMI trust fund and invested in U.S. Treasury securities (HCFA, 2001b).

Part B must be applied for at age 65 when enrolling in Medicare Part A. The monthly Part B premium is automatically deducted from the person's Social Security check (HCFA, 2001b).

Medicare Part B pays for a wide range of medical services and supplies. Medically necessary services of a physician are covered no matter where the enrollee receives them, whether at home, in the physician's office, in a clinic, nursing home, or hospital. Part B benefits have special requirements, and some are more strictly limited than others. The Medicare Part B premium covers physician services, hospital outpatient care, and durable medical equipment.

Ambulance services is one of the benefits that is strictly limited. Medicare Part B will pay for an ambulance when the ambulance, equipment, and personnel meet Medicare requirements and if the transportation in any other vehicle could endanger the enrollee's health. Coverage is generally restricted to transportation between the enrollee's home and the hospital or the enrollee's home and a skilled nursing facility.

The enrollee is responsible for paying 20% of whatever the hospital charges, not 20% of a Medicare-approved amount. For some outpatient mental health services, the enrollees share can be as much as 50% of the Medicare-approved amount. See Table 6-3 for a summary of Medicare Part B benefits. A further discussion of Medicare can be found later in this chapter.

Medicaid

Medicaid is a program funded by federal and state taxes and administered by the states. Medicaid pays for the health care of low-income persons. Services and eligibility differ from state to state; however, all states must provide certain federally mandated services in order to qualify for federal matching funds. Medicaid does not cover all people below the federal poverty line. Those mandated for coverage by the federal government are the following:

1. Recipients of Aid to Families with Dependent Children (AFDC)

2. Those people who are over age 65, blind, or totally disabled and who receive income from Supplemental Security Income (SSI)

3. Pregnant women with incomes up to 133% of the federal poverty line

4. Children born after 1983 to families with incomes at or below the federal poverty line

A more detailed discussion of Medicaid can be found later in this chapter. Both Medicare and Medicaid rely on

DRGs to finance and reimburse services they cover (HCFA, 2001c).

FACTORS CAUSING INCREASED HEALTH CARE COSTS

Issues related to health care costs underlie all aspects of the U.S. health care system and greatly influence all policy questions. Lee and Estes (1994) cite three basic reasons for the tremendous expenditure on health care in the United States:

1. Rising cost per volume of service

2. Per-capita increase in volume of services

3. Growth in specific population groups such as elderly persons

A number of experts would additionally cite the introduction of advanced technology, rising administrative costs, client complexity, excess capacity, uncompensated care, and health care fraud as driving forces in the rapid and sustained increase in health care costs in the United States (Lamm, 1994). A brief discussion of these factors follows.

Cost per Volume of Service

Cost per volume of service (CPVS) is the cost associated with a particular volume of service. For example, a community health agency knows the cost of doing a certain number of home visits for a particular type of client, such as a postoperative hip replacement. The costs associated with the care of the hip replacement client are supplies (dressings and drugs), equipment (bedside commode, trapeze, wheelchair), and staff salaries. The agency can calculate the cost of care for a particular volume of clients and then staff the agency accordingly. The staffing procedure is directly linked to the amount of reimbursement an agency will receive for a particular diagnosis. The cost of that volume minus the rate of reimbursement is considered profit for the agency.

Per-Capita Increase in Volume of Services

Per-capita increase in volume (PCIVS) is the increase in client days in the hospital, client visits in the ambulatory clinic, or home visits in the community health agency calculated over a one-year period. It is important to know exactly which services are increasing or decreasing so resources can be properly allocated to that service.

Growth in Specific Populations

Growth in specific population groups is a vital piece of information for any health care agency. Federal, state, local, and private agencies need to know the types of individuals they are serving to better plan service delivery.

Population-based programs for specific groups such as the elderly or pregnant teenagers have very specific needs, and programs must be planned and financed with these needs in mind.

Advanced Technology

The introduction of advanced technology may or may not decrease the cost of care. In one example, Bodenheimer and Grunback (1998) note that the introduction of the laparoscopic cholecystectomy increased both the cost per volume of service and the number of procedures. They point out that laparoscopic technology shortened the operation time, decreased postoperative pain, and decreased length of hospital stay and recuperation. At first review this seems like a win-win situation for the client, the health care organization, and the physician. However, on closer examination, the actual cost of the surgery increased. This technology greatly decreased the dangers of conventional surgery and drove up the per-capita volume of cholecystectomies, and the total cost of this increased volume actually increased the cost of the cholecystectomy 11%.

Rising Administration Costs

Administration costs associated with the management of health care are expressed as a percentage. Rising administration costs have been a concern because every dollar spent on administration costs is a dollar not available for direct patient care. Bodenheimer and Grunback (1998) note that administration costs have typically risen at a higher percentage than the cost of providing the care itself.

Client Complexity

Client complexity also adds to the cost of care. The more complex the client's needs, the more costly the care. For instance, a middle-aged man who has had a myocardial infarction and is also a brittle diabetic is likely to consume more health care resources than that same man without diabetes. Clients with complex needs are particularly suited for case management.

Uncompensated Care

Uncompensated care refers to the personal health care rendered by hospitals or other providers without payment from the client or a government-sponsored or private insurance program. It includes both charity care, which is provided without the expectation of payment, and bad debts, for which the provider has made an unsuccessful effort to collect payment due from the client (Prospective Payment Assessment Commission, 1997).

Over the past two decades, whenever hospitals have complained that Medicare payments for services provided to beneficiaries are too low, administrators have asserted that they will be unable to continue providing charity care at the same level. The threat of further limited access to care for certain vulnerable populations has resulted in Congress's creating certain additional payments to hospitals that serve a relatively large volume of low-income clients (called the disproportionate share adjustment) (Prospective Payment Assessment Commission, 1997). Uncompensated care has also been raised by critics of for-profit hospitals who have argued that these hospitals have lower uncompensated care levels and hence provide less care to low-income people and those without health insurance. However, the evidence on this issue is mixed and far from conclusive. Nonetheless, in the years ahead, community health nurses can anticipate that as payments to hospitals become tighter and prospective payment systems are applied to nonhospital providers, the level of uncompensated care provided by community and other nonhospital providers will probably rise and threaten the financial stability of these organizations. As this occurs, the issue of uncompensated care will gain increasing attention by policymakers and community health agencies.

Health Care Fraud

The Medicare program defines fraud as the intentional deception or misrepresentation that an individual knows to be false or does not believe to be true and makes, knowing that the deception could result in some unauthorized benefit to himself or herself or some other person. The most frequent kind of fraud arises from a false statement or misrepresentation concerning payment under the Medicare program. Violators include physicians and other practitioners, hospitals and other institutional providers, clinical laboratories and medical device suppliers, employees of providers and billing services, and beneficiaries or people in a position to file a claim for Medicare benefits. Examples of the most common forms of fraud include billing for services not furnished; misrepresenting the diagnosis to justify payment; soliciting, offering, or receiving a kickback; unbundling or "exploding" charges; and falsifying certificates of medical necessity, plans of treatment, and medical records to justify payment. Because each year the Medicare program makes several billion dollars in fraudulent payments, Congress and the Clinton administration passed legislation aimed at identifying and severely penalizing those who commit fraud. In the years ahead, community health nurses can expect their employers to be increasingly cautious to avoid engaging in any fraudulent activities or risk the appearance of fraud.

GOVERNMENT'S ROLE IN HEALTH CARE

The question of the proper role of government in health care as well as the relative distribution of power among federal, state, and local governments has been the subject of heated philosophical debates in health care reform circles. The rising costs of health care have overwhelmed third-party payors, leading them to decrease the total number of covered citizens. This has left a staggering 16.3% of the U.S. population—or an estimated 44.3 million people—without insurance (U.S. Census Bureau, 2000, Tables 172, 174, 177). The underinsured constitute an estimated additional 15 million people (U.S. Census Bureau, 1997). The uninsured and underinsured often seek health care through the most expensive and least effective avenue of the U.S. health care system: hospital emergency departments. Episodic care coupled with a lack of follow-up services may exacerbate both the person's illness and the financial woes of the health care system. An additional contributing factor to the numbers of uninsured and underinsured people is the inability of small and medium businesses to offer health insurance. As the price of providing health care insurance has increased, so has the inability of small to medium business owners to afford the cost of providing employee health insurance (Levit et al., 1992).

Data from the U.S. Census Bureau (Table 6-4) reveals that lack of insurance affects ethnic groups differently. In 1998 the percentage of the total Hispanic U.S. population without health insurance was 35.5%, followed by blacks at 22.2%, and the percentage of whites without health insurance was 15.0%. In 1998 the federal government included Asian and Pacific Islanders, and the percentage without health insurance was just below blacks, at 21.1% (U.S. Census Bureau, 1998, Table 2). Data such as these that are also available by state can help the community health nurse plan programs tailored for specific populations within their community. As resources become more and more scarce, it is imperative that community health programs are planned in such a way as to diminish the chances of planning and implementing programs not suited for their communities (see Table 6-4). For additional information on related topics, see Chapters 13, 15, and 16.

Race and ethnicity continue to be associated with lack of health insurance. In 1996, minority workers, especially Hispanic workers, were far more likely than Caucasians or African Americans to be uninsured. As illustrated in Table 6-4, 38% of Hispanic workers and 25.7% of African-American workers were uninsured in 1996, compared with 14.7% of Caucasian workers (HCFA, 1997a).

Concomitantly, federal and state governments have also reduced health benefits covered by Medicare and Medicaid and state-sponsored programs, via reform of laws governing hospital and physician reimbursement policies. Additionally, employers have attempted to control the skyrocketing costs of health care by developing strategies that reduce cost, such as offering incentives for employees to reduce their use of health care services or charging a copayment for services consumed. Walsey (1992) notes an alarming and growing trend among many employers, especially those in the service sector, of simply not providing access to health insurance coverage. (Service sector jobs are those generally associated with low or minimal wage, such as retail store clerk and fast-food service worker.)

In terms of health and welfare, generally the U.S. system of government provides for the government to do only that which private institutions either cannot or will not do. The role of the government has therefore historically been to intervene only when a remedy was needed for a failure of the private sector to provide a service. This rule of exception rather than of primary intervention on the part of government has led to the current uncoordinated, piecemeal health care system that, while currently consuming 13% of the U.S. gross national product (GNP) (HCFA, OA, 2001a, Table 1), does not provide comprehensive care for at least 44 million citizens who have no insurance (U.S. Census Bureau, 2000, Table 172).

Over the past 200 years, the role of the U.S. government in the policy, organization, financing, and destiny of health care has evolved from that of a highly constricted provider of services and protector of public health to that of a major financial underwriter of an essentially private enterprise. Government policies and procedures have increasingly encroached on the autonomy of providers as a means to control costs (Levit et al., 1992; Walsey, 1992). As costs began to spiral upward and out of control, the government increasingly became the agency of cost control, access, and quality via programs such as Medicare and Medicaid.

Litman (1994) cites several distinct characteristics of government's role in the U.S. health care system:

1. Paying vendors to ensure availability of care
2. Policing the system to ensure standards
3. Providing direct funding to upgrade systems and educate the health care practitioner

THE CHANGING CLIMATE IN HEALTH CARE

Between 1961 and 1969, the federal government's role and responsibility began to change in relation to health care. During the Kennedy and Johnson presidencies, federal health care aid moneys were channeled through the state systems. The federal government began to direct federal support for local governments, nonprofit organizations, and private businesses and corporations to provide health care, health education, social services, and community development programs focused on the health of its citizens. Davis (1994) notes that with the passage of the Great Society legislation, and specifically Medicare and Medicaid, the federal government ushered in a new era of commitment to improving the health and well-being of the poor and elders, including increasing their access to health care services. In 1966, 19.1 million people were enrolled in Medicare; in 1986 that number climbed to 31.7. And in 1999 the total number of Medicare

TABLE 6-4 Persons without Health Insurance for Entire Year 1999 by Selected Characteristics (in thousands)

	TOTAL POPULATION	NUMBER UNINSURED	PERCENT
	271,743	44,281	16.3
Males	132,764	23,014	17.3
Females	138,979	21,266	15.3
By age			
Under 18	72,022	11,073	15.4
18–24	25,967	7,776	30.0
25–34	38,474	9,127	23.7
35–44	44,744	7,708	17.2
45–64	58,141	8,239	14.2
65 years and over	32,394	358	1.1
By race			
White	223,294	33,588	15.0
Non-Hispanic white	193,074	22,890	11.9
Black	35,070	7,797	22.2
Asian and Pacific Islander	10,897	2,301	21.1
Hispanic	31,689	11,196	35.3
By Education (18 years +)			
No high school diploma	34,811	9,294	26.7
High school graduate only	66,054	12,094	18.3
Some college, no degree	39,087	6,211	15.9
Associate degree	14,114	1,730	12.3
Bachelor's degree	45,655	3,880	8.5
By Work Experience (age 18+)			
Worked during year	137,003	24,655	18.0
Worked full time	113,683	19,244	16.9
Worked part time	23,365	5,411	23.2
Did not work	30,323	8,194	27.0

From U.S. Census Bureau, Health Insurance Coverage: 1998 Table 2: Persons without Health Insurance for the Entire Year. By Selected Characteristics. *[On-line]. Available: www.census.gov/hhes/hlthins/hltin98/hi98t2.html.*

enrollees was 36.1 million, almost doubled from 1966 (U.S. Census Bureau, 1999, Table 4).

In 1960, life expectancy at age 65 was 69.7 years for all races. In 1998, the figure was 76.7 years, an increase of more than 7 years. Data for the same year indicate that females of all races have the longest life expectancy at 79.5 years, compared with 73.8 years for males of all races (Centers for Disease Control and Prevention, 2001).

During the 1970s, President Nixon began his program of New Federalism and, with that, the move to a system that transferred revenues for state and local use with as few strings and regulations as possible. This sys-tem became known as block grants. Under President Nixon, block grants were given so that states and communities could use the monies for broad purposes that met their specific needs. President Nixon additionally believed that the federal government should play a significant role in providing health care and, thus, sought the direct support of both private and public institutions and systems that provided care (Litman, 1994).

The administrations of presidents Reagan and Bush accelerated the degree of change in health care policy that began with Nixon. The Reagan-Bush agenda had several specific aims, specifically to:

1. Reduce federal funding for domestic social welfare programs.
2. Decentralize programs to states using block grants.
3. Emphasize greater market forces to shape the health care system.
4. Implement the DRG prospective payment system.

Reagan and Bush attempted a variety of cost control strategies at the federal, state, and local levels of government. Despite their efforts, however, health care costs continued to escalate (Enthoven, 1994; Litman, 1994).

During his first presidential campaign, President Clinton proposed that employers pay for much of the cost of health care and that federal subsidies be used for the purchase of insurance for low-income citizens. Clinton also wanted the federal government to provide subsidies to small-business owners for whom the universal mandate would be overly burdensome (Kronick, 1993; Enthoven, 1994). Without governmental subsidies, neither low-income people nor small-business owners would have been able to afford the Clinton mandate for employer-based health care coverage.

The Clinton administration advocated universal coverage through managed care, health alliances, and employer health care mandates. The Clinton plan included a guaranteed comprehensive health care package encompassing hospital and physician services, prescription drugs, and laboratory services. The plan also called for long-term care and expanded in-home services as well as prevention services for prenatal care, immunizations, and annual examinations (Enthoven, 1994; Enthoven & Kronick, 1994; Lundberg, 1994).

Although the Clinton plan failed as a total package, certain features of the plan were adopted in 1996 by the 104th Congress. Senators Kennedy and Kasselbaum drafted and the Congress passed a health care bill that prevents persons who change jobs from losing their health care benefits. The major disadvantages of the Kennedy-Kasselbaum bill were that mental health benefits were not covered and no limitation was placed on the percentage of premium increase when a person transfers from one carrier to another.

As major payors, providers, and regulators of health care, the states are playing an ever-increasing role in the health care system. At no time in the history of the United States has this been truer than in the current throes of health care reform. Despite the fact that health care reform failed in 1994 in the 103rd Congress, several states have implemented their own health care reform measures. Moreover, states have come to regard fundamental changes in both the financing and delivery of health care as necessary to control costs and ensure access (Berrand & Schroeder, 1994). Potential health care reform measures include increasing the number of Medicare enrollees in managed-care insurance plans, increasing the amount of copay for services and medications, and, perhaps, introducing means testing for level of coverage within the

Medicare system. Means testing is a mechanism for determining the amount of money an enrollee might pay for services on the basis of his or her annual income (White House Fact Sheet, 1998).

President Clinton's 1998 budget contained proposals to continue to provide Medicare and Medicaid enrollees with both managed-care and fee-for-service plans. Clinton also proposed to extend the Kennedy-Kasselbaum health portability plan to people in Medicare and Medicaid programs and, further, to improve access to medigap coverage (private health insurance that pays certain costs not covered by fee-for-service Medicare, such as Medicare copayments and deductibles). President Clinton also proposed a series of new efforts to enroll uninsured children in health insurance programs. Of the 11 million uninsured children in 1999, nearly 90% had parents who worked but who did not have access to or could not afford health insurance (U.S. Census Bureau, 2000, Table 172). In response, President Clinton proposed an investment of $900 million over 5 years in children's health outreach programs (U.S. Census Bureau, 2000, Table 172).

President George W. Bush (see U.S. Office of Management and Budget, 2002) has proposed to the 107th Congress that the United States will spend an estimated $193 billion on federal health care in 2002, with 84% of that money to finance or support direct health care services to individuals. President Bush has proposed a new program he calls Immediate Helping Hand (IHH) to provide critical assistance to the most vulnerable senior citizens for the cost of their prescription drugs. IHH will provide $46 billion for 2001–2005 to states to help nearly 9.5 million low-income Medicare beneficiaries pay for their prescriptions. IHH will cover the full cost of drug coverage for individual Medicare beneficiaries with incomes up to $11,600 per year who are not eligible for Medicaid and for married couples with incomes up to $15,700 per year. IHH will also provide catastrophic drug coverage for all Medicare beneficiaries, giving them financial security against the risk of very high out-of-pocket prescription expenditures ("Senior Rx," 2001).

Modernizing and saving Medicare ranks very high on President Bush's priorities. One of the greatest flaws in the Medicare program is its failure to cover outpatient prescriptions. Approximately 98% of private health insurance plans offer a prescription drug benefit or a cap on out-of-pocket expenses as an integral part of the package. President Bush notes that drugs can often be cost-effective therapies preventing the need for more expensive hospitalizations or other intensive therapies (U.S. Office of Management and Budget, 2001).

Of particular interest to community health nurses is President Bush's proposal to the 107th Congress to strengthen the health care safety net. There are approximately 44 million people without health care. Many of the uninsured and medically underserved live in the inner city and rural communities where there are few or no physicians and health care services, and these Americans have a lower life expectancy and high death rates from cancer and heart disease compared to the general population. To strengthen the health care safety net for those most in need, President Bush has made an additional budget proposal for $124 million for community health. He hopes to increase community health centers by 1200 to deliver health care to approximately 11 million patients, 4.4 million of whom are uninsured. For additional information concerning the President's health care agenda, visit www.whitehouse.gov/news/usbudget/blueprint/bud21.html.

Medicaid has constituted the fastest growing component in state budgets. The number of Medicaid recipients increased from approximately 10 million in 1967 to 40.6 million in 1998. The number of enrolled dependent children rose from 9.8 million in 1985 to 26.9 million in 1998 (U.S. Census Bureau, 2000, Table 172).

For over four decades, health care spending has far outpaced economic growth in the United States. Between 1960 and 1999, national health expenditures increased twice as fast as did the GDP. As a result, the share of GDP devoted to health care grew from 5.1% in 1960 to 12.0% in 1990 and to 13.2% in 2000 (HCFA, OA, 2000a).

For this reason, the cost of health care continues to attract the attention of the public, employers, insurance companies, federal and state governments, and policymakers. In 1960 the United States spent $143 per capita (per person) for health care, and in 1999 the United States spent $4,358 (HCFA, OA, 2000a).

One of the most dramatic increases by the federal government to reduce Medicaid expenditures, the Balanced Budget Act of 1997 (BBA) was signed into law by President Clinton in August 1997 (Iglehart, 1999; Center for Budget and Policy Priorities, 1997). The legislation was projected to achieve gross federal Medicaid savings of $17 billion over the next 5 years and $61.4 billion the next 10 years. The BBA also represented the most significant structural changes to the Medicaid program since 1991. This legislation greatly expanded the already substantial discretion that states enjoyed in administering their Medicaid programs, such as the State Children's Health Insurance Programs (S-CHIP). It eliminated minimum payment standards that states must currently meet in setting reimbursement rates at hospitals, nursing homes, and community health centers. Further, it also allowed states to require Medicaid beneficiaries to enroll in managed-care organizations (MCOs) that do business only with Medicaid. According to the U.S. Census Bureau (2000), the total number of Medicaid recipients enrolled in MCOs increased from 29.4 million in 1995 to 53.6 million in 1998. Another provision of the BBA was to provide an additional $20.3 billion in new federal funds over the next five years for the purpose of reducing the number of uninsured low-income children. According to the National Center for Health Statistics, a division of the Centers for Disease Control and Prevention (CDC), 15.4% of the children under the age of 18 were without health insurance in 1998. (U.S. Census Bureau, 1998, Table 4). The most up-to-date information on Medicare and Medicaid can be found on the web, at www.whitehouse.gov/news/usbudget, www.omb.gov (the Office of Management and Budget, which analyzes the financial impact of all federal programs), www.cms.hhs.gov (the Centers for Medicare & Medicaid Services, formerly the Health Care Finance Administration), which collects and analyzes statistics on health care spending, insurance coverage, and the cost of the U.S. health care system), www.nih.gov (the National Institutes of Health), and www.census.gov (a federal agency that takes the census of the United States and identifies trends in population, health insurance coverage, and work-related issues).

COST CONTROLS

A myriad of initiatives designed to curb increases in health care expenditures have met with generally limited success (Kronick, 1993). Some such initiatives—such as prospective payment systems (DRGs), increased governmental regulation, audits, and controls on access to care—are meant to drive down costs. Other initiatives include managed care and the publishing of comparative pricing information to assist individuals and employers in selecting health care providers.

Cost controls are of two primary types: finance controls and reimbursement controls. **Finance controls** attempt to limit the flow of funds into public or private health care insurance plans. The intention is to force the plans to reduce the outflow of reimbursement. Finance controls can be further subdivided into two types: regulation and competition (Enthoven, 1993; Kronick, 1993).

Regulatory finance controls for public systems rely primarily on restricting the amount of state or federal tax revenues deposited into programs that fund health care programs such as Medicare or Medicaid. Another finance substrategy is to introduce competition into the market system. This strategy is used primarily in employment-based systems and takes advantage of market forces to constrain costs. Market forces rely on microeconomic principles to drive down costs. Competition forces providers and insurance plans to hold down costs in order to attract enrollees to their services (Enthoven, 1993; Kronick, 1993).

Reimbursement controls take several forms: price controls, utilization controls, and client cost sharing. The state and federal governments as well as insurance plans have enacted price control mechanisms such as usual and customary reimbursement. In **usual and customary reimbursement,** the provider agrees to provide a service for a predetermined level of reimbursement (Enthoven, 1993). In **client cost sharing,** or copay, the client is required to pay for a portion of his or her health care. The intention is to make the consumer aware of the cost of care in the hope of driving down cost (Kronick, 1993).

Utilization controls are primarily geared toward controlling the supply side of the health care market. The primary strategy is to monitor the clinical activities of providers for the purpose of controlling costs (Enthoven, 1996). The provider is evaluated against other providers who offer similar services to determine the cost of care in relation to quality and outcomes. Providers who fall outside the preestablished norm are often sanctioned by the insurance plan. Sanctions can take many forms. Decreased referrals are one form of sanction, reimbursement made at the predetermined level regardless of the cost to the provider is another.

Actions to Control Costs

Although the introduction of the 1983 Medicare prospective payment system, known as DRGs, provided some respite from double-digit health care cost inflation, the majority of savings resulted from the decrease in the rates of hospital admissions under the DRG system. With the DRG system, Medicare established a fixed schedule of regionally appropriate fees paid for the treatment of each of the 475 DRGs. If the actual cost to the provider is lower than the DRG fee, the provider keeps the difference. If the cost of providing care is higher than the DRG fee, however, the provider absorbs the loss. The purpose

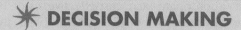

✳ DECISION MAKING

The Nurse's Role in Controlling Health Insurance Costs

Employer-subsidized health insurance costs are increasing, which may result in increasingly fewer employers being able to offer health insurance to their employees.

◆ How can nurses help employers control insurance costs while enhancing the health of employees?

◆ What role can nurses take in an organization, and what programs might they design, to help create a healthier work environment with the concomitant benefit of curbing the rising costs of employer-based health insurance?

of the prospective payment system was to encourage price sensitivity and, thereby, galvanize providers to control costs. The consumer and physician, however, did not feel price sensitivity, because the majority of savings were realized in decreased admission rates rather than in

RESEARCH FOCUS

A Randomized Trial of Early Hospital Discharge and Home Follow-up of Women Who Have Unplanned Cesarean Section

Study Problem/Purpose

To determine whether early discharge after unplanned cesarean section is safe and cost effective.

Methods

Participants included 122 women randomly assigned either to early discharge with home follow-up care by a nurse specialist or to usual discharge time frame of 2–3 days.

Findings

Women in the early discharge group went home 30.3 hours earlier than did those in the other group. Women discharged early expressed greater satisfaction with their care, and the charges for their home care were

29% lower than the charges for women discharged within the usual time frame.

Implications

Women who have had unplanned cesarean sections can be discharged early without compromising, and, in some cases, increasing satisfaction while at the same time controlling the cost of care. Reducing the cost of care and maintaining a quality service as judged by the client is thus a reachable goal. Maintaining quality while reducing the cost of care requires planning and client postdischarge support and education. Nurses have a responsibility to control costs whenever possible, and this study clearly indicates that this can be accomplished. To do so, nurses and other members of the health care team must continually undertake critical examination of the care process.

Source: Brooten, D. (1994). A randomized trial of early hospital discharge and home follow-up of women who have unplanned cesarean section. Obstetrics and Gynecology, 84, 832–834.

more efficient, appropriate, and cost-effective care. By the end of the third year of the DRG system (1986), the yearly increase in health care spending had risen to 10.7% of the GDP (Mechanic, 1994). In 1999, national health care expenditures as a percentage of GDP (see Table 6-2) had increased to 13.0%. However, it is worth mentioning that between 1992 and 1999 the health care expenditures expressed as a percentage of GDP peaked at 13.4% in 1993 and 1995. It decreased to 13.2% in 2000 (HCFA, OA, 2000a).

Issues related to health care cost underlie all aspects of our system of health care and they greatly influence all policy questions. Lee and Estes (1994) note that there are three basic reasons for the U.S. tremendous expenditure on health care: (1) rising cost per volume of service, (2) per-capita increase in volume or services, and (3) growth in specific population groups such as the elderly. In 2001, these same issues are operational. A number of other experts would add the introduction of advanced technology, rising administrative costs, patient complexity, and excess capacity as driving forces for rapid and sustained cost increases in health care in the United States (Lamm, 1994, p. 150).

An example of cost controls that takes into account most of the variables mentioned above is to control the types, rather than the numbers, of providers. Enthoven (1996) notes that increasing the proportion of generalist physicians may lead to savings for two reasons. First, generalists earn lower incomes than specialists. Second, generalists appear to practice less resource-intensive care and thus generate overall lower health care expenditures. Additionally, Enthoven notes that studies indicate nurse practitioners can effectively perform many tasks of the primary care physician at lower cost and of equal quality. Therefore, the combination of increasing the number of generalists and the addition of nurse practitioners as primary care providers may drive down cost while maintaining access and quality. According to the Office of Management and Budget, nurse practitioners and physicians are offered scholarships by the National Health Insurance Service Corp. in exchange for their service to communities that lack health services and has placed over 20,000 professionals in communities that lack access to care (U.S. Office of Management and Budget, 1998).

subsidized via federal and state taxes (Levit et al., 1992). In 1960, the per-capita personal health care expenditures were $143, with $69 (48%) of that being out-of-pocket expenses. In 1999, per-capita health care expenditures had increased to $4358, with $622 (15%) as out of pocket. Note that the out-of-pocket expense decreased from 56% to 18% from 1960 to 1966 (HCFA, 2001a, Table 4). This dramatic decrease is due to the federal government and private and employer-based insurance programs taking a larger and larger role in financing of health care in the United States.

At first glance, the employment-based system seems to provide employees and dependents with insurance at very low costs, because employers generally pay most of the premium. Careful analysis, however, demonstrates that the employer's cost is largely shifted back to the employee in the form of lower wages and reduced benefits (Levit et al., 1992; Congressional Budget Report, 1993).

One of the most troubling developments in recent years is the increase in the number of employees and their dependents who do not have health insurance even though they are employed full time. This lack of coverage constitutes a particularly acute problem among certain groups of employees, such as those who work for small businesses or those who work for low wages, especially in the growing service sector of the U.S. economy. This expanding pattern is not accidental; rather, it reflects inherent weaknesses in the current system of employment-based insurance. As health care costs continue to grow unchecked, the disparity between those traditionally enjoying employment-based coverage and those uninsured in the small-business and service sectors will continue to grow.

According to the U.S. Census Bureau statistics for 1998, of the 274.5 million total U.S. population, 194.5 million were covered by private health insurance, and 66.2 million were insured by government programs. Also in 1998, there were 11 million children without health insurance (U.S. Census Bureau, 1998, Table 2).

According to the Agency for Health Care Policy and Research (1996), three primary factors influence the growing number of uninsured and underinsured citizens. First, employment-based insurance is voluntary. Second, insurance companies practice risk sorting and restrictive

ACCESS TO HEALTH CARE INSURANCE

No single nationwide system of health insurance guarantees access to health care in the United States. The United States relies primarily on employers to voluntarily provide health insurance coverage to their employees and dependents. Although the popularity of employment-based insurance plans can be explained, in part, by their cost advantage over individual plans, the major reason for their dominance is that such plans are

---

REFLECTIVE THINKING

Our Nation's Values in Health Care

If each nation's health care system is a reflection of its values, what values are being reflected in the U.S. health care system?

underwriting. Under these practices, employers are assessed premiums on the basis of the health experience of their employees. Employers with high-risk employees, such as smokers or employees with preexisting health conditions, pay higher premiums than do employers with low-risk employees. Third, some people rely on subsidized health care provided in the emergency rooms of public hospitals. The growing numbers of people who fall into this category are those who work 40 hours per week and do not have access to health care insurance, those who have been laid off, and the increasing numbers of homeless.

Health insurance obtained through the workplace is the primary source of private coverage for most Americans. Data from the 1997 Medical Expenditure Panel Survey (MEPS) (HCFA, 1997b) indicate that during the first half of 1996, on average, nearly two-thirds of nonelderly Americans (64.1%, or 148.5 million persons) obtained employment-related health insurance. The MEPS data also indicate that nearly one-fifth of nonelderly workers ages 16–64 (18.4%, or approximately 23 million persons) were without health insurance.

The importance of the workplace as a source of private health insurance, the incentives for inefficient health plan choice associated with the employment-based insurance system, and the size and composition of the employed uninsured population have constituted ongoing public policy concerns. Specific issues receiving attention have included availability disparities, out-of-pocket costs, and tax treatment of employment-based coverage for workers in different employment circumstances. The inability of some workers or their dependents with health problems to obtain such coverage and the gaps in the continuity of work-related health insurance during employment transitions will constitute major areas of focus of Congress over the next five years (White House Fact Sheet, 1998).

HEALTH CARE PROGRAMS

Health insurance mandated and subsidized by the federal and state governments and offered via employers is getting increased attention by the federal and state governments as a means of access to health care providers. For several decades, the United States has been faced with the problems of increasing numbers of uninsured and underinsured persons and rising health care costs. Options for insuring the growing numbers of uninsured and underinsured have become an increasingly important issue to policymakers, employers, and individuals as health care costs have skyrocketed in the last quarter of the 20th century. The projected health care costs for the last decade of the 21st century offer no comfort to these groups in the foreseeable future.

The uninsured and underinsured are affected by these facts because the lack of health insurance may create a bar-

rier to health care and thereby exacerbate or create health care problems that potentially are most costly and certainly detrimental to the health and well-being of this group. For the insured, the continually rising costs of health care may make insurance unaffordable at some point, thereby forcing them into the ranks of the uninsured.

There are more than 1200 private health insurance companies providing health insurance with various levels of coverage (HCFA, 2000c). Only state insurance commissioners regulate these companies; the federal government does not regulate insurance companies. This lack of national attention has led to a loosely structured delivery system organized at the local level and lacking federal or interstate influence on planning and coordination. There is little coordination between private and public programs.

Employment-Based Programs

The importance of the workplace as a source of private insurance, the incentives for inefficient health plan choice associated with the employment-based insurance system, and the size and composition of the employed uninsured population have been ongoing public policy concerns. These concerns have focused primarily on disparities in the availability, out-of-pocket costs, inability of some workers or their dependents with health problems to obtain coverage, and gaps in the continuity of work-related health insurance during employment transitions (HCFA, 2000c).

Nearly three-quarters (73.7%) of working adults ages 18–64 were covered by employment-related health insurance. However, working adults comprised half (50.4%) of the uninsured population under age 65 in 1998. Of all children uninsured throughout the first half

---

REFLECTIVE THINKING

Consumers' Understanding of Our Health Care System

- What do you think is the proper role of the federal government in meeting the health care needs of its citizens?
- How would you educate the public regarding what to expect from a health care system operated via managed care?
- How can nursing help the public understand that the resources available to provide health care to U.S. citizens are finite?

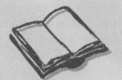

Out of the Box

City of Escondido, California

Health Care and Community Service Program

The goal of this innovative Health Care and Community Service Program is to reduce the harmful effects of alcohol and drug use in the community of Escondido. The program seeks to integrate a cross section of community services, including law enforcement, hospital emergency rooms, community health agencies and community health nursing. Unlike most alcohol and drug control programs, which target individuals already dependent on alcohol and drugs, the Escondido program seeks to identify users who are at risk of becoming dependent. Community health nurses (CHNs) play an active role in screening and referral services for this program. CHNs are ideally suited for this role because their role is to coordinate and integrate a wide range of acute and community health services for clients and communities.

Source: Institute of Medicine. *(1996). Using performance monitoring to improve community health: Conceptual framework and community experience.* Washington, DC: Author. ■

REFLECTIVE THINKING

Health Care Access and the Unemployed

Perhaps you have known persons who have lost a job and, therefore, health insurance coverage for themselves and/or dependents. Describe the ways that these individuals or families were able to meet health care needs.

- Did the provision of health care become a central focus?
- Did the individuals or families outwardly express concern over the possibility of someone's getting ill?

---

of 1998, about 90% were in households with a working adult. Working women were more likely than men to be covered by employment-related health insurance and were less likely to be uninsured. Minority workers, especially Hispanic workers, were far more likely than white workers to be uninsured. In work settings with fewer than 10 employees, 58.8% of wage earners had employment-related coverage and 30.4% were uninsured. In work settings with 500 or more employees, 91% of wage earners had employment-related coverage and only 6.7% were uninsured (U.S. Census Bureau, 2000, Table 177).

There were three primary reasons for the shift in who would be covered by health insurance. First, because the costs of providing health coverage rose at such alarming rates, the total number of employers who could offer this benefit decreased. Second, as copayments were introduced as a means of controlling and sharing health insurance coverage, the number of employees who could afford coverage decreased. Third, the distribution of work shifted from manufacturing to the service sector, the latter of which traditionally has not provided health

insurance coverage even for full-time work (U.S. Census Bureau, 1997).

Government Programs

Two governmental health care programs provide coverage for the aged, disabled, or poor: Medicare Parts A and B and Medicaid.

Medicare

Medicare is a national health insurance program for the aged and for some disabled persons. It is the largest health insurer in the United States. As of January 1999, Medicare covered 39.1 million people, including virtually all the elderly over age 65, or 34.1 million people, and certain persons with disabilities that included an additional 5.2 million people. The program is financed by a combination of payroll taxes, general federal revenues, and premiums (U.S. Census Bureau, 2000, Table 174). Table 6-3 lists the Medicare benefits for Parts A and B.

Medicare expenses are increasing faster than revenues, which, if expenditure controls are not enacted, could bankrupt the program early in the 21st century (Congressional Budget Office, 1995). There are numerous reasons for this path to bankruptcy, but primarily it is due to the fact that there will be fewer workers contributing to the program as our country's population ages. In 1960, there were five workers for each beneficiary and currently there are three (White House Fact Sheet, 1998). There has been rapid growth in Medicare payments from 1960 to 1999. In 1960 Medicare paid $7.3 billion, and in 1996 that figure had increased to $197.8 billion, or a $205.9 billion increase (HCFA, OA, 2000b).

Medicaid

The 2001 HCFA *Medicaid Bulletin* indicates that Medicaid is a health insurance program for certain categories of the poor and is administered by the states with federal matching funds. States have administered the program based on broad federal policies that govern the scope of services, the level of payments, and group eligibility. Federal Medicaid law (Title XIX of the Social Security Act) authorizes federal matching funds to assist the states in providing health care for certain low-income persons. The states have considerable flexibility in structuring their programs. For the most up-to-date information regarding Medicare and Medicaid, visit www.cms.hhs.gov.

EMERGING TRENDS

The trends in health care economics, those either enacted or under consideration, are put forth in great part to improve access, control costs, control the rapid implementation of technology so that costs and benefits can be assessed, and improve quality. Most would agree, however, that controlling costs is the paramount reason that employers, employees, third-party payors, and the federal and state governments are examining new mechanisms to provide health care.

Managed Care

Managed care has been a limited feature of the U.S. health care system for decades. The history of managed care shows the approach to have produced demonstrable savings over the better known fee-for-service system. Managed-care systems integrate the delivery of services and the financing of those services (Heshmat, 2001; Enthoven, 1993; Enthoven & Kronick, 1994). Iglehart (1994) notes that managed care is characterized by several factors:

1. Contracts with selected physicians and hospitals that furnish comprehensive health services exclusively to their members
2. Care delivered for a predetermined premium
3. Predetermined control over utilization
4. Members receiving financial incentives for receiving care from a single provider
5. Some associated financial risk on behalf of the contracting physicians

Examples of such programs are HMOs and the Medicare prospective payment program known as DRG. Among HMOs, Group Health of Puget Sound (1945) and Kaiser Permanente Medical Program (1940) have been very successful for over 50 years at providing prospectively financed health care with outcomes matching those of other health care delivery systems. These early HMOs met with such success in part because they were prepaid systems (managed care), they experienced very little competition given that the majority of health plans were fee for service, and they focused primarily on wellness (Heshmat, 2001; Finkler & Kovner, 2001; Enthoven & Kronick, 1994).

Managed Care in Medicare and Medicaid

Since 1993, the number of Medicare and Medicaid beneficiaries enrolled in managed-care plans has grown considerably. As a result, the Centers for Medicare & Medicaid Services (CMS), which administers these two programs, is the largest purchaser of managed care in the country, representing 36.5 million Americans (HCFA, OA, 2000c, Table 174).

As of February 1, 1999, almost 4 million Medicare beneficiaries—more than 10% of the total Medicare population—were enrolled in managed-care plans. This represents a 67% increase in managed-care enrollment since 1993. In 1995, an average of 68,000 Medicare beneficiaries voluntarily enrolled in HMOs each month. Medicare beneficiaries can enroll or disenroll in a managed-care plan at any time and for any reason with 30 days notice (HCFA, 1996). By 1996, of the 35.2 million recipients of

---

REFLECTIVE THINKING

Medicare and Medicaid

Do you know persons on Medicaid or Medicare?

- Are their health care needs being met?
- Do they fear hospitalization in terms of their financial viability? If so, what are they doing about it?

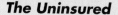

REFLECTIVE THINKING

The Uninsured

- How many persons or families do you know without health insurance?
- Of those persons or families, how many have full-time jobs but are still unable to afford health insurance?
- How do they meet their health care needs?
- Where and how do they seek health care?

Medicare, over 60% were enrolled in managed care (HCFA, 1997a).

Medicaid managed-care enrollment has grown even more. As of June 30, 1999, 17.8 million Medicaid beneficiaries were enrolled in managed-care plans, representing 55.6% of all Medicaid beneficiaries (HCFA, 1999).

The federal government grants two types of Medicaid waivers: Section 1915(b) "free choice" waivers and Section 1115 demonstrations. Freedom-of-choice waivers permit states to require beneficiaries to enroll in managed-care plans. To receive such a waiver, states must prove that these plans have the capacity to serve Medicaid beneficiaries who will be in the plan. States often use freedom-of-choice waivers to establish primary care programs and other forms of managed care. In 1995, five freedom-of-choice waivers were approved by HCFA, CMS's predecessor (HCFA, 1997a).

Section 1115 demonstrations allow states to test new approaches to benefits, service eligibility, program payments, and service delivery, often on a statewide basis. The approaches are frequently aimed at saving money so as to allow states to extend Medicaid coverage to additional low-income and uninsured people. Since January 1, 1993, comprehensive care reform demonstration waivers have been approved for 12 states, and 8 such waivers have been implemented. When all 12 have been implemented, 2.2 million previously uninsured individuals are expected to receive health coverage (HCFA, 1997a).

Managed Competition

Heshmat (2000) and Enthoven (1993) note that the precursor of the managed competition scheme is the prepaid group practice association such as Kaiser Permanente Medical Care Program and other HMOs. Enthoven defines managed competition as "a strategy whereby consumers and employers reap maximal value for each dollar spent" (p. 27).

Managed competition, based on microeconomic principles, focuses on providing the best care while also restraining costs, improving quality, and satisfying consumers and their employers. President Clinton's national health care reform movement relied heavily on the concept of managed competition. He envisioned organizing the competition around health insurance purchasing cooperatives (HIPCs) that would compete with each other to attract consumers and employers on the basis of value, outcomes, and satisfaction. Value, outcomes, and satisfaction would be accomplished via the HIPCs' providing a standardized health care package at a fixed, per-capita rate.

President Bush, in an interview with the *Economist* (September 30, 2000), prior to the presidential election, stated that he would rely on health insurance companies to compete in offering insurance to the public. As of August 2001, President Bush has been largely silent on this issue of managed competition since taking office in January 2001.

REFLECTIVE THINKING

Your Health Care Coverage

- How would managed care affect your access to health care?
- Would belonging to an HMO change your perspective of quality, cost, and access with regard to care?
- How has rationing of health care services affected your own state of health and well-being? Someone else's?

Rationing

In one form or another, the U.S. health care system has used rationing to control access and cost. In general, **rationing** takes two forms. Implicit rationing limits the capacity of a system and places specific dollar targets to that system so that the system may not exceed that amount. This usually requires the rationed system to prioritize services to be offered. A system would predetermine the services to be provided and the rate of reimbursement. This type of rationing is similar to the ethical concept of utilitarianism. Finite health care resources should be deployed so that they can do the greatest good for the greatest number of people. Explicit rationing, or the ability-to-pay scenario, is the most obvious strategy in the United States. The United States generally looks at health care as any other commodity or service to be purchased, which has made explicit rationing the dominant form of rationing in the United States. In an economic democracy, like the United States, as opposed to a social democracy, like Canada, a citizen's ability to obtain a service is determined by personal ability to pay for that service or by ability to obtain some sort of assistance (Medicaid) to obtain the service. Rationing of health care services and dollars is a very contentious topic in the United States. As the federal and state governments, insurance companies, HMOs, employers, and consumers attempt to control health care costs, the mechanism by which resources are allocated must change; however, some form of rationing will be necessary.

HEALTH CARE FINANCE AROUND THE WORLD

Containing the cost of health care has become a goal of virtually all countries. Abel-Smith (1992) studied the ways that European nations control the cost of health care and concluded that it is technically possible to control health care cost via governmental policies that regulate supply rather than demand. According to World Health Organization (WHO) statistics, in 1999, the United States outspent all European countries in per-capita health care expenditures. In terms of GDP, the United States outspends all other Western nations on health care.

In providing social services such as health care, the U.S. government historically has become involved when no remedy from the private sector could be found. In Europe, conversely, governments establish a level of health care for all citizens ("Patients or Profits," 1998).

In Europe, governments use finance controls as a means of controlling health care costs. Finance controls limit the flow of funds into health care, effectively placing a ceiling on spending with each fiscal year budget. European governments are also beginning to experiment with copayments as a means to increase consumers' awareness of the cost of their care (Enthoven, 1994). Moreover, utilization controls are used in Europe to control the supply of health care services (WHO, 1998).

The methods used by various countries to control costs differ according to the ways those countries organize and finance health care. Control is more easily attained when the government owns health care facilities and pays health care professionals on a salaried basis. Controlling cost is made more difficult when health care providers are under contract with the government and bill for services they provide. Many European countries use rationing as a means of controlling health care expenditures. Implicit rationing limits the capacity of the health care system, and the Europeans clearly use implicit rationing at every level of their health care systems (Reinhardt, 1993; Enthoven, 1994; "Patients or Profits," 1998).

As compared with the U.S. government, European governments take a much more active role in the provision and financing of health care. The primary reason for this is that most European democracies are social democracies, in sharp contrast to the economic democracy of the United States. Social democracies typically provide some level of cradle-to-grave health care subsidized by a heavy personal tax base.

Many Americans view the level of taxes paid by people in western European countries as oppressive. In many European countries, such as Sweden, France, England, Germany, and Norway, the federal tax liabilities of citizens can reach 50%–57% of total annual income, whereas in the United States our tax liability generally does not exceed 38% ("America's Bubble Economy," 1998).

The World Health Organization Report 2000

The WHO conducted the first analysis of the world's health systems, as discussed in Chapter 5. Two of the five indicators used to evaluate the 191 countries (members of WHO) included fairness of financial contribution (the fraction of household's capacity to spend money on its health care) and per-capita health expenditures. The report noted that there was wide variation in performance, even among countries with similar levels of income and health expenditures. The report also stated that the impact of failures in health care systems is most

severe on the poor everywhere and the poor are driven deeper into poverty by the lack of financial protection against illness. Moreover, the poor are treated with less respect, given less choice of service providers, and offered lower quality care (WHO, 2000). For additional information regarding the WHO World Health Report, visit www.who.org.

The WHO report goes on to say that the main failings of many health care systems are that (1) many governments fail to prevent a black market in health, where widespread corruption, bribery, and low income of health workers further undermine those systems, and (2) many health ministries and departments fail to enforce regulations that they themselves have created or are supposed to implement in public interest. For additional information on the WHO World Health Report, see Chapter 5.

HEALTH CARE ECONOMICS AS AN EXPRESSION OF CARING

With the advent of the national health care reform debates of the mid-1990s, the United States appears to be on the verge of associating the economics of health care with what some have called a moral imperative to provide basic health care services to *all* citizens of this country. As pointed out in Chapter 1, Fry (1994) defines caring as a moral concept whereby efforts of caring are directed toward meeting human need and caring is perceived as a *duty* to respond to that need. As indicated in the current chapter, European countries have long ago established that they have a moral obligation to provide basic health care service to their citizens, health care service that ensures access and quality while controlling costs.

Nurses in the United States are in a unique position to help ensure that the economics of health care in this country reflects the ways that neighborhoods, communities, cities, states, and the federal government *care* for themselves and for their most vulnerable citizens. For nurses, this represents a nationally focused expression of caring. Nursing organizations such as the American Nurses Association (ANA) have called for federally defined minimum standards for essential health care services. The central premises of ANA's health plan are as follows:

1. All citizens must have equitable access to essential health care services.

2. Primary care should play a more prominent role in health care in the United States.

3. Consumers must assume more accountability for their care.

4. A better balance must be created between the traditional illness and cure model and a wellness and care model.

5. Consumers must be protected from the costs of catastrophic illness (ANA, 1995).

As discussed in Chapter 8, Leininger (1981) posits that a culture guides decisions and actions. For nurses to be effective in changing the U.S. health care system so that it provides services to vulnerable populations, they must first understand the historical reasons for the establishment of that system. Knowing the traditional roles of the state and federal governments gives the nurse the historical perspective needed to take action without returning to past federal policies that no longer meet the health care needs of millions of U.S. citizens. The U.S. health care system has rarely changed quickly in relation to need; rather, it has changed incrementally. Enthoven (1994) notes that legislated change, while being necessary, fundamental, and far reaching, cannot be sudden and bear no resemblance to the past. Change that is so radical as to totally negate the past is much more difficult to accept than change that is balanced with some of the old and the new.

Nurses make up the single largest group of professional health care providers in the United States. United and coordinated efforts on the part of professional nursing organizations could bring about the needed change within our health care system via the paradigm of caring. However, it is necessary to first fully understand the source and evolution of the current "you're on your own" paradigm and the ways that the paradigm of caring (the moral duty to meet human needs) can be initiated to bring about desired changes. Specifically, all nurses must have a clear understanding of the economics of care. Without understanding the ways that our economic democracy operates, nurses stand little chance of influencing it. Nurses must also learn ways to be political at every level of health care—institutional, local, state, and federal. Politics has been described as the art of the possible. Without active and informed participation, however, nothing is possible.

A paradigm is a model or a way of thinking (Barker, 1992) and is amenable to change if certain conditions exist. New paradigms appear and are considered for implementation when old ways no longer serve the intended purpose. In other words, less effective paradigms take increasingly more time, money, and effort to solve increasingly fewer problems. This accurately describes the present condition of the U.S. health care system. How can nurses effect the paradigm shift from economics of overspending and serving increasingly fewer people to economics as an expression of caring for *all* citizens?

First, nurses must understand the theories of macro- and microeconomics as applied to health care. Economics should be a part of undergraduate education to facilitate a broad understanding of the U.S. health care system and its spending habits. At the undergraduate level, students should study the economic as well as the social bases of health care. They should prepare budgets and analyze budget reports for positive and negative variances and the causes of those variances. No student should graduate from an undergraduate program if he or she cannot prepare and analyze a budget and understand and document the cost of the care that health professionals provide. Furthermore, nursing undergraduates should have gained a clear understanding of the macro- and microeconomic pressures that influence the allocation and spending of health care dollars at the institutional and local levels.

At the graduate level, particularly in nursing leadership and management programs, economics should be required for a minimum of one semester and, ideally, two semesters. These courses should focus on macro- and microeconomics as applied to managed care, managed competition, and global budgets. The usefulness of economic theory as a means of better understanding the ways that the U.S. health care system is financed should also be emphasized. At the graduate level, nursing students must be able to prepare and defend a workable business plan for any health care service or institution.

✳ DECISION MAKING

Your Curriculum and Health Care Economics

◆ How could your school of nursing better prepare you to manage the health care resources in community health nursing?

◆ Make a formal recommendation to your faculty on how they could incorporate contemporary health care financing trends into the curriculum at your school.

REFLECTIVE THINKING

Is the Government Responsible for Providing Health Care?

• Does the U.S. government have a moral obligation to provide health care for its citizens?

• Given that limited amounts of money are available to spend on health care, to whom would you give care first? Last? State the rationale for each of your answers.

• How does your community express its desire to care for its vulnerable citizens?

Perspectives... ✳

"Your Money or Your Life," "Patients or Profits," and "Where Has the 'Caring' in Health Care Gone?"—all headlines from U.S. publications and all referring to managed care. About 10 years ago, a few hospitals and health systems in California tried to curb costs by rationing health care. The momentum grew, and currently, 160 million U.S. citizens are insured by a managed-care insurance policy. The managed-care industry has become one of the newest, largest, least understood, and perhaps most reviled aspects of the U.S. health care system.

As managed-care companies continue to squeeze out traditional health insurance, clients are often caught unaware of newly placed restrictions on access and treatments, and nurses and physicians are concerned about both the state of health care for their clients and the health of their practices. Meanwhile, politicians are scrambling to introduce changes in managed care that please everyone—especially the voting public.

It is hard to dispute that managed-care companies are very unpopular. The news is not all bad, however. Before managed care came to the United States, health care costs were rising at an alarming rate. The United States spends more money per capita on health care than does any other Western nation, yet it does not rank number one in numerous outcome measures. Under managed care, the rate of inflation with regard to health care costs slowed somewhat, a feat achieved without a measurable drop in the quality of care. The best HMOs—and, yes, there are good HMOs—have devised techniques to allocate resources and measure outcomes, techniques that the rest of the world might replicate.

There is little doubt that terrible mistakes have been made under managed care; however, a question that must be asked is whether such mistakes also happened under other forms of insurance and care. Because the emphasis in managed care appears to be strictly cost instead of cost *and* quality, many Americans believe that cheaper health care equates with poor-quality health care. The evidence suggests, however, that the HMO movement has saved money while maintaining previous standards of care.

Standards of care are much harder to measure than is money. For instance, it is impossible to demonstrate a link between health care delivery and life expectancy. Lifestyle choices such as diet, exercise,

stress reactions, smoking, and substance abuse are not under the control of the HMO; yet poor choices in these areas greatly contribute to morbidity and mortality in the United States. Diet, level of stress, and whether to exercise, smoke, or abuse substances constitute individual choices—choices about which far too many Americans still seem to make poor decisions. If we are ever to change the way Americans view their part in maintaining their health and in promoting wellness, HMOs may be a route to doing so because they emphasize not only treatment of episodic illness but, more importantly, prevention.

The inability of the traditional fee-for-service systems to provide effective preventive care may contribute to the fact that the average American is no fitter than citizens in countries where far less is spent per capita on health care. Diabetes is a good basis on which to compare the health of Americans with that of citizens of other nations. In 1990, Americans with diabetes were twice as likely as their British counterparts to go blind or to have a limb amputated. Why? The British Health Service, which operates on a limited budget per citizen, appears to be more effective in ensuring that clients take their insulin, have regular eye exams, and generally manage diet and insulin more effectively.

Our government may play a very large role in what appears to be variation in health care quality across the nation. For Medicare alone, the federal government imposes over 22,000 pages of rules and regulations. Via overwhelming numbers of regulations that are at times more confusing than helpful, the government is attempting to micromanage health care. Many of these micromanagement regulations mandate specific treatments for specific conditions. This essentially forces the practitioner, whether nurse practitioner or physician, into a boiler plate or cookie cutter approach to health care. Many nurse practitioners and physicians feel these regulations interfere with the client-provider interaction.

Instead of the government (local, state, or federal) being seemingly always at battle with HMOs, providers, and the employers who purchase health care plans for their employees, we desperately need to develop a national health care policy that takes into account the nature of our economic system. We believe that Oregon and Hawaii are on the right track. These two states have decided that there is indeed enough money to cover the

(continues)

Perspectives...

health care costs of their citizens and have engaged their citizens, insurers, governmental agencies, and employers in dialogue regarding meeting the health care needs of their citizens. The jury is still out on whether their efforts will be effective in the long run, but Oregon and Hawaii have instituted important changes that we should watch with an open mind.

The American health care system must continue to change. The types of change and the effectiveness of the changes should be guided by all of us—insurers, providers, citizens, and governments. Rather than holding on to a health care system that has served to maintain a lifestyle for a select number of providers at the expense of far too many citizens of this great country, our priority should be engaging in open, collaborative dialogue that focuses on system and individual accountabilities to ensure quality health care for all.

—Robert Geibert, RN, EdD
Wendy Smith, RN, DNS

COMMUNITY NURSING VIEW

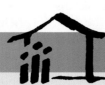

Mrs. Yu has been referred to you for home care. She lives alone and has just left the hospital after two weeks, including three days in intensive care. She had been on a drinking binge for a week before her admission and was admitted to the hospital for severe esophageal and rectal bleeding. She was diagnosed with esophageal varices and rectal cancer. As soon as her esophageal bleeding was controlled, the rectal cancer was removed and she was given a colostomy. She was sent home with instructions for colostomy care and a warning that continued drinking would lead to further esophageal bleeding. You are making your first visit to her to supervise her colostomy care. The first question she asks is, "How much is all this going to cost me? I have no health care coverage and I'm afraid the cost will clean me out!" You know that her finances are good and she is expecting to pay for her hospital and home care. You realize that she speaks little English and will not understand her hospital bill, nor will she be able to easily contact the hospital and home care agency to get her questions answered. You want to help Mrs. Yu find answers to her questions.

Nursing Considerations

Assessment

◆ What information do you need to help Mrs. Yu understand the costs of her care?

◆ What agencies can you contact that can give you the information you need—not just for Mrs. Yu but for clients who use other agencies?

◆ If you can't get the data from the agencies, who else can you ask?

◆ What other information do you need to know about costs?

Diagnosis

◆ Is there a diagnosis that would apply in this situation?

Outcome Identification

◆ What is the outcome you expect to achieve?

Planning/Interventions

◆ How will you calculate the health care finance information you will need?

Evaluation

◆ How would you evaluate your results?

Graduate students must have a better understanding of economics in general. For advanced-practice nurses to fully participate in the economic health of their organizations, they must be able to actively and intelligently participate with other financial professionals. Nurses must learn that they can advocate simultaneously for the wellness of the client and the wellness of the organization.

A second means of effecting the paradigm shift is for nursing organizations and places of employment to further their efforts at getting nurses involved in the political aspects of the economics of the U.S. health care system. All economic policies are the result of a political process, a process that generally eludes most nurses. It is therefore imperative that nurses become familiar with and involved in the political process of health care policy formation, implementation, and evaluation (see Chapter 18).

Third, nurses must make their concerns known to candidates, office holders, and lobbyists who shape the national and, therefore, state and local health care systems. Such involvement on the part of nurses is central to bringing about a health care system that operationalizes caring in a financially responsible manner.

Economics will play an ever-increasing role in professional nursing. Because health care policy and economics are linked, nurses must increase their knowledge regarding economic principles and the ways that those principles affect the health of the nation. Community health nurses have long been committed to maintaining and improving the health of U.S. citizens. In order to fulfill this commitment, nurses must become health care economists who insist on full participation in the policies that shape the systems in which they work.

Because health care in the United States is a dynamic process, students should visit government web sites to obtain the latest information. Throughout this chapter there are web addresses that will facilitate your search.

This author encourages readers to become active participants in health care policy. According to the U.S. Census Bureau, in 1998 there were 2.2 million nurses with active licenses and only 678,649 physicians with active licenses, yet physicians appear to have more influence in policy development than do nurses. For additional information on how and why nurses need to be more politically active, see Chapter 18. Also, by using an Internet search engine such as Lycos or Google, you can search the web for health care public policy sites that contain additional information, such as www.aarp.org (the American Association of Retired Persons), www.ana.org (the American Nurses Association), or www.ons.org (the Oncology Nursing Society).

KEY CONCEPTS

- Nurses must thoroughly understand how the U.S. health care system functions in order to affect it in ways that promote wellness.

- Reasons for the rise in health care costs include rising cost per volume of service, per-capita increase in volume of services, growth in specific population groups, advanced technology, rising administrative costs, client complexity, excess capacity, uncompensated care, and health care fraud.

- The major financial trends in the U.S. health care system are primarily focused on controlling increases in health care expenditures at the local, state, and federal levels.

- Government has become the agency of cost control, access, and quality through programs such as Medicare and Medicaid.

- Cost control mechanisms include DRGs, managed care, managed competition, global budgeting, and rationing.

- These cost controls primarily use three strategies: finance controls, reimbursement controls, and utilization controls.

- There is no nationwide system of health insurance that guarantees access to health care in the United States. Thus, many people do not have any health insurance or are underinsured.

- Three primary factors influence the growing number of uninsured and underinsured: Employment-based insurance is voluntary, insurance companies practice risk sorting and restrictive underwriting, and some people go without insurance because they are relying upon subsidized health care provided in the emergency rooms of public hospitals.

- Our health care system is divided into private and government sectors.

- Most European governments establish a level of health care for all citizens. They use financial and utilization controls to control spiraling health care costs. Their citizens bear the burden of high taxes to finance the health care system.

- Caring and economics are not antithetical concepts.

- Nurses must be aware of and active in politics and policy formulation, and they must understand how our health care systems are funded in order to change them.

RESOURCES

Centers for Medicare & Medicaid Services (formerly the Health Care Financing Administration): www.cms.hhs.gov
Office of Management and Budget: www.omb.gov/budget
U.S. Census Bureau: www.census.gov
National Institutes of Health: www.nih.gov
White House: www.whitehouse.gov

Unit

III

FOUNDATIONS OF COMMUNITY HEALTH NURSING

The foundational knowledge required for application of caring in all community settings in which nurses serve aggregates is discussed in Unit III. The knowledge includes the study of philosophical, cultural and spiritual, and environmental perspectives, communication, teaching and learning, and health promotion and disease prevention.

IN THIS UNIT

Chapter

7

PHILOSOPHICAL AND ETHICAL PERSPECTIVES

Nancy Kiernan Case, RN, PhD

MAKING THE CONNECTION

The ethically preferred world is one in which creatures are caring and cared for. Its institutions support and sustain caring while simultaneously reducing the need for care by eliminating the poverty, despair, and indifference that create a need for care.

—Manning, 1992, p. 29

COMPETENCIES

Upon completion of this chapter, the reader should be able to:

- Cite major ethical theories and principles that apply to community health nursing practice.
- Discuss the effect of a caring perspective on ethics in community health.
- Describe the essential components in an ethical decision-making model.
- Demonstrate the application of an ethical decision-making model in a dilemma that may occur in community health nursing.

KEY TERMS

autonomy	moral obligation
beneficence	nonmaleficence
best interest judgment	principlism
deontology	substituted judgment
ethics	teleology
fidelity	utilitarianism
justice	veracity
moral agency	

Chapter 1 clearly presented caring as an essential feature of community health nursing practice. Caring is also an essential feature of evolving models of health care ethics (Gastmans, Dierckx de Casterle, & Schotsmans, 1998; Leininger, 1990; Manning, 1992; Sherwin, 1992; Taylor, 1998). Such models incorporate traditional theories and principles in the search for guidelines to live morally good lives and to develop ethical professional practice. **Ethics** is the study of the nature and justification of principles that guide human behaviors and are applied when moral problems arise. The role of the professional community health nurse demands practice that bears moral responsibility for individuals, families, and communities as they grow toward full health potential.

This chapter discusses clients' rights and professional responsibility in community health, summarizes applicable classical ethics theories and principles, sets the ethical framework within caring, provides guidelines for ethical decision making, and examines some of the ethical issues unique to community health nursing practice.

CLIENT RIGHTS AND PROFESSIONAL RESPONSIBILITIES IN COMMUNITY HEALTH

The recognition of a client's rights concerning health care is considered one of the extensions of basic human rights (Annas, 1978). The right to health care is one of the basic human rights of clients recognized by the health care delivery system, in particular the public health system (Christoffel, 2001). Public health ethics "critiques current practices and suggests ways to construct healthy societies without stigmatizing individuals or groups" (p. 341). Of course, there are other client rights that are important, such as the rights to informed consent, to privacy, and to refuse treatment. However, the major focus of this discussion will be on the right to health care.

The right to health care is a right to goods and services to improve and maintain the health that exists. It refers to a client's claim against the state or its agencies to provide certain types of health care services (Daniels, 1979). The right to health care has stimulated a considerable amount of discussion and debate in the United States, such as what the government should provide, how access can be assured, and what services should be provided and by whom (Munson, 2000). Even with these debates the issues have not been resolved.

In the 21st century, these discussions will continue with greater focus on the role of the government and of the private sector in the allocation of health services. Societal obligations to citizens regarding basic health services and the responsibilities of health care providers in response to the client's right to health care must be explored. Equitable access to health care will continue to be a challenge for both the public and private health care sectors.

In response to client rights, community health nurses have responsibilities or duties that they are obligated to perform. In addition to caring, advocacy, and veracity, one of the major responsibilities is accountability. Moral accountability is addressed in the American Nurses Association (ANA, 1985) *Code for Nurses*. Moral accountability in nursing practice means that nurses are answerable for how they promote and protect health, as well as prevent disease and injury, while respecting client rights to self-determination in health care.

In community health nursing, whose primary emphasis is on aggregates rather than individual clients, moral accountability means that nurses are accountable for how the health of population aggregates is promoted, protected, and met. The moral accountability requires a consideration of "what we, as a society, do to collectively assure the conditions in which people can be healthy" (Darragh & McCarrick, 2000, p. 339). In community health nursing, nursing actions are guided not only by the professional ethic of nursing but also by the public health ethic, which places emphasis on the provision of accessible and available health services to maximize the health of the community. Thus, the need to explore ethical issues related to the right to health care is not new but has gained importance recently, particularly since the U.S. health care system continues to undergo major transformation due in part to factors associated with the high cost of health care, burgeoning technology, increased awareness by a population informed in part through easier access to the Internet, and a rapidly growing aging population whose longevity is also increasing.

CLASSICAL ETHICAL THEORIES AND PRINCIPLES

Rapid advances in science and health care technology have precipitated a dramatic rise in the ethical dilemmas confronting health care professionals and the people to whom they provide care. The identification of vulnerable populations, such as those with HIV or AIDS, the poor and under- or un-insured, increasing numbers of immigrants with little understanding or acceptance of the U.S. health care system (Fadiman, 1997), or the growing population of elderly without health care services, also contributes to current ethical dilemmas in health care. Ethical dilemmas occur whenever ethical principles conflict. In such dilemmas, more than one resolution may be justifiable, but no one resolution satisfies all of the perspectives involved. Regardless of the setting, every nurse must anticipate ethical dilemmas in professional practice. Each nurse must be prepared to address the dilemmas by acquiring a thorough understanding of the theories, principles, decision-making models, and mechanisms to facilitate sound ethical decisions. Community health nurses face ethical dilemmas specific to their area of practice. Basic theories and principles provide universal guidelines for an underlying approach to ethical issues regardless of the setting for health care.

Basic Ethical Theories

Understanding ethical theories and principles is helpful to nurses in approaching ethical issues and decisions. It is important to remember that ethical theories are guides that are useful only in providing meaning for moral experience. Ethical decisions in health care are guided primarily by two classical ethical theories: deontology and teleology or, more specifically, one form of teleology called utilitarianism.

Deontology

Deontology is the classical ethical theory based on moral obligation or duty. **Moral obligation** refers to the duty to act in certain ways in response to moral norms. This theory suggests that the moral rightness or wrongness of human actions is determined by the principle or the motivation on which the action is based. From the deontological perspective, the consequences of an action neither drive ethical decisions nor serve as guides for ethical justification (Beauchamp & Childress, 1994; Beauchamp & Walters, 1999; Monagle & Thomasma, 1998; Munson, 2000). Beauchamp and Childress (1994) indicate that the determination of rightness or wrongness of human actions may be based on religious traditions, an appeal to divine revelations, or intuition and common sense.

Utilitarianism

Utilitarianism is one form of teleology. **Teleology** is the ethical theory that determines rightness or wrongness solely on the basis of an estimate of the probable outcome. Unlike deontology, **utilitarianism** is based on usefulness or utility rather than moral obligation or duty. According to utilitarianism, the rightness or wrongness of human actions is determined by an assessment of outcomes. The utility of an action is decided on the basis of whether that action would bring about the greatest number of good consequences and the least number of evil consequences and, by extension, greater good than evil in the world as a whole (Beauchamp & Childress, 1994).

To assist in distinguishing between the two theoretical positions, consider the issue of lying or withholding the entire truth concerning an issue. A deontologist's perspective suggests that lying, under any circumstances, is wrong because it violates the moral duty of veracity (truth telling). According to deontology, humans have a moral obligation to tell the truth regardless of the consequences. On the other hand, the utilitarian might argue that there are known circumstances in which lying would

---

REFLECTIVE THINKING

What Is Your Code of Ethics?

- Do you believe that some actions are absolutely wrong in all circumstances? Give examples.
- Do you believe that you have an innate knowledge of right and wrong?
- How did you learn right and wrong? What was the influence of your parents? Society? Other forces?
- What are your thoughts about the ways that beliefs concerning right and wrong originate? To what degree do you believe that rules about right and wrong originate from a universal source? From within oneself?

Adapted from *Ethics and Issues in Contemporary Nursing,* by M. A. Burkhardt and A. K. Nathaniel, 1998. Clifton Park, NY: Delmar Learning.

bring greater good and fewer evil consequences. Consider the circumstance of lying to an evildoer, one who would do unwarranted harm to an individual. If one lied to conceal the whereabouts of the individual, the utilitarian would evaluate the action as moral because of the greater good consequences. The utilitarian would argue that a world of such decisions would promote greater good than evil, despite the violation of the moral duty to tell the truth. The deontologist, however, would focus on the violation of the duty of veracity, declaring the act of lying ethically unjustifiable.

Another example to illuminate the differences between deontology and utilitarianism is the issue of abortion. Abortion, even to save the life of the mother, remains unjustifiable to the deontologist because the action violates the moral duty to preserve life and to avoid killing. To the utilitarian, however, preserving the life of the mother may be justified by the greater number of positive (good) consequences. Preventing the death of the mother by aborting the fetus may allow the woman to return to her family, spouse, and other children or to contribute to society in general. The abortion of the fetus, while tragic to the utilitarian, represents fewer bad consequences than allowing the mother to die.

Although many health care professionals consider themselves utilitarians, an understanding of deontology is particularly helpful when ethical principles conflict. The ability to establish priorities among ethical principles or to establish the moral weight of ethical principles is fundamental to deontology. When confronted with ethical dilemmas, most health care professionals operate from a perspective carefully derived from aspects of both major classical theoretical positions.

Basic Ethical Principles

Several ethical principles that evolve from ethical theory apply in conflicts that occur in health care ethics. Beneficence, nonmaleficence, justice, and autonomy are among the ethical principles that influence decisions in health care ethics. Ethical rules represent another level of ethical perspective beyond theories and principles. Fidelity, veracity, and accountability are three ethical rules that exert a strong influence in community health nursing.

Beneficence

Beneficence is the principle of promoting the legitimate and important aims and interests of others, principally by preventing or removing possible harms (Beauchamp & Childress, 1994; Beauchamp & Walters, 1999; Monagle & Thomasma, 1998; Munson, 2000). Because promoting the welfare of clients is explicit in the role of the professional nurse, beneficence becomes a complicated issue when benefit to one client conflicts with other ethical requirements, such as benefit to another client, agency goals,

and other ethical principles such as client autonomy or the fair distribution of resources. Nurses must also consider whether client benefit should reflect overall benefit or be limited to health benefit.

As an example, a nurse's insistence on a low-sodium diet for an elderly client provides the greater health benefit for that client yet denies the client control over dietary choices and, thus, may deny the client pleasure, a sense of life quality, and autonomy (the experience of control over one's destiny). Underlying these considerations are significant questions regarding the meaning of benefit and who should define benefit in real-world treatment decisions. Is it the responsibility of the care provider, the client, or the client's family to decide the importance of dietary restrictions? In community health, the partnership between client and provider in decision making is essential (Ladd, Pasquerella, & Smith, 2000).

Nonmaleficence

Nonmaleficence is the ethical principle that requires the care provider to do no harm. From an ethical perspective, nonmaleficence carries greater moral weight than does beneficence. A nurse must first be assured of doing no harm (nonmaleficence) before being ethically justified in trying to help or promote the legitimate interests of the client (beneficence). In illustration, consider a community health nurse who wishes to respect the right of a client to confidentiality regarding information about a disease state such as HIV status. That nurse must first be assured that keeping such information confidential for one client will not put other clients or the community at risk.

The avoidance of harm also seems inherent in the provision of professional nursing care. In practice, however, the nurse must constantly reflect on the multiple definitions and meanings of harm as well as on who is defining the term, remembering that the care provider's definition of harm may not coincide with that of the care recipient or the community.

Recent changes in the health care environment, particularly critical shortages of nurses in many parts of the United States, mean that nurses may be confronted with increased client loads in the face of reductions in time and resources. In such instances, the nurse must first be convinced that the reduction of resources has not also compromised the quality of care in a manner that exposes the client to increased risk. When safety and quality of care are affected, the nurse is morally justified in providing care (beneficence) only after being assured that no harm (nonmaleficence) will come as a result of the reduction in resources.

A less complex example of the moral weight of nonmaleficence over beneficence is the common ethical struggle of the nurse who becomes mildly ill and debates the benefits and burdens of seeing clients and, therefore, exposing them to the ailment or staying home to prevent such exposure but thereby denying care for those clients on that day.

Justice

Justice is the principle of fairness that is served when an individual is given that which is due, owed, or deserved. The principle of justice or fairness may be examined from two different perspectives. That which individuals feel is their due or is owed them, such as the political right to vote or the economic right to a fair wage, is evaluated or perceived as a benefit (entitlement theory). Responsibility owed by individuals to society, such as military conscription or taxes, may be evaluated or perceived as a burden. Both benefits and burdens are thus incorporated within the principle of justice.

In the current atmosphere of health care reform and increased recognition of the limitations of health care resources, the principle of justice, especially the more focused principle of distributive justice, takes on great importance. Distributive justice refers to the fair distribution and allocation of resources within the population. The importance of the principle of justice must be evaluated in light of benefits and burdens to individuals, groups in the community, and society in general.

The principle of justice, especially when applied to the allocation of scarce resources, is extremely complex. Although justice fundamentally suggests that equals should be treated equally (egalitarian theory), there are examples in which unequal treatment is more just. In such an instance, an individual or group with a greater need receives a greater share of the resource under consideration. Competing interests are thus treated unequally but, perhaps, more fairly. An example of unequal but fair treatment occurs when a child with a chronic disease, such as cystic fibrosis, receives more of the available health care resources, such as home visits or access to necessary medications, than does a child with no chronic disease.

In a situation where the equal distribution of agency resources, such as personnel or time, results in care for all agency clients that is below a minimal standard of care, justice may be served better by the unequal distribution of the agency's resources. In other words, if the even distribution of a nurse's time leaves insufficient time at each visit for appropriate wound care for all clients, justice and client care may be served better by dividing the nurse's time on the basis of clinical criteria such as acuity of the wound or availability of other resources for each client than by simple division of the nurse's time. The requirement to prioritize resources according to need may be judged as unfair by those whose access to those resources is limited as a result. Careful allocation of an agency's resources within established guidelines may ultimately provide the greatest benefit to the most clients. Policy decisions regarding environmental needs within a community constitute other examples of allocation decisions made under the principle of justice.

The determination of that which is owed may be based on individual effort, merit, need, societal contribution, rights, or simple equal division (Beauchamp, 2001; Beauchamp & Childress, 1994). Justice is a particularly important consideration in community health, an environment increasingly characterized by care limitations imposed by third-party payors. Limitations such as an arbitrary number of days of care for a given diagnostic category often do not coincide with individual disease trajectories or healing patterns and may not take into account the plans or policies within a specific community. In such instances, the community health nurse must discover a mechanism to perpetuate needed care for each client without jeopardizing the care available to all clients.

Autonomy

Autonomy, the principle of respect for persons, refers to an individual's right to self-determination. This principle of self-rule honors the right of competent individuals to make free, uncoerced, informed decisions while respecting the rights of others. Under the principle of autonomy, humans are recognized as unconditionally worthy, regardless of any special circumstances or that which they bring to others. Beauchamp and Walters (1994) emphasize the importance of the principle of autonomy:

> To respect the autonomy of self-determining agents is to recognize them as entitled to determine their own destiny, with due regard to their considered evaluations and view of the world, *even if it is strongly believed that their evaluation or outlook is wrong and even potentially harmful to them.* (p. 29)

Although in recent years the principle of autonomy has been influential in health care ethics, its influence is beginning to wane somewhat. Autonomy will likely remain a pivotal principle in community health ethics, however, primarily because of the shift in power that oc-

---

REFLECTIVE THINKING

Nonmaleficence and Beneficence

What should happen when the goal of the agency where you work is to provide a high level of care to all clients but one of your clients requires a greater percentage of your time and resources than the agency guidelines allow, or that is reimbursable?

curs when care is provided in the client's home or immediate environment rather than on the "turf" of the provider. Community health practice has led the way in developing partnerships between care providers and care recipients, especially for the purpose of making care decisions. Requirements for an adequate moral framework in community health nursing "must recognize the patient's decision-making authority and autonomy, . . . must allow the exercise of the nurse's moral rights, and . . . must recognize the patient's relationships to significant others" (Ladd et al., 2000, p. 105). Autonomy is thus a pivotal ethical principle in community health nursing.

Issues surrounding the harms that come from unhealthy lifestyles highlight ethical conflicts regarding autonomy. Clients who continue to smoke, eat poorly, refuse to exercise, or demonstrate inconsistency relative to medication or treatment routines may challenge the community health nurse's commitment to honoring the right of each client to make decisions (autonomy).

Informed consent, fidelity (promise keeping), and veracity (truth telling) all rely on the acceptance and exercise of autonomy. Informed consent requires that clients be given "the opportunity to choose what shall or shall not happen to them" (National Commission for the Protection of Human Subjects of Biomedical and Behavioral Research, 1978, p. 10); "affirming that every human being of adult years and sound mind has a right to determine what happens to his or her own body" (Teays & Purdy, 2001). This means that clients must be provided with the necessary information to make decisions about their health care. The information provided to them must be at a level that they understand, and the consent must be voluntary and free of coercion (Beauchamp & Childress, 1994). The rules of *confidentiality*, so important in community health, also receive moral weight from the principle of autonomy. Clients maintain the right to full, accurate information and to protection of intimate and private information necessarily shared in the health care setting. All information regarding a client belongs only to that client, and only that client may grant permission for that information to be released publicly. Respect for each person dictates meticulous attention to the handling of client and family information.

Fidelity and Veracity

Fidelity, or promise keeping, is a rule of ethics that is fundamental to nursing practice in community health. Caring practice is based in large part on the development of a trusting relationship between care provider and care recipient. The expectations inherent in such trusting relationships are based on fidelity. **Veracity,** or truth telling, may be considered a type of promise keeping and is also essential to a trusting relationship. When care is delivered in the community, balance within the relationship may shift to the care recipient, but fidelity and ve-

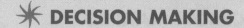

✳ DECISION MAKING

Outcomes of Client Empowerment

Upholding the view that clients know what they need opens nurses to the probability that some clients will make decisions that are inconsistent with what the nurse or other health team members think is best. Such decisions may have a relatively minor impact on a client's or family's health and well-being or may be judged to have potentially serious outcomes for the client or family.

◆ What factors must be considered when making decisions involving differing values between clients and nurses?

◆ Give examples of situations in which client empowerment might potentiate an ethical dilemma for you.

◆ If you thought that a client was making an unwise decision, how would you respond?

◆ Discuss your view regarding any limits or constraints on client empowerment.

Adapted from *Ethics and Issues in Contemporary Nursing,* by M. A. Burkhardt and A. K. Nathaniel, 1998, Clifton Park, NY: Delmar Learning.

racity remain the moral responsibility of the care professional. This is true despite the fact that the care recipient may have greater control than in an agency setting simply because care is provided in the recipient's home or immediate environment. It is helpful for the community nurse to foster, acknowledge, and honor this shift in the balance of power between professional care provider and care recipient.

Accountability

According to the ANA (1985), "accountability refers to being answerable to someone for something one has done. [It is] . . . grounded in the moral principles of fidelity and respect for the dignity, worth, and self-determination of clients" (p. 8). Safe, autonomous practice is ensured through various processes of nursing accountability. Accountability is related to both responsibility and answerability (Leddy & Pepper, 1998). Because of the trust accorded nurses by society (gained through recognition of nurses' expertise) and the right given the profession to regulate practice (professional autonomy), individual clinicians and the profession must be both responsible and accountable.

Related to the principle of autonomy and the concept of authority, accountability is an inherent part of

✳ DECISION MAKING

Ethics and Confidentiality

◆ What would you do with confidential information regarding substance abuse or potential domestic violence on the part of a family member who is not your client and is not under your care?

◆ What is the professional and *ethical* response of the community health nurse?

everyday nursing practice. Each nurse is responsible for all individual actions and omissions. The ANA *Code for Nurses with Interpretive Statements* makes it clear that each nurse has the responsibility to maintain ethical and competent practice regardless of circumstances, stating that "neither physicians' orders nor the employing agency's policies relieve the nurse of accountability for actions taken and judgments made" (1985, p. 9). The courts have tended to support this claim.

Many situations in community health care magnify the dilemmas that occur when the rights of some individuals conflict with the rights of other individuals, an agency, the community, or society or when ethical principles conflict with each other. "Increased recognition has been given to the fact that the health of individuals is intertwined with the health of their communities, the community's ability to provide preventive and primary

care services, and a multiplicity of related socioenvironmental factors that underlie health" (Higgs, Bayne, & Murphy, 2001, p. 3). Consider a situation in which a nurse providing care believes that as long as sufficient money is unavailable for full immunization programs, no money should be spent on organ transplantation programs, even to benefit a client. Further suppose that one of the clients to whom this nurse provides care is trying to raise public money for lung transplantation. The nurse's beliefs may interfere with his or her ability to provide adequate care to this client if those beliefs are not acknowledged and addressed.

Another situation often encountered in the community is that of disagreement among family members regarding the intensity of intervention in long-term care. If the client desires continued high-level intervention but the family feels unable to sustain such care, the nurse provider may feel caught in the conflict (Ladd et al., 2000).

Finally, the community health nurse may become involved in a case in which another agency is unable or unwilling to honor client decisions. A terminally ill teenager, for example, may have negotiated end-of-life decisions such as do-not-resuscitate (DNR) with family members, health care providers, and local emergency services but may find that school personnel are unwilling or unable to honor such an order while the teen is in school (Kuehl, Shapiro, & Sivasubramanian, 1992; Scofield, 1992; Strike, 1992; Younger, 1992).

Throughout health care, ethical principles sometimes conflict. A client's right to decide for self (autonomy) may conflict with the care provider's interpretation of that which is best for the client (beneficence) or what may ac-

TABLE 7-1 Ethical Principles Influencing Health Care Decisions

ETHICAL PRINCIPLE	DEFINITION	EXAMPLE
Beneficence	The principle of doing or promoting good that requires abstention from injuring others and promotion of the legitimate interests of others primarily by preventing or removing possible harms.	Teaching an elderly client about safety features in the home.
Nonmaleficence	The principle of doing no harm.	Not leaving a client in acute distress.
Justice	The principle of fairness that is served when an individual is given that which he or she is due, owed, deserves, or can legitimately claim.	Providing nursing services regardless of ability to pay.
Autonomy	The principle of respect for persons that is based on recognition of humans as unconditionally worthy agents, regardless of any special characteristics, conditions, or circumstances.	Allowing a client to refuse a home visit.
Fidelity	The principle of promise keeping. The duty to keep one's promise or word.	Making a home visit at the agreed-upon time.
Veracity	The principle of truth telling. The duty to tell the truth.	Being honest; being authentic.

tually harm the client (nonmaleficence). The allocation of scarce and precious resources on the basis of fairness (justice) may harm individuals or groups with lesser claims to those resources (nonmaleficence) yet provide the greatest good to the greatest number (utilitarianism).

Consideration of risks, benefits, and burdens must be an integral part of discussions surrounding these conflicts. Another challenge in the consideration of ethical rules, principles, and theories revolves around the question of whose rights prevail. Do the rights of a group or community automatically supersede the rights of an individual? The complexity of ethical issues demands a thorough, organized approach to adequately utilize ethical theories and principles in a context of care to facilitate appropriate resolution of conflicts. Table 7-1 summarizes some of the ethical principles influencing health care decisions.

PERSPECTIVES IN ETHICAL DECISIONS

Historically, ethical decisions in health care (bioethics and medical ethics) have relied almost exclusively on the formal application of ethical principles to resolve dilemmas. This system of theory and practice in ethics is known as principlism. In the past, **principlism** provided nurses, physicians, and the public with a simple and direct language and a structure within which to discuss the conflicts arising out of the rapid advances in health care technology that have spread to every aspect of the health care environment (DuBose, Hamel, & O'Connell, 1994).

Currently, health care ethics in the United States is moving toward the incorporation of broader perspectives in ethical dilemmas and decisions. Feminist, cross-cultural, and caring perspectives are among those moving health care ethics beyond principlism. There is great hope that the integration of these perspectives—especially the caring perspective—with principlism will promote greater understanding and acceptance of the meaning of the web of relationships that each individual brings to situations of ethical conflict. The diversity and complexity of the individuals, groups, and situations in the changing health care environment further highlight the need for broader perspectives. In an integrated ethical system, the principlist emphasis on autonomy and individual rights may become muted by the incorporation of community and societal values as well as by the interdependent relationships of the individual.

The caring perspective may help neutralize one criticism frequently directed toward principlism, that it "does not make space for emotion or take sufficient account of the notion of care in relationships" (DuBose et al., 1994, p. 3). Caring maintains the focus on the support, development, and importance of relationship. Therefore, the ethics of caring incorporates attention to specific, contextual relationship rather than to the abstract principles on which the principlist approach to ethical conflict and decision making is founded. In a feminist analysis of the limits of principlism, Gudorf (1994) points out that "more

social principles—mutuality, community, solidarity, empathy, nurturance, wholeness or integrity, and relationality itself—are not lifted up, despite our knowledge of their importance for individual as well as community growth, health, and healing" (p. 167). New approaches to health care ethics seek to incorporate perspectives from caring and feminism in a manner that modifies "both the body of relevant principles and their interpretation," recognizing the "need to connect the use of principles with an examination of the concrete situation of those most at risk" (Gudorf, 1994, p. 168) in the ethical debate.

THE DECISION-MAKING PROCESS

Ethical dilemmas occur when principles conflict with one another or when the duties, rights, beliefs, and values of an individual conflict with those of another individual, of an agency, or of the greater society (Mitchell, 1990). Understanding ethical theories, principles, and rules is only a first step in reaching ethically defensible resolution to conflict situations arising in community health. Conflicts regarding community health care revolve around issues such as the actual or potential abuse of clients or care providers; the continuation of care when reimbursement for that care is no longer available; obvious differences in lifestyle values such as diet or substance abuse; and demonstration by the client of values different from those of the professional care provider, particularly in relation to levels of intervention or to the determination of futility of care.

Application of ethical theories and principles must be made in a manner that facilitates the creation of moral space, or an environment in which the formation, discussion, and application of moral standards can occur (Walker, 1993). An environment that provides moral space and that respects the values of all of the participants is essential. It is vital to acknowledge the effects of the multiple allegiances that nurses hold, the types of decisions being made, and the perspectives driving the decisions.

A decision-making process should be established for every setting where there exists potential for ethical conflict. A large number of ethical decision-making models are available in the literature (Benjamin & Curtis, 1992; Aiken & Catalano, 1994; Husted & Husted, 1995; Monagle & Thomasma, 1998; Beauchamp & Walters, 1999). Regardless of the model, however, six components are essential for adequately addressing ethical dilemmas (see Figure 7-1).

Essential Components of Decision-Making Models

Six essential components contribute to the adequacy of ethical decision-making models. Prior to encountering an actual dilemma requiring urgent resolution, every nurse should select and practice the application of an ethical

---

FIGURE 7-1 Decision Model Components

Each model should have a means of determining:

- Those who are involved in the issue, the decision, and the outcome
- All relevant information—medical, physical, social, spiritual, psychological, economic, emotional, and relational
- Options for potential resolution of the issue
- A process for reaching resolution
- A plan for acting on the resolution
- A method of evaluating the process, the decision, and the outcome

---

decision-making model to gain facility in using a decision-making process.

Determining Involvement

Any decision-making model should provide a means of determining those who are involved in the decision making *and* in the outcome of the decision. Determining involvement requires a thoughtful approach to uncovering all those even subtly touched on by the issue under discussion. For example, nurses who may not be providing direct care to the client and family involved in the dilemma but have provided care to similar clients may still provide important insights and options based on prior experience. In addition, the outcome of the dilemma may have a direct effect on other nurses who provide similar care. It is very important to involve team members from each discipline in the process, especially in the collection of important information and the determination of appropriate actions.

Gathering Data

Decision-making models must also provide means of gathering all relevant information. Information gathered should be factual and should encompass medical, psychological, spiritual, social, economic, resource, and emotional data. Information should be obtained beyond the obvious diagnosis, prognosis, and treatment options.

The development of an adequate database is essential to making "good"—that is, ethically justifiable—ethical decisions. Data collection provides an opportunity for the nurse to identify, define, and refine issues and to determine ownership of the problem, of the consequences, of the information, and of the decision itself. The nurse must be instrumental in the determination of all of these facets of data gathering.

Outlining Options and Consequences

Outlining options to reach potential resolution of the dilemma is the third component of any adequate decision-making model. Inherent in this component is an exami-

nation of the likely consequences of each option under consideration. In order to remain open to all practical options, especially to options that represent opposing viewpoints, a mechanism to identify and temporarily set aside values is helpful. The importance of considering divergent views cannot be overemphasized in the context of caring. Divergent views may encompass differing values regarding such things as life quality, standards of cleanliness in the home, aggressiveness of care, alternative therapies, the meaning of spirituality, or lifestyle in general.

The ability to recognize values as components in the decision-making process is critical when a nurse is engaged in ethical decision making. Although values initially must be set aside to accommodate consideration of all potential options, values return to the discussion before a choice is made. Without a discussion of the values of all persons involved, the resolution sought may be ethically justified but remain acontextual.

Process for Resolving Conflict

The fourth component of an adequate decision-making model is an identified process for resolving conflict. A number of practical issues must be addressed within the scope of this component. In order for conflict resolution to occur, issues such as ultimate responsibility and accountability for decisions, ways to reach consensus, ways to communicate the consensus, and steps to take if agreement is impossible must be considered and agreed upon. A review of driving and restraining forces as well as the benefits, risks, and burdens of each option is also part of this process. The likelihood of a successful outcome also must be considered for each option. Selecting an option that cannot be acted upon within the confines of the law, for instance, would be counterproductive.

Planning for Action/Implementation

The fifth component of an adequate decision-making model is a plan for enacting the resolution. How is the decision to be carried out and by whom? Outlining options and consequences, resolving conflict, and enacting the resolution constitute the decision making itself.

Evaluation

The sixth and final essential component of an adequate decision-making model is a method of evaluation. This component encompasses evaluation not only of the decision but also of the consequences of the decision and of the decision-making process itself.

Together, then, these six components contribute to the adequacy of any decision-making model or framework, guiding whether the model is likely to foster ethically justifiable decisions. It should be clear that the process that occurs in ethical decision making parallels the nursing process utilized in clinical practice: gathering data—assessment; synthesizing data—analysis and diagnosis; outlining and selecting the options—planning; acting on the options—implementation; and evaluating the process and the decision—evaluation. On the basis of their experience in clinical decision making, nurses should thus feel confident in their ability to engage in ethical decision making. Figure 7-2 portrays an ethical decision-making model.

External Factors That Affect Decision Making

A number of factors affect the nurse's ability to make ethical decisions, even with an adequate decision-making model and experience in clinical decisions in place. Among these factors are the multiple allegiances that encumber the nurse in practice; the type of decision being made—medical, legal, or ethical; environmental factors, or the atmosphere of the work setting; resources for decision making, such as the presence of and access to a formal decision-making system or process; and personal and professional values. All of these factors reflect the medical, legal, economic, and societal schema within which health care ethical decisions are made.

Multiple Allegiances

Nurses in all clinical settings are subject to the complexities of multiple allegiances. Multiple allegiances affect the interpretation of ethical conflicts as well as the decision-making process itself. As care managers, most professional nurses consider their role as client advocate to be fundamental. As members of interdisciplinary care teams, nurses practice in various levels of collegial relationships with a diverse group of other care providers. In some community situations, particularly in home health or hospice, nurses depend on physicians' orders for part of the care they deliver. Many nurses in community health also provide independent care, engaging the client as an active participant in the care decision-making process. As clients and families become more active participants in the health care team, additional role definitions and allegiances evolve for the nurse in clinical practice. The caring relationship based on trust, integrity, and genuine presence on the part of the nurse is fundamental to the partnership between nurse and client.

 DECISION MAKING

Ethical Decision Making

◆ What would you do if a client did not tell the truth or withheld some information regarding care issues?

◆ Would your response be the same if the lack of truthfulness affected another family member? Another care provider? The client, but not in a manner related to the care you provide?

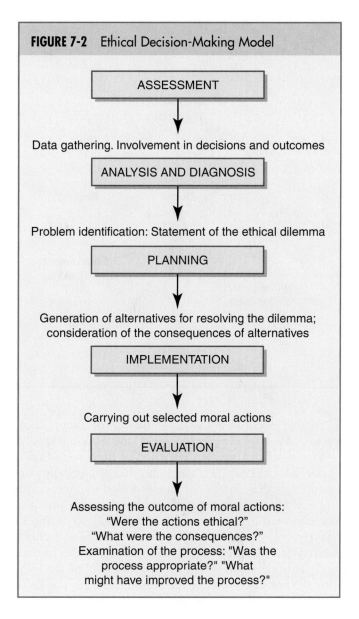

FIGURE 7-2 Ethical Decision-Making Model

ASSESSMENT

Data gathering. Involvement in decisions and outcomes

ANALYSIS AND DIAGNOSIS

Problem identification: Statement of the ethical dilemma

PLANNING

Generation of alternatives for resolving the dilemma; consideration of the consequences of alternatives

IMPLEMENTATION

Carrying out selected moral actions

EVALUATION

Assessing the outcome of moral actions:
"Were the actions ethical?"
"What were the consequences?"
Examination of the process: "Was the process appropriate?" "What might have improved the process?"

The nurse is usually an employee of an agency or institution. Nurses therefore owe additional allegiance to their employers. In the community or in independent practice, the professional nurse may owe yet another type of allegiance, that to third-party payors. Personal, professional, community, and societal allegiances also place demands on the nurse in practice. It is therefore critical that each nurse maintain clarity regarding the effects of each allegiance on ethical issues, inherent values, and decision making. Figure 7-3 illustrates the multiple allegiances of the nurse that may affect decision making.

Decision Types

In the face of ethical conflicts, clarity regarding the nurse's allegiances should accompany a similar clarity regarding the type of decision being made. Health care (or medical), legal, and ethical aspects of conflicts are inextricably intertwined. A "good" or justifiable decision according to the standards of one discipline may not be

FIGURE 7-3 Example of Multiple Allegiances That Affect Decision Making

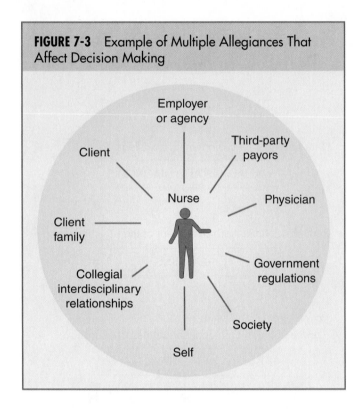

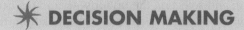

DECISION MAKING

Conflicting Duties

Ms. Washington is director of a local hospice service. Unrelated to her work with hospice, she serves on a statewide advisory board that makes recommendations about allocation of Medicaid services. In response to a dramatic decrease in federal appropriation, the board is mandated to recommend funding cuts to specific programs. Ms. Washington and other board members are asked to choose between eliminating funding for adolescent well-child screening programs that serve tens of thousands of youth or eliminating a single costly program that provides catastrophic assistance to only a few individuals. Because of her experience with hospice care, Ms. Washington recognizes the importance of programs to help with catastrophic illness; however, she is hesitant to advise eliminating a program that is proven to help large numbers of children.

◆ To what degree does Ms. Washington have a primary duty to see that catastrophic programs benefiting her hospice patients continue to be funded?

◆ As an advisory board member, what is Ms. Washington's responsibility to the large number of adolescents who would be denied health care if the well-child program for adolescents were no longer funded?

◆ What basis should Ms. Washington use for making her decision?

◆ How would you decide what to do in this situation?

Adapted from *Ethics and Issues in Contemporary Nursing*, by M. A. Burkhardt and A. K. Nathaniel, 1998, Clifton Park, NY: Delmar Learning.

justifiable according to the standards of other disciplines. As an example, consider the Hmong family, whose newborn son is diagnosed at birth with Down syndrome (trisomy 21). The infant has a surgically correctable cardiac defect commonly found in clients with trisomy 21. Without surgical intervention, the infant is not expected to live into early childhood. According to the Hmong's religious, spiritual, and cultural beliefs, surgery is forbidden; intentional cutting of the human body is understood to kill the spirit or soul of the individual. (For discussion of the Hmong culture, see Fadiman, 1997.) From a *medical* perspective, denying a simple, highly successful surgical repair of a cardiac defect represents a poor, unjustifiable decision.

From a legal perspective, Baby Doe rules and regulations should be considered. These regulations provide for the protection of handicapped infants against nontreatment decisions based on actual or potential handicap. (For a complete review, interesting discussion, history, and summary of the Baby Doe rules and regulations see Pence, 1990.) Babies with Down syndrome may face both mental and physical handicaps as a result of their genetic aberration and are therefore given protective consideration under the Baby Doe regulations. Although not legally binding, the regulations provide strong legal direction for health care decisions regarding infants with potential handicaps. From the legal perspective, decisions regarding care must not be made based on actual or potential handicaps. In the case of the Hmong infant, careful investigation must be undertaken to determine the motivation for refusing the surgery. From a *legal* perspective the decision is unclear, at best.

From an *ethical* perspective, sound decisions incorporate the significant values of everyone involved in the decision, particularly those who bear the greatest burden of the decision. Allowing the Hmong family to refuse surgery for their son because of their spiritual and cultural values represents an *ethically* justifiable decision that is *medically* unsound and *legally* in need of clarification. Supporting the genuine decision to love and care for their son within the confines of their own culture as an intact family committed to the natural consequences of refusing surgical intervention represents a contextual, caring, ethically justifiable decision. To suggest that the more desirable health care outcome resulting from surgery would be worth the ostracism and spiritual death of the Hmong family is to deny their moral experience and, furthermore, is based on values to which they do not ascribe.

Another example of the need to clarify the decision type involves the discipline of law. Numerous examples of legally sanctioned continued life support are questionable from the medical perspective and ethically unjustifiable or, at the very least, unsound. Without question, quality-of-life issues remain among the most poignant and complex ethical questions for care providers and recipients alike. Whenever confronted with an ethical dilemma, the community health nurse would be wise to seek clarity regarding the type of decision being made. It is inappropriate to claim ethical justification for a decision derived solely from the standards or values of another discipline—most often the discipline of law. Nursing practice requires adherence to the law, but actions dictated by law should not automatically be assumed to be justifiable ethically.

As conflicts arise—as they are bound to in our pluralistic, culturally diverse world—it is critical that participants in the conflict and the decision-making process openly acknowledge the various perspectives that drive decisions. Each individual's perspective must be respected because it affects the understanding and use of ethical theories, principles, and rules and the decision-making process.

Environmental Factors

Agency and institutional constraints continue to be imposed on nursing practice, affecting the nurse's ability to participate in ethical decision making. Although early discussions of such constraints implicated acute-care institutions, community care agencies have been shown to impose similar constraints. Since the late 1970s, nursing authors have identified some of the classic constraints on nurses. Sadly, many of these constraints still exist in the acute-care setting and have extended to other practice settings such as community health.

These constraints include the roles and social positions of the nurse, physician, and care administrator, particularly as they exist within bureaucratic settings; the role and power of nursing leadership within the health care system; sexism; paternalism; and any limitations imposed on nursing practice that prevent moral agency in the nurse. **Moral agency** is the ability of the nurse to act according to professional moral standards. Each of these factors may be found to varying degrees within the community health practice setting.

Because of the more independent nature of practice in the community, the community health nurse may be less constrained by bureaucracy than is the nurse in the acute-care setting, but agency administrators or governmental regulations may still inhibit the community health nurse in practice. Rules, regulations, policies, or procedures may assist in the smooth operation of an agency yet may present barriers to appropriate care for an individual client or be poorly suited to the needs of the community itself.

In community health, the role relationship within the bureaucracy may be focused on nonphysician care providers, family members, or third-party payors as well as on physicians. Support from nursing colleagues, leaders, or supervisors may not be available to the nurse in community practice, particularly as community practice models continue to grow and restructuring of the delivery system moves forward. As awareness has increased regarding the potential harm of sexism and the inappropriateness of paternalism in health care, the signs and symptoms of both have become ever more subtle. Addressing ethical dilemmas in community health demands a keen awareness of even subtle environmental factors that may affect the nurse's ability to create, maintain, and enhance caring within that environment.

The development of collegial interdisciplinary relationships must continue in order to meet the needs of all clients in community health. Again, the multiple allegiances that encumber nurses are reflected among the interdisciplinary relationships that influence the caring environment and decisions within that environment. Conditions may exist within the care environment that affect professional relationships and, therefore, the nurse's ability to care. Administrative regulations, organizational constraints, and power structures within the environment are among those conditions and should be of primary concern to the nurse. It is important for the nurse to acknowledge, understand, and, in some cases, change those environmental factors that adversely affect the nurse's ability to maintain and enhance caring.

Resources for Decision Making

Closely related to environmental factors are the resources available to the community health nurse to facilitate ethical decision making. The presence of and access to a formal decision-making process has much to do with the nurse's ability to make and implement effective ethical decisions. Whereas most large acute-care institutions have formal ethics committees in place, community agencies have only recently begun to develop formalized approaches to ethical decision making.

Bioethics committees in the United States were initially established to review policies and procedures; provide ethics education to committee members, the respective institution or agency, and the community at large; and supply active and retrospective case review and consultation when ethical conflict occurred (President's Commission, 1983; Smith & Veatch, 1987). The 1991 Joint Commission on Accreditation's (JCAHO) manual for hospital standards directed agencies seeking accreditation to demonstrate access to a formal ethical decision-making process and to have nurses represented in that process (Joint Commission, 1990).

More recent guidelines (Joint Commission, 1994; Joint Commission, 1996; Joint Commission, 2000) directed agency ethics committees to become more responsible for the ethical environment. These regulations call on institutional ethics committees and, by implication, community agency ethics committees to set the ethical tone of the agency, to

Perspectives...

COMMUNITY VALUES AND CARE IN A COMMUNITY

In a rural area of the southwestern United States, a researcher, studying the influence of Hispanic religion and culture on decisions about their children who were diagnosed with a genetic disorder, uncovered the power of a "network of nurses" who provided health care services to the local communities. Initially, health services were provided intermittently from a large city to the north. Providers traveled to the community for assessments, but the provision of the care offered remained in the urban area, several hours away. Individuals with significant health challenges, especially children, were either denied care or unable to take advantage of services available because their parents lacked transportation, money for the services, or the ability to leave work and other family members to travel to the large city to access needed care. As an alternative, the researcher reported the emergence of a network of nurses in the community, not only locally available, but whose caring behaviors were consonant with the cultural patterns of the community. These nurses relied heavily on established social networks and an in-depth knowledge of the people. This network preceded the delivery of goods and services while also establishing the foundation for effective care.

When the state established regional offices for the care of children with disabilities, officials supported this model of networking by the county public health nurses as appropriate for this region, in contrast to models based upon local health departments from other areas. The collaboration that developed among care providers was based, in large measure, on the nurses' personal knowledge and respect for families and their distinctive cultural community. Relationships based upon trust and

care between the county health nurses and the community reflected the cultural patterns and values of the community. Individuals, families, and the community worked together, bringing health services closer to the clients in need. The services supported each family's ability to deal with illness and health care access in the context of their local community. Negotiating the cultural terrain, seen as natural by the county health nurses, relied on a community network.

Respect for the values of the community, especially the "incredible valuing of children," provided a motivation and priority for services in spite of severely limited facility and financial resources. Religious and cultural traditions influenced family decisions, choices about care, and the patterns of care that were successful within the community. One of the nurses told the story of a mother who was advised by a visiting physician to terminate her pregnancy based on the negative outcome of a prenatal screening test. The doctor suggested that it was "best for society," but the mother responded, "What is this child but society?" Many health care providers from the community understood the fundamental influence of cultural values and beliefs on the delivery and acceptance of care. The ability of the nurses to understand and respect local values and beliefs, to respond authentically, and to approach each family in a manner that allows them to decide how to access appropriate care is essential to the success of culturally sensitive and meaningful care.

—Deborah Blake, Professor of Religious Studies, Regis University, Denver, Colorado

establish and implement a code of ethical behavior for members of the agency, and to integrate ethics into the daily life of the agency. Under these guidelines, the ethics committee is responsible for the ethical environment of the agency itself. The institutional bioethics committee is being asked to support an environment of ethical practice: "The goal of the patients' rights and organization ethics function is to help improve patient outcomes by respecting each patient's rights and conducting business relationships with patients and the public in an ethical manner" (Joint Commission, 2000). Community-based bioethics committees are developed in response to the need for formal decision-making processes to respond to ethical challenges outside the acute-care setting. Although most community health care agencies do not come under

JCAHO review, it seems prudent for community-based ethics committees to be appropriately sensitive to these important JCAHO guidelines.

Community-based bioethics committees have been termed "third-generation" ethics committees (Mason, 1995). First-generation committees evolved as care review committees, abortion review committees, institutional review boards, prognosis committees, and dialysis patient selection committees. Second-generation committees are familiar to many as those that developed in the 1980s in acute-care settings. Community health care agencies often have found it impossible to develop from within the resources needed for a formal ethics committee on the order of the second-generation hospital-based ethics committees that blossomed in the 1980s (Ross, Glaser,

Rasinski-Gregory, McIver, Gibson, & Bayley, 1993). The need for ethics education, policy review, and case consultation exists within community health agencies just as it does in the acute-care setting. To address this need, third-generation community-based ethics committees that combine and share resources across agencies have been initiated. Such committees, when available, may provide community health nurses with a formal process to address ethical conflicts encountered within the practice setting.

One example of a community-based ethics committee is the Denver Community Bioethics Committee. This committee is a model for community-based ethical review of health care decisions, primarily in long-term care facilities. As a noninstitutional volunteer committee, the members meet monthly and as needed for emergency consultation, to address issues and dilemmas involving long-term care clients or residents who lack decisional capacity. The committee was established through the Denver Department of Social Services with assistance from the Guardianship Alliance of Colorado to help agencies, facilities, and family members in the Denver metropolitan area negotiate difficult ethical issues related to the care of Social Service Department wards and long-term care clients or residents. Membership consists of 25 individuals including nurses, physicians, attorneys, social workers, clergy, adult protection administrators, nursing home ombudsmen, health care administrators, and an ethicist. All members have received ethics education. The committee focuses on issues related to the care of individuals who lack decisional capacity, including questions about life support and treatment termination. Access to the committee is by request through committee members. Anyone facing difficult health care decisions may access the committee (Mason, 1995).

A similar committee, the Montgomery County Department of Social Services' Ethics Committee in Rockville, Maryland, assists with difficult issues for clients with public guardians. On some occasions, the county committee has collaborated with a hospital ethics committee to resolve issues. The county committee has 17 members, including nurses, physicians, clergy, social workers, and members of the community. This committee makes recommendations to the director of the Department of Social Services, who, in turn, makes recommendations to the court. Members of this committee also receive training in ethics and ethical decision processes: "Training encompasses ethical, religious, moral, and value implications of providing services to children and vulnerable adults" (American Health Consultants, 1994, p. 115).

In the absence of a community-based ethics committee, the nursing leadership within each agency as well as the individual nurse practicing in the agency bears the responsibility to investigate the possibility of developing such a committee. At the very least, access to other formalized assistance with ethical decision making should be sought. Individual community health nurses should understand those mechanisms that are available and the process to access those mechanisms.

Values

Personal and professional values significantly influence the community health nurse's ability to make and effect ethical decisions. The values that the individual nurse brings to the care setting as well as the values of everyone involved in an ethical conflict must be addressed. The nurse's values must remain clear in order to avoid confusing the nurse's personal or professional values with those of other care providers, the client, the family, and the community. Unless each nurse maintains clarity regarding values, the very real danger exists that one set of values will inadvertently supersede another set of values in the conflict.

Knowledge about and respect for the values of all participants in a conflict situation is critical to reaching ethically justifiable resolution to ethical conflict. Understanding one's own values may facilitate remaining open to the values of others. Caring, as a core value in professional nursing, may enhance the ability of the practicing nurse to remain open and genuine in the face of differing and conflicting values. Health promotion and disease prevention, core values in community health, may not be

---

REFLECTIVE THINKING

How Have Your Values Developed?

Think of three ideals or beliefs that you prize in your personal life. Try to trace each belief or ideal back to the earliest time in your life when you were aware of its importance or presence.

- When and how did you learn to view each belief or ideal as important?
- How have your beliefs and ideals changed or evolved over time?
- Where do you find your support for them?
- How prevalent do you think these beliefs or ideals are among other people?
- What do you think of people who hold different beliefs or ideals?
- Think of a time in your life when one of these beliefs or ideals has been challenged. How did you feel? How did you react?

Adapted from *Ethics and Issues in Contemporary Nursing*, by M. A. Burkhardt and A. K. Nathaniel, 1998, Clifton Park, NY: Delmar Learning.

shared by all those seeking care. Budget limitations, a client's or agency's orientation to the present rather than the future, and an interest in curing disease instead of taking measures to prevent the onset of disease represent the kind of value conflict encountered in community health.

Ethical Codes

Several nursing organizations have developed codes as guidelines for ethical conduct. The ANA delineates the nurse's obligations to clients: "A code of ethics indicates a profession's acceptance of the responsibility and trust with which it has been invested by society" (ANA, 1985). The ANA code of ethics can be found in Figure 7-4. The International Council of Nurses has also developed a code of ethics (see Figure 7-5).

FIGURE 7-4 American Nurses Association Code for Nurses

1. The nurse, in all professional relationships, practices with compassion and respect for the inherent dignity, worth, and uniqueness of every individual, unrestricted by considerations of social or economic status, personal attributes, or the nature of health problems.

2. The nurse's primary commitment is to the patient, whether an individual, family, group, or community.

3. The nurse promotes, advocates for, and strives to protect the health, safety, and rights of the patient.

4. The nurse is responsible and accountable for individual nursing practice and determines the appropriate delegation of tasks consistent with the nurse's obligation to provide optimum patient care.

5. The nurse owes the same duties to self as to others, including the responsibility to preserve integrity and safety, to maintain competence, and to continue personal and professional growth.

6. The nurse participates in establishing, maintaining, and improving health care environments and conditions of employment conducive to the provision of quality health care and consistent with the values of the profession through individual and collective action.

7. The nurse participates in the advancement of the profession through contributions to practice, education, administration, and knowledge development.

8. The nurse collaborates with other health professionals and the public in promoting community, national, and international efforts to meet health needs.

9. The profession of nursing, as represented by associations and their members, is responsible for articulating nursing values, for maintaining the integrity of the profession and its practice, and for shaping social policy.

From the *Code for Nurses*, 2001, © American Nurses Association, Washington, D.C.

FIGURE 7-5 International Council of Nurses Code for Nurses

The fundamental responsibility of the nurse is fourfold: to promote health, to prevent illness, to restore health, and to alleviate suffering.

The need for nursing is universal. Inherent in nursing is respect for life, dignity, and rights of man. It is unrestricted by considerations of nationality, race, creed, color, age, sex, politics, or social status.

Nurses render health services to the individual, the family, and the community and coordinate their services with those of related groups.

Nurses and People

The nurse's primary responsibility is to those people who require nursing care.

The nurse, in providing care, promotes an environment in which the values, customs, and spiritual beliefs of the individual are respected.

The nurse holds in confidence personal information and uses judgment in sharing this information.

Nurses and Practice

The nurse carries personal responsibility for nursing practice and for maintaining competence by continual learning. The nurse maintains the highest standards of nursing care possible within the reality of a specific situation.

The nurse uses judgment in relation to individual competence when accepting and delegating responsibilities.

The nurse, when acting in a professional capacity, should at all times maintain standards of personal conduct that reflect credit upon the profession.

Nurses and Society

The nurse shares with other citizens the responsibility for initiating and supporting action to meet the health and social needs of the public.

Nurses and Coworkers

The nurse sustains cooperative relationships with coworkers in nursing and other fields. The nurse takes appropriate action to safeguard the individual when his care is endangered by a coworker or any other person.

Nurses and the Profession

The nurse plays the major role in determining and implementing desirable standards of nursing practice and nursing education.

The nurse is active in developing a core of professional knowledge.

The nurse, acting through the professional organization, participates in establishing and maintaining equitable social and economic working conditions in nursing.

From *ICN Code for Nurses: Ethical Concepts Applied to Nursing*, by the International Council of Nurses, 1973, Geneva, Switzerland: Imprimeries Populares. Reproduced with permission.

ETHICAL DILEMMAS IN COMMUNITY HEALTH

Ethical dilemmas are universal in health care. The uniqueness of each health care setting, however, makes it appropriate to examine ethical dilemmas from the perspective of respective health care settings. Ethical issues in community health cover a spectrum as diverse as the agencies, client populations, and care providers in the community itself. Issues of client abandonment through care limitations, decisional capacity and competence, potential and actual client or provider abuse, lifestyle diversity, and compliance or cooperation with treatment regimes are addressed next.

Client Abandonment

The increasingly limited health care resources characteristic of the changing health care environment, increasing numbers of nurses entering retirement, and decreasing numbers of individuals entering the nursing profession create issues of client abandonment, common in community health nursing centers. Although some have expressed concern regarding characterizing limitations imposed on care as abandonment, community health nurses understand the terminology well. Restrictions and limitations on client care services have undeniably grown in response to the ever-increasing number, type, and complexity of payment systems and the significant limitations on health care resources.

Increasingly, coverage ends before the need for care ends. Nurses may be faced with critical decisions regarding the reporting of client care needs in order to place the client in the most advantageous light for continued receipt of coverage for needed care services. The nurse may also face conflict regarding the provision of care for which payment will not be forthcoming, thus potentially jeopardizing the economic stability of the employing agency or the level of care available to other clients.

It often happens that when Medicare coverage expires, clients need ongoing care but are unable (or unwilling) to pay out of pocket for additional services. Rather than discharge such clients from care (and be liable to regulatory rebuke and legal challenge, not to mention moral quandary), an agency may continue care without reimbursement—at its own fiscal peril. . . . Agencies often have to choose between insufficient care and no care. When an agency assesses a client at a level of care for which funding is denied, the agency can offer a lower (but reimbursed) level of care or it can refuse to initiate or continue care. But refusing clients—or, worse, discharging them—can negate the whole purpose and mission of the agency. . . . Moral commitments bind the agency to the client in ways that wreak havoc with the autonomy of the agency and its commitment to the client's autonomy and well-being. (Collopy, Dubler, & Zuckerman, 1990, p. 5)

Nurses in the community most often choose to compromise regarding the care provided rather than abandon the client. The challenges are enormous for the nurse trying to provide optimal care within an atmosphere of cost containment, limited time, and restricted resources.

Decisional Capacity

Given the focus on the care provider–care recipient partnership in making care decisions in community health settings, community health nurses must assess the client's ability to make informed, uncoerced, competent decisions. In community health, the client is most often encountered at home or in the immediate community. Resources and collegial support that are available in an acute-care setting are less accessible to the community health nurse who needs assistance in determining the client's capacity and competence to make appropriate health care decisions. The terms *competence* and *capacity* are often used interchangeably, although by definition, decisional competence is determined formally through the court system and capacity is usually determined more informally by the professional care providers in the health care system. Here, the term *capacity* is used to refer to the client's ability to make health care decisions. Capacity for making health care decisions assumes the ability to understand the nature, consequences, and alternatives of such decisions (Devetere, 2000). In U.S. society, adults are presumed to have decisional capacity. Decisional capacity may be limited, however, according to the gravity of the decision and the weight of the consequences. Physicians are most often charged with the determination of health care decisional capacity. When a client has been judged incapable of making his or her own decisions, two models

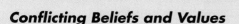

REFLECTIVE THINKING

Conflicting Beliefs and Values

Consider a diabetic client who has progressed in the knowledge of self-care but who still requires further teaching, supervision, and practice in self-care skills.

- How will you manage personal beliefs and professional values that conflict with corporate practice or agency policy?
- How will you feel about having to cease care provision to this client when funding runs out?
- What will you do?

RESEARCH FOCUS

Crisis Nature of Health Care Transitions for Rural Older Adults

Study Problem/Purpose

A study that culminated 10 years of ethnographic research within the "culture and context of the rural western United States" examined the experiences of older adults as they transitioned across differing levels and types of health care. Based on the notion that changes in the American health care system and socioeconomic and environmental problems place older adults and their families at high risk for disease and disability and that distance, geography, and poor distribution of services and health care providers restrict access for rural elderly, Magilvy and Congdon (2000) added to community nursing's knowledge base in their analysis of data gathered on the effectiveness of community-based care in assisting rural families and other informal caregivers to provide and coordinate care for rural elders. Prior research indicates that rural elders "may have lower health expectations and be reluctant to seek care until they are acutely symptomatic, expressing resistance to outside help." In addition, "strong rural values of hardiness, independence, and family support" (p. 336) have been identified as factors that may attenuate or exacerbate the problems of rural elderly.

Methods

To further study the experiences of rural older adults transitioning across differing levels and types of health care, Magilvy and Congdon interviewed older adults (including patients, families, and older community residents), health care providers, and community leaders over a period of four years in 13 counties in two rural areas in one western state in the United States. The researchers asked three primary research questions:

- What is the experience of transitioning across health care services for rural elders and their families?
- What aspects of the rural health care delivery system are most problematic?
- What interventions or models are needed to support community and individual strengths and address problems?

One hundred seventy-five people were included in the sample for the minimally structured, ethnographic, audiotaped interviews.

In addition to the interviews, observations were conducted in the community; in health care settings, including hospitals, homes, nursing homes, and clinics; health and social service agencies; and senior centers. The researchers found

the people in the rural areas . . . physically active, friendly, and caring toward each other. They were independent and self-reliant, and willing to share with us their experiences, stories, and recommendations about aging and health care. We observed that churches or other faith communities and religions were essential institutions in community life. Older persons were especially connected to their faith communities and perceived churches to be places of safety, community support, and spiritual fulfillment. (p. 338)

Photographs, slides, and prints were used to illustrate and provide insights into culture, rural environment, context, and health care practices. Artifacts such as local newspapers, magazines, and historical items were also examined. Data were analyzed for categories, domains, patterns, and themes.

Findings

The major cultural theme that emerged from the analysis of data from transcripts, field notes, photographs, and articles was the crisis nature of health care transitions experienced by rural older adults and their families and observed by rural nurses and other health care providers:

We found that seeking health care or transitioning across health care settings, such as from hospital to nursing home, home to nursing home, or hospital to home, involved difficult decisions for our older participants and were most often experienced as crises. The rapidly changing health care system and changing availability of health care services in rural areas led to inconsistencies in care and transition decisions. Decisions about the most appropriate care settings were often made hastily. . . . Our older participants . . . had not anticipated acute or chronic illnesses or planned for long-term care either in their home or an institution. Inconsistent distribution of health care services, closing of some facilities exacerbated the problems. The transition decision, therefore, frequently precipitated confusion and crisis. (p. 339)

(continues)

Notably, Magilvy and Congdon found that limited knowledge of resources by providers, elders, and families alike compounded the problems; inconsistent discharge planning disrupted the transitions; and changing family support necessitated admission to nursing homes. Positive findings identified rural home health care as a strength and found that continuity of care in nursing home discharge lessens the transition crisis.

Rural elders tend to remain at home until a crisis point, such as an accident, acute illness or chronic illness complication, is reached. The researchers found little evidence of transition planning and recognized that for some elders and their families accessing any type of assistance was intimidating.

A lack of collaborative decision making existed among patient, family, and nurse. Although the nurses displayed an intimate knowledge of the patients and families in their care, nurses also displayed a limited knowledge of local resources that tended to exacerbate the transition crises. The lack of knowledge of resources was attributed, in part, to a lack of career development opportunities. Nurses who were born, raised, and worked in the local community often had to move to other communities for career advancement. In such instances, the knowledge of patients, families, and community resources was diminished.

Not surprisingly, when discharge planning was consistent, timely, and appropriate, transitions were less disrupted:

> Care management services by nurses or social workers available in . . . large urban health care systems, were not observed in these rural areas. . . . Little collaborative decision making was observed, and no time was allotted for deliberation and exploration of resources. . . . Lack of knowledge of community health and social service resources on the part of lay people and health care providers led to fragmentation of care. (pp. 341, 343)

Implications

This study emphasizes the importance of formal and informal circles of care as well as nurses' knowledge of community care resources. Older persons need support, especially when accidents, falls, acute illness, worsening chronic illnesses, or general frailty lead to deterioration of health and functional ability: "A care manager or PHN [public health nurse] working with rural elders should be cognizant of and develop resources within the two circles of care" (p. 343). The formal circle of care provides essential services but needs the circle of informal support to overcome the burdens of geography, transportation, and access or distribution problems in rural communities.

Magilvy and Congdon indicate that there is a need for "comprehensive care management" provided by a variety of community nurses, nurse consultants, public health nurses, or parish nurses to rural older persons and their families: "Essential interventions toward improving quality of life and health care decision making would include: providing appropriate information and referrals; anticipatory guidance; respecting whole-person health including physical, psychosocial, cultural, and spiritual aspects; and understanding complex age-related health needs and transitions" (p. 344). The researchers conclude that

> nursing interventions are necessary to facilitate smooth transitions and insure coordinated quality health care across diverse settings congruent with local culture and values. . . . Older persons and their families need well-organized, consistent, community-based care management and public health nursing interventions to facilitate desired results of optimal health; accessible, appropriate, and acceptable health care; independence; and quality of life." (p. 344)

The ethical dimensions of this study relate to the principles of autonomy, beneficence, and justice. The importance of a solid understanding of community and individual values is underscored.

Source: Magilvy, J. K., & Congdon, J. A. (2000). The crisis nature of health care transitions for rural older adults. Public Health Nursing, 17(5), 336–345.

of surrogate decision making can be used: substituted judgment and best interest judgment.

Substituted judgment refers to a decision made on behalf of another who is unable, due to age, developmental status, or medical condition, to make the decision on her or his own behalf. Substituted judgment is made "as if" the individual were making the decision. Such a surrogate decision is based on knowledge of the history, lifestyle, desires, prior decisions, and values of the individual for whom the decision is being made. Advance directives are particularly helpful in substituted judgment. Written statements about desires, decisions to be made, and values provide useful guidance to those attempting a substituted judgment (Devetere, 2000).

Best interest judgment is a less personal surrogate decision based on what a reasonable person in similar circumstances would decide. Best interest decisions differ from substituted judgment in that the standard for the decision is an unknown other rather than the known history and past decisions of the individual for whom the decision is being made (substituted judgment). A best interest judgment may very well not represent what the individual would decide were he or she able to do so.

The distinction between these two models is a particularly salient reminder to the nurse to acknowledge whose values are driving a surrogate decision—those of the client for whom the decision is being made (as in substituted judgment) or those of the individual making the decision (e.g., a family member or professional who is trying to determine what is in the best interest of the client). Caution must also be exercised in determining the need for a surrogate decision maker in the first place. To exercise such caution, one must understand individual state statutes regarding the process of assigning surrogates, the legal rights of surrogates, any formal review of surrogates, and the presence and status of any advance directives.

In examining a client's decisional competence or capacity, there is always the danger of the client being judged incompetent purely on the basis of the client's making decisions that differ from those the health care provider would make. It is unjust for health care professionals to award decisional capacity only to those with whom they agree. The right to make decisions for oneself (autonomy) is highly valued in our society. It is difficult to honor that right, however, when the client lacks the knowledge or skill to make decisions. In complicated medical situations, such as when religious or cultural beliefs conflict with prevailing medical opinion (as may be the case with Jehovah's Witnesses or Christian Scientists, whose religious beliefs forbid the use of specified medical treatments) or when family members disagree with

each other, it is especially difficult to adequately evaluate the appropriateness of autonomous decisions.

Decisions regarding quality of life issues, made for another who is suffering from increased pain or progressive dementia, may be blurred by the values of the person making the decision. The blurring of values has the potential to affect the response of the care provider, who may have values different from the client or family. To the care provider who values life at all costs, the decision of a client or family to stop aggressive treatment may be viewed as incompetent. A care provider who holds quality of life in high esteem, however, may not question the competence of the client or family who makes such a decision.

Client/Provider Abuse

The awesome burdens of providing care to a relative in the home may lead to frustration that develops into some form of abuse. Providing intense care "represents a major commitment of time and energy to tasks that are mundane, unglamorous, repetitive, and labor intensive" (Collopy et al., 1990, p. 4). Neglect and abuse may be inherent consequences of such care. Significant demands on family members related to employment outside the home or geographic distances between family members compound the stress of providing care to a relative in the home. Families in which violence or abuse have occurred in the past are unlikely to change because of the presence of the community nurse in the home. The community nurse is thus challenged to positively influence care provided in the home and seek additional resources to provide family members with appropriate respite. The safety of the nurse, the client, and the family members must always be considered.

Legal guidelines in cases of potential or actual client, family, or provider abuse are beyond the purview of this chapter. The professional responsibility of every nurse requires full knowledge and understanding of the law as it affects nursing practice. Beyond the law, however, the community health nurse should reflect on ethical responsibility in cases of actual or suspected abuse. It is important to consider the risks and benefits to client, provider, and family. Abuse may be physical, psychological, or financial. Providing care to clients in their daily surroundings renders the nurse vulnerable to physical or verbal abuse from clients or family members. Fazzone, Barloon, McConnell, and Chitty (2000) recommend that all agencies provide ongoing education and training programs to professional and nonprofessional staff regarding personal safety while providing care in the home. In addition, results of their research demonstrated the need for comprehensive personal safety policies and procedures to be developed, implemented, and reviewed by all staff several times a year. Threats to provider's safety, particularly, may compromise client care. Administrative support for those providing care in

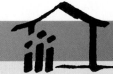

COMMUNITY NURSING VIEW

The following excerpt is fictional, although the elements of the case are extracted from actual practice. Any resemblance to real individuals is purely coincidental.

Ms. Y. is a 47-year-old African American woman who for two years has received home health services under the auspices of the Public Health Visiting Nurse Agency. As a result of progressive symptoms of multiple sclerosis, she requires maximum assistance with activities of daily living (ADL), including personal care and hygiene, dressing, feeding, toileting, transfers, and exercise. On "good" days, she is able to ambulate with a walker. Home health aides provide most of her care during daily visits. On weekly visits, the RN provides medication assistance as well as ongoing assessment of nutritional status, skin integrity, ability to maintain care regimens, overall health status, and a monthly catheter change. Physical therapy visits are also provided through the agency. Most of her medical care is provided through a regional Multiple Sclerosis Center located in the next town. Despite the progression of her disease, Ms. Y. has remained communicative, with a bright personality and warm, smiling responses to her caregivers. Her home is located in a high-risk neighborhood where multiple assaults, murders, thefts, and acts of vandalism have occurred. Her husband, the only family care provider, is described as loud, belligerent, and verbally abusive. He also has documented alcohol and drug problems that appear to magnify his emotional responses. He has verbally and physically intimidated young female caregivers, has refused to allow male caregivers into the home, and has threatened staff with a gun on two occasions. Concerns have been expressed regarding actual or potential abuse of Ms. Y. She is considered to be competent to make decisions regarding her own care. Arrangements have been made for two-week respite periods during which Ms. Y. would be cared for out of her home. Mr. Y. receives money for providing care to her at home and is anxious to keep that source of financial support for them. Ms. Y. has been unwilling to leave her home or her husband.

Nursing Considerations

Assessment

◆ What are the nurse's responsibilities to the client? The agency? Mr. Y.? The community? Self and family?

◆ Does safety of the client or of the care provider come first? How might the safety of both be balanced in the situation described?

◆ What should be included in the assessment of the situation?

Diagnosis

◆ State the ethical dilemma faced by the nurse.

Outcome Identification

◆ What outcomes would you anticipate that would help you determine if you had made an ethically justifiable decision?

Planning/Interventions

◆ What alternatives are possible in this situation?

◆ Is it fair to assign staff to provide care to a client who has demonstrated need but whose care may compromise the safety of the staff?

◆ Is transfer to another agency ethical? If yes, under what circumstances?

◆ Discuss the relationship between client abandonment and the principles of nonmaleficence and beneficence?

Evaluation

◆ How did you decide which alternatives were possible?

◆ Did you have the information you needed to make an ethically justifiable decision?

◆ What principles did you use to arrive at your decisions?

---

situations of potential or actual abuse is also essential for the well-being of providers, clients, and families. Resolution of situations involving abuse is difficult and complicated. Abuse by a family member of the client threatens the safety of both client and nurse. It is often impossible to bring another provider into the situation, and abandonment of the client not only puts the client at greater risk for potential abuse but also exposes the client to a lack of care. Transfer of care to another

provider or agency may be considered but must be done in conjunction with full disclosure (veracity) of the risk to the safety of others. It is appropriate to question any agency policy requirement that places the nurse, the client, or a family member at risk.

Unreasonable risk to the safety of oneself or others should never be acceptable in community practice. No benefit will accrue if the care recipient or the care provider is harmed.

Lifestyle Diversity and Compliance

As discussed earlier in this chapter, the community health nurse may become intimately engaged in conflicts with clients regarding differing lifestyle beliefs. Clients who demand care but who are unable or unwilling to make lifestyle modifications to enhance and facilitate positive outcomes from care truly challenge health care providers. Clients who do not cooperate with medication and treatment regimens may likewise frustrate care providers. The nurse may begin to question the appropriateness of providing care to clients who do not accept responsibility for their own behaviors in the plan of care. Frustration may be magnified in situations where resources are limited and decisions about those who are to receive available care must be made.

Similarly, clients or families who demand care that is deemed unnecessary by the nurse highlight differing values among family members, clients, and care providers. Trying to understand the motivation for and desired outcome from the demanded care may help the nurse educate the client and family about more appropriate levels of care. The nurse must be assured, however, that such education is neither coercive nor directed toward changing the client's request merely because the client does not agree with the nurse or family. If this kind of disagreement is not resolved or if it is a true source of conflict, the nurse must involve others in a review of the conflict.

Review by an ethics committee may provide the nurse, the client, and the family with the knowledge and confidence that care options are offered in an unbiased manner, that the voices of all of the participants are respectfully heard, and that all options are carefully considered. Such committee review should be obtained to facilitate discussion of conflicts in an open, safe environment where all participants have equal power and voice in the discussion. Ideally, the ethics committee functions as facilitator of good decisions rather than as arbitrator of intractable conflicts.

Community health nurses face unique ethical challenges with far fewer resources and sometimes diminished collegial support as they seek to provide optimal care to clients, families, and populations throughout the community. Nurses must seek and seize opportunities for building multidisciplinary approaches both to providing

care and to resolving the ethical conflicts that inevitably arise in the course of providing care. The role of nursing in influencing community values and health care policies must continue to expand to facilitate access to appropriate levels of care for all clients.

▨ KEY CONCEPTS

- ◆ A caring perspective enhances the nurse's ability to resolve ethical conflict in a contextual way.
- ◆ Ethical theories, principles, rules, and values are important in the resolution of ethical conflicts in community health nursing.
- ◆ Analysis of any ethical issue must incorporate components of a decision-making process that allow for resolution of the acknowledged conflict.
- ◆ Six components are essential in any ethical decision-making model used to guide the resolution of ethical dilemmas: (1) a means of determining those who are involved in the decision and the outcome; (2) a means of gathering all relevant information; (3) a process for outlining potential options for resolving the dilemma; (4) a process for resolving any conflict that arises; (5) a plan for implementing the selected resolution to the dilemma; and (6) a means of evaluating the decision, the process, and the resolution.
- ◆ Despite the development of the best possible database, complete data may not be available, and disagreements regarding the facts may occur.
- ◆ Both the direct and the indirect consequences of ethical decisions to all participants should receive attention before a resolution is selected.
- ◆ There are important distinctions among medical, legal, and ethical decisions.
- ◆ A multidisciplinary approach to ethical conflicts lends broad support and diverse perspectives to attempts at conflict resolution.
- ◆ Limited resources affect ethical decisions as well as the nurse's ability to provide optimal care.

✳ DECISION MAKING

Lifestyle Diversity and Compliance

You are caring for a client who refuses to modify lifestyle habits related to diet and exercise yet continues to demand goods and services such as medication, hospitalization, nursing care, and adjunctive therapies.

- ◆ What must you consider before acting?
- ◆ How would you respond?

▨ RESOURCES

Center for Bioethics at the University of Minnesota:
www.bioethics.umn.edu
Center for Biomedical Ethics:
www.hsc.virginia.edu/medicine/inter-dis/bio-ethics
CWRU's Center for Biomedical Ethics:
www.cwru.edu/med/bioethics.html
National Reference Center for Bioethics Literature:
www.georgetown.edu/researcher/nrcbl
Program in Biomedical Ethics and Medical Humanities:
www.medicine.uiowa.edu/bemh

Chapter
8

SPIRITUAL AND CULTURAL PERSPECTIVES

Phyllis E. Schubert, DNSc, RN, MA

MAKING THE CONNECTION

Imagine how it [would feel] to always belong—belong in a diversified community, for it is the diversity in nature that gives the web of life its strength and cohesion. . . . Imagine being able to relax into our connectedness—into a web of mutually supportive relations with each other and with nature. . . . Imagine a world where what is valued most is not power but nurturance, where the aim has changed from being in control to caring and being cared for, where the expression of love is commonplace. . . . The very fact that you can imagine these things makes them real, makes them possible.

—Adair, 1984, p. 284

COMPETENCIES

Upon completion of this chapter, the reader should be able to:

- Explore linkages among spirituality, culture, health beliefs, and health practices.
- Explore the human search for purpose and meaning in life.
- Identify elements of spiritual assessment used in clinical practice.
- Discuss the importance of cultural understanding to community health nursing.
- Explore the effects of ethnocentrism and related concepts in nursing practice.
- Examine issues related to cultural differences between the nurse and the client.
- Discuss the meaning of culturally appropriate health care.
- Examine transcultural nursing theory as an interpretation of caring.

KEY TERMS

acculturation	folk health system
bicultural	healing practices
biracial	historical religion
chakras	homogeneity
cultural assessment	locus of control
cultural compatibility	minority
cultural competence	pattern appraisal
cultural diversity	primal religion
culturally diverse care	race
cultural sensitivity	religion
cultural values	spiritual assessment
culture	spirituality
culture bound	stereotyping
enculturation	transcultural nursing
ethnicity	universalistic argument
ethnocentrism	

Spirituality and culture are aspects of life that bring beauty and joy to human beings when differences among people are appreciated but that lead to conflict and misery when differences are met with disrespect. The community health nurse must have not only knowledge about spiritual and cultural beliefs and practices but also, and more important, understanding and wisdom in the implementation of that knowledge. Cultural issues continue to challenge the nurse, and continuous learning throughout one's professional life is essential because the beliefs that originate from cultural and spiritual life determine lifestyle, health, and **healing practices.** Healing practices are those intended to facilitate integration of one's whole self and relationships.

Spirituality is defined by Dossey and Guzzeta (2000) as "a unifying force of a person; the essence of being that permeates all of life and is manifested in one's being, knowing, and doing; the interconnectedness with self, others, nature, and God/Life Force/Absolute/Transcendent" (p. 7). Religion, on the other hand, is quite different. Burkhardt and Nagai-Jacobson (2000) define **religion** as "an organized system of beliefs shared by a group of people and the practices, including worship, related to that system" (p. 92). Religion is an aspect of culture (see Leininger's sunrise model in Figure 8-7) which provides structure and tools for spiritual life. Religion bridges culture and spirituality in the search for the meaning and purpose of life, a major determinant of health (Frankl, 1959).

Leininger (1991) defines **culture** as the values, beliefs, norms, and practices of a particular group that are learned and shared and that guide thinking, decisions, and actions in a patterned way. Building on this definition, Giger and Davidhizar (1999) further define culture as "a patterned behavioral response that develops over time as a result of imprinting the mind through social and religious structures and intellectual and artistic manifestations" (p. 3). **Cultural values** are those desirable or preferred ways of acting or knowing something that over time are reinforced and sustained by the culture and ultimately govern one's actions or decisions.

The aims of the chapter are to (1) advance cultural competence in community health nursing practice, (2) promote understanding and respect for the vast diversity of meanings represented in the health beliefs and practices of clients and nurses, and (3) introduce some useful tools for cultural and spiritual assessment. Transcultural nursing theory is presented as the framework for

---

REFLECTIVE THINKING

Spirituality and Philosophy of Nursing

- What is your philosophy of nursing?
- How would you define spirituality as it is reflected in your philosophy?

application of the previously mentioned concepts because this model is built on the practice of caring (discussed in Chapter 1). Caring is to cultivate, to nurture, and to support growth and is a major thread running through most cultures.

The chapter begins with a discussion of spirituality. We have elected to separate culture and spirituality, emphasizing that culture reflects our diversity whereas spirituality reflects that which unites us. A discussion of frameworks for understanding spirituality and culture in turn provides the framework for nursing assessment and intervention.

SPIRITUALITY: A UNIVERSAL NEED

Spirituality is the essence of our being and reflects our wholeness; it permeates our lives and directs our unfolding awareness of who and what we are, our purpose for being, our inner resources, and the shape of our life journey (Burkhardt & Nagai-Jacobson, 2000). It reaches the deeper aspects of an individuals capacity for love, hope, and meaning. Spirituality is basic to nursing because it is essential to human life, yet spirit is not understood because it is intangible (Burkhardt & Nagai-Jacobson,

2000), experienced beyond the limits of the senses, ego, space, or time. We resort to metaphors, paradox, and parables to speak of things that have no words (Canda & Furman, 1999).

Spirituality is considered in nursing and other health professions to be an aspect of human experience along with biological, psychological, and sociological aspects. In addition, spirituality is described as the irreducible wholeness of human beings. In Figure 8-1 Canda and Furman (1999) depict spirituality in relation to the biopsychosocial model using three metaphors: spirituality as the wholeness of the person, spirituality as the center of the person, and spirituality as the spiritual aspect of the person. The spiritual aspect impels us to give meaning and purpose to our bodies and biological functions, our thoughts and feelings, and our relationships with other people and the rest of the universe. Spirituality, as the wholeness of being human, addresses the sacredness of every person, demanding that each person be treated with respect and care regardless of any particular qualities or conditions.

Religion addresses values and beliefs related to spirituality; religion, however, is a matter of choice and spirituality is not. Religion, an aspect of culture (Leininger,

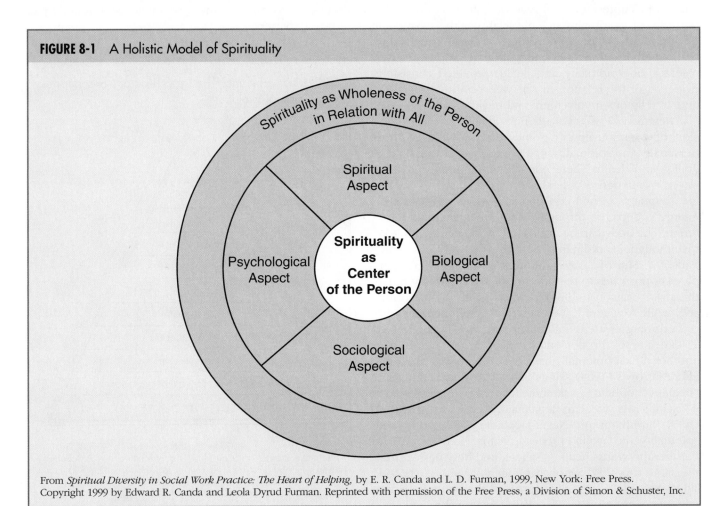

FIGURE 8-1 A Holistic Model of Spirituality

From *Spiritual Diversity in Social Work Practice: The Heart of Helping,* by E. R. Canda and L. D. Furman, 1999, New York: Free Press. Copyright 1999 by Edward R. Canda and Leola Dyrud Furman. Reprinted with permission of the Free Press, a Division of Simon & Schuster, Inc.

1991), creates diversity in human life and spirituality the wholeness and unity of all that is. Vivekananda, the great Hindu monk speaks of this relationship: "Unity in variety is the plan of the universe" (*Complete Works of Swami, Vivekananda,* 1989, Vol. II, p. 396) and "When we perceive the diversity, the unity has gone, and as soon as we perceive the unity, the diversity has vanished" (Vol. V, p. 273).

Burkhardt and Nagai-Jacobson (2000) conclude from their review of the literature that spirituality is the cornerstone of nursing practice. They found consensus that spirituality is a broader concept than is religion; involves a personal quest for meaning and purpose in life; is related to the inner essence of a person; is a sense of harmonious interconnectedness with self, others, nature, and an ultimate reality; and is the integrating factor of the human personality. Nursing has traditionally held the position that spirituality is at the core of health and healing, the nature of person and environment, and the nurse-client relationship.

Conceptual Foundations for Spiritual Assessment

Miller and Thoresen (1999) reviewed studies of the relationship of spirituality to physical health, to mental health, and to alcohol and drug problems. They found that, whether correlational, longitudinal, or prospective, research on spirituality and health provided consistent evidence of the relationship between spiritual practices and/or religious involvement and health.

Newman (1994), who defines health as the expansion of consciousness, assumes that individuals grow personally and spiritually as they experience disease, disability, and death. These conditions, then, are included in one's experience of health.

Neuman's (1995) conceptual position suggests that energy is depleted through illness, grief, pain, and suffering. The body can be nourished by the spirit with positive thoughts and diminished with negative ideas (Isaia, Parker, & Murrow, 1999). Stevens Barnum (1996) compares approaches to the concept of spirituality by nurse theorists. "Watson's (1988) view envisions a developing self, while Newman (1994) describes a self merging with or becoming aware of its participation in a larger whole. In either case, the person is conceived as entering yet another developmental phase beyond rational maturity, after Maslow's (1968) self-actualization, onto a transpersonal level of being or to some level of participation in a consciousness we can legitimately label as spiritual" (p. 7). Burkhardt and Nagai-Jacobson (2000) addressed spirituality and healing processes: "it is useful to remember that the words healing, whole, and holy derive from the same root: Old Saxon hal, meaning whole" (p. 99). Thus, healing is a spiritual process that attends to the wholeness of a person. The shared relationship and connectedness between the nurse and the client, basic to healing, is in itself a manifestation of spirituality.

According to Travelbee (1971), the purpose of nursing is to assist the individual, family, or community in preventing or coping with illness and suffering and, if necessary, in finding meaning in these experiences. Nurses' perceptions of the ill individual and their beliefs about human beings are related directly to the quality of care that the client receives. The result is healing through the experience of caring and finding meaning regardless of whether curing occurs.

In Schubert and Lionberger's (1995) view of the person, healing is the process of self-transformation during which one experiences a sense of becoming, or movement toward self-realization of potential and sense of oneness with absolute reality. Figure 8-2 depicts this potential as emerging from within as tension and conflict are released. Whereas symptoms of physical or mental distress, at the base of the triangle, are often the presenting problem, healing responses usually involve other aspects of the self. The phases of healing may occur in any order and may overlap. The lines of demarcation in the figure are included only to help the reader grasp the complexity and general direction of the process. Nevertheless, there seems to be a general pattern of experience.

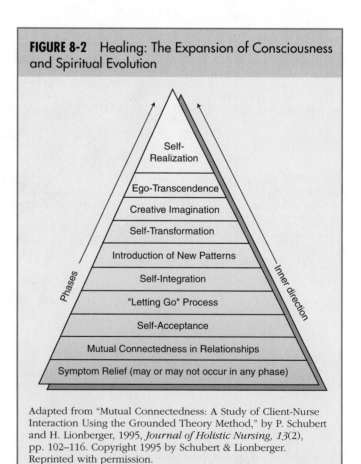

FIGURE 8-2 Healing: The Expansion of Consciousness and Spiritual Evolution

Adapted from "Mutual Connectedness: A Study of Client-Nurse Interaction Using the Grounded Theory Method," by P. Schubert and H. Lionberger, 1995, *Journal of Holistic Nursing, 13*(2), pp. 102–116. Copyright 1995 by Schubert & Lionberger. Reprinted with permission.

Spiritual Health Indicators

Spirituality is basic to an understanding of health as a state of wholeness. According to Pender (2002), spiritual health includes finding meaning and purpose in life; experiencing love, joy, peace, and fulfillment; and achieving one's highest potential. Other dimensions of spiritual well-being include a sense of trust that one has the inner strength and guidance and the needed support of others as needed (Dossey & Guzzetta, 2000).

Life Meaning and Purpose

Frankl (1959), a psychiatrist who survived the Nazi concentration camps of World War II, notes that those who could find reasons for living beyond the experience were better able to cope and survive. He developed an approach to help people identify meaning and purpose in their lives, because he found this to be critical to health.

Frankl believes that it is possible to preserve spiritual freedom even under terrible conditions and that spiritual freedom allows the person to make choices about how one perceives any experience. The power to choose how one perceives an experience provides the inner way of strength, courage, love, wisdom, and understanding. He writes, "Meaning is something to be found, rather than given; man cannot invent it but must discover it" (Frankl, 1959, p. 51).

Sense of Connectedness

Spirituality is both deeply personal and interrelational in nature. The depth of connectedness to one's inner self, to one's God, or however one names and defines ultimate reality, to nature, and to others is reflected in being connected to one's own values, being in meaningful relationships with others, and being committed to God and humankind in a way that provides a reason for living. These relationships are grounded in expressions of love, forgiveness, and trust (Hover-Kramer, 2000).

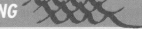

REFLECTIVE THINKING

What Gives Life Meaning and Purpose?

- What is the meaning of life for you?
- What gives your life meaning and purpose?
- What do you do to stay in harmony with yourself, with others, and with nature?
- How do these activities affect your state of health and/or facilitate your healing processes?

Prayer, meditation, reading of spiritual literature, and practicing hope, forgiveness, and trusting in the power of grace are used to maintain connectedness with oneself, others, the natural world and one's ultimate reality.

Sense of Joy, Peace, Inner Strength, and Mystery and Love of Beauty

Feelings based in a sense of joy, peace, inner strength, and mystery and love of beauty are reflections of spiritual health. A nurse's sense of peace is very helpful to recipients of care. Kunz (1992) states, "It is far more important to send peace to someone than to send thoughts that you love them." The thoughts of a man with AIDS as he struggled with the disease are represented in Figure 8-3.

Human beings are spiritually nourished by the beauties of color, sound, and form found in both nature and created art forms (music, sculpture, and painting) (Schubert, 1989). Beauty, although culturally defined, is often enjoyed across cultures by those who are spiritually inclined. Religious rituals and art forms reflect beauty as it is perceived by various cultures as well as the shared

---

FIGURE 8-3 An Experience of Holistic Healing

Finding Peace and Inner Strength

I am much more at peace and much healthier when I listen chiefly to my own body signals and hardly at all to the messages from the media, medical experts, or even social activists and alternative healing groups. . . . One of my first acts when in danger is to reach out for help to mother or father, to doctors, to friends, to pills and potions, to books, anything to hold on to or lean upon, like the drowning man to straws. The real source of my strength and healing is from within and it is important for me to go there, stay there, live there, see from there, meet and make peace with whatever comes from there and do my reaching from there from my body. I think when some of my friends got sick, the fear and desperation took them a long way out from their bodies in search of a cure. So much of their hope was invested in external possibilities that they almost abandoned their bodies—as if they could flee what is happening inside. I think it is necessary to go back down and deep within yourself to face and feel and own your own experience. I realize I can't send something else down to do battle in my place. No miracle, no surgeon's knife, no megavitamin, no medicine or macrobiotic diet, no crystal energy, no faith healer's touch, or shaman's prayer—nothing is of any value at all unless I am there fully present . . . Without one foot in the past, the other in the future. I think of healing a little differently than I used to—it's not about living forever or curing disease. It is about living and feeling fully the whole spectrum from joy to sadness, however long that is, dying with a sense of peace, whenever that comes.

Anonymous.

FIGURE 8-4 Spiritual Assessment

To facilitate the healing process in clients/patients, families, significant others, and yourself, the following reflective questions assist in assessing, evaluating, and increasing awareness of the spiritual process in yourself and others.

MEANING AND PURPOSE These questions assess a person's ability to seek meaning and fulfillment in life, manifest hope, and accept ambiguity and uncertainty.

- What gives your life meaning?
- Do you have a sense of purpose in life?
- Does your illness interfere with your life goals?
- Why do you want to get well?
- How hopeful are you about obtaining a better degree of health?
- Do you feel that you have a responsibility in maintaining your health?
- Will you be able to make changes in your life to maintain your health?
- Are you motivated to get well?
- What is the most important or powerful thing in your life?

INNER STRENGTHS These questions assess a person's ability to manifest joy and recognize strengths, choices, goals, and faith.

- What brings you joy and peace in your life?
- What can you do to feel alive and full of spirit?
- What traits do you like about yourself?
- What are your personal strengths?
- What choices are available to you to enhance your healing?

- What life goals have you set for yourself?
- Do you think that stress in any way caused your illness?
- How aware were you of your body before you became sick?
- What do you believe in?
- Is faith important in your life?
- How has your illness influenced your faith?
- Does faith play a role in regaining your health?

INTERCONNECTIONS These questions assess a person's positive self-concept, self-esteem, and sense of self; sense of belonging in the world with others; capacity to pursue personal interests; and ability to demonstrate love of self and self-forgiveness.

- How do you feel about yourself right now?
- How do you feel when you have a true sense of yourself?
- Do you pursue things of personal interest?
- What do you do to show love for yourself?
- Can you forgive yourself?
- What do you do to heal your spirit?

These questions assess a person's ability to connect in life-giving ways with family, friends, and social groups and to engage in the forgiveness of others.

- Who are the significant people in your life?

(continues)

---

consciousness of the many people who long for the spiritual. Peace, joy, inner strength, and life harmony are characteristics that seem to be nurtured by the beauty of sound, color, and form.

Signs of Spiritual Distress

Spiritual distress (distress of the human spirit) is defined by the North American Nursing Diagnosis Association (NANDA), (1999) as "a disturbance in the belief or value system that provides strength, hope, and meaning in life" (p. 852). Spiritual distress may be experienced when there is loss and/or confusion related to the meaning and purpose of life, death, and suffering; loss of connection with self and others; or conflicts related to beliefs, values, or spiritual practices. Govier (2000) identified signs and symptoms of spiritual distress: fear, doubt, depression, and despair. Causes of spiritual distress include concerns about the meaning or purpose of life, death, and suffering; conflicts in beliefs and values;

and participation in religious rituals. Families and communities may suffer spiritual distress as a result of disasters. Interventions include helping the client (individual, family, or community) to find hope and to mend disrupted relationships.

Spiritual Assessment Tools

Spiritual assessment, the collection, verification, and organization of data regarding the client's beliefs, feelings, and experience related to life meaning and purpose, goes beyond inquiring about a client's membership in a particular religion and taps deeper beliefs and feelings about the meaning of life, love, hope, forgiveness, and life after death. Connectedness is an important part of spirituality, including being connected with one's inner self and understanding one's values, being connected with others in meaningful relationships, and being connected with a larger purpose in life. Religious or philosophical beliefs, such as commitment to humankind or

FIGURE 8-4 (continued)

- Do you have friends or family in town who are available to help you?
- Who are the people to whom you are closest?
- Do you belong to any groups?
- Can you ask people for help when you need it?
- Can you share your feelings with others?
- What are some of the most loving things that others have done for you?
- What are the loving things that you do for other people?
- Are you able to forgive others?

These questions assess a person's capacity for finding meaning in worship or religious activities and a connectedness with a divinity or universe.

- Is worship important to you?
- What do you consider the most significant act of worship in your life?
- Do you participate in any religious activities?
- Do you believe in God or a higher power?
- Do you think that prayer is powerful?
- Have you ever tried to empty your mind of all thoughts to see what the experience might be like?
- Do you use relaxation or imagery skills?

- Do you meditate?
- Do you pray?
- What is your prayer?
- How are your prayers answered?
- Do you have a sense of belonging in this world?

These questions assess a person's ability to experience a sense of connection with all of life and nature, an awareness of the effects of the environment on life and well-being, and a capacity or concern for the health of the environment.

- Do you ever feel at some level a connection with the world or universe?
- How does your environment have an impact on your state of well-being?
- What are your environmental stressors at work and at home?
- Do you incorporate strategies to reduce your environmental stressors?
- Do you have any concerns for the state of your immediate environment?
- Are you involved with environmental issues such as recycling environmental resources at home, work, or in your community?
- Are you concerned about the survival of the planet?

Source: Based on Margaret Burkhardt: Spirituality: An Analysis of the Concept, *Holistic Nursing Practice,* Vol. 3, No. 3, p. 69. 1989. 1999. From *American Holistic Nurses' Association (AHNA) Core Curriculum for Holistic Nursing,* by M. Burkhardt, 1997, pp. 46–47. Also appears in Spirituality and Health, by M. Burkhardt and M. Nagai-Jacobson, 2000, in B. Dossey, L. Keegan, and C. Guzzetta, 2000, *Holistic Nursing: A Handbook for Practice* (3rd ed., pp. 91–117), Gaithersburg, MD: Aspen. Reprinted with permission of M. Burkhardt.

trust in God, put life in perspective and provide a reason for living (Pender, 1996). See Figure 8-4 for an assessment guide.

Healing Practices for Restoring Wholeness

Arrien (1993), in her studies of health beliefs across cultures, found several universal agreements regarding behaviors that support health and healing. One such agreement is that food and its rituals sustain health and well-being. Gathering the food, cooking, sitting down, breaking bread, communing with each other, and celebrating life together are as important as are the food nutrients. The foods eaten as children in our own families and cultural traditions are found to be the most healing for us throughout our lives.

All cultures utilize some form of communication with a God-force: meditation, prayer, contemplation, or ritual. Music, singing, and dancing also are important in all cultures. Native Americans believe that when one does not

sing, one loses life and experiences soul loss. Hindus use mantras and sonics to waken the **chakras** (energy centers within the energy fields) and elevate consciousness. The universal instruments of drums, bells, rattles, and silence are used in rituals to honor Spirit (Arrien, 1993).

All or most cultures hold the following to be essential for good health and healing: positive affirmations, imagery, and avoidance of negative thinking or judgments; being with nature; beauty and order in the home; and being in right relationship with self, family, friends, and community.

Spiritual Self-Care for the Community Health Nurse

The community health nurse must practice spiritual self-care in ways addressed by Burkhardt and Nagai-Jacobson (2000). These ways include pausing for reflection on what is happening within as well as outside the self; taking time for oneself, for one's relationships, and for whatever builds and restores energy; and being mindful of the need to nourish one's own spirit.

RESEARCH FOCUS

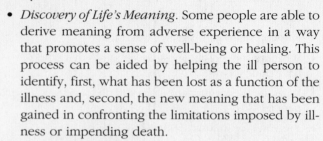

Spirituality and Healing

Study Problem/Purpose

To reveal the influence of spirituality and spiritual experiences on the health and well-being of chronically ill individuals with life-threatening illnesses. It was found that although health care providers seemed to be concerned about the role of spirituality in healing, a survey of the literature had indicated that healing effects attributed by clients and health professionals to spirituality were not reflected in scientific journals.

Methods

A team of researchers conducted interviews, each lasting from one to two hours, with 162 people suffering from serious chronic illnesses. Participants suffered from coronary artery disease, cancer, HIV, chronic obstructive pulmonary disease, and chronic mental illness. Ages ranged from 25 to 96 years with a mean age of 59 years. Symptoms ranged from mild to severe and near death. Although the study focused on spirituality, there was no requirement for participants to have any religious background, and efforts were made to include those with a wide range of spiritual belief perceptions.

Each participant interviewed was asked about their beliefs, thoughts, and experiences related to the following questions: (a) "Could you help me understand what gives your life meaning?" (b) "How does this (referring to the first question) impact your everyday life?" (c) "Does a higher power or guiding force (God, Spirit) play a significant role in your life? What role is that?" (d) "How do you express your belief in God or a higher power?" They were also asked questions concerning their views of the connection between spirituality and health and well-being, such as "What brings you peace?" and "Describe a time when you felt at peace." They were asked about various elements of spiritual care, such as "What do you need to feel your inner strength at this time?" and questions about changes in their spirituality over the course of their illness.

The data were analyzed in two stages: (a) responses to selected questions regarding their views on the meaning of life, the existence of a "higher power," the relationship (if any) between spirituality and health, and their personal hopes for improved health and (b) emergent themes that reoccurred regardless of the questions asked.

Findings

Five major findings emerged from the analysis of the interviews:

- *Discovery of Life's Meaning.* Some people are able to derive meaning from adverse experience in a way that promotes a sense of well-being or healing. This process can be aided by helping the ill person to identify, first, what has been lost as a function of the illness and, second, the new meaning that has been gained in confronting the limitations imposed by illness or impending death.

- *Role Played by Religious History.* A person's religious upbringing—whether it was experienced as a comfort or as an obstruction—strongly influences the way one copes with life-threatening illness. Some people find religion to be a spiritual path to acceptance, but others find no peace in their religious experience. Caregivers can help clients reach acceptance and peace by respecting their spiritual and cultural diversity, helping them embrace what is life giving about their religious heritage, and helping them achieve closure for that which was wounding and in need of healing in their lives.

- *Participation in Religious Activities.* Seriously ill people often lose the ability to participate in formal religious activities. Caregivers need to plan rituals and activities with their clients to determine what would bring the most comfort. Often, a quiet touch is what is most needed.

- *Value of Storytelling.* People with chronic illnesses need to tell their story in their own way and in their own time. Storytelling gives the client a means for (a) organizing and shaping personal experience and thought, to help make sense of life; (b) sharing personal experiences with another person, thus facilitating connectedness and intimacy; and (c) contributing to something larger than oneself and understanding the relationship between spirituality and healing.

- *Gift of Relationship.* Relationships are the key to providing care and healing for people with chronic or life-threatening illnesses. Health care providers can best establish a relationship with a client by paying close attention to what she or he is saying. Open-

(continues)

RESEARCH FOCUS (continued)

ended questions, careful listening to the replies, and expressed compassion and respect are the tools for building healing relationships.

Spirituality is also expressed in many ways other than through religious activities. People experience God, for example, in relationships, nature, music, art, and pets. Effective spiritual care providers integrate these expressions of spirituality.

Implications

Spiritual care is intended not just for people who believe a certain way or who define God according to a particular doctrine. Spiritual care is for everyone, and each of us expresses his or her own spirituality in a unique way.

Source: Skogan, L., & Bader, D. (2000). Spirituality and healing. Health Progress, January–February, pp. 38–42.

Nursing Interventions for Restoring Wholeness

Providing spiritual care to clients is a professional nursing responsibility and essential to holistic nursing. Nurses are sometimes reluctant to accept this responsibility because of fear of imposing beliefs and values on others. Burkhardt and Nagai-Jacobson (2000) encourage spiritual care by saying:

Nurses who integrate spirituality into their care of others need to recognize that, although each person acts out of and is informed by her or his own spiritual perspective, acting from this foundation is not the same as imposing these beliefs and values on another. In fact, many practitioners believe that the more grounded they are in their own spiritual understandings, the less likely they are to impose their values and beliefs on others. (p. 101)

A reason for including spirituality in nursing practice is knowing the client (individual, family, or community) in their wholeness with all its complexities. Clinical research regarding this knowledge is more easily obtained through qualitative studies, but researchers continue to attempt quantitative approaches because they tend to be more acceptable to the scientific community. Yet, Burkhardt and Nagai-Jacobson (2000) warn that reliance on quantitative measurements tends to promote the use of diagnostic reasoning over listening and building healing relationships.

Attentive listening and focused presence are essential for caring of the spirit. These therapeutic communication skills are discussed in Chapter 10. The practice of various spiritual disciplines such as prayer, centering, awareness, and meditation help nurses to develop the ability to be fully present and to listen with full attention. Such listening provides a deep sense of safety for the client, helping them to hear themselves with greater clarity and self-understanding. Burkhardt and Nagai-Jacobson maintain that such listening and presence fosters "authenticity in the nursing process" (p. 102). See Figure 8-5.

FIGURE 8-5 Listening in Healing Ways

- Be intentionally present.
- Maintain focus on the patient/client as a whole person.
- Set aside the need to "fix," "answer," or "correct."
- Learn to be with another in silence.
- Interrupt as little as possible, recognizing that even what is not said at a particular time has meaning and that the way and sequence in which a story is told are part of the story.
- View the other as embodied spirit, in an ongoing and unfinished story.
- Hear the journey, the relationships, the meanings in the story.
- Listen with all your senses.
- Do not prematurely diagnose.
- Let the conversation flow, being with silence as well as words.
- Breathe!

From *Spirituality: Living Our Connectedness,* by M. A. Burkhardt and M. G. Nagai-Jacobson, 2002, Albany, NY: Delmar. Copyright 1997 by Mary Gail Nagai-Jacobson and Margaret A. Burkhardt. Used with permission.

Stories and metaphors are very useful in spiritual care. Since spirituality is multidimensional and extremely complex, the language is difficult. Stories and metaphors often provide a language and form for conveying the richness of one's spirituality when factual statements of experience fail to do so. Stories bring enjoyment while teaching and solving problems. Listening and encouraging people to share their stories are very important in spiritual care.

Burkhardt and Nagai-Jacobson (2000) suggest that both client and nurse explore the question "Who am I?" in all its ramifications. The nurse is encouraged to view the myriad assessment data (physical, mental status, and laboratory) within the context of beginning to know the client and to promote the client's self-knowledge. In this way, the nurse helps the client make sense of all the information in terms of personal meaning.

THE NEED FOR CULTURAL UNDERSTANDING AND SENSITIVITY

People of various cultural backgrounds create a tapestry of color and form, reflecting cultural diversity worldwide. The advancement of technology has led to increased contact among people of various cultures through travel and sophisticated communication systems. Native Americans and Mexicans, indigenous to the United States, have been joined by people of cultures from around the globe. People living together in the United States have created a blend of culture often addressed in metaphor: originally it was the melting pot, then a set of tributaries, a tapestry, and a garden salad. The "melting pot" idea has not proved accurate because the many cultural groups have adapted to one another and accommodated and/or taken on practices of other groups while holding their own unique heritages. Neither has the tributary metaphor survived because we now think of each distinct culture as important in its uniqueness rather than rivers merging in an ocean where all cultures merge into one. The tapestry and garden salad metaphors seem to be more acceptable although the tapestry seems to reflect the quality of changelessness; and cultural groups in the United States are more fluid. The garden salad idea allows for no stability and indicates a constant flux, which does not accurately describe the situation either (Lustig & Koester, 1999).

The U.S. census data for the year 2000 reveals a racially diverse population. For the first time, persons had the option of identifying themselves as belonging to more than one race. The following are percentages of the 274.6 million people who reported only one race:

White	75.1%
Black or African American	12.3%
American Indian and Alaska Native	0.9%
Asian	3.6%
Native Hawaiian and other Pacific Islander	0.1%
Some other race	5.5%

Hispanics, who may be of any race, represented about 13% of the total population count. The following information was obtained from a separate question on His-

panic or Latino origin. Hispanics accounted for 97% of those who reported "some other race" only. The questions on race for the 2000 census was different from the race question used in 1990, making direct comparisons between the two censuses difficult.

Of the 6.8 million people who reported more than one race, 93% reported two races. The most common combinations were:

White and some other race	32%
White and American Indian and Alaska Native	16%
White and Asian	Nearly 13%
White and black or African American	About 11%

Of all respondents who reported more than one race, about 7% indicated three or more races (U.S. Department of Commerce News, March 12, 2001; (see http://www.census.gov/press-release/www/2001/ cb01cn61.html).

Projections based on current census data indicate increasing percentages in "minority" populations. These projections also indicate increasing numbers of foreign-born people. These figures reflect an increasingly diverse and culturally complex population. Such diversity requires that those working with people of various cultures be culturally competent in the care of others. These challenges also require that the nurse understand her own culture and develop self-awareness of cultural beliefs and behaviors (see www.census.gov/population/projections/nation/summary/).

Cultural diversity, the great variety of cultural values, beliefs, and behaviors, is expanding rapidly, requiring nurses to view health, illness, and nursing care from different perspectives (Grossman, 1994). Cultural diversity is recognized and accepted in theory, but in reality, intolerance for and prejudice against those with differing beliefs, values, and lifestyle practices often exist. Respect for such differences can help to create a healthier environment for humankind.

The community health nurse is confronted daily with clients and colleagues whose values differ from those of the nurse. The nurse who supports clients and colleagues within their own belief and value systems will be more likely to experience cooperation in the nurse-client or nurse-community relationship. In contrast, the nurse who insists on imposing her values on clients or colleagues will meet with resistance, conflict, and little or no progress toward resolution of the problems at hand. The work of health promotion and disease prevention in culturally diverse settings requires the nurse to be knowledgeable about various cultures, be respectful of all persons, and have insight regarding personal cultural beliefs. The following paragraphs provide some foundation for understanding the concept of culture and some related issues.

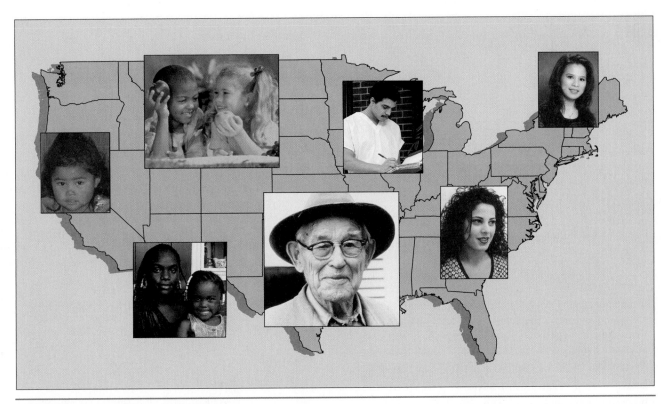

The many faces of the United States.

CULTURAL COMPETENCE IN COMMUNITY HEALTH NURSING

Since the relationship between the community health nurse and the client determines the outcomes of intervention, it is necessary to examine how differences in the cultural beliefs and practices affect the relationship. The development of relationship includes three levels: conceptual, behavioral, and cultural. The conceptual level could include client and nurse perception of sincerity, openness, honesty, motivation, empathy, sensitivity, inquiring concerns, and credibility. The behavior level may include the client's perception of the nurse's professional competency and the nurse's perception of the client's ability to follow directions and to use the skills needed to self-implement the treatment plan (Paniagua, 1998).

The cultural level includes two hypothesis: the first being the **cultural compatibility** hypothesis, which suggests that assessment and intervention within multicultural groups would be enhanced if racial and ethnic barriers between client and nurse are minimized. In other words, the ideal situation would be if the nurse and client were both from the same culture (Paniagua, 1998). Since cultural compatibility is often not practical for many reasons, a second hypothesis has been proposed: the **universalistic argument** (Dana, 1993; Paniagua, 1996, 1998; Tharp, 1991). This argument states that effective assessment and intervention will be the same across all multicultural groups independent of client-nurse racial

and ethnic differences or similarities and proposes that what is relevant in the assessment and treatment of multicultural groups is evidence that the nurse can display both **cultural sensitivity** (i.e., awareness of cultural variables that may affect assessment and treatment) and **cultural competence** (i.e., translation of this awareness into behaviors leading to effective assessment and treatment of the particular multicultural group). Thus, white nurses are as effective as African American nurses in the assessment and intervention of African American clients as long as these two qualities (sensitivity and competence) are manifested in the clinical practice of white nurses working with African American clients. This hypothesis also suggests that when a nurse and client share the same race and ethnicity, effectiveness of care is not guaranteed. The nurse must show evidence of sensitivity and competency to enhance effectiveness of assessment and treatment strategies, regardless of the shared race and ethnicity dimension in the client-nurse relationship (Paniagua, 1998).

Cultural competence is defined by Purnell and Paulanka (1998) as a conscious process of creating awareness of one's existence, sensations, thoughts, and environment in order to understand and accept clients of different cultures. Cultural competence requires continuous seeking of skills, practices, and attitudes that move the client toward positive health outcomes. Giger and Davidhizar (1999) address cultural competence as "a dynamic, fluid, continuous process whereby an individual,

---

FIGURE 8-6 Andrews/Boyle Transcultural Nursing Assessment Guide: A Summary

Cultural Identification

To what cultural group(s) does the client say he or she belongs? How strong is the client's identification with the group?

Values

What are the client's values and beliefs about life events such as birth and death, health, illness, and health care providers?

Cultural Behavior and Expression

In what ways does the client's cultural group express emotion and feelings, spirituality, and religious beliefs? What are culturally appropriate ways to express grief and loss?

Communication

What language(s) does the client speak or read? In what language does the client prefer to communicate? Does the client speak and/or write English? Is an interpreter needed? What patterns of communication are used by the client?

Health-related Beliefs and Practices

What are the client's beliefs about the cause(s) of illness and disease? What does the client believe promotes health and healing? What is acceptable behavior for one who is sick?

Nutrition

How does the client's cultural background influence nutrition? What are the beliefs of the client about which foods promote health and which ones do not? Do religious beliefs and practices influence the client's diet?

Socioeconomic Issues

What persons are involved in the client's social network? How do they influence the client's health status? How do they define caring? How does the client's economic status impact lifestyle, living conditions, and the ability to obtain health care?

Health Care Organizations and Cultural Support

How do ethnic/cultural organizations impact the client's access and response to health care?

Education

What is the client's highest level of education? Does the client's education level affect his or her understanding of the health care delivery system, knowledge of how to obtain needed care, experience of the teaching-learning process, and ability to use written material he or she is given?

Religion

To what religion does the client belong? How does the client's religious beliefs affect health and illness? Are there healing rituals or practices the client believes can promote well-being or hasten recovery from illness? Who performs these?

Culture and Disease Incidence

Are there any specific genetic or acquired conditions that are more prevalent for a specific cultural group? Are there socioenvironmental diseases more prevalent among a specific cultural group?

Developmental Considerations

Are there any distinct growth and development characteristics that vary with the client's cultural background? What factors are significant in assessing children of various ages from the newborn period through adolescence? What is the cultural concept of aging? What are culturally acceptable roles for the elderly? (Andrews & Boyle, 1999).

---

system, or health care agency finds meaningful and useful care-delivery strategies based on knowledge of the cultural heritage, beliefs, attitudes, and behaviors of those to whom they render care" (p. 8).

Campinha-Bacote (1998) and Purnell and Paulanka (1998) have established four levels of cultural competency: (1) unconscious incompetence, in which caregivers are unaware of cultural differences in their relationships with clients; (2) conscious incompetence, in which caregivers are aware of cultural differences but lack practical skills in dealing with the health needs of diverse populations; (3) conscious competence, in which caregivers attempt to remedy deficits in knowledge and awareness of cultural differences and begin to provide culturally relevant care; and (4) unconscious competence, in which caregivers automatically provide culturally sensitive care to clients of diverse populations. Community health nurses should evaluate at what stage of the continuum she or he is beginning (Rankin & Stallings, 2001).

General baseline knowledge of different cultural group beliefs, values, and health practices is a good place to start, but such knowledge must be used cautiously because it can lead to stereotyping. **Stereotyping** occurs when an assumption is made that all people of a cultural racial or ethnic group are alike and that they all share the same values and beliefs. This assumption can lead to faulty data gathering and faulty assumptions because each person is culturally unique—a product of past experience, cultural beliefs, and cultural norms. Cultural expressions become patterned responses giving each individual a unique identity which creates diversity within as well as between cultural groups. Competent nursing in this culturally diverse society requires great skill; a cookbook approach will simply not work. So how does the nurse learn the cultural beliefs and values of an individual, a family, the community? The nursing process must be applied through a cultural lens to illicit knowledge of the client. See Figure 8-6 for a list of questions to help the nurse.

CONCEPTUAL FOUNDATIONS FOR TRANSCULTURAL NURSING

Culture, the full product of human concerns, helps us define who we are and what we believe, value, think, and feel. Culture dictates the way we address certain life events, including birth, death, puberty, childbearing, childrearing, illness, and disease, and it influences our language, dietary habits, dress, relationships, and health behaviors. Culture shapes our personalities, families, and social organizations. It is a dominant force in the determination of health-illness caring patterns and behaviors. Because life transitions and health behavior are major focuses of nursing, it is imperative that cultural differences be a central issue in nursing practice. **Culturally diverse care** refers to the great variability in nursing approaches needed to give culturally appropriate care to a rapidly changing, heterogeneous client population (Giger & Davidhizar, 1999). Culturally diverse nursing care employs appropriate variability to meet the needs of more than one aggregate (Giger & Davidhizar, 1999).

Understanding health and illness behavior is crucial to nursing care because behavior both affects and is affected by health status and healing processes. The nurse acknowledges that behavior is meaningful and that meaning is communicated through behavior. When behavior is examined from a cultural perspective, it becomes obvious that the client makes choices on the basis of his or her life meaning and view of the illness.

Transcultural nursing theory in community health nursing practice reflects knowledge, understanding, and sensitivity to diverse cultural values and meanings. **Transcultural nursing,** as defined by Leininger (1991), is "a learned humanistic and scientific area of formal study and practice which is focused upon differences and similarities among cultures with respect to human care, health (or well-being), and illness based upon the people's cultural values, beliefs, and practices" (p. 55). The goal of transcultural nursing practice is to use relevant knowledge to provide care that is culturally specific and congruent. Figure 8-7 is a model reflecting Leininger's sunrise model (1991) of transcultural nursing theory. This model of cultural care reflects influences of one's worldview on the cultural and social structure dimensions which influence language and environment. These factors, then, influence the folk, professional, and nursing systems. This model has served as a prototype for other transcultural nursing models and tools (Giger & Davidhizar, 1999).

A transcultural nursing assessment is necessary to determine those cultural factors, ranging from religious views to folk cures, that may influence the client's health or illness behavior. An important part of this assessment is to determine the client's basic beliefs about the nature of health and disease (Andrews, 1999a). For example, in some cultures, health is considered a gift from God and illness a punishment for sin. In other cultures, illness is thought to result from exposure to the elements, to witchcraft, or to evil spirits. In yet other cultures, health is understood as the balance of feminine (yin) and masculine (yang) energies, and a disharmony in this balance is thought to disturb body functioning. Members of other cultures believe that hot and cold forces are thrown out of balance during illness; these people will eat in a manner and exhibit behavior that they believe will balance these forces.

Cultural assessment is an essential aspect of the nursing process because understanding of culture gives context to behaviors that might otherwise be judged negatively. If cultural behaviors are not recognized as such, their significance may be misunderstood by the nurse.

Two models for cultural assessment are presented here. The Leininger (1991) model is broad in scope and provides a systems approach to cultural understanding. Giger and Davidhizar (1999) propose a model that provides a basis for understanding culturally determined behavior.

The Leininger Sunrise Model

A culture is made up of educational, economic, political, legal, kinship, religious, philosophical, and technological systems. Each of these identified systems affects health.

Health needs are biological, psychosocial, and cultural and are met within a combination of two subsystems: a folk health system (primarily related to religious beliefs and practices) and the professional health system. Leininger (1991) points out that the greater the differences between folk and professional care practices, the greater the need for nursing care accommodations.

The **folk health system** refers to traditional or indigenous health care beliefs and practices. These are performed by local practitioners, are well known to the culture, and have special meanings and uses to heal or assist people to regain well-being or health or to face unfavorable circumstances (Leininger, 1991). *Professional health system* refers to those cognitively learned and practiced modes of assisting others that are obtained through formal professional schools of learning.

Folk medicine systems vary, but they often explain illness in terms of balances between the individual and the physical, social, and spiritual worlds and focus on personal relationships, perhaps involving many persons. Folk medicine classifies illness and disease as natural or unnatural. Natural illnesses are based on logical cause-and-effect relationships. Unnatural events are believed to occur when the harmony of nature is upset. They are unpredictable and may be considered a result of evil forces.

FIGURE 8-7 Leininger's Sunrise Model to Depict Theory of Cultural Care Diversity and Universality

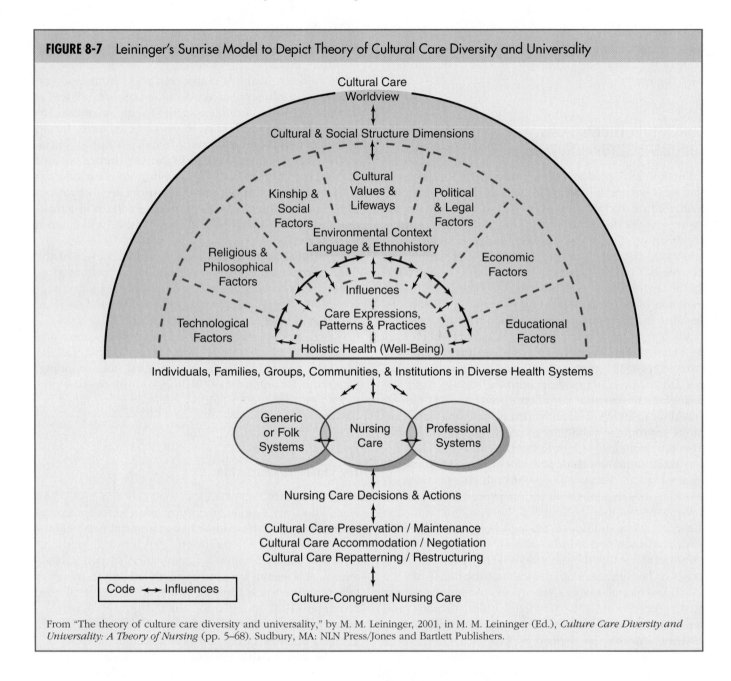

From "The theory of culture care diversity and universality," by M. M. Leininger, 2001, in M. M. Leininger (Ed.), *Culture Care Diversity and Universality: A Theory of Nursing* (pp. 5–68). Sudbury, MA: NLN Press/Jones and Bartlett Publishers.

Unnatural illness may be attributed to punishment for an evil act of some kind, for example.

Although the cultural systems identified by Leininger represent all cultures within and outside the United States, discussion in this text addresses cultures only as they exist within the United States. This textbook is written from the perspective of the dominant culture looking at other cultures. Philosophical and religious systems and their impacts on values, beliefs, and health practices in general are discussed very briefly in this chapter. The reader is referred to Internet web sites for more information on health practices specific to different cultures. Philosophy involves the search for theoretical and analytical knowledge of the nature of the universe and religion the intuitive knowledge obtained through religious and spiritual practices.

The Giger and Davidhizar Model

The Giger and Davidhizar (1999) model proposes that culturally diverse nursing care take into account six cultural phenomena that vary with regard to application and use yet are in evidence among all cultural groups: communication, space, time, social organization, environmental control, and biological variations. These phenomena vary not only across cultures but also with regard to caregiver response, recipient response, context of care, and goals of care. The six phenomena are discussed next.

Communication

Communication implies the entire realm of human interaction and behavior and is the means by which culture is

REFLECTIVE THINKING

Language Barriers

Imagine that you are in another country where few people speak your language. You are well educated and speak the language of the land well but with a heavy accent. You realize people are pretending to understand you rather than asking you to repeat what you say. How do you feel? What might you do to deal with this situation?

transmitted. It provides the way we connect with each other, share information, and send messages and signals related to ideas and feelings. We affect each other by communicating with written or spoken language, gestures, facial expressions, body language, personal space, and symbols. Approximately 100 languages are spoken in the United States (Grossman, 1994), and interpreters are often necessary in community health nursing practice (see Chapter 10).

Communication may present barriers to the client-nurse relationship when the participants are from different cultural backgrounds. These barriers exist when the languages spoken and/or the communication styles, patterns, and understandings are different, leading to feelings of helplessness and alienation for one or more participants. These issues and suggestions for minimizing such barriers are further discussed in Chapter 10.

Space

An individual's comfort level is related to personal space—the area that surrounds a person's body and the objects in that area. Discomfort is experienced when this area is invaded. Personal space is an individual matter and varies not only with the situation but also across cultures. According to Giger and Davidhizar (1999), although some individual variations do exist, persons in the same cultural group tend to exhibit similar spatial behavior.

Because individuals are usually unaware of their own personal space needs, they often have difficulty understanding those of people from different cultures. What one person experiences as a physical expression of friendship, thus, may be interpreted as a threatening invasion of personal space by another. Individuals who step back from the nurse, do not directly face the nurse, or pull their chairs back from the nurse are nonverbally requesting more personal space. Because subtle variations in nonverbal signals can lead to misunderstanding, knowledge of cultural variations in nonverbal behavior is helpful to the community nurse.

Social Organization

The social organization of a culture provides the structure within which **enculturation,** or the process whereby children acquire knowledge and internalize values and attitudes about life events, occurs. A child learns by watching adults and other children while they make inferences about what is appropriate behavior. The resulting values tend to persist for life.

As individuals experience enculturation, they tend to become **culture bound,** meaning they become limited to their own view of reality and are unable to consider the views of other cultures or persons, unable to alter their own beliefs and values, and unable to learn from others. Nurses are culture bound when they insist that the scientific method or nursing process is the only way to solve problems, whereas clients may feel some of their problems can be solved in other ways.

Ethnocentrism refers to the belief that one's own lifeway is the right way or is at least better than another. The outcome of ethnocentrism is cultural imposition. The nurse, for example, might impose her beliefs and values on the client. The client, in turn, might perceive such ethnocentrism as demeaning, possibly resulting in client dysfunction, noncompliance, anger, and/or feelings of inferiority. Such outcomes can be avoided when the nurse has an attitude of openness and the desire to learn from others.

Homogeneity is the assumption that all persons from a particular ethnic group or culture share the same beliefs and values. Variations within a culture or family occur because of age, religion, dialect or language, gender identification and roles, socioeconomic status, geographic location, history of the subcultural group, amount and type of contact between younger and older generations, and degree of adoption of values by the subgroup. It is necessary, therefore, to instead assume that each individual person holds unique beliefs, values, and health care practices.

A person is considered **bicultural** who crosses two cultures, lifestyles, or sets of values. **Ethnicity** refers to a group whose members share a common social and cultural heritage passed on to successive generations. Members of an ethnic group feel a bond and a sense of identity. **Race** implies biological characteristics, such as skin color and bone structure, that are genetically transmitted from one generation to another. A person is **biracial** who crosses two racial and cultural groups. A person who is both bicultural and biracial is in an extremely difficult situation and may not be accepted by any group. **Minority** is a label applied to race, ethnicity, religion, occupation, gender, or sexual orientation. The term carries a variety of potential meanings but in general implies fewer in number than the general population. It may, however, refer to those who lack power or have characteristics perceived as undesirable by those in power.

Acculturation refers to the change of cultural values over time when the influence of another culture is experienced. In the United States, many cultures are represented, and people are influenced by each other. This process accounts, to a large extent, for the great variety of cultural beliefs and practices within any group of people.

The Leininger and the Giger and Davidhizar models provide frameworks for assessing cultural issues involved in nursing relationships where value conflicts exist (see also Chapter 10 on transcultural communication).

Time

Giger and Davidhizar (1999) differentiate social time (duration, time passing) and clock time (points in time). Social time refers to patterns and orientations that are related to social processes and to the conceptualization and ordering of social life. Cultural patterns acknowledge social time such as dinner time, time for bed, prayer time, and gathering time. Whereas most cultures acknowledge social time, attention to clock time varies greatly across cultures. In some cultures, clock time dictates most aspects of life, whereas in others, clock time is ignored or even scorned.

The temporal orientation of a group refers to a focus on either past, present, or future. Cultures or individuals who have a past orientation are generally resistant to change, whereas those with a future orientation tend to change more easily, as long as the existing order is not seriously threatened. Present-oriented persons or cultures tend not to adhere to strict, time-structured schedules. Those who are living in crisis and those who face homelessness, poverty, lack of transportation, and health problems tend to have a present temporal orientation, focusing on moment-to-moment survival. Such people often have difficulty keeping appointments in the health care system. Future orientation is requisite to disease prevention efforts such as immunizations, use of condoms, and efforts toward earthquake safety. A future orientation, thus, dictates activities of the present, and knowledge of past efforts and their consequences provides information for planning the future.

Clock time is of paramount importance in the U.S. culture. Accordingly, time management is important to the economics, effectiveness, and efficiency of health care delivery in the United States. The varying temporal orientations of those served by the U.S. health care system may conflict with the prevailing clock time orientation. Clients may interpret provider behaviors stemming from such conflicts as lack of caring.

Environmental Control

Beliefs about humankind's relationship with nature are important to health care. Cultural beliefs and values regarding the nature of the human-environment relationship vary on a continuum, from humans must dominate to humans must live in harmony with to humans are subjugated to nature. For example, a fatalistic attitude of "if I'm going to get cancer, I'll get it no matter what" will deter preventive care. Such beliefs determine one's perceived **locus of control** as being either internal or external, depending on whether one feels one's health is controlled by one's own behaviors and choices or by factors outside one's self. Specific examples of how these beliefs affect family health behavior are discussed later in this chapter.

Biological Variations

Biological variations are differences among people that are attributed to heredity, including body structure, skin color, and other visible physical characteristics; enzymatic and genetic variations; electrocardiographic patterns; susceptibility to disease; nutritional preferences and deficiencies; and psychological characteristics. People of different races tend to vary in height, body size, skin color, and other physical characteristics such as mongolian spots on the skin of African American, Asian, Native American, or Mexican newborns. Enzymatic variations make some health conditions more likely among people of certain races. For example, lactose intolerance is a problem for many Japanese, and inverted T waves in the precordial leads of an electrocardiogram is a common finding among African Americans but is considered abnormal among Caucasian Americans.

Susceptibility to disease is considered to have genetic or environmental origins or a combination of the two. Sickle cell anemia is found predominantly in the African American population. Systemic lupus erythematosus is fairly common among women in general but is considered extremely rare among Asians, including Asian women.

Nutritional patterns also affect biological variation. Cultural differences in nutritional intake are addressed in Chapter 11. Nutritional patterns most likely affect body structure, susceptibility to disease, and many of the biological variations found among races and cultural groups.

Psychological characteristics also vary among racial groups. Feelings of insecurity may be related to cultural background. For example, psychological adjustment may be difficult for a Native American who has lived on a reservation but goes to a college where there are few, if any, other Native Americans. Mental health may be defined as a balance in a person's internal life and the person's adaptation to the outer reality. Normal behavior, then, is culturally determined, and psychological characteristics are based on enculturation processes. Other variables affecting mental health are family relationships, childrearing practices, language, attitudes toward illness, social status, and economic status. Racism may be a major factor in the mental and physical health of minority groups.

CULTURAL BELIEFS AND VALUES OF PROFESSIONAL NURSING AND THE NURSE

Cultural awareness and understanding apply not only to the cultural beliefs and practices of the client but also to those of the nurse. Self-awareness and careful identification of one's own values as cultural phenomena facilitate understanding in transcultural settings and relationships. The values the nurse may explore include those shared with the culture of the nursing profession, those shared with the dominant culture, ethnic values shared with family, and individual values shared with select peers and friends.

Cultural Beliefs and Values of Professional Nursing

Value conflicts often occur between clients and nurses and/or between clients and others who work in health care. A look at some of the shared beliefs held not only by nurses but also by others within the health care system may be helpful. These beliefs are related to a standardized definition of health and illness and to the omnipotence of technology. Persons are usually considered ill only when medical diagnostic tests indicate disease. Certain procedures are used during birth and death, and rituals surround events such as the physical examination, surgical procedures, and visitors and visiting hours in institutions (Spector, 1996).

Disease prevention is encouraged via the use of immunizations and annual physical examinations involving certain diagnostic procedures. A systematic approach and problem-solving methods are valued. Health promotion activities are linked with diet, exercise, and stress management. As a rule, health care professionals approve of clients who are prompt, neat, clean, and organized and who have a high degree of compliance. More significance is placed on biological processes than on psychological or social processes. The U.S. culture values independence and self-responsibility. Financial dependence on others for health care is therefore met with a certain attitude of disapproval on the part of care providers and shame or embarrassment on the part of indigent care receivers.

Disease is a condition clearly defined in biomedical sciences. Illness, on the other hand, involves a perception of being sick on the part of the person involved. Illness is culturally shaped because it is individually perceived. Human response to perceptions of illness is considered the domain of nursing.

The biomedical approach of contemporary health care has served well but has needed the balance of nursing to promote and nurture positive health and holistic healing. Nursing traditionally has addressed the wholeness of persons. Rogers (1990), an early theorist, defines the person as more than the sum of his or her parts and as "an irreducible, indivisible, multidimensional energy field identified by pattern and manifesting characteristics that are specific to the whole and which cannot be predicted from knowledge of the parts" (p. 7). Furthermore, person and environment are perceived in this paradigm as inseparable, functioning as interpenetrating processes. These notions contrast markedly with the culture of the United States but fit well with many others and tap into a long-standing theme of nursing theory and practice. According to Rogerian nursing theory, organizational patterns of the human-environment interrelationship determine health. Thus, this philosophy or conceptual model for nursing practice uses the term **pattern appraisal** for health assessment.

Nursing theories provide a holistic view of the person that fits with the human need for respect of one's wholeness.

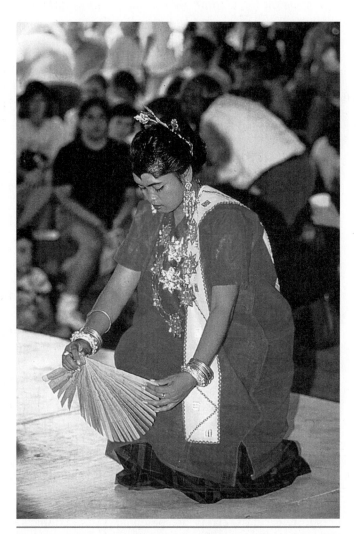

Respect for and interest in the client's cultural background are very important in transcultural assessment. Photo courtesy of the Smithsonian Institution.

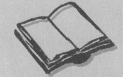

Out
of the Box

Developing Cultural Competence

Cultural competence is achieved not only by knowing about the culture of another person, but by understanding one's own cultural values and beliefs as well as those of clients. Self-examination is required. Grossman's (1994) guidelines serve as the basis for this exercise. Journal your thoughts as you reflect on your own cultural beliefs and values and how they are expressed in your life.

- *Know yourself. Examine your own values, attitudes, beliefs, and prejudices before trying to help people from other cultures.*
- *Keep an open mind. Look at the world through the perspectives of culturally diverse people by reading books and seeing movies that reflect different cultural perspectives.*
- *Respect differences among peoples. Recognize and appreciate the inherent worth of diverse cultures (including your own), valuing them equally with your own.*

- *Be willing to learn. Learn by getting to know culturally diverse peoples through traveling, reading, attending events held by local ethnic or cultural organizations, and talking with clients and colleagues.*
- *Learn to communicate effectively. Study another language. Be sensitive to the nuances of language and expression, affect, posture, gestures, body movements, and use of personal space. Cultivate trust in your relationships with clients.*
- *Do not judge. Refrain from making judgments about cultural behaviors and practices that seem strange to you.*
- *Be resourceful and creative. Remember that there are many ways to attain the same goal. Tailor your nursing interventions to fit people of different cultures.*

Adapted from "Enhancing Your Cultural Competence," by D. Grossman, 1994, American Journal of Nursing, July, pp. 58–62. Copyright 1994 by D. Grossman. ■

Cultural Beliefs and Values of the Nurse

Cultural competence requires nurses to provide an environment in which the values, customs, and spiritual beliefs of clients will be respected. Nurses, to meet this requirement, must first understand their own values and beliefs before they can respect those of clients. Values clarification processes require self-reflection and deep self-understanding related to personal values and beliefs. Personal values provide a foundation for the development of professional values. These values do change over time through education and exposure to new ideas, new people, and new life situations. Value clarification processes have been developed to help individuals identify their beliefs and values and to gain self-understanding (Lustig & Koester, 1999). (See Out of the Box.)

Exploring one's own beliefs and values is very important in working with those of different cultures. Understanding one's own beliefs and values from a cultural perspective lends clarity to potential value conflicts. Leininger (1978) identifies the values and preferences of U.S. culture: independence; equality; individuality; justice; privacy; materialism; competition; efficiency; and freedom of speech, enterprise, action, and worship. These values, as dear as they are to many in the United States, are often in direct opposition to the values held by other cultures. For example, independence among family members—a valued trait in white, middle-class America—may be viewed negatively in a culture that values cooperation among group members.

FAMILY FOLK HEALTH PRACTICES

Although variation in health beliefs and practices exists among people of any culture, there are many shared beliefs and practices within any given culture and also across cultures. This section outlines some beliefs and practices (grouped according to stage of development) that, though often unfamiliar to the nurse, the nursing profession, and the dominant culture being served, are found in many cultures. A word of caution, though, is necessary; since there is wide variation within any cultural belief system, the nurse must not assume that a person practices any particular belief or health behavior.

Pregnancy, Birth, and the Postpartum Period

In all cultures, many beliefs and practices exist that are related to pregnancy, birth, and the postpartum period. Figure 8-8 offers examples of cultural beliefs about pregnancy.

Beliefs surrounding birth have to do with whether the culture defines the birth process as an achievement, a defilement, or a state of pollution necessitating ritual purification. Differences also exist with regard to whether the partner should be present at the birth. In some cultures (Mexican American, Cambodian, Native American), the partner is expected to be present in the birthing room. Other cultures (Orthodox Jewish, Islamic, Chinese, and Asian Indian backgrounds) have prohibitions against the man's viewing the woman's body or require the separation of the husband and wife once the bloody show or cervical dilation has occurred. Thus, the nurse cannot assume that a partner is uninvolved or uninterested in the birth process just because he is absent from the birth (Lauderdale, 1999).

Many cultural groups have beliefs that postpartum vulnerability is due to *imbalance* (disharmony caused by the processes of pregnancy and birth) or to *pollution* or *being unclean* (bleeding at birth and in the postpartum period). Restitution of balance and purification are achieved through certain behaviors. These include dietary restrictions or prescriptions, ritual baths, seclusion, activity restriction, or other ceremonial events (Lauderdale, 1999). If the nurse does not understand certain observed behaviors, it is important to inquire about them to ascertain their relevance to the client's situation. For instance, pregnancy is considered a "hot" physical state in the theory of hot/cold practiced by Hispanics and African Americans and in the yin/yang theory practiced by the Chinese and some other Asian cultures. Heat is thought to be lost during the birthing process, so postpartum practices focus on restoring the balance between cold/hot or yin/yang. To this end, clients will eat foods that are considered hot but not those that are considered cold. When providing nutritional information in such instances, the nurse should find out which foods will be acceptable to the client and her family (Lauderdale, 1999; Spector, 1996).

Infants and Small Children

In many Middle Eastern cultures, children are covered with multiple layers of clothing even in warm temperatures, because it is believed that young children become chilled easily and die from exposure to the cold.

Mal ojo (evil eye) is feared throughout much of the world, and it is believed to be caused by "an individual who voluntarily or involuntarily injures a child by looking at or admiring him or her. The individual has a desire to hold the child, but the wish is frustrated, either by the parent or the infant or by the reserve of the individual"

FIGURE 8-8 Family Folk Practices about Pregnancy

Prescriptive Beliefs

- Remain active during pregnancy to aid the baby's circulation (Crow Indian).
- Remain happy to bring the baby joy and good fortune (Pueblo and Navajo Indians, Mexican, Japanese).
- Sleep flat on your back to protect the baby (Mexican).
- Keep active during pregnancy to ensure a small baby and an easy delivery (Mexican).
- Continue sexual intercourse to lubricate the birth canal and prevent dry labor (Haitian, Mexican).
- Continue daily baths and frequent shampoos during pregnancy to produce a clean baby (Filipino).

Restrictive Beliefs

- Avoid cold air during pregnancy (Mexican, Haitian, Asian).
- Do not reach over your head, or the cord will wrap around the baby's neck (African American, Hispanic, Caucasian, Asian).
- Avoid weddings and funerals or you will bring bad fortune to the baby (Vietnamese).
- Do not continue sexual intercourse, or harm will come to you and the baby (Vietnamese, Filipino, Samoan).
- Do not tie knots or braid or allow the baby's father to do so because it will cause difficult labor (Navajo Indian).
- Do not sew (Pueblo Indian, Asian).

Taboos

- Avoid lunar eclipses and moonlight, or the baby may be born with a deformity (Mexican).
- Do not walk on the streets at noon or five o'clock because doing so may make the spirits angry (Vietnamese).
- Do not join in traditional ceremonies such as Yei or Squaw dances, or spirits will harm the baby (Navajo Indian).
- Do not get involved with persons who cast spells, or the baby will be eaten in the womb (Haitian).
- Do not say the baby's name before the naming ceremony, or harm might come to the baby (Orthodox Jewish).
- Do not have your picture taken because it might cause stillbirth (African American).

From "Transcultural Nursing Care of the Childbearing Family," by J. Lauderdale and D. Greener (1999), in M. M. Andrews and J. S. Boyle (Eds.), *Transcultural Concepts in Nursing Care* (3rd ed., pp. 81–106), Philadelphia: J. B. Lippincott. Copyright 1995 by J. B. Lippincott. Adapted with permission.

(Andrews, 1999b, p. 127). Several hours after this experience, the child cries and develops symptoms of fever, vomiting, diarrhea, appetite loss, eyes rolling back in the head, and listlessness. Mal ojo can be prevented by "touching or patting the child when admiring him or her" (p. 127). The services of a *curandera* (traditional healer) are usually sought to pray and to massage the child with oil. An unbroken raw egg may first be passed over the child's body and then cracked and placed in a bowl of water under the crib. This process is believed to draw the fever from the child and to poach the egg (Andrews, 1999b). From the nurse's perspective, the child's symptoms are indicative of dehydration. Without interfering with the curandera's treatment, however, nurses can teach the family how to treat and prevent dehydration.

In most cultures, symptoms are identified in a culturally unique way. In the Hispanic culture, *susto* (nervousness, loss of appetite, and loss of sleep) is believed to be caused by a frightening experience. Treatment is relaxation. *Pujos* (grunting sounds and protrusions of the umbilicus) is believed to be caused by contact with a woman who is menstruating or by the infant's own mother if she menstruated before 40 days after delivery. The cure is achieved by tying a piece of fabric from the woman's clothing around the baby's waist for three days (Andrews, 1999b; Spector, 1996).

Caida de la mollera (fallen fontanel symptoms including crying, fever, vomiting, and diarrhea) is believed to be caused by a variety of things such as falling on the head, abrupt removal of the nipple from the infant's mouth, and failure to place a cap on the infant's head. People of many cultures see it as synonymous with deshidratacion (dehydration), with which the symptoms correspond. Families do not always recognize the need to seek medical help, so the nurse's assessment is very important (Andrews, 1999b; Spector, 1996).

Children

Female genital mutilation, a ritual found primarily in many African countries, is potentially devastating and is viewed with disdain by many people outside the countries where it is practiced. This ritual is carried out on girls between 4 and 12 years of age. The procedure ranges from *clitoridectomy* (cutting away part or the whole of the clitoris), to *excision* (amputation of the clitoris and the inner lips of the labia), to *infibulation* (removal of the clitoris and the labia minora, with the labia majora being stitched together and a small opening being created for the passage of urine and menstrual flow). This procedure results in lifelong physical, sexual, and psychological problems. The practice continues because it is believed to be necessary for cleanliness and for becoming a real woman. It is also believed that a woman cannot be married without the completion of the ritual (Touba, 1995). In these countries, being unmarried is an economic

calamity. Although outlawed, this ritual continues to be practiced not only by those in the home countries but also by families who have emigrated to the United States or other countries. In addition to the extreme physical danger in which this practice places the female child, marital and childbirth problems continue throughout life.

Empacho (stomach pains and cramps) is believed to be caused by a ball of undigested food clinging to some part of the gastrointestinal tract or by lying about the amount of food eaten. Treatment is to rub and gently pinch the spine. This treatment can be problematic if the cause of symptoms is something serious such as appendicitis (Andrews, 1999b; Spector, 1996).

A health treatment used by many Chinese to treat mumps or convulsions is *moxibustion*. The moxa plant is ignited and placed near specific areas of the body. After this treatment, tiny craters can be observed on the skin. Similarly, *skin scraping* (applying special oil to a symptomatic area and rubbing the area with the edge of a coin in a firm, downward motion) may be used for treating colds, heatstroke, headache, and indigestion, and *cupping* (creating a vacuum inside a cup by burning a special material in the cup and then placing the cup immediately on a selected area and keeping the cup there until it is easily removed) may be used for treating headaches, arthritis, and abdominal pain. Skin scraping can result in multiple bruises on the skin, and cupping appears as circular bruises with burns to the skin (Giger & Davidhizar, 1999). The nurse must understand these practices in order to assess whether they are harmful, neutral, or beneficial to the client. Education can be directed toward supporting beneficial and neutral practices and finding alternatives to those that are harmful. It is important to assess the intention of the family. Practices such as those just described may cause slight physical damage but should not be construed as intentional child abuse.

All Ages

Food Patterns

Nutrition is a most important consideration in nursing care, and cultural heritage is a major determinant of food intake. Nurses focus much of their care on teaching proper nutrition and encouraging their clients to improve their eating habits. Good nutrition helps people, not only physically and psychologically, but in sharing food with others, they experience sociocultural values and lifeways. Sharing a meal is usually a sign of affection and friendship, whereas refusal to eat with someone reflects anger, hostility, rejection, punishment, or mistrust (Andrews, 1999b).

Other related factors determining food intake patterns include lifestyle, socioeconomic status, religion, education, and individual factors such as nutritional requirements for age, gender and body size, health status, and taste physiology. In many cultures, people are concerned with maintaining balance in their food intake. For instance, some cultures believe in hot/cold theory and some follow an ancient system of yin/yang balance. In the hot/cold system, health is considered to be a state of balance among the body humors (blood, phlegm, black bile, and yellow bile) manifesting in a wet, warm body. Illness is thought to result from a humoral imbalance that results in a body that is dry, cold, hot, wet, or a combination of these states. Balance in the yin/yang theory maintains harmony in the universe. Yin represents female, cold, and darkness, whereas yang represents male, hot, and light. Foods are yin, yang, or neutral in nature and imbalances in these types of food cause disease (Andrews, 1999b). Nutritional guidance for health promotion, maintenance, and restoration must be given within the cultural framework of the individual and/or family client.

Herbal Remedies

Other beliefs are related to natural healing and herbal practices. Many families believe in using certain herbs for particular illnesses while also making use of Western medicine (Giger & Davidhizar, 1999). Native Americans use herbs because they believe the basis of therapy lies in nature. Only proper plants are picked, and specific rituals are followed meticulously. Some herbs that have the same effects as pharmaceuticals could result in harmful interactions or overdoses if used along with certain pharmaceuticals. It therefore is important for the nurse to identify all drugs and herbs being used by the client so that potentially harmful results can be avoided. See Chapter 12 for further discussion.

Traditional Practitioners

Many families are likely to use traditional practitioners prior to or in conjunction with Western medicine. Native Americans have tribal practitioners who use their knowledge of prevention, health maintenance, and treatment and who interweave religious beliefs and healing practices to attain total healing of the mind, body, and spirit. Clients of Hispanic descent may use the services of a curandera. For many African Americans, the church serves as a support, with the minister helping to reinforce health beliefs and practices. Other cultural healers in African American culture are older women who have herbal knowledge, the spiritualist who has received the gift of healing from God, the voodoo priest or priestess, and the root doctor (Boyle, 1995; Andrews & Herberg, 1999). In the dominant North American culture, many religious groups incorporate religious leaders into healing practices.

Treatments

Clients may use a wide variety of folk remedies prescribed or administered by family members or folk healers. Some clients, for example, treat respiratory congestion by rubbing the chest with warm, camphorated oil and wrapping

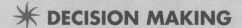

✳ DECISION MAKING

Family Health Beliefs

You are visiting a Hispanic family who has lived in the United States for six months, having moved here from Mexico. When you enter the home, Leticia, the mother, is rubbing the stomach of her crying, one-month-old child, Roberto. She tells you he has empacho.

♦ How would you begin a discussion about combining a medical perspective with Leticia's cultural perspective?

♦ How would you identify a possible cause of the problem from your perspective and at the same time respect Leticia's perspective?

♦ How can you work with Leticia to teach her how to manage the situation and also respect her health beliefs and practices?

up in a warm blanket. They may also apply poultices to painful or inflamed areas to draw out the cause of the infection.

The nurse must not forget that the dominant U.S. culture, composed of Caucasians of European descent (primarily German, Irish, English, Italian, French, Polish, and Dutch), has family folk health beliefs of its own. Some such beliefs are applying a bag of camphor around the neck prevents the flu (Irish); drafts cause irritation that can lead to a cold and then pneumonia (Italian); sleeping with the windows open prevents illness (German); and illness is caused by poor diet (Polish) (Spector, 1996). These and many other beliefs are held by families throughout the United States, prompting health behaviors that may be different from those of the nurse. Each country has its own predominant health beliefs that are powerfully meaningful to the people who practice them. It is important for the nurse to consider the intent behind related behaviors and to work with families in the best interests of positive health outcomes.

RELIGION: BRIDGING CULTURE AND SPIRITUALITY

The search for the meaning of life has provided the impetus for the formation of religion. Every religion has three aspects: philosophical, mythological, and ritualistic. Among the various religions, the fundamental philosophical principles are very much alike; the mythology is in some ways similar and in some ways different; and the rituals and practices are quite different (Viswananda, 1938/1992). All religions purport that there is an ultimate being who is creator, and most purport that the ultimate being has sent at least one (and, in some cases, several)

Primal Religions of the World

Smith (1991) has classified the world religions as either **primal** or **historical. Primal religions** are those that have existed as oral traditions for millions of years within tribal groups or communities. The numbers of people practicing primal religions are decreasing, yet tribal traditions are practiced in Africa, Australia, Southeast Asia, the Pacific Islands, Siberia, and North and South America. The sacred traditions honor the spoken word, as opposed to recorded scriptures; the sacred place, which is the symbol for a particular setting such as that provided by nature; and time, in that the past is honored as being closer to the source of all divine creation. These foundational beliefs provide the foundation for the use of rhythms, intonations, accents, pauses, animal postures, sounds, and silence performed as religious rituals of chanting, storytelling, and theater arts. Members of these groups believe that one life pervades all form, that all are one, and that all life is sacred. The life goal of these peoples is to live in constant consciousness with the sacred. A dynamic sense of harmony with the earth and her cycles permeates all life, and a spiritual force surrounds art, ritual, and ceremony (Heinberg, 1989).

Historical Religions of the World

The **historical religions,** formed over the past 4000 years or so, almost blanket the earth. These religions are founded not on abstract principles but in concrete events, actual historical happenings. They have sacred texts to teach and guide the followers, and their cumulative traditions have developed over time (Smith, 1991).

In this section some of the major religions of the world are briefly described. The purposes of the discussion are to promote understanding and appreciation for the similarities in their philosophical positions and to foster awareness of the great variances in health care practices and rituals within each religion, branch, denomination, group, or practicing family. The community health nurse determines specific health beliefs and values by engaging each client in a thorough cultural assessment.

Hinduism

The Hindu religions are thought to be the oldest of the historical religions. Hinduism reflects a metaphysical understanding and way of life—defining morals, customs, medicine, art, music, and dance—and comprises a vast range of beliefs and practices. It is believed that "underlying the human self and animating it is a reservoir of being that never dies, is never exhausted, and is unrestricted in consciousness and bliss" (Smith, 1991, p. 21). This infinite center, the hidden Self, is one with Brah-

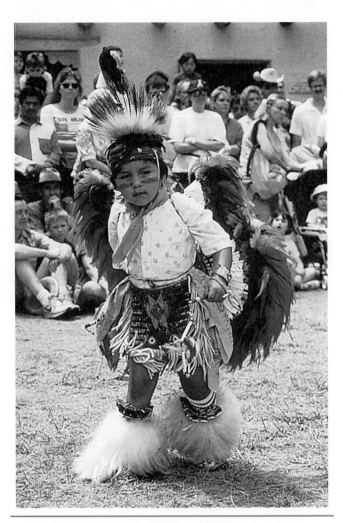

This young Native American celebrates an ancient tradition. Photo courtesy of the Smithsonian Institution.

great teachers to the earth to help humankind in some way. Some believe their religion to be the only true way, and others believe that all of the world's great religions lead to truth.

A common theme in religious mythology is that, in the beginning, a great sea of unfathomable chaos—a profound darkness—covered a vast potential having no beginning and from which emerged the One from which all creation is manifested. These mythological stories purport to reveal the origin of the world. Though the stories differ from culture to culture, the sacred theme reveals the underlying search for the meaning and purpose of life and death. Stories, symbols, and rituals provide guidelines for happy and productive lives. When the inevitable suffering occurs, legends guide the search for meaning. These stories form the foundation for cultural beliefs from which individuals derive meaning. The quest for spiritual understanding is as universal as are stories and can be seen as guiding the unfolding of our lives.

man, the underlying force of all that is. Although the ultimate purpose of life is to fully realize that Oneness or enlightenment, one moves through various stages. The path of the Hindu may be one of intuitive knowledge, love for God, work with no thought of reward, or meditation.

Hinduism accepts all religions as paths to God. The Vedas, the ancient scripture of the Hindus, declare that "Truth is One; sages call it by different names" and "It is possible to climb life's mountain from any side, but when the top is reached the trails converge" (Smith, 1991, p. 73). Hindus believe that the universe is in constant change but there is order and meaning in which one must participate for health and well-being. The purpose of life is seen as attainment of enlightenment through union with Brahman or God. Although one may not reach Oneness or God-realization in this life, any spiritual development attained is not wasted but, instead, is brought back for use in the next life.

Health practices in the Hindu culture are based on an understanding of prana, the life force energy of the human being. Chakras (energy centers) are associated with consciousness and body function. Health results when these primary forces are in harmony. Disease or illness is thought to result when there is a break in this system. Disease reflects the whole of one's life, so diet, relationships, environment, season, thoughts, attitudes, and lifestyle are considered in diagnosis and treatment.

Buddhism

The Buddha, born Siddhartha Gautama in 563 B.C. in present-day Nepal, was considered a reformer of Hinduism. In fact, many of Buddha's reforms were instituted by Hinduism, and Buddha is considered to be an incarnation of God by Hindus (Smith, 1991). Known as the Enlightened One, or Awakened Being, he taught his followers lessons on right living for 45 years and died of dysentery at the age of 80. He taught his followers how to live a balanced life in which a body is given just what it needs to function optimally and no more.

Buddha observed and stated his Four Noble Truths. First, life lived in a typical way is filled with suffering due to birth trauma, sickness, morbidity and related fears, fear of death, inability to get rid of unwanted conditions, and separation from what we love. Second, personal desires are a cause of suffering, while desires for others or for the whole of humanity are liberating. The Third Noble Truth addresses the Second Noble Truth in this way: since the cause of torment in life is personal desire, the cure lies in overcoming craving for personal desire. The Fourth Noble Truth contains the prescription for eliminating the craving for personal desire and for bringing relief from suffering. The Eightfold Path begins when right association is established and is followed by (1) right views, (2) right intent, (3) right speech, (4) right conduct,

(5) right livelihood, (6) right effort, (7) right mindfulness, and (8) right concentration. He taught followers to seek *nirvana,* the release of boundaries of the finite self, manifesting boundless life and bliss, the highest destiny of the human spirit.

Buddhist teachings deny the existence of a personal Creator-God and emphasize personal responsibility and intense self-effort for right living (Smith, 1991). Many schools of thought and numerous sects exist within the Buddhism; the teachings presented here are core beliefs. Teachings encourage living a healthy lifestyle of moderation and balance. Buddhists teach nonkilling, are vegetarians and do not drink intoxicants.

Judaism

Judaism is best understood through the historical experience of the Jewish people. In fact, the meaningfulness of history is considered very important because (1) the context in which life is lived affects the way life is lived, creating problems, delineating opportunities, and conditioning its outcomes; (2) since contexts are crucial for life, social action is required; (3) history, then, provides a field of opportunity for service to God and for learning; and (4) each of these life opportunities are unique and challenging, but some are particularly decisive in the course of history, requiring timely attention since opportunities pass and may never return (Smith, 1991). The prophets, those persons who are considered to speak by authority of God, are also significant in that they teach that the future of any people depends primarily on justice within the social order and that individuals are responsible for the social structure of their society as well as for their own direct personal dealings. Social justice is required for political stability, yet mercy is also a requirement of Yahweh's (a name for God) limitless love:

REFLECTIVE THINKING

Honoring a Jewish Family's Death Rituals

How can you show respect for a Jewish family at the time of death?

- The rituals surrounding death are complex and important aspects of Jewish tradition. How would you learn about these rituals?
- How would you provide support to the family as they honor their traditions?
- How would you share in these traditions if you are Jewish? If you are not?

A king had some empty glasses. He said: "If I pour hot water into them they will crack; if I pour ice-cold water into them they will also crack!" What did the king do? He mixed the hot and the cold water together and poured it into them and they did not crack. Even so did the Holy One, blessed be He, say: "If I create the world on the basis of the attribute of mercy alone, the world's sins will greatly multiply. If I create it on the basis of the attribute of justice alone, how could the world endure? I will therefore create it with both the attributes of mercy and justice, and may it endure!" (Quoted by Smith, 1991, p. 292)

Judaism represents not only the faith and culture of a people but also observance of numerous laws and basic rituals such as the Sabbath, dietary laws, daily prayers, and the like. Judaism also represents a nation of people. Jews vary greatly in their beliefs; there are Jews who believe that every letter and punctuation mark in the Torah was dictated by God and there are others who do not believe there is a God. Actions define the religious and spiritual practices of the Jewish people in a more consistent way than do thoughts or beliefs (Smith, 1991).

The core beliefs of Judaism are there is but one God and only the sins of humankind separate people from the divine. Central to Jewish faith is that humans are to love, praise, and serve God above all else. The Torah holds the laws and sacred traditions (Steinberg, 1974).

The family is seen as the basic unit of society; it has sacred obligations to maintain integrity and purity in relationship with God. The Sabbath is the central day of the week. There are regulations regarding permitted and forbidden foods, including regulations against eating flesh cooked with milk, certain animal parts, an animal that has not been killed in accordance with the law, and the like (Steinberg, 1974). Many laws regulate caring for the sick and dying. Specific prayers are uttered while loved ones lie on their deathbeds and at synagogue services for 11 months after death. Spirit and body are considered separated at death, with the spirit entrusted to God and the body returned to the earth.

Christianity

Christianity emerged with the birth of Jesus around the year A.D. 5. Jesus Christ, the healer-teacher-visionary and the revealer of God's laws, came to fulfill and transform the old laws of Judaism. Christianity teaches of one God consisting of a trinity: the Father, the Son, and the Holy Spirit—the spirit of love and grace that descends upon humanity for relief of suffering. God is found within, and the search provides the purpose and meaning of life.

The Christian church has split into three branches: Roman Catholicism focuses on the Vatican in Rome and spreads from there and is dominant through central and southern Europe, Ireland, and South America. Eastern Orthodoxy has its major influence in Greece, the Slavic countries, and the Soviet Union. Protestantism dominates northern Europe, England, Scotland, and North America. The deepest differences in Protestantism today are not denominational but cut across denominational lines: fundamentalist, conservative-evangelical, mainline, charismatic, and social activist. These differences have developed recently and are only mentioned here to demonstrate the complexity of the divisions in Protestantism. Eighty-five percent of Protestants belong to 12 denominations, yet the 4 major groups—Baptist, Lutheran, Calvinist and Anglican—have subdivided into some 900-odd Protestant denominations in the United States alone (Smith, 1991). The ecumenical movement is the stimulus for the merger occurring among some of these denominations. Health beliefs and practices vary widely. The Bible is the source of inspiration for Christians, although interpretation and understanding vary.

The writings about Jesus contain many examples of his healing the sick through laying on of hands, faith healing, and releasing demons. These practices continue in certain Christian churches. Common to most denominations, if not all, is the use of prayer in support of those who are ill or suffering (Mitchell, 1991).

Islam

The prophet Muhammad was born in Mecca around A.D. 570 and became the channel through which the nature of God as the Absolute was made known. In his middle years, after being married and raising a family, Muhammad spent his time praying in a cave. In the silence, he heard the revelation "Thou art the messenger of God, and I am Gabriel" (Azzam, 1964, p. 30). The teachings channeled through Muhammad by the archangel Gabriel while Muhammad was in the cave are recorded in the Koran. The historical teachings share roots with Judaism and Christianity in the stories of Abraham in the Old Testament and theological concepts are similar in the three religions. Smith (1991) describes the progression of teachings in relation to the three religions and their prophets: First, God revealed the existence of one God through Abraham; then God revealed the Ten Commandments through Moses; and Jesus taught, "Love God with all your heart and mind and strength" and the Golden Rule—"Do unto others as you would have them do unto you." The question left in this process was "How does one love God? How does one love their neighbor?" The answer came through the prophet Muhammad and was recorded in the Koran.

The meaning of the word *Islam* is "the peace that comes when one's life is surrendered to God" (Smith, 1991, p. 222). *Allah* is the word used for the Absolute Reality or God. Those who adhere to Islam are known as Muslims. The Koran is central to Islamic life, and portions of this book are chanted at births, weddings, and deaths.

The Koran proclaims repeatedly that there is no God but Allah and warns against worship of idols (Nasr, 1975). Muhammad established a political, social, and religious structure based on his understandings of the teachings.

Like all world religions, the Law of Islam orders that one do good and reject all that is reprehensible. Rituals of faith associated with Islam are prayer, giving of money or food, fasting, and making the pilgrimage to Mecca at least once in one's life. Specific rules govern the way of death and proper burial.

Core Beliefs Shared by World Religions

All these religious traditions have similar belief systems and contain a strong message of love for a divine nature of ultimate reality and for others. It is important to note that extremists of any religion do not reflect the mainstream and, as such, may be dangerous and oppressive to others (Viswananda, 1938/1992).

Religion serves as a vehicle for expressing spirituality through a framework of values, beliefs, and rituals and, for some, provides answers to essential questions about life and death issues. Nurses must acknowledge, honor, and respect the fact that people choose their own form of religion. The forms may not always be those accepted by recognized world religions such as those discussed here. Many people experience a blurring of boundaries and a blending of various religious traditions in relation to their own spirituality. Some experience their spirituality best within a particular religious tradition. Others address their spirituality through blending different religious and philosophical traditions; and still others experience their spirituality outside organized religious systems. People express, experience, and nurture their spiritual selves in many ways and cultural assessment tools provide a means to obtain knowledge for giving relevant nursing care (Burkhardt & Nagai-Jacobson, 2000).

Although religion does not provide specific information about health care practices, it does provide a basis for understanding people and their behaviors. Other cultural health care practices may be specific to a certain locality or ethnic group, but even these practices can vary greatly with education, acculturation, and social contacts.

PRACTICE APPLICATIONS IN TRANSCULTURAL NURSING

Culturally diverse nursing care is characterized by variability in nursing approaches. Because intercultural differences in care beliefs, values, and practices do exist, nursing practice must reflect these differences. Nurses must provide clinically appropriate care while supporting health behaviors based on the client's beliefs, religion, and cultural practices. The nurse is thus required to step back, see the client's perspective, and work to bring the best of both the professional system's and the folk system's approaches to the situation. Case management can provide a framework for facilitating culturally appropriate care. In this way, the nurse can meet the needs of each client by marshaling resources, interventions, activities, and services.

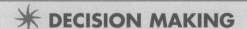

DECISION MAKING

Cultural Conflict

You are case manager for an elderly woman with breast cancer who has been told that her condition is terminal. Family members tell you of a plan to take their dying mother on a pilgrimage to Mecca against medical advice.

♦ How would you proceed?

♦ What resources would you use?

♦ How would you evaluate the client's wishes in this matter?

♦ What goals of care would influence your intervention?

♦ What factors of care and prognosis would you consider most important?

Assessment Tools for Transcultural Nursing Practice

A variety of assessment tools help uncover the meaning of health behaviors. Leininger (1978) defines cultural nursing assessment as a "systematic appraisal or examination of individuals, groups, and communities as to their cultural beliefs, values, and practices within the cultural context of the people being evaluated" (p. 86).

Perspectives...

INSIGHTS OF A COMMUNITY HEALTH NURSE

I work for a public health department, providing care to people who have communicable diseases. This work has given me a lot of field experience teaching people about bacteria and "bugs." Sometimes, my teaching falls on deaf ears. The population we serve is culturally diverse: Vietnamese, Laotian, Cambodian, Eretrian, Filipino, Korean, Japanese, and Spanish-speaking. I am bilingual in Spanish and English, so much of the teaching I do is with the Spanish-speaking community.

Our staff of public health aides reflects a smattering of our client population, and they are superhelpful to we Caucasian nurses regarding the culturally sensitive issues of our clients. Even so, my interventions are not always heeded, and I get disappointed. I tell myself not to have expectations—to go with the flow—but it is easy to assume that people will act how I think they should . . . and when they do not, I get really disappointed. Other times, I think the people are a certain way—so I think they live in a certain kind of house, and it ends up different than what I expected. So I am often surprised because I have expectations, and things are often different than what I think they will be. I will give you a couple of examples.

A Vietnamese public health aide helped us to understand why a young Chinese woman refused to have blood drawn around the time of the Chinese New Year. He explained that it is a bad omen to take blood out of the body at any time, but especially at the New Year.

We could, then, understand why—no matter how easy we made it for this educated Chinese student—she did not follow through with our instructions. One nurse was able to use a lot of coaxing to get her to do her blood test.

Another time, I was doing follow-up on an active TB case who was Hispanic. I went to a lumbermill where the contact was the only woman who worked in the mill, a middle-aged Caucasian woman who does cleanup. She wore a hard hat, flannel jeans, work pants, and boots, and even after washing her hands, they looked dirty. The dirt was embedded in her skin. When she came to clinic appointments, she dressed the same, except without the hard hat. Her 12-year-old daughter (who could not stop talking) was also a contact. The girl was given a PPD test at the clinic and came back three days later to have it read. When the repeat PPD was done three months later there were transportation problems. I ended up taking the mom home from the clinic so I could read the girl's skin test. My expectation (I cannot get away from them) was that they would live in some sort of shack or very low-income apartment or cottage. As I pulled up to this large, modern, ranch home, I was surprised. The home was very much one you would find in any middle-class suburb. The furnishings were simple and plain.

—Anonymous

REFLECTIVE THINKING

Solving a Dietary Problem

Suppose your cultural assessment reveals that a (child) client is diabetic and the family is unwilling to provide a prescribed diet.

- Which cultural standard is most likely to be met?
- How could you discover a potentially successful intervention?
- Is there a way you could alter the health care system's standard in this case?

Table 8-1 presents an overview of cultural assessment components (Boyle, 1999). These components can be used to assess diverse cultural groups within a community. Boyle (1999) notes that the concept of culture may be more easily applied to a community or group of persons than to an individual. Cultural and spiritual assessments are a part of the nursing process and are performed to identify patterns that may assist or interfere with a nursing intervention or planned treatment regimen.

Questions related to spiritual assessment are best asked toward the end of the interview, when the client and nurse are more at ease with each other. Clients should be informed that assessing their spiritual well-being is integral to evaluating their overall health (Pender, 1996).

TABLE 8-1 Components of the Cultural Assessment

CULTURAL COMPONENT	DESCRIPTION
Family and kinship systems	Is the family nuclear, extended, or "blended"? Do family members live nearby? What are the communication patterns among family members? What are the role and status of individual family members? By age and gender?
Social life	What is the daily routine of the group? What are the important life-cycle events such as birth, marriage, death, etc.? How are the educational systems organized? What are the social problems experienced by the group? How does the social environment contribute to a sense of belonging? What are the group's social interaction patterns? What are its commonly prescribed nutritional practices?
Political systems	Which factors in the political system influence the way the group perceives its status vis-à-vis the dominant culture: that is, laws, justice, and "cultural heros"? How does the economic system influence control of resources such as land, water, housing, jobs, and opportunities?
Language and traditions	Are there differences in dialects or language spoken between health care professionals and the cultural group? How do major cultural traditions of history, art, drama, etc. influence the cultural identity of the group? What are the common language patterns with regard to verbal and nonverbal communication? How is the use of personal space related to communication?
Worldview, value orientations, and cultural norms	What are the major cultural values about human nature and humankind's relationship to nature and to one another? How can the group's ethical beliefs be described? What are the norms and standards of behavior (authority, responsibility, dependability, and competition)? What are the cultural attitudes about time, work, and leisure?
Religion	What are the religious beliefs and practices of the group? How are these related to health practices? What are the rituals and taboos surrounding major life events such as birth and death?
Health beliefs and practices	What are the group's values, attitudes, and beliefs regarding health and illness? Does the cultural group seek care from indigenous health (or folk) practitioners? Who makes decisions about health care? Are there biological variations that are important to the health of this group?

From "Culture, family & community," by J. S. Boyle, 1999, in M. M. Andrews and J. S. Boyle (Eds.), Transcultural Concepts in Nursing Care *(3rd ed., p. 322), Philadelphia: J. B. Lippincott. Copyright 1999 by J. B. Lippincott. Reprinted with permission.*

Caring and Cultural Diversity

In a study of 30 cultures, Leininger (1978, 1984) found a universal desire for and expression of caring, respect, and cherishing, even though caring practices varied from culture to culture. She notes that caring for oneself and for others seems to be significant to the survival of a culture. Indeed, care values, behaviors, and beliefs are considered essential to human growth, living, and survival. Human beings across time have sought ways to care and be cared for, to relate, and to express caring. These same needs are reflected in today's world.

Ethnocentrism often creates barriers in client-nurse relationships and is a deterrent to effective health care. The constructive power of diversity increases as alternative views are valued. Diversity is honored when we:

- Stop to consider another's point of view, especially when our immediate response is to reject it.
- Take deliberate action to keep ourselves open to differences.

Caring is the spiritual process through which we seek to understand our individual place within the whole of our society. Suffering is a human given; caring is the antidote. Found within one's culture are the supports for emergence to wholeness (Arrien, 1993).

COMMUNITY NURSING VIEW

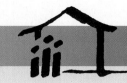

Nancy is a 19-year-old Native American woman who grew up on the reservation in a family of alcohol- and drug-addicted relatives. Physical and sexual abuse started early in her life, and she became an alcohol abuser at age 14. She moved to the city at age 16, lived with a boyfriend who battered her, and was a member of a gang in which relationships were violent. The nurse first saw Nancy after she had been raped by a stranger. She had kept the shame to herself and had told no one. Pattern appraisal (a Rogerian nursing assessment) revealed isolation, hopelessness, low self-worth, feelings of powerlessness, and no future goals except to have a baby. She had been trying to have a baby for three years. The nurse started slowly teaching her about addiction, domestic violence, choices, and basic human rights, including suggestions to help maintain her safety. In addition, the nurse provided counseling support and therapeutic touch treatments that were consistent with Nancy's cultural beliefs.

Each time the nurse saw her, Nancy's expressions of health and self-confidence had grown. As her interests and social patterns grew more diverse and her self-esteem increased, she started making plans to return to school and work. She retold her life experiences with insight and expanding awareness. She was making changes for the better, at her own pace.

Her action plan included incorporating traditional Native American spirituality, healing, and ritual. Nancy and the nurse explored the female aspect within the Native American culture. In the past, Nancy's personal role models had included only women from her family who reflected a picture of subservience, chemical addiction, and domination by male partners. These role models were in direct conflict with traditional Native American female characterizations. She found that, actually, women had always been the power figures and leaders of tribal spirituality and law. Each visit included discussion of a role model chosen from among her women ancestors to emulate and an exploration of available choices.

The nurse stated that she believes that when she sees one person from the Native American community, she is working with at least 50 people. Discuss the following questions regarding the client-nurse relation-

ship and what you would do if you were the community health nurse in this situation.

Nursing Considerations

Assessment

◆ What would be your plan for cultural assessment?

◆ How would you know whether the client has decided that she can trust you?

Diagnosis

◆ What is the relevancy of a pattern appraisal perspective for nursing diagnosis in this situation?

Outcome Identification

◆ Give one expected treatment outcome identified by the client.

◆ Give one expected treatment outcome identified by you, the nurse.

◆ Is it possible to identify expected outcomes in a way that is philosophically consistent with the Rogerian concept of pattern appraisal?

Planning/Interventions

◆ How would you involve Nancy in a mutual planning process for her treatment?

◆ On the basis of your knowledge of Native American cultural beliefs about health and healing, what interventions might be appropriate for Nancy?

Evaluation

◆ How would you evaluate Nancy's progress?

◆ What do you think the nurse meant when she said, "When I work with one person, I believe I am working with at least 50 people"? (From Barrington, 1997).

KEY CONCEPTS

◆ Increased cultural diversity demands that nurses expand their views of health, illness, and nursing care.

◆ Transcultural nursing involves understanding and supporting different meanings among diverse health values and beliefs.

◆ Ethnocentrism presents barriers in the client-nurse relationship and is a deterrent to caring practice.

◆ Nurses should encourage cultural health practices unless such practices are known to be dysfunctional.

◆ Spiritual assessment focuses on the client's inner strength, awareness of life meaning and purpose, and sense of peace and harmony with the universe.

◆ Culture represents the infinite variety of beliefs and lifeways reflected in our differences.

◆ Cultural assessment tools help the nurse understand the meaning of client health behaviors.

◆ All cultures express caring, but in different ways.

RESOURCES

SPIRITUALITY

Dictionary of universal spiritual terms: http://innerself.com/ Magazine/Spirituality

Becoming spiritual, by Wayne Dyer: http://www.innerself.com/newsletter/Spirituality/becoming

Spirit—Finding hope in a world of uncertainty: http://hopeandspirit.com

Joan Borysenko: http://www.joanborysenko.com

CULTURAL UNDERSTANDING AND COMPETENCE

The Spanish language and cultural competency—Latino healthcare: http://www.hhcc.arealahec.dst.nc.us

Asian Pacific Health Care Venture: http://aphcv.apanet.org

Global Intercultural Services: http://globalintercultural.com

History of biomedicine—Indigenous cultures: http://www.mic.ki.se

Folk medicine in Hispanics in the southwestern United States: http://riceinfo.rice.edu/projects/HispanicHealth

African cultures: http://africancultures.about.com/culture

Southeast Asian Archive: http://www.lib.uci.edu/rrsc/sasian.html

Cultural diversity, alternative medicine, and folk medicine: http://www.temple.edu

Health of native people of North America: http://wings.buffalo.edu/publications/mcjrnl/v1n2/gray

Native American foods, culture: http://www.go2net.org

Native American culture: http://www.ewebtribe.com/NACulture

Culturally diverse childrearing practices: Abusive or just different? http://hunter.cuny.edu

International home remedies: http://www.otan.dni.us/webfarm

India parenting: Home remedies: http://www.indiaparenting.com/homeremedies

Traditional health, medicine and healing—Alaska native people: http://www.ankn.uaf.edu/health.html

Traditional medicine—WHO: http://www.who.int

Curanderismo: Folk healing in the southwest: http://soundprint.org/radio/display_show

State Department of Health warns about dangerous Mexican folk remedies: http://www.doh.wa.gov

RELIGION

Taoism as an Earth-based tradition: http://www.apocryphile.net/jrm/articles/taoism.html

Religion & spirituality: http://home.about.com/religion

Religion and ethics—Judaism: http://www.bbc.co.uk/religion

Understanding Islam and Muslims: http://islam.org/Mosque/uiatm/ un_islam.htm

Chapter

9

ENVIRONMENTAL PERSPECTIVES

Phyllis Schubert, DNSc, RN

What nursing has to do . . . is to put the patient in the best condition for nature to act upon him. Generally, just the contrary is done. You think fresh air, and quiet and cleanliness extravagant, perhaps dangerous, luxuries, which should be given to the patient only when quite convenient, and medicine the sine qua non, the panacea. If I have succeeded in any measure in dispelling this illusion, and in showing what true nursing is, and what it is not, my object will have been answered.

—Nightingale, 1860/1969, p. 133

Upon completion of this chapter, the reader should be able to:

- Discuss environmental hazards—those related to air, water, and soil—and concomitant health effects to communities.
- Discuss the Institute of Medicine's recommendation that nurses address environmental concerns in nursing practice, education, and research.
- Identify five dimensions of environment and their significance for application of the nursing process to environmental problems.
- Examine the works of nurse theorists to understand the person-environment relationship and its impact on health.
- Consider how five human responses interact with the five dimensions of environment.
- Review the characteristics of a healing environment and how they are related to caring.
- Summarize ways to apply the systematic nursing process to environmental issues and concerns.

█ **KEY TERMS**

advocacy role
beauty
bioaccumulative
biodiversity
biomonitoring
biopersistent
bioterrorism
chemical terrorism
consciousness
cultural competence
dimensions of environment
ecological balance
educator role
environment
environmental hazards
environmental health
environmental justice
general systems theory
healing environment

health determinant
health risk communication
helicy
human aggregate dimension
human field pattern
human responses
integrality
internal dimension
interpenetrating processes
investigator role
ionizing radiation
nurturance
occupational health
order
organizational dimension
person-environment interrelationship

physical dimension
policy framework
quantum mechanics
repetitive-motion injuries (RMIs)
resonance
respect

safety
social dimension
social support
subenvironments
Superfund site
Sustainable environment

As we enter the new millennium, there is cause for grave concern: Environmental issues are threatening the life of the earth, at least life on the earth as we know it. Because life essentially depends on air, soil, and water, human health and the **environment,** that which is perceived as being outside the self, are inextricably woven, and because nursing is involved with human health, environment is central to nursing. Conceptually, health can be thought of as the manifestation of the **person-environment interrelationship,** the whole of the interpenetrating, inseparable process that makes up the person and environment.

The World Health Organization's (WHO, 1997) definition of **environmental health** is used in the *Healthy People 2010* objectives:

> In its broadest sense, environmental health comprises those aspects of human health, disease, and injury that are determined or influenced by factors in the environment. This includes the study of both the direct pathological effects of various chemical, physical, and biological agents, as well as the effects on health of the broad physical and social environment, which includes housing, urban development, land-use and transportation, industry, and agriculture. (Draft)

This definition includes not only the air, water, and soil often used to define the physical environment provided by the earth but also the man-made environment created by society.

DETERMINANTS OF HEALTH

Human health depends, to a very large extent, on environmental health. National, state, and local efforts to ensure clean air and safe food and water supplies, manage sewage and municipal wastes, and control or eliminate vector-borne illnesses have greatly contributed to improvements in public health. Yet, poor environmental quality is estimated to be responsible for 25% of illness in the world. New knowledge of the interaction between individual genetic variations and environmental factors provides opportunity for health promotion and disease prevention for life on the earth. More research is needed to determine how public health programs affect the health status of people exposed to environmental hazards (USDHHS, 2000a).

This chapter addresses a full range of environmental influences on health, including environmental hazards in various settings, conceptual understandings of the person–environment–health nursing relationship, conceptual models for nursing practice and implications of environmental health efforts for community health nursing. A major emphasis is on physical and social areas of concern addressed by international, national, state, and local governments for health promotion and disease prevention. The learner is referred to other chapters where certain specific concerns are discussed. Because environmental influences on the health of individuals, families, and populations and related linkages are so complex and pervasive, environmental issues are discussed throughout the book.

Major determinants of health include biological, behavioral (see Chapter 11), and environmental factors. Environmental and behavioral factors together determine about 70% of all premature deaths in the United States (USDHHS, 2000b). Development and implementation of policies which address the determinants of health can reduce illness, enhance quality of life, and increase longevity. Efforts are being made to control the impact of environmental hazards. The major environmental health concerns addressed by *Healthy People 2010* related to the physical environment at the community aggregate level are, primarily, contamination of air, water, soil, and food supply.

ENVIRONMENTAL CONCERNS BY SETTING

All dimensions of environment in various settings where human beings live, work, and play—homes, workplaces, schools, communities, and the world at large—are determinants of health. Dimensions of the external environment may be identified as physical, social, and organizational. Physical determinants of environmental health include not only chemicals, biologicals, allergens, and traditional toxicants but also light, noise, odors, and particulate matter [Institute of Medicine (IOM), 1999]. Stressors such as limited access to health care and education, low socioeconomic status, racial and ethnic minority status, and political disenfranchisement reflect organizational and social influences on environment. WHO (1974), as discussed in Chapter 1, has defined health as "a state of complete physical, mental and social well-being and not merely the absence of disease or infirmity" (p. 1). These definitions are broad in scope, but definitions are even broader when conceptually defined for the nursing profession (discussed later in this chapter). Available online: www.oms.ch/aboutwho/en/definition.html

Because they work in homes, workplaces, schools, and various community settings, community health nurses

have repeated opportunities to detect possible environmental disease and underlying etiology. Residents seek counsel from the nurse about birth defect risk, drinking water safety, cancer risk from chemical exposure in the workplace, the effects of residential lead or radon, workers' compensation claims, and the costs of rectifying such problems. The IOM (1995) recommends that nurses be aware of environmental hazards and work as investigators, educators, and advocates for individuals and the community at large to identify environmental disorders and to eliminate the causes.

Environmental Concerns in Homes and of Families

Economically disadvantaged people, most often served by community health nurses, are at increased risk for exposure to hazardous environmental pollutants. Low-income and minority populations often live near or work in or near heavily polluting industries, hazardous waste dump sites, or incinerators. Such populations live in substandard houses with friable asbestos and deteriorating lead paint and have contaminated soil in their yards. They may be exposed to toxic chemicals through diets of seafood or fish taken from local waters designated unfit for swimming and fishing. Nurses serving these populations must serve as educators to and advocates for the people to solve these problems (IOM, 1995, 1999).

The U.S. Environmental Protection Agency (EPA) reports that more than 40 million people live within four miles of **Superfund sites,** known hazardous waste dumps designated by the EPA as threats to human health, and approximately 4 million people reside within one mile of such sites. In addition, home environmental hazards that carry documented health risks include "radon, environmental tobacco smoke, pesticides, carbon monoxide and airborne particulate from wood-burning stoves, nitrogen dioxide from natural gas stoves, formaldehyde and other chemicals . . . from new carpets, blown-in foam insulation, and the synthetic materials that cover the indoor surfaces of many mobile homes" (IOM, 1995, p. 25).

Environmental Concerns in Workplaces

Occupational safety is one of the 28 priority concerns of the *Healthy People 2010* project (USDHHS, 2000). Work-related injury, deaths, and nonfatal injuries decreased during the past decade, indicating progress toward meeting *Healthy People 2000* objectives. The objective for reducing hepatitis B infection among occupationally exposed workers was exceeded. Statistical evidence related to other objectives indicates increasing problems; however, it is suspected that the numbers have increased due to improved surveillance, reporting, and diagnosis. A major emphasis planned for the next 10 years is to establish tracking systems to document cost-effectiveness and impact on worker health. The lack of evidence indicating intervention effectiveness blocks introduction of new programs and threatens continuation of ongoing programs. Corporate safety and health programs, regulatory requirements and voluntary consensus standards, workers' compensation policies and loss control programs, engineering controls, and educational campaigns are among the types of programs being recommended by the Centers for Disease Control and Prevention (CDC) for development, implementation, and evaluation (CDC, 2000b).

Exposure to toxic chemicals and other environmental hazards in occupational settings is well documented. The U.S. Department of Labor (Bureau of Labor Statistics, 2000) reports 5.7 million work-related illnesses and injuries having occurred in 1999. Sprains and strains predominantly involving the upper body were the most frequent injuries. High-incidence work-related illnesses included repetitive-motion injuries and long-term latent diseases, such as skin cancer following exposure to arsenic or to the transfer of energy via electromagnetic waves or subatomic particles, which is known as **ionizing radiation.** A total of 6,037 fatal work injuries occurred in 1999, the most common work-related deaths being traffic accidents and homicides (Bureau of Labor Statistics, 2000).

Healthy People 2010 (CDC, 2000) reports progress since 1992 in the decrease of hepatitis B and occupation-related lung disease but a dramatic increase in cumulative trauma disorders such as **repetitive-motion injuries (RMIs)** and occupational skin disorders. Homicides in the workplace have become a major area of concern since the original document was developed.

Job stress, a significant risk factor for a number of health problems such as cardiovascular disease, musculoskeletal disorders, and workplace injury, is addressed in the occupational health objectives for 2010. Research indicates that up to one-third of all workers report high levels of job stress. Worksite programs to reduce stress adopt either stress management or coping skills as primary prevention strategies. Again, more research is needed to determine which programs are most effective (CDC, 2000).

Environmental Concerns of Local Communities and of Cities

Environmental hazards affecting communities and cities are generally classified as chemical, physical, biological, or psychosocial. The first three types may occur naturally, such as radon emitted from materials of the earth and ultraviolet light emitted from the sun, or they may be man made, such as particulates and gases released into the environment as exhaust fumes from automobiles, industrial waste, or tobacco smoke (IOM, 1995; USDHHS, 2000). Psychosocial hazards, including

racism, prejudice, crime, and violence, are addressed later in this chapter as well as in Chapter 30.

The Healthy People 2010 (USDHHS, 2000) project of the United States set priority goals and objectives to achieve a healthier nation by the year 2010. Environmental concerns for homes and communities include indoor allergens, office air quality, radon in homes, environmental hazards in schools, lead-based paint testing, substandard housing, and disaster preparedness. These objectives must be met at the local community or city level but are supported by and fit within the structure of state and federal environmental programs and funding. Lead agencies charged with the responsibility of meeting these goals are the Agency for Toxic Substances and Disease Registry (ATSDR), CDC, and the National Institutes of Health (NIH). These agencies agree that substantial efforts to meet these goals must be made by federal, state, and local health and environmental agencies; private citizens; professional organizations; and community leaders if the goals and objectives are to be met. A lengthier discussion of *Healthy People 2010* can be found in Chapter 11.

Healthy People 2010: (USDHHS, 2000a) evaluates progress made toward meeting the objectives at mid-decade. Indicators from 1998–1999 show that *Healthy People 2000* objectives were met in the following areas: (1) outbreaks of water-borne diseases, (2) solid waste, and (3) toxic substances released through industrial processes. Substantial progress was made involving (1) the proportion of people living in counties that meet EPA air standards for air pollution, (2) the number of states requiring radon disclosures with real estate transactions, and (3) recycling household hazardous waste. There has been moderate progress in the areas of radon and lead-based paint testing in homes, asthma hospitalizations, and states with laws to track environmental diseases. Mixed progress or reversals have been seen related to impaired surface waters (rivers, lakes, and estuaries). Data regarding cleanup of hazardous waste sites are difficult to assess. There has been progress in blood lead levels in children, although the objective has not been met (CDC, 2000).

National and International Concerns

Improving access to clean water and sanitation is probably the single most effective means of alleviating human suffering. Such action could increase the average life expectancy in developing countries by 15 years. Poor sanitation ranks as one of the highest contributing factors to the global burden of disease and injury discussed in Chapter 3. Diarrheal diseases kill nearly 3 million persons a year in developing countries as a result of poor sanitation and consumption of contaminated drinking water (ATSDR, CDC, NIH, 2000).

Environmental quality is a global concern. Health risks such as infectious diseases and chemical hazards in the form of pesticides are increasingly transferred across national borders. Imported fruits, vegetables, and seafood may carry pesticides that are restricted or illegal in the United States (ATSDR, CDC, NIH, 2000).

Bioterrorism, the use of infectious agents as weapons by terrorists to further personal or political agendas, is of concern for public health officials. Biological agents of concern include those that can produce mass casualties, are relatively easy and inexpensive to produce, cause death or disabling diseases, and can be aerosolized and distributed over large geographic areas, i.e., anthrax, plague, brucellosis, smallpox, viral encephalitis, and viral hemorrhagic fevers (McDade & Franz, 1998). **Chemical terrorism,** the use of chemicals as weapons, poses an additional threat to public health. Methyl parathion is one of many chemicals which threaten environmental health whether contamination is intentional or by accident. Public health strategies have been focused, primarily, on laboratory testing for chemicals in people as well as in the environment (Jackson, 1998).

The Center for Disease Control and Prevention (CDC) (2001) has identified the following public health problem related to bioterrorism:

- Bioterrorism is a significant public health threat facing the United States
- Response to a bioterrorism event will require rapid deployment of scarce public health resources
- The nation's public health infrastructure currently is not adequate to detect and respond to a bioterrorist event

The CDC has established a Bioterrorism Program plan to ensure the rapid development of federal, state, and local capacity to address bioterrorism if it occurs. Health departments at all levels will:

- Continue to enhance public health infrastructure
- Continue to develop response capacity
- Provide training in bioterrorism preparedness and response for the public health workforce
- Continue to enhance the pharmaceutical stockpile and information systems (CDC, September 20, 2001).

Online. Available: *www.bt.cdc.gov/documents/btinitiative.asp*

Dr. Jeffrey Koplan, Director, CDC (Koplan, 2001) has outlined areas of priority for development of an infrastructure that can better protect public health in the United States. These areas of priority are:

- A well-trained, well-staffed, fully prepared public health workforce
- Laboratory capacity to produce timely and accurate results for diagnosis and investigation
- Epidemiology and surveillance systems with the ability to rapidly detect health threats

- Secure, accessible information systems which facilitate the ability to communicate rapidly, analyze and interpret health data, and provide public access to health information
- Communication that is swift, secure, and facilitates a two-way flow of information. This includes the ability to provide timely, accurate information to the public, advice to policy-makers in public health emergencies, and the ability to routinely translate scientific information and provide health information
- Effective policy and evaluation capability. Effectiveness of public health programs must be routinely evaluated and priorities established for planning and ongoing program development
- Maintenance of preparedness and response capability

Online. Available: *www.cdc.gov:* Building Infrastructure to Protect the Public's Health.

There are a number of issues requiring global attention. These include burning of fossil fuels, which causes air pollution and global warming along with other climatic changes; use of chlorinated compounds that do not decay **(biopersistent)** and tend to accumulate as a result of their nondecaying nature **(bioaccumulative),** thereby disrupting endocrine and immune functioning; mining and distribution of uranium and its by-products, resulting in radioactive waste; and overdevelopment, which diminishes **biodiversity,** the variety of life that now exists, thereby destabilizing the **ecological balance,** the relationship among living things and between a specific organism and its environment, and creating unknown consequences (Raven, 1998).

ENVIRONMENTAL JUSTICE

The United States and other industrialized nations produce large quantities of goods and technologies that make modern life comfortable, convenient, and efficient. The processes that create the nation's power, manufacture its goods, and provide transportation, however, produce by-products that pollute the environment and are hazardous to human health (IOM, 1999). These environmental health hazards have been a concern for the past 30 years; but more recently there has been a growing concern that these environmental burdens and hazards are being borne by those in lower income communities, especially those of ethnic and racial minorities. Efforts to correct these disparities is based on a concern for environmental justice.

Environmental justice is defined by EPA (1998) as the fair treatment and meaningful involvement of all people regardless of race, ethnicity, income, national origin or educational level with respect to the development, implementation, and enforcement of environmental laws, regulations, and policies. Fair treatment means that no population, due to policy or economic disempowerment, is forced to bear a disproportionate burden of the negative human health or environmental impacts of pollution or other environmental consequences resulting from industrial, municipal, and commercial operations or the executive of federal, state, local and tribal programs and policies. (p. 2)

Environmental justice is also a significant concept in occupational health since low-income and minority workers in the United States suffer disproportionately from work-related illnesses and are employed in occupations with higher levels of exposure to health hazards (Frumkin & Walker, 1997; IOM, 1999). **Occupational health** is the study and prevention of environmental problems in worker populations within the workplace. National and global occupational health objectives address environmental conditions in the workplace.

A major challenge for this time is to balance the use of the earth's resources with human needs for development within a very complex world of infinite possibilities. **Sustainable development** refers to the growth and development within a society that is intended to meet the needs of the present without compromising the ability of future generations to meet their own needs (ATSDR, CDC, NIH, 2000). Society must not sacrifice the earth's natural resources for comfort and pleasure. A **sustainable environment** is one in which health is maintained for future generations.

ENVIRONMENTAL HEALTH: A NEW ROLE FOR COMMUNITY HEALTH NURSING

Environmental health efforts present critical challenges at this time. The IOM (1995) challenges nurses to take responsibility for serving aggregates and populations and working to create healthy environments. Basic environmental health principles for community health nursing are listed in Figure 9-1. Related competencies required for community health nursing practice as identified by the IOM are shown in Figure 9-2. The IOM report encourages more population-focused practice, education, and research by the nursing profession. Given that there are an estimated 2.2 million nurses in the United States, the nursing profession could have a tremendous influence on the environmental health of this nation and the world. Chapter 13 addresses population-focused practice.

Neufer (1994) states that although environmental health issues are central to the historical and theoretical perspectives of nursing, application has been limited to individuals and families. However, the critical state of environmental health now requires that community health

---

FIGURE 9-1 General Principles of Environmental Health for Community Health Nursing

- Humans may be exposed to chemical, biological, and radiological risks in all of the "environments" in which they live, work, play, and learn. Human health can be impacted by these exposures.

- Many factors influence the relationship between environment and health. Host factors such as age, gender, genetic makeup, and underlying diseases can affect disease outcomes.

- Chemical and radiological exposures can be cumulative. Nurses must assess a person's total exposure to environmental risks in order to understand and address potential health threats.

- Environmental (and occupational) health is based on a public health model with an emphasis on prevention. Prevention in environmental health includes pollution prevention, product design, engineering controls, and education.

- Although U.S. standards are "health based," they often are not sufficiently protective of our most vulnerable populations. Like occupational standards, they are based on the health risks to an otherwise healthy, 70-kilogram (154-pound) white male. This may not provide sufficient protection to pregnant women and fetuses, young children, the frail, the elderly, as well as the immunocompromised.

From *Nursing, Health, and the Environment: Strengthening the Relationship to Improve the Public's Health,* by the National Academy of Sciences, 1995, Washington, DC: Author. Copyright 1995 by the National Academy of Sciences. Reprinted with permission.

---

nurses adapt their assessment and diagnostic skills and play a proactive role in the treatment of environmental health hazards.

Community health nursing has historically merged public health and nursing in applying the nursing process to primary, secondary, and tertiary situations that involve individuals, families, and communities. At this time, nurses are being asked to take more responsibility for assessing environmental health risks and serving in the roles of investigator, educator, and advocate for those at risk. Nurses with graduate preparation are expected to assume leadership positions in environmental health.

School nurses, occupational health nurses, and public health nurses must work to improve environmental health conditions in schools, workplaces, and the general community, respectively. All nurses, in fact, are being encouraged to address environmental health factors in their work with individuals and families (IOM, 1995). Public health functions identified by the Public Health Service (1994) are given in Figure 9-3. All can be seen as within the realm of nursing.

FIGURE 9-2 General Environmental Health Competences for Nurses

I. *Basic Knowledge and Concepts*

All nurses should understand the scientific principles and underpinnings of the relationship between individuals or populations and the environment (including the work environment). This understanding includes the basic mechanisms and pathways of exposure to environmental health hazards, basic prevention and control strategies, the interdisciplinary nature of effective interventions, and the role of research.

II. *Assessment and Referral*

All nurses should be able to successfully complete an environmental health history, recognize potential environmental hazards and sentinel illnesses, and make appropriate referrals for conditions with probable environmental etiologies. An essential component of this is the ability to access and provide information to patients and communities and to locate referral sources.

III. *Advocacy, Ethics, and Risk Communication*

All nurses should be able to demonstrate knowledge of the role of advocacy (case and class), ethics, and risk communication in patient care and community intervention with respect to the potential adverse effects of the environment on health.

IV. *Legislation and Regulation*

All nurses should understand the policy framework and major pieces of legislation and regulations related to environmental health.

From *Nursing, Health, and the Environment: Strengthening the Relationship to Improve the Public's Health,* by the National Academy of Sciences, 1995, Washington, DC: Author. Copyright 1995 by the National Academy of Sciences. Reprinted with permission.

FIGURE 9-3 Public Health Functions

- Prevent epidemics and the spread of disease.
- Protect against environmental hazards.
- Prevent injuries.
- Promote and encourage healthy behaviors.
- Respond to disasters and assist communities in recovery.
- Ensure the quality and accessibility of health services.

In addition to these traditional functions, contemporary threats require responsible action for prevention and intervention related to:

- Chronic diseases
- Violence
- Emerging pathogens
- Threats of bioterrorism
- Social contexts that influence health disparities

Adapted from *Public Health in America,* by Public Health Service, 1994, Washington, DC: Author; and "Foreword: Framework for Program Evaluation in Public Health," by J. Koplan, 1999, *Morbidity and Mortality Weekly Report, 48*(11), pp. 1–40.

Community health nursing has traditionally been considered a synthesis of the public health perspective and nursing perspectives. What the public health perspective brings to nursing is a focus on prevention as opposed to one on illness, the focus inherent in traditional care-and-cure models. Although the nursing discipline deals with environment and health, most nurses are unprepared to deal with such issues except on an individual basis. The IOM (1995) report states:

Public health issues must be approached from a population-based, primary-prevention perspective. Yet, most nurses practice their profession from a curative perspective that focuses on ill individuals. This mismatch creates conceptual and practical difficulties for nurses involved with environmental health issues. They may feel that they lack the authority to take a public health approach or that they lack the skills to analyze health issues in population-based terms. . . . In light of the controversy that sometimes surrounds public health issues, nurses may feel safer caring for individuals because this is the task with which they are more familiar; caring for individuals allows nurses to stay solidly within the boundaries of the health care system without stepping into the social, legal, and political arenas important for disease prevention. (p. 18)

Many nurses, though, do have the skills and knowledge required to assess and assist individuals, families, and communities in primary, secondary, and tertiary prevention of environment-related illness. They are able to elicit an environmental health history, conduct a community assessment, educate, and serve as advocates. Application of these skills in social, legal, and political arenas is a challenge that nurses can meet.

PERSON-ENVIRONMENT THEORIES

More than any other nurse theorist, Florence Nightingale (1860/1969) emphasized the importance of environment to health and healing. She clearly established that it is within the realm of nursing to create a healing environment. Her work in lowering morbidity and mortality rates in hospitals demonstrated the strong link between environment and health and healing. These events firmly established environment as a central concept of nursing theory. Nurse theorists have continued to study and to increase understanding of the conceptual linkages among health, environment, person, and nursing.

Einstein's Theory

Since Nightingale's time, scientific breakthroughs have changed our understanding of the nature of the person-environment relationship. Einstein's work during the early 1900s challenged the idea that the world of nature, including human beings, consists of parts that fit together in a machinelike manner. Conventional wisdom had been that we could understand the whole by studying the parts in isolation from the rest and that, in learning about the parts, the whole would become known. Applied to health, the belief was that we could study health and illness separately and could understand environment apart from its relationship to persons. Within this understanding, the whole was thought to be the sum of the parts. Einstein's work, however, refuted those notions of separateness and, instead, proposed ideas of process, relationship, and organizational pattern as significant areas for the study of nature.

Einstein's work in **quantum mechanics,** that branch of physics concerned with the energy characteristics of matter at the subatomic level, is now approximately 100 years old, yet there is still little general understanding or acceptance of how this work applies to health and healing. Some theorists believe that when Einstein's work is interpreted to apply to the nature of the human being, activities to promote health and healing will change dramatically (Herbert, 1987).

Systems Perspectives

Influenced by Einstein, von Bertalanffy (1968) attempted to apply Einstein's ideas to social systems. He developed **general systems theory,** in which he supported the view of system theorists that the whole is more than and different from the sum of the parts. This work has greatly influenced nursing theory and understanding of the human-environment interrelationship. General systems theory has served as a foundation for organizational knowledge used in working with families, communities, and environmental health. See Chapter 24 for more on systems theory and its application to family processes.

Whitehead (1969), a contemporary of Einstein, argued not only that the whole is more than and different from the sum of the parts but also that all consist of **interpenetrating processes** of energy patterns that are totally inseparable from all else. His work and that of others provided a foundation for understanding the oneness of person and environment, leading to the study of consciousness and caring in health and healing. Today,

physicists, theologians, philosophers, and scientists of many disciplines are studying what mystics of both the East and the West have taught for ages. This is part of the shift toward understanding patterns of wholeness as related to health and healing (as discussed in Chapter 12).

Nursing Theories

The work of Nightingale, Einstein, Whitehead, and von Bertalanffy greatly influenced Martha Rogers, a major nurse theorist. In the 1970s, who argued that humans and environment are inseparable and brought about renewed interest in environment as a central phenomenon of nursing (Newman, 1994).

Rogers (1990) uses Einstein's theory to define the universe as an energy field in which person-environment fields are identified by pattern and organization. Her descriptors of resonancy, helicy, and integrality characterize these field patterns and their related principles. **Resonancy** refers to a continuous change from lower to higher frequency wave patterns (the evolutionary principle); **helicy** refers to the unpredictability, diversity, and innovation of human and environmental field patterns (the complexity principle); and **integrality** refers to the continuous mutual process of these field patterns (the spirituality principle). In Rogers' construct, **human field patterns** are irreducible, indivisible, and pandimensional. They are identified by characteristics specific to the whole and cannot be predicted simply from knowledge of the parts.

Newman (1994), was influenced by physical scientist David Bohm's (1980) work concerning quantum realities. Newman defines health as the expansion of consciousness and consciousness as the informational capacity of the person-environment system. Components of this system include the nervous system, the endocrine system, the immune system, and the genetic code, to name a few. Knowledge of these systems indicates the inherent complexity in the person-environment response (Newman, 1994).

Mutual connectedness theory utilizes concepts of caring and consciousness to address client-nurse relationships within healthy and healing environments (Schubert & Lionberger, 1995). Both the client and the nurse experience health and healing in such a relationship. Caring in practice requires a balance of many responsibilities in demonstrating caring for the nurse's self and family, clients and their families, the community, the country, and the world. Expanding consciousness parallels an increasing sense of responsibility (see Figure 9-4); being centered and at peace with oneself requires the nurse to focus attention on what is at hand while maintaining an awareness of the whole. The admonition, thus, is to *think globally but act locally.*

Caring and concern for the well-being of people and environment must be balanced with caring for oneself.

FIGURE 9-4 Expanding of Caring, Consciousness, and Responsibility in the Creation of Healthy and Healing Environments

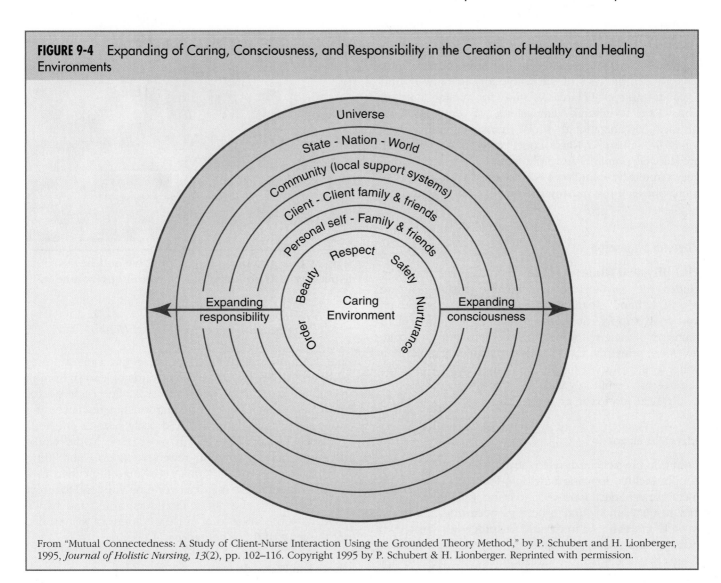

From "Mutual Connectedness: A Study of Client-Nurse Interaction Using the Grounded Theory Method," by P. Schubert and H. Lionberger, 1995, *Journal of Holistic Nursing, 13*(2), pp. 102–116. Copyright 1995 by P. Schubert & H. Lionberger. Reprinted with permission.

Staying centered helps one practice caring within the limits of what is possible for one human being to accomplish. Dass (1993) provides some additional guidelines that can help community nurses avoid overextending themselves and becoming exhausted from too much responsibility and overwork. He suggests that the helper act from deep intuitive appreciation of what is appropriate in the moment by asking whether each act undertaken:

- Is in harmony with the helper's personal values
- Uses the helper's particular skills, talents, and personality characteristics
- Makes use of opportunities
- Acknowledges liabilities as well as assets
- Takes into account existing responsibilities
- Honors the diverse roles the helper is called on to fulfill in the moment

A CONCEPTUAL FRAMEWORK FOR ASSESSING ENVIRONMENTS

A model for applying the nursing process to environmental issues is proposed in this section. The process involves assessing the five **dimensions of environment**—physical, organizational, social, human aggregate, and internal—identifying **human responses** to environmental issues, and proposing an intervention that will alter the environment in a health-promoting way.

The model provides a conceptual framework for assessing environmental issues and is intended to provide the student not with all that needs to be known about environment but, instead, with one way of thinking about the person-environment interrelationship.

Although this model provides a broad look at environmental concerns in all five dimensions, particular emphasis is placed on the physical dimension of the community aggregate. The nurse is encouraged to use this model conceptually and creatively for assessment at all levels and dimensions of environment.

Kim (1983) suggests the use of **subenvironments** to approach analysis of the whole and to draw boundaries around specific areas of study for nursing intervention. Five structural dimensions of environment—physical, organizational, social, human aggregate, and internal—similar to Kim's concept of subenvironments are derived primarily from the work of Moos (1979) and are adapted by Puntillo (1992) to assist with the assessment phase of the nursing process.

Physical Dimension

The **physical dimension** of environmental health includes the elements of architecture design, climate, sound, lighting, cleanliness, and adequacy of water, air, and food supply. Concerns related to the physical dimension of the environment at the community aggregate level are, primarily, those related to contamination of air, water, soil, and food supply. The physical environmental hazards are commonly classified and are discussed here as physical, chemical, or biological.

Physical Hazards

Common physical hazards to the air, water, soil, and food supply include ionizing radiation, lead and other heavy metals, mechanical hazards, and noise. Ionizing radiation can result from natural processes occurring inside and outside the earth or from artificial processes created by human beings, such as those associated with medical x-rays or nuclear events. Radiation has both positive and negative outcomes.

Ultraviolet radiation, a natural by-product of sunlight, helps to produce vitamin D when the skin is exposed to the sun but also causes sunburn and acts as a causal factor in basal and squamous cell carcinomas and malignant melanomas. The ozone layer of the atmosphere protects against this radiation, but with the loss of this layer as a result of chemicals being released into the atmosphere, skin cancer is increasing significantly.

Infrared radiation, produced by the sun and molten metals, causes burns to the skin and eyes, potentially causing cataracts. Radon occurs naturally in the materials of the earth: When inhaled as dust, radon can damage lung tissue.

Lead and other heavy metals (mercury, arsenic, and cadmium) contaminate air, water, and soil. Sources of lead are vehicle emissions, burning of coal, industrial processes, lead-based paint, and solid-waste decomposition. The reduction of blood lead levels in children, however, has been one of the most significant achievements in environmental health in recent years. A unified approach among all levels of government and the private sector contributed greatly to this major public health suc-

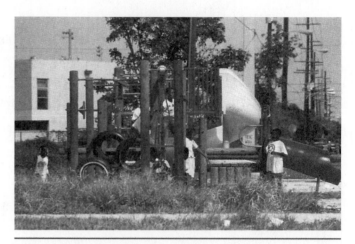

Review this photograph. List positive and negative aspects of this children's playground environment.

cess (*Progress Review: Environmental Health,* March 12, 1997). The *Healthy People 2010* target is to totally eliminate lead poisoning in children of the United States (ATSDR, CDC, NIH, 2000). The hazards of lead poisoning in children are discussed in Chapter 22. See Table 9-1 for information regarding other hazardous agents, including sources, exposure pathways, and body systems affected.

Mechanical hazards occur most often in the workplace and include vibration, repetitive motion, and lifting in various cumulative-trauma situations. Repetitive motion and lifting cause injuries over time and tend to affect the upper body: the neck, shoulders, arms, and hands (CDC, 2000b). Noise can cause a variety of symptoms, not the least of these being loss of hearing.

Chemical Hazards

Chemical and gaseous hazards constitute another category of toxins that harm body tissues and are found in the air, water, and soil. Insecticides, herbicides, fungicides, and rodenticides all contain chemical poisons. Health effects of pesticide poisoning include dizziness, nausea, lymphoma, leukemia, bladder cancer, and neurotoxicity. Exposure occurs when working with the chemicals or by ingesting them through food and water. Another environmental hazard is accidental poisoning of children who ingest household chemicals. The community health nurse should always check for these hazards on the home visit (see Chapter 21).

Pesticide residues on fruits and vegetables and the bioaccumulation of chemicals and other pollutants in fish and seafood are other areas of concern. Community health nurses can educate people regarding eating fish from contaminated waters and proper cleaning of fresh vegetables and fruits (IOM, 1995).

The diseases and conditions known to have strong links to the physical environment are cancer, reproductive disorders such as infertility and low birth

TABLE 9-1 Agency for Toxic Substances and Disease Registry 1993 Priority List of Rank-Ordered Top 10 Hazardous Substances

HAZARDOUS AGENT	SOURCES	EXPOSURE PATHWAYS	SYSTEMS AFFECTED
Lead	Storage batteries; manufacture of paint, enamel, ink, glass, rubber, ceramics, chemicals	Ingestion, inhalation	Hematological, renal, neuromuscular, GI, CNS
Arsenic	Manufacture of pigments, glass, pharmaceuticals, insecticides, fungicides, rodenticides; tanning	Ingestion, inhalation	Neuromuscular, skin, GI
Metallic mercury	Electronics; paints; metal and textile production; chemical manufacturing; pharmaceutical production	Inhalation, percutaneous and GI absorption	Pulmonary, CNS, renal
Benzene	Manufacture of organic chemicals, detergents, pesticides, solvents, paint removers	Inhalation, percutaneous absorption	CNS, hematopoietic
Vinyl chloride	Production of polyvinyl chloride and other plastics; chlorinated compounds; used as a refrigerant	Inhalation, ingestion	Hepatic, neurological, pulmonary
Cadmium	Electroplating, solder	Inhalation	Pulmonary, renal
Polychlorinated biphenyls	Formerly used in electrical equipment	Inhalation, ingestion	Skin, eyes, hepatic
Benzo(a)pyrene	Emissions from refuse burning and autos; used as laboratory reagent; found on charcoal-grilled meats and in cigarette smoke	Inhalation, ingestion, and percutaneous absorption	Pulmonary, skin, eyes (BaP is a probable human carcinogen)
Chloroform	Aerosol propellants, fluorinated resins; produced during chlorination of water; used as a refrigerant	Inhalation, percutaneous absorption, ingestion	CNS, renal, hepatic, mucous membrane, cardiac
Benzo(b) fluoranthene	Cigarette smoke	Inhalation	Pulmonary

From Nursing, Health, and the Environment *(pp. 36-37) by the National Academy of Sciences, 1995, Washington, DC: National Academy Press. Copyright 1995 by the National Academy of Sciences.*

Note: CNS = central nervous system; GI = gastrointestinal.

weight, neurological and immune system impairments, and respiratory conditions such as asthma. A major focus of attention at present is breast cancer, the second leading cause of cancer death in women. This disease results from a complex interaction of genetics, hormonal, and, possibly, environmental factors. Environmental hazards currently being studied—including pesticides, radiation, and toxic chemicals—enter the body through air, water, and food. These hazards are being evaluated to determine whether they do in fact contribute to disease or other disruptions in health (ATSDR, CDC, NIH, 2000).

Authors of the *Healthy People 2010* project (USD-HHS, 2000b) recognize the interrelationship between human beings and environment. They state:

To be successful, programs to improve environmental health must be based on scientific evidence. The complex relationship between human health and the acute and long-term effects of environmental exposures must be studied so prevention measures can be developed. Surveillance systems to track exposure to toxic substances such as commonly used pesticides and heavy metals must be developed and maintained. To the extent possible, these systems should use **biomonitoring** [emphasis added] data, which provide measurements of toxic substances in the human body. A mechanism is needed for tracking the export of pesticides restricted or not registered for use in the United States. (p. 10).

Health concerns play a huge part in the efforts of the U.S. government to foster a safe physical environment.

RESEARCH FOCUS

Prevalence of Headache among Hand-Held Cellular Telephone Users in Singapore: A Community Study

Study Problem/Purpose

Present knowledge of the health effects on humans by the frequency band (870–995) used within hand-held cellular telephones is limited. Anecdotal reports of symptoms experienced by persons using hand phones (HP) include headaches, dizziness, warmth or tingling around the ears and face, and difficulties concentrating. This study was done to study the prevalence of specific central nervous system (CNS) symptoms among HP users compared to non-HP users and to determine the association of risk factors and CNS symptoms among HP users.

Methods

A cross-sectional study in a sector of Singapore composed of 800 persons ages 12–70 years was conducted. Participants were told the study was to obtain data about headaches; they were unaware of any relationship to HP use. A two-tier interview was used, first to obtain data about any headache problems (frequency, nature, and severity) or other CNS symptoms such as dizziness, difficulties in concentration, loss of memory, unusual drowsiness or tiredness, sense of warmth behind the ear and face, tingling sensation to the face, and visual disturbances (e.g., flashes). They were asked how often they experienced the symptoms during the past year, frequency of each symptom, and if they used an HP. The HP users were defined for the study as those who use an HP at least once a day.

Statistical analysis involved descriptive summary measures of central tendency, frequencies, and associations with tests of significance where appropriate. Bivariate analysis was carried out to determine the association between CNS symptoms among HP users and various predictor variables, age, sex, occupations, and exposure to video display terminals.

Findings

Three percent of the studied population had a history of CNS problems (e.g., brain surgery, stroke, posttrauma headache); data from these respondents were removed from the analyses. Headache was the most prevalent symptom among the HP users as compared to non-HP users. After using the proportional hazards model and adjusting for age, sex, ethnic group, use of video display terminals and occupational group, the adjusted prevalence rate ratio was 1.31 (95% confidence interval, 1.00–1.70). The prevalence of headache was significantly associated with the duration (minutes) of using the HP per day. Headache was prevalent in 60.3% of HP users and in 54% of nonusers. There was a significant increase in the prevalence of headache with increasing duration of use (in minutes per day). The prevalence of headache was reduced by >20% among those who used hand-free equipment compared to those who never used the equipment. An explanation for this result is that the equipment would reduce the exposure to radio frequency radiation by keeping the antenna farther from the head.

Implication

Researchers report no knowledge of another community study on the prevalence of CNS symptoms related to the use of the HP. There has been a dearth of studies of environmental hazards and their effects on humans. The study has limitations, i.e., the collection of data was done by those administering the study, the overall participation rate was low, and the cause-and-effect relationship cannot be determined by such a study. A causal relationship is theoretically possible, however, and other studies have shown effects of these frequencies on the blood-brain barrier in rats.

Source: Chia, S.-E., Chia, H.-P., & Tan, J.-S. (2000). "Prevalence of headache among handheld cellular telephone users in Singapore: A community study". Environmental Health Perspectives, 108(11), 1059–1062.

Nursing research on environmental health is rare, but nurses may turn to related research carried out in other health disciplines, for instance, epidemiology. The accompanying Research Focus Box demonstrates some of the problems of epidemiological research.

Biological Hazards

Biological hazards in the environment include infectious agents, insects, animals, and plants. Infectious agents are most often found in water. Water-borne diseases are occurring less often in the United States (ATSDR, CDC, NIH, 2000) but are a serious problem in many areas of the world. Contamination of the water supply generally results from problems related to sewage and to solid waste disposal methods. Rainwater that runs through waste disposal sites carries organisms into water supply systems. Wastewater must be carefully monitored because it is often recycled for irrigation and may contaminate fruit and vegetable produce. Improper disposal of medical supplies such as needles and syringes that have been contaminated with human blood or other body fluids constitutes another major biological hazard. Infectious organisms are also transmitted in the air, including indoors, by unclean air-conditioning and heating systems, which serve as breeding grounds for pathogenic organisms [National Institute of Environmental Health Sciences (NIEHS), 2000].

Insects and animals breed in solid waste and spread communicable diseases. Feces provides a breeding ground for insects that transmit disease. Plants also pose a biological hazard because some are poisonous when ingested or touched, and some are allergens.

In addition to these physical environmental hazards, assessment of any setting requires a careful look at its structures and neighborhoods and how they function. The community health nurse, upon entering a home,

school, or workplace, checks for adequate heating and cooling systems with vents to prevent air poisoning, adequate food and water supply, a functioning sewage system, appropriate clothing, and other physical things needed for health. Community assessment requires many of the same observational skills but involves more input from and involvement with other community workers in assessment, planning, intervention, and evaluation. The nurse must be aware of the total community and how its structure affects the well-being of individuals, families, schools, workplaces, and the general community.

All systems of community—from individual and family to local, state, national, and international—have a physical dimension that affects health. These physical hazards are closely linked to other aspects of environment as discussed earlier. Social concerns related to environmental health are also complex, but a major issue is that certain segments of society are more likely to experience exposure to physical hazards in various settings. Nurses are involved in all these levels of community. Many examples are discussed in later chapters.

Organizational Dimension

Assessing the **organizational dimension** of environmental health involves looking at the structural and functional effectiveness of any particular person, family, community, or population. A careful family assessment will certainly reveal how community organization has affected the family at hand. Community organization comprises all the various community structures—political, economic, public assistance, legal and judicial, health care, schools, transportation, housing, and recreational.

Organizational patterns may be formal (officially recognized by those involved) or informal (not officially part of the organizational plan). Informal patterns are often more powerful than formal ones—and more difficult to change. If the community health nurse finds that families are having difficulty because of a problem in community organization, the nurse may serve as an advocate and take action to change the organizational system of the community. (See Chapters 4 and 6 regarding health care delivery and health care economics, respectively.)

Salmon (1995) maintains that the **policy framework** (policies structured to meet the needs of society and individuals within that society) for health care delivery is a **health determinant** that either enhances or detracts from the health of the people. Assessment of that policy framework indicates that the United States is "rich in knowledge and technology but currently poor in the public health policies that mobilize these assets on behalf of the public's health" (p. 2). She advocates a system in which public health rather than illness, individual medical care, and technology is the foundation, pointing out that a very small portion of the aggregate amount for all health care in the United States is spent on population-based

---

REFLECTIVE THINKING

Physical Environmental Hazards

There are three common categories of physical environmental hazards: physical, chemical, and biological.

- Think about recent news reports regarding any of these three types of hazards in the community.
- How might you, as a nurse, have become involved in the events?
- How might you have worked to prevent one of the events?

REFLECTIVE THINKING

Community Organization

Imagine that you serve on the board of supervisors or the equivalent structure of a county or township. The group is currently making preliminary plans for reorganizing how families on welfare will be helped by the community.

- What concerns might you have for protecting and promoting the health of the citizens?
- Might you experience any conflict between the needs of the community and the needs of the families involved?
- What organizational resources might you look to for conflict resolution?

✳ DECISION MAKING

Social Health and Community Planning

Imagine that you live in a community comprising three very distinct social groups. Wealthier property owners, some of whom work outside the community, constitute one group. Another group is made up primarily of families who provide services to the wealthier group. The third group is composed of some homeless people and some families who receive public assistance. Recently, vandalism has increased sharply, and graffiti have appeared downtown for the first time.

- ◆ Develop a plan for gathering data needed for an environmental assessment.
- ◆ What segments of the population would you involve in the assessment and in the planning? In the implementation of the plan?
- ◆ How would you evaluate the efforts to solve the identified problems?

---

public health activities. Public policy provides the organizational aspect of environment, which affects health at the local, state, and national levels.

Just as the organizational structure of the family is assessed by the community health nurse (see Chapters 21 and 24), community structure and organization are the focus of community assessment (see Chapter 15).

Social Dimension

The **social dimension** of the community environment comprises the attitudes of various groups and cultures regarding age, race, ethnicity, religion, socioeconomic status, and lifestyle. Prejudice affects the health of individuals, families, the group being attacked, and the community as a whole.

The social dimension of environment embodies relationships among people within a setting, personal growth or goal orientation, and variables related to system maintenance or system change. The quality of the relationships among immediate family members, extended family members, friends, neighbors, community groups, and health care workers all contribute to **social support,** a perceived sense of support from a complex network of interpersonal ties and from backup support systems for nurturance. Social support is a necessary ingredient of a healthy and healing environment.

Theory and research regarding social support and its relationship to health have been a part of nursing science since 1976 (Powers, 1988). The role of self-esteem in health status emerged in several studies (Weiss & Louquist, 2000; Rowe & Kahn, 1998). In 1981, the California Department of Mental Health undertook a major educational project to encourage its citizens—in the name of improving their health—to strengthen their social support systems. This project was based on numerous studies indicating that social support improved physical and mental health.

Human Aggregate Dimension

The **human aggregate dimension** refers to certain composite characteristics of people within a specific environment—age range, educational level, areas of knowledge, values, culture, communication style, and self-care practices. The human aggregate dimension of environment is addressed from the perspective of the group as a whole and from the personal perspective of the involved individuals. Community assessment includes a description and analysis of the human aggregate (as outlined in Chapter 15). Program planning is determined by this description and analysis (see Chapter 16).

Cultural values held by the human aggregate constitute a significant factor in environmental health issues and all public health concerns. Cultural values in the United States have played a significant part in the efforts to reform health care (Lum, 1995; Williams, 1995). A report by an interdisciplinary group at the Center for Bioethics (1992) at the University of Minnesota offers the perspective that cultural values prevent the United States from building a health care system that would provide universal access to health care and make a serious commitment to the mission of public health. Data indicate

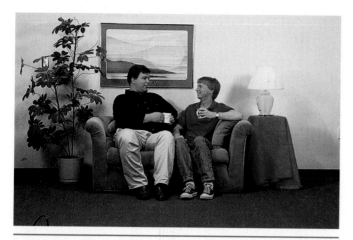

Social support is an important part of a healthy and healing environment.

REFLECTIVE THINKING

Person and Environment

- Where do you as a person end and your environment begin?
- Are your thoughts a part of the environment, thereby interacting with you as a person, or are they an aspect of you as person?
- What is consciousness? Are your thoughts a part of the person-environment bridge that determines health?

that the United States, although sharing similar culture, philosophy, democratic tradition, and demographics with other Western countries, stands alone as a country, lacking universal access to health care and a commitment to public health. The group concludes that "the United States stands alone with its non-universal, patchwork health care system, in part, because of its embrace of individualism, its establishment of provider autonomy as the preeminent value, and its neglect of community oriented values" (Center for Bioethics, 1992, p. 15). Williams (1995) states that recognition of these underlying cultural values is important and that acknowledgment simply clarifies the nature of the challenges related to values and political context. See Chapter 8 for a discussion on cultural perspectives.

Lum (1995) also recognizes the difficulties involved in building a strong environmental health and public health program. He encourages nurses to serve as educators of the public and emphasizes the importance of **cultural competence** (the ability to communicate with people of various cultures, beliefs, and values to promote a positive outcome) and of **health risk communication** (informing people about environmental health hazards and health risks) in bringing about exchange of information and clarification of values. The IOM has also emphasized the need for nursing competency in the field of environmental health (IOM, 1995).

Internal Dimension

The **internal dimension** of environment comprises the biological, psychological, and spiritual attributes of the person. Modern psychology supports the notion that perception determines boundaries of person and environment and that perception changes with developmental processes and consciousness. For example, the infant perceives its mother and itself as one being. The growing child learns to differentiate the self and the mother, to perceive the body as the self and everything outside

the body as separate. Further into adulthood, the person may perceive the body as environment for the self. At some point, the perceived outer environment may include aspects of **consciousness,** such as thoughts and feelings, in which case the self is equated with the soul or spirit, and thoughts, feelings, and perceptions are experienced as environment. These aspects of consciousness, then, are considered to be one's internal environment. Consciousness therefore plays a profound role in this relationship and in health or healing. This model treats the outer environment as that which is outside the mind and body.

The internal dimension of community environment is considered here as the individual inner experiences of the people within the community. Although the sum of these experiences makes up the human aggregate, the internal dimension speaks to the individual and to the individual's attitudes, beliefs, values, and internal experiences.

An assessment of internal environment addresses the biological, psychological, and spiritual attributes of individuals and the unique ways individuals relate to the outer environment. The internal and external environments are interrelated and are involved in constant interaction, influencing and being influenced.

Figure 9-5 depicts both process and structure within the environmental model, with the structure comprising the five dimensions described previously. The process components are permeability and transaction. Permeability, denoted by overlapping of the circles, refers to the inseparability of person and environment. Transaction, denoted by bidirectional arrows, refers to an integrative relationship between person and environment and between dimensions—that is, person and environment affect and are affected by each other, and both change as a result of an encounter.

The nurse is required not only to assess each of these dimensions of environment for health hazards and strengths but also to determine the human response to the myriad environmental factors in these dimensions.

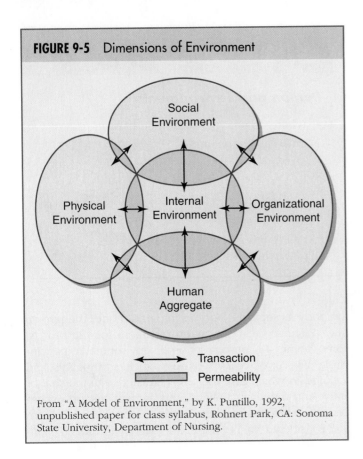

FIGURE 9-5 Dimensions of Environment

From "A Model of Environment," by K. Puntillo, 1992, unpublished paper for class syllabus, Rohnert Park, CA: Sonoma State University, Department of Nursing.

REFLECTIVE THINKING

The Human Response of a Community

When a child is kidnapped or missing, the pain and loss can be felt at many levels of the community. Consider the case of Polly Klass, a California youngster who was kidnapped and later found murdered.

- What levels of community might experience response to such an event?
- How might you be involved as a community health nurse? If you knew Polly, how would that fact affect your ability to focus?
- In what dimensions of environment might you consider intervention?

Remember, the aim of nursing has been identified as the study of human responses to health and illness (American Nurses Association, 1995).

HUMAN RESPONSES

Human responses to environment are often determined during health assessment of individuals and families. Problems are identified and interventions devised on the basis of those findings. Among the many common examples of human responses that may indicate a need for nursing intervention are failure to thrive, altered immunocompetence, loss, conflict, pain, illness, injury, disability, and technology dependence. Human response phenomena cross clinical sites and conditions and are balanced by varying strengths that facilitate self-sufficiency.

Physical findings may provide clues to environmental health hazards in the person's life. Epidemiological studies using morbidity and mortality statistics and investigation of possible causes help identify environmental factors involved.

Human responses, however, are numerous and may be determined in large part by the internal dimension of the environment. The very young, elders, and those who are in weakened conditions may be more dramatically affected by environmental health hazards than are members of the general population. For instance, children are

especially vulnerable to chemical poisoning because of rapid growth and cell division, high metabolic and respiratory rates, and dietary patterns that differ from those of adults (NIEHS, 2000). Elders tend to experience progressive deterioration in cardiac, renal, pulmonary, and immune system function and in the ability to detoxify chemicals. Studies of drug therapies for the aged, in fact, reveal a decline in blood flow to both liver and kidney, making it increasingly difficult for the aged to rid the body of drug residues and, most likely, environmental toxins (IOM, 1995; NIEHS, 2000).

In practice, individuals' responses are often analyzed and treated as the focus of intervention, yet a shift of focus toward environment can often provide a more appropriate approach to relieving certain responses. For example, pain might be lessened by increased social support or immunocompetence may be strengthened by lessening environmental stress in some way. Studies in the field of psychoneuroimmunology indicate that attitudes affect the ability of the body to deal with stressors (Aden, Felten, & Cohen, 2000). Depression and despair weaken the immune system and increase vulnerability.

Community Responses

Human responses can be understood as community as well as individual phenomena. Thus, mental health teams respond to communities where earthquakes, floods, and other disasters occur, helping these aggregates deal with their losses, regroup, and move on with their lives as quickly as possible. In this way, the severity of the response is mitigated. On an even larger scale, the Chernoble nuclear disaster had worldwide effects—loss, pain, and conflict felt at many levels of community.

Certainly, technology dependence and altered immuno-competence have been results, and years later, communities worldwide continue to act in response to the event.

Societal Responses

Human responses to factors related to the social dimension of environment are addressed as indicators of social health. Social health in the United States has been measured using the Index of Social Health, developed by researchers at Fordham University in New York City (Brink & Zeesman, 1997). Indicators include 16 measures of well-being, and data have been collected and analyzed from 1970 to the present. Miringoff (1999) examined measurement of economic well-being as reflected by the gross domestic product (GDP), generally used as the indicator of progress, and measurement of well-being as reflected by the Index of Social Health. The Index of Social Health accounts for well-being during different stages of life. Each measurement is compared with a standard, the highest measurement achieved in that particular area since 1970.

Figure 9-6 shows the total GDP steadily rising and the Fordham Index of Social Health steadily falling. Since the mid-1970s, 11 measures have declined and 5 have risen. Improvements have been seen in infant mortality, high school dropout rate, poverty among those over age 65, and life expectancy. Indicators that have worsened over time are children in poverty, child abuse, teen suicide, average weekly wage, violent crime, health insurance coverage, and inequality. Indicators of shifting performance are teenage drug use, teenage births, alcohol-related traffic fatalities, affordable housing, and unemploy-

ment. The results indicate that social health in the United States has fallen from 76 out of a possible 100 points in 1973 to 43 points in 1996.

The Human Response to Disaster

Although the human spirit is strong, certain events can be so overwhelming that people lose hope and sink into despair. When disaster strikes and others come with help, people are better able to cope and rebuild their lives. When a whole community or country falls, as in a war or other devastating act of violence, the resulting despair can render people helpless and unable to go on. At such times, help is essential but often difficult to find. Agencies such as the Red Cross help by furnishing necessary items to sustain physical life and nurture the human spirit.

Natural disasters, such as floods, earthquakes, or hurricanes, often cause great stress in all dimensions of environment. Nurses are often involved in community efforts to provide needed assistance and to help people find the strength and ability to cope in such situations. The nursing model described in this section provides a framework for disaster nursing in the community. Application of the nursing process to the environment requires assessment of each dimension of environment and the associated human responses. The base of the triangle in Figure 9-7 represents the five dimensions of environment

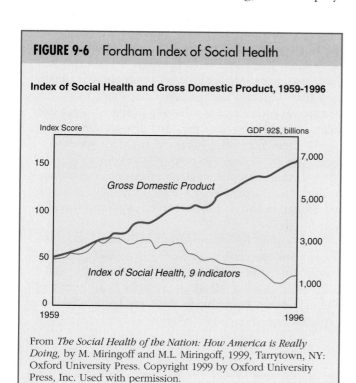

FIGURE 9-6 Fordham Index of Social Health

Index of Social Health and Gross Domestic Product, 1959-1996

From *The Social Health of the Nation: How America is Really Doing*, by M. Miringoff and M.L. Miringoff, 1999, Tarrytown, NY: Oxford University Press. Copyright 1999 by Oxford University Press, Inc. Used with permission.

✳ DECISION MAKING

Nursing Process in Disaster Nursing

Imagine yourself in the situation described by the public health nurse in the accompanying perspectives box. Consider each of the various dimensions of environment—physical, organizational, social, human aggregate, and internal—and how each might be affected. Consider the potential human responses of the victims to the needs identified.

♦ Identify the needs related to each dimension of environment.

♦ Identify what is being done to meet the needs in each dimension?

♦ List the areas of need according to the level of priority.

♦ List the needed resources currently available.

♦ How are internal dimension needs being assessed?

♦ Make a plan for application of the problem-solving process to the situation by using the model provided in the triangle of Figure 9-7: dimensions of environment.

FIGURE 9-7 Conceptual Linkages: Creating a Caring Environment to Support Health and Healing Processes

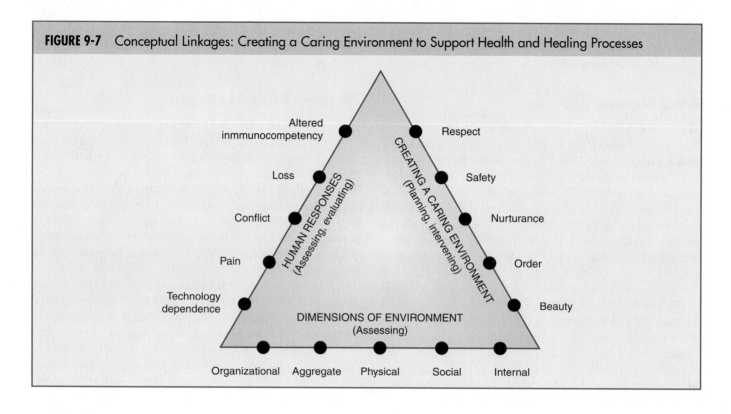

Perspectives...

INSIGHTS OF A COMMUNITY HEALTH NURSE

I work as a public health nurse in a county where a major river floods every few years, leaving at least one small town, hundreds of homes, and highways and roads under several feet of water. The flood relief plan is put together by the county EMS (emergency medical services). That agency is an umbrella group for coordinating with county departments—the Red Cross and other flood relief agencies. The EMS assists in setting up shelters at county veterans' buildings. In Guerneville, the old and defunct Bank of America is used as a center where agencies set up tables and send their workers to help people of the community get what they need to cope with the flood and to restore their homes and lives. So, flood victims can do "one-stop shopping" at the center.

At the center, one can apply for emergency Aid to Families with Dependent Children (AFDC), Medicaid, and delay of tax payment and can get a free lunch, cleaning supplies, water, and other basic supplies from the Red Cross.

I help answer telephone calls that the other agencies cannot help with and vice versa. I assist the Red Cross volunteers, do triage, and teach hand washing, food handling, and kitchen precautions to prevent the occurrence and spread of infection. I offer advice, assist victims with finding resources, and give tetanus shots.

Workers represent agencies such as social services, the Red Cross, the county tax department, and county environmental health inspectors. The mental health department offers resources and crisis counseling. Mental health and social service workers are available to clients.

The public health nurse in this setting works the shelters and the centers where flood victims seek help. I am involved in all multidisciplinary meetings, and I help with planning. Meetings are held at the start and end of the day. I am able to share my knowledge and expertise regarding the community with my colleagues.

—*Susan Miller, PHN*

FIGURE 9-8 Nursing Responsibilities to Prepare for and Respond to Disasters

- Participate in national/local predisaster planning.
- Cooperate in international programs in case of disasters in other countries.
- Assist communities in their action on environmental health problems.
- Work with community programs to reduce harmful pollutants (chemical, biological, or physical, e.g., noise) in air, soil, water, and food by industries or other human efforts.
- Improve nutrition.
- Encourage family planning.
- Assess environmental factors in work situations and pursue activities for the elimination or reduction of hazards.
- Educate the general public and all levels of nursing personnel in environmental and other health hazards, especially those related to unacceptable levels of contamination.

- Participate in research providing data for early warning and prevention of deleterious effects of the various environmental agents to which man is increasingly exposed.
- Participate in research conducive to discovering ways and means of improving living and working conditions.
- Serve as principal investigator, or in collaboration with other nurses or related professions, carry out epidemiological and experimental research designed to provide data to measure the impact of nursing intervention on environmental health: i.e., hazards, early warning for prevention of health hazards, improving living and working conditions, and monitoring the environmental levels of pollutants.

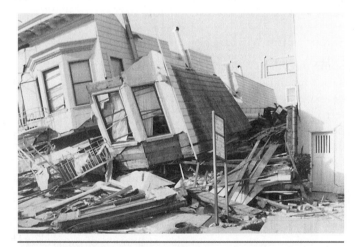

The community health nurse can provide assistance and help people cope with difficult situations.

to be assessed; the left side depicts the human responses to the environment. Planning for intervention requires linking these two sets of concepts with a third set—creating a caring environment (one that supports health and healing)—in order to alter the environment to increase its propensity to promote health and healing. Nursing activities for disaster preparation and intervention are listed in Figure 9-8.

CREATING A CARING ENVIRONMENT

Using qualitative research methods, Schubert (1989) identified five elements provided by nurses in creating an

environment supportive of health and healing processes: respect, safety, nurturance, order, and beauty. The nurses' efforts were grounded in both science and their intuitive knowledge of natural healing processes. Thus, the right side of the triangle in Figure 9-7 can serve as a goal for proposal development and nursing intervention related to environment.

Caring in modern nursing can be applied through the nursing process to create environments that promote health and healing. The idea of using the nursing process to create healthy and **healing environments** that are safe, nurturing, respectful, orderly, and beautiful is applicable to the world, nations, populations, communities, families, and individuals. Communities, however, are where grassroots actions take place—where families and individuals who are touched by environmental problems and feel strongly about these issues demand action. None of these entities operates independently of the others because each either comprises or is a component of other levels, or both.

Caring with intent to promote health and healing is the motivational force that provides guidance as the nurse identifies appropriate environmental health interventions. It is the integrative force that underlies safety, nurturance, respect, order, and beauty in an environment that supports natural healing processes. Focused intention to help and to facilitate healing provides direction for nursing activities related to environment. Thus, nursing practice is extended to issues of environmental health in all dimensions, levels, and settings.

Safety

Client safety can be classified as physical, mental, emotional, or spiritual. **Safety** is that component of environment that protects and keeps a person secure, unharmed, and free from danger. Nursing commonly involves protection of clients from external forces, but it also involves protection from internal forces, as in the case of suicide attempts and self-abuse. Specific safety issues vary with the setting. Safety issues in various settings are discussed in the following sections.

Safety in the Home

It is sometimes easiest for nurses to see the client's safety as a concern at the individual level. When working with families in the home, the nurse would likely be especially aware of the presence or absence and the appropriate placement and maintenance of fire alarm units, as well as avenues of escape in case of emergency. In both individual and family care, safety concerns tend to center on an identified problem. For example, in providing care to clients with diminished ability to walk, a concern might be obstacles to safe movement around the home. Climbing stairs or performing other types of physical exertion may be of concern for the client who has circulatory or respiratory problems.

Similarly, a visit to a family with a member who is experiencing allergies includes a search for allergens in the environment. In the case of food allergies, the concern is foods, items used in meal preparation, and sources of products used; in the case of allergies related to inhalation, sources of dust, animal dander, fibers, and pollens are investigated, as is evidence of efforts to restrict levels of these allergens.

Safety in Communities

We can carry the example of an allergy related to inhalation a step further. Some communities have higher than average levels of air pollution. Efforts to intervene might include involvement in a community action group aimed at controlling either emissions from local industries or by-products of community waste disposal systems.

Safety in Populations

Both damaging emissions and rising consumption leading to waste disposal problems can be seen as results of growing populations' making ever greater demands on the environment (Raven, 1998). Because of this, populations constitute an important stratum in the environmental impact on health. Obviously, when such broader reaching strata are involved, it no longer makes sense to limit health advocacy to narrow concerns. With this recognition, some individuals in various populations—for example, different countries or varying segments of communities—band together and begin to work toward change. As is the case with other groups, some nurses will become political activists and some will not, but it is important that all nurses be aware of the broader implications. Membership in state, national, and international nursing organizations is one way that individuals can support interventions in the larger context.

Even in smaller communities, populations may constitute a stratum of concern when minority aggregates are at risk for certain health problems or have less access to health care than do other community members. Frequently, these groups are also less likely to be in a position to advocate change. It then becomes the responsibility of health care professionals to identify the problems and seek solutions.

Safety in Nations

Often when we think of populations, we think at the national level. With the emergence of rapid-communication systems, it has become easier than in the past to share information about health care, whether that information concerns disease-specific treatments, common habits or activities that affect health, or conditions that threaten the quality of air, water, housing, and the like. Many threats to health must be confronted at the national level, simply because local measures lack sufficient scope to maintain healthful conditions, even locally. Air quality is one example; whatever changes are instituted locally, the problem is likely to be aggravated by conditions beyond local control.

Safety in the World

Some threats to individual safety are being recognized as so far-reaching that only international interventions can be expected to reduce the danger. In addition to war and terrorism, the global issues identified (Raven, 1998) as posing the severest environmental crisis in history are rising consumption and damaging technology. The need for research to determine health and safety is great. See the Research Focus box for an examination of some challenges inherent in environmental research efforts.

We have only a few decades' worth of oil supplies left, the world's rain forests are shrinking, species are being extinguished at a rapid rate, and much of the world's farmland is deteriorating. Air pollution, acid rain, ozone depletion, and rising carbon dioxide concentrations are destroying the atmosphere.

The community health nurse can have an impact on all levels of physical safety by increasing consciousness of the issues through example. By contributing to others' awareness, the nurse may influence individual and group attitudes, leading indirectly to healthier environments.

Mental, Emotional, and Spiritual Safety

Mental safety related to values and beliefs was discussed in Chapter 8 and will not be explored at length here. Beliefs and values stem primarily from culture and religion and are sometimes altered by experience and education. Freedom and individual responsibility are important values in the free world, where it is generally assumed that

---

REFLECTIVE THINKING

Environmental Health Behavior

- Why is nursing concerned with recycling? Waste disposal? Air pollution?
- At what environmental level or levels might these issues trigger concern?
- At what level or levels would intervention be appropriate?
- Who or what might the client be?

FIGURE 9-9 Characteristics of a Respectful Environment

- The client identifies the problem.
- The nurse plays a supportive role as the client learns, develops, and fulfills the solution to the problem.
- Problems are opportunities.
- The nurse acknowledges the client's ability to take advantage of the opportunity.
- The nurse cannot independently solve the problem.

---

safety to believe as one chooses is a right as long as behavior does not threaten the safety of oneself or of others. Again, the student is reminded that respect for various beliefs and values contributes to environmental safety.

Tending to mental and emotional safety often begins with the nurse's attitude when addressing physical issues. Knowing that someone cares and will listen seriously to one's problems can make it easier for the client to think clearly and can reduce client stress related to uncertainty. Treating the client as a partner in health promotion enhances this feeling. As clients take more responsibility for their feelings, they will be more in control and will perceive less threat in the relationship with environment. Clients learn to think more positively about themselves while progressively feeling safer in their respective environments. Specific issues vary with the setting and the client's basic needs.

It is sometimes necessary to make clients aware of how the nurse's activities will promote safety, reassuring them that their safety is a concern. Families often feel threatened when visited by someone in an official capacity, such as a community health nurse, but when the nurse's attitude is one of genuine caring, the client usually is able to enter into a working partnership.

Spiritual safety can also imply confidence to follow one's religious beliefs or spiritual discipline without criticism or persecution. More subtly, it can imply an environment that allows clients to repattern the energy of fear engendered by feelings of being physically or emotionally unsafe. Fears may occur in response to external or internal stimuli and might include fear for physical safety, fear of rejection, or fear of being judged as incompetent or as having little value, among other fears. Such fears may be traced to ideas about oneself, as in suicidal ideation, or to one's perceptions of others' judgments, as in low self-worth.

Respect

Respect is an aspect of caring (see Chapter 1) and has also been identified by Schubert (1989) as a crucial element of environments that support health and healing.

Respect includes consideration and concern for others, as well as trust in others' capability and potential for growth and healing. A respectful environment provides support as the individual or aggregate experiences increasing order, organization, and ability to be interactive, independent, and interdependent. As indicated in Figure 9-9, the client may make mistakes and learns from those mistakes.

This attitude toward the client requires the nurse to encourage each person, family, or group to assume self-responsibility. The nurse supports the client's efforts but does not take over and try to *fix* the problem. Within a relationship of mutuality and partnership, the nurse exhibits patience as the client learns to take charge.

Colodzin (1993) suggests that in environments where disrespect is the rule, it becomes a habit and is taken for granted. If the opposite is also true, we can assume that when nurses model and teach caring at all practice levels, they contribute not only to a more balanced society but also to a world that can more effectively promote and protect health.

Nurturance

Nurturance is the provision of materials discussed by Nightingale (1860/1969), such as nourishing food, proper temperature, quiet, light, fresh air, cleanliness, and shelter. To this list, the authors would add respectful touch.

Nurturance in the Home and Family

The home and family are major sources of nurturance in all cultures. The family provides shelter and protection from the weather, food, furnishings for comfort, and affection and respectful touch. When families fail to provide nurturance, the deprivation is destructive to physical and emotional health. Their young members may suffer from addictions, nutritional disorders, or physical or mental chronic illness. The community nurse works to strengthen the family's ability to provide nurturance and, thus, to prevent these problems.

Nurturance in the Community

The family and community share resources to provide individuals with food, clothing, shelter, and necessities for

✳ DECISION MAKING

A Respectful Environment

Imagine that a family in the small, rural community where you work as a community health nurse is one of three African American families in the community. One of the children has been hurt in a fight on the way home from school. Use the triangle in Figure 9-7 to assess the situation by considering the following:

◆ The various dimensions of environment
◆ The human responses
◆ Those characteristics, if any, that need work
   How would you intervene?

health and healing. When the family and community are both strong, mutual sharing occurs; when the family is in some way weakened, the community must absorb more responsibility for the family. For example, if a parent becomes jobless, extended family, friends, churches, and other organizations that provide food, clothing, and shelter may become involved. When the specific community is significantly weakened and these resources become unavailable, malnutrition, homelessness, and disease bring suffering. Governmental and private agencies often assume responsibility for helping those in distress.

Ingenuity and creativity are useful in finding community resources for a family. The nurse serves as client advocate in approaching organizations designed to help in certain circumstances. The nurse can identify available services and help the client contact resources. The nurse can sometimes help by guiding the family back to lost social supports such as extended family, friends, and church groups.

Nurturance in World Populations

Nurturance is a major problem for the world at large. Much of the problem can be traced to exploding population, growing at the staggering rate of 100 million people each year and thereby doubling the earth's population every 40 years (Raven, 1998).

This population explosion is fostering disparities between the rich and the poor, both within and outside the United States. Income per person in developed countries is approximately 30 times that in the poorest countries. The worst devastation related to this poverty is starvation and malnutrition.

These problems create great concerns for community nurses who work to provide a nurturing community and world environment. Nurses are joining the ranks of poli-

cymakers and international health workers who attempt to guide the world's population to greater health by working to create an environment that supports health and healing.

Order

Order, or the methodical and harmonious arrangement of time, space, and objects in one's life, is another aspect of a healing environment. Its presence or relative absence can be observed in physical, psychological, time-related, or other aspects of a client's situation. The harmony and rhythmic patterns of a productive nurse-client interaction require creative sensitivity and can themselves contribute to order—an esthetic quality of the environment. For example, the sensitivity of the nurse to the client's time and activity schedule is important, and, in the United States, the client is apt to feel disrespected if the nurse does not keep appointments on schedule. This is true whether the nurse is visiting a family at home or has a speaking engagement at a community service group meeting.

Individuals and organized groups have varying degrees of tolerance for the unexpected, and when a client experiences dislocation for any reason, the nurse's assistance may be necessary to help bring about or guide and support the process of restoring order. Sorrell (1994) describes esthetic knowing as an aspect of the art of nursing that includes synthesis of scattered details of perception into a coherent whole. The understanding that emerges from this synthesis is what helps the nurse work with discordant issues that arise in the community.

The structure of time and activity and the arrangement of things in the home, workplace, school, or other community setting very definitely influence ability to function, whether the focus is the individual, the family, or a larger aggregate. In the home involved, individuals may need the nurse's assistance to regain order and the ability to function. In society, more people and planning are required to restore the infrastructure and the organizational structures that establish and maintain optimum order.

A word of caution is necessary here. Just as lack of order may interfere with one's ability to function, so may an overemphasis on maintaining order. On one hand, order is a friend and facilitates living processes; on the other, an obsession with order may interfere with functioning. Individuals, families, or groups who cannot tolerate disorder may stifle activity and functioning. For example, a home or classroom that is never cluttered may be the setting for a family or group of students whose creativity and freedom to grow and develop according to their human potential are stifled and limited.

Human attempts to control the forces of nature seem to have created more disorder in the world; cooperation with and respect for natural forces could potentially promote more order and less destruction. Order, as a characteristic of a healthy and healing environment in communities and the world, is influenced by natural forces. Nature also provides the beauty of color, sound, form, and rhythm, which support health and healing.

Beauty

Most people have certain places they associate with peace, solitude, relaxation, rejuvenation, restoration, and/or some form of physical, mental, and/or spiritual healing. Physical environmental factors work together with individual and societal factors in the healing process. Place is understood as being influenced not only by the physical and built environment but also by the human mind and material circumstances, reflecting both human intentions and actions and the constraints and structures imposed by society. Places of beauty create a sense of peace and rest, and are used by many to achieve physical, mental, and spiritual healing. The tranquility of rural settings and nearness to the beauty of nature are well known as places to seek healing of the body, mind, and spirit.

Aesthetic **beauty** is experienced through the senses and either exists naturally in or is developed as a part of the environment. The components of beauty are sound, color, and form. Form is expressed as patterns or rhythms of matter and energy and often is intimately associated with sound and color. Those forms found in nature seem to have healing qualities. At the same time, each person manifests his or her own unique pattern such that not everyone experiences the same form of beauty as healing.

Gardens, beaches, and forest walks may be used when possible for nurse-client interaction and as an environment for health and healing. In addition to benefiting from the incredible beauty found in nature, persons need to create things of beauty. Artistic creation and the enjoyment of others' work can serve as media for inner healing from deep emotional and spiritual wounds. Artistic self-expression through movement and other art forms demonstrates healing in the interpenetrating processes and pattern reorganization of the person-environment interrelationship. Many cultures use the beauty of dance to restore balance and harmony and to promote health and wholeness.

Certain sounds, such as those of ocean waves, a waterfall, or a breeze in the trees, can restore a sense of balance and harmony for some individuals. A Bach fugue, with its interweaving and integration of parts, can be very healing for others who feel confused and helpless. Clients themselves are the best sources of ideas regarding those things that enhance their sense of beauty.

Color is used by some nurses to stimulate healing. Perhaps the wave frequencies of colors promote healing for persons of different energy patterns or resonances. Appreciation of beauty depends on one's ability to perceive it and on one's level of awareness, but these are difficult to assess. Maslow (1962) referred to appreciation of beauty as a self-actualizing process. It is unlikely, however, that only those persons whose basic needs have

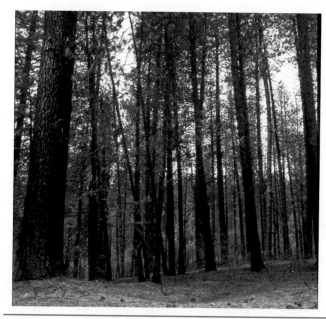

The sights and sounds of a forest may bring about healing to a client. What enhances your sense of beauty?

been met can respond therapeutically to beauty, as Maslow's hierarchy of needs might suggest.

Beauty in Communities

Beauty in larger communities can be achieved through order, discussed previously, and through development of the resources of the community itself. These resources are both material and personal. In relatively rare cases, the nurse may be involved in planning or implementing the aesthetic aspects of a physical community. Nevertheless, all of the work that community health nurses do at the level of larger communities can be seen as addressing beauty in some way. One such example is the harmony that grows out of a community's increasing understanding of itself and its responsibilities.

Proposals for Creating Healthy and Healing Environments

The triangle in Figure 9-7 may be used in the development of proposals for creating and maintaining healthy and healing environments. For instance, a problem found in the assessment of the physical dimension and indicating the presence of an environmental hazard associated with the human response of a related skin disorder indicates a possible physical safety issue. Thus, the nurse would design her proposal to increase safety in the questionable dimension of environment and would protect the client through education and appropriate treatment to prevent further disability. Primary, secondary, and tertiary prevention are applied, then, not only to the person involved but also to the environment.

The IOM advanced nurse specialists Josten, Clarke, Ostwald, Stoskopf, and Shannon (1995) encourage development of advanced nurse specialists in the public health specialist role, wherein nurses with graduate degrees would work to create healthy environments in the community and to educate and guide the populace toward positive health behavior. In this model, community health nurses participate in activities to create healthy environments; at present, however, the major focus of the community health nurse is providing individual or family care in community settings such as a home or a workplace.

APPLICATION OF THE NURSING PROCESS TO ENVIRONMENT

The nursing process—assessing, diagnosing, planning, implementing, and evaluating—is a deliberate, logical, and rational problem-solving process whereby the practice of nursing is performed systematically. Assessment of potential environmental hazards in the lives of individuals and families should include questions about exposure to chemical, physical, or biological hazards and about temporal elements between environmental events and symptoms (see Figure 9-10).

Although the nursing process was developed for use in the care of individuals, it has been expanded for use in the care of families, communities, and larger populations. The IOM (1995) report suggests that new methods may be required for application of the nursing process to environmental health issues (see Figure 9-11). The nursing process is compatible with the California Public Health

Foundation, currently known as the Public Health Institute (1992) framework, an approach utilizing investigator, educator, and advocate roles to address environmental health issues. The **investigator role,** the gathering of data and formulation of a nursing diagnosis, is equivalent to the assessment and evaluation phases; the **educator** and **advocacy roles** constitute the intervention phase. The educator role involves helping others gain knowledge, skills, and characteristics needed for good health; the advocacy role involves speaking or acting in behalf of those who are unable to do so for themselves. Policy making and program planning are among the skills needed for the intervention phase.

FIGURE 9-10 Questions to Assess Exposure to Potential Environmental Hazards

- What are your current and past longest-held jobs? (For children and teenagers, the question can be modified to, "Where do you spend your day, and what do you do there?")

- Have you had any recent exposure to chemicals (including dusts, mists, and fumes) or radiation?

- Have you noticed any (temporal) relationship between your current symptoms and activities at work, home, or other environments?

From *Nursing, Health and Environment,* by the National Academy of Sciences, 1995, Washington, DC: Author. Copyright 1995 by the National Academy of Sciences. Reprinted with permission.

FIGURE 9-11 Application of the Nursing Process for Environmental Action

Assessment

- Get an *exposure history* of the individual, family or community.

- Do a *visual inspection* for additional assessment data.

- Gather *risk assessment* data by reviewing existing health effects information.

- Identify *patterns of comorbidity* among family/community members which suggest environmental etiologies.

- Be alert for *sentinel events.*

- Obtain *continuous input* from individuals, families, and communities.

- Make a nursing diagnosis using the North American Nursing Diagnosis Association (NANDA) for individuals, families, and communities.

Planning/Outcomes

- Establish health optimal outcomes for individuals, families, and communities.

Interventions

- Provide education about hazards and ways to protect from hazards.

- Advocacy by developing, enforcing environmental regulations.

- Referrals to medical experts, nursing colleagues, public health agencies, etc.

- Case management by coordinating activities to reduce/eliminate exposure.

Evaluation

- Consider health outcomes.

- Evaluate hazard abatement.

From *Nursing, Health and Environment,* by the National Academy of Sciences, 1995, Washington, DC: Author. Copyright 1995 by the National Academy of Sciences. Reprinted with permission.

An aggregate focus for community health nursing requires additional skills and reinterpretation of the nursing process. Neufer (1994) offers a method for application of the nursing process to aggregates when environmental issues are concerned. First, data from federal, state, and local resources are collected (see Table 9-2). Major federal

TABLE 9-2   Sources of Environmental Health Data

FEDERAL	STATE	LOCAL
EPA studies and ATSDR public health assessments for NPL sites	State environmental agencies (priority lists, environmental monitoring data, other studies)	Community health concerns
ATSDR public health assessments, consultations, studies	State health agencies (health advisories, disease registries, epidemiologic studies or surveys)	Community action groups
Toxic chemical release inventory database		Health screening programs and surveys
		Local health departments

From "The Role of the Community Health Nurse in Environmental Health," by L. Neufer, 1994, Public Health Nursing, 11*(3), p. 157. Copyright 1994 by Blackwell Science, Inc. Reprinted with permission.*

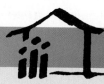

COMMUNITY NURSING VIEW

A public health nurse (PHN) works as an environmental scientist at ATSDR, assisting communities affected by hazardous waste releases. ATSDR is contacted by an activist group concerning a creek in the group's local area, and the resulting report is forwarded to the PHN for follow-up. The report indicates that the creek is grossly polluted with dangerous industrial wastes. The group is especially concerned because, although there are warning signs posted, children and adults continue to play and fish in the creek (Phillips, 1995).

Nursing Considerations

Assessment

◆ Where would the nurse look for clues of potential sources of pollution?

◆ What steps would the nurse take to determine the level of contamination?

◆ What other factors besides the contaminated water would the nurse consider when formulating the assessment?

◆ What resources would the nurse have to use to obtain assessment data?

Diagnosis

◆ Who in the community may be at risk?

◆ Can a significant potential for injury be identified?

◆ What are the host and environmental factors related to diagnosis?

Outcome Identification

◆ What outcomes would be identified for people who have already been exposed to the creek? For those who have potential for exposure?

Planning/Interventions

◆ What interventions would the nurse employ to minimize further exposure to the creek?

◆ How would the nurse identify those who have been exposed?

◆ What type of educational programs would the nurse devise to encourage full community awareness of treatment methods for those already exposed?

◆ What types of agencies would the nurse notify to aid in cleanup efforts?

Evaluation

◆ What factors would indicate that the nurse's plan is successful?

If the plan were not successful, what amendments could be made?

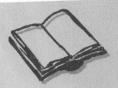

Out of the Box

Betsy Beam had served as School Nurse at Jefferson Forest High School for two years. She had kept meticulous records of the students' complaints and the classrooms in which they were enrolled. After a year, she realized the records had tracked a pattern of health complaints that could be related to air quality problems. She asked for air quality testing and was told that testing had been done the previous year and that there were no problems. When she asked to see the report, she was told the report could not be found.

Ms. Beam said she recorded every visit a student made to the school clinic, with dates, times and results. She recorded everything from serious illnesses to requests for bandaids. She had been on the job a few months when she noticed a large increase in the number of students with headaches. The noticeable increase prompted her to send out a questionnaire to the faculty. The questionnaire revealed similar results, with teacher reports of not feeling well and suffering from headaches. She, then, asked for air quality testing.

She continued to gather data regarding the number of students carrying inhalers and frequency of use. She provided the school administrator with the data gathered each month. At the end of each semester she gave the information to the county school nursing coordinator who was unable to draw clear conclusions from the data.

A complaint was filed with OSHA after a second year. Preliminary testing revealed that four classrooms out of the 30 that were checked had elevated levels of mold. School officials then closed the school for the rest of the year while engineers continued to collect data and make decisions for intervention.

Used with permission of *The News and Advance,* Lynchburg, VA, and Marcia Apperson, reporter. ■

FIGURE 9-12 Formulating Nursing Diagnoses for an Environmental Health Assessment

Nursing diagnosis in an environmental health assessment provides answers to the following questions:

- Who in the community is at highest risk?
- Can a significant potential for injury be identified?
- What are the host and environmental factors related to the diagnosis?
- Do data substantiate the nursing diagnosis?

From "The Role of the Community Health Nurse in Environmental Health," by L. Neufer, 1994. *Public Health Nursing, 11*(3), pp. 155–162. Copyright 1994 by Blackwell Scientific Publications. Reprinted with permission.

---

volve consultation with environmental activists and experts on specific topics as well as with the people at risk.

Next, an environmental health nursing diagnosis should be formulated (see Figure 9-12). This diagnosis identifies the potentially unhealthful response for a community. It is aimed at a specific aggregate of people, a "collection of individuals who are not part of an interdependent group, but who share some health risk or health-seeking behavior" (Neufeld & Harrison, 1990, p. 252). When the aggregate has been identified, the potential for injury and the factors (both host and environmental) related to the health problem are determined. Data gathering should continue to monitor results.

KEY CONCEPTS

- ◆ Community health nursing perspectives include both public health and the environmental focus of nursing.

- ◆ The Institute of Medicine report recommends that nurses address environmental health concerns.

- ◆ Assessment of the environment can be facilitated by analyzing the various dimensions of the environment and the human responses of the client.

- ◆ Nurse theorists since the time of Florence Nightingale have emphasized the creation and maintenance of healthy and healing environments as the goal of nursing.

- ◆ Proposals for intervention link assessment data from the various dimensions of environment and the human responses of the client with actions to enhance health or healing qualities of the environment.

- ◆ A healthy and healing environment reflects caring and is characterized by safety, nurturance, respect, order, and beauty.

---

resources are the EPA; the ATSDR; the national priorities list (NPL), which includes identified hazardous toxic waste sites; and the toxic chemical release inventory database, which lists all reported substances by city, county, or zip code. Environmental laws are available through the EPA and other state and local agencies. Applicable state and local agencies and groups vary. Data gathering should in-

◆ The nursing process—assessing, planning, intervening, and evaluating—can be applied to the environment to promote client health and healing.

RESOURCES

U.S. GOVERNMENT AGENCIES— ENVIRONMENTAL HEALTH

Center for Disease Control and Prevention (CDC): http://www.cdc.gov

National Institute of Environmental Health Sciences (NIEHS): http://www.niehs.nih.gov

National Library of Medicine Environmental Health Directory: http://www.nlm.nih.gov/medlineplus

Environmental Protection Agency (EPA): http://www.epa.gov

Environmental Protection Agency—Office of Children's Health Protection (OCHP): http://www.epa.gov/children

Environmental Protection Agency—Superfund Health and Safety: http://www.epa.gov/superfund/health

Environmental Protection Agency—*How to report environmental violations*: http://www.epa.gov/epahome/violations

Environmental Protection Agency—*Pesticides and food*: http://www.epa.gov/pesticides/food

Environmental Protection Agency—*Environmental justice:* http://www.es.epa.gov/oeca/main/ej

National Institutes of Health (NIH): http://www.nih.gov

National Association of County and City Health Officials (NACCHO): http://www.naccho.org

Agency for Toxic Substances and Disease Registry (ATSDR): http://www.atsdr.cdc.gov

INTERNATIONAL AGENCIES—ENVIRONMENTAL HEALTH

United Nations Environment Programme (UNEP): http://www.unep.org

Global Change Research Information Office: http://www.gcrio.org

Pan American Health Organization (PAHO): http://www.paho.org

Center for Health Communications of the Harvard School of Public Health: http://www.worldhealthnews.harvard.edu

World Health Organization (WHO): http://www.who.int/whosis

Environmental indicators: Environment Canada, Pacific and Yukon Region: http://www.ecoinfo.org

NONGOVERNMENTAL AGENCIES— ENVIRONMENTAL HEALTH

Indigenous Environmental Network: http://www.ienearth.org

International Health News: http://www.yourhealthbase.com

Environment News Service: http://ens-news.com/ens

University of Maryland School of Nursing: http://www.envirn.umaryland.edu

CARING COMMUNICATION AND CLIENT TEACHING/LEARNING

Phyllis E. Schubert, DNSc, RN, MA

MAKING THE CONNECTION

Talking with [clients] is easy when the nurse treats the [client] as a chum and engages in a give-and-take of social chitchat. But when the nurse sees her part in verbal interchanges with [clients] as a major component in direct nursing service, then she must recognize the complexity of that process. Social chitchat is replaced by the responsible use of words which help to further the personal development of the [client].

—Peplau, 1960, p. 964

COMPETENCIES

Upon completion of this chapter, the reader should be able to:

- Name one factor that sets health care models apart from other models of communication.
- List at least five concepts defined in nursing communication theory.
- Describe and explain two possible levels of client responsibility in developing the client-nurse relationship.
- Demonstrate four forms of active listening.
- Compare and contrast information sharing and therapeutic interviews.
- Identify the phases of group development.
- Identify a goal of *Healthy People 2010* that is related to health education and describe how the characteristics of andragogy can be used to help meet the goal.
- Identify nine factors that are important to the physical learning environment.
- Describe the five components of the learning process.
- Describe the three stages that form the basis of an empowering community education program.
- Identify elements of a win-win conflict resolution strategy.

KEY TERMS

active listening

affective learning
   objectives

andragogy

behavioral learning
   objectives

centering

clarity

client centered

closed questions

cognitive learning
   objectives

cognitive organization

communication

conflict

conflict management

conflict resolution

content-oriented
   groups

continuity

critical thinking

directive approach

empathy

empowerment
   education

energy field

feelings reflection

formal teaching

informal teaching

interpersonal systems

intrapersonal systems

learning process

lose-win approach

meanings reflection

midrange groups

negotiation

nondirective approach

nonverbal behaviors

open questions

open systems

pedagogy

principled negotiation

process-oriented
   groups

psychomotor learning
   objectives

self-care

self-efficacy

social systems

strategic planning

summative reflection

teaching/learning
   process

telecommunications

telehealth

telenursing

warmth

win-lose approach

win-win approach

Communication, the process of using a common set of rules in order to share information, is the core of client-nurse work, dictating its quality and effectiveness. **Communication** is required of nurses in all situations, especially in the home and community settings, and may take the form of information gathering, therapeutic communication, or teaching. Whether the job at hand is teaching parenting skills, completing an infant health assessment, counseling a discouraged or rebellious adolescent, or planning and implementing a health education program, the nurse must be able to communicate caring in a way that is helpful to clients.

Efficient and effective communication is also a necessity in professional relationships, whether one is making referrals, reports, or suggestions; leading groups; chairing meetings; or participating in conflict resolution activities. This chapter focuses on health care communication skills, adult learning theory, and teaching skills and how these apply in the helping relationship.

HEALTH-RELATED COMMUNICATION

Health communication is communication centering on health-related issues of individuals and groups. It encompasses feelings and attitudes as well as information and is carried out by the use of symbols and language. Transactions are verbal or nonverbal, oral or written, personal or impersonal, issue oriented or relationship oriented.

Contexts for community nurses' communication include **intrapersonal systems, interpersonal systems,** and **social systems,** the latter including small-group, organizational, and public systems. The intrapersonal context is our inner thoughts, beliefs, and feelings, as well as our "self-talk" about issues that influence our health-directed behaviors and attitudes toward our clients and colleagues. Interpersonal contexts include client-nurse, nurse-nurse, and nurse-other professional situations. In small groups, nurses are involved with client family constellations and in group teaching, treatment or education planning, staff reports, and health team interactions. Organizational health communication occurs in contexts such as administration, program planning, staff relations, and dialogue with institutions involved in a client's care. Public communication encompasses presentations, speeches, and public addresses made by individuals on health-related topics such as national and world health programs, health promotion, and public health planning.

Carl Rogers' Client-Centered Model

Carl Rogers (1951), a psychologist, set the stage for therapeutic models of communication, which emphasize the important role that relationships play in assisting clients to adjust to their circumstances, move toward health and away from illness, or learn to cope with the illness. When used by health professionals, therapeutic communication can be defined as a skill that helps others find the strength to do what they need to do. It is used to help clients learn to deal with stress, get along with other people, adapt to situations they cannot change, and overcome emotional and mental blocks to achieving their potential.

Health Communication Model

The Health Communication Model (HCM) (Northouse & Northouse, 1998) focuses specifically on transactions between health care participants about health-related issues. Figure 10-1 shows the variables and directions of communication in this model. The focus is communication that occurs in various kinds of relationships in health care; the three major variables of the health communication process are relationships, transactions, and contexts.

Relationships are of four major types: professional-professional, professional-client, professional-significant other, and client-significant other. Transactions are interactions between participants in the health communication process over the life span and involve both content and relationship dimensions. The spirals in the model reflect the ongoing, transactional nature of the process. In community nursing, the context is usually outside the hospital, typically in homes, clinics, schools, and workplaces. The nature of these settings and the number of people involved also affect health communication.

NURSING INTERACTION MODELS

Nursing scholars have developed a progression of theories to account for the unique focus of nursing as it applies to interactions with clients and to other health care disciplines. These efforts began when Peplau (1952) identified communication and client-nurse interaction as nursing concerns.

Peplau defines nursing as a therapeutic, interpersonal process requiring supportive communication, including **nonverbal behaviors** which communicate attitudes, meaning, or content to another, either intentionally, through gestures, or unintentionally, through body language. She defines supportive communication as being characterized by **clarity** and **continuity;** that is, the meaning is understood and agreed upon by sender and receiver, and the nurse picks up on threads of the client's meaning in the process of conversation.

Influenced by Peplau, Orlando (1961, 1972) identifies the nursing process as consisting of three basic elements:

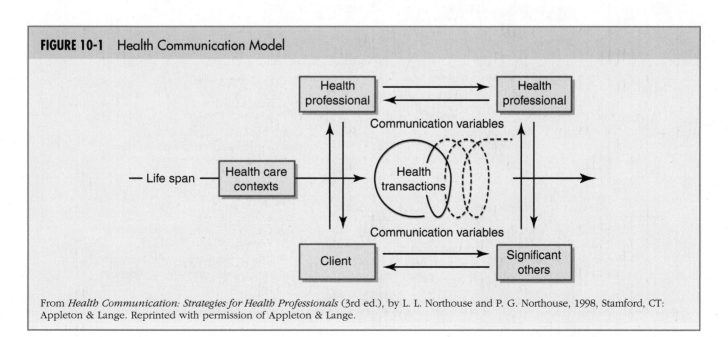

FIGURE 10-1 Health Communication Model

From *Health Communication: Strategies for Health Professionals* (3rd ed.), by L. L. Northouse and P. G. Northouse, 1998, Stamford, CT: Appleton & Lange. Reprinted with permission of Appleton & Lange.

client behavior, the reaction of the nurse, and nursing actions designed for the client's benefit. Into this framework, Travelbee (1963, 1964, 1971) introduces the concept of **empathy** (understanding the subjective world of another and then communicating that understanding) and the importance of the nurse's caring for the client.

King (1981) depicts client-nurse interactions as acknowledging the influence of perceptions, responsibility for sharing information, and the client's right to participate in decisions influencing his or her health. King places the client-nurse interaction in an open-systems framework (**open systems** are systems, such as human beings, that exist in interrelationship with their environment, taking in and assimilating energy and eliminating waste).

Rogers' Science of Unitary Human Beings (Rogers, 1990) is based on the premise that human beings and environment are inseparable open systems. This premise enables us to see the nurse as one aspect of the client's environment and vice versa. Thus, anxiety, fear, anger, or nonjudgmental acceptance, for example, is expressed in the nurse's **energy field** (the whole of a person's being as seen in one's presence through observation, sensing, and timing) and is communicated to the client. The reverse is also expected, with the nurse able to sense changes in the client's field, especially when the nurse has sensitized herself to perception of energy (Krieger, 1993).

Rogers' energy field is one way of understanding the phenomena that are at the heart of interpersonal theories of nursing. Empathy, for example, increases awareness of feelings in the other person and communicates a healing atmosphere. With her notions of energy exchange, Rogers' theory complements traditional definitions of interpersonal interaction.

INFLUENCES ON CLIENT-NURSE COMMUNICATION

King's (1981) model, mentioned earlier, introduces the concepts of mutual goal setting and goal attainment in the client-nurse relationship. Successful outcomes depend, to a large extent, on client-nurse bonding, which is based on caring and trust, as shown in Figure 10-2. Table 10-1 gives a conceptual framework for understanding the dynamics of the client-nurse relationship reflecting mutual connectedness and how formation of work roles and healing outcomes are affected (Schubert & Lionberger, 1995). Follow the arrows in the model to understand the flow of the process. Before discussing communication skills themselves, one must understand the three aspects of the client-nurse relationship that influence communication in modern nursing: namely, mutual problem solving, the client's evolving level of responsibility in that process, and shifting roles in the client-nurse relationship.

Mutual Problem Solving in the Client-Nurse Relationship

Mutual problem solving depends on the use of validation. The validation process serves to keep the nurse focused on the rights and obligations of the client to their own health-related decisions. Validation of the client's opinions and feelings is sought at each step and phase of the process. Implicit in validation are unearthing questions or concerns about plans for health care and securing understanding and willingness to proceed to the next step (see Figure 10-3) (Balzer-Riley, 2000).

Contracts or agreements between the client and nurse constitute useful tools in the mutual problem-solving process. The contract outlines the activities and responsibilities for which each will be accountable.

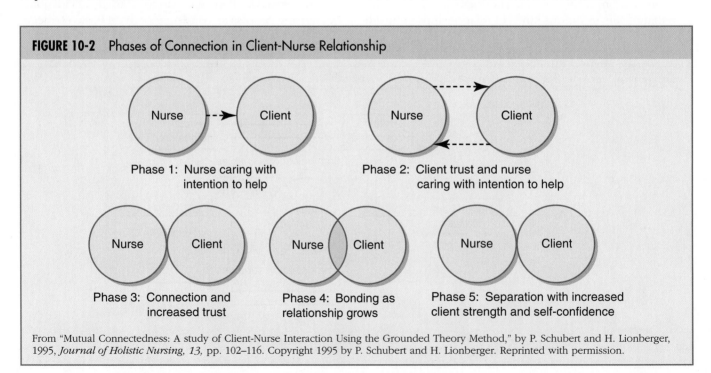

FIGURE 10-2 Phases of Connection in Client-Nurse Relationship

Phase 1: Nurse caring with intention to help

Phase 2: Client trust and nurse caring with intention to help

Phase 3: Connection and increased trust

Phase 4: Bonding as relationship grows

Phase 5: Separation with increased client strength and self-confidence

From "Mutual Connectedness: A study of Client-Nurse Interaction Using the Grounded Theory Method," by P. Schubert and H. Lionberger, 1995, *Journal of Holistic Nursing, 13,* pp. 102–116. Copyright 1995 by P. Schubert and H. Lionberger. Reprinted with permission.

TABLE 10-1 Theory of Mutual Connectedness: Categories and Conceptual Linkages

MAJOR CATEGORY	CARING ENVIRONMENT	MUTUAL CONNECTEDNESS	NURSING THERAPY	HEALING
Properties	Safety Nurturance Respect Beauty/order	Trust Compassion Shared consciousness	Identification and enhancement of health patterns	Inner directed Unpredictable Nature's time frame
Conditions	Nurse readiness Client comfort with intimacy	Intimacy and trust become bonding	Works roles formed	Releasing old and introducing new patterns
Strategies	Nurse centering Client inner negotiation for trust	Both parties listening and opening	Nursing interventions	Self-acceptance worked on by each party
Outcomes	Intimacy Client decision to trust and bond	Roles formed for further work	Releasing old and introducing new patterns	Transformation Evolution of self-potential Creativity

Adapted from "Mutual Connectedness: A Study of Client-Nurse Interaction Using the Grounded Theory Method," by P. Schubert and H. Lionberger, 1995, Journal of Holistic Nursing, 13, pp. 102–116. Copyright 1995 by P. Schubert and H. Lionberger. Reprinted with permission.

FIGURE 10-3 Mutual Problem-Solving Process Model

1. Assess
   A. Collecting data
   B. Analyzing data
   C. Validating interpretation of data with the client
   D. Identifying actual or potential problems with the client
   E. Validating the nursing diagnoses with the client
2. Plan
   A. Setting priorities for resolution of identified problems with the client
   B. Determining expected and desired outcomes of nursing actions in collaboration with the client
   C. Deciding on the nursing strategies to achieve these outcomes in collaboration with the client
3. Implement
   A. Implementing nursing actions with assistance from the client
   B. Encouraging client participation in carrying out nursing actions to meet the outcomes
4. Evaluation
   A. Evaluating the outcomes of nursing care in consultation with the client.

From *Communication in Nursing* (4th ed.), by J. Balzer Riley, 2000, St. Louis: Mosby. Used with permission.

Client's Evolving Level of Responsibility

In all interactions with a client, the nurse must be alert for indications of how much responsibility the client wants or is willing to assume. The nurse's communication skills are crucial as changes occur. Clients who have a clear understanding of their health problems and those things that they and their nurse can do about those problems will expend less energy worrying and more energy doing something constructive. Having clarity regarding nursing diagnoses and having a say in the best ways to handle the diagnoses give clients a sense of control.

Consumers today are speaking up, asking questions, seeking second opinions, demanding alternative health care options, and forming self-help groups. This assertiveness and independence reflect the true meaning of the label "client"—one who claims the rights and privileges of partnership in health care (Balzer-Riley, 2000). Figure 10-4 lists client privileges.

Balzer-Riley (2000) encourages nurses to transform all client-nurse relationships into relationships of mutual problem solving and participation by calling on the strengths of the clients and inviting—even requesting—their full participation as partners in the process. Active listening, discussed below, is a useful tool for accomplishing this goal.

Shifting Roles in Client-Nurse Relationship

The importance of communication skills is evident in Schubert's (1989) study of private community nursing clients. Interviews revealed diverse and shifting patterns of roles taken by the nurse and client over time. Clients reported a parent-child or a teacher-student relationship, a partnership, or they saw the nurse as serving as the catalyst for growth. Some nurses were particularly adept at shifting their roles as their clients were able to take more responsibility for their health and healing. These roles were experienced in alternating rhythms by both nurses

FIGURE 10-4 Client Privileges in Helping Relationships

Clients, as consumers of our health care services, have a right to:

- Expect a systematic and accurate investigation of their health concerns by thorough and well-organized nurses.
- Be informed about their health status and have all their questions answered so that they clearly understand what nurses mean.
- Receive health care from nurses who have current knowledge about their diagnoses and are capable of providing safe and efficient care.
- Feel confident they will be treated courteously and that the nurses have genuine interest in them.
- Trust that any issues of personal confidentiality will be respected.
- Be informed about any plans of action to be carried out for their benefit.
- Refuse or consent to nursing treatments without jeopardizing the relationship with their nurses.
- Secure help conveniently and without hassles or roadblocks.
- Receive consistent quality of care from all nurses.

From *Communication in Nursing* (4th ed.), by J. Balzer Riley, 2000, St. Louis: Mosby. Used with permission.

✳ DECISION MAKING

Mutual Problem-Solving Process

The school principal has referred 14-year-old Juan to the clinic where you work. The principal says the boy complains of stomachaches every day and refuses to participate in physical education activities. You interview Juan and learn that there are many problems. First of all, he has received major orthodontic treatment and has braces on his teeth. This work was financially supported by a migrant health program provided by the school nurses in the area. Juan says the orthodontist told him not to get hit with a ball. Juan had imagined that if he got hit anywhere on his body, his teeth would fall out. You reassure him and explain the dentist's instruction. You ask Juan about his family, and, as you ask questions and he hesitantly answers, you get an idea about the family. There are nine children, of which he is the third; his father is out of work; they have no money to buy food; and Juan is afraid his father is going to kill a neighbor.

As you talk about all of Juan's concerns, you ask, "What is your biggest worry?" He responds, "I do not know how to work my combination lock at school. I have to find someone to help me all the time, and I am always late for class. The teachers are mad at me."

- ◆ What would you do first?
- ◆ Develop a plan including support for Juan at school, a home visit, and potential community resources for the family.

---

and clients as clients took more or less responsibility in the different areas of their lives.

COMMUNICATION SKILLS

A nurse's abilities to comprehend the client's needs and to successfully exchange information are always crucial. In community health nursing, the process is complicated by the variety of situations wherein communication occurs. In every instance, active listening enhances the process. A discussion of this skill is followed by discussions of a number of applications including interviewing, group process, teaching, conflict management, translating in cross-cultural communication, and public speaking.

Active Listening

Active listening, also called reflective listening, focuses on feelings and thoughts, demonstrating the inherent value of the client's needs as compared with those of the health care world. The nurse first focuses attention on the client and then shifts the focus back to processing knowledge of the client's feelings in order to develop a plan of things to say or do that will be in the client's best interest.

In active listening, the nurse verbally reflects as closely as possible the content of the client's statement, any feel-

ings heard or observed, the nuances and strength of those feelings, and the reasons for those feelings. Four kinds of reflection are commonly used: paraphrasing, feelings reflection, meanings reflection, and summative reflection.

Parroting the same words back is irritating and implies lack of understanding. Paraphrasing, on the other hand, lets the client know how much has been understood and invites clarification if the nurse has missed an important part of the message. The following is an example of this skill:

Client: We get a little further behind financially every month. I'm thinking about taking a job helping to serve lunches at school, but it will take almost all the free time I have now. And I don't know what I'll do if one of the kids gets sick.

Nurse: You want to help out by earning some extra money, but you are not clear yet how getting a job will affect your responsibilities at home.

REFLECTIVE THINKING

Passive or Active Client Role?

- Put yourself in the role of a person seeking health care. Would you choose a passive role or a more active and responsible role as client? Why?
- As the nurse, how might you support your client in taking a more active and responsible role in the relationship?

Sometimes a client's difficulties are related more to his or her feelings about a situation than to the situation itself. Words or body language or both may alert the nurse to such a situation, especially if the two are incongruent. In such a case, **feelings reflection** can be used to help the client recognize and deal with feelings. The nurse might say, for example, "You seem tense as you talk about that," giving the client an opportunity to clarify.

In feelings reflection, the words chosen by the nurse must match the feelings expressed by the client verbally or otherwise Balzer-Riley (2000). For any given feeling, the nurse may have many corresponding words from which to choose. For instance, the corresponding empathic word for *feeling afraid* might be any of the following: *afraid, agonized, alarmed, anxious, apprehensive, cautious, concerned, disturbed, in dread, fearful, fidgety, frightened, hesitant, ill at ease, in a cold sweat, jittery, jumpy, nervous, on edge, panicky, petrified, quaking, quivering, restless, scared, shaken, tense, terrified, trembling, troubled, uncomfortable, uneasy, wary,* or *worried.*

In addition to the actual verbal message, the sender and receiver constantly exchange emotionally laden nonverbal communication signals through facial expression, tone of voice, choice of words and gestures, emphasis, omissions, and timing of the communication. These factors all play a part in the formation, preservation, and termination of a client-nurse relationship and determine whether the nature of the relationship promotes healing or is destructive to the client (Arnold & Boggs, 1999, p. 67).

Meanings reflection is a response that addresses meanings and facts together in one phrase. Suppose, for example, that a client describes satisfaction regarding a new job that a family member has just found in another town but at the same time is frowning and is hunched in the shoulders. Upon hearing the information being communicated and witnessing the incongruent body language, the nurse might respond, "You're proud of your child's success but a little fearful about being separated for the first time."

A **summative reflection** groups the topics discussed in a foregoing conversation into several categories so that the client and nurse can have a clear idea of those things that have been accomplished and those things that remain to be done. For example:

> We have talked about how you are caring for your colostomy and how your relationships have been affected since the surgery. You asked about relaxation exercises and whether they might help with your nervousness about what is happening; so, unless you have some other questions, we can do some work on that before I go.

The community nurse's use of active listening can facilitate some of the client privileges listed in Figure 10-4. Figure 10-5 lists some characteristics and tools of effective helpers that either enhance or are enhanced by active listening. Although this significant body of work was originated by Truax and Carkhuff (1967) for the

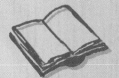

Out of the Box

Try Role Playing to Improve Your Communication Skills

Ask a classmate to role play some ways nurses communicate with clients. First, imagine a situation and the type of communication you consider helpful in that situation. Then imagine the same situation and a type of communication you consider not helpful. Then role play both ways of communicating and ask your partner for feedback. Also, try adding touch to each situation and receive feedback. Imagine the following:

- *A situation which requires the nurse to do most of the talking to the client.*
- *A situation which requires the nurse to be quiet most of the time and to listen.*
- *A situation which requires both the nurse and client to talk.*
- *A situation in which the nurse and client are together and both are silent.*

Were you surprised by any of your partner's responses? In what situations might you tend to talk too much and to listen too little? When was the touch most helpful? What kind of touch seemed most helpful? When was silence most helpful? ∎

FIGURE 10-5 Characteristics of Effective Helper

Warmth: Showing warmth to others means conveying that you like to be with them and accept them as they are. It is usually displayed nonverbally by subtle facial expressions, body language, and gestures. Culturally prescribed rules for displaying warmth are related to factors such as the need, occupation, status, role position, and gender of the people involved. Touch can be a way to transmit warmth. It may be a brief touch on the shoulder, an embracing hug, or an extended hand. Warmth through touch is communicated only when one is truly comfortable and sincere in the expression of caring and extended comfort. Since the acceptability of touch varies with the culture (see Chapter 8), knowledge of client cultural beliefs and values are necessary.

Respect: Respect means accepting others for who they are rather than on condition of certain behaviors or characteristics. Behaviors characteristic of respect are looking at the client, giving undivided attention, maintaining eye contact (in some cultures), moving toward the client, determining how the client likes to be addressed, making contact by handshaking or gentle touching, making it clear who you are and what your role is, and being clear about how you can help. In some situations, a deeper respect based on belief in the client's ability to learn and to change requires that the nurse challenge the client in different ways.

Genuineness: Genuineness is behavior congruent with thoughts and feelings. If we pretend our thoughts and feelings are different from what they are, we say things we do not believe. If we act on thoughts and feelings we do not have, we give the wrong impression about ourselves. We tend to lack genuineness when we feel at risk for rejection.

Specificity: Being specific involves giving concrete details so that communication is focused, clear, and logical. When the nurse helps the client to address concerns specifically, clarity and self-understanding are increased for both parties.

Empathy: Empathy is the act of communicating understanding of the client's feelings (see active listening discussion) and is nonjudgmental and accepting. The benefit to the client often is tremendous relief because the need to struggle to be heard or to justify reactions is eliminated.

Self-disclosure: Self-disclosure is one's willingness to be known to others. Thoughts, feelings, and experiences should be revealed only for the sake of the client. The nurse self-discloses to show understanding that derives from similar thoughts and experiences. Consider two questions before self-disclosing: Is the disclosure likely to demonstrate understanding? Will I feel safe from repercussions and embarrassment—that is, legally, morally, and emotionally secure—if I reveal this information to my client? Each question should get a clear affirmative answer before proceeding with self-disclosure.

Confrontation: Confrontation is pointing out incongruities or discrepancies between beliefs, attitudes, thoughts, and behaviors. It is an invitation for persons to examine their behavior honestly when that behavior invades the rights of the nurse or others or is destructive to the client or others. Confrontation encourages change by placing respectful emphasis on positive outcomes.

Spirituality: Spirituality of the nurse is reflected to others as being at peace with herself, being calm and quiet, being totally present for a client and connected. Those who are comfortable with silence and stillness while being totally present communicate acceptance in a way that is very therapeutic. It is not necessary, or even helpful, to be talking and doing all the time. Balzer-Riley (2000) states, "If you don't know what to say, just be quiet and stay there. Try saying, 'I don't have any words to help, but I will stay with you a while' " (p. 223). Communication is much more than the verbal and nonverbal behavior. The ability to stay present in the moment requires conscious effort. Such effort is sometimes difficult but makes moments of connection possible. These moments of connection demonstrate the movement from Buber's (1958) concept of I-It to I-Thou while moving from the routines of teaching and caring to a deep intimacy and knowing.

Humor: Humor can help to make connections between people and provide an attitude that brings relaxation and relief. When we can laugh at our own shortcomings, we are freed to learn and to be creative. But humor can be healing or destructive, and it is necessary to know the difference. Positive humor is associated with love, hope, joy, creativity, or a gentle sense of playfulness. Its intent is to bring people closer together. Negative humor isolates and alienates people by putting them on the defensive and making them feel put down (Balzer-Riley, 2000).

Adapted from *The Skilled Helper: Model, Skills, and Methods for Effective Helping* (2nd ed.), by G. Egan, 1982, Monterey, CA: Brooks/Cole Publishing; *Toward Effective Counseling and Psychotherapy: Training and Practice*, by C. Truax and R. Carkuff, 1967, Chicago: Aldine. Spirituality and humor have been added from *Communication in Nursing* (4th ed.), by J. Balzer-Riley, 2000, St. Louis: Mosby.

counseling profession, it provides a theoretical foundation for all the helping professions today. In fact, effective helping theory is currently being used to teach communication skills to nurses (Balzer-Riley, 2000). The characteristics and associated skills are applicable whether the nurse is teaching or counseling individuals, families, or groups; facilitating or participating in committee- or work-related meetings; engaging in public speaking; or presenting educational materials for mass media.

INTERVIEWING

Northouse and Northouse (1998) define the interview as purposeful, goal-directed, and focused interpersonal communication, usually involving questions and answers, with the goal of sharing information or facilitating therapeutic outcomes. Effective questioning saves time and elicits pertinent and useful information. Figure 10-6 lists guidelines for asking questions. Helping

FIGURE 10-6   Guidelines for Asking Questions

- The client is the best person to interview, when it is possible. When it is necessary to ask for information from family members, it is best to conduct the interview in the presence of the client or to get the client's permission.

- A suitable place must be found where there is privacy without interruptions.

- Clients are more likely to answer your questions more openly if they understand why you are asking the questions.

- Privacy is most important and the client needs to know how the information will be used and with whom it will be shared.

- Give the client enough time to answer one question before going on to another question or giving your own opinions, beliefs, and advice.

- Phrase your questions clearly and sequence them in a logical progression.

- Avoid "why" questions because they tend to be intimidating or threatening.

- Use language the client understands; avoid medical jargon.

- Keep the client informed by giving feedback on the data collection or problem-solving process (Balzer-Riley, 2000).

Adapted from *Communication in Nursing* (4th ed., pp. 178–191), by J. Balzer-Riley, 2000, St. Louis: Mosby. Used with permission.

interviews are of two types: information sharing and therapeutic.

INFORMATION-SHARING INTERVIEWS

Information-sharing interviews center on the request for and provision of information, with the focus being on content rather than on relationship or feelings. This type of interview is useful for admission and history taking, relies primarily on closed questions, and assumes a **directive approach,** meaning that the nurse defines the nature of the client's problem, prescribes appropriate solutions, and provides specific, concrete information needed for problem solving. **Closed questions** restrict the client to providing specific information; **open questions** (addressed in the discussion of therapeutic interviews, in the next section) do not restrict the client's responses. Closed questions, used in health care to gather demographic data, medical histories, or diagnostic information, often ask for a "yes" or "no" answer. For example:

"Have you ever had surgery?"
"Is there a history of heart problems in your family?"

The directive approach is efficient; interviews focus on the problem and take less time than other approaches. There are, however, disadvantages, to the directive approach. Assessment information known only to the client is missed. The nurse may then, in turn, give the client erroneous information or make decisions before getting necessary information about the client's situation. Ineffective or misdirected solutions may in turn result.

Therapeutic Interviews

Therapeutic interviews are designed to help clients identify and work through personal issues, concerns, and problems. Clients feel free to express their personal thoughts and feelings, gain new insights, develop new problem-solving strategies, and find better ways of coping with their experiences. Therapeutic interviews frequently involve open questions and either a directive or a nondirective approach. A **nondirective approach** encourages clients to seek solutions to their own problems and to express thoughts and feelings.

The nondirective approach is more flexible and client focused than the directive approach. Rather than having the client answer a lot of questions, the nurse encourages the client to tell his or her story with interruptions for clarification only. Information is elicited about clients' feelings regarding their health or illness situation by using open questions (discussed below). Consistent with the active role of clients, this approach provides more complete data on which to base a nursing diagnosis, allows for a more comfortable health care assessment encounter, and affords the client more control during the encounter. As a result, clients often disclose more, feel freer to ask questions, and more readily reveal their concerns and levels of knowledge.

Open questions do not restrict the client's responses; rather, they allow extended and unlimited answers. Open questions are a means of providing an opportunity for clients to freely disclose their situations and problems. For example:

> "You seem concerned. Tell me what is bothering you."
> "Describe what you think might happen to you."
> "How do you think we are doing in meeting our contract?"

The nondirective approach is based on the assumption that the client is the person best able to identify and resolve his or her problems (Gleit, 1998). Advantages of this approach are interrelated. Inherent in the nondirective approach is acknowledgment of the client's potential for identifying and solving problems; thus, one advantage is increased opportunity of identifying and therefore addressing the problem experienced by the client. Furthermore, the enhanced sense of control associated with being an active participant increases probability of client follow-through on making necessary changes.

Phases in the Interview Process

Interviews take place in clinics, homes, schools, meeting houses, hospitals, public places—every place that people go and live. The length of an interview depends on the goal of the interview, the severity of the client's problem, the skills of the clinician, and the number of problem areas that emerge. Less time is needed when the goal is information sharing rather than therapeutic change, when the client's personality is well integrated as opposed to severely disorganized, and when there is a single problem rather than several. In the following discussion, Northouse and Northouse's (1998) interview phases for health professionals are adapted for community health nurses.

Preparation Phase

The preparation phase involves anticipating and planning for the interview. In a community health setting, a nurse who receives a referral from another agency may have considerable information about the client before the initial meeting with the client. Likewise, the client often seeks information about a nurse before the initial meeting by consulting with friends, relatives, or other professionals. Nurse preparation may include researching recent treatment advances, preparing assessment forms and educational materials, or locating an appropriate place to meet. The nurse also arranges for a comfortable setting by, for example, ensuring that there are enough chairs to accommodate a family.

A second task of this phase is self-assessment (Stuart & Laraia, 1997). Self-assessment means that the nurse sorts through personal feelings and biases and, if necessary, seeks help in resolving personal anxieties related to problem areas. **Centering** oneself in the present moment and focusing attention on the well-being of the client are another part of preparation. They can be accomplished by sitting quietly and taking a breath or two while drawing one's attention inward and focusing on the task at hand.

Initiation Phase

The initiation phase begins with the first face-to-face client-nurse contact. After reconciling initial expectations of each other, the first task is to establish a therapeutic, nonthreatening climate that will foster trust and understanding. A brief period of commonplace talk gives participants time to adjust to the setting and to each other (e.g., "Did you have any trouble finding the clinic?" or "Your directions were excellent; I had no problem finding you").

The next task is to clarify the purpose of the interview. A community health nurse on a first home visit, for example, might say, "We talked on the phone about my coming to share ideas on home care for your baby when your baby comes home from the hospital next week" or "I know you have some concerns about caring for the colostomy. We can talk about those concerns today and tomorrow I can come back to teach you how to do colostomy care." At this point, the contract can be formulated and mutual goals established. Northouse and Northouse (1998) identify common initiation-phase errors: a vague explanation of the interview purpose by the nurse, a premature attempt to elicit personal information from the client, or a drifting on the part of either party into social conversation to avoid feelings of discomfort.

Exploration, or Working, Phase

The exploration phase is the time to confront, analyze, and work on the client's problems. The nurse tries to help clients master anxieties, increase their sense of independence and responsibility, and acquire new coping abilities (Stuart & Laraia, 1997). Clients often will first introduce a lesser problem and decide whether to trust the nurse with a more important problem on the basis of how the lesser problem was handled. A second task in this phase is to help clients manage feelings generated by the discussion of issues. In an atmosphere of acceptance and support, the nurse can help clients manage and express their feelings.

Common errors by nurses in this phase are loss of focus and changing the topic or giving insufficient feedback to help the client continue the discussion. Other errors include giving inappropriate advice, approval, or reassurances and responding in stereotyped ways such as the overuse of reflective statements.

Termination Phase

The termination phase is a time to acknowledge that the purpose for the interview has been met and that it is time to end a meaningful relationship. Termination is often difficult because, along with the feelings of joy associated with meeting goals, termination can evoke feelings of sadness, fear, or uncertainty. The major task, thus, is to plan for closure. This is a part of the contract and should therefore be a part of the discussion throughout the entire interview or set of interviews. Finally, the nurse helps the client express feelings about termination. Feelings are often mixed; although termination may be desired, it is common for the client to also feel sadness, anger, abandonment, guilt, and helplessness (Northouse & Northouse, 1998).

Community nurses who make home visits to families over a period of time often find it very difficult to simply say goodbye to their clients and sometimes instead say things like "I will stop to see you now and then" or "I will

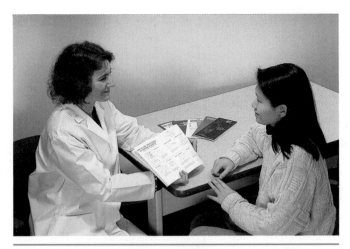

The exploration phase is the time to confront, analyze, and work on the client's problem.

call to see how you are." These ways of saying goodbye leave expectations that often go unfulfilled, causing unnecessary pain and disappointment. At the other extreme, nurses must guard against feeling uncertain and quickly terminating the interaction. They may allow too little time to deal with the feelings, bring up emotional issues that should have been dealt with earlier, or avoid termination issues, feeling that they have not been helpful to the client. It is useful to anticipate these feelings in order to effectively negotiate them.

COMMUNICATION BARRIERS

Communication barriers are responses that affect communication in a negative way. Gordon (1970) identifies three general categories of barriers: judgment, sending solutions, and avoidance of others' concerns. Most likely to be destructive when one or more involved persons are interacting under stress, barriers can diminish self-esteem and trigger defensiveness, resistance, and resentment. Barriers can also lead to withdrawal, dependency, and feelings of defeat or inadequacy, and they can decrease the likelihood that the client will find a solution to the problem. Further, each barrier can reduce the probability that all parties will constructively express their true feelings. Over time, these negative effects can cause permanent damage to relationships.

GROUP MEMBERSHIP AND LEADERSHIP

During the past decade, groups have been used for many discussion and therapy functions that once were performed on an individual basis (or not at all). A small group is a collection of individuals who influence one another, derive some satisfaction from maintaining membership in the group, interact for some purpose, assume specialized roles, are dependent on one another, and communicate face to face. A small group will meet some but not necessarily all of these criteria. The primary group, or the basic social unit to which one belongs, is the family; the social group, in which one socializes with others, may (for example) consist of classmates. Other examples are education groups, that is, those joined for the purpose of learning together, such as in a book club, and work groups, which have specific goals to be achieved. Work groups are often required within the context of one's job (Tubbs & Moss, 2000).

The number of self-help groups has increased dramatically in recent years, and many other types of groups are now being formed to teach clients how to maintain health and to overcome or cope with illness. There are fitness groups, relaxation groups, nutrition groups, health education groups, and support groups. Groups among health professionals are also more plentiful. Interdisciplinary groups, advisory groups, task forces, management groups, stress reduction groups, and care-for-the-caregiver groups are some of these professionally oriented problem-solving groups (Northouse & Northouse, 1998).

The community nurse is often called on to be a group member or leader in one or several such groups. It is imperative, therefore, that the nurse understand how groups work and how members communicate within groups. Communication is the process that connects members to one another and enables them to work interdependently.

Small-group communication refers to the verbal and nonverbal communication that occurs among three or more individuals who are interdependent to some degree. **Content-oriented groups** focus on tasks and goals. **Process-oriented groups** focus on relating to and getting along with people. **Midrange groups** focus on a blend of process and content or tasks (Loomis, 1979). Some major components of groups are goals, norms, cohesiveness, leader behavior, member behavior, and curative factors that influence group functioning. Because they are concerned with how the group works, the first three components are considered here under the general heading of group behaviors. The last three components are treated separately. The phases of group development are then reviewed. It should be noted that these discussions are necessarily brief and that the student is encouraged to seek more in-depth training in small-group leadership.

Group Behaviors

Its goals provide the reason for the existence of the group. Group goals and individual goals exist simultaneously in any group and must be compatible in order for the group to succeed. Norms are the rules of behavior established and shared by group members. Overt norms are those verbally agreed-on rules known to the members; covert norms are not usually verbally acknowledged by the group members. An example of a covert norm might be that when one person talks, the others listen. Cohesiveness is a sense of "we-ness," the cement that holds groups together. High cohesiveness is frequently associated with increased participation, consistent attendance, and high member satisfaction.

Leader Behaviors

Leadership is the process whereby one person attempts to influence others in order to attain some mutually agreed-on goal. In groups, leader behavior has a strong effect on member interactions. An effective leader selects communication methods that are likely to have a positive

---

FIGURE 10-7   Group Task Roles

- **Initiator-contributor:** Suggests new ideas or a new way of viewing the group task.

- **Information seeker:** Asks for clarification or for additional information about the problem being discussed.

- **Opinion seeker:** Asks for clarification of values that may be involved in the goal or task that the group is discussing.

- **Information giver:** Offers facts or personal experiences that are related to problems being discussed by the group.

- **Elaborator:** Expands on ideas being discussed by offering an example or the rationale for a suggestion.

- **Coordinator:** Pulls together various ideas and suggestions made by group members or tries to coordinate group activities.

- **Orientor:** Defines the present position of the group in relation to its goals or raises questions about the direction in which the discussion is moving.

- **Evaluator-critic:** Considers the practicality or logic of suggestions offered in the group.

- **Energizer:** Stimulates the group toward an action or a decision.

- **Procedural technician:** Assists group movement by carrying out routine tasks for the group.

- **Recorder:** Writes down suggestions or activities decided on by the group.

From "The Process of the Basic Encounter Group," by C. Rogers, 1972, in R. Diedrich and H. A. Dye (Eds.), *Group Procedures, Purposes, Processes and Outcomes,* Boston: Houghton Mifflin. Used recently by Marquis & Huston (2000), Arnold & Boggs (1999), Northouse & Northouse (1998). Used with permission.

---

impact on followers and will move the group toward its goals. Emergent leaders are verbally active and fluent and express their thoughts articulately in group interaction. They initiate new ideas in conferences, seek opinions from others, and express their own opinions with firmness but not rigidity (Northouse & Northouse, 1998; Marquis & Huston, 2000).

Member Behaviors

Member behavior is just as important as leader behavior. Some member behaviors are constructive to the group process, and some are destructive. Constructive member behaviors are listed and defined as group task roles (see Figure 10-7) or group-building and maintenance roles (see Figure 10-8). These roles promote cohesion among group members. The role names reflect constructive participation in the work of the group. Individual roles represent destructive member behaviors and are named for behaviors that reflect the participant's psychological needs rather than the needs of the group. These behaviors are listed in Figure 10-9. (Arnold & Boggs, 1999; Marquis & Houston, 2000; Northouse & Northouse, 1998; Rogers, 1972).

Curative Factors

Curative factors exert a therapeutic influence on the group members. Yalom (1983) identifies these positive factors as (1) instillation of hope as members realize others

---

FIGURE 10-8   Group-Building and Maintenance Roles

- **Encourager:** Accepts and praises all contributions, viewpoints, and ideas with warmth and solidarity.

- **Harmonizer:** Mediates, harmonizes, and resolves conflict.

- **Compromiser:** Yields his or her position in a conflict position.

- **Gatekeeper:** Promotes open communication and facilitates participation by all members.

- **Standard setter:** Expresses or evaluates standards to evaluate group process.

- **Group commentator:** Records group process and provides feedback to the group.

- **Follower:** Accepts the group's ideas and listens to discussion and decisions.

From "The Process of the Basic Encounter Group," by C. Rogers, 1972, in R. Diedrich and H. A. Dye (Eds.), *Group Procedures, Purposes, Processes and Outcomes,* Boston: Houghton Mifflin. Used recently by Marquis & Huston (2000), Arnold & Boggs (1999), Northouse & Northouse (1998). Used with permission.

FIGURE 10-9 Individual Roles of Group Members

- **Aggressor:** Attacks or disapproves of others' suggestions, feelings, or values.

- **Blocker:** Resists, without good reason, or becomes extremely negative to others' suggestions.

- **Recognition seeker:** Calls attention repeatedly to own accomplishments and diverts the group's attention.

- **Self-confessor:** Uses the group's time to express personal, non-group-oriented feelings or comments.

- **Playboy/playgirl:** Plays around and displays other behavior that indicates that he or she is not involved in the group process.

- **Dominator:** Tries repeatedly to assert own authority and often interrupts other group members.

- **Help seeker:** Tries to elicit sympathy from other group members.

- **Special interest pleader:** Speaks for a particular group or person (e.g., the union, the unemployed, the American people) but is really using the group to meet personal needs and to cloak personal biases and prejudices.

From "The Process of the Basic Encounter Group," by C. Rogers, 1972, in R. Diedrich and H. A. Dye (Eds.), *Group Procedures, Purposes, Processes and Outcomes,* Boston: Houghton Mifflin. Used recently by Marquis & Huston (2000), Arnold & Boggs (1999), Northouse & Northouse (1998). Used with permission.

have succeeded or overcome similar issues; (2) universality, with the realization that one is not alone; (3) information sharing with each other; (4) altruism as members help each other; (5) corrective recapitulation of the primary family group as parallel relationships occur in the group and in the member's family; (6) development of socializing techniques or development of needed social skills; (7) imitative behavior as the leader and other members model desirable behavior; (8) interpersonal learning as members provide one another with feedback regarding interpersonal behavior; (9) catharsis as members learn to express feelings appropriately coupled with interpersonal learning; and (10) existential factors as members realize that life is sometimes not fair and we must take responsibility for the way we live our lives.

Phases of Group Development

One popular version of group development phases was presented by Tuckman (1965): forming, norming, storming, and performing. This model is still in use today (Arnold & Boggs, 1999). Yalom (1975) conceives of these phases as orientation, conflict, cohesion, and working and adds termination. Short-term and ad hoc groups may move through these phases in a single session, whereas long-term groups may spend weeks in a single phase.

Orientation

In the orientation period, the task is to assess the members' purposes for joining the group and to figure out where they fit in the group. Communication during this phase is often stereotypic and restricted. Leadership during this phase is directed toward helping members satisfy their needs for belonging. This involves helping them to feel a part of the group but also to feel a sense of privacy and independence. In addition, the leader provides structure, establishes group guidelines, shapes norms, and assists members in understanding their roles in the overall functioning of the group.

Conflict

The conflict phase occurs as members become interested in control issues such as how they are influencing the group. Each wants to be perceived by others as a competent group member with something to offer. Conflicts arise in this struggle for control, and the work of the leader is to help the members accept and work through group conflicts. As members satisfy their needs for control, conflicts lessen, and the group moves on.

Cohesion

The cohesion phase occurs as members realize that time is moving on and work needs to be done; they become more understanding and accepting of one another, and there surfaces a desire to move closer to one another but not too close. The leader has only to provide guidance and direction as needed and, thus, plays a lesser role during this time.

Working

The working phase is similar to the cohesion phase but is longer. The members actually perform the work they set out to do. Group spirit and a feeling of unity among members are often high during this time. The work of the leader is similar to that in the cohesion phase.

Termination

The termination phase occurs when the work has been completed or the allotted time is running out. The end of the group is a loss, and this phase is a time for sharing the whole range of emotions, from guilt to fear, depending on each person's experience with termination. The leader must summarize the work of the group, emphasize goals that have been achieved, and help group members find a sense of closure as they confront their feelings about the approaching end of the group meetings and member relationships.

TEACHING/LEARNING

The **teaching/learning process** involves all the communication skills described previously and is a part of almost every nursing intervention, whether with individuals or groups. As hospital stays become shorter and nurses increasingly care for clients in ambulatory and home settings, the importance of the nurse's role in assisting clients to understand their health care needs and to care for themselves takes on additional importance.

The mandate from *Healthy People 2010* emphasizes aggregate client education (U.S. Department of Health and Human Services, 2000). Health education is a key component of health promotion programs and is emphasized as the major strategy for achieving the global target of health for all by the year 2010. (Velsor-Friedrick, 2000). Health education depends upon teaching and learning processes to promote health and healing.

Models for health promotion and disease prevention, discussed in Chapter 11, provide an overall perspective for community health nursing practice. Teaching/learning theories are conceptually linked to health promotion models and play a pivotal role in all nursing practice since health teaching is a major nursing role function in all practice settings (discussed in Chapters 19 and 20).

Adult Learning Theory

Learning involves a "persistent change in behavior as a result of experience" (Gleit, 1998, p. 66). Thus, behavior change is the foundation for learning theory. Learning theories are of three types: cognitive, behavioral, and humanistic. All three maintain that we learn by experiencing interaction with our environment and that learning creates change. In health teaching, health beliefs, attitudes, and behaviors are the targets of this change. Be-

haviorists believe learning has occurred when there is a change of behavior; cognitive theorists believe learning is an internal process in which information is integrated or internalized into one's cognitive (intellectual) structure; and humanists stress integration of attitudes, feelings, and interests as well as cognition and taking responsibility for behavioral changes.

Knowles, Holton, and Swanson (1998) share a perspective that each theoretical viewpoint has its place in teaching/learning. The level of complexity of the learning task and client learning ability interact to determine the appropriate approach, the behaviorist approach being the least complex and the humanistic being the most highly complex since it requires integration of the self (Gleit, 1998).

Conceptual models for nursing practice depend largely on humanistic perspectives for health education. The person is seen from a holistic view with interrelated qualities, characteristics and experiences that make up the individual human being. Self-concept is emphasized and teaching/learning processes include feelings about, attitudes toward, and evaluation of oneself, one's ideas, and how one fits into one's world. These perceptions are considered very significant in the learning process.

A humanistic, nondirective approach focuses on the teacher as a facilitator of learning rather than a provider of information. Communication skills, i.e., active listening, addressed earlier in this chapter are helpful skills in this type of teaching. The primary goal involves client reorganization of the inner self for greater personal integration, effectiveness, and realistic self-appraisal. The learning environment plays an important role and requires warmth, openness, acceptance, and trust. Clients take responsibility for their own learning. They examine their values. They are not required to change their outward behavior but rather are required to understand and clarify their values so that they can direct their own learning. These ideas are based on the work of Carl Rogers discussed earlier.

Teaching models in nursing focus on self-care and self-efficacy. **Self-care** is the care performed by oneself for oneself, upon reaching a state of maturity or wellness in which one can take consistent control in health situations. **Self-efficacy** is the belief that a person responds best to difficult situations if they feel capable and confident in performing available and appropriate skills.

Nursing theoretical models have provided these perspectives, yet traditional teaching/learning methods (**pedagogy**) tend to emphasize passive learning (often through short-term lecture methods), even though current knowledge indicates that **andragogy** is a more appropriate approach to health education. Andragogy, which addresses the learner's need to be a part of the process rather than a passive recipient, fits well with humanistic approaches and teaching self-care. Table 10-2 clarifies the differences between the two approaches (Knowles et al., 1998). Gleit (1998) provides support for

TABLE 10-2   Comparison of Pedagogy and Andragogy

PEDAGOGY	ANDRAGOGY
1. Learners must learn what the teacher teaches—not how it applies to learners' lives.	1. Learners need to know why they need to learn.
2. Learner's concept of self reflects teacher's concept of learner—that of a dependent personality.	2. Learners have self-concept of being responsible for own decisions and lives.
3. Learner's experience of little worth. What counts are the individual experience of the teacher and the media used for teaching.	3. Quality of experience: individual differences, life experiences, biases, self-identity derived from experiences.
4. In order to pass, learners become ready to learn what the teacher tells them to learn.	4. Ready to learn what they need to know to cope with life situations.
5. Subject-centered orientation: learning is acquiring subject-matter content.	5. Life-centered (or task-centered or problem-centered) orientation to learning.
6. Learners motivated to learn by external motivators.	6. Most potent motivator is internal pressure to learn.

Adapted from The Adult Learner: The Definitive Classic in Adult Education and Human Resource Development *(5th ed., pp. 61–70), by M. Knowles, E. Holton, and R. A. Swanson, 1998, Houston: Gulf.*

the belief that the **client-centered** approach is self-empowering for the learner.

The role of the teacher in this model is outlined in Table 10-3 by Knowles (1990; Knowles et al., 1998) and is built upon the principles of warmth, indirectness, cognitive organization, and enthusiasm. **Warmth,** as defined in Figure 10-5, conveys to someone that he or she is liked and accepted. Indirectness is the way of guiding the learner to find his or her own way rather than supplying pat answers to problems. Knowles notes, though, that the andragogical model does allow for the provision of directed information when necessary. For instance, it is appropriate to give a mother instructions about how to change her daughter's dressing as long as time is provided for her to practice the skill and ask questions about the procedure.

Cognitive organization refers to an intellectual grasp of the material required of any effective teacher, and enthusiasm refers to interest and excitement about the subject being taught (Knowles et al., 1998). These teaching behaviors are congruent with the nursing profession's concept of caring.

Approaches to Client Education

Three dimensions of client education must be considered. They are client education models, types of teaching, and modalities for teaching.

Models

Client education models provide frameworks that help the nurse understand client motivation for participating in health care practices that promote healthier lifestyles. Two such commonly used models are the health belief model and Pender's health promotion model (see Chap-

ter 9). They represent compliance models focusing on the variables that motivate clients to follow or not to follow recommended behaviors that facilitate health. These models tend to emphasize professional, rather than personal, health expectations.

On the other hand, the self-regulation model suggests that personal meanings and responses to illness may be the critical factors in client decision making related to health (Rankin & Stallings, 2001). It does not, however, address how emotions and social activities are affected or how "valued social activities (e.g., meals with family members) affect emotional adjustment to illness, health definitions, and health practices" (p. 37). The self-regulation model involves consideration of numerous factors in the life of the client and requires critical thinking skills by the nurse. Critical thinking skills utilize logical/analytical and intuitive/creative approaches to solving problems.

Critical thinking involves looking at a situation from multiple perspectives. The purpose is to help clients make use of the knowledge they already have and be able to reason through difficult problems.

Empowerment education, another approach that reflects **self-efficacy** (the power to produce effects and intended results on one's own health and in one's own life), is particularly applicable to community health education (Rankin & Stallings, 2001). **Empowerment education** is based on Freire's (1983) ideas. Wallerstein and Bernstein (1988) describe this process as "the collective knowledge that emerges from a group sharing experiences and understanding the social influences that affect individual lives" (p. 382). The purpose of empowerment education is human liberation so that learners are a part of their own destinies. Freire's ideas are similar to health education's guiding principles; that is, start with the

TABLE 10-3 The Role of the Teacher

CONDITIONS OF LEARNING	PRINCIPLES OF TEACHING
The learners feel a need to learn.	1. The teacher exposes students to new possibilities of self-fulfillment. 2. The teacher helps each student clarify his own aspirations for improved behavior. 3. The teacher helps each student diagnose the gap between his aspiration and his present level of performance. 4. The teacher helps the students identify the life problems they experience because of the gaps in their personal equipment.
The learning environment is characterized by physical comfort, mutual trust and respect, mutual helpfulness, freedom of expression, and acceptance of differences.	5. The teacher provides physical conditions that are comfortable (as to seating, smoking, temperature, ventilation, lighting, decoration) and conducive to interaction (preferably, no person sitting behind another person). 6. The teacher accepts each student as a person of worth and respects her feelings and ideas. 7. The teacher seeks to build relationships of mutual trust and helpfulness among the students by encouraging cooperative activities and refraining from inducing competitiveness and judgmentalness. 8. The teacher exposes her own feelings and contributes her resources as a colearner in the spirit of mutual inquiry.
The learners perceive the goals of a learning experience to be their goals.	9. The teacher involves the students in a mutual process of formulating learning objectives in which the needs of the students, the institution, the teacher, the subject matter, and the society are taken into account.
The learners accept a share of the responsibility for planning and operating a learning experience and therefore have a feeling of commitment toward it. The learners participate actively in the learning process.	10. The teacher shares his thinking about options available in the designing of learning experiences and the selection of materials and methods and involves the students in deciding among these options jointly. 11. The teacher helps the students to organize themselves (project groups, learning-teaching teams, independent study, etc.) to share responsibility in the process of mutual inquiry.
The learning process is related to and makes use of the experience of the learners.	12. The teacher helps the students exploit their own experiences as resources for learning through the use of such techniques as discussion, role playing case method, etc. 13. The teacher gears the presentation of her own resources to the levels of experience of her particular students. 14. The teacher helps the students to apply new learning to their experience and thus to make the learning more meaningful and integrated.
The learners have a sense of progress toward their goals.	15. The teacher involves the students in developing mutually acceptable criteria and methods for measuring progress toward the learning objectives. 16. The teacher helps the students develop and apply procedures for self-evaluation according to these criteria.

Adapted from The Adult Learner: The Definitive Classic in Adult Education and Human Resource Development *(5th ed., pp. 93–94), by M. Knowles, E. Holton, and R. A. Swanson, 1998, Houston: Gulf.*

community's concerns, use active learning methods, and engage clients in determining their own needs and priorities. It is up to the group to raise its themes for mutual reflection and for the health educator to contribute information afterward.

Three stages to establishing an empowering education program are as follows:

1. Listen so as to understand the felt issues or themes of the community. Community members and health providers are equal partners in identifying problems and determining priorities. Community members are active in all program stages.

2. Institute a problem-posing dialogue about issues. This process is called *problem posing* rather than

problem solving because the problems explored through this process are complex, do not have immediate solutions, and, in any case, are slow to change. Problem posing reflects the recognition of the complexity of the problems and of the time needed for solutions. Problem posing can be therapeutic as people explore visions and work on their problems (Wallerstein & Bernstein, 1988). The group describes those things that they see and feel, defines the many levels of the problem, shares similar experiences from the individual members' lives, questions why the problem exists, and develops action plans to address the problem.

3. Take action toward positive changes that people envision during their dialogue. Solutions emerge from an exploration of the problems in the real world. This action provides new information that leads to further reflection on the problem at a deeper level, enabling people to learn from each other in their efforts to change and to surmount cultural, social, or historic barriers (Wallerstein & Bernstein, 1988, p. 383).

All of these models contribute information about client variables and dynamics that is important to health education. Nurses must consider which models are most appropriate to their particular teaching needs. The critical challenge is to remember that the client is the center of the health care team. It is the responsibility of the health professional both to work with people in the community to facilitate their abilities to identify their problems and solutions and to create the conditions under which professionals and communities can collaboratively engage in empowering practice (Wallerstein, Sanchez-Merki, & Don, 1996).

Types of Teaching

Teaching may be formal or informal. **Informal teaching** occurs during interactions with individual clients and families in spontaneous, one-to-one teaching sessions or family conferences (Arnold & Boggs, 1999). **Formal teaching** usually occurs in a group setting or at a prearranged individual or family appointment. For instance, during a family visit, a nurse might schedule another visit specifically to discuss parenting skills with a mother and father. Another example would be a weekly seniors group in a day care center wherein various health topics are discussed.

Modalities

Boyd (1998) encourages a variety of modalities for teaching: workshops, lectures, support groups, computer-assisted instruction, self-help groups, and interactive videotapes. In general, learning is enhanced when more than one modality is used, for instance, by including media as part of a workshop or lecture. In addition to using these formats, nurses also create educational videotapes, infor-

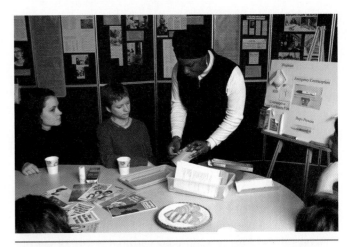

In this formal setting, the nurse teaches prenatal nutrition to these soon-to-be mothers.

mation pamphlets, or other written or spoken material to be distributed to the public. Nurses also participate at local, state, national, and international levels in the development of broad-based education programs that use all of these modalities.

Health-Oriented Telecommunications

Telecommunications use wire, radio, optical, or other electromagnetic channels to transmit or receive signals for voice, data, and video communications. Computers and telecommunications networks are used to compose, store, deliver, and process communication. These systems support the ability to exchange, edit, store, broadcast and copy written material, to send information and documents instantly, and to consult electronically. Applications include e-mail, computer conferencing, and long-distance blackboards and bulletin board systems. **Telehealth**, the use of telecommunications, has become a major part of the health care delivery infrastructure (Skiba & Barton, 2000). Telehealth services provide health care services and access to medical information for both health care professionals and consumers; increase awareness of health-related issues; educate the public regarding health; and facilitate care related to medical issues (Anderson, Anderson, & Glanze, 1998). **Telenursing** is a form of telehealth in which nursing practice is delivered via telecommunications, and interactive transmissions of voice, data, and video [American Nurses' Association (ANA), 1997].

Voice communication developments over the past decade now provide for telephone conferencing, voice mail, fax machines, computer communication, and picture phones. The use of telephones in nursing is expanding rapidly, especially in primary care settings and in discharge planning. Kinsella (1998) categorizes telephone care as "keeping in touch" calls, nurse-initiated calls, client-initiated calls, computer-generated single-purpose calls, and computer-generated interactive calls. Telephone intervention during the 21st century is expected to include social and emotional support, anticipatory guidance, education, advocacy, and consultation.

Data communication is being shared as consumers, businesses, and professionals connect with each other through the use of a computers, telecommunications software, and modems. Health information is now widely available on the Internet and the World Wide Web. According to a 1999 Louis Harris & Associates poll, 74% of the estimated 97 million U.S. adults now on-line have used the Internet to search for health and medical information. Numerous Internet support groups have been formed by and for clients who share a particular diagnosis. Klemm, Pepper, and Visich (1998) did a content analysis of messages exchanged within a group of clients with colorectal cancer. The messages were categorized as information giving/seeking, personal opinions, encouragement/support, personal experience, thanks, humor, prayer, and a miscellaneous area.

Interactive health communication (IHC) involves the interaction of a consumer, client, caregiver, or professional through communication technology to relay information, enable informed decision making, promote healthful behaviors, promote peer information exchange and emotional support, promote self-care, and manage demand for health care services (Robinson, Patrick, Eng, & Gustafson, 1998). The number of applications available to consumers and professionals is accelerating; consumers are expected to have access to all information used by health care providers.

Video communications is most commonly one-way transmission, i.e., television, but may also include interactive video and conferencing systems. Videophones, personal computers, and television sets are commonly used in home care to make "video visits." These video visits may also include blood pressure cuffs, glucometers, and transtelephonic electrocardiograph monitors (Kinsella, 1998). The possibilities and potentialities for health teaching/learning seem to be limitless at this time.

Teaching/Learning Environment

Elements of physical learning environments that affect the teaching/learning experience include space; temperature; visual, auditory, and olfactory stimuli; equipment; resources; furniture arrangement; physical comfort; and time. If the space in which the teaching is to take place is too small, clients may find the closeness uncomfortable, or, if instruction is to occur in a public place, such as a waiting room, privacy may be lacking and noise intrusive. In the latter case, it would be important to find a room that has fewer distractions and would therefore facilitate confidential discussion. An environment that is too hot or too cold would constitute a distraction in the form of the related physical discomfort. Likewise, the visual, auditory,

and olfactory distractions could impede learning in a home where the television is on and dinner is cooking.

In groups or at home, if a VCR is available, the nurse may use a videotape that illustrates a procedure. Written material can explain or reinforce aspects of the teaching. Audio- and videotapes may be left with clients to reinforce learning but should not take the place of client-nurse interaction. Such materials are supplemental and must be discussed with the individual, family, or group so that clients understand and can use the information.

When teaching a group of people, arranging chairs in a circle rather than in rows will facilitate interaction among group members. If a meeting with a family takes place in the home, part of the assessment is to notice where family members arrange themselves in relation to one another. For instance, do they line themselves up to face the nurse (thereby facilitating interaction with the nurse rather than among each other), sit facing one another (thereby facilitating family interaction), or keep a distance between one or more family members (thereby suggesting barriers to family interaction)?

In today's health care system, time is often limited. Teaching should be planned so that there is not too much content relative to the time available. More than one session may be necessary to convey the necessary information. Written, audio, or visual material may reinforce a verbal presentation and discussion of the subject, particularly if the information can be studied by the learners at their leisure.

The nurse can solicit the help of the client in creating a suitable learning environment, for instance, by asking a group to put their chairs in a circle or asking a family member to turn off the television. Explaining the reasons for such a request itself constitutes an element of teaching. Creativity and flexibility are needed to provide an optimal environment.

✳ DECISION MAKING

Teaching/Learning Environments

You are visiting a family for the second time. Your plan is to discuss parenting skills with the mother and father as they had requested during your first meeting. When you enter, the two children are watching television in the room where you will be meeting, and the father is not home. The mother says she will tell him about what is discussed.

◆ Can you continue with your teaching plan?

◆ How do you deal with the children and the television?

◆ How do you address the issue of the absent father?

LEARNING PROCESS

Regardless of where the teaching/learning takes place, the learning process is the same. That pattern is discussed next.

Phases of Learning Process

The **learning process** parallels the nursing process in that both are based on the problem-solving model. Learning involves cognitive, affective, and psychomotor components. In some cases, assessment and diagnosis are treated as one step. Here, assessment, diagnosis, planning, implementation, and evaluation are each presented as they pertain specifically to the learning process.

Assessment

The assessment determines the health-related needs of the client by way of identifying health problems, those things that the client knows about or wants to know about these problems, and the client's readiness to learn (Whitman, 1998). Additional factors to assess are the most acute needs to be met, unmet learning needs (the gaps between the information an individual knows and the information the individual needs to know in order to perform a function or to care for himself), and life-threatening problems (Rankin & Stallings, 2001). It is always important to consider the degree to which an individual's, family's, or group's cultural practices may influence client teaching. Some considerations are (1) immigration issues, including recency of immigration, whether it was forced, how different the client's culture is from that of the United States, and whether the client came from an urban or a rural area; (2) cultural norms and behaviors, such as whether religious, social, and recreational activities are within the cultural group, whether the client maintains traditional dietary habits and dress and speaks the native language exclusively or only in the home, and whether the client stays within the neighborhood; (3) support systems—specifically, whether the client's friends are from the same ethnic group and whether the client lives in an ethnoculturally diverse or homogeneous neighborhood; (4) use of folk medicine or traditional healers; and (5) existence of discrimination against the client's ethnocultural group that may make acculturation more difficult (Rankin & Stallings, 2001). Such information will help the nurse identify learning needs and determine teaching methods.

The client's education and reading levels must also be assessed. Literacy levels are usually three to four grades below the grade completed in school (French & Larrabee, 1999). If material is hard to read or is not understandable to the client, no learning can take place. One assessment tool that has been developed and is being used in a preventive medicine clinic at Louisiana State University Medical Center in Shreveport is called Rapid

Estimate of Adult Literacy in Medicine (REALM). In this test, clients are asked to read a series of 66 common medical words that become progressively more difficult. Testing of the tool has shown that the scores can be interpreted as estimates of literacy; as such, the scores can be used to identify clients who are nonreaders and those who have trouble reading medical words. Although this test focuses on reading recognition rather than on reading comprehension, it alerts health care providers to clients who have limited reading skills due to a wide variety of factors and will probably have difficulty comprehending most client education materials. Unfortunately, the test has been proved useful only for

Perspectives...

INSIGHTS OF A PUBLIC HEALTH NURSE

I am a public health nurse and receive referrals for 13- to 14-year-old (and sometimes younger) pregnant girls and substance-abusing women in their twenties. I make home visits, connect individuals and families with care providers and community resources, and serve as an advocate when needed. I take weights and measures, teach child development and infant and child care, promote bonding, and give emotional support.

The child mothers are in a developmental crisis and need extra support. Actually, they are in this situation because they need attention and affection. The mothers turn to their babies to get their needs met. They give their babies adult characteristics. For instance, the mother tends to interpret the baby's crying as rejection of herself, as illustrated by remarks such as "She doesn't like me" or "He doesn't want me." When the baby cries to eat every little bit, the mother often says, "She is greedy," or when the baby watches her with normal curiosity the mother may say, "She is so nosy."

I enjoy my work even though I often feel frustrated and overwhelmed. In the beginning, I did a lot more for clients. Now I do more teaching. The mothers are actually strengthened and empowered when they learn to do things themselves. When they learn to care for their babies, they do not abuse or neglect their babies; when they learn about normal developmental milestones, they do not abuse their children later on; and when they get appropriate emotional support, they do not reject their babies.

—Paula, PHN

English-speaking clients. For clients who do not speak English, the nurse must perform reading comprehension tasks, such as observing whether clients have difficulty reading and understanding medical instructions (Fisher, 1999).

As in all communication, active listening and observation of nonverbal language are critical. Watching and listening to family and friends as well as to the client are vital. Individuals or groups with whom the client routinely interacts can be supportive or may create barriers to learning and applying new behaviors. Family feedback is also important in evaluating teaching effectiveness.

Arnold and Boggs (1999) provide a framework for the kinds of information the nurse must obtain to complete an assessment (see Figure 10-10). They note that it is best to begin with the least threatening questions and to move to more sensitive topics only after rapport (a close, harmonious relationship between or among human beings) is established. Sample questions might be:

"What has this illness been like for you?"
"Have you had any previous experiences or heard any information about other people with similar health problems?"
"Can you tell me what your doctor has told you about your treatment?" (p. 376)

A summary of significant points identified during the assessment serves two purposes: it helps clients identify critical factors relevant to their learning, and it illuminates misinformation the nurse may have about any of the collected data (Arnold & Boggs, 1999).

FIGURE 10-10 Learning Needs Assessment

- What does the client already know about his or her condition and treatment?
- In what ways is the client affected by it?
- In what ways are those intimately involved with the client affected by the client's condition or treatment?
- To what extent is the client willing to take personal responsibility for seeking solutions?
- What goals would the client like to achieve?
- What will the client need to do to achieve those goals?
- What resources are available to the client and family that might affect the learning process?
- What barriers to learning exist?

Adapted from *Interpersonal Relationships* (3rd ed., p. 377), by E. Arnold and K. Boggs, 1999, Philadelphia: W. B. Saunders. Reprinted with permission by W. B. Saunders and Company.

Nursing Diagnosis

The most common NANDA nursing diagnoses in relation to learning needs are likely to have to do with a knowledge deficit or with ineffective coping. It is not enough to simply identify the deficit or the coping problem; it is most meaningful to know (*not* to assume) the reasons behind the problem. A knowledge deficit may be due to a variety of factors, i.e., lack of experience or interest, cultural values, misinformation, or organic deficits. Actually, all nursing diagnoses should have related client/family teaching as one aspect of the nursing intervention (Carpenito, 1997, pp. 216–217).

Planning

With the assessment performed and learning diagnosis determined, teaching tools and objectives can be established, priorities identified, and content and teaching methods selected. It is important to organize the content in manageable amounts appropriate to the time available. All such activities are subject to the basic rules of teaching: for instance, developing measurable objectives, structuring the environment to foster learning, considering the client's readiness and motivation to learn, identifying the client's learning style (see Table 10-4), and selecting strategies that meet the needs of the client. The reader is referred to any basic client education text for more detail regarding these components of teaching.

Teaching strategies that help strengthen teaching and that encourage client involvement include set induction, stimulus variation, reinforcement, use of examples and models, questioning, and closing. Definitions, specific

✳ DECISION MAKING

Planning and Implementing a Teaching Strategy

You are visiting a 65-year-old woman in her home. She is hypertensive and lives with her husband, who is diabetic. As you are talking with her in her kitchen, you notice the groceries on her shelves. They include several cans of soup, chocolate, cereal, fruit, and hot dog rolls.

- What nursing diagnoses might you consider regarding the family's educational needs about nutrition?
- How would you initiate a discussion with her about your concerns?
- Would you include her husband in your discussion? Why or why not?

TABLE 10-4 Characteristics of Different Learning Styles

VISUAL	AUDITORY	KINESIC
Learns best by seeing.	Learns best with verbal instruction.	Learns best by doing.
Likes to watch demonstration.	Likes to walk through things.	Likes hands-on involvement.
Organizes thoughts by writing them down.	Likes to have ideas explained or to explain.	Needs action and likes to touch, feel.
Needs detail.	Detail not as important.	Loses interest with detailed instruction.
Looks around and examines situations.	Talks about situations—pros, cons.	Tries things.

Adapted from Interpersonal Relationships *(3rd ed., p. 382), by E. Arnold and K. Boggs, 1999, Philadelphia: W. B. Saunders. Reprinted with permission of W. B. Saunders.*

purposes, and examples of these strategies are listed in Table 10-5. By planning ahead for the use of these strategies, the nurse prepares for a focused and meaningful learning experience.

Behavioral learning objectives are set by the nurse educator to ensure that learning interventions are tailored to client's unique situation and needs. These objectives describe the behaviors or actions the client will perform to meet the educational goal. **Cognitive learning objectives** refer to knowledge gained; **affective learning objectives** refer to attitudes; and **psychomotor learning objectives** refer to skills. Behavioral objectives have three components: performance, conditions, and criteria. Performance indicates any activity in which the client will engage. An action verb is used and must be measureable in some way so that competency can be shown. In other words, what does the client have to do to show that learning has been achieved? Conditions are spelled out to indicate any special circumstances to be included in the client's performance, i.e., use of special equipment. Criteria are those factors that show both the nurse and the client that learning has been accomplished, i.e., how will the client know when the task is done well enough? (Rankin & Stallings, 2001).

Learning activities are selected by the nurse educator according to which ones work best in each situation. Rankin and Stallings (2001) recommend the following:

- Match learning activities with learning objectives.
- Keep clients and family involved in the discussion; activities should include role-play, games, and a variety of media.
- Test the client's new abilities to nurture a sense of achievement and accomplishment.
- Make learning fun by using humor and support to increase client comfort and decrease anxiety.
- Allow ample time to practice skills and do not wait until the end of the session for practice time.

- Do not depend on lecture alone to teach skills and attitudes. The combination of a variety of teaching activities works the best for most clients. (p. 281)

Teaching people with low literacy skills requires special approaches and planning. Written, audio- or videotaped, or other materials and verbal strategies must be simple and clear and must be presented in an orderly, logical sequence that allows time for the client to process the information. The message should be short, direct, and specific because clients with low literacy skills tend to have short attention spans (Rankin & Stallings, 2001).

Health education material should be simple and consistent and use appropriate terminology and illustrations. It should be relevant to the specific needs of the population. Fisher (1999), Doak, Doak, and Root (1996), and Miller and Bodie (1994) recommend writing health education material at the fifth- to eighth-grade levels. Doak et al. (1996) indicate that clients with higher reading levels also prefer health-related material written at lower levels because it is shorter, takes less time, and is easier to comprehend. For easier reading, the print size should be large and the text sharply contrasted with the background. Written materials should be pretested on a sample of the intended population before making them available for general distribution (Fisher, 1999).

Audiotape instruction is useful for clients who are visually impaired or who learn better by listening than by reading (Boyd et al, 1998). It is also useful for standardized or introductory material and in cases of a foreign-language or dialect problem (if the tape can be made in the language or dialect in question). Audiotapes can also be used in conjunction with written material or pictures.

Implementation

Nurses must have knowledge about and confidence in the content they are teaching. However, mastery of content is useful only in concert with good communication

TABLE 10-5 Selected Teaching Strategies

STRATEGY	PURPOSE	EXAMPLE
1. *Set Induction:* Sets the tone for the session.	• Prepares for what will be learned • Provides framework for organization of teaching • Creates curiosity and readiness to learn	• Begin teaching by reading a poem pertinent to the subject to be presented. Use the ideas from the poem to show connections to the ideas to be taught.
2. *Stimulus Variation:* Different types of learning activities and approaches to teaching are used.	• Keeps students interested in the subject • Increases attention span	When teaching a family the components of a diabetic diet: • Show models of portion size of selected foods. • Provide written information about the subject. • Show a short videotape that demonstrates how to measure food amounts.
3. *Reinforcement:* Instructor or student, or both, repeat information verbally or through actions.	• Strengthens learning	When demonstrating how to bathe a baby at home: • Ask the mother to return the demonstration. • Also, provide written material or a videotape that shows the steps of bathing.
4. *Examples and Models:* Provides an illustration to explain content verbally and visually.	• Foster a common language between teacher and learner	• *Example:* When explaining the mechanism of the heart, compare it to something familiar to the student, such as a car motor. • *Model:* When discussing the various forms of birth control with a group, provide samples of each type for the group members to look at and touch.
5. *Questioning:* Raises issues about content for learner to think about.	• Encourages learner to pay attention • Encourages critical thinking • Clarifies issues • Refocuses or redirects discussion	• When teaching about any health topic, ask the students to tell you what they know about the subject before giving any information. • During the teaching, ask students to problem solve a situation. For instance, what are the symptoms of an infected incision, and what would they do if they had these symptoms?
6. *Closing:* Reviews or summarizes content; can include application to similar or new situations.	• Facilitates retention of content • Organizes content through review of major points and application to situations	• Summarize, or have the client review with you, the major points of the session. • Point out how this information can be used in other situations as well as in the one discussed.

From unpublished class notes of J. Hitchcock, Sonoma State University, Rohnert Park, CA. Based on Strategies for Teaching Nursing, *by R. Detornyay, 1971, New York: John Wiley & Sons.*

✳ DECISION MAKING

Developing Teaching Strategies

You are working in a clinic that serves homeless men and women. You have found that many of the clients have severe foot problems and little understanding of how to identify symptoms and the need to seek treatment early.

◆ How might you go about planning a group to teach foot care?

◆ How would you facilitate the clients' readiness and motivation to learn?

◆ What teaching strategies would you consider using to facilitate learning? Why?

FIGURE 10-11 Strategies for Teaching People Who Are Partially Fluent in English

- Use a caring tone of voice and facial expression to help alleviate the client's fears.
- Speak slowly and distinctly, but not loudly.
- Use gestures, pictures, and play acting to help the client understand.
- Repeat the message in different ways if necessary.
- Be alert to words the client seems to understand and use them frequently.
- Keep messages simple and repeat them frequently.
- Avoid using medical terms and abbreviations that the client may not understand.
- Use an appropriate language dictionary.

Adapted from *Transcultural Nursing: Assessment and Intervention* (3rd ed., p. 34), by J. N. Giger and R. E. Davidhizar, 1999, St. Louis: Mosby.

---

and assessment skills to identify client learning needs. In addition, the nurse must be able to engage the client in learning by working in partnership with the client (Rankin & Stallings, 2001).

The content being taught is often emotionally charged, as when discussing prenatal care with a pregnant teen and her family or when presenting a class at a senior citizens' center about how to care for a family member diagnosed with Alzheimer's disease. Such situations require a combination of teaching and support. It is important to acknowledge the client's anxiety and to support needs if learning is to take place (Rankin & Stallings, 2001). For example, a nurse who is giving information to a family about community resources available for a family member who has Alzheimer's disease may note reluctance on the part of the family to consider these options. In this case, the nurse should take the time to explore with the family their concerns and their sense of inadequacy in providing the necessary care. This discussion might reveal some knowledge deficits about the course of the disease, in which case the nurse would provide needed information and clarification with the goal of reducing the family's worries and thereby facilitating the family's emotional readiness to consider the community supports initially described to them by the nurse.

Other persons who must be included in the teaching have to be identified. For instance, Kelley and Fitzsimons (2000) explain that when a health care worker is teaching Native Americans, identifying incongruities between the health beliefs and practices of the Native American culture and of the health provider's culture is not enough to ensure cultural relevance. They caution that the tribal authority and other members of the community must be involved in securing approval for the intervention.

Accessing knowledge by reasoning through problems is particularly difficult when teaching people who are partially fluent in English. Giger and Davidhizar (1999) recommend strategies for doing so when no bilingual persons are available to facilitate communication (see Figure 10-11).

When a client is being taught in the home, reimbursement mechanisms usually require that visits be time limited. Thus, the nurse must be well organized to ensure that necessary teaching for both the client and caregivers as well as other necessary activities are performed (Graham & Gleit, 1998). Teaching the elderly client requires slower presentation of information, careful observation for tiring or for lapsed attention, and accommodation to sensory deficits. Follow-up evaluation of learning outcomes is always crucial.

Using an Interpreter

Nearly 32 million people in the United States speak a language other than English at home. One of the greatest challenges in cross-cultural communication occurs when you and your client speak different languages. Interviewing or teaching a non-English-speaking client requires a bilingual interpreter, ideally a trained medical interpreter who knows interpreting techniques, has a health care background, understands patients' rights, and is knowledgeable about cultural beliefs and health practices (Andrews & Boyle, 1999). While it is tempting to ask a relative, friend, or whoever is readily available and wants to help, it is much more helpful to make arrangements for a bilingual member of the health care team. Clients often have information about personal health matters they do not want to share with family members

REFLECTIVE THINKING

Assessing the Problem

You are visiting Mrs. Sayer, a 70-year-old woman with severe emphysema, and her husband. Mrs. Sayer is continuously on oxygen. On her table, you notice an ashtray holding several half-smoked cigarettes.

- What is your first reaction to this observation?
- What issues of your own must you address before approaching the client regarding this observation?
- How would you develop your teaching goal? Why?
- How would you include Mr. Sayer in your teaching?

FIGURE 10-12 Evaluating a Teaching Intervention

- Did the objectives clearly state observable client behaviors?
- Were the objectives realistic for the client?
- Was the original assessment complete?
- Did the client perceive the identified problem as important? Did he or she want to change?
- Did new problems pose obstacles to behavioral change?
- Did the client participate in goal setting?
- Were the interventions tailored to meet the objectives?
- Was behavioral change measured and documented accurately?
- Is there a skill deficiency? Should there be changes in the nursing interventions?

Adapted from *Patient Education: Issues, Principles, Practices* (4th ed., p. 330), by S. H. Rankin and K. D. Stallings, 2001, Philadelphia: Lippincott. Used with permission.

---

or friends. An interpreter must have transcultural sensitivity, understand how to impart knowledge, and understand how to be a client advocate to represent the client's needs to the nurse. Clients may find it difficult to get their deeper concerns and fears adequately communicated even when an interpreter is involved; it is recommended that the interpreter meet with the client beforehand to establish rapport and to obtain basic descriptive information about the client such as age, occupation, educational level, and attitude toward health care, thus easing the interpreter into the relationship.

Both you and the client should speak only a sentence or two and then allow the interpreter time. Use simple language, not medical jargon. Summary translation by the interpreter may be used for teaching simple health techniques while the nurse watches for nonverbal cues (Andrews & Boyle, 1999).

Evaluation

Evaluation is linked to assessment and to the learning objectives, and it is ongoing. With the learning objectives as a guide, the nurse can judge the results of teaching. How have the objectives been met? Determining the answer to that question can be difficult. Some change in behavior is usually the desired outcome. Thus, the nurse may ask clients to describe their behavior or may question clients about their knowledge and activities (Giger & Davidhizar, 1999). Figure 10-12 lists suggested questions to guide the nurse in the evaluation process.

Another aspect of evaluation is to review the teaching module itself. How effective was it? How could it be changed to be more effective? Is the source of a given problem the client, the teacher, or the teaching plan?

Child as Learner

Children have different learning needs than do adolescents or adults. Teaching children demands ingenuity on the part of the nurse teacher. Growth and developmental levels must be assessed as well as the cognitive level of each child learner. Children, in general, have shorter attention spans and greater needs for support and nurturance and learn even more easily through active participation than do adults. The material should be presented in an abbreviated format over short periods. Children learn more quickly and enthusiastically when their teacher shows warmth and affection for them. Also, when children are actively involved in the learning process, they more readily assimilate the information. Children learn through play, and play becomes the means for learning about their health problem, what will happen, and how best to care for themselves. Play helps the child to deal with unresolved feelings and to ask questions about problems.

Adolescents are able to use abstract thinking as a learning tool and, like adults, are able to reason deductively. Learning processes at this stage, though, are different in that social development and the peer group are very significant aspects of learning. The nurse teacher re-

RESEARCH FOCUS

Relationships among Educational Material Readability, Client Literacy, Perceived Beneficence, and Perceived Quality

Study Problem/Purpose

Relationships between measurements of participant reading levels, self-reported years of education completed, and readability of an educational pamphlet were studied to determine how learning is affected when individual literacy levels do not match the educational readability level of the written material. While literacy is the ability to read and write at about the sixth-grade level, the median grade reading level of the U.S. population is estimated at eighth grade and client education programs generally use educational materials geared to about the twelfth grade.

Methods

Variables measured in this study included (1) estimated grade reading level, (2) educational literature readability, (3) client-perceived beneficence, (4) client-perceived quality, and (5) demographic characteristics. Reading levels were determined by using a simple screening tool, The Slossan Oral Reading Test-Revised (SORT-R), for assessing a person's reading level based on his or her ability to recognize and pronounce words. Educational literature used was a widely used, commercially published pamphlet for teaching about hypertention. Readability was estimated using the McLaughlin SMOG readability formula in which a count of words with three or more syllables is taken from each of 10 sentences in the beginning, middle, and end of a text. A conversion table or a mathematical formula is then used to calculate the grade level. Client-perceived beneficence was determined by using an instrument, the Visual Analogue Scale (VAS) to assess how much help the pamphlet was for client learning about personal health, with scores ranging from "not helpful" to "very helpful." Client-perceived quality was measured by using an instrument, the Visit-Specific Satisfaction Questionnaire (VSQ), created to measure client satis-

faction immediately following a provider's office on a scale of 1–5, with 5 being excellent and 1 being poor. Data were also collected related to age, gender, ethnic origin, occupation and job status, annual income, years of schooling completed, and self-assessment of health status.

Findings

The mean reading level was substantially lower than mean years of education, and there was a high correlation between the measured reading level and client-perceived beneficence. The higher people's measured reading level was, the more benefit they derived from reading the twelfth-grade level hypertension pamphlet, and conversely those with lower literacy levels perceived less benefit from reading the same pamphlet. As anticipated, the measured reading levels were found to be lower than the stated years of education.

Implications

Providers must evaluate the readability of each written document they distribute, revise or prepare documents appropriate for the mean reading level of their population, and consider use of alternatives to written material for nonreaders. Several formulas for identifying grade level are available and are considered to provide estimates of readability based on complexity of words and sentences, sentence length, and diversity of words. In general, the more polysyllabic words and the longer the sentences, the higher the readability level of written material. Lack of cultural sensitivity may also reduce readability for certain groups. Awareness of cultural differences should help local health providers prepare culturally sensitive written educational materials.

Source: French, K. S., & Larrabee, J. H. (1999). Relationships among educational material readability, client literacy, perceived beneficence, and perceived quality. Journal of Nursing Care Quality, *13(6), 68–82.*

alizes that an adolescent develops identity in relation to peers; the best learning most often occurs when the parents are not present. Teens enjoy being with others of their own age who have similar health problems. They enjoy being in groups together in which they can share their experiences and learn from one another. Developmental readiness for learning requires integration of maturation, learning, and cognition before teens can enter into meaningful learning experiences about their health issues (Rankin & Stallings, 2001).

RELATED HEALTH EDUCATION AND COMMUNICATION ISSUES

The focus of community health education is on health promotion for population aggregates. Such education may take place at the local, state, national, or international level. People of all ages and socioeconomic and sociocultural backgrounds are included. Education occurs in such places as schools, clinics, prisons, occupational settings, homeless shelters, and community forums. Education programs may be directed toward a specific population, such as diabetic pregnant women, or toward a specific community, such as a village in Cambodia where people want to learn about immunizations. Programs may range from one-time presentations to long-term, state-initiated, multifaceted programs that involve the cooperative planning of health, governmental, environmental, and other community systems.

The same process of assessment, diagnosis, planning, implementation, and evaluation used in individualized teaching is used in large community health education programs. There are additional considerations, however. In large programs, many people and departments are involved. Thus, the nurse must use good communication, group process, and community organization skills to coordinate the various components of program planning. Furthermore, a large project requires time to arrange and to obtain community support. It also involves working with different cultural groups and with people with opposing interests. Political and legal influences are other significant factors to be considered. Decision makers, such as legislators or special groups, with interests in such things as tobacco or drugs can influence the direction of a program by effecting legislation that addresses these issues or by providing money for programs that promote their interests but not necessarily the needs of the community. Rankin and Stallings (2001) have summarized the factors that affect health promotion programs. These include socioeconomic status, educational level, culture and language, formal and informal power structures, occupation, and marketing forces.

Conflict Resolution

Conflict arises when persons hold seemingly incompatible ideas, interests, or values. Conflict is inevitable in any relationship; in fact, it has been said that without conflict there is no relationship. Although conflict is inevitable, it is also rich with opportunity for mutual gain arising from cooperation and collaboration. Cushnie identifies four categories of conflict: intrapersonal, interpersonal, intragroup, and intergroup.

There are three ways to approach **conflict resolution** (efforts to resolve conflict by expressing concerns and differences of opinion until clarity and resolution are achieved); one is constructive and two are destructive. The **win-win approach** is constructive and requires self-assertion and responsibility. This approach results in a solution with which all participants are satisfied. **Conflict management** refers to those efforts to work together while at the same time recognizing and accepting the conflicts inherent in the relationship. See Figure 10-13 for the steps involved in an integrative problem-solving approach, a win-win conflict management strategy rec-

---

✳ DECISION MAKING

The Child As Learner

Ann Parlo is a 14-year-old newly diagnosed diabetic who has just returned home from a one-week course on how to manage her diabetes. Her parents and her 12-year-old sister participated in a one-day seminar for relatives of diabetics. Her mother tells you that the whole family is still trying to absorb all they have learned. She is worried that she will not cook the right foods, and Ann still finds it difficult to self-administer her insulin, so the mother has been doing it for her.

Consider the following in developing a teaching plan with the family:

◆ What goals and objectives would you want to develop with the family?

◆ What assessment data do you need?

◆ What is your learning diagnosis?

◆ What plan would you want to make? What teaching strategies would you use? What environmental considerations would be relevant?

◆ How could you evaluate the outcome of your teaching?

FIGURE 10-13 Win-Win Conflict Resolution Strategy

- Identify the problem (including values, purposes, goals).
- Encourage free exchange of ideas, feelings, attitudes, and values in an atmosphere of trust.
- Search for alternative ways to resolve the problem.
- Ask for help from outside sources as needed.
- Set up means for evaluation of solutions.
- Keep interacting until all members want and value the solution.

Adapted from *What You Need to Know about Today's Workplace: A Survival Guide for the Workplace*, by American Nurses Association, 1995, Washington DC: Author.

REFLECTIVE THINKING

Assessing Conflict-Resolution Skills

- Examine your own conflict resolution skills.
- Which conflict resolution skills do you use well?
- Which conflict resolution skills do you need to improve?
- What steps do you need to take to use the win-win strategy?

FIGURE 10-14 Guidelines for Negotiation

- Establish a cooperative tone at the outset.
- Strive for a win-win outcome.
- Ask lots of questions and really listen to the answers. Knowledge of the other person's needs, expectations, preferences, pressures, and strategies will help you reach an understanding.
- Find a line of reasoning that meets your needs while also meeting the other party's needs at the least cost to you.
- Know your "bottom line." Don't give away more than your maximum or accept less than your minimum.
- Stay calm. If you feel you are losing your temper, call for a break.
- Don't appear too anxious for a solution. Avoid snap judgments.
- If you reach an impasse, either suggest a recess or restate the consequences of not reaching an agreement. You may also suggest a trade of items from each party.

From *Yes, You Can!* by S. Deep and L. Sussman, 1996, Reading, MA: Addison-Wesley. Copyright 1996 by Sam Deep and Lyle Sussman. Reprinted with permission of Perscus Books Publishers, a member of Perscus Books, LLC.

ommended by the ANA (1995). In the **lose-win approach** to conflict resolution, one person allows resolution of the conflict at his or her own expense. This approach is nonassertive and nonresponsible. The **win-lose approach** is the opposite; one person resolves the conflict in a way satisfying to him- or herself but in the process "bulldozes" the rights of the others. This is an aggressive and irresponsible approach.

Methods of conflict resolution (Kilmann & Thomas, 1975) most often used are (1) avoidance by not dealing with it at all; (2) competition and the use of aggression or power to win; (3) compromise, in which each person has to give in a bit in order to reach a solution but may not yield the best solution that might be found with a more creative approach; (4) accommodation, which requires one person to give up their needs in order to smooth things over and ease the tension; and (5) collaboration, which requires the highest level of commitment to the relationship of any of these styles. Collaboration involves a high degree of concern for achieving the goals of both parties and for the relationship between parties. This style is hard work but, in the best cases, the relationship can be strengthened in the process. Yet, collaboration can only work if both parties are willing to participate in it.

Negotiation strategies are useful when groups or corporations are involved in conflict and are seeking resolution. **Negotiation** is defined by Walker and Harris (1995) as "the process of resolving differences through mutually acceptable tradeoffs" (p. 2). Guidelines for this process are outlined briefly in Figure 10-14. Negotiation is a highly complex set of communication skills yet offers opportunity to experience win-win situations for all concerned.

Principled negotiation involves decision making based on the merits of an issue rather than by taking positions and trying to get the other party to come to our own position. There are four rules of thumb in principled negotiation: separate people from the problem, focus on

interests, not positions; invent various options for mutual gain; and use objective criteria (Tubbs & Moss, 2000).

Public Speaking

Throughout this chapter we have discussed intrapersonal communication, or "self-talk" in the process of self-awareness, and interpersonal communication, or interacting and sharing information with others. Public speaking is the act of using spoken words to communicate with many individuals at one time. Nurses can expect to be involved in this activity, particularly with regard to community education and to involvement in community health issues.

The goals of public speaking with regard to health teaching are to reach large numbers of people with information about health topics that affect the community and to urge adoption of healthy behaviors. Effective speakers use strong critical thinking skills and strategic planning. Critical thinking is defined as "the ability to form and defend your own judgments rather than blindly accepting or instantly rejecting what you hear or read . . . a conscious, systematic method of evaluating ideas wherever you encounter them" (p. 48). Critical thinking emphasizes reflective judgment, the acceptance of ideas through a considered and thoughtful approach to determine if an

COMMUNITY NURSING VIEW

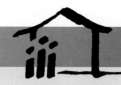

A 17-year-old girl who is six months pregnant and living in a temporary shelter for homeless women has been referred to you. The referral states that she must leave in four weeks and that she has not made any effort to find another place to live. Further, she made one prenatal visit to a local clinic but has missed the last three appointments. You make a home visit to the shelter to interview the girl and to assess the situation. She seems friendly and receptive to you and your visit. She appears to be underweight and states that she has gained only five pounds since she got pregnant and just does not feel like eating. She is worried because she does not want to get fat. When you encourage her to eat, explaining why it is so important, she responds by saying that she will try to eat more. You express your concern that she must get prenatal care and find another place to live. She says the most important thing for her to do is get a job. You make an appointment for a follow-up visit in two days to do a physical assessment, get a complete health history, formulate a treatment plan, and make a contract with her. When you arrive at the designated time, she is not home. A staff person says she went out to look for a job.

Nursing Considerations

Assessment

♦ How will you assess her physical condition? Where will you do the examination? What equipment will you need? What records will you keep?

♦ The psychosocial situation indicates serious problems. What questions will you ask to gain further information about her situation? How will you assess strengths in her environment? Why is it important to assess for potential support systems (i.e., family, church, friends, or groups)?

♦ What are her inner strengths? Beliefs? Values? Cultural health care practices?

Diagnosis

♦ What diagnoses would be appropriate for her?

♦ What issues are related to the diagnoses?

Outcome Identification

♦ What behaviors could serve as indicators of progress?

♦ What psychological indicators might reflect positive treatment outcomes?

♦ What psychological outcomes could reflect positive treatment outcomes?

Planning/Interventions

♦ When will you make a return visit? Will you notify her of your intention to visit? If so, how will you notify her?

♦ What is your plan of action for when you do next meet with her? How will you learn what she is willing to do for herself? How will you address your concerns for her?

♦ Do you think a contract might be helpful? Would you do it verbally or would you put it in writing, complete with signatures?

♦ What information does she need to empower her to take more responsibility for herself and her unborn child? How will you know when she is actively participating in the teaching/learning process? Is she interested in learning some relaxation techniques for stress management and for labor?

♦ How does your listening help motivate her to do what she needs to do for herself?

♦ What referrals may be appropriate? How can you serve as an advocate for her?

Evaluation

♦ How will you evaluate the success of your plan and interventions? Will you measure success by physical findings? Her keeping of appointments? Her follow-through on contracted responsibilities?

---

idea merits acceptance and support. Effective speakers use **strategic planning** by identifying their goals and then by determining how best to achieve them (Zarefsky, 1999). These skills together lay a strong foundation for success in public speaking. Public speaking is a power-

ful tool, the necessary skills of which take time and effort to develop. Great speaking skills are respected and, in general, are a mark of successful men and women. For a summary of 10 steps to making a public speech, see Figure 10-15.

FIGURE 10-15 Tips for Making a Public Speech

1. Select a topic that is important to you and to your audience.
2. Create an outline for your speech so that it has an introduction, a body, and a conclusion.
3. Organize your thoughts, keeping in mind your personal experience, what you bring to the topic, what your audience already knows, and what you can tell them.
4. Give special attention to planning the introduction and conclusion of the speech.
5. Outline the major points you wish to make in the body of the speech and the supporting statements for each point.
6. Rehearse your speech aloud and use a VCR for feedback.
7. Concentrate on making your ideas clear to the audience.
8. Use only a one-page outline as notes. Rehearse with the outline and maintain eye contact with the audience.
9. Present yourself to your audience by dressing in a way that does not call attention to itself and by approaching the podium with confidence and purpose.
10. Choose your words carefully; use colorful and appropriate language while avoiding jargon, technical terms, and excess verbiage to achieve clarity, rhythm, and vividness.

Adapted from *Public Speaking: Strategies For Success* (2nd ed.), by D. Zarefsky, 1999, Boston: Allyn & Bacon.

KEY CONCEPTS

◆ Communication is the core of client-nurse work in the community, dictating its quality and effectiveness in serving the best interests of the client.

◆ The interactionist nurse theorists emphasize the client-nurse relationship, particularly with regard to its serving to meet the health needs of the client.

◆ Client-nurse communication embodies the sharing of information, feelings, thoughts, beliefs, values, and behaviors related to client health and healing processes as the client assumes increasing responsibility.

◆ Active listening, a powerful tool in communicating empathic understanding, calls for the qualities of effective helping: warmth, respect, genuineness, specificity, empathy, self-disclosure, and confrontation.

◆ The contract is often helpful as a tool for goal attainment in the therapeutic process, defining nurse and client responsibilities in solving a problem.

◆ All groups follow a predictable developmental pattern, whether their goals are related to work planning or the therapeutic process.

◆ Education is necessary in meeting many of the *Healthy People 2010* objectives, and andragogy is the most appropriate approach because it emphasizes client self-efficacy.

◆ Various factors, including space; temperature; visual, auditory, and olfactory stimuli; equipment; resources; furniture arrangement; physical comfort, and time, affect the teaching/learning environment.

◆ The learning process uses the same steps as the nursing process; a child's learning process differs from an adult's only with regard to level of educational readiness.

◆ Empowerment community education encourages the community to find solutions to its own problems by starting with the community's concerns, using active learning methods, and engaging clients in determining their own needs and priorities.

◆ Conflict is inevitable in any relationship, and resolution can bring about closeness and shared understandings.

◆ Negotiation is a very complex communication skill and a powerful tool for resolving differences while offering opportunity for win-win situations for all concerned.

◆ Effective speakers lay the foundation for public talks by using critical thinking skills and strategic planning.

RESOURCES

HEALTH COMMUNICATION

Communication skills for health professionals:
   http://www.medinfo.ufl.edu
Up Front: Journal of Health Communication: http://gwu.edu
Harvard School of Public Health Center for Health
   Communication:
   http://www.hsph.harvard.edu/Organizations/chc

HEALTH EDUCATION

*ATSDR—Evaluation primer on health risk communication
   programs:* http://www.atsdr.cdc.gov/HEC/primer.html
Health skills for life—Comprehensive school health program:
   http://www.healthskills.com

National Center for Education in Maternal and Child Health:
http://www.ncemch.org/

*Community development: Promoting health through
empowerment and participation:* http://www.hc-
sc.gc.ca/hppb/wired/community.html

Center for Community Health, Education and Research, Inc.:
http://www.ccher.org

Project for Rural Health Communication and Information
Technology (PRHCIT):
http://www.med.monash.edu.au/mrh/research/prhcit

HEALTH PROMOTION AND DISEASE PREVENTION PERSPECTIVES

Phyllis E. Schubert, DNSc, RN, MA

MAKING THE CONNECTION

Life is. . . .
To endure
The ebb and tide of keeping life's balance,
To care. . . .
Not just to procure.
Disease or illness is. . . .
To prevent with the power of knowledge,
To accept things that cannot be altered,
To travel the road with leverage.
Death is. . . .
To accept transition. . . .
To respect the rose with petals falling,
To ease the change of time or place. . . .
Not just to say good-bye, but to heed the calling.

—Mary Jo Starsiak

COMPETENCIES

Upon completion of this chapter, the reader should be able to:

- Trace the recent history of the efforts to move national and international health care toward a focus on disease prevention and health promotion in addition to treatment of disease.
- Discuss theoretical perspectives related to health promotion, disease prevention, health behavior choice, and health education.
- Discuss moral and ethical issues related to social and individual responsibilities for health.
- Recount recommendations related to diet, exercise, sleep, and stress management.
- Discuss philosophical issues related to research in the areas of health promotion and disease prevention.
- Explain a conceptual model for application of caring in the clinical practice of health promotion.
- Discuss clinical application to nursing practice of disease prevention and health promotion in the community.

KEY TERMS

aerobic conditioning	leading health indicators
biotechnology	ovovegan diet
community nursing centers (CNCs)	paradigm
created environment	promotional indicator
deep relaxation	psychoneuroimmu-
determinants of health	nology
disease prevention	risk factors
energy	self-esteem
health behaviors	social support
health education	story telling
health promotion	stress
health protection	stress response
integrative models of health	stressors
lacto-ovovegan diet	traditional indicators
lactovegan diet	vegan diet
	wellness

G reat strides in the treatment of disease have been made over the past few decades causing the average life span to lengthen. Consequently, qual-

ity of life in the added years has become an important consideration.

Health as a state of well-being resulting from harmonious interaction of body, mind, spirit, and environment was defined for community health nursing in the first chapter. Based on this definition, it is clear that individual health is "almost inseparable from the health of the larger community and that the health of every community in every state and territory determines the overall health status of the Nation" [U.S. Department of Health and Human Services (USDHHS), 2000, p. 3]. Figure 11-1 reflects the many interrelated factors which determine health. Recognition and understanding of these factors and influences provide the foundation for goals and objectives for health promotion and disease prevention programs represented in the *Healthy People 2010* vision for the United States.

The purpose of this chapter is to explore nursing issues and implications related to national and international political efforts to promote health and prevent disease. Because both individual responsibility and social responsibility are required in these efforts, a synthesis of individual health behavior choice and societal efforts to provide a healthy environment for all is emphasized. (Application of these concepts to populations is more fully developed in other chapters, with population-focused strategies for health promotion and prevention serving as the major focus of Chapter 13.) The material related to individuals may serve as content for health education programs. **Health education** is defined as obtaining self-awareness, information, and support for changing problem health behaviors through the teaching/learning process. Because to a large extent health behavior is taught via modeling, some features in this chapter focus on the health behavior of the nurse. A brief overview of theoretical perspectives related to health promotion and wellness, disease prevention, health education, and health behavior choice is also included. These models provide a basis for research and the application of health education and clinical programs.

HEALTHY PEOPLE 2010: A NATIONAL PLAN

Theoretical frameworks and research have long indicated the need for emphasis on health promotion and disease prevention in order to reduce health care costs and to improve the quality of life internationally and nationally. In 1978, the Declaration of Alma Ata [World Health Organization (WHO), 1981], which addressed worldwide concerns about health and health care, emphasized the need to shift from a disease care focus to a focus on health. Health for All (HFA) by the Year 2000 became the guiding slogan for the work at the WHO conference in Ottawa, Canada, where the historic Ottawa Charter for Health Promotion (WHO, 1986) was developed. This charter identified the factors fundamental to community health: peace, shelter, education, food, income, a stable ecosystem,

FIGURE 11-1   Factors That Influence Health Status

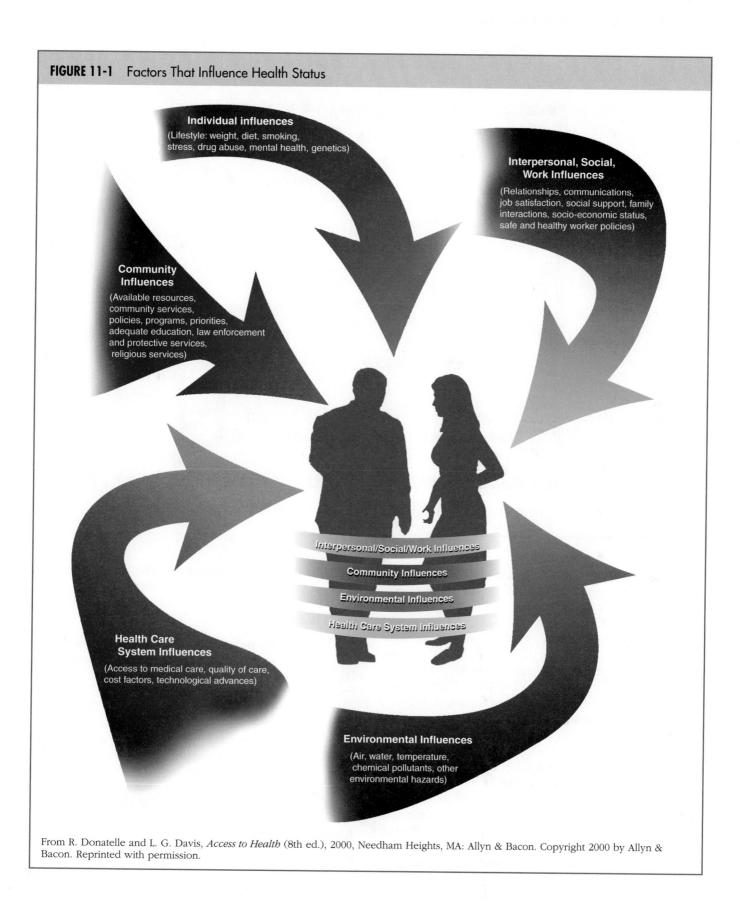

From R. Donatelle and L. G. Davis, *Access to Health* (8th ed.), 2000, Needham Heights, MA: Allyn & Bacon. Copyright 2000 by Allyn & Bacon. Reprinted with permission.

FIGURE 11-2 Determinants of Health

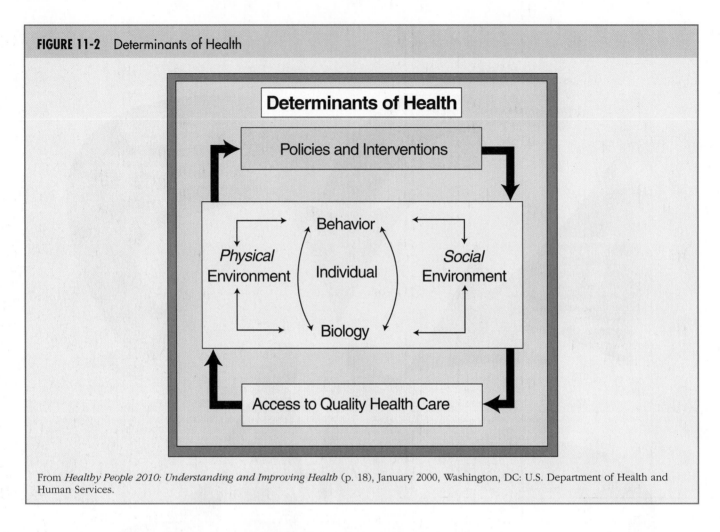

From *Healthy People 2010: Understanding and Improving Health* (p. 18), January 2000, Washington, DC: U.S. Department of Health and Human Services.

sustainable resources, social justice, and equity. In the United States, a need for emphasis on the promotion of health rather than on the treatment of disease was also addressed. The Office of Disease Prevention and Health Promotion, a division of the USDHHS, has accepted the responsibility for overseeing the nation's Healthy People projects during the past 20 years (USDHHS, 1980, 1990) and for the next 10 years (USDHHS, 2000). Great progress has been made over the last decade to improve the nation's health. Statistics from the year 2000 indicates a significant reduction in infant mortality; an increase in the percentage of children immunized against childhood diseases; a decrease in the number of teenagers becoming parents; a decrease in the use of alcohol, tobacco, and illicit drugs; decreasing unintentional injuries; and declining death rates for coronary heart disease and stroke. In addition, progress had been made in the diagnosis and treatment of cancer.

Yet, there has been a lack of progress in some areas. Statistical indicators reveal increased diabetes and other chronic conditions, obesity, violence and abusive behavior, and undiagnosed and untreated mental disorders. Indicators also reflect decreased physical activity and increased smoking among adolescents. HIV/AIDS remained a serious health problem, especially among women and communities of minority peoples (USDHHS, 2000).

Goals and Objectives

The overarching purpose for *Healthy People 2010* goals and objectives is to promote health and prevent illness, disability, and premature death. The goals are (1) to increase quality and years of healthy life and (2) to eliminate health disparities (USDHHS, 2000). These goals serve as guidelines for developing objectives which identify activities and measurement of health status. Health status is measured by using figures related to birth and death rates, life expectancy, quality of life, morbidity from specific diseases, risk factors, use of health delivery services, and financing (USDHHS, 2000).

Determinants of Health

Critical influences that determine the health of individuals and communities are known as **determinants of health.** These determinants include biology, behavior, social and physical environments, policies and interventions, and access to quality health care. Figure 11-2 depicts relationships between determinants of health and

Out
of the Box

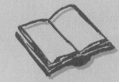

Preventing Child Abuse and Neglect in At Risk Families

The field of health care still focuses mainly on treatment of existing problems and sometimes on prevention. Some programs, especially in the area of family support and child development, are designing programs based on a promotion model. This is an approach that optimizes positive growth and functioning of each family rather than the more traditional preventive approach (to forestall the occurrence of specific problems) or the medical/treatment approach (to provide care after a problem has occurred) (Dunst, Trivetta & Deal, 1995). A characteristic of promotional programs which differentiate them from other types of programs is the quality of universal access—being open to all families. Families do not have to have a particular risk factor or problem to participate. Also, families determine for themselves the resources that will strengthen their families and ultimately result in sustained gains in family functioning and childhood development. Having them decide for themselves what they need is empowering for families.

One example of this kind of program is the Young Children and Families (YCF) program in Moscow, Idaho. I worked with this program during the first two years of its operation as an Americorps VISTA volunteer. YCF offers First Steps, a national program started by the Georgia Council on Child Abuse. YCF trains volunteers to visit each family of a newborn born in Latah County and offers a program of support, education, and resource connection. A welcome baby bag is given to each family, whether they decide to participate or not. The bag contains a resource directory, published by YCF, a developmental milestones calendar, a pocket of baby's first books donated by the county library, and information about parenting classes. First Steps volunteers make regular phone calls to participating families to provide the support, educational information, and information about resources they need at the time. Although YCF's First Steps program was not specifically designed to target families at risk for child abuse and neglect, data indicate that among comparison counties, Latah County (where

YCF is located) showed the most significant decrease in the number of valid/verifiable child abuse reports and percent of newborns who are low-birthweight babies. YCF's First Steps program is the first of its kind in the northwest. YCF is planning to expand this service to families during the prenatal period.

New parents are also offered the opportunity to participate in a developmental screening program through the Ages and Stages Questionnaire (ASQ). Beginning at four months and every two or three months after that through age five years, an age-appropriate questionnaire is mailed to the family, who fills it out and mails it back to a YCF child development specialist who scores it and gives feedback to the family. This feedback usually includes some information about this stage of development and specific activities that are appropriate for this age. The questionnaire focuses mainly on motor and cognitive development. Recently, social-emotional scales have been developed as well and YCF will incorporate these into the program. Families report that using the ASQ is an excellent way for them to learn about early childhood development as well as tracking their child's growth. During the first 15 months of operation, the number of children receiving developmental screening in Latah County has increased by 250%—from 70 in 1998 to more than 180 in the year 2000. At present over 400 families are participating in this process.

YCF also manages Baby Tracks, an immunization postcard reminder program. County immunization rates increased from 76% to 88% within the first year of operation. YCF annually publishes the Community Compass, a family friendly resource guide. Since its inception, 48% of parents asked indicated they have used the Community Compass to locate child care, parenting resources, and recreation activities for themselves and/or their young children.

Because promotional programs are relatively new and because their success relies on a broad array of complex factors, indicators of progress are in the beginning stages of development. **Traditional indicators** are measures of reduction or elimination of

(continues)

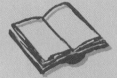

Out
of the Box (continued)

diseases or dysfunctional or at-risk behaviors and conditions. These traditional indicators, such as the incidence of child abuse and the immunization rates for a county or state, make it much easier to identify and maintain records that show, for example, "percent of parents or caregivers who have appropriate knowledge of child development and have realistic expectations for their children," an example of a promotional indicator. A **promotional indicator** is defined as a measure of positive growth or enhanced functioning of a child, youth, family, or community.

Since appropriate knowledge of child development and having realistic expectations for children have been found to be key factors in allaying incidence of child abuse, this is an important measure and worth the effort of developing ways to do it.

A cross-state work team of representatives from eight states, facilitated by the Family Resource Coalition of America (FRCA), has identified three interrelated reasons why promotional indicators are needed:

- To bring a strength-based approach to measure condition of well-being for children, youth, families, and communities
- To identify intermediate markers of growth development and functioning that are highly consistent with successful long-term outcomes for children and families
- To demonstrate the value of family support strategies (Lepler et al)

The cross-state work team recommends a mix of traditional and promotional indicators at the policy and practice levels.

–Joan Heron, RN, PhD

Sources: Dunst, C., Trivette, C. & Deal, A. (Eds.). (1995). *Supporting and strengthening families: Methods, strategies and practices.* Cambridge, MA: Brookline.

Lepler, S., Rosenkrantz, R., Diehl, D., Koser, G. (1999). *Promotion indicators for children and families: A concept paper.* Paper submitted by the Family Resource Coalition of America at a Symposium on Promotional Indicators, May 11–12, 1999, Minneapolis, MN. ■

---

health status (USDHHS, 2000). According to the USDHHS (2000), individual behaviors and environmental factors are responsible for about 70% of all premature deaths in the United States.

Healthy People 2010 calls for a multidisciplinary approach to health by communities, states, and national organizations, involving health, education, housing, labor, justice, transportation, agriculture and the environment (USDHHS, 2000). Fielding (1999) reflects this mandate as follows:

In this quest, health promotion is adopting many professionals who might not have considered themselves in the business of health promotion. Yet the lawyers working to increase tobacco taxes through public referenda are health promotion practitioners. So are the politicians who work to reduce poverty, and the community organizers who seek to reduce the attractiveness of gang life to youth and those who fight for high-quality child care that promotes social and mental development. Of course, the formal education and skill set of health promotion practitioners who regulate food ingredients or use the law to get lead abated in housing may differ from those teaching breastfeeding to new mothers or conducting exercise classes at a worksite. (p. 940)

BALANCING SOCIAL AND INDIVIDUAL RESPONSIBILITY FOR HEALTH

Health promotion in community health programs involves both individual and community efforts at various levels. A theme that runs through all health promotion and health protection/disease prevention efforts is shared responsibility. Success depends on (1) individual efforts toward health behavior; (2) the community's efforts to provide a support structure for these voluntary actions; and (3) collaborative efforts of health professionals at all levels, sharing responsibility for the health of individuals. This collaboration involves providing support for primary preventive actions when the individual is basically healthy; secondary prevention interventions to identify problems; and tertiary prevention strategies to minimize the effects of disease after it has occurred (Wilson, 1999). (See Chapter 1 for definitions and discussion of primary prevention, secondary prevention, and tertiary prevention strategies.)

Health promotion definitions vary, as discussed in Chapter 1 of this book. Fielding (1999) identifies the mission of health promotion as changing conditions so that health of individuals and populations is improved. His operational definition of health promotion programs are those which combine educational, organizational, eco-

Individual versus Social Responsibility for Health

In the United States, third-party payment most often extends to those who need medical care: for example, those who are hospitalized for drug therapy or surgery. Educational programs for those with addictions and destructive health behaviors are less often funded. Drug rehabilitation programs have long waiting lists. Emphasis on nutrition, sleep, and exercise is seldom a part of prevention and treatment programs, and health promotion programs are almost nonexistent.

- What changes would you make to provide a more economical, effective, and efficient system?
- Give examples of appropriate individual responsibility for health promotion.
- Give examples of appropriate societal responsibility.
- How would you avoid a "blame the victim" perspective and still require individual responsibility for health behavior choice?

nomic, and environmental supports for individual behavior and conditions of living conducive to health.

In Chapter 9, Schubert proposes that individual responsibility starts with providing the best environment possible for oneself to be healthy or to heal. As health and expanding consciousness occur and awareness regarding needs at various levels of environment— family, local, state, national, international, planetary, and universal— increases, social responsibility for the world at large also increases. With heightened awareness and responsibility, people can make decisions appropriate to their situations, whether that means recycling waste in the home or making proposals on the floor of the U.S. Senate or in the WHO.

This perspective also presumes a caring environment for growth and development of human potential, health, and healing. When an individual, family, or community is in a situation where basic needs cannot be met, help and assistance are essential until caring, nurturance, respect, safety, and order (beauty) can be reestablished. Obviously, caring for others and oneself requires services necessary for disease prevention and health promotion.

Health promotion activities depend on acceptance of oneself and others, with each person being viewed as whole and as perfect in the present phase of spiritual growth and development. Then, and only then, can helping serve the needs of both the giver and receiver.

LEADING HEALTH INDICATORS

Leading health indicators, those major health concerns in the United States identified by *Healthy People 2010* organizers, were selected on the basis of their ability to motivate action, the availability of data to measure progress, and their importance as public health issues. The group of 10 indicators are listed in Figure 11-3 with related public health priorities.

THEORETICAL PERSPECTIVES OF HEALTH AND WELLNESS

Nurse theorists and authors on the whole conceptualize health as adaptation, self-actualization, or some combination thereof and address health as either a state of being or a process of evolving potentiality. Because all these theories reflect health as being determined by the person–environment relationship, all provide strong foundations for health promotion programs. The theoretical models discussed in this section represent these three categories.

Neuman Systems Model

Figure 11-4, represents the major nursing concepts in the Neuman systems model: client/client system (person/s), environment, health, and nursing. Client/client system and health are both reflected as "basic structure energy resources." In addition to its basic energy structure, environment both applies stress and protects from stress as flexible lines of defense serving all three systems interact with each other. Nursing in Neuman's model is presented as interventions related to primary, secondary, and tertiary prevention. The model is useful in numerous community health nursing settings, including those settings where client aggregates and geopolitical communities are served (Beddome, 1995).

The Neuman systems model (Neuman, 1990) is one nursing theory that addresses health as a process of adaptation and achievement of equilibrium. Neuman's model focuses on the concepts of energy and created environment. **Energy** is defined as "the pervasive force within the client that empowers and regulates all systemic functions from cellular to motor" (p. 129). Energy, then, may be thought of as a resource for system empowerment and achievement of wellness. A state of health or wellness is facilitated by conservation of energy through increasing awareness of environmental stressors as risk

FIGURE 11-3 Leading Health Indicators

- **Physical activity:** Regular physical activity throughout life is important for maintaining a healthy body, enhancing psychological well-being, and preventing premature death. Regular physical activity decreases the risk of death from heart disease, lowers the risk of developing diabetes, and is associated with a decreased risk of colon cancer. Regular physical activity helps prevent high blood pressure and plays a role in decreasing existing high blood pressure. *Public health priority:* Promote daily physical activity.

- **Overweight and obesity:** Overweight and obesity raise the risk of illness from high blood pressure, high cholesterol, type 2 diabetes, heart disease and stroke, gallbladder disease, arthritis, sleep disturbances and problems breathing, and endometrial, breast, prostate, and colon cancers. Obese individuals may also suffer from social stigmatization, discrimination, and lowered self-esteem. *Public health priority:* Promote good nutrition and healthier weights.

- **Tobacco use:** Cigarette smoking is the single most preventable cause of disease and death in the United States. Smoking is a major risk factor for heart disease, stroke, lung cancer, and chronic lung diseases. Smoking during pregnancy can result in miscarriages, premature delivery, and sudden infant death syndrome. Environmental tobacco smoke (ETS) increases the risk of heart disease and significant lung conditions, especially asthma and bronchitis in children. ETS is responsible for an estimated 3000 lung cancer deaths each year among adult nonsmokers. *Public health priority:* Prevent and reduce tobacco use.

- **Substance abuse:** Alcohol and illicit drug use are associated with many of this country's most serious problems, including child and spousal abuse, sexually transmitted diseases including HIV infection, teen pregnancy, school failure, motor vehicle crashes, rising health care costs, low worker productivity, and homelessness. Alcohol and illicit drug use also can result in substantial disruptions in family, work, and personal live. *Public health priority:* Prevent and reduce substance abuse.

- **Responsible sexual behavior:** Unintended pregnancies and sexually transmitted diseases (STDs), including infection with the human immunodeficiency virus (HIV) that causes AIDS, can result from unprotected sexual behaviors. Abstinence is the only method of complete protection. Condoms, if used correctly and consistently, can help prevent both unintended pregnancy and STDs. *Public health priority:* Promote responsible sexual behavior, including abstinence.

- **Mental health:** Mental health is a state of successful mental functioning resulting in productive activities, fulfilling relationships, and the ability to adapt to change and cope with adversity. Mental health is indispensable to personal well-being, family and interpersonal relationships, and one's contribution to society. Approximately 20% of the U.S. population are affected by mental illness during a given year; no one is immune. Major depression is the leading cause of disability and is the cause of more than two-thirds of suicides each year. *Public health priority:* Promote mental health and well-being.

- **Injury and violence:** More than 400 Americans die each day due primarily to motor vehicle crashes, firearms, poisonings, suffocation, falls, fires, and drowning. The risk of injury is so great that most persons sustain a significant injury at some time during their lives. *Public health priority:* Promote safety and reduce violence.

- **Environmental quality:** An estimated 25% of preventable illnesses worldwide can be attributed to poor environmental quality. In the United States, air pollution alone is estimated to be associated with 50,000 premature deaths and an estimated $40 billion to $50 billion in health-related costs annually. Two indicators of air quality are ozone (outdoor) and environmental tobacco smoke (indoor). *Public health priority:* Promote healthy environments.

- **Immunization:** Vaccines are among the greatest public health achievements of the 20th century. Immunizations can prevent disability and death from infectious diseases for individuals and can help control the spread of infections within communities. Immunizations against influenza and pneumococcal disease can prevent serious illness and death. Pneumonia and influenza deaths together constitute the sixth leading cause of death in the United States. *Public health priority:* Prevent infectious disease through immunization.

- **Access to health care:** Strong predictors of access to quality health care include having health insurance, a higher income level, and a regular primary care provider or other source of ongoing health care. Persons with health insurance are more likely to have a specific source of care and to have received appropriate preventive care. *Public health priority:* Increase access to quality health care.

From *Healthy People 2010: Appendix A.* [On-line]. Available: http://health.gov/healthypeople/Publications/HealthyCommunities2001/appendices.htm.

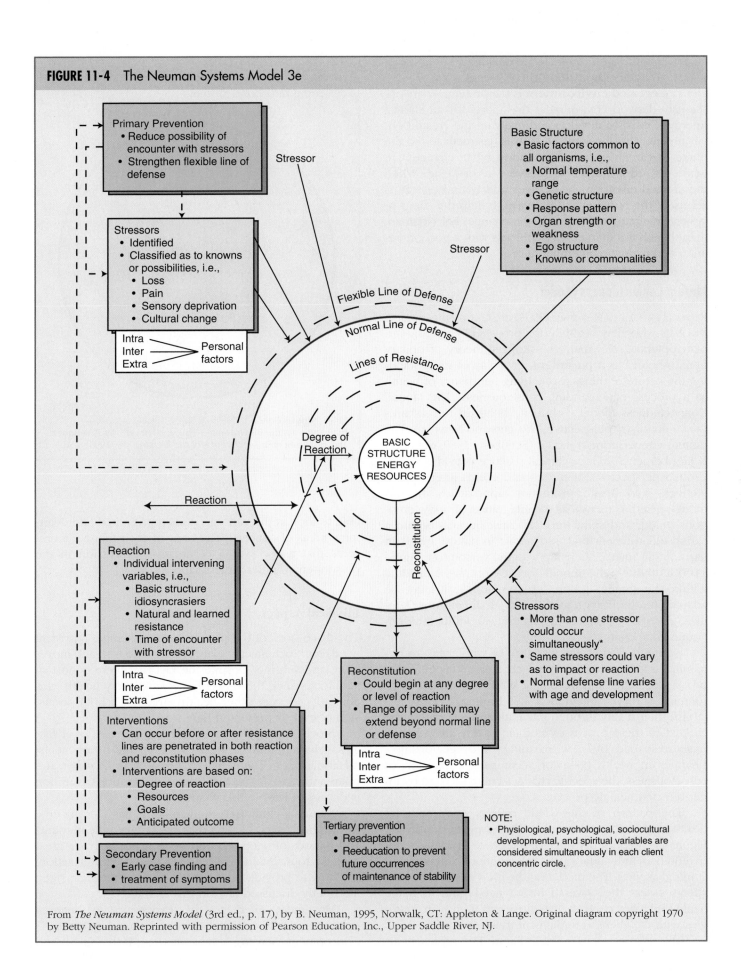

FIGURE 11-4 The Neuman Systems Model 3e

Primary Prevention
- Reduce possibility of encounter with stressors
- Strengthen flexible line of defense

Stressors
- Identified
- Classified as to knowns or possibilities, i.e.,
  - Loss
  - Pain
  - Sensory deprivation
  - Cultural change

Intra
Inter   Personal
Extra   factors

Stressor

Stressor

Basic Structure
- Basic factors common to all organisms, i.e.,
  - Normal temperature range
  - Genetic structure
  - Response pattern
  - Organ strength or weakness
  - Ego structure
  - Knowns or commonalities

Flexible Line of Defense

Normal Line of Defense

Lines of Resistance

Degree of Reaction

BASIC STRUCTURE ENERGY RESOURCES

Reaction

Reconstitution

Reaction
- Individual intervening variables, i.e.,
  - Basic structure idiosyncrasiers
  - Natural and learned resistance
  - Time of encounter with stressor

Intra
Inter   Personal
Extra   factors

Interventions
- Can occur before or after resistance lines are penetrated in both reaction and reconstitution phases
- Interventions are based on:
  - Degree of reaction
  - Resources
  - Goals
  - Anticipated outcome

Secondary Prevention
- Early case finding and
- treatment of symptoms

Reconstitution
- Could begin at any degree or level of reaction
- Range of possibility may extend beyond normal line or defense

Intra
Inter   Personal
Extra   factors

Stressors
- More than one stressor could occur simultaneously*
- Same stressors could vary as to impact or reaction
- Normal defense line varies with age and development

Tertiary prevention
- Readaptation
- Reeducation to prevent future occurrences of maintenance of stability

NOTE:
- Physiological, psychological, sociocultural developmental, and spiritual variables are considered simultaneously in each client concentric circle.

factors that threaten or challenge health and by increasing or strengthening existing client strengths.

The **created environment** is the protective, unconsciously derived environment that exists for all clients. Energy is used to develop and maintain the created environment. This mechanism often is destructive, and the nurse or caregiver provides support while changes are made toward a more constructive way of being. When the created environment changes and bound energy is released, the nurse must find ways to help the client or system integrate and adjust to the change. For Neuman, then, health is a living energy process with a goal of creating and maintaining equilibrium.

Mutual Connectedness Model

Rogers (1990) and Newman (1994) are among those nurse theorists who view health as the process of emerging human potential. Newman uses Rogers' theory of unitary human beings as a **paradigm,** or a way of understanding the nature of things, in building her theory of health as a process of expanding consciousness. The Mutual Connectedness Model (Schubert, 1989), in turn, shares the evolutionary perspective of Rogers and Newman. The mutual connectedness model (Schubert, 1989; Schubert & Lionberger, 1995) for clinical practice provides a conceptual perspective for nurses and clients interested in wellness and health promotion approaches. In this model, health is treated as the integration of body, emotions, mind, and spirit through consciousness within a caring environment that is dynamic in nature and is in harmonious interrelationship with the person (see Figure 11-5). Although the model focuses on the individual within the family, group, or community, it may be adapted for application to clients of all dimensions (families, groups, populations, communities) within their environmental contexts.

Figure 11-5 indicates a pattern of wholeness—a dynamic, moving, constantly changing evolutionary process of being and becoming wherein a caring environment supports integration and healing. Persons establish their reality through integration of self within the context of these processes as their worlds are continuously reshaped by new meanings and relationships. Changes in health behavior accompany expansion of consciousness, the specific changes being dictated by inner directed healing processes.

The pattern of the whole reflects one's state of health. Although separation of these aspects is artificial, Figure 11-6 represents some of the needs likely to be inherent in an individual's physical, emotional, mental, and spiritual aspects. The model can be used as a tool to help clients assess their overall health needs and to make health behavior choices. The nurse can then plan strategies with the client to implement those choices.

The sides of the triangles in Figure 11-6 represent areas of need affecting health behavior choice. Clients are

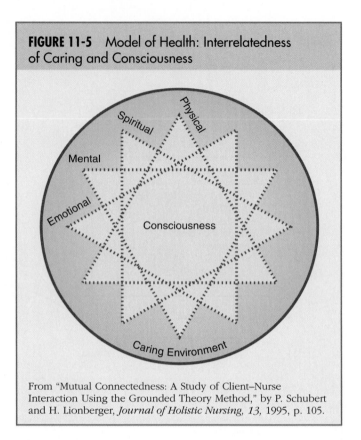

FIGURE 11-5 Model of Health: Interrelatedness of Caring and Consciousness

From "Mutual Connectedness: A Study of Client–Nurse Interaction Using the Grounded Theory Method," by P. Schubert and H. Lionberger, *Journal of Holistic Nursing, 13,* 1995, p. 105.

able to look at the various needs represented and determine areas of concern. The base of each triangle represents that aspect's area of creative expression in the person–environment interrelationship.

Physical Aspect

The three sides of the physical aspect triangle represent needs for biochemical balance, sleep and rest, and movement and sensing. Despite the fact that there is no real way to separate these needs (because every health variable affects every other health variable), a brief discussion of each is presented here.

Biochemical balance encompasses a variety of factors including nutrition intake via food and supplements; metabolism; environmental factors such as air, water, and pollutants or toxic substances; and medications. Nutrition is discussed later in this chapter.

Nature, including the human body, has a strong urge toward health and healing. The body, given the nutrients and periods of deep rest and sleep it needs, has a great capacity to maintain health and to heal itself. Relaxation, as a way to provide brief periods of deep rest, and sleep are briefly discussed later in this chapter.

Movement refers to the experience of internal rhythms and to the integration of body–mind and person–environment. Sensing—sight, hearing, taste, smell, and touch—also are a part of this experience. When one

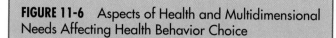

FIGURE 11-6 Aspects of Health and Multidimensional Needs Affecting Health Behavior Choice

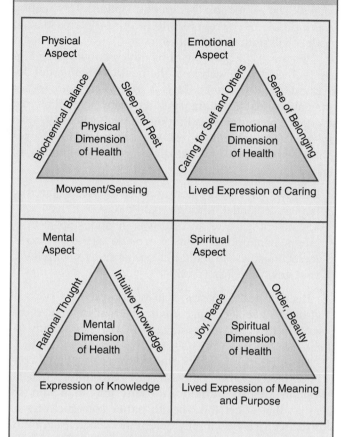

Adapted from "Mutual Connectedness: A Study of Client–Nurse Interaction Using the Grounded Theory Method," by P. Schubert and H. Lionberger, *Journal of Holistic Nursing, 13,* 1995. p. 105.

sense is missing, others become more acute. Physical exercise is addressed later in this chapter, and the student is encouraged to pursue further study in the area of expressive arts and dance for understanding of body–mind integration.

Emotional Aspect

Emotions affect the physical body, mental capacity, and spiritual development. Health behavior choice involves one's relationships with self and others. The emotional aspect of health includes caring for and being cared for by others and a sense of belonging. **Social support** (resources provided to a person by others, such as affection, indications of belonging, emotional support, and actual material goods, when needed) has been shown to be fundamental to health (Gullette & Blumenthal, 1999).

Holding oneself and others in high esteem is a hallmark of good emotional health. **Self-esteem** (feelings about oneself and how one measures up to that which one expects) is important in health behavior choice; in fact, lack of self-esteem is a major motivating factor in

self-destructive behaviors. The need to belong—to be a part of a couple, a family, or a group—is also key. Feeling isolated, alone, and without social support contributes to both physical and mental illness.

Expression of caring is necessary for harmony and balance in the person–environment interrelationship. Lack of such expression creates conflict and disharmony in relationships. An open heart reveals qualities of caring and nourishes relationships as well as one's own health and the health of others.

Mental Aspect

The mental aspect refers to a person's need to learn and to express knowledge gained from the person–environment experience. Knowledge is gained through both intuition and rational thought processes. Knowledge also seeks expression in the person's lived experience. The mental aspect shapes information provided by the physical, mental, emotional, and spiritual aspects into thoughts, beliefs, values, and understandings that shape belief systems upon which lives are built.

Intuitive knowledge refers to direct knowing or learning of something without the conscious use of rational thought or reasoning. Much knowledge from the everyday world is obtained in this way. Although some of this knowledge is tested by logical, rational thought, more goes unquestioned because it is simply recognized and accepted.

Rational thought is based on reasoning. For example, careful consideration is given to the events leading to an unexpected outcome in order to determine the thing or things that change the expected outcome. This kind of careful consideration of cause and effect is highly valued in science and in Western culture as a whole. Although scientific thought is based on reason, reasoning is limited to a single cause and effect. In an orientation to integrated wholeness, such thought becomes increasingly difficult because there are limitless variables in the life experience. Reason is also valued highly in Eastern cultures, but in these cultures, reasoning involves the holistic, or integrated, perspective that allows for many causes and effects.

Critical thinking requires both intuitive and rational skills. All information obtained from any source is considered. Intuition and reasoning are equally important, with each providing a valuable means of testing knowledge and understanding.

Because knowledge is shared through activities such as building, teaching, communicating, sharing, and writing, expression of knowledge is also valued as a means to interrelatedness and person–environment integration.

Spiritual Aspect

Spirituality lifts daily experience into a higher dimension of consciousness. Spirituality, as discussed in Chapter 8, actually permeates all of one's being; in addition to being an aspect of oneself, spirituality is the core and the essence of being. It is therefore reflected as both a part or aspect of the person and the whole. Emotional aspects of health, discussed previously, nurture one's spiritual growth through the lived experiences of caring, compassion, and belonging as they lead to an experience of unity.

Spiritual health is reflected in a sense of deep joy and peace that may or not be related to external events. Faith in a higher order, a sense of oneness with all that is good or divine, and a belief that there is purpose in this life and that the individual's life is in harmony with that purpose are characteristic of the spiritual aspect. Joy, beauty, and life meaning and purpose seem to be areas of need experienced by all persons regardless of belief in a Supreme Being.

The mutual connectedness model for clinical practice seems to be consistent with the assumptions and conceptual frameworks of Martha Rogers (1990) and Margaret Newman (1994). These models encourage intervention strategies wherein the nurse gives appropriate support and assistance to the client as the client sets his or her own goals and works to meet them. The nurse who views health as a developmental process is less apt to rely on the practice of giving advice and information and instead will emphasize caring support and encouragement. The client is thus empowered, and creativity is strengthened.

Creativity is the expression of one's unique way of being in the world. The expression of one's totality—of one's blueprint of experience—is reflected in the creative act. Creativity is not limited to art, music, poetry, sculpture, or pottery. It means drawing upon one's own resources, capacities, and roots. It means facing life directly and honestly, courageously searching for and discovering while experiencing grief, joy, suffering, pain, struggle, conflict, and inner solitude.

Although health behavior choice is only one of the many complex factors that determine health status, it is a significant determinant. Because health education programs are established to influence health behavior choice, and because nurses develop and teach such programs, some potentially useful conceptual frameworks are presented next.

Pender's Health Promotion Model

Pender's (2002) model of health promotion encourages the use of **integrative models of health** (see Figure 11-7), which take a broad biopsychosocial view of human health phenomena. Clinical indicators in such models are numerous and include interpersonal behavior, social support, socioeconomic status, mood state, cognitive efficiency, symptom complaints, hormone levels, neurotransmitter breakdown products, neurochemical sub-

strates, immunoglobulin status, or any combination of the preceding. Human response patterns may be identified to determine predictors of healthy or unhealthy outcomes. The scope of therapeutic options for treating health problems or responses to health problems in such models will undoubtedly enlarge.

Pender's (2002) model of health promotion (see Figure 11-7) is a modification of the health belief model developed by Rosenstock (1966) to predict the use of preventive health actions such as going to a clinic for screening procedures and modified by Becker (1974) to predict other preventive behaviors. Pender (1996) integrates stabilization and actualization in a definition of health:

> Health is the actualization of inherent and acquired human potential through goal-directed behavior, competent self-care, and satisfying relationships with others while adjustments are made as needed to maintain structural integrity and harmony with relevant environments. (p. 22)

Because health is reflected in the context of the person–environment relationship, environmental influences are pivotal in health processes. Figure 11-1 reflects many influences on health status.

Health is increasingly being viewed as a cultural concept defined in various ways according to cultural beliefs. Although **health behaviors** (behaviors exhibited by persons that affect their health either constructively or destructively) are culturally determined, increasing numbers of people are seeking **wellness** (a state of health accompanied by a sense of exuberant well-being) through commitment to lifestyles that promote health and, thereby, reduce risk of premature death and disability.

Although the same positive health behaviors are employed for both **health promotion** and **health protection (disease prevention),** definitions of these terms differ. Pender (1996) defines disease prevention as health protection:

> Health protection is directed toward decreasing the probability of experiencing health problems by active protection against pathologic stressors or detection of health problems in the asymptomatic stage. Health protection focuses on efforts to move away from or avoid the negatively valanced states of illness and injury. . . . Health promotion is directed toward increasing the level of well-being and self-actualization of a given individual or group. Health promotion focuses on efforts to approach or move toward a positively valanced state of high-level health and well-being. (Pender, 1996, p. 34)

Pender's (1996) model provides a tool for "exploring complex biopsychosocial processes that motivate individuals to engage in behaviors directed toward the enhancement of health" (p. 51). Whereas in the Rosenstock

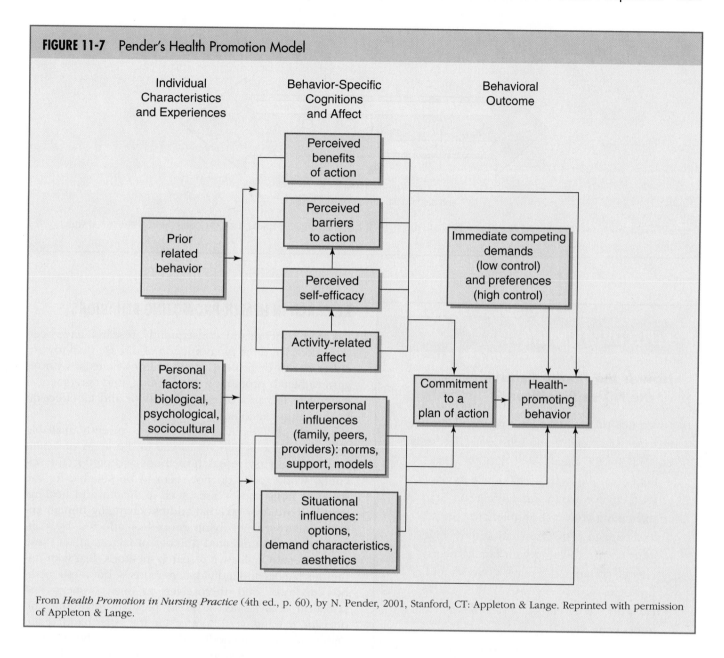

FIGURE 11-7 Pender's Health Promotion Model

From *Health Promotion in Nursing Practice* (4th ed., p. 60), by N. Pender, 2001, Stanford, CT: Appleton & Lange. Reprinted with permission of Appleton & Lange.

model, perceived threat was viewed as a motivator, Pender argued that although immediate threats to health may serve to motivate action, threats in the distant future lack the same motivational strength. Because adolescents and young adults tend to see themselves as invulnerable to illness, perceived threat has been replaced in Pender's model by perceived potentiality. And given that the Pender model relies on perceived potentiality as a motivator for health behavior choice, the model has applicability throughout the life span.

Pender's efforts to test and refine the health promotion model strengthen nursing science by broadening knowledge of health and health behavior choice. Refinement increases the model's potential use in prediction and intervention with regard to health behavior choice.

Travis's Wellness Model

Ryan and Travis (1981) address a continuum of health, ranging from high-level wellness at one end to premature death at the other end. In the middle of the continuum (see Figure 11-8) is a state void of physical signs and symptoms *and* of a sense of well-being. The center is where "many people lack physical symptoms but are bored, depressed, tense, anxious or generally unhappy with their lives. These emotional states often lead to physical disease through the lowering of the body's resistance" (p. 2).

This illness-wellness continuum was adapted by Edelman and Mandle (1998) to reflect differences between illness- and wellness-oriented care. As the client moves to the right of the neutral point, increasing levels of health and well-being are experienced; as the client

FIGURE 11-8   Wellness-Illness Continuum

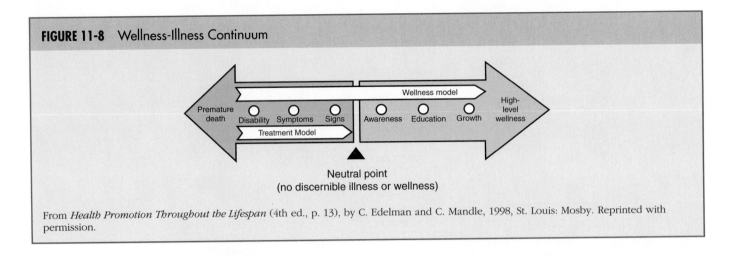

From *Health Promotion Throughout the Lifespan* (4th ed., p. 13), by C. Edelman and C. Mandle, 1998, St. Louis: Mosby. Reprinted with permission.

REFLECTIVE THINKING

How Is the Health Behavior of the Nurse Significant?

Given that role modeling is a powerful teaching tool (see Chapter 10) and self-care is necessary not only for the client but also for the nurse:

- Reflect on the circle of influence in your own environment (see Figure 11-1). Start by examining your responsibility to yourself and expand your examination to include your responsibility to your family, peers, clients, communities, nation, world, and universe.
- How does your choice of health behaviors affect your client?

moves toward the left, decreasing health and disease-oriented care are experienced (Edelman & Mandle, 1998).

It is important to realize that many people, especially elders and those who are disabled, live in states of wellness yet are physically handicapped, chronically ill, or dying. Thus, wellness does not depend solely on physical functioning. In wellness-oriented care, the focus is on awareness, education, and growth, whereas in disease- or illness-oriented care, the focus is on treating signs, symptoms, and disability. Although the wellness model does take symptoms into account, the overall perspective is one of education, healing, and wholeness. This model is frequently used as a conceptual model for health promotion services.

The haiku in Figure 11-9 reflects an understanding of health as the total experience of life and living.

RESEARCH IN HEALTH-PROMOTING BEHAVIORS

Far more concern and, consequently, research have been directed toward the phenomenon of disease than toward either health or healing. Many unknowns exist with regard to health promotion and healing, and agreement is lacking in the area of health behavior and its effect on health status outcomes.

Some philosophical issues make currently available research methods difficult to use in the areas of health and healing. First, research methods accepted in the scientific world today do not seem to be suitable for the study of holistic processes such as health and healing. Required are methods that address changing human energy patterns as evolving processes affected by consciousness. An unlimited number of factors affect these phenomena. Qualitative research methods deal with numerous factors and individual responses, but these methods do not lend themselves to measurement and statistical analysis as those in program planning and decision making would prefer. On the other hand, quantitative research methods ordinarily used in health studies depend on isolation of one or several variables that can be measured and analyzed statistically. See the Research Focus box for an assessment of research methods used to study health behavior changes over the past decade.

Second, guidelines for health behavior choice have been developed for application to whole populations and large numbers of people, even though individuals differ in their responses to any variable or set of variables. In this sense, each person is his or her own experiment in health and healing. For example, whereas most persons seem to do well by eating whole-grain products, others who have allergic responses to gluten or to a certain grain do poorly.

Thoughtful and creative use and development of research methods are needed, especially in the areas of health promotion and healing. Personal experience and

---

FIGURE 11-9   Health: A Haiku

Health is well-being,	Health is fulfillment,	Health is here and now,
Self-actualization,	Ability to perform,	Yesterdays and tomorrows,
Ever-unfolding.	Aggregate powers.	Time continuum.
Health is potential,	Health is adapting,	Health is holistic,
Soaring to greater heights,	Balance with environment,	Integration of oneself,
Becoming one's best.	Equilibrium.	Higher awareness.
Health is energy,	Health is expression,	Health is one's wholeness,
Dynamic and ongoing,	Of one's source and direction,	A process of functioning,
Continuous flow.	Of values and goals.	A state of being.

From Gwen Frostic Prints (undated). Reprinted with permission of Gwen Frostic.

 DECISION MAKING

Clinical Applications of Health and Wellness Models

You are working with a 43-year-old Caucasian male who became quadriplegic as a result of a diving accident 10 years ago. He lives with his wife and two adolescent boys. He has been referred to you because of irritability, sleeplessness, and frequent respiratory infections.

◆ Select one of the wellness and health promotion models described in this section to develop an appropriate plan for application of the nursing process.

---

anecdotal evidence indicate that a positive attitude, playing, having fun, practicing deep relaxation, exercising, and other such activities have a positive effect on health and stimulate healing. On the other hand, depression, guilt, anger, fear, worry, and pretense negatively affect health and healing. Research in this area is currently being conducted in **psychoneuroimmunology** (Friedman, Thomas, Klein & Friedman, 1996), a field of study focusing on the manufacture of neurotransmitters, specifically endorphins and enkephalins, by the brain. Studies have shown that these brain hormones increase with certain behaviors such as laughing, running, meditating, and hugging and that increased hormone levels are accompanied by feelings of well-being and peace (Hardman, Limbrid, Molinoff, Rudder, & Goodman-Gilman, 1996).

These findings are rich in potential for application to health promotion and healing.

HEALTH BEHAVIORS FOR HEALTH PROMOTION AND DISEASE PREVENTION

Behaviors related to nutrition, exercise, sleep, and stress management are significant in preventing disease and disability. Because accidents often happen when people are stressed or sleep deprived, preventive behaviors also include those that address safety. Stressed people are often hurried and distracted and may ignore safety precautions and regulations made by society to protect human health. A distracted mind and a lack of concentration or mindfulness in the present may also contribute to accidents. The practice of meditation helps to focus the mind, develop concentration, and promote calmness.

Health behavior change is generally considered an area of personal responsibility, yet social responsibility for health behavior change is also important and includes provision for educational information and programs, equipment, and social support to encourage positive health. Some of the most common problem health behaviors are related to consumption of unhealthy diets, overeating, lack of exercise, smoking, abusing drugs and alcohol, inadequate sleep, poor stress coping, and maintaining dysfunctional relationships. Many individuals make frequent attempts to change their behavior or lifestyle but eventually return to former habits.

The transtheoretical model of change (Velicer, Prochaska, Fava, Norman, & Redding, 1998), a theory of behavior change, has served as an integrative model for the development of effective health behavior change. The central organizing construct of the model is the Stages of

RESEARCH FOCUS

Impact on Health of Workplace Health Promotion Programs and Methodologic Quality of Research Literature

Study Problem/Purpose

To conduct a comprehensive review of the published research literature on health promotion programs in workplace settings. The purpose was (1) to determine the impact of health promotion programs and (2) to assess the quality of the research methods used for such study.

Methods

Published reports related to workplace health promotion programs were found by searching databases. The search identified 383 studies published between 1968 and 1995 and were distributed to and critiqued by experts. Studies of health behavior programs addressed smoking, hypertension, stress, weight control, nutrition and cholesterol, exercise, safety belt use, health risk appraisals, alcohol use, HIV and AIDS, and multicomponent programs. Study methods were rated conclusive, acceptable, indicative, suggestive, or weak according to a set of criteria.

Findings

Outcome measures revealed that health promotion programs *usually* produce short-term changes in knowledge, *often* produce changes in behavior, and *sometimes* produce changes in health, but there was little evidence of permanent behavior change. The researcher concluded from the studies that it is realistic to expect short-term changes and maintenance of adopted behaviors only as long as participants are enrolled in the programs.

Evaluation of the study methods revealed that 27% of the studies were conducted with randomized control groups and 21% were properly conducted with nonrandomized comparison groups. This finding was considered by the authors as comparable or superior to the body of literature supporting outcomes of medical interventions, although rankings were low in studies related to HIV and AIDS, alcohol use, health risk appraisal, seat belt use, and exercise programs.

Implications

A similar review and study of the health promotion literature in 1986 had received a much less favorable rating. The authors of this study were quite encouraged to find that the quality of health promotion research had made such progress during the last decade.

The author of this report encourages studies that include comparison groups (quasi-experimental design), and especially randomly assigned control groups (experimental design). Studies were ranked according to their designs: experimental (five stars), quasi-experimental (four stars), and nonexperimental (two to three stars). The differences in rigor significantly impacted outcome measurements. Outcomes for the nonexperimental groups measured 100% mostly positive, the quasi-experimental groups 56% mostly positive, and the experimental groups 26% mostly positive. To achieve this level of success, nonexperimental studies had to show only statistical significance in most of the outcome measures. The success rate determined for the quasi-experimental studies was less because the programs not only had to show some improvement in most of the outcome measures, but improvement had to be statistically more significant than the improvements seen in a comparison group. The success rate was lowest for experimental studies because people were randomly assigned to both the intervention group and the control group and to show some improvement in most outcome measures. Improvement in the experimental groups had to be statistically more significant than those improvements seen in a control group.

Source: O'Donnell, M. P. (1999). The impact on health of workplace health promotion programs and the methodologic quality of the research literature. In J. Rippe (Ed.), Lifestyle medicine (pp. 920–927). Malden, MA: Blackwell Science.

Change (see Figure 11-10 for a description of the five stages). The research related to the use of this model and behavioral outcomes is extensive. Health behaviors studied are smoking cessation, exercise, low-fat diet, radon testing, alcohol abuse, weight control, condom use for HIV protection, organizational change, use of sunscreen, drug abuse, medical compliance, mammography screening, and stress management. (See related websites for more information.)

Smoking and drug and alcohol use and abuse are addressed in Chapter 31 and other problem behaviors in Chapter 27. Health behaviors related to dietary intake,

FIGURE 11-10 The Five Stages of Behavioral Change

- **Precontemplation** is the stage in which people are not intending to take action in the foreseeable future, usually measured as the next six months. People may be uninformed or underinformed about the consequences of their behavior. Or they may have tried to change a number of times and become demoralized about their ability to change.

- **Contemplation** is the stage in which people are intending to change in the next six months. They are more aware of the pros of changing but are also acutely aware of the cons. This balance between the costs and benefits of changing can produce profound ambivalence that can keep people stuck in this stage for long periods of time.

- **Preparation** is the stage in which people are intending to take action in the immediate future, usually measured as the next month. They have typically taken some significant action in the past year and have a plan of action.

- **Action** is the stage in which people have made specific overt modifications in their lifestyles within the past six months. People must attain a criterion that scientists and professionals agree is sufficient to reduce risks for disease.

- **Maintenance** is the stage in which people are working to prevent relapse but they do not apply change processes as frequently as do people in action. They are less tempted to relapse and increasingly more confident that they can continue their change.

From "Detailed Overview of the Transtheoretical Mode," adapted for Cancer Prevention Research Center website from "Smoking Cessation and Stress Management: Applications of the Transtheoretical Model of Behavior Change," by W. F. Velicer, J. O. Prochaska, J. L. Fava, G. J. Norman, and C. A. Redding, 1998, pp. 2–3, *Homeostasis, 38*, pp. 216–233. Available: http://www.uri.edu/research/cprc/TTM/detailedoverview.htm.

exercise, sleep, and stress management are included in this chapter. Overweight and obesity are discussed as risk factors for children and adults in Chapters 22 and 23. See the *Healthy People 2010* website for objectives related to health behavior of U.S. citizens.

Nutrition in the U.S. American Diet

Eating habits affect almost every aspect of one's life—appearance, energy, stamina, resistance to illness, mental outlook, stress level, and academic and social success. Healthy eating, then, requires not only knowledge of nutrition but also an understanding of oneself and an awareness of how different foods affect one's sense of wellness. Dysfunctional eating may be the result of social, emotional, or educational barriers.

Although a nutritionally adequate diet is not difficult to accomplish for most people in the United States, many

who have the necessary resources to do so just do not get the nutrition they need. This seems to be a cultural issue in that people do not plan their meals for adequate nutrition. U.S. Americans tend to eat whatever is fast, convenient, and affordable, even though this diet is associated with poor health status.

The U.S. Department of Agriculture (USDA) Center for Nutrition Policy and Promotion studies (1998) revealed that only 12% of U.S. Americans eat a diet close to the recommendations made in the *Dietary Guidelines for Americans* (USDA/DHHS, 2000a) (see Figure 11-11) (a score above 80%). Twelve percent eat a poor diet (a score below 51%) and 71% have diets that need improvement (a score between 51% and 80%) based on these guidelines. People score lowest on the fruits component (17%) of the *healthy eating index (HEI)* and the milk component (26%). They found that women generally eat a healthier diet than men; older people eat a healthier diet than younger people; and people with more education eat healthier than those with less education. Their findings clearly illustrate the importance of nutrition education as a tool to help improve people's diets (Lino, Basiotis, Anand, & Variyam, 1998).

The USDA guidelines and corresponding pyramid encourages consumption of more grains and fewer meats, sweets, and fats, with a broad area representing grains and a narrow area representing sweets and fats to emphasize the relative importance of those foods and the others that were placed between them on the pyramid. See Figure 11-12 for serving size recommended for use with the Food Guide Pyramid.

The Daily Food Guide used in Canada takes the form of a rainbow but conveys essentially the same information as that on the Food Guide Pyramid. Both the Daily Food Guide and the Food Guide Pyramid can be easily adapted to include foods from different cultures. (Although fruits, vegetables, and grains as well as the way foods are prepared may vary across cultures, they still correspond to these food guides.)

Vegetarian Diets

A planned vegetarian diet can easily provide the body's nutritional needs. There are four types of vegetarian diets: a **lacto-ovovegan diet,** which includes both dairy products and eggs; a **lactovegan diet,** which includes dairy products but no eggs; an **ovovegan diet,** which includes eggs but no dairy; and a **vegan diet,** which consists solely of grains, legumes, nuts, seeds, fruits, and vegetables and must be supplemented with vitamin B_{12}.

People choose to be vegetarians for various reasons, including:

- Religious and philosophical concerns related to killing or abusing animals.

- Environmental concerns. It takes approximately 10 pounds of livestock feed to produce 1 pound of

FIGURE 11-11 The Food Guide Pyramid: A Guide to Daily Food Choices

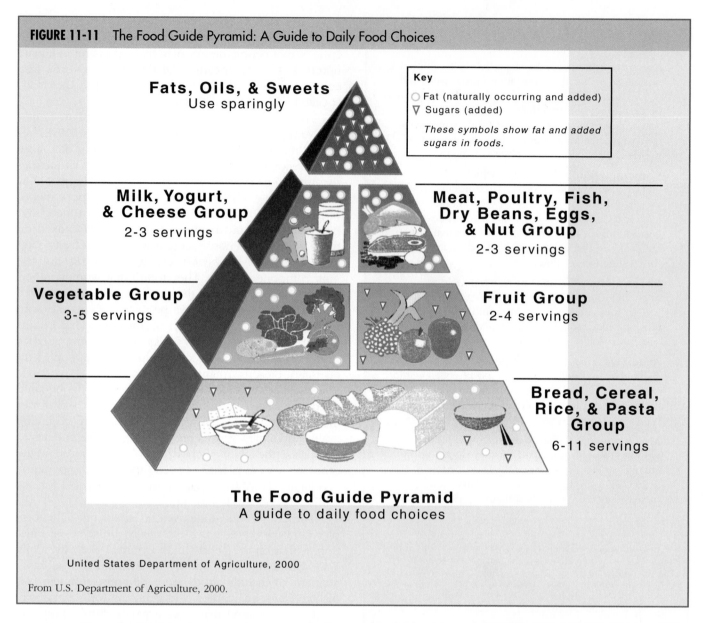

Fats, Oils, & Sweets
Use sparingly

Key
○ Fat (naturally occurring and added)
▽ Sugars (added)

These symbols show fat and added sugars in foods.

Milk, Yogurt, & Cheese Group
2-3 servings

Meat, Poultry, Fish, Dry Beans, Eggs, & Nut Group
2-3 servings

Vegetable Group
3-5 servings

Fruit Group
2-4 servings

Bread, Cereal, Rice, & Pasta Group
6-11 servings

The Food Guide Pyramid
A guide to daily food choices

United States Department of Agriculture, 2000

From U.S. Department of Agriculture, 2000.

meat. Thus, the food it takes to make 1 pound of meat would serve several people in this time of world hunger being so great.

- Health benefits. When foods are balanced and nutrients are combined from a variety of foods, the result is a very healthful vegetarian diet. Health benefits of a vegetarian diet are (1) a lower intake of saturated fatty acids, (2) a higher intake of dietary fiber, and (3) a higher intake of antioxidant nutrients (Old Ways Preservation & Trust, 1999–2001).

Although there are nutritional benefits to the vegetarian diet, potential complications include (1) iron deficiency anemia in women; (2) vitamin B$_{12}$ deficiency for vegans (those using no eggs or dairy products); (3) vitamin D deficiency, or rickets, for vegans; and (4) bulky diets (too much fiber) to the extent that many nutrients are

not able to be absorbed from the small intestine. These potential complications are applicable to all persons of all races and genders. When other factors are taken into consideration, additional measures must be taken to ensure adequate nutrition. For example, pregnant or lactating women need more nutrients such as calcium, iron, and folate (Old Ways Preservation & Trust, 1999–2001).

The HEI, discussed earlier, which is determined by how well persons are following the guidelines reflected in the Food Guide Pyramid, was found to be higher for vegetarians than for any other group (USDA/CNPP, 1998). This measure indicates greater care taken by vegetarians to follow a healthy diet.

Vegetarian diets rely mainly on plant foods: grains, vegetables, legumes, fruits, seeds, and nuts. Vegetarians can use food guides but must select meat alternates to fulfill meat requirements (i.e., legumes, seeds, nuts, and tofu). Soy products provide nutrients similar to dairy

---

FIGURE 11-12 What Counts as a Serving

Bread, cereal, rice, and pasta group (grains group)—whole grain and refined

- 1 slice of bread
- About 1 cup of ready-to-eat cereal
- ½ cup of cooked cereal, rice, or pasta

Vegetable group

- 1 cup of raw leafy vegetables
- ½ cup of other vegetables—cooked or raw
- ¾ cup of vegetable juice

Fruit group

- 1 medium apple, banana, orange, pear
- ½ cup of chopped, cooked, or canned fruit
- ¾ cup of fruit juice

Milk, yogurt, and cheese group (milk group)*

- 1 cup of milk** or yogurt**
- 1½ ounces of natural cheese** (such as Cheddar)
- 2 ounces of processed cheese** (such as American)

Meat, poultry, fish, dry beans, eggs, and nuts group (meat and beans group)

- 2–3 ounces of cooked lean meat, poultry, or fish
- ½ cup of cooked dry beans# or ½ cup of tofu counts as 1 ounce of lean meat
- 2½ ounces of soyburger or 1 egg counts as 1 ounce of lean meat
- 2 tablespoons of peanut butter or ⅓ cup of nuts counts as 1 ounce of meat

*This includes lactose-free and lactose-reduced milk products. One cup of soy-based beverage with added calcium is an option for those who prefer a nondairy source of calcium.

**Choose fat-free or reduced-fat dairy products most often.

#Dry beans, peas, and lentils can be counted as servings in either the meat and beans group or the vegetable group. As a vegetable, ½ cup of cooked, dry beans counts as 1 serving. As a meat substitute, 1 cup of cooked, dry beans counts as 1 serving (2 ounces of meat).

From U.S. Department of Agriculture/Department of Health and Human Services, 2000a.

---

products, especially if they have been fortified with calcium, vitamin D, and vitamin B$_{12}$. A vegetarian diet requires the use of vegetable protein sources, such as soybeans and grains, to prevent protein deficiency (Old Ways Preservation & Trust, 1999–2001).

Nutritional Supplements

Controversy surrounds the supplemental use of vitamins and minerals generally provided by fruits, vegetables, and whole grains. Conventional wisdom holds that a well-balanced diet consisting of plenty of whole foods—whole-grain breads, fresh fruits, and vegetables—supplies the necessary variety and amounts of vitamins and minerals. In this view, supplementation should be necessary only for those people who primarily eat processed foods, in which vitamins and minerals have been destroyed.

Many nutritionists and researchers, however, believe that the recommended dietary allowances (RDAs) for many vitamins and minerals are too low and that it is probably wise to take a well-balanced daily vitamin supplement in addition to following a well-balanced diet. They furthermore contend that other supplements may be needed for treatment and prevention of health problems. Use of nutritional supplements for treatment purposes seems to be increasing, and ongoing research will continue to add to the knowledge base.

Food Safety Concerns

Safe food is addressed in the *Dietary Guidelines for Americans* (USDA/DHHS, 2000a) as food that poses little risk of foodborne illness. Food safety, then, means "safe from harmful bacteria, viruses, parasites and chemical contaminants" (p. 24). See Figure 11-13 for related recommendations for protection of food safety.

The Center for Food Safety and Applied Nutrition of the FDA (January 2001) adds the following as major areas of concern: additives, dietary supplements, food biotechnology, and environmental pollutants such as pesticides. These concerns are introduced as environmental concerns in Chapter 9. The student is referred to the appropriate websites for further details.

Additives

American food manufacturers use thousands of artificial colorings, preservatives, flavorings, and emulsifiers in their products to make foods less expensive, safe to eat, more visually appealing, and easier to store. Certain additives

---

FIGURE 11-13 Food Safety Guidelines

- Build a healthy base by keeping food safe to eat.
- Clean. Wash hands and surfaces often.
- Separate. Separate raw, cooked, and ready-to-eat.
- Cook. Cook foods to a safe temperature.
- Chill. Refrigerate perishable foods promptly.
- Check and follow the label.
- Serve safely. Keep hot foods hot and cold foods cold.
- When in doubt, throw it out.

From U.S. Department of Agriculture/Department of Health and Human Services, 2000a.

help prevent food poisoning. Whereas some additives may be safe, others have not yet been sufficiently tested. Some are associated with allergic reactions and increased risk of cancer (USDA/DHHS, 2000a).

Pesticides in Food

Part of Chapter 9 was devoted to a discussion of environmental pollution and its effect on the food supply. Synthetic pesticides are subject to the approval of the Environmental Protection Agency (EPA) and are applied to fruits and vegetables to kill insects that could damage the crops. Fungicides, the class of pesticides of greatest concern, are applied to extend shelf life and to make produce picture perfect. The EPA (2000) sets tolerance levels for pesticide residues, and the Food and Drug Administration (FDA) enforces the residue-monitoring program.

Food Biotechnology

Agricultural **biotechnology** involves the use of certain scientific techniques, including genetic engineering, to create, improve, or modify plants, animals, and microorganisms. Modern techniques enable scientists to move genes and enhance desirable traits. Intentions guiding such efforts include (1) combating human diseases by developing medicines, (2) promoting human health by boosting nutritional value of foods, (3) combating animal diseases by developing vaccines, (4) fighting hunger by increasing crop yields and developing disease-resistant plants, and (5) helping the environment by reducing pesticide use (USDA, 1999).

The community health nurse must have in-depth knowledge not only of nutritional processes but also of

human responses to the many psychological and cultural issues surrounding food and eating. Because nutrition is a major factor in health and healing, the nurse uses such knowledge daily, when teaching and counseling individuals, families, and groups. Because much is still to be discovered, the nurse's educational process with regard to nutrition should be lifelong.

Physical Exercise

It is essential that our society move from being a sedentary one to one that is more active. At the same time that more and more people are sitting in front of computer screens at work and at schools, schools and universities have cut back on their physical education programs. When budgets are stretched, communities have less money to build and staff parks, recreational areas, and playgrounds. Children and youth find it easier to watch television or play video games than to engage in individual or group physical activity (USDA/DHHS, 2000a). One of the greatest challenges encountered by the

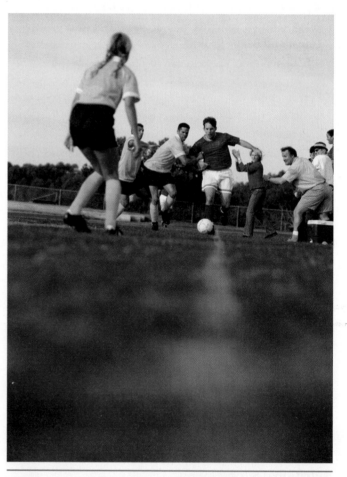

Regular physical activity coupled with proper nutrition and adequate sleep promotes wellness. Examine your own activity, nutrition, and sleep patterns. How could you improve them?

Healthy People 2010 project is getting people to exercise. Although more worksites have workout rooms and exercise programs, the exercise objectives with regard to children and youth are losing ground.

The USDA/DHHS (2000) included exercise guidelines as part of their dietary recommendations. Exercise was stressed in this way because of its role in weight management. An increase in physical activity allows for greater caloric and nutrient intake without weight gain. People are encouraged to apply the principles of variety, balance, and moderation in their selection of activities. Participating in many different physical activities exercises many muscles. The activities chosen should provide an exercise balance, focusing on cardiovascular endurance, muscular strength, bone strength, and flexibility. One should exercise to stay fit without overdoing. Thirty minutes or more of moderate daily exercise most days of the week is generally advised.

Culture is a major determinant of the quantity and quality of exercise. In the past, hunting for food and traveling met this human need in some cultures and civilizations. In more recent times, work on farms and in industrial settings required physical exercise. Recreational activities often involve movement and exercise. Culturally based dances have traditionally offered rich opportunities to be physically active while enjoying the spiritual benefits of dance rituals. African dance, for example, can be aerobic, work upper body muscles, and improve coordination.

In the Western European cultures, walking, jogging, running, bicycling, dancing, and aerobic workouts have become favorites of the middle class. Aerobic exercise practiced according to cardiovascular training principles provides an efficient and effective way to achieve the exercise needed for optimum health.

The best known benefit of physical exercise is **aerobic conditioning,** wherein the heart and lungs are subjected to a *planned* series of exercises that forcefully cause heart and respiration rates to rise rapidly and thus deliver large volumes of blood and oxygen to the cells of the body. See Figure 11-14 for beneficial outcomes of regular aerobic exercise.

People who exercise regularly often report psychological and spiritual benefits such as reduced anxiety, tension, and fatigue and increased vigor and ability to cope with stress. Regular exercise also tends to eliminate depression and improve self-image and self-esteem (Rose & Keegan, 2000).

Sleep and Health Behavior Choice

Adequate sleep is known to enhance attentiveness, concentration, mood, and motivation. Lack of sleep impairs judgment and makes one irritable. Research has shown that sleep deprivation may also play a major role in automobile accidents and in some chronic health condi-

FIGURE 11-14 Benefits of Regular Exercise

Aerobic workouts are used by many to accomplish their fitness goals. Short of planned aerobic workouts, Donna Shalala, Secretary of U.S. Health and Human Services (1995), encouraged citizens to garden, play golf, walk briskly, and use the stairs instead of elevators. These activities can help control weight, improve health, and prevent disease.

The benefits of a regular exercise program include:

- A healthy heart and blood vessels.
- Maintenance of body weight within generally accepted normal limits.
- Prevention and alleviation of chronic low-back pain.
- Improved sleep.
- Greater energy reserve for work and recreation.
- Improved posture, which leads to improved physical appearance and the ability to withstand fatigue.
- Greater ability of the body to cope with illness or accidents.

From *Nutrition and Your Health: Dietary Guidelines for Americans* (4th ed.), U.S. Department of Agriculture/Department of Health and Human Services, 1995, Washington, DC: Author.

tions [National Institute of Neurological Disorders and Stroke/National Institutes of Health (NINDS/NIH), 2000].

Sleep researchers believe that to make more time for other things that crowd their lives the majority of Americans sleep 60–90 minutes fewer a night than is necessary for optimum functioning. Sleep is considered expendable, and less sleep is culturally valued as a sign of ambition and drive (Lindsley & Stephenson, 1999).

When body energy is low and the nervous system is fatigued, the immune system is affected, resulting in more infections and allergies and impaired cognitive functioning and coping ability. The nurse can promote the client's health by teaching and encouraging constructive sleep behavior. Figure 11-15 lists suggestions for addressing sleep problems.

Coping with Stress

Stress is the body's reaction to any stimulant. **Stressors** are the environmental pressures that activate one's **stress response.** These pressures can be either desirable, thereby providing opportunity, or undesirable, thereby posing obstacles to progress. The stress response presents as behavior changes and changes in the autonomic nervous and immune systems. Chronic stress response may precipitate a variety of physical disorders.

Stress has been shown to lead to illness in three different ways: by directly damaging tissues, by leading to self-destructive habits as means of coping (e.g., drug and

FIGURE 11-15 Tips for a Good Night's Sleep

- Set a schedule. Go to bed at a set time each night and get up at the same time each morning.

- Exercise. Try to exercise 20–30 minutes a day 5–6 hours before going to bed.

- Avoid caffeine, nicotine, and alcohol. Sources of caffeine include coffee, chocolate, soft drinks, nonherbal teas, diet drugs, and some pain relievers.

- Relax before bed. A warm bath, reading, or another relaxing routine can make it easier to fall asleep.

- Sleep until sunlight. If possible, wake up with the sun, or use very bright lights in the morning. Sunlight helps the body's internal biological clock reset itself each day.

- Don't lie in bed awake. If you can't get to sleep, don't just lie in bed. Do something else, like reading, watching television, or listening to music, until you feel tired.

- Control your room temperature. Maintain a comfortable temperature in the bedroom.

- See a doctor if your sleeping problem continues. If you have trouble falling asleep night after night, or if you always feel tired the next day, then you may have a sleep disorder and should see a physician. Most sleep disorders can be treated effectively.

Adapted from "When You Can't Sleep: The ABCs of ZZZs," by the National Sleep Foundation, in *Brain Basics: Understanding Sleep,* website for the National Institute of Neurological Disorders and Stroke (NINDS, June, 2000). [On-line]. Available: http://www.ninds.nih.gov/health_and_medical/pubs/ understanding_sleep.

REFLECTIVE THINKING

Stress

- How do you experience stress?
- Which stressful situations in your life can you influence so that they are less stressful?
- Which stressful situations do you believe cannot be changed? How can you better cope with these situations?
- Are you aware of a time when you became ill due to stress? What early signals might you have noticed? What might you have done differently to alter your stress level or your ability to cope?
- How can you distinguish between stress sufficient to provide a challenge for growth and stress sufficient to make you ill?

alcohol use), and/or by failure to recognize the need for lifestyle changes or assistance. During stress, tissue function is altered and neurohormonal changes occur. Tissue changes associated with short-term stress are temporary. Alterations in tissue resulting from long-term stress are often permanent.

Plotnikoff & Faith, (1998) have contributed greatly to the understanding of how stress affects the body and how certain coping behaviors alter stress and its effects. The positive health behaviors discussed here and in other chapters have been found to improve coping ability. These behaviors include a healthy diet; exercise; **deep relaxation** (a state intentionally induced to promote inner-healing processes and rejuvenation) and sleep; conflict resolution; enjoying the beauty of nature; living creatively with joy, meaning, and purpose; and maintaining a strong support system. See Table 11-1 for a comparison of personal characteristics that make one less prone or more prone to stress. See Figure 11-16, tips to help reduce and control stress.

A good social support system depends on the availability of other people who offer care and support, positive social climate (absence of prejudice, racism, and expectations), and institutional support and services. Necessary resources for those who seek help in stressful

TABLE 11-1 Personal Characteristics as Indicators of Proneness to Stress Response

LESS PRONE	MORE PRONE
• Believe they can control their environment	• Believe they lack control
• Perceive life changes to be opportunities for growth	• Feel helpless in the face of change
• Ready and willing to respond to challenges	• In the face of challenges, hold little hope for favorable outcomes
• Optimistic about their ability to succeed	• Seek permission from others prior to acting

Adapted from Health and Wellness: A Holistic Approach *(4th ed., p. 216) by G. Edlin and E. Golanty, 1992, Boston: Jones & Bartlett. Copyright 1992 by Jones & Bartlett.*

FIGURE 11-16 Tips for Reducing or Controlling Stress

Some of these suggestions may help immediately, but if your stress is chronic, it may require more attention and/or lifestyle changes. Determine *your* tolerance level for stress and try to live within these limits. Learn to accept or change stressful and tense situations whenever possible.

- **Be realistic.** If you feel overwhelmed by some activities (yours and/or your family's), learn to say NO!
- **Shed the "superman/superwoman" urge.** No one is perfect, so don't expect perfection from yourself or others.
- **Meditate.** Just 10–20 minutes of quiet reflection may bring relief from chronic stress as well as increase your tolerance to it. Use the time to listen to music, relax, and try to think of pleasant things or nothing.
- **Visualize.** Use your imagination and picture how you can manage a stressful situation more successfully.
- **Take one thing at a time.** For people under tension or stress, an ordinary workload can sometimes seem unbearable. The best way to cope with this feeling of being overwhelmed is to take one task at a time.
- **Exercise.** Regular exercise is a popular way to relieve stress. Twenty to 30 minutes of physical activity benefits both the body and the mind.
- **Hobbies.** Take a break from your worries by doing something you enjoy.
- **Healthy lifestyle.** Good nutrition makes a difference. Limit intake of caffeine and alcohol (alcohol disturbs regular sleep patterns), get adequate rest, exercise, and balance work and play.
- **Share your feelings.** A conversation with a friend lets you know that you are not the only one having a bad day, caring for a sick child, or working in a busy office. Stay in touch with friends and family. Let them provide love, support, and guidance. Don't try to cope alone.
- **Give in occasionally. Be flexible!** Not only will you reduce your stress, you may find better solutions to your problems.
- **Go easy with criticism.** Help may be as close as a friend or spouse. It may be helpful to talk with your doctor, spiritual advisor, or employee assistance professional. They may suggest a visit with a psychiatrist, psychologist, social worker, or other qualified counselor.

From "Stress—Coping with Everyday Problems," Leading the Way for America's Mental Health, by the National Mental Health Association. [On-line]. Available: http://www.nmha.org/infoctr/factsheets/41.cfm. Used with permission.

REFLECTIVE THINKING

Social Support

- List the people you have warm feelings for and feel comfortable with and who nurture you. Think of long-standing friends—friends from school, work, classes, churches, and social or political groups.
- Look at your list of friends. Are there some with whom you would like to reconnect, even in the form of a long-distance relationship?
- Some names may trigger a feeling of wanting to do something for those people—to send a card, a note, a tape, a gift. Note these feelings on another list.
- Make your lists into a diagram—or place the names of the people on a map of the world wherever the people live.
- Put this map in a prominent place. When you glance at it, imagine those people and send them a warm thought or a beautiful color. Do not be surprised if you hear from someone on your list.

CLINICAL IMPLICATIONS

Health promotion is not a primary focus in most nursing settings. Primary prevention is the major emphasis of health education programs. Community health nurses in certain settings such as schools and workplaces do have opportunities to teach individuals and groups in health promotion efforts. Creative, energetic, and entrepreneurial nurses in private practice have more opportunity to practice health promotion.

Preventive work often is done by nurses in homes, schools, workplaces, and community clinics. Community health nursing practice is primarily based on the prevention model. Activities involve primary, secondary, and tertiary care work. This work includes identifying health risks, screening for potential health deviations, providing updated information and general health education, and counseling to gain participation. Although health education programs are multidisciplinary, the community health nurse is crucial to prevention programs.

Community nursing centers (CNCs) have existed since Lillian Wald established the Henry Street Settlement in 1893. These centers are based on nursing models that

situations include appropriate income, food, and shelter; access to information and helping services; and, perhaps, tools and equipment. These are all resources the nurse may be able to offer.

Perspectives...

A COMMUNITY HEALTH NURSE LIVES A HEALTHY LIFESTYLE: IS IT POSSIBLE?

When I was 40 I had a total hysterectomy because of endometriosis. I was given hormone replacement therapy. The effects of this experience on my body, mind, and spirit were negative and severe. About six months later, my joints became swollen and painful. A rheumatologist told me I had rheumatoid arthritis, prescribed aspirin, 80 grams a day, and told me I would have this for the rest of my life. I had been suffering with frequent migraine headaches since I was 11 years old and lived in fear of these regular occurrences; with the only relief coming from prescribed narcotics. In my mid-forties my blood pressure became elevated, another cause for concern.

Now I am 67 and have none of these problems. People have asked me how I got rid of migraines or arthritis and I often have the feeling they are looking for a single, simple solution. It is really a story of long-term lifestyle changes, implemented one at a time as I investigated various healing strategies. The first thing that helped was my belief that I didn't have to live with these ailments and taking such strong medicines. Some of the other things I've done over the years are:

- Consulted health practitioners who had knowledge of alternative—often ancient—therapies (see Chapter 12), e.g., use of herbs, various forms of massage, acupuncture, medical intuition.
- Gradually assuming more responsibility for learning about various aspects of self-care, including increasing awareness of my body's needs and attending to those needs.
- Regular prayer, meditation, and other ways of honoring spirit.

- Spending time in nature regularly.
- Adjusting my work schedule to meet my health needs; some of these are small things like having buffer time between meetings and appointments.
- Starting and being part of a codependency group for four years; I am now much more powerful about my relationships.
- Becoming very proactive in order to better manage my life including being able to develop transformative changes rather than just more or less of the same thing.
- Consulting a counselor whenever I feel I need help with an issue or situation confronting me. Some examples of this are during divorce, after my son and grandson's deaths, before going to the Peace Corps, after returning home, while dealing with an alcoholic daughter.
- Learning and practicing Reiki, an integrative energy balancing therapy (Chapter 12).
- Changing dietary patterns and incorporating a variety of supplements.
- Focusing on becoming a healing presence rather than being concerned with changing others. I have noticed that I carry a peaceful aura with me that seems to change the ambience in different settings.
- Developing interpersonal skill to a high art—group process, collaboration, conflict negotiation, risk taking in the service of learning and greater intimacy—so that interaction, based on love with little fear, becomes tremendously rewarding and joyful and in work situations MAGIC happens!

—Joan Heron, RN, PhD

include nursing services for health promotion and disease prevention. A holistic, client-centered approach with direct access to professional nursing services is provided. Program administration as well as nursing care are provided by professional nurses (usually advanced practice nurses). Nursing models of care are used to "diagnose and treat human responses to potential and actual health problems, and promote health and optimal functioning among target populations and communities" [American Nurses' Association (ANA), 1987]. The centers, in most cases, provide care for underserved populations and are usually connected with schools of nursing (Neuman, 1995). The Community Nursing Center (CNC) of the

University of Rochester School of Nursing was created using the Neuman systems model as its conceptual model (see website). Services include (1) those associated with life transitions such as birthing, parenting, puberty and adolescence, midlife changes, aging, divorce, and death; (2) those designed to enhance quality of life for individuals and families experiencing chronic illness, physical and/or developmental disabilities, and aging; (3) expert consultation, clinical case management services, staff development and health education programs, and employee wellness programs for community organizations, businesses, and health care providers; and (4) those designed for informal caregivers in life-altering crises such as Alzheimer's patients and survivors of trauma (Hinton Walker, 1991; in Neuman, 1995). These nursing centers will, hopefully, take a larger role in the health care delivery of the future.

Primary Prevention

Primary prevention refers to those activities carried out to prevent disease, disability, and injury. Health education is a major strategy in primary prevention. Research has indicated that health education affects health behavior choice and change under certain conditions (O'Donnell, 1999). Multifaceted programs are needed to address varied needs. Colorful, fast-moving, and interactive presentations appeal to a public accustomed to television and telecommunication. Learning within the context of a caring relationship, though, is important because health behavior is personal. Chapter 10 discusses effective social environments for learning.

Community health nurses are seeking ways to be increasingly creative in their approaches to health education. Some ideas are offered here to stimulate imaginative and creative strategies to make teaching and learning fun for clients and groups of clients.

The therapeutic use of story is an enjoyable and effective tool in health education programs. **Story telling** is the sharing of stories from one person to another. Clients naturally tell their stories as they give their life histories, and nurses convey stories of how other clients have coped or experienced success with challenges they have faced. Stories also provide myth and metaphor for the unconscious mind as it seeks healing through symbolic meanings. People create their own meanings in relation to the stories they hear, making stories powerful tools for healing. Appreciation of cultural diversity and cultural understanding is effectively taught through story telling (Rew, 2000).

Television offers a powerful tool for education of the general public. There has been grave concern in recent years that children are being taught to value violence through television's use. It seems likely that life-affirming values could also be taught on television. Such values might be equally influential in society and help to teach positive health behaviors. To this end, creative and artistic nurses can offer educational programming for health education.

Local television stations offer opportunities for innovative programming. Nurses can take advantage of such opportunities to deliver primary prevention to large and targeted populations. A children's puppet show, for example, could tell the tale of Cindy's strep throat, or a health education program could include a community health nurse and a primary physician or nurse practitioner as cohosts. Because many families have access to video cassette recorders (VCRs), video production also provides opportunities.

The nurse may also use creative abilities to write for magazines or develop pamphlets, comic books, television scripts, or plays. For example, Kaiser Foundation Health Education in California developed a play in which teens demonstrate how lack of openness and knowledge can contribute to the spread of sexually transmitted diseases.

Computer communication is an increasingly valuable resource for health education as more and more people acquire this technology. The computer-savvy nurse can write educational computer programs and use graphic design software to develop visual teaching aids. The opportunities for community health education are great. Community health nurses must continue working with public health and volunteer agencies such as the American Cancer Society, the American Heart Association, American Lung Association, the American Red Cross, and the American Diabetes Association to reach people at health fairs, classes, and counseling. At the same time, nurses must address the technological influences in society through creative development of educational programs using today's technology (Rankin & Stallings, 2000).

Finally, nurses teach by modeling healthy behavior; exhibition of destructive health behaviors undermines credibility of the teacher. Modeling is a powerful tool, as the nurse goes beyond "illness" or "disease" care and guides clients to health and high-level wellness. This extension is necessary as social awareness shifts from a disease orientation to one of health and wellness and as costs of disease care rise.

Secondary Prevention

Secondary prevention refers to those activities related to early detection and treatment. It focuses on clinical screening to detect disease in its early stages and involves in-depth interviewing, history taking, and physical examination. While engaged in these processes, the well-educated, alert, psychologically astute, and culturally sensitive nurse uses observational skills to detect persons who are either at risk or show early signs of disease. Identification of **risk factors** (precursors to disease that increase one's risk of the disease) is a crucial aspect of community health nursing practice.

History taking provides the foundation for identification of risk factors, and this process continues for the length of the nurse–client relationship. With the deepening of relationship, client comfort increases. Concomitant sharing of private health beliefs and lifestyle facilitates continued revelation of risk factors. Ignorance of risk factors greatly increases the risk of developing certain diseases (Thibodeaux & Patton, 1997). When a client is identified as being at risk, appropriate laboratory tests are then conducted. Data from the history and laboratory tests are then combined to determine the need for further intervention or referral. When a client is found to have a

COMMUNITY NURSING VIEW

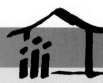

Eiswari Osler is a divorced, 57-year-old woman. Her two daughters are grown, live in distant cities, are busy with families of their own, and call their mother approximately once a month. Eiswari works in a very busy accounting office, shouldering heavy responsibilities and working long hours. She is also active in several community organizations, filling her time with activities.

Eiswari attended a community nursing clinic for a routine physical because one of her friends worked there as a nurse. She completed a computerized health risk appraisal and was interviewed by the nurse, who took a thorough health history. The nurse identified and recorded the following lifestyle factors that placed Eiswari at risk for certain health conditions.

Physical: Walks one block each morning from her car to the office. She has a very full schedule and has not planned for further exercise. She says she enjoys these brief walks and enjoyed swimming when she was younger.

Psychological: Feels intense pressure from being in a middle-management position at work. States she feels angry a lot but tries not to lash out, and she does not have a good way to express her anger. States she has been thinking about joining a support group for women in management positions.

Sociological/physical: Has four or five female friends who exchange phone calls and meet her for lunch from time to time. Attends many social events associated with work and her community-organization activities. Tends to eat fatty, salted foods with others at work and at social events because these snack foods are always available. Smokes one pack per day and drinks scotch and water after work and at social events. Takes Valium three or four times a day for stress.

Spiritual: States she has not identified her life meaning or purpose. She simply wants to save enough money for her older years so that she will not be a burden to her children.

Environmental: Lives in the inner city and states she is concerned about traffic and safety in the streets. She carries a beeper that makes a loud noise in her purse in case of attack.

Nursing Considerations

Assessment

♦ You find that her physical examination is essentially negative. What, if any, tests (other than physical) might be indicated in her assessment?

Diagnosis

♦ Based on the information you have, what nursing diagnoses might you identify?

♦ What risk factors are inherent in Eiswari's situation?

♦ For what diseases and/or conditions would you expect her to be at risk?

Outcome Identification

♦ What are the client's goals for health behavior change?

♦ How can you help her set realistic goals?

♦ What are signs of accomplishment? Discouragement?

♦ How can you encourage and support her progress?

Planning/Interventions

♦ What strategies would you use for building a therapeutic relationship with Eiswari?

♦ How might you initiate development of a treatment plan and a contract with her?

♦ What is she choosing to work on?

♦ Does she wish to change any of her health behaviors?

♦ How will you introduce your concerns, or will you introduce them? (Refer to Chapter 10 for the mutual problem-solving process nursing checklist and follow the suggestions there.)

♦ What specific nursing therapies could you use?

♦ How would you use teaching? Counseling? Deep relaxation or guided imagery? Touch therapies?

♦ Where would you start with an educational program?

♦ What medical or community health programs might be appropriate referrals for Eiswari?

Evaluation

♦ What indicators might help you determine whether the plan is working for Eiswari?

♦ How will you know whether the plan is successful?

subclinical communicable disease, a case-finding interview to determine the number and type of contacts provides information leading to new cases.

Tertiary Prevention

Tertiary prevention is directed toward preventing chronicity and disability in the light of full-blown disease. It is appropriate in acute diseases such as pneumonia and in degenerative diseases such as diabetes, which can lead to breakdown of organ systems and other body tissues and, thus, impede performance and functioning. Degenerative diseases can be caused by genetic factors (cystic fibrosis), continuous infection (chronic ear infections), toxins (lung cancer and smoking), repeated injuries (arthritis), and/or aging or the "normal" wear and tear of life (decreased muscle size and bone density).

Nursing activities include health education related to taking medication, receiving or self-administering treatments and procedures, and follow-up care. In counseling and educative roles, the nurse reexplains, reinforces, and redirects health promotion as well as rehabilitation, or limiting disability to the lowest possible level. Assessment of temporary and permanent damage guides appropriate interventions. Rehabilitation addresses not only the physical but also the spiritual/psychological need to become whole again. Rehabilitation and wellness efforts might include meditation, healthful nutrition, exercise, and psychological/spiritual healing. Prostheses and equipment may be necessary, and self-help support groups, such as Special Olympics for physically and mentally disabled persons, may provide a social tie and reduce feelings of victimization.

Using an integrated model of health promotion (Chapter 12), the community health nurse can help the client identify particular health needs. What are the nutritional needs? Is equipment needed for movement or sensing? Is a stronger support system needed? Is there life meaning and purpose? A need for expression? How can all these needs be met? The client and nurse work together to promote health and healing within a safe, nurturing, caring, and orderly or aesthetically pleasing environment. The aim is to help the client experience higher levels of wellness even when disease is progressive.

KEY CONCEPTS

- A shift is occurring in health care policy that could change the health care delivery system from one focused on disease care to one focused on prevention and health promotion.
- Health promotion is more than the prevention of disease; its focus is to expand consciousness and human potential.

- Lifestyle issues and health behavior choice are major responsibilities of individuals in society.
- Environmental issues and social policy are areas of social responsibility for disease prevention and health promotion.
- Core lifestyle issues and health determinants are related to nutrition, exercise, sleep, and stress management.
- Current methods for health-related research are challenged by the definition of health as a process.
- Health promotion and disease prevention research is limited because current quantitative methods are designed to measure intervention outcomes based on single cause and effect rather than on processes of organization or dynamic wholeness.
- Community health nurses work to help enhance the health status of clients who may fall anywhere along the illness/wellness continuum.
- Nursing serves as a critical link in community health education programs and provides much-needed services to help individuals, families, and populations meet their health needs.

RESOURCES

U.S. GOVERNMENT AGENCIES

Healthy People 2010: http://health.gov/healthypeople,
   http://health.gov/dietaryguidelines,
   http://www.health.gov/healthypeople/Publications/Healthy
   Communities2001
U.S. Department of Health and Human Services (USDHHS):
   http://www.hhs.gov
U.S. Department of Health and Human Services—Mental Health:
   http://www.surgeongeneral.gov/library/mentalhealth
Agency for Healthcare Research and Quality (AHRQ):
   http://www.ahrq.gov
National Institutes of Health: http://www.nih.gov,
   http://www.osteo.org/health
National Institute of Neurological Disorders and Stroke:
   http://www.ninds.nih.gov
Food and Nutrition Information Center:
   http://www.nutrition.gov
U.S. Department of Agriculture (USDA): http://www.usda.gov
U.S. Department of Agriculture Center for Nutrition Policy and
   Promotion: http://www.usda.gov/cnpp
Centers for Disease Control and Prevention (CDC):
   http://www.cdc.gov
National Center for Health Statistics: http://www.cdc.gov/nchs
National Center for Chronic Disease Prevention and Health
   Promotion: http://www.cdc.gov/nccdphp
Administration on Aging: http://www.aoa.dhhs.gov
National Food Safety Programs: http://www.cfsan.fda.gov
National Institute for Occupational Safety and Health:
   http://www.cdc.gov/niosh/stress99.html
Healthfinder: http://www.healthfinder.gov

Environmental Protection Agency (EPA): http://www.epa.gov
Food and Drug Administration (FDA)—Food Safety Programs:
   http://www.FoodSafety.gov
Food and Drug Administration (FDA): http://www.fda.gov

United States Agency for International Development:
   http://www.usaid.gov/pop_health

INTERNATIONAL GOVERNMENTAL HEALTH-RELATED ORGANIZATIONS

World Health Organization: http://www.who.int
Healthy people: Other nation's health:
   http://health.gov/healthypeople/Implementation
Office of Global Health: http://www.cdc.gov/ogh
Office of International and Refugee Health:
   http://www.globalhealth.gov/oirh

NONGOVERNMENTAL HEALTH-RELATED AGENCIES

American Academy of Sleep Medicine: http://www.aasmnet.org
Mayo Clinic: http://www.mayoclinic.com
Old Ways Preservation and Trust: http://oldwayspt.org
Cancer Prevention Research Center (CPRC):
   http://www.uri.edu/research/cprc/TTM
National Mental Health Association (NMHA): http://nmha.org
National Sleep Foundation: http://www.sleepfoundation.org
Internet Healthcare Coalition: http://www.ihealthcoalition.org

Chapter

12

INTEGRATIVE HEALTH CARE PERSPECTIVES

Phyllis E. Schubert, RN, DNSc, MA

MAKING THE CONNECTION

(S)chools of thought that are currently based on seemingly incommensurate world views may well turn out to be closer than seems apparent at present.

—Patel (1987)

COMPETENCIES

Upon completion of this chapter, the reader should be able to:

- Define integrative health care and identify integrative therapies.
- Examine the historical and social perspectives of integrative health care therapies.
- Compare and contrast allopathic health care perspectives with integrative health care perspectives.
- Examine scientific theories thought to provide a foundation for understanding integrative therapies.
- Explain nursing theories that provide a foundation for understanding integrative therapies.
- Delineate safety and effectiveness issues related to frequently used integrative therapies.
- Explain the reasons community health nurses should be knowledgeable about the various integrative therapies and related research.
- Delineate nursing implications for use of integrative health care therapies in nursing.

KEY TERMS

acupoints	integrality
acupressure	integrative therapies
acupuncture	Interactive Guided Imagery
biofeedback training	Jin Shin Jyutsu
centering	Krieger-Kunz method of Therapeutic Touch
chakra	
chi (qi, ki)	
complementary and alternative medicine (CAM)	meridians
	orthomolecular therapies
curing	paradigm
deep relaxation	paradigm shift
guided imagery	quantum theory
healer	relaxation response
healing	resonancy
helicy	safety energy locks
holistic healing therapies	touch therapies
hologram	visualization
human energy field pattern	yang
	yin
imagery	

During the past 30 years or so there has been an emerging interest in **integrative** or **holistic healing therapies** in the Western world. The aim of such therapies is to stimulate healing of the whole person by integrating body, mind, and spirit. The groundswell of interest in these therapies has come from the lay public with gradual acceptance by the medical and other related professions. Nursing has been cautious in its acceptance of integrative therapies yet has embraced the possibilities because its theoretical and conceptual frameworks are concomitant with the aims of these practices. Schools of nursing and of medicine offer courses in integrative therapies under the term **complementary and alternative medicine (CAM).**

CAM is generally defined as those treatments and health care practices not taught widely in medical schools, not generally used in hospitals, and not usually reimbursed by medical insurance companies [National Center for Complementary and Alternative Medicine (NCCAM), 2001a]. The term *alternative* is used when received without medical care and *complementary* when used in conjunction with mainstream medical care.

The term *integrative* is used throughout this chapter to emphasize the nursing perspective that the aim is wholeness, an integration of body, emotions, mind, and spirit. CAM is used as needed when governmental programs and perspectives are addressed. Discussion of integrative therapies is included in this textbook because of the need for community health nurses as well as other health workers to:

- Increase their knowledge related to integrative therapies used by clients.
- Obtain awareness of the legal/regulatory/insurance issues.
- Gain knowledge and ability to advise clients and make decisions about the use of integrative therapies.
- Assist clients by making appropriate referrals and selecting practitioners (NCCAM, 2001b).
- Be familiar with how to use certain integrative therapies as therapeutic tools with individuals and educate families and aggregates in self-care appropriate for individuals, families, and communities.
- Understand the needs of clients for approaches that reflect caring for the whole person.

This chapter addresses the increasing use of integrative therapies, provides an overview of the thought traditions and perspectives for health care and related research issues, and addresses issues of nursing theory, use of integrative therapies in community health nursing, and implications for practice.

The concepts and language used in this chapter reflect perspectives not always consonant with Western thought and culture. Western thought is reflected in a language that emphasizes the relationship between cause and effect, while other perspectives represented here emphasize relationships within systems which include the whole or oneness of everything (Chapter 8). The reader may find the concepts difficult at times and will be challenged to understand the different perspectives.

NATIONAL INTEREST IN COMPLEMENTARY HEALTH CARE

Surveys in 1990 and 1997 reveal that the number of U.S. Americans using CAM rose from about 33% in 1990 to 42% in 1997. Therapies that were reported used most often were herbal medicine, massage, megavitamins, self-help groups, folk remedies, energy healing, and homeopathy. A survey published in 1994 found that more than 60% of doctors from a wide range of specialties had recommended CAM for their clients at least once. In addition, 47% of the physicians in the study reported using CAM themselves. In 1997, U.S. Americans spent more than $27 billion on these therapies, exceeding out-of-pocket spending for all U.S. hospitalizations (Eisenberg et al., 1998).

Astin's (1998) study of why clients are seeking integrative therapies reveals increasing numbers of people doing so, not because they are unhappy with conventional care, but because integrative therapies mirror their own values, beliefs, and philosophical orientations toward health and life. More people seem to be seeking a more holistic orientation to health and are looking for ways, not just to cure their diseases and disorders, but to heal their lives (body-emotions-mind-spirit). Most integrative therapies are used to promote healing of the whole person.

REFLECTIVE THINKING

Why People Are Turning to Integrative Therapies

- Increasing concern with health promotion and wellness as opposed to disease care.
- Distrust and disillusionment with mainstream health care.
- The experience of comfort and peace felt with many such therapies.
- A sense of taking responsibility for oneself.

What do you think? What suggestions would you add to this list?

National Center for Complementary and Alternative Medicine

In 1993 Congress established the Office of Alternative Medicine (OAM) located within the National Institutes of Health (NIH) with an annual budget of $2 million and charged with the responsibility of promoting and supporting research related to the safety and effectiveness of CAM and to disseminate the results to health care providers and public citizens. In 1998, the agency became the National Center for Complementary and Alternative Medicine with an annual budget of $68.7 million in the year 2000 and is expected to exceed $100 million in 2002. This funding increase reflects the public's growing interest and need for information and knowledge of integrative therapies based on rigorous scientific research (NCCAM, 2001c). Director Stephen E. Strauss MD described the purpose of the program thus:

> Many Americans turn to these practices to relieve or prevent disease symptoms or the side effects of their treatment, despite a lack of clear and compelling data about them. We have the scientific tools, the commitment, and the resources to begin to guide their decisions regarding these practices. Consistent with our mandate, we have identified priority areas that warrant more immediate action due to pressing public health needs and either a dearth of valid scientific information or sufficient maturation of the science (NCCAM 2001d).

CAM is a new area for scientific inquiry, and there is great need for both basic and applied or clinical studies. Basic research refers to investigations taking place under controlled conditions in scientific laboratories, and clinical research refers to studies of treatments given in health care settings. CAM research centers are funded by NCCAM and focus on the following public health needs: drug addiction, aging and women's health, arthritis, craniofacial disorders, cardiovascular diseases, neurological disorders and pediatrics. Information about the research centers may be found on-line at http://nccam.nih.gov/nccam/fi/research/centers.html.

NCCAM has grouped CAM practices into five major domains: (1) alternative medical systems, (2) mind-body interventions, (3) biologically based treatments, (4) manipulative and body-based methods, and (5) energy therapies (NCCAM, 2001e). See Figure 12-1 for examples of each domain.

Safety and Effectiveness

Concerns regarding safety and effectiveness of integrative therapies apply to three areas: safety and effectiveness of the treatment, expertise and qualifications of the practitioner, and quality of the service delivery. Although efforts are underway to gather systematic data relevant to

FIGURE 12-1 Major Domains of Complementary and Alternative Medicine

- Traditional oriental medicine: acupuncture, herbal medicine, Oriental massage, qi gong
- Ayurvedic medicine: diet, exercise, meditation, herbs, massage, exposure to sunlight, and controlled breathing
- Other traditional medical systems: Native American, Aboriginal, African, Middle Eastern, Tibetan, Central and South American
- Homeopathy
- Naturopathy: diet and clinical nutrition; homeopathy; acupuncture; herbal medicine; hydrotherapy; spinal and soft-tissue manipulation; physical therapies involving electric currents, ultrasound, and light therapy; therapeutic counseling; pharmacology
- Mind-body interventions: meditation; certain uses of hypnosis, dance, music, and art therapy; prayer and mental healing
- Biological-based therapies: dietary supplements—herbal, special dietary, orthomolecular, and individual biological therapies
- Manipulative and body-based methods: chiropractic manipulation, osteopathic manipulation, massage therapy
- Energy therapies: qi gong, reiki, therapeutic touch
- Bioelectromagnetic-based therapies: pulsed fields, magnetic fields, alternating current or direct current fields

From NCCAM, 2000b.

these areas of concern, few data are currently available to help clinicians and clients make appropriate decisions.

A major issue of concern is that clients do not tell their conventional health professionals that they are using alternative therapies. In fact, one survey revealed that over 75% of those who use integrative services did not tell their physicians (Eisenberg et al., 1998; Spiegel et al., 1998). Although clients tend not to share this information, neither do health professions ask if they are using integrative therapies. Health professionals are becoming increasingly comfortable, though, with making referrals for integrative care when there is likelihood the client will benefit from the treatment and the practitioner is experienced and licensed.

Health professions in the West must have a body of literature based on rigorous scientific study of integrative therapies before integrative therapies can be approved and accepted into mainstream health care. A sense of fairness requires that clients have access to alternative therapies known to be safe, effective, and appropriate for specific conditions. However, clinical research has been quite limited and there are few data available to support

requests for fair access. For example, there is great concern related to safety and efficacy of unproven practices, especially when used with children and pregnant women (Sugarman & Burk, 1998).

Strauss, Director of NCCAM (2000a), shared his vision for the future of integrative medicine in this way:

> I am confident that NCCAM's leadership will stimulate both conventional and CAM communities to conduct compelling scientific research. Several therapeutic and preventative modalities currently deemed elements of CAM will prove effective. Based on rigorous evidence, these will be integrated into conventional medical education and practice, and the term "complementary and alternative medicine" will be superseded by the concept of "integrative medicine." The field of integrative medicine will be seen as providing novel insights and tools for human health, and not as a source of tension that insinuates itself between and among practitioners of the healing arts and their patients. Modalities found to be unsafe or ineffective will be rejected readily by a well-informed public. (p. 4)

HISTORICAL PERSPECTIVES

During the past few hundred years, conventional medicine has become increasingly mechanical in its treatment approaches, i.e., treating symptoms, diseases, and disorders of body parts. Holistic treatment within this context has included referral to medical specialists for treatment of diseased body parts, to a psychiatrist or psychologist for a troubled mind out of touch with reality, and to a minister for spiritual care. Consumers are turning to integrative therapies that focus on healing and wholeness.

Cultural foundations for integrative therapies are based in ancient cultural beliefs of indigenous people of India, Egypt, Greece, and China (Graham, 1999). These ancient traditions as well as those of modern medicine, the new physics of the past century, and those of Eastern cultures have contributed to these new/old systems of care termed integrative health care.

Ancient Cultural Traditions

Ancient mythology and various teachings reveal a belief that human beings have the inherent capacity to be attuned to nature with instinctive understanding of fundamental life forces and the ability to live in accordance with them. This wisdom is considered intuitive in nature and not a matter of intelligence or reasoning. There is a belief among some modern mystical groups that this wisdom still exists but is limited because the knowledge is beyond the five senses. They believe a much greater reality exists beyond what is immediately apparent. Visionaries, with insight into the true nature of the universe and its mysteries, perceive "an infinite, ever-changing, expanding, indivisible and ultimately indescribably universe of harmonious relationships and interrelationships of which man is part, and which can only be perceived by those so attuned" (Graham, 1999, p. 22).

Western Perspectives

Hippocrates, known as the father of modern medicine, was inspired by this same mystical vision. He viewed health in terms of harmony and adaptation to the environment. He saw disease as an imbalance in the elements of earth, fire, water, and air, which he associated with the qualities of coldness, heat, wetness, and dryness, as affected by thoughts, feelings, emotions and behaviors, climate, polluted water, over- and underactivity, lack of sunlight, and other environmental factors. Thus, health and illness were considered in Hippocratic philosophy to be natural biological phenomena responding to environment, lifestyle, and other factors which can be influenced by therapeutic procedures and wise management of one's life (Graham, 1999).

Since the time of Hippocrates, Western thought moved increasingly toward a belief system very different from that of the ancient traditions, while Eastern culture has continued to evolve from within the ancient worldview. Hence, these perspectives are very different. Integrative therapies are a reflection of the ancient worldview and of the new physics.

Supporters of the Eastern worldview and the new physics express concerns related to Western scientific thought. Some of these concerns involve health and health care perspectives in the United States. Not only has acceptance of science as the purveyor of truth made belief in a Creator increasingly difficult and respect for the Divine gradually disappear from the scientific worldview, but the view of person has become separate from sickness and professional interest has shifted from the person to the disease. Hospitals tend to focus more on the study and treatment of disease processes than on caring for the sick, and nearly all talk about health has actually become about disease. The goals of conventional medicine have become focused on repairing, removing, or replacing parts.

Quantum View of Universe: New Physics

Newtonian theory of physics has provided the theoretical foundation for modern science, medicine, and health care, but this worldview was greatly undermined during the early part of the 20th century. Scientific discoveries, led by Albert Einstein, shifted the worldview, **paradigm,** of the universe from one in which the universe is perceived as a machine, predictable and unchanging, to one in which the universe is interconnected, interrelated, with constant and unpredictable changes. Einstein's theory includes use of the formula $E=mc^2$ (where E is en-

ergy, m mass, and c the speed of light), which indicates that mass and energy are the same thing and that mass is simply bound energy which is constantly changing. This "new physics" is often used to support the use of integrative therapies for health, healing, or "wholeness." The concepts addressed in these theories are baffling and astounding to the Western mind, which is geared to a Newtonian understanding and worldview.

Table 12-1 provides a comparison of classical Newtonian and quantum perspectives of Einstein and others.

Quantum theory, the branch of physics which studies the energetic characteristics of matter at the subatomic level, is a very practical branch of physics in that it has yielded the laser, the electron microscope, the transistor, the superconductor, nuclear power, and is the basis of modern chemistry and biology (Graham, 1999). Newtonian theory also remains useful in the everyday realm of experience. Predictions made within the Newtonian framework are generally similar to those made using quantum theory, and there is an advantage in that the former is simpler to understand in the Western cultural perspective. Yet, those interested in healing processes and integrative therapies must look to relativity and quantum theories for scientific understanding.

It is now recognized that the new physics restates mystical descriptions of reality common to ancient traditions throughout the world still emphasized in Eastern cultures. Acceptance of this **paradigm shift** (changing of worldviews) is helping many Westerners to understand and accept the Eastern worldview of healing. Physicists have been shocked by comparisons between the descriptions of new physics and mysticism. Some, however, have realized that mysticism provides a philosophical background to Western science, unifying and harmonizing scientific discoveries and human spiritual beliefs.

Western scientists and thinkers who have made great contributions in the move to understand the impact of relativity and quantum perspectives include David Bohm (1980), who examined the role of consciousness in the energy-matter relationship; Prigogine & Stengers (1984), who argued that order evolves from chaos; and Karl Pribram (1971), who proposed the hypothesis that the brain works similarly to a hologram within a universe that functions in the same way similar to a hologram.

Eastern Perspectives

Just as knowledge of the natural world is obtained in Western culture through scientific theories and research, Eastern and indigenous cultures gain knowledge through intuitive ways of knowing. Eastern metaphysical philosophies, although derived from intuitive and subjective ways of knowing over thousands of years, describe perspectives on reality similar to those of relativity and quantum theories of physics developed over the last century (Capra, 1977; Gerber, 1988; Graham, 1999; Herbert, 1987; Hunt, 1995; Zukav, 1979).

TABLE 12-1 Assumptions of Classical and Quantum Mechanical Views Compared

CLASSICAL VIEW	QUANTUM VIEW
• There is an objective world independent of the observer, and our bodies are an aspect of this objective world.	• The physical world, including our bodies, is a response of the observer.
• The body is composed of clumps of matter separated from one another in time and space.	• In their essential state, our bodies are composed of energy and information arising from the universe.
• Mind and body are separate and independent from each other.	• The mind and body are inseparably one. This unity I experience as the subjective stream—thoughts, feelings, and desires—and the objective stream—my body. At a deeper level, however, the two streams meet at a single creative source from which we are meant to live.
• Materialism is primary; consciousness is secondary. We are physical machines who have learned to think.	• The biochemistry of the body is a product of awareness. Beliefs, thoughts, and emotions create the chemical reactions that uphold life in every cell.
• Human awareness can be completely explained as the product of biochemistry.	• Perception appears to be automatic, but in fact it is a learned phenomenon. If you change your perception, you change the experience of your body and your world.
• As individuals, we are disconnected, self-contained entities.	• Impulses of intelligence create your body in new forms every second. Change your understanding of their patterns and you will change.
• Our perception of the world is automatic and gives us an accurate picture of how things really are.	• Although each person seems separate and independent, all of us are connected to patterns of intelligence that govern the whole cosmos. Our bodies are part of a universal body, our minds an aspect of a universal mind.
• Time exists as an absolute, and we are captives of that absolute. No one escapes the ravages of time.	• Eternity exists as an absolute. Time does not. Time is quantified eternity, timelessness chopped up into bits and pieces (seconds, hours, days, years) by us.
• Our true nature is totally defined by the body, ego, and personality. We are wisps of memories and desires enclosed in packages of flesh and bones.	• Each of us inhabits a reality lying beyond all change. Deep inside us, unknown to the five senses, is an innermost core of being, a field of nonchange that creates personality, ego, and body. This being is our essential state—it is who we really are.
• Suffering is necessary—it is part of reality. We are inevitable victims of sickness, aging, and death.	• We are not victims of aging, sickness, and death. These are parts of the scenery, not the seer, who is immune to any form of change. This seer is the spirit, the expression of eternal being.

From Ageless Body, Timeless Mind, by D. Chopra, 1993, Harmony Books. Copyright by Deepak Chopra. Used by permission of Harmony Books, a division of Random House, Inc., New York.

According to the Taoist view, health reflects harmony between external and internal forces. The universal energy or life force (called **chi** or **qi** or **ki**) nourishes the mind and body and is produced through action of the body. Illness results when there is an excess, deficiency, or blockage in the flow of chi (Pelletier, 2000).

Yin and Yang

Concepts of **yin** and **yang** as well as the five elements illustrate this view. Yin and yang are complementary and opposing forces. Yin is the negative, small, dark, earthly nature that represents the internal and the right side of the body. Yang, on the other hand, represents light, large, positive and expansive forces, the left side, external, and heavenly nature. Body organs are assigned either yin or yang, as are herbs and foods used to nourish the body. Illness occurs when these forces are out of balance (Pelletier, 2000).

The Five Elements

The five elements of nature have yin and yang qualities and consist of wood, fire, earth, metal, and water. Organs also reflect the five elements. For example, the heart is a fire organ while the liver is a wood organ. A problem with the heart may be related to a problem in the liver, just as a fire cannot burn without its fuel (wood). Thus, intervention based on this understanding may be directed at the liver, rather than at the heart itself. Relationships among the organs indicate the direction in which chi flows through pathways called **meridians.** Balance is restored by influencing the flow of chi, often at **acupoints** along the meridians. Figure 12-2 reflects the pattern of this energy flow in comparison with drawings representing Western and ancient Indian perspectives.

Traditional **acupuncture** originated in China about 5000 years ago and is a complex system of examination, diagnosis, and treatment. It is based in an understanding of balance between internal and external forces, for example, yin and yang and the five elements. According to Chinese medicine theory, more than 2000 acupoints exist on the human body and connect with 12 main and 8 secondary pathways. These meridians conduct energy, or qi,

---

FIGURE 12-2 Concepts of the Human Body

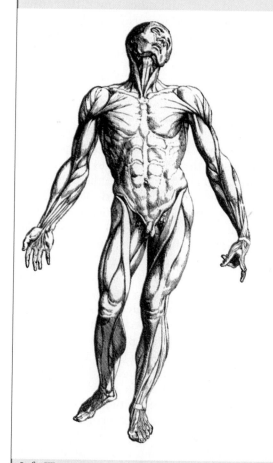
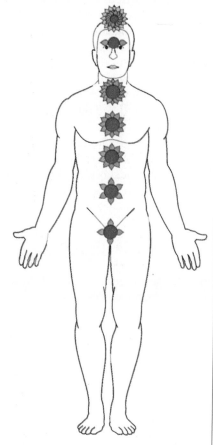

| Left: Western scientific concept of the human body as made up of interrelated systems of muscles, tissues, bones, nerves, blood vessels, cells, and organs. | The drawing shown was done by Vesalius in the 16th century, and is based on anatomical observations obtained by dissection of the human body. | Center: Eastern philosophical concept of the human body as a complex network of meridians, which are pathways for distributing vital energy, called Qi. | The drawing shown is a meridian map dating from 200 B.C. Ancient Eastern healers did not concern themsleves with the actual physical makeup of the body. | Right: Indian spiritual concept of the human body as a complex of energy centers and channels that distribute vital energy, called Prana, throughout the body. | The drawing shown is a modern depiction. While India possesses many ancient medical texts, it has virtually no ancient tradition of illustrative medical drawings. |

From *Essential Anatomy: For Healing and Martial Arts* (p. 9), by M. Tedeschi, 2000, Trumbull, CT: Weatherhill. Reprinted with permission of Weatherhill.

throughout the body. Acupuncture uses fine stainless steel needles inserted at the acupoints to stimulate the central nervous system to release chemicals into the muscles, spinal cord, and brain. These chemicals either change the experience of pain or release other chemicals, such as hormones, that influence the body's self-regulating systems. Qi regulates spiritual, emotional, mental, and physical balance and is used to balance yin and yang, keep the normal flow of energy unblocked, and restore health to the body and mind (NCCAM, 1999). **Acupressure** uses pressure applied with the thumbs on the acupoints to accomplish the same thing.

Human Energy Field Model

Energy field patterns are acknowledged by ancient cultures. Energy centers related to the human body are reflected in drawings from 5000 years ago in ancient Egypt (Hover-Kramer, 1993). Hippocrates, the father of modern medicine, acknowledged the human energy field in 500 B.C. A sample of names for this energy field and the cultures from which they come is given in Table 12-2.

According to Vedanta (Rama, 1978), a system of Eastern philosophy based on teachings from 2000 to 500 B.C., the human energy field is organized in and around seven major sheaths of vibratory energy that permeate and surround the physical body—the most dense and slowest vibratory level. Each layer from the physical body outward is a successively more expansive version of the self, and each layer is associated with a major energy center called a **chakra.**

The seven chakras are located near the coccyx, sacrum, lumbar region, heart, throat, brow, and crown. Each chakra mediates the flow of universal energy into local energy fields associated with parts of the body's metabolic, neurohormonal, and organ systems. According to this construct, disease processes occur when flows of energy are blocked or disrupted, affecting associated physical structures or physiological processes (Slater, 2000).

In this theory, the subtle body is made up of the first three layers of the human energy field described above. This aspect of the energy field is important to Therapeutic Touch (discussed later) and other **touch therapies,** those treatment systems used to balance and harmonize the energy field by the use of the hands applied to the area surrounding the body but not necessarily touching the skin.

A SYNTHESIS OF EAST AND WEST

Graham (1999) observes that increasing recognition of the "whole of things" in the West has led to the advocacy of integrative medicine. Many integrative theories, called holistic therapies in the past, have existed alongside conventional treatments, and now integrative medicine is taking its place alongside conventional medicine. The principle held by Graham (1999) is that integrative medicine may consist of many systems that are not in conflict with one another. These various systems can be seen as fully consistent with the principles of modern science, understandable in terms of the related principles of time and energy. The premise developed is that all forms of healing can be understood as either modifications of the time sense or of energy, factors which determine the energy-matter phenomenon, as stated in Einstein's formula $E = mc^2$. Therapies that promote relaxation or modify the individual's relationship to time may facilitate greater mobilization or utilization of energy. Energetic treatments, on the other hand, may work directly with subtle energies in and around the individual and by so doing indirectly influence the individual's experience of time by producing relaxation. Patel (1987) predicted that the various schools of thought that seemingly hold such different worldviews might be closer to each other than it appears to be possible at present.

Subtle energy fields around the body have eluded scientific measurement until recently. Because these forces are not easily detected by physical instruments in the orthodox scientific world, they are considered by Western science to have no physical reality. Research studies have been carried out, though, which reveal the existence of the human energy field. Two examples are given here.

TABLE 12-2 Some Equivalent Terms for the Energy Field	
ENERGETIC NAME	**CULTURAL SOURCE**
Ankh	Ancient Egypt
Arunquiltha	Aborigine (Australia)
Bioenergy	U.S./England
Gana	South America
Ki	Japan
Life force	General usage
Orenda	Iroquois
Pneuma	Ancient Greece
Prana	India
Qi (chi)	China
Sila	Inuit
Subtle energy	U.S./England
Tane	Hawaii
Ton	Dakota
Wakan	Lakota

From "The Re-emergence of Biofield Therapeutics within Complementary Medicine," Caduceus, 30, *pp. 36–38.*

Japanese physicist Motoyama (1986) developed technology to detect and measure the human energy field. His findings indicate the existence of the chakras and of the meridian system in human beings. He compared the chakra activity of people who had practiced meditation for years to that of people who did not meditate or who were beginners and discovered that the chakra energy of advanced meditators measured far greater in frequency and amplitude than did that of the other group. Motoyama concluded from his studies that the energy systems underpinning traditional Chinese and Indian medicine are fundamentally the same, despite differences in terminology (Graham, 1999).

Valerie Hunt (1995) also conducted a basic research program to study energy field patterns, using telemetry instruments. Her studies indicate chakra activity in response to thoughts, movements, and activities. Further, she found improved performance, emotional well-being, excitement, and advanced states of consciousness with enhanced chakra activity. Motor, sensory, and intellectual capabilities diminish with increased anxiety and emotion when there is electromagnetic field deficit (Hunt, 1995). Physiological research related to the human energy field by Hunt and others supports the growing interest in health promotion and use of integrative touch therapies.

The next section provides a look at theoretical perspectives related to the scientific and philosophical foundations that support the various touch therapies, **imagery** (the use of the imagination) and **visualization** (the use of visual images with the imagination) to reach the deeper intuitive knowing of oneself with intention to promote physiological changes for health promotion and healing. These theories reflect a mixture of Western science and Eastern philosophy. The theories discussed here contribute to nursing's understanding of integrative therapies and interventions. Additional theoretical material is presented within the sections on relaxation and imagery.

RESEARCH METHODOLOGY

Research methods appropriate for the study of integrative therapies constitute another major area of controversy. One side of the argument maintains that a different kind of science is needed, one based on the perspective of the new physics, rather than on Newtonian physics, which provides the perspective of current research methods. Cherkin (NCCAM, 2001b) argues for the other side of the controversy. While he acknowledges significant challenges for those conducting scientifically rigorous studies of integrative therapies, he believes conventional methods can work if they are applied creatively and take into account the broad context within which they are provided. He gives suggestions such as formulating com-

parison (control) groups and blinding (as seen in the Research Focus box of this chapter). He insists that new research methodology is not the answer and predicts that good science in the study of these therapies will occur when conventional researchers and integrative care providers collaborate in a manner that is based on mutual respect and the common goal of helping clients (NCCAM, 2001b).

NURSING THEORIES AND NATURE OF HEALING

Quinn (2000) contrasts **curing** and **healing** in her discussion of conventional and integrative worldviews:

Curing and healing are two different processes in that curing is the elimination of the signs and symptoms of disease; while healing of the person includes the emergence of right relationship at one or more levels of the body-mind-spirit system. Cure may not be possible, but there is always potential for healing. For example, death means failure in the curing model and is avoided at all cost, while from a perspective of healing, "death is part of the natural unfolding of the life process." (p. 42)

Historically, the topic of healing has been outside the domain of nursing research or literature. It is found in the health-related literature as wound healing and in the anthropological and philosophical literature as a transformative process encompassing body, mind, and spirit (Dossey & Keegan, 2000). We refer here not only to healing of the body after illness or injury but also to a process that moves one toward fulfillment of the highest human potential. Healing is seen as an evolutionary process toward integrated wholeness.

Healing is defined in *Merriam-Webster's Collegiate Dictionary* as "to make sound or whole." Dossey and Keegan (2000) define healing as "a process of bringing all parts of one's self together at deep levels of inner knowing, leading toward an integration and balance, with each part having equal importance and value; also referred to as self-healing or wholeness" (p. 361).

In Schubert and Lionberger's (1995) view of person, healing is the process of self-transformation during which one experiences a sense of becoming or movement toward one's realization of potential. Figure 8-2 in Chapter 8 depicts this potential emerging from within as tension and conflict are released. While symptoms of physical or mental distress, at the base of the triangle, are often the presenting problem, healing responses usually involve other aspects of the self. For example, a person seeking relief from a pounding sensation in her ears following a car accident came to a nurse for integrative therapy. Conventional medicine had provided no relief for three years. She connected in a very strong way with the nurse and soon focused her attention on managing the stress in her life. She continued to come to the nurse for treatment as she received counseling support and **Jin Shin Jyutsu,** a touch therapy for balancing and harmonizing the subtle energy of the whole self. Over a period of three months, the intensity of the pounding had decreased significantly and was no longer considered a problem. Her attention had shifted to other life issues considered by her to be more important to her life.

Rogerian Science of Unitary Human Beings

According to Rogers, a nursing theorist, the healing process can be explained as movement of energy toward harmony of the person/s-environmental field/s (Rawnsley, 1985). Healing occurs as a natural internal process within a caring environment (see Chapter 9). Thus, the **healer** (or person doing the treatment) does not bring about healing but merely provides elements of caring and facilitates the inner process. Holistic perspectives of life and the universe hold that every part exists throughout the whole and the whole is reflected in every part, such as in a **hologram,** a photographic method that uses laser light to produce three-dimensional images, in which each fragment contains the picture of the whole.

Rogers' (1970, 1980, 1981, 1983, 1985–1987, 1990) principles of homeodynamics describe **human energy field patterns** as always interacting with others and with the environment in entirety. She uses the term **resonancy** to represent continuously increasing complexity of one's relationship with the environment; **helicy** to describe the relationship's diversity and unpredictability; and **integrality** to indicate that interaction is ongoing and mutual, whether we are aware of these phenomena or not. She describes the interaction as occurring in many ways in nature, forming ever new patterns.

She states the practice of nursing is evolving to include noninvasive modalities such as Therapeutic Touch, meditation, imagery, relaxation, the teaching of unconditional love, hope, and humor. These methods are considered representative of nursing therapies of the future and consequently the focus of nursing research.

Newman's Theory of Health as Expanding Consciousness

Margaret Newman (1994) notes that "[t]he focus of nursing is the *pattern of the whole,* health as pattern of the evolving whole, with caring as a moral imperative" (p. xix). In the development of her ideas on health as the expansion of consciousness, she is influenced in part by relativity, quantum, and systems theorists, all of whom made significant contributions to the development and/or interpretation of Einstein's theories of relativity and quantum mechanics as applied to human experience.

The Newman (1994) model—which defines health as the expansion of consciousness in a universe of undivided wholeness and nursing as the promotion of health—supports a nursing practice model that does not aim to produce a particular result. She holds that the particular form expansion of consciousness will take cannot be known. In place of the usual result-oriented intervention practice model, she proposes a nursing intervention based on a "relational paradigm that directs the professional to enter into a *partnership* with the client, often at a time of chaos, with the mutual goal of participating in an authentic relationship, trusting that in the process of unfolding, both will emerge at a higher level of consciousness" (p. 97). She suggests that the aim of the nurse is to provide support as clients move through the process depicted in the Prigogine model (Figure 12-3).

Newman (1994) suggests that one may view the human/environment energy field pattern in the following way. The figure represents, first, the seemingly predictable fashion in which a system such as one's normal daily life proceeds until some unexpected event occurs. This event, which could be an illness or a misunderstanding at work, for example, precipitates disorganization and uncertainties that force the person to reassess the situation and perhaps make changes. Resolution of the situation then leads to a new way of being in the world and life emerges with a new pattern and a higher level of organization. Quantum theory and human field theory described above provide support for addressing the human energy field as the fundamental unit of consideration for health promotion and healing.

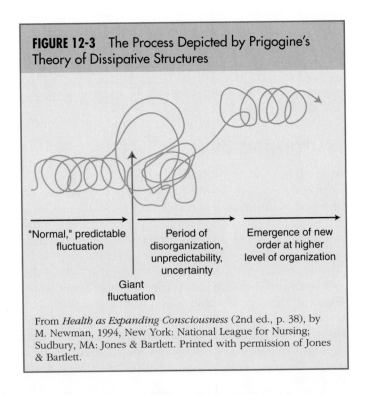

FIGURE 12-3 The Process Depicted by Prigogine's Theory of Dissipative Structures

"Normal," predictable fluctuation

Giant fluctuation

Period of disorganization, unpredictability, uncertainty

Emergence of new order at higher level of organization

From *Health as Expanding Consciousness* (2nd ed., p. 38), by M. Newman, 1994, New York: National League for Nursing; Sudbury, MA: Jones & Bartlett. Printed with permission of Jones & Bartlett.

Model of Mutual Connectedness

Schubert's (1989) mutual connectedness model for nursing practice identifies nursing therapies for promotion of health and healing as touch therapies, visualization, imagery, teaching, and counseling within the context of caring and the intention to help and heal. The work of Rogers and Newman as well as the scientists and philosophers who influenced these theorists is also used in the presentation of this clinical practice model (Schubert & Lionberger, 1995).

Integrated nursing therapies used in the mutual connectedness model are selected because of their abilities to release physical, emotional, mental, and spiritual tension, which in turn facilitate inner healing. Physical letting go creates relaxation of the body; emotional letting go, release of emotion; mental letting go, release of beliefs that impede one's movement toward fulfillment of potential; and spiritual letting go, release of the need to control and willingness to surrender to those things beyond one's control.

Properties of these integrative therapies also aid in identifying and enhancing health patterns. They include counseling to aid release of emotional tension, teaching to help the client recognize destructive health patterns and form new health behaviors, visualization and imagery to introduce new patterns through use of the imagination, and touch therapies to release and balance energy field patterns. Together with a caring relationship and the nurse's intention to promote the client's fullest potential, these therapies form a set of interventions and way of clinical practice that allows working with the client toward healing. See Figure 12-4 for a pictorial representation of the mutual connectedness model for nursing practice.

INTEGRATIVE NURSING THERAPIES

Touch therapies are intended to balance energies by deliberate use of the hands on the body or near it. Keegan (1994) identified and described a variety of touch therapies practiced by nurses (see Table 12-3). Of these, Therapeutic Touch (TT) and Jin Shin Jyutsu (JSJ) are briefly discussed in this chapter as an introduction to integrative therapies practices.

Therapeutic Touch (Krieger-Kunz Method)

TT was developed in the early 1970s by Dolores Krieger (1979, 1993), Professor of Nursing at New York University, and Dora Kunz, a noted healer who believes that anyone with the capacity to care for others can facilitate healing. The practitioner uses the hands in a consciously directed process of energy exchange to facilitate healing (Cugelman, 1998). See Figure 12-5 for the underlying assumptions of TT practice.

FIGURE 12-4 Nursing Practice in the Mutual Connectedness Model

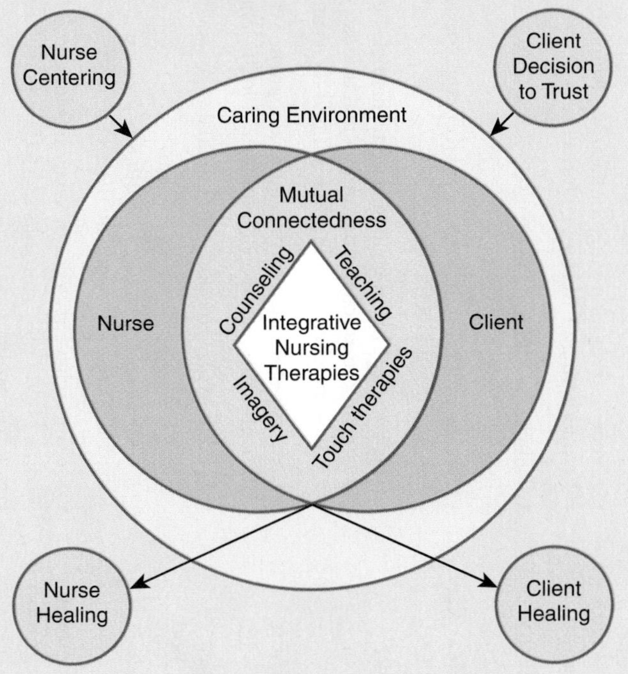

Original copyright 1994 by Phyllis Schubert and Harriett Lionberger.

FIGURE 12-5 Basic Assumptions Underlying Therapeutic Touch Practice

- Healing is a natural human potential.

- Human beings are open, complex, and pandimensional energy systems that are not bound by their skin (Rogers).

- Open energy systems express dynamic wholeness and synergy (Rogers).

- The universal healing (energy) field is a dynamic force that underlies the life process (Kunz).

- Practitioners of Therapeutic Touch act as instruments for the universal healing field (Kunz).

- Human energy fields display patterns of growth, organization, and rhythmicity (Rogers).

- Balance, harmony, and symmetry characterize a healthy energy field, whereas illness creates disorder, disharmony, and imbalance in the field (Kunz).

- Healing is an intrinsic movement toward order that facilitates human transformation and/or transcendence (Krieger).

- Life energy follows the intent to heal (Krieger).

From *Nurse Healers—Professional Associates, International. (NH-PAI) Basic Core Curriculum* (p. 201), 1998. Reprinted with permission of NH-PAI, 3760 South Highland Dr. #429, Salt Lake City, UT 84106, 801-273-3399, Fax 509-693-3537, nh-pai@therapeutic-touch.org, Website: www.therapeutic-touch.org.

TABLE 12-3 Touch Therapy Modalities

TECHNIQUE	RATIONALE	PRACTICE
Acupressure	Ancient Chinese technique based on the principles of acupuncture.	Practitioners use finger pressure on specific points along body meridians.
Alexander technique	Based on the idea that poor posture is responsible for energy imbalance and distortion of the flow.	Practitioners teach simple, efficient movements designed to improve balance, posture, and coordination to provide symptomatic relief by providing hands-on guidance and verbal instruction.
Deep-tissue bodywork	Based on the idea that manipulation encourages tissues to function properly.	A range of therapies to massage or manipulate deep connective tissues and muscles.
Feldenkrais	To help create freer, more efficient movement through functional integration and awareness through movement.	Combines movement training, touch, and discussion to improve the client's breathing and body alignment and to help client relearn the proper ways to move the body.
Infant massage	Designed to enhance bonding between parent and child.	Taught to new parents as preventative therapy, and as an aid to relaxation for both infants and parents.
Jin Shin Jyutsu	Based on the belief that attitudes of anxiety, fear, anger, depression, and pretense can create tension, fatigue, and illness by blocking the energy flow through the body.	Practitioners hold their hands lightly on two of the "safety energy locks" at a time to open the energy flows to restore harmony and balance. There are 26 pairs of these points on the body.
Kinesiology	A diagnostic system based on the premise that individual muscle functions can provide information about a client's overall health.	Practitioners test the strength and mobility of certain muscles to determine needed changes in lifestyle such as diet and exercise.
Massage therapy	A general term for a range of therapeutic approaches with roots in both Eastern and Western cultures.	It involves kneading or otherwise manipulating a person's muscles and other soft tissue.
Polarity	To help balance the energy flow of the person environment to support healing processes.	Bodywork, dietary guidance, exercise, and lifestyle are thought to release blocked energy.
Reflexology	Specific points on the hands and feet correspond with organs and tissues throughout the body.	With fingers and thumbs, the practitioner applies pressure to these points to treat a wide range of stress-related conditions.
Reiki	This ancient Tibetan healing system channels healing energies to the recipient to treat emotional and mental distress, chronic and acute, and to assist the client in achieving spiritual focus and clarity.	Practitioners vary widely in technique and philosophy, generally using light hand placements for treatment.
Rolfing	Used to restore the body's natural alignment, which may become rigid through injury, emotional trauma, and inefficient movement habits.	Uses deep manipulation of the fascia in a process involving 10 sessions, each focusing on a different part of the body.
Rosen method	Used to evoke emotion with the goal of achieving relaxation and self-awareness.	Combines gentle touch with verbal communication.
Shiatsu	A form of Japanese acupressure, this practice has been used for more than 1000 years to stimulate the vital energy.	Practitioners use a series of techniques to apply rhythmic finger pressure at specific points on the body.
Structural integration	Seeks to relieve patterns of stress and impaired functioning in order to correct body misalignments created by gravity or physical and psychological trauma.	In a series of 10 sessions the practitioner uses hands, arms, and elbows to apply pressure to the connective tissue while the client participates through directed breathing techniques.

(continues)

TABLE 12-3 Touch Therapy Modalities (continued)

TECHNIQUE	RATIONALE	PRACTICE
• **Therapeutic Touch**	• Based on the premise that the body is an open system of energies in constant flux and that illness is caused by deficit or imbalance in these patterns.	• The TT practitioner "assesses" where the person's energy field is weak or congested and then uses the hands to direct and balance it.
• **Touch for Health**	• A system of balancing the body's energy to improve overall health and strengthen resistance to common ailments and physical complaints.	• Practitioners apply gentle pressure to contracted muscles and other points along the body.
• **Trager**	• Used to loosen joints and ease movement, to retrain the body's old patterns of movement and prevent problems from recurring.	• The practitioner uses rocking and shaking motions while cradling and moving the client's still limbs.
• **Trigger point myotherapy**	• Trigger points are tender, congested areas on muscle tissue that may radiate pain to other areas. This technique is similar to shiatsu or acupressure, yet uses Western anatomy and physiology as its basis.	• Application of pressure to specific points on the body to relieve tension.

In The Nurse as Healer *by L. Keegan (1994). Published by Delmar.*

Indications for the use of TT include promoting relaxation, altering the perception of pain, decreasing anxiety, accelerating healing, and promoting comfort in the dying process. TT has also been used to alleviate symptoms such as dyspnea, coughing, hiccups, diarrhea, cramping abdominal pain, constipation, and fever (Egan, 1998).

Phases of Therapeutic Touch

Lionberger (1985) summarized the phases of TT as follows:

1. **Centering** oneself physically and psychologically, that is, finding within oneself an inner calm focus of attention

2. Using the tactile sensitivity of the hands to assess the energy field of the client for cues to differences in the quality of energy flow

3. Mobilizing areas in the client's energy field that the nurse may perceive as sluggish, congested, or static, that is, lacking in effective energy flow

4. Consciously influencing body energy through the use of the hands to assist the client to repattern his or her own energy

5. Reassessing the field and eliciting feedback from the client and giving the person an opportunity to rest and integrate the process

Steps 1 and 2 are described below as *centering* and *assessment*. Steps 3 and 4 are combined as *treatment;* and step 5 constitutes *evaluation*.

Centering

This is a critical phase of TT practice. It consists of bringing body, mind, and emotions to a quiet, focused state of consciousness. It brings about an inner sense of quieting the body, mind, and emotions as well as a feeling of being in harmony with the client, and "attuning with his or her well-being, inner strength, and peace; being nonjudgmental" [Nurse Healers—Professional Associates (NH-PA), 1992, p. 2]. Centering is a valuable tool to use in any situation to make your work more effective and contribute to your health.

Research in Therapeutic Touch

An extensive body of research on the effects of TT has accumulated over the past 25 years providing evidence that it promotes relaxation, decreases pain, and reduces anxiety [Clark, 2000; Hover-Kramer 1993; National Healers—Profession Association, International (NH-PAI), 1998; Quinn, 1992]. It has been found to accelerate wound healing (Wirth, 1990) and contribute to positive psy-

---

REFLECTIVE THINKING

Try It: An Exercise to Help You Learn to Center

- Sit comfortably and close your eyes.
- Inhale and exhale deeply.
- Focus your mind on some image in nature, such as a tree or a mountain, which brings you a sense of peace. If you become distracted, gently bring your mind back to your image of peace. Remember not to tighten up or try to force your mind to be still. Just maintain a calm but firm intent to keep focused on the image.
- Were you able to center? Describe your experience.

---

choimmunologic changes (Quinn & Strelkauskas, 1993). Gordon, Merenstein, D'Amico, and Hudgens (1998) studied the effects of TT on clients with osteoarthritis of the knee and found significant improvement in function and pain levels. Ireland (1998) studied the effect of TT on anxiety levels of HIV-infected children and found much lower mean scores in anxiety than in those who received sham treatments. Turner, Clark, Gauthier, and Williams (1998) studied the effect of TT on pain and anxiety in burn patients. See the Research Focus box for an overview of this study and its outcomes.

TT research depends on Rogers' Science of Unitary Human Beings for theoretical support. In spite of a 30-year history of clinical experience, literature, and research, the effectiveness of TT is seriously challenged. A major deficit in the body of literature is the dependence on qualitative evaluation by TT practitioners. Another major concern is that there is no accepted evidence in Western science concerning the existence or nature of energy fields. Urgently needed is research to determine the scientific basis of TT in terms of the existence, nature, and modulation of a personal energy field, as is collaboration with scientists—engineers and biophysicians and experts in biofeedback, autonomic physiology, and electrophysiology—to seek empirical validation (University of Colorado Health Sciences Center, 1994).

Jin Shin Jyutsu

Jin Shin Jyutsu uses hand contact at specific points on the body to promote energy flow to improve health and well-being. An ancient art rediscovered in this century by

RESEARCH FOCUS

Effect of Therapeutic Touch on Pain and Anxiety in Burn Patients

Study Problem/Purpose

The purpose of this single-blinded randomized clinical trial was to determine whether TT versus sham TT could produce greater pain relief as an adjunct to narcotic analgesia, a greater reduction in anxiety, and alterations in plasma T-lymphocyte concentrations among burn patients.

Methods

Data were collected at a burn center in southeastern United States. The subjects were 99 men and women between the ages of 15 and 68 hospitalized for severe burns who received either TT or sham TT once a day for five days. TT treatments were provided by one of three experienced TT practitioners trained in the **Krieger-Kunz method of Therapeutic Touch.** Sham treatments were administered by research assistants (RAs) who had no previous knowledge of TT. RAs were trained to make the same hand movements as the TT practitioners and were not allowed to perform the sham treatment until uninformed observers could not tell whether TT or sham TT was being performed in a staged demonstration. Baseline data were collected on day 1, data were collected before and after treatment on day 3, and postintervention data were collected on day 6. Instruments used to measure outcomes were the McGill Pain Questionnaire, Visual Analogue Scales for Pain, Anxiety and Satisfaction with Therapy, and an Effectiveness of Therapy form. Blood was drawn on days 1 and 6 for lymphocyte subset analysis. Medication usage for pain in mean morphine equivalents, and mean doses per day of medication for sleep, anxiety and depression were given and recorded.

Findings

Subjects who received TT reported significantly greater reduction in pain and greater reduction in anxiety than did those who received sham TT. Only 11 subjects were available to receive the blood test both at the beginning and at the end of the treatment period and gave their consent, but those who received TT had a decrease in CD8+ cells and those receiving the sham treatment an increase, indicating a possible increase in immunity for those receiving TT. There was no statistically significant difference between groups on medication usage.

Implications

Anxiety is severe with burn injuries because of the great pain associated with debridement and the lengthy healing process. Pain and anxiety are major issues in the nursing care of the burn patient, with the pain of the therapeutic procedures often being more intense than that of the injury itself. Although limited research has been done on nonpharmacological interventions to reduce pain and anxiety in severely burned patients, studies have shown a decrease in pain and anxiety with **biofeedback training** (a technique of learning to control certain emotional states, such as anxiety, by training oneself, with the aid of electronic devices, to modify involuntary body functions, such as blood pressure or heartbeat), teaching patients coping skills, showing videos, relaxation training, and deep-breathing exercises. Another major problem for burn patients is suppression of the immune system with resultant infections, slowing healing and contributing to the protracted pain. Although the number of subjects who received blood testing for lymphocytes was very small, the results are similar to that of another study by Quinn and Strelkauskas (1993), indicating the need for further research in that area.

Source: Turner, J., Clark, A., Gauthier, D. & Williams, M. (1998). The effect of therapeutic touch on pain and anxiety in burn patients. Journal of Advanced Nursing, 28(1), 10–20.

Master Jiro Murai in Japan, it has been taught in the United States by Mary Burmeister since the 1950s. Her students now lead workshops attended by nurses and other health professionals as well as by lay people.

According to this system, there are 26 JSJ **safety energy locks** located on each side of the body (see Figure 12-6). They are so called because they are understood to lock as a safety mechanism when they

FIGURE 12-6 Location of 26 Safety Energy Locks. Used in Jin Shin Jyutsu®

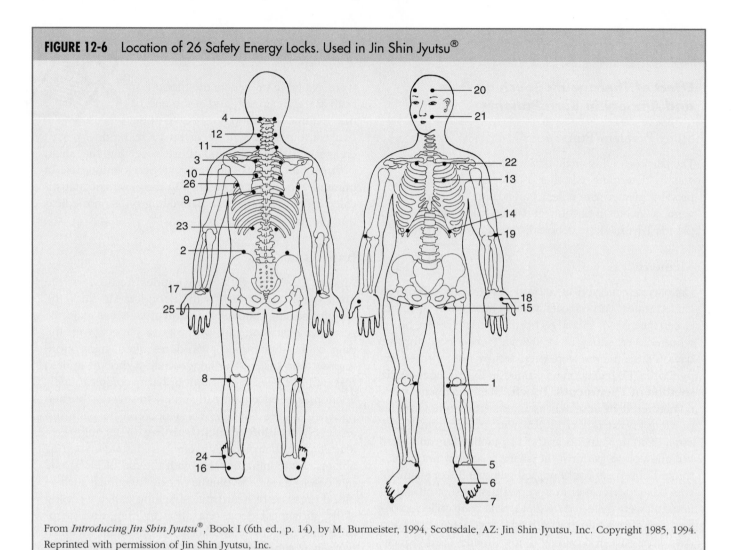

From *Introducing Jin Shin Jyutsu*®, Book I (6th ed., p. 14), by M. Burmeister, 1994, Scottsdale, AZ: Jin Shin Jyutsu, Inc. Copyright 1985, 1994. Reprinted with permission of Jin Shin Jyutsu, Inc.

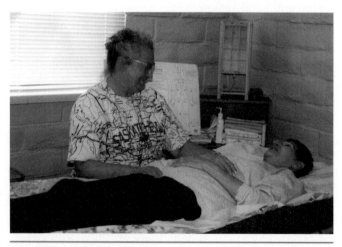

Rose Murray, RN, MSN, Jin Shin Jyutsu practitioner, listens to the 12 pulses of her client in her integrative nursing practice.

become overloaded by such factors as lifestyle excesses, tensions, habits, emotional anxieties, accidents, or hereditary characteristics (Burmeister, 1981). Resulting alterations in energy flow produce discomfort, letting us know when attention needs to be paid to the body.

The goal of a JSJ session is to facilitate harmony and balance in the client's energy patterns. The role of the practitioner is to use the hands to help restore the natural flow and rhythm of the universal revitalizing energy along the client's energy circulation pathways (Burmeister, 1980). JSJ assessment and treatment are done with the client fully clothed, lying on a comfortable cot. The process generally takes 45 minutes to 1 hour. However, there are brief treatments that can be done by the nurse or taught to the client for self-help. Try the flow given for self-help in Figure 12-7.

FIGURE 12-7 Jin Shin Jyutsu® Self-Help Flow: Main Central

Right hand on top of head

Left hand between eyebrows

Left hand on tip of nose

Left hand between the breasts

Left hand at base of sternum

Left hand on top of pubic bone

Right hand at base of spine (coccyx)

Hold fingers of the right hand on top of the head and hold fingers of the left hand between the eyebrows. Hold the two areas for a minute or two or until a pulse is felt in both hands and comes into its own harmony. Continue to hold the right hand on top of head while you hold each of the other areas listed above. Move your right hand to the coccyx while keeping your left at the top of the pubic bone to complete the flow. Do this flow every day to feel a difference in your well-being.

From *Introducing Jin Shin Jyutsu*®, Book I (6th ed., p. 14), by M. Burmeister, 1994, Scottsdale, AZ: Jin Shin Jyutsu, Inc. Copyright 1985, 1994. Reprinted with permission of Jin Shin Jyutsu, Inc.

MIND-BODY THERAPIES

Mind-body interventions are designed to facilitate the mind's capacity to affect bodily function and symptoms. Some of these therapies now have a well-documented theoretical basis and are considered a part of conventional health care practice, i.e., client education. Others such as meditation, prayer, hypnosis, dance, music and art therapy, visualization, and imagery are considered complementary and alternative (Academy for Guided Imagery, undated).

Persons from many cultures practice meditation in some form. There are many different forms of meditation, but all hold a common purpose: a conscious attempt to focus attention and still the mind (Graham, 1999). Meditation is a common spiritual practice in Eastern cultures and involves a shift of attention from the external world to the inner one. Since Western cultures hold an external focus and emphasize action and doing, direction and control, meditation may seem strange to many Westerners.

Other mind-body interventions increasingly familiar to nurses are relaxation therapies, imagery and visualization, and art and music therapies. A brief discussion is included here as an introduction to these potentially useful tools.

Deep Relaxation

Relaxation as a state is usually defined as the absence or lessening of tension. It affects heart rate, respiratory rate,

and blood pressure and reflects psychological and physiological conditions such as anxiety and muscle tension. The concept came into general use as an intervention when Benson (1975) coined the term **relaxation response** to denote the state of **deep relaxation** produced by an exercise that came to be known as a technique.

Benson (1975) identified four essential ingredients of a technique to bring about the relaxation response: (a) decreased environmental stimuli; (b) a mental device such as an object to dwell on (word, sound, object, or feeling); (c) a passive attitude; and (d) a comfortable position, so that minimal muscular work is required.

Relaxation exercises are often employed as an adjunct to other therapies and are used in numerous classes, groups, home visits, hospice, and private practice where community health nurses often work with those clients who are experiencing fatigue, tension, and distress. Pain and other symptoms that result from muscle tension and insomnia caused by emotional stress are often relieved by relaxation exercises. In general, application opportunities are similar to those of imagery, discussed below.

Guided Imagery

Relaxation and imagery are used together to influence a person's physiology, mental state, and behavior. Such therapy can counter chronic distress and promote more positive self-perceptions and a stronger sense of well-being. Chronic distress can precipitate physiological damage resulting in heart disease, ulcers, and other disorders or it may manifest in such emotional difficulties as depression and chronic anxiety (Anselmo & Kolkmeier, 2000). Rossman and Bresler (2001) have found that imagery affects almost all major physiological systems of the body: respiration, heart rate, blood pressure, metabolic rates in cells, gastrointestinal mobility and secretion, sexual function, cortisol levels, blood lipids, and immune response. When the body/mind is deeply relaxed, a healing process inherent in nature is triggered. In this way **guided imagery** is a significant alternative to pharmacotherapy, with greater safety and far fewer complications. In guided imagery a guide suggests to a client or group of clients what to imagine and how to move through the process and the clients use their imaginations to respond silently in their own way (Rossman & Bressler, 2001).

Imagery involves mental pictures, as in visualization, and/or mental representations of hearing, touch, smell, taste, and movement. Such representations may be of reality, fantasy, or both. The body responds physiologically to imagery in the same way it would respond to an external event. In our minds, "we can hear the sound of our child's voice, see a loved one's face, smell a fish, taste a lemon, feel our feet buried in warm sand, and sense our bodies swimming in cool water" (Zahourek, 1988, p. 53). Imagining any of these stimuli can evoke noticeable responses.

Schaub and Dossey (2000) note that there have been a number of nursing research studies that indicate imagery promotes the healing process. Nurses often find imagery to be a very practical tool because it is noninvasive and always available for use and "demonstrates the application of esthetic knowledge in healing" (Rew, 1996, p. 79). Moreover, clinical reports show that imagery helps clients work with a wide range of conditions, including chronic pain, allergies, high blood pressure, irregular heartbeats, autoimmune diseases, cold and flu symptoms, and stress-related gastrointestinal, reproductive, and urinary complaints (Rossman & Bresler, 2001; Schaub & Dossey, 2000). It also seems to help speed healing after injuries such as sprains, strains, or broken bones. Much of the benefit may be due to the client becoming deeply relaxed.

Visualization is based on the ability to see an image in the mind's eye and is the most common form of imagery, although all the senses may be involved. One might imagine lying on the beach, feeling the warm sand, listening to the ocean, and smelling the sea air. Rossman (1993) suggests that persons who are unable to visualize "may be able to relax by imagining the warmth of the sun, recalling a favorite tune, or conjuring up the aroma of brewing coffee or the taste of freshly baked bread" (p. 12). Often, a person who is not ordinarily aware of

REFLECTIVE THINKING

Try Relaxing with the Help of Imagery

To get a taste of how relaxing imagery can be, try a simple, quick exercise:

- Keep your eyes closed while you take a few deep, easy breaths, and imagine yourself in the most peaceful, beautiful, serene place possible. Think of a time when you felt relaxed and peaceful—perhaps a walk in the park, a day on a sunny beach, or an evening at a concert—and focus intently on the sights, smells, and physical sensations associated with that event. Focus on this image for about 5 minutes.

- Come back to everyday reality and notice how you feel. You may feel calmer, more alert, and refreshed—as if you had a long rest.

REFLECTIVE THINKING

Nursing Process and Imagery

- Remember that Margaret Newman (1994) recommended a model for nursing practice that is not based on specific outcome criteria. Do you think the model by Schaub and Dossey is consistent with Newman's intention? Give the reasons for your decision.

visual images will experience them when doing an imagery exercise.

Nurses' interest in imagery has grown in recent years due to the desire to provide noninvasive and nonchemical support to clients seeking help for physiological or psychosocial difficulties. Schaub and Dossey (2000) provide a model for application of the nursing process through the use of imagery. This process model includes (a) assessment (appropriateness of intervention for the client, patterns/problems/needs), (b) planning and carrying out the intervention (treatment and mental rehearsal), and (c) evaluation (feedback and planning). Highly individualized and based on an adequate understanding of the client's needs and goals, the process is built on a thorough understanding of the problem or disease; the client's cultural beliefs and values; the client's coping skills, past and present; the client's method of processing information; and an assessment of the client's unique imagery system.

There are three levels of interactivity in guided imagery techniques: (a) noninteractive communication in which the client is a passive recipient of suggestion (often used with large groups), (b) one-way (linear) or partial interactive communication in which the client(s) indicate when they are ready to go on, and (c) two-way or full interactive communication in which the client directs the interaction. The client is thus self-empowered by using unconscious processes to direct and guide the therapeutic intervention. Rossman and Bresler (1994) have developed the latter as a system of **Interactive Guided Imagery** in which the client guides the process while the guide (nurse) provides the support and helps to direct the flow of the process.

Nursing therapies discussed in this chapter share the goal of helping clients meet their individual needs. Skills are achieved by careful training and practice and are acquired through postbasic education.

BIOLOGICAL-BASED THERAPIES

This category of integrative therapies includes herbal remedies (plants used for their therapeutic value), special diet therapies (those believed to prevent disease and promote health), **orthomolecular therapies** (the use of chemicals such as magnesium, melatonin, and megavitamins to treat diseases), and individual biological therapies (such as laetrile, bee pollen, and shark cartilage) (NCCAM, 2000b).

The body of knowledge about herbal and medicinal drugs is growing but still is rudimentary. It is important for health care professionals to stay abreast of the current research findings being provided by the NCCAM research centers on the Internet. Some common concerns related to the use of herbs are listed in Table 12-4.

The possibility of untoward reactions are particularly dangerous to those who are frail and on other medications, i.e., the very young, the frail elderly, and those who

are in poor health. Certain herbal and biologically based therapies, however, may be found to be safer and more effective than those pharmaceuticals being used presently. See Figure 12-8 for guidelines to help determine safe and effective use of herbal therapies.

CLINICAL IMPLICATIONS

Nurses often use integrative therapies in their self-care regimens and find that very simple practices bring significant results in many ways. For instance, Jin Shin Jyutsu self-help techniques include sitting quietly and holding each finger with the fingers of the other hand wrapped around it, each finger in turn. When practiced over time,

TABLE 12-4 Commonly Used Herbs		
HERB	**USE OR ACTION**	**CLINICAL CONSIDERATIONS**
Echinacea: *E. purpurea, E. pallida,* and *E. angustifolia*	Immune stimulant, anti-infective	Contraindicated in patients with immune system disorders; hepatotoxic with persistent use
Feverfew: *Tanacetum parthenium*	Migraines, menstrual irregularities, arthritis	May increase clotting time; hypersensitivity reaction in those allergic to ragweed, asters, chrysanthemums, or daisies; abrupt cessation can result in withdrawal syndrome
Garlic: *Allium sativum*	Antihypertensive, antibiotic, lowers cholesterol	May increase clotting time; large amounts (> 5 cloves) can cause gastrointestinal upset; may decrease blood glucose levels
Ginger: *Zingiber officinale*	Antinauseant, antispasmodic, prevents motion sickness	May increase clotting time; should not be used for morning sickness
Ginkgo: *Ginkgo biloba*	Increases cerebral blood flow; decreases symptoms of peripheral vascular disease; relieves vertigo, tinnitus, and symptoms of intermittent claudication; antioxidant	May have inhibitory effect on platelet-activating factor; may interact with antithrombotic therapy
Ginseng root: *Panax ginseng* (Asian); *P. quinquefolius* (American); *Eleutherococci radix* (Siberian)	Decreases fatigue; increases stamina	Ginseng abuse syndrome, which is characterized by insomnia, hypotonia, and edema; Siberian ginseng may falsely elevate digoxin levels; may potentiate monoamine oxidase inhibitors (MAOIs)
St. John's wort: *Hypericum perforatum*	Antidepressant and anxiolytic (mild to moderate symptoms)	Not to be combined with MAOIs or selective-serotonin reuptake inhibitors; may cause photosensitivity; unsafe when combined with ephedra
Valerian: *Valeriana officinalis*	Sedative, hypnotic, muscle relaxant	Not to be combined with sedatives or anxiolytics; not to be used regularly; may cause excitatory effects; may cause hepatotoxicity when combined with other herbs (skullcap, mistletoe)

Source: Blumenthal, M., & Busse, W. R. (Eds.). 1998. The complete German Commission E monographs. Austin, TX: American Botanical Council; (1998). PDR for herbal medicines. Montvale, NJ: Medical Economics; Tyler, V. E. (1993). The honest herbal: a sensible guide to the use of herbs and related remedies (3rd ed.). New York: Pharmaceutical Products Press.

FIGURE 12-8 Guidelines for the Safe Use of Herbs

- Always inform your health care provider of herb use so that all agents—whether nutraceutical or pharmaceutical—will be documented.

- Remember that "natural" does not mean safe.

- Discontinue the use of any herb if you develop side effects or unusual symptoms, and report these effects to your health care provider.

- Herb-drug interactions do occur, and they can be serious; therefore, it's best to let your primary care provider determine the safety of combining herbs and drugs.

- Purchase herbal products that have been standardized—that is, products for which there are known effects for a given dosage and for which the manufacturer ensures consistency from batch to batch.

- Purchase products that have the following on the label: the scientific name of the herb; a statement confirming that the product has undergone scientific testing and that the manufacturer has adhered to good manufacturing practices; a lot number, the date of manufacture, and an expiration date; and the address of the supplier.

- Buy from reputable sources; ask your provider for help in determining where to purchase herbs.

- Avoid herbs during pregnancy and lactation or when attempting to become pregnant.

- Herbs should not be used in larger-than-recommended dosages or for more than several weeks (unless approved by your provider).

- Infants, children, and the elderly should not take herbal treatments without professional supervision.

From "The Proverbial Herb," by T. Hatcher, 2001, *American Journal of Nursing, 101*(2), pp. 41–42. Reprinted with permission of Lippincott Williams & Wilkins.

Out of the Box

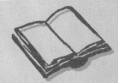

Practice of Reiki for Self-Help

Reiki has been an important part of my life for 12 years. Reiki is an ancient form of hands-on healing originating in Japan. In 1989, I experienced the deaths of a 3-year-old grandson and a 28-year-old son and a divorce after 37 years of marriage, all within a 13-month period. A nursing student offered to give me Reiki sessions at her house. Along with other practices such as massage, prayer, and meditation, Reiki helped with my healing process. A few months later I took a Reiki workshop and became a first-degree Reiki practitioner myself. While continuing my own healing process, I also used Reiki in my summer work as a volunteer at a retreat center where I served as nurse and cook. I remember an occasion when a man had fallen down the side of a mountain and injured his knee. I was amazed to feel the inner parts of his knee rearranging themselves when I was doing Reiki on him. I was present during my daughter's labor and home delivery of my grandson and used Reiki throughout the process.

A few years later I received more training and became a second- and then a third-degree practitioner and then a Reiki master. An important part of a Reiki master's responsibility is to teach others. While I was a Peace Corps volunteer in Turkmenistan, I used Reiki with clients', families and Turkmen colleagues. Then I taught Reiki to colleagues and brought them through all stages of training, so that by the time I left, there were two Reiki masters in Turkmenistan.

Now I am part of a Reiki circle which meets regularly for each other's healing. This has been very helpful to me while working in a different part of the country for two years as an Americorps VISTA volunteer. ■

—Joan Heron, RN, PhD

---

results may include a sense of balance and harmony, peace and contentment, as well as gradual healing of chronic conditions.

Integrative therapies are entering mainstream health care, and many clients are selecting these therapies, practitioners, and products even though there is very little or no scientific study to support their decisions. Well-informed community health nurses are in a good position to stay abreast of basic and clinical research through Internet communications and to share scientific information about safety and effectiveness of various therapies with clients—individuals, families, and aggregates. Other issues involve the choice of a practitioner and service delivery.

NCCAM (2001e) provides the following guidelines for the selection of a practitioner. These guidelines may be shared with clients requesting guidance in the selection process:

- Assess the practitioner's background, qualifications, and competence. A state or local regulatory agency with authority over those who practice the therapy sought may be contacted to determine whether the practitioner holds the appropriate license, education, and accreditation for the therapies practiced and if there have been any complaints filed against the practitioner. Most integrative practices have national organizations representing practitioners which provide information about laws related to state licensing, certification, and registration. Some organizations also provide referrals and information about specific practitioners.

- Talk with those who have had experience with this practitioner—both health practitioners and clients—to determine competence and whether there have been complaints by clients.

- Visit the practitioner and ask about the level of education, additional training, licenses, and certifications, both conventional and nonconventional.

- Assess the practitioner's openness to talk about technical aspects, possible side effects, and potential problems with the treatment sought. Choose a practitioner who is easy to talk with and who seems comfortable answering these questions.

- A sense of trust and a caring connection with the practitioner are essential.

Assessment of the service delivery is also important even though these factors may not affect the safety or effectiveness of the treatment being considered. Suggestions for this assessment include the following:

✳ DECISION MAKING

Choosing an Interactive Guided Imagery Practitioner

You are a public health nurse and an organization in your community has asked you to recommend a health practitioner to speak on the therapeutic uses of Interactive Guided Imagery at a health fair the group is sponsoring in the spring. You know nothing about Interactive Guided Imagery and its practitioners.

◆ What do you need to know about the practice? Where will you look for this information?

◆ How will you proceed with your search for a qualified practitioner? What are the qualifications?

◆ You decide to meet the practitioner. What questions will you ask?

◆ Are there other issues you need to explore for making your decision? What other information do you need? How will you obtain the information?

- During the visit to the practitioner's office, clinic, or hospital, ask how many clients are seen in a day or week and how much time the practitioner spends with the client. Note the conditions of the office or clinic. Determine whether costs are excessive for the service and if the service sought is covered by insurance. Also check to see if the service delivery is according to regulation standards for safety and care.

- Discuss all issues concerning treatments and therapies with the primary care provider. It is essential for competent health care management that practitioners have a complete picture of the client's treatment plan.

Community nurses serve in various roles, as discussed in Chapters 19 and 20. They intervene in many ways: counseling, teaching, consulting and collaborating with other care providers, making referrals, gathering data, assessing, diagnosing nursing problems, planning, intervening, and evaluating. Clients include individuals, families, aggregate groups, and the community at all levels. These levels of care apply also with integrative therapies. Education and training are available along with certification to practice. Professional organizations provide training, support, standards of practice, and assistance with marketing. Some community health nurses work in private practice, giving integrative care to individual clients, teaching families to work together for health promotion and healing of their family members, speaking at public events, consulting with community leaders and collaborating with other health professionals, and serving on health boards and in community organizations.

Nurses in private practice may choose to focus in one area of practice, i.e., giving TT or JSJ treatments along with health counseling and teaching to individuals with chronic health problems and their family members. Most integrative therapies are applied directly to those in need. They provide self-help mechanisms that may be taught in a myriad of situations unique to the individual or family. The nurse may go into a home finding someone in pain—physical, emotional, mental, or spiritual—and decide to offer TT. A TT treatment for someone dying of a painful illness may help to bring peace and comfort in that process.

Jin Shin Jyutsu provides a host of self-help techniques that can be applied by the client or by family members. These tools also help people deal with addictions and other psychological stressors. Family members may be taught to do the treatments and find comfort in their own ability to help their loved one. Similarly, these and other health enhancers are brought to larger populations through presentations at established facilities in the community, such as senior centers and youth programs.

Interactive Guided Imagery helps those who wish to change their health habits and who are experiencing

Perspectives...

INTEGRATIVE THERAPIES IN COMMUNITY HEALTH NURSING

Several years ago, I was invited to join a small group of nurse colleagues in creating a private nursing practice which would provide integrative nursing therapies: Jin Shin Jyutsu, Therapeutic Touch, Interactive Guided Imagery, health counseling, and health education. These services were given to individuals, families, and groups interested in various aspects of health. Individual clients came for Jin Shin Jyutsu treatments, and each of us had a number of clients, some who came quite often and some who came occasionally.

Clients came who had rejected conventional medical therapies and were seeking alternative therapies; others came for complementary holistic therapies to assist with the medical therapy they were receiving. They also came to prevent illness and to have supportive care as they made alterations in their health behaviors.

We networked with various community groups and participated in community health education projects and health fairs. We supported research projects by students from the local university. Weekly Therapeutic Touch clinics were held for those in the community who wished to participate. Self-help classes and continuing education classes for nurses and other health professionals were held.

Community health nurses participated in classes offered at the center and applied them in their various work roles: home visits, hospice settings, community clinics, and everywhere they worked. Clients and nurses took the self-help classes and learned to focus on being well and increasing wellness. Although the clinic was seen simply as a setting for nurses in private practice, it reached into the community through free clinics open to all who came and worked with the local university and other community agencies to sponsor various programs. It is described here as a model, not for exact replication, but as an idea to encourage others to be creative in offering community health nursing to segments of the population that may not be reached in other ways.

—Phyllis Schubert, RN, DNSc, MA

barriers to their success. Nurses skilled in the use of guided imagery find numerous situations for application. It has been widely used as an adjunct to cancer treatment, helping clients find meaning in the healing and/or dying process, for example. Some self-help techniques can be taught to groups within the community.

Professional and Ethical Implications

All community health nurses are confronted daily with ethical dilemmas, some more serious than others. Some are very complex, with long-term and serious consequences for those in our care. Keegan (2000) encourages the use of a case analysis process developed by Jonsen (1998) for consideration in an ethical dilemma. The case analysis process holds four components: (1) medical indications, (2) patient preferences, (3) quality of life, and (4) contextual issues. In addition, for holistic or integrative approaches, Keegan (2000) adds questions of relationship for consideration. These include "Who am I? What is my relationship to others? What other factors are contributing to my decisions? Am I wise and courageous enough to perceive and respect others' differences and honor them as I would honor my own beliefs?" (p. 166).

Guidelines for transcultural communication and the mutual process given in Chapters 8 and 10 should also be reviewed. It is essential to remember that the nurse always works within the framework of the client's belief and value system. The client's verbal (if possible) or nonverbal (when the client does not have speech) permission is sought as part of the treatment when appropriate for the client, as is noted in the descriptions below.

> ## ✳ DECISION MAKING
>
> ### Request for Permission to Give Therapeutic Touch
>
> Imagine that you have learned to do TT and would like to give a treatment to your client. He is dying of cancer and in great pain. You need to determine if the client and family are comfortable with you doing TT and will give permission. How will you approach the subject? What will you say to him? To the family? To anyone else present? What will you put in the record?

COMMUNITY NURSING VIEW

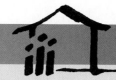

Irene, a 47-year-old single Caucasian woman, came to the nursing clinic for Jin Shin Jyutsu treatments. She came in response to a presentation by one of the nurses at the agency in which she worked as an administrative assistant.

Medical history: Her history involved a diagnosis of thyroid cancer at the age of 17 years and treatment of a thyroidectomy and radiation. During the past three years there had been formation of scar tissue in the area and she had suffered from obstruction of the esophagus and larynx. Since that time she has received two laser surgeries to open her airway and release her esophagus so she could breathe and swallow.

Presenting symptoms: She was experiencing shortness of breath, severe coughing and choking episodes, difficulty swallowing, and deep fatigue and could only talk in a whisper due to paralysis of the vocal cords. Her physician had advised surgery to do a permanent tracheotomy and stated that laser surgery would no longer be helpful.

Intervention: Jin Shin Jyutsu treatments were started immediately and were applied daily for two weeks, then gradually decreased as she learned the self-help applications. She was also being monitored by her physician. Counseling for work stress became a major part of treatment as she was able to return to her job.

Outcomes: The client immediately started breathing more easily without the coughing and choking, and within two weeks she could swallow soft foods. Her progress was constant over the nearly one and a half years she received weekly treatments. She now sees the nurse less frequently but applies the self-help daily. Her voice is sporadic, sometimes stronger than others but usually much stronger than at the beginning of the treatments. She continues to maintain her job and to help teach Sunday School at her church. She expresses amazement that something so simple could have such profound effects on her health and helped her to avoid surgery. The nurse believes this client's commit-ment to self-help practice has contributed greatly to her healing.

Nursing Considerations

Assessment

◆ What measures would you use to determine whether the client is obtaining the care essential to her health?

◆ On what observations would you base your decisions for care?

◆ How would you assess her work stress levels and what would you suggest for relief?

Diagnosis

◆ On what information and observations, in addition to the energy pulses, do you base your nursing diagnosis?

◆ Give an example of pattern appraisal as a nursing diagnosis for this person.

Outcome Identification

◆ What does the client hope to accomplish with the treatment?

◆ How do you implement the mutual problem-solving process?

Planning/Interventions

◆ How do you implement planning in this integrative treatment situation?

◆ What observations would you make as you work together in the planning and treatment phase?

Evaluation

◆ How will you evaluate her progress?
◆ How will you evaluate your working relationship with her? Her physician? Her family?

Legal Implications

Community health nurses must be familiar with the law of their state and with the regulations of the institutions where they are employed. In addition, all nurses are responsible and accountable to the Nursing Practice Act and Rules and Regulations of the Board of Nurse Examiners for their state. Standards for professional practice require that the nurse practice within his or her skill level. The nurse must know the law and practice within it. Further, although the practices discussed here are within the average nurse's abilities, additional training for specific interventions is necessary. For example, certification is offered by the professional association for those who have received training in the method, e.g., Jin Shin Jyutsu, Inc. or the Academy for Guided Imagery.

In general, TT is within the legal framework of nursing and need not be mentioned specifically in the Nurse Practice Act. The nursing practice of offering comfort measures legally covers integrative therapies such as TT.

KEY CONCEPTS

◆ Modern energetic healing methods are rooted in ancient cultural healing methods and beliefs.

◆ The underlying purpose of holistic healing modalities such as touch therapies, relaxation exercises, and imagery interventions is to promote health and healing.

◆ The conceptual models of nursing that form a foundation for holistic healing modalities are rooted in the quantum mechanical view of the universe.

◆ Healing is self-transformation, a continuous life process toward integration and harmony.

◆ Health is one's state of being or integrated wholeness at a given point in time.

◆ Therapeutic Touch, Jin Shin Jyutsu, relaxation exercises, and imagery are examples of a broad range of therapies available to nurses to aid clients in their healing processes.

◆ Community health nurses use their knowledge of integrative therapies in a variety of ways while promoting health and healing of their clients.

RESOURCES

GOVERNMENT AGENCIES

National Center for Complementary and Alternative Medicine: http://nccam.nih.gov

National Library of Medicine—PubMed: http://www.ncbi.nlm.nih.gov, http://www.nlm.nih.gov/medlineplus

National Institutes of Health: http://www.nih.gov/health

PROFESSIONAL ORGANIZATIONS

Academy for Guided Imagery: http://www.interactiveimagery.com

Nurse Healers—Professional Associates International: http://www.therapeutic-touch.org

International Society for the Study of Subtle Energies and Energy Medicine: http://www.issseem.org

Unit

IV

CARING FOR THE COMMUNITY

The primary aim of community health is to serve aggregate populations. This emphasis on the total population, while challenging, does reinforce the necessity to consider aggregate needs. This includes the considerations of distribution of resources, community involvement, a multisectoral approach, and an emphasis on primary health care. These considerations are discussed in Unit IV. This unit also includes a discussion of quality management and the use of power, politics, and public policy in creating and maintaining new health care delivery systems.

IN THIS UNIT

Chapter

13

POPULATION-FOCUSED PRACTICE

Eileen M. Willis, BEd, MEd
Anne L. Biggins, RN, RM, Psych, BN, MPHC
Jenny E. Donovan, RN, RM, MCHN, DipApp/Sci, BN, MSC

MAKING THE CONNECTION

Give a man a fish, and you feed him for a day. Teach a man to fish, and you feed him for a lifetime.

—*Chinese proverb*

COMPETENCIES

Upon completion of this chapter, the reader should be able to:

- Discuss the history of population-focused health care.
- Identify the key concepts contributing to a theoretical understanding of a population approach, e.g., primary health care, intersectoral collaboration, multidisciplinary teamwork, new public health, equity in health, sustainability, social models of health, social capital, and capacity building.
- Examine the need to develop partnerships across all sectors: private for profit, nonprofit, and public—national and global.
- State the mission and core functions of public health as a population-focused practice.
- Examine the issues surrounding population-focused health care.
- Discuss social science theories that provide insights into population-focused nursing care.
- Examine key practice approaches to population-focused health care.
- Discuss population-focused practice as the foundation for community/public health nursing.
- Consider the practical benefits and political implications of community participation and collaboration in health care.

KEY TERMS

assessment	needs assessment
assets assessment	policy development
assurance	population approach
capacity building	population-focused
empowerment	health care
intersectoral	primary health care
collaboration	social capital

The landmark Ottawa Charter for Health Promotion [World Health Organization (WHO), 1986] identified the prerequisites for Health for All as peace, shelter, education, food, income, a stable ecosystem, sustainable resources, social justice, and equity. This is a change in the definition of health from a traditional focus on the absence of disease to a social model of health and calls for a shift in health care practice (WHO and Com-

monwealth Department of Community Services and Health, 1988). It is a recognition that the struggle for better health happens primarily outside of the medical care, or sick care system as it is sometimes called. This shift also has implications for nursing practice and is a shift to promoting health for all.

A **population approach** to health promotion requires a shift from a focus on individuals to a focus on communities or aggregates of populations. It is an approach that builds on sound epidemiological research, assets and needs assessment, program planning, and evaluation. A population approach to health care is about sound management and service provision to communities, regions, nations, and the international community. A population approach focuses on strategies for health promotion, health maintenance, and disease prevention, taking into account the sociopolitical context in which community problems exist and are resolved.

ORIGINS OF POPULATION-FOCUSED CARE

The term **population-focused health care** can have many different meanings depending on the contextual framework within which it is being used. At the global level WHO has discussed population-focused health care as a concept in a number of documents and international conferences on health promotion. Action by the WHO has tended toward selective population primary health care such as EIP (extended immunization program) and GOBI (growth, oral rehydration therapy, and breast feeding). These programs tend to focus on specific population groups or specific conditions and attempt to eradicate the condition through technical and medical intervention. Comprehensive population-focused care, on the other hand, deals with social, political and environmental issues. A more contemporary term refers to **social capital** and **capacity building.** At first sight these words appear to be earlier ideas with new names; however, there are subtle differences between these two approaches which are discussed later in this chapter.

The documents, conferences, and programs related to health promotion that give shape to what the WHO understands by population-focused health care are presented in its Global Strategy of Health for All by the Year 2000 (WHO, 1993). This section examines the strategies recommended and provides an overview of primary health care and health promotion as population-focused principles and strategies.

The Global Strategy of Health for All

The idea for a global strategy of Health for All by the Year 2000 arose from a study conducted by the WHO released in 1973 (WHO, 1978b). This study identified universal worldwide dissatisfaction with health services and a correlation between the health status of the population and the social and economic development of a country. With that study, health became recognized as more than the provision of health services (Newell, 1988).

The WHO initiated a global strategy of Health for All by the Year 2000 at the 30th World Health Assembly in 1977. The target of Health for All set by WHO for governments and member nations was defined as "the attainment by all citizens of the world that will permit them to lead a socially and economically productive life" (WHO, 1978b, p. 3).

The seven principles of Health for All outlined by the WHO are (Bastian, 1989, p. 15):

- The right to health
- Equity in health
- Community participation
- Intersectoral collaboration
- Health promotion
- Primary health care
- International cooperation

These seven principles are seen as a framework for guiding health care workers working with groups of people whether at an international level or at the level of an individual country or community. The global strategy of Health for All by the Year 2000 was adopted by WHO in 1991. The very term "Health for All" suggests a focus on the total population rather than on individuals.

Table 13-1 provides an overview of the Health for All movement. Different phases of the movement are identified, beginning with the primary health care phase; the lifestyle phase based on the European lifestyle movement; the new public health phase, which is discussed in this chapter; and the ecological public health phase, which focuses on creating and maintaining sustainable environments through healthy public policy and more recently the social capital phase, which positions many of the strongly held principles of previous phases against economic rationalism. Social responsibility and mutual responsibility are two of the new terms reflecting the increased partnerships with the private sector, government calls for accountability, and the need for individuals to be engaged in their own health. These various initiatives and principles provide a framework for the current Health for All movement.

In order to take positive steps to maintain and improve the health status of populations, the WHO recognized the need for implementation strategies. If the target was to be reached, national and international actions at both operational and policy levels were required. Part of the challenge was to make widespread the recognition

---

TABLE 13-1   Overview of the Health for All Movement: Initiatives and Phases

YEAR	MAJOR INITIATIVES AND MOVEMENTS	PHASE
1977–1979	Target of Health for All by the Year 2000 Alma Ata Declaration on Primary Health Care WHO global strategy	Primary health care phase
1980	European Lifestyle Movement	Lifestyle phase • Behavioral approach • Focuses on individual
1980–1990	WHO Charter for Health Promotion: Ottawa WHO Healthy Cities Healthy public policy	New public health • Intersectoral collaboration • Empowerment • Community participation
1990–2000	Ecology for Health Jakarta Declaration	Ecological public health phase Social responsibility Partnerships for health Global health promotion
2000 and beyond	Enhancing social capital within a climate of economic rationalism Mexico health promotion conference	Evidence-based outcomes Investments in health Capacity building to enhance social capital

Sources: Adapted from McPherson, P. (1992). In H. Gardner (Ed.), Models of the Health for All movement. *Health Policy: Development, Implementation, and Evaluation in Australia. Australia: Churchill Livingstone and New South Wales Department of Health; capacity building: www.health.nsw.gov.au/public-health/health-promotion/hpss/capacitybuilding/questions/cbdefinitions.htm. (February 8, 2001).*

that health is a fundamental right for all people and includes the right and duty to participate in the planning as well as implementation of health care. Including other sectors that impinge on health such as welfare, transportation, and education was understood as an important feature of the strategy. This planning strategy has been termed **intersectoral collaboration.** The role that the individual, family, and community could play in health development was also emphasized (WHO, 1978b, p. 6).

In 1993, the WHO released an evaluation report that analyzed the progress of the Health for All strategy in 151 of the 168 countries involved in the strategy (WHO, 1993, p. 1). The report identified trends and challenges for a new framework for sustainable development and argued for the following:

- Mobilizing resources for high-priority population groups and health needs

- Ensuring equity in health through more effective collaboration and intersectoral health promotion and protection

- Pursuing equality in access to primary health care

The Health for All global strategy continues to emphasize the importance of a population-focused approach at all levels but has begun to be more selective in the way in which the strategy targets specific population groups. Two strategies emphasized in the document are those of primary health care and health promotion, both of which have a population focus.

Primary Health Care As a Strategy toward a Population Approach

In 1978 in Alma Ata, in the former Soviet Republic of Russia, the WHO proclaimed primary health care as the strategy to achieve the target of Health for All by the Year 2000. The Alma Ata Declaration defined **primary health care** as health care that is

> based on practical, scientifically sound and socially acceptable methods and technology made universally accessible to individuals and families in the community and at a level the country can afford to maintain at every stage of their development in the spirit of self-reliance and self-determination. (WHO, 1978a, p. 3)

Primary health care includes a comprehensive range of services, such as public health, prevention, and diagnostic, therapeutic, and rehabilitative services. Primary health care was endorsed by the international community. A number of governments and many health professionals saw it as the answer to the health problems of both developed and developing nations. The use of this model of health care, which epitomized a social view of health, however, required changes in the way governments and communities understood and implemented health care.

The Alma Ata Declaration viewed the health problems in terms of inequalities in health care between nations and between individuals within nations. The Health for All strategy was the approach selected to overcome this inequality. Consequently, primary health care was seen not only as the first level of care but also as an approach to health care, incorporating the following principles (WHO, 1985):

- Building self-reliance at personal and community level

- Supporting community participation in the development of health care programs

- Intersectoral collaboration in working to establish environments that are supportive for health and in which "healthy choices are the easier choices"

- Integration of health services to facilitate continuity of care and efficiency in resource use

- Providing special attention to high-risk and vulnerable groups, as a precondition for equity in health outcomes and health care access

- Use of appropriate technology

As Baum, Fry, and Lennie (1992) note, primary health care was viewed both as a level of health care and as an approach. As an approach, it is a reorientation of

---

✳ DECISION MAKING

Health Care Financing Through Taxation

The *World Health Report* (2000) analyzed the world's health systems using five performance indicators to measure the health systems of 191 member states, as discussed in Chapter 5. Interestingly, the United States ranked 37th, although it spends a higher percentage of its gross domestic product (GDP) than any other country. The United Kingdom, which spends 6% of its GDP, ranked 18th.

The report suggests that while progress has been made in the past decade, virtually all countries are underutilizing the available resources, leading to unnecessary deaths and illness. The report also discussed the form of "prepayment" health care, whether in the form of insurance, taxes, or social security. In Great Britain health care is universally free to all and is funded through taxation. In the United States health care is not universally free, except for the very poor, the elderly, and disabled. In Australia those in private insurance receive tax rebates. What are the implications for governments if health care is financed through taxation?

the health care system from its present concentration of expensive late-stage, high-technology hospital services to community and preventive services. It is in effect a framework for policy development. Primary health care, as a policy approach, goes beyond policies directed specifically to health promotion and disease prevention to consider how the principles can be applied to the acute-care sector. It calls into question approaches to health financing, management of services, and health evaluation (National Centre for Epidemiology and Population Health, 1991).

Health Promotion and a Population Approach

The concept of a population approach was formally endorsed in 1986 at the first International Conference on Health Promotion, held in Ottawa, Canada. A focus on the health of the public is not new; however, the processes are. At Ottawa, a shift was made from focusing on primary health care to including healthy public policy, and the term "new public health" emerged. The new public health concept builds on the traditional or the "old public health" concerns that had begun to focus mainly on physical environments. The intention was to broaden this to include environmental, political, social, and economic factors in analyzing and devising strategies to deal with public health issues (Ashton & Seymour, 1988).

The original public health movement of the 19th century had a strong political and social focus, but by the 1970s the medical model, which focused on cure of illness, became paramount. Public health was often associated with "sewerage, rats and adulterated food" (Baum et al., 1992, p. 304). Public health was seen to be a poor cousin of high-status acute care in clinical hospital settings. According to Baum et al. (1992), the new public health sought to involve citizens, as well as health professionals and government, in policy development in all sectors that had implications for health and illness.

Primary health care came to be seen as the operational tool by which improvements to the health status of the community at the local level could be achieved. Creating healthy public policy became the strategy for regional and national organizations, with primary health care as the means of operationalizing public policy. Five health promotion action areas were advocated at Ottawa: building healthy public policy, creating supportive environments, strengthening community action, developing personal skills, and reorienting health services (Gardner, 1992).

In the last five years a series of international conferences on health promotion have reinforced the Ottawa Charter. Priorities for health promotion in the 21st century were identified in Jakarta in 1997: "(1) promote social responsibility for health, (2) increase investments for health development, (3) consolidate and expand partnerships for health, (4) increase community capacity and empower the individual and (5) secure an infrastructure for health promotion" (WHO, 1993, p. 3–4). The Jakarta Declaration called for the building of global health promotion alliances. The building of global health alliances was promoted, and a key role for the WHO was seen to be "to engage governments, non governmental organizations, development banks, UN agencies, interregional bodies, bilateral agencies, the labour movement and cooperatives as well as the private sector in advancing the action priorities for health promotion" (WHO, *Jakarta Declaration on Health Promotion into the 21st Century*, 2001, p. 4).

The Fifth Global Conference on Health Promotion held in Mexico in June 2000 took up the challenge to examine the difference health promotion makes in the quality of life and health of people living in adverse circumstances. Two other objectives for the conference were to place health high on the development agenda of international and local agencies and to stimulate partnerships for health between different sectors and levels of society. Again, the globalization of health promotion, increasing social capital, community capacity, and further increasing participation in health promotion at all levels and sectors of the community, both public and private, were stressed. Key principles included a commitment to investment in research and evaluation; the development of indicators; the interaction, cooperation, and participation between researchers; and the need for policymakers, practitioners, and the community to have their needs served.

Other issues that were highlighted included the ability to assemble, synthesize, and communicate findings

---

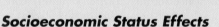

REFLECTIVE THINKING

Socioeconomic Status Effects

One of the guiding principles of the focus on populations in health care is the recognition that the health status of individuals and of nations is linked to socioeconomic status.

- In what way does your socioeconomic status affect your health?

- Does your socioeconomic status affect your health behavior? Explain.

- Does your socioeconomic status prevent you from changing behaviors that are not health promoting? Explain.

- Can you think of examples of social or cultural groups whose health status is clearly linked to their economic status?

- Do you think culture or class is the best indicator of health status? Why?

from ongoing research and evaluation; the ability to develop socially and politically relevant ways to communicate research evidence; and to develop solidarity among practitioners and activists and encourage networks. It was agreed that there was a need to recognize that the mobilization of resources of all kinds from all sources, both public and private, was necessary. In addition, it was also agreed that governments should ensure that the necessary resources are available for the development of community capacity and human resources. Other principles that were promoted included the creation of networks and associations of health promotion practitioners with the view that practitioners and associations should be able to work with and through existing political systems and structures. In many ways these principles are seen as a second wave of health care reform (*Fifth Global Conference on Health Promotion,* 2001).

DEBATES SURROUNDING THE HEALTH FOR ALL MOVEMENT AND POPULATION-FOCUSED HEALTH CARE

Challenges to the Health for All movement and the strategies that inform population-focused health care come from a variety of sources. The Alma Ata Declaration itself is not without its critics. The Alma Ata Declaration argues that primary health care should be defined in a manner that is specific to each country's health needs and that reflects the sociopolitical and cultural requirements of that particular society (Peterson, 1994; Cheek & Willis, 1998). This attempt to be politically and culturally sensitive is problematic. If primary health care is to be used as the strategy for reframing health care services globally, then it needs to be both a cultural and political agent of social change at all levels of health care (globally, nationally, and locally). Some cultural practices are detrimental to a social model of health: for example, cultural beliefs that hinder women from attaining literacy skills. But whether and how community health nurses should challenge such beliefs and practices is another question.

Further, resources are not distributed equally, and equity is not universal. Questions need to be asked about what resources are available in each country and how wealthy nations participate in the redistribution of resources so that the world population has acceptable and accessible health care. In dealing with these issues, the international community has yet to come to terms and work with the fact that nations come to the negotiating table with different political and sociocultural knowledge and that the questions address the core of the economic systems.

Population-Focused Care and Risk

McPherson (1992) argues that initially the primary health care concepts of self-reliance and community participation had a narrow focus that concentrated on primary prevention. This focus, as McPherson suggests, occurred when the Health for All movement joined with the "lifestyle movement" in the early 1980s. During this phase health was seen to be determined by the individual, plus social factors related to interpersonal behavior. Ill health, therefore, resulted from faults in either or both of these two factors and was the responsibility of the individual. Prevention depended on reducing identified health risk factors at the individual level and in changing individual behavior. The role of health education was to help people identify their risk factors and modify their "faulty" behavior. The problem with this approach was that there was a potential for blaming the victim, with little recognition of the social, political, environmental, and economic forces that act on individuals and are outside their control.

More recent interaction between social scientists and health professionals has resulted in a realization that many risk factors are outside the control of individuals. Risk is now viewed as a part of the local, national, and global food chains, the atmosphere, and political systems. Decisions on environmental toxins made in one country, for example, affect citizens in another. These issues call for multisectoral, international collaboration (Beck, 1989).

Selective versus Comprehensive Approaches

The international journal *Social Science and Medicine* published a series of articles by Warren (1988), Wisner (1988), Mosley (1988), and Walsh (1988) debating the topic selective versus comprehensive primary health care. The crux of the debate was that the approach to health care taken with particular populations should be comprehensive rather than selective. Proponents of comprehensive primary health care argued that health programs should involve the entire population in health-promoting activities utilizing community development approaches that work on identifying health problems and solutions in conjunction with the population concerned. This approach was argued to be truly participatory, with ideas and solutions emerging from within the entire population. Further, solutions developed within the group would be culturally congruent, and the technologies and skills needed would be affordable. In this approach the underlying cause of ill health was seen to be economic and social inequality. Improvements in health care called for structural, political, cultural, social, and economic reform, including democratic forms of health service management.

Those representing the case for selective primary health care argued that the WHO and UNICEF had had a number of successes in eradicating specific diseases, such as smallpox, by dealing with these diseases exclusively or by identifying specific at-risk groups within populations, such as women or people with disabilities, and concentrating resources on those groups.

Comprehensive primary health care was not viewed as cost effective or efficient. The debate regarding comprehensive versus selective primary care continues although the names may have changed.

Consider the following case example. In Australia in the 1970s and 1980s, the Women's Health Movement was instrumental in bringing over one million women together in focus groups across the entire nation to discuss the proposed National Women's Health Strategy. This strategy was bolstered by a national network of stand-alone women's health centres funded by the federal government but run by community boards of management. Women's health in Australia was highlighted, bolstered by a social movement and a consultative approach. Policy focused on broad issues that saw women's health directly linked to their social, economic, and political status. In the wake of a conservative backlash against the women's movement, genuine gains made by women, and a shift toward policy decision making based on economic outcomes, women's health policy has shifted toward targeting specific populations, those with specific complaints. In addition, success is determined based on the numbers of those who are screened. Hence policy is now directed toward body parts, such as breasts, rather than women's social and political issues, and women's health centres in many states are now incorporated into government health departments. This is an example of a shift from a comprehensive approach that saw all women involved to a selective approach where policy focuses on selective populations and selective body parts (Willis, 1999). The downside of this selective approach has been a loss of social networks.

To counter this change in focus in women's health policy, many community health professionals are now working from a position where they have incorporated the language and strategies of the Ottawa Charter for Health Promotion with the principles underlying the nurturing of social capital. In effect, they see their role as capacity building across the whole community or with particular population groups. Social capital is a term that is much debated. It is often reduced to terms such as *networks, clubs, teams,* and *trust* but is more than the sum of these terms (Foley & Edwards, 1999). Individuals are said to have social capital when they can access economic resources via social relationships. For example, people in a community may belong to a choir because they love to sing. Membership in the choir opens up opportunities for them that enhance their access to economic resources. The important issue in this definition is that individuals do not join the choir in order to access economic resources. The access simply arises out of the choir networks. Hence social capital is not the number of clubs or telephones in the area, or the number of friends individuals have, or their trust in institutions. It is directly linked to the economic resources that can be accessed through information obtained in their social networks. Capacity building enhances community development

through a focus on the whole community or with particular population groups that address both social isolation and poverty. As an approach it comes close to comprehensive primary health care or to community development, but it should not be seen as a radical socialist approach. It is still very much within the framework of consensus politics.

PUBLIC HEALTH PRACTICE: HEALTHY PEOPLE IN HEALTHY COMMUNITIES

Public health practice in the United States, as well as in most other industrialized nations, has significantly improved the health status and life expectancy of the population over the past 200 years (Keck & Scutchfield, 1997). Most of these improvements have come from measures used to protect the public from environmental hazards (for example, food supply, water safety, sewage disposal, injury control) and to pursue health promotion activities (for example, changes in tobacco use, hypertension control, dietary patterns, injury control, automobile safety restraint). The public, however, has been largely unaware of the many contributions of public health. In the Institute of Medicine (IOM, 1988) report to the United States, *The Future of Public Health,* the IOM Committee for the Study of the Future of Public Health described agreement across the United States as "public health does things that benefit everybody" and "public health prevents illness and educates the population" (p. 3).

In an effort, however, to further clarify the role of public health's population-focused services, the IOM committee proposed a public health mission statement and a set of core functions. The committee defined the mission of public health as "fulfilling society's interest in assuring conditions in which people can be healthy" (IOM, 1988, p. 7). The core functions of public health agencies at all levels of government were identified as "assessment, policy development, and assurance" (p. 7). **Assessment** refers to systematic data collection on the health of the community; monitoring the population's health status, health needs, and health problems; and making information available on the health of the community. **Policy development** refers to the provision of leadership in developing comprehensive public health policies, including the use of a scientific knowledge base in decision making about policy. **Assurance** refers to the role of every public agency in assuring that high-priority personal and community-wide health services are available, which may include the direct provision of high-priority personal health services for those who are not able to afford them. Assurance also refers to making sure that a public health and personal health care work force is competent and available.

The proposed mission statement and core functions generated a great deal of discussion and action in the United States, with positive responses received. In the

RESEARCH FOCUS

British Whitehall Study 11

Study Problem/Purpose

Socioeconomic conditions play a significant role in morbidity and mortality patterns. What has been difficult is to know how to accurately measure socioeconomic status or how the various demographic factors of age, gender, marital status, and race interact or what impact they have in countries like Britain, Norway, and Australia, where even the poorest person has access to free universal health services. The British Whitehall 11 study provides an example of research which focuses on the relationship between socioeconomic class, health status, and control over work. Marmot and his colleagues examined the relationship between social class, psychosocial work conditions and cardiac disease, psychiatric illness, and absenteeism for over two decades for British civil servants across all grades of employees from senior executives to white collar clerks.

Methods

Marmot et al. examined morbidity and mortality patterns for a variety of conditions, collecting their data from successive national censuses, self-reporting, and employer data bases. In Britian the national census provides information on socioeconomic class linked to employment. Five social classes were identified, and more recently seven have been identified. Within the civil service employees, white collar jobs were spread across four grades from administrative to executive/professional, clerical, and other, with a number of classifications within these grades. In their earlier research the Whitehall team examined the relationship between social class, civil service grade, and behavioral factors such as smoking, weight, and leisure activities for a range of diseases. The characteristics of the work such as monotony, intensity, and interest were found to have more impact on mortality ratios than other factors. This led them in subsequent studies to examine *work demand* and *control over work* as two factors significant to mortality and morbidity patterns. The research has

been detailed with study requiring civil servants to measure their own blood pressure at home and at work for differences across social domains.

Findings

Several significant findings have emerged from the Whitehall 11 study. For example, in the study that asked civil servants to record their blood pressure at home and at work, it was found that both the highest and lowest grade of worker had similar readings at work and at home; however, the highest grade of workers had lower readings for home. Marmot et al. concluded that social domain impacts on physiological reactions with high-grade workers experiencing stress at work but not at home while low-grade workers experience stress in both environments.

In addition, it was found that high-grade civil servants with high demand but high control over their work have lower rates of self-reported sickness and absent days than those with high demand and no control or low demand and no control over their work day.

Implications

The findings suggest that perceptions of *power* and *control* are factors intimately linked to mortality and morbidity rates for all grades of workers and all classes of citizens. The higher the grade of employment, the more likely that workers perceive themselves as having power, although this is not always so. The health promotion implications point to the need to enhance democratic work practices, trust, team building, and security in the work place. Capacity building may very well promote the development of sound industrial relations legislation.

Sources: Marmot, M., & Theorell, T. (1988). Social class and cardiovascular disease: The contribution of work. International Journal of Health Services, 18(4), 659–674. North, F., Syme, L., Feeney, A., Shipley, M., & Marmot, M. (1996). Psychological work environment and sickness absence among British civil servants: The Whitehall 11 Study. American Journal of Public Health, 86(3), 332–340.

state of Washington, for example, the Washington State Department of Health and its core governmental Public Health Functions Task Force developed a definition of the IOM core functions and the role they play in improving a community's health. Following this activity, the state's Public Health Improvement Plan Steering Committee developed in 1994 a "Public Health Improvement

Plan" intended to improve the health status in the state through prevention and improved public health services delivery (Washington State Department of Health, 1994).

In July 1994, the National Association of County Health Officers (NACHO, 1994) published its *Blueprint for a Healthy Community: A Guide for Local Health Departments,* in which it examined the core public health functions in terms of the services needed to create and maintain a healthy community. Health departments are charged with the responsibility of assuring that 10 essential elements are provided by some community-based agency or program. The 10 essential elements identified by NACHO included:

1. Conduct a community diagnosis—analyze data for the purpose of information-based decision making.
2. Prevent and control epidemics and injuries.
3. Provide a safe and healthy environment—clean and safe air, water, food, and facilities.
4. Measure performance, effectiveness, and outcomes of health services.
5. Promote healthy lifestyles—provision of health education to individuals and communities.
6. Provide laboratory testing—identify disease agents.
7. Provide targeted outreach and form partnerships—assure access to services for vulnerable populations and the development of culturally congruent care.
8. Provide personal health services ranging from primary and preventive care to specialty and tertiary treatment.
9. Promote research and innovation.
10. Mobilize the community for action—initiate collaborative efforts and provide leadership to improve the community's health.

Because of public health's importance in influencing population health and in providing a foundation for the

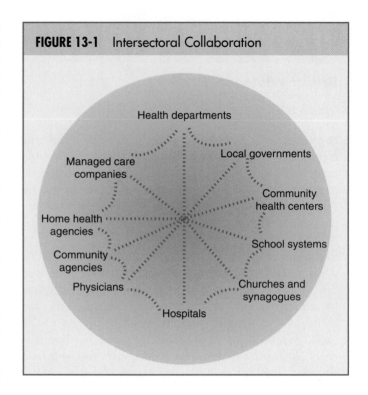

FIGURE 13-1 Intersectoral Collaboration

health care system, the U.S. Public Health Service and other groups are advocating a renewed emphasis on population-focused services. To ensure that all citizens will receive the effective services they need in the future, public health departments in the United States will need to build collaborative public-private partnerships with other community health agencies and with the illness care systems in the community, including other health departments, other departments of local governments, community health centers, school systems, churches, and other community agencies. Such collaboration is imperative for effectively improving population health not only in the United States but in other industrialized nations as well. Service and referral linkages with hospitals, physicians, home health agencies, managed-care companies, and other illness-based services are necessary also in order to provide a seamless system of services that promote population health, prevent illness, diagnose disease early, and provide treatment within a culturally sensitive, caring, healing environment. See Figure 13-1 for an illustration of intersectoral collaboration.

SOCIAL SCIENCES AND POPULATION-FOCUSED CARE

The shift from a health care system that primarily focuses on acute hospital-based services to one of preventive and population-based care is a direct result of social science research. The social model of health arises from social epidemiology and sociological research that has established clear links between socioeconomic status and health status (Black, Townsend, & Davidson, 1982). In

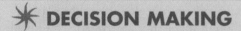

✳ DECISION MAKING

Community and Social Capital

◆ What is your experience of community? Consider this experience in terms of class, ethnicity, race, religion, gender, geography, age, sexual preference, or interests.

◆ What issues brought this community together and how did it come together?

◆ Can you list clubs, networks, and associations in your community that people join for social or cultural reasons that also bring them economic gains? How is this made possible?

◆ Can these community groups be seen as increasing **social capital** for its members? If so, how?

◆ If you were a community/public health nurse working in this community, how would you facilitate **capacity building** in this group?

short, mortality and morbidity rates of countries, and of groups within countries, mirror the socioeconomic conditions of these groups or nations. What is not clear is why or how political, economic, and social factors influence health status. The most debated factors are those in the Black Report (Black et al., 1982) commissioned by the British Labour government in the 1970s. The Black Report argued that inequalities in health are a result of one of four factors: artifact explanations, natural selection, materialist or structural explanations, or cultural or behavioral explanations.

Artifact explanations deal with problems inherent in the research tools that establish the links between morbidity and mortality patterns and the socioeconomic status of the population being studied. The problem of how to measure the relationship between social class and health status remains an issue for social scientists and health planners. One of the difficulties is in defining social class. This measure is often referred to as socioeconomic class and may also include age, disability, gender, and isolation or, as the Research Focus indicates, *power and control over one's work.* Another major issue linked to socioeconomic status in many countries is access to health care. This is particularly an issue where services must be purchased through insurance. For example, in the United States, "people aged 18–24 were the most likely to lack a usual source of ongoing primary care. Only 80 percent of individuals below the poverty level and 79 percent of Hispanics had a usual source of ongoing primary care" [U.S. Department of Health and Human Services (USDHHS), p. 45]. Class, race, gender and access to care intersect. Some measures defined social class as simply a matter of income. Others seek to incorporate social status, prestige, occupation, and even residence.

Natural selection refers to the suggestion that healthy individuals do well economically in any society, while those who are not healthy or able bodied will not do well economically (Powles & Salzberg, 1989). This theory was originally based on the belief that some groups in the population were biologically healthier than others. What this fails to explain is why certain morbidity and mortality patterns are found in occupational, ethnic, and gender groups, as well as geographic areas. Lundberg (1991) and Vagero (1991) argue that those born with certain chronic diseases are more likely to have inferior education and fewer employment opportunities. As a consequence, they are more likely to be poor and hence lack access to adequate health care resources.

Materialist or structural explanations argue that morbidity and mortality are a result of material conditions. Simply stated, those born into poor families are more likely to live in substandard houses and poor neighborhoods, have inferior health care services or no health care resources at all, have limited access to education and hence fewer opportunities for employment or be employed in low-skilled, low-paid occupations that are

highly dangerous. The cultural explanations have been linked to materialist explanations, suggesting that people who live in poverty have behaviors and cultural beliefs that are illness producing. An example of this is the high rate of diabetes, hypertension, and renal failure among Australian Aborigines (Anderson, 1996). While it is no doubt true that different groups in a society have different habits and beliefs that may not be health enhancing, one needs to ask whether these behaviors are based on cultural beliefs or poverty exacerbated by racism. It may be that poverty, rather than cultural beliefs and habits, creates certain unhealthy ways of being in the world.

Cultural explanations place the problem with the at-risk groups, while materialist explanations situate the problems with inequalities in the society, including inequalities in access to health care. The WHO promotes the view that universal free health care is a prerequisite for primary health care. This debate has been further enriched by what is known as the McKeown thesis. Thomas McKeown (1962), a medical researcher, stated that improvements in the health of the population in Britain following the industrialization in the 19th century was not the result of advances in medical science primarily but was the result of improvements in living conditions. McKeown argued that the decline in the death rate in Britain between 1870 and 1914 was the direct result of improvements in nutrition.

Others have argued that the improvements in the health of the population were a result of improvements in the living conditions of the poor, a direct result of improved working conditions, better housing, and increased wages achieved by working-class people better positioned to negotiate with employers (Blane, 1987). Scheyner, Landefeld, and Sandifer (1981) pointed out that the proponents of the old public health movement had begun the process of reform through the regulation of sanitation, water supply, food control, and town planning. However argued, the McKeown thesis supports preventive health over curative measures and materialist and structuralist explanations over cultural explanations.

More recently, social scientists have offered a post-structural critique of health promotion directed at specific populations. This critique is based on the work of the French social critic Michel Foucault (1980), who addressed both the self-help, individually based behavioral change approach to public health and the more broadly based population-focused campaigns. Foucault's argument was that the rise of medicine coincided with the emergence of the social sciences and that the fundamental aim of both is the control of the population. The old forms of social control such as death and torture gave way to prisons, asylums, and institutions for those who were deemed deviant. Those who were institutionalized came under the control of wardens, psychiatrists, social workers, and nurses. In the late 20th century new forms of social control have emerged. Asylums are no longer necessary to separate deviants from those who are perceived as normal. We do this for ourselves by embracing ideologies of what constitutes normal developmental stages and behaviors or what constitutes appropriate health-enhancing behaviors. We now regulate our own health through diets, exercise, and annual visits to our physician for pap smears, cholesterol checks, and mammograms, for example. At the macro level, the health behaviors of the population are regulated through legislation (e.g., antismoking laws), gathering of disease statistics, and identifying at-risk and high-risk groups. Population-focused health care runs the risk of focusing on control rather than on the concept of empowerment. Empowerment enhances community participation in health promotion efforts, and community health nurses play a vital role in the empowerment process. Empowerment of communities to participate in the process of health promotion is critical.

Clearly these theoretical explanations have implications for nursing actions. Cultural explanations lead to health promotion activities based on individual and group behavioral change, while materialist and structural explanations lead to health promotion activities based primarily on identifying community needs, deficits, or impediments to health. A variety of approaches is needed.

POPULATION-FOCUSED PRACTICE

A population approach suggests that a regional approach to health planning be aimed at providing a comprehensive health service across the three levels of health care: primary, secondary, and tertiary. A population approach provides management with directions for service provisions. Community assessments based on the use of epidemiology and biostatistics, community needs surveys and focus groups, as well as community involvement all help to determine those priorities and subsequent planning of services for the community. Managers provide the directions for services that are consistent with the identified needs. A needs- and assets-based approach also enables the identification of disadvantaged groups who might otherwise be neglected. Chapter 15 includes further discussion of community assessment.

Assets (Strength Building) and Needs Assessment

Program planning is essential to meet local, state, and national government mandates for funding, as well as philanthropic organization funding guidelines. Planning programs and planning for program evaluation are two critical activities for community health nurses in order to implement successful programs. These important skills are discussed further in Chapter 16.

The two key ingredients in the planning process are assets and needs assessment. **Needs assessment** is de-

fined as the systematic appraisal of the type, depth, and nature of health needs/problems as perceived by clients, health providers, or both in a given community. Prior to implementing any program, a needs assessment should be conducted to ensure that the program is meeting client and not the service provider needs. The data gathered from a needs assessment, as well as an assets assessment, should be the basis and rationale for program planning. It is important to understand the process involved in needs assessment and the different types of needs.

Hawe, Degeling, Hall, and Brierley (1990) outlined the following needs as necessary to identify:

- Normative needs—needs of a community defined by experts who judge what a community needs on the basis of their expert experience

- Expressed needs—needs that have been expressed by members of the community

- Comparative needs—those needs that emerge when one community lacks services that are provided in another community

- Felt needs—those needs that the members of the community say they want, via a community survey, for example

Hawe et al. (1990) also outlined the following nine steps, divided into two stages, that should be followed to ensure accurate assessment of client needs:

Stage I: Identification of the health problem/need, (1) consultation, (2) data collection, (3) presentation of findings, and (4) determining priorities

Stage II: Analysis of the health problem/need, (5) literature review, (6) description of the target population, (7) exploration of the health problem/need, (8) analysis of factors contributing to the problem/need, and (9) reassessment and strengthening of community resources

Assets assessment, initially recommended by John McKnight (1986), is also a very important ingredient in the planning process. McKnight argued that health professionals should view communities and populations in terms of the resources (assets) that they possess and that these resources should be acknowledged and utilized. Strength building, similar to "empowerment" (Rapport, 1987), is about building social support and building community. This means engaging in health-promoting activities that build strengths (skills, knowledge, competencies, self-esteem, power, and social support) (Raeburn & Rootman, 1998, p. 14). Where the opposite exists, poor health will be the result (Syme, 1989). Professionals should therefore abandon the tendency to define communities only by what they lack. By focusing only on need, health professionals lose touch with the rich capability of communities and the people in them. Thus, population-focused practice includes both assets and needs assessment in the planning process.

Population-Focused Practice in Community/Public Health Nursing

Population-focused practice is historically consistent with public health philosophy and is reflected in the American Public Health Association, (APHA, 1996) definition of public health nursing: "the practice of promoting and protecting the health of populations using knowledge from nursing, social, and public health sciences" (p. 1). Of particular importance is the APHA statement about public health nursing practice, which "includes assessment and identification of sub-populations who are at high risk of injury, disease, threat of disease, or poor recovery and focusing resources so that services are available and accessible" (p. 4). The APHA goal of public health nursing is "to improve the health of populations through ongoing assessment, coordinated interventions; and care management, working with and through relevant community leaders, interest groups, employers, families, and individuals; and through involvement in relevant social and political actions" (p. 4).

Public health nursing in the United States is viewed as a specialty in the broad field of community health nursing (Williams, 1996). According to the APHA (1996), "public health nurses integrate community involvement and knowledge about the entire population with personal, clinical understandings of the health and illness experiences of individuals and families within the population" (p. 2). Public health nurses "translate and articulate the health and illness experiences of diverse, often vulnerable individuals and families in the population to health planners and policy makers, and assist members of the community to voice their problems and aspirations" (p. 2).

Population-level decision making is different from clinical care decision making. At the clinical level the focus is on the individual client—assessing the health status, planning care with the client, and evaluating the effects of care. At the population level, the focus includes, for example, questions that address the incidence and prevalence of health conditions among various age, race, economic, and gender groups in the community. Obtaining information regarding the community's perceived health needs and assets is also included. Planning includes the development of programs in the community through coalition building and partnerships to lower the risk of certain conditions. Program evaluation is also included as part of the process. Table 13-2 outlines some of the distinctions between population-level and clinical care decision making.

The current changes occurring in the health care delivery system, as well as projected changes, will require nursing leaders, in addition to those in the public health nursing specialty, to think in population terms. This focus on populations and preparation in the use of population-oriented methods (e.g., epidemiology, biostatistics, demography, and community building) is necessary to make evidence-based practice decisions in program development. There is a need for nurses with skills in population assessment, management, and evaluation. In addition, there is a need for nurses prepared to participate in coalition building and partnership efforts to improve the health of populations.

Community Development

One of the major strategies for health promotion in population-focused health care, which emerged for example in Australia, Canada, and New Zealand, is community development, where the focus is empowerment through participation and equity (Jackson, Mitchel, & Wright, 1989; Labonte, 1990). Currently within community health practice, a tension exists between the perceived value of one-to-one casework and community development with its group action focus. This tension has led some community nurses to situate good practice primarily in group-focused activities. The concept of the community development continuum proposed by Jackson et al. (1989) has attempted to overcome this tension (Willis,

---

TABLE 13-2 Population-Level Decision Making versus Clinical Care Decision Making

POPULATION LEVEL	CLINICAL CARE
• Consider the incidence and prevalence of health conditions among various age, race, economic, and gender groups within community.	• Focus on individual client. (a) Assess health status. (b) Plan care with client. (c) Evaluate the care.
• Obtain information regarding the community's perceived health needs and assets.	
• Develop programs with the community through coalition building and partnerships that would lower the risk of certain conditions.	
• Perform program evaluation.	

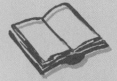

Out
of the Box

A Community-Based Prevention Model

A free public health urban and rural pilot screening program has been started for people at risk of lymphoedema following the removal of lymph nodes during surgery to control breast, prostate, and other cancers and injury. The need for raising public awareness of this condition was prompted by the experience of one of the team involved in the project, a nursing academic who developed lymphoedema following surgery for breast cancer. Heralded a world first, this program was made possible through combined collaborative efforts of the Schools of Nursing and Midwifery and Medicine at Flinders University in Adelaide, Australia, in conjunction with the Surgical Oncology Unit, Flinders Medical Centre, the Lymphoedema Support Group SA, and the Lions Club who funded the idea. Venues were provided by shopping centers in Adelaide. It is believed that the program has the potential to become a national community-based model for the prevention and early treatment of lymphoedema.

About 30% of all women who have an axillary clearance and radiotherapy to the chest or axilla to control breast cancer will develop chronic secondary lymphoedema during their life. Approximately 30% of all men and women who have a groin clearance and groin area radiotherapy to control cancer of the cervix, cancer of the bowel, and cancer of the prostate and other structures will develop chronic secondary lymphoedema. The risk is high but statistically unknown for melanoma excisions. Conservative estimates indicate there are currently about 150,000 sufferers of chronic secondary lymphoedema in Australia and an at-risk group of some 300,000. Another form of lymphoedema exists called primary lymphoedema of which there are three types, and they occur at birth, puberty (mainly in girls), or in later life (30–40 years). These represent about 3%–10% of all lymphoedemas.

Once the swelling (lymphoedema) is present in secondary lymphoedema, it is difficult to control and requires a lifetime of treatment, which may cost approximately $2500 per year. The client also has to deal with social and psychological issues, including changes in body image and loss of work productivity. The purpose of the community screening program, therefore, is to detect individuals at risk of developing lymphoedema and to provide information on precautions to prevent or delay its onset. Those individuals with signs and symptoms of lymphoedema are also assisted by increasing their knowledge of treatment and management options. Longer term outcomes were a possible reduction in the prevalence of chronic secondary lymphoedemas and the design of a working template for the start of a national screening program.

The first urban program was sponsored by the Lions Club. It was anticipated that among a population of approximately 50,000 in a designated area (Glenside), approximately 500 persons could potentially manifest lymphoedema and another 1000 persons could potentially be at risk. Publicity strategies to promote the program included television, a letter drop, newspaper articles, and radio interviews. Lions Club members assisted with setting up and running the project and nursing academics, and members from other agencies interviewed participants and assisted them in completing a risk assessment questionnaire. Following the completion of the risk assessment questionnaire, the score determined whether the person was at a low, moderate, or high risk for developing lymphoedema. Moderate- and high-risk participants and those with established lymphoedema were invited to undertake a bio-impedance measure of the fluid distribution in the at-risk or affected limb(s). Written information was provided to the participants, especially that which alerted them to the need to wear medi-alert bracelets to ensure that their at-risk or affected limb was not subjected to pressure from intravenous fluids or medical monitoring equipment that might trigger a lymphoedema. A follow-up assessment was organized for clients who had been identified as having a moderate- to high-risk chance of developing lymphoedema. Other preventive and referral options were also discussed.

The provision of information and the raising of awareness among those who attended the program should lead to the adoption of strategies to reduce lymph load and increase transport, both of which are important in reducing risk and controlling lymphoedema. These in turn will improve a client's quality of life and be a cost benefit to society as a whole. Many participants involved in this early program traveled hundreds of kilometers to attend this program because funding bodies do not currently recognize lymphoedema. Further initiatives will include collecting and analyzing data from the initial participant group to determine if there is a reduced rate of the appearance of lymphoedema in this group compared with a nonscreened group.

—Jenny Donovan, 2001 ■

✳ DECISION MAKING

Community Development Continuum

Examine the community development continuum presented in Table 13-3.

◆ How helpful do you think this model is for understanding the community development process?

◆ Do you think the representation of the continuum should be circular, given that in reality people might enter at one or several points?

1990). The five points on the continuum defined by Jackson et al. (1989) are:

1. Developmental casework
2. Mutual support
3. Issue identification and campaigns
4. Participation
5. Control of services and social movements

Jackson et al. (1989) suggest that health workers can work through the continuum in the course of their work and can be engaged in several points at any one time. As can be seen from the points identified in Table 13-3, individuals ideally move along the continuum toward greater levels of control over areas of their own lives,

joining with other people who hold similar interests to assume more social and economic power, forming communities of interest. The continuum provides a variety of possibilities for community health nurses in a variety of settings. The continuum supports actions which include advocacy for a single client of family, client education, and comprehensive discharge planning as well as group work and social action.

Moving forward from the community development continuum, governments are also realizing they do not have all of the answers or cannot solve the problems of communities alone. It is here that the social movement of the community development continuum and the new term *capacity building* have some similarities. Both are based on the realization that local communities are often the best at identifying and responding to local problems and that real solutions will only emerge if governments work in partnership with communities to find them (Department of Family and Community Services, 2000).

Empowerment

Each stage in the community development continuum is characterized by empowerment and an opening to the possibilities of further action along the continuum. **Empowerment** is the process whereby individuals feel increasingly in control of their own affairs. Generally, the process begins with one or more motivational triggers, such as a crisis, frustration, or outrage. In most cases, the motivational trigger leads to change because individuals learn that they have a voice and that there are people

TABLE 13-3 Community Development Continuum

DEVELOPMENTAL CASEWORK	MUTUAL SUPPORT	ISSUE IDENTIFICATION AND CAMPAIGNS	PARTICIPATION	CONTROL OF SERVICES AND SOCIAL MOVEMENTS
• Casework emphasizing self-help	• Promoting self-help support groups	• Community education and public awareness	• Collective participation	• Control
• Liaison and networking	• Creating mutual support networks	• Formation of action groups to deal with the issues		• Intensifying advocacy
• Information collection and dissemination	• Linking isolated individuals with existing social groups	• Support of action groups to raise profile of issues to the conscious level		• Participating in policy and legislative changes
• Referral	• Strengthening neighborhood networks	• Encouraging critical profile/community action		
• Linking to family and friends	• Improving social support			
• Advocacy				

Adapted from Jackson, T., Mitchel, S., & Wright, M. (1989). The community development continuum. Community Health Statistics, *13(1).*

REFLECTIVE THINKING

Empowerment

- What does empowerment mean to you?
- What do you think about the criteria for empowerment proposed by Labonte?
- How do you experience empowerment both personally and professionally in your own life?

who will listen and understand (Lord & McKillop, 1990, p. 4). The criteria for empowerment identified by Labonte (1990) are improved status, self-esteem, and cultural identity; the ability to reflect critically and solve problems; the ability to make choices; increased access to resources; increased collective bargaining power; the legitimating of people's demands by officials; and self-discipline and the ability to work with others.

The role of nurses is not to do unto others but to assist others by working with them and functioning as resources, supporting their right to make decisions for themselves (Labonte, 1993; Friedman, 1992). An empowering practice requires that we view clients as equal

Perspectives...

INSIGHTS OF A NURSING PROFESSOR

Nursing from a primary health care perspective requires that nurses understand the health care issues for populations and how these impact on the individuals and groups receiving their care. As a nursing faculty member, I believe that nursing students need to know about and understand the society in which they work. Such an understanding ensures that nurses view "health" as a sociopolitical and economic issue—and that nurses do not work in a vacuum. Bringing nursing students to an understanding of how the "social" impacts on their practice and the wider society's health care is key to ensuring that they have a far wider view than merely the health of an individual. Such a view would ensure that nurses understand how individual choice is affected by the power structures in which people live. Such knowledge also ensures that nurses can work with groups and individuals with an understanding of how these individuals and groups make their health care decisions.

Over the years of my practice as a nurse, I have found that challenges, for individuals and groups, are more apparent where different sectors of government meet. For instance, where various health agencies, government departments, and competing interests of business coincide, implementation of health care policies become complex matters indeed. For example, a recent study in Australia into the "Burden of Disease" suggests that depression will be a major mental health issue. Research about depression and the funding of treatment programs are now a governmental priority. From a population perspective, then, an emphasis on depression makes sense. But as a mental health practitioner, I wonder what will happen to those people who do not have a diagnosis of depression, but whose quality of life and access to care are reduced because

we now have a new priority. Such a reprioritization constrains community health and mental health nurses' practices everyday.

As a health professional interested in the mental health of workers, I believe a focus on depression is important. We live in a world that is influenced globally by a culture of "risk" management, heightened individual responsibility, and insecure employment. In such an environment, employee insecurity leads to unsafe practices, work-related stress, and mental health issues. In linking the trend in disease burden to rates of depression diagnoses and the insecurities of late industrial employment, I am highlighting, from a population perspective, that it is important to recognize that the entire social fabric needs to be taken into account if we are to achieve health for all.

Indeed, worker insecurity and other social issues mean that rates of diagnosed depression are likely to increase. But are we likely to see changes to employment security where global economics and technological developments encourage such practices? Does empowering workers or community/mental health service users provide the answer? A brief answer would probably be no. However, a nurse who is aware of these issues will be able to identify where a person or group of people are coming from. The nurse's practice is likely to be more responsive at both the individual and group level and, in collaboration with clients, will make practice more political in its intent. Nursing from a primary health care perspective is political, enabling nurses to have a greater say in social and health care reform. Knowledge and power are everything: The result is strategic nursing!

—Trudy Rudge, RN, RPN, BA (Hons), PhD

COMMUNITY NURSING VIEW

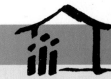

In the state of South Australia, the Child Adolescent and Family Health Service, a government-funded service, works with families who have new babies and young children. Under the affirmative action policy, after the birth of a child, some families are visited in their own homes. Others are contacted by an interagency with the maternity hospital concerned. In rural areas, all new mothers are visited in the local hospital.

At the clinic visit, clients initially experience one-to-one developmental casework, health assessment, and anticipatory guidance whereby the professional enables consumers of that service to draw on their own experiences and look for their own solutions (WHO, 1986). This is in contrast to the more traditional approach wherein people depend on the health workers (Jackson et al., 1989). Women and men are supported to make informed choices during their current experiences as new parents; however, the numbers of fathers who attend the clinics is slowly increasing (Russell et al., 1999).

In 1989, a universal parent education program was developed for all parents with new children. Topics focused on issues such as pregnancy, birth and homecoming, settling babies and nutrition, when to call the doctor, child development, play ideas, discipline and safety, and self-esteem for parents and their children. The new movement is toward topics that focus on attachment and the importance of the early years.

Parents gain valuable information about their babies' normal behavior and find that they experience similar issues. They are invited to attend new parents courses or coffee mornings, to see how they might help and support each other. By meeting together, parents establish more realistic, attainable standards that can be adapted to individual preferences and needs. Being accepted as a member of the group is an important factor for many people. Group education has the added bonus of empowering parents, who, while sharing their ideas, discover that their parenting is satisfactory and that their feelings about parenting, both positive and negative, are normal. The participants gradually gain more confidence in themselves and their own ability to make decisions.

Small groups, particularly self-help groups, can be empowering because they normalize people's experience of powerlessness. Once trust and acceptance have been established with others, participants feel more able to contribute and to move on to broader community issues. This is considered to be the successful transition from reliance on one-to-one contact with a professional to recognizing the value of mutual support and being able to build links with each other.

Facilitators can enhance the parents' sense of competence and control by assisting them to develop a support network within and outside the group. Research by Telleen, Herzog, and Kilbane (1989) showed the effectiveness of educating parents about the use of social support as a means of coping and enhancing their problem-solving capabilities.

It is intended that the groups be in an environment that is socially, culturally, and geographically acceptable to all clients and that a primary health care focus is maintained. The programs encourage the development of friendships and social networks to bring people together who are dealing with common issues and similar life circumstances. "This point marks the transition from participation for survival to participation to achieve change" (Jackson et al., 1989, p. 70). The program has positive effects on the mothers' attitudes toward their children and reduces the sense of social isolation in their parental role (Telleen et al., 1989; Lord & McKillop, 1990).

As parents move from participation for survival to participation to achieve change, collective participation occurs and they take a more active role in assisting others. The outcomes for people moving along the community development continuum are similar to some of the areas identified in the Ottawa Charter for Health Promotion. A supportive environment is created when people form mutual support groups. Community action is strengthened when people identify and campaign for change. By being involved, people are able to develop personal skills such as the ability to work out health-promoting solutions, contribute as an active team member, and encourage others to think about options for change.

Nursing Considerations

Having read the scenario about the community development continuum, consider how empowerment, community development, and community participation were utilized in the example given. Were the strategies of the Ottawa Charter for Health Promotion apparent? What would you have done differently?

Assessment

◆ What data would you need to begin to plan a parent education and support program?

◆ What are some of the barriers that might prevent parents from attending child health clinics or family-centered health centers?

(continues)

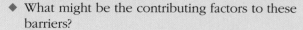

COMMUNITY NURSING VIEW (continued)

◆ What might be the contributing factors to these barriers?

◆ How would you distinguish the needs of parents from differing socioeconomic groups?

Diagnosis

◆ What should be considered in formulating nursing diagnoses related to parents who participate in a parent program?

Planning/Interventions

◆ If you were organizing parent education and support groups for parents, how would you establish them? What process would you use?

◆ What problems might occur in the process of organizing parent education groups within an organization, given the different needs of clients?

◆ How might you work collaboratively with parents in program planning?

◆ How might you work collaboratively with other organizations to maximize the health professionals' input?

◆ Since the social movement stage of the continuum was not discussed in the scenario provided, what would you suggest that would demonstrate this movement?

Outcome Identification

◆ What expected outcomes would you formulate specific to the development of a parent education and support program?

Evaluation

◆ Who should be involved in developing the evaluation process and methods?

◆ What evaluation methods would you recommend?

---

community members, as persons capable of and responsible for their own empowerment. A critical element in the empowerment process for the individual or family is someone characterized as a "good listener," an "equal," a "guide," and as a person "who really cares" (Lord & McKillop, 1990, p. 5). Stacey (1988) states that "the goal of empowering and enabling must be to make it unnecessary to enable or empower, because people will understand what of value we have to offer" (p. 321).

Empowerment enhances community participation. An essential ingredient for effective population-focused practice is community participation in assessment, planning, and policy development. Active involvement of the people who are affected by health programs and policies is a shift to community responsibility in planning, for either preventive or curative services.

Empowerment provides for the creation of new ways of being, doing, and living. It promotes the creation of caring communities, the possibility of establishing an equitable, just society in which community members have an opportunity to develop their unique contributions regardless of age, race, gender, culture, sexual orientation, or economics.

This chapter discusses population-focused practice and health care, highlighting that a population approach is one element of health promotion. A discussion of population-focused practice in community/public health nursing and in public health provides an opportunity to examine strategies that foster the development of healthy communities, strategies such as needs- and assets-based planning, community development, and empowerment.

KEY CONCEPTS

◆ The focus of population-focused health care is the health of communities or aggregates of populations.

◆ Primary health care as a policy model emphasizes community participation, intersectoral collaboration, integration of health services, and health care access and equity for all.

◆ Primary health care has a key role to play in reducing the current inequalities in the health status between different sections of the population and in providing equal opportunities for access to health care for the whole population.

◆ The core functions of public health in the United States are assessment, policy development, and assurance.

◆ Needs and assets assessment is about collecting information that will give a good indication of the needs and assets of a community, laying the foundation for creating healthy, caring communities.

◆ Community development is a construct that describes the actions intended to change the aspects of the environment that promote ill health, inequity, poverty, and powerlessness. Community participation promotes the philosophy of the World Health Organization that people have a right and duty to participate in the planning and implementation of health care.

◆ Empowerment is the process whereby individuals and families feel increasingly in control of their own affairs.

◆ Strengthening community action with information, education, and support is about empowering communities and individuals to work toward ownership and control of their issues. It is about communities acting in partnership to enhance opportunities for social change.

◆ Reorienting health services includes sharing the responsibility for health decisions and services between individuals, community groups, community leaders, health professionals, and governments while working to promote health.

Community health nurses have a vital role to play in this process.

◆ Building healthy public policy by raising awareness beyond the health care system includes acting as advocates at all levels of the health system in cooperation with a wide range of agencies. It includes developing social policies that foster greater equity and access to health care for everyone, aiming to provide the opportunity for people to make choices that will promote health and healing.

RESOURCES

Australian government: http://www.aihw.gov.au
New South Wales Department of Health:
   http://www.health.nsw.gov.au
New South Wales Department of Health:
   http://www.health.nsw.gov.au

Chapter

14

EPIDEMIOLOGY

Janice A. Young, RN, MS

Lindsey K. Phillips, RN, MS

MAKING THE CONNECTION

The potential for preventing or alleviating illness has grown at an astounding rate. This may be attributed to the rapid pace of discovery, aided by public confidence and willingness to support research, and to the decreasing lags between scientific discovery and its practical application.

—*Freeman, 1963, p. 13*

COMPETENCIES

Upon completion of this chapter, the reader should be able to:

- Define epidemiology.
- Examine the historical development of epidemiology.
- Identify key concepts in the epidemiological approach.
- Discuss the significance of the epidemiological approach in community health nursing.
- Describe the types of epidemiological investigations and study designs.
- Identify key population measures and vital statistics used in epidemiology.
- Discuss the uses and application of the epidemiological approach in community health nursing practice.

KEY TERMS

agent

analytic epidemiological studies

attack rate

attributable risk percentage (AR%)

bias

case fatality rate

case reports

case series

case-control study

cause-specific death rate

chemical agents

cohort study

correlational study

cross-sectional survey

demography

descriptive epidemiological studies

disease frequency

ecology

environment

epidemic

epidemiology

false-negative test

false-positive test

host

incidence rate

infectious agents

intervention studies

levels of prevention

maternal mortality rate

measures of association

morbidity rate

mortality rate

natural history of a disease

nutritive elements

observational studies

odds ratio (OR)

pellagra

physical agents

point prevalence

PRECEDE-PROCEED model

prevalence rate

prevention trials

prospective study

relative risk

retrospective study

risk

sensitivity

specificity

surveillance

therapeutic trials

vital statistics

The science of epidemiology is important to community health nurses because its methods provide for the assessment and understanding of health, disease, and injury in a community or target population. **Epidemiology** is a population-focused applied science that uses research and statistical data collection methodology to find answers to the following questions:

- Who in a population is affected by a disease, disorder, or injury?
- What is the occurrence of this health problem in the community?
- Can the causative factors and risk factors contributing to the problem be determined?

The epidemiological approach provides community health nurses with the methodology and language to describe and analyze health concerns in population-based care. Related community health disciplines such as public health, occupational health, and the environmental sciences also use epidemiology in everyday practice. The use of epidemiological techniques also alerts community health nurses to the possible etiology of health problems in a neighborhood or district.

This chapter serves as an introduction to the epidemiological concepts, methods, and measures that enable the community health nurse to examine aggregate health concerns in a neighborhood, community, or township.

DEFINITION AND BACKGROUND

Green (1996) describes community health as a triad of applied sciences that includes epidemiology, human ecology, and demography. Community health goes beyond the individual to focus on the health problems of populations. This group focus is the distinguishing difference between community health nursing and clinical nursing, which focuses on the individual or family.

Ecology in community health, according to Green (1996), refers to the interrelationship between the individual and his or her physical, cultural, and social environments. Ecology in this sense, then, may include climate, geography, industry, and religious and cultural factors influencing a community. **Demography** is an analytic tool used to measure a population by recording births, deaths, age distribution, and other vital statistics. Epidemiology is a companion science to demography in that it also uses analytic tools to find causes, frequency, and distribution of health problems in a community. A clear and concise definition of epidemiology is provided by Last (1995): "Epidemiology is the study of the distribution and determinants of health-related states or events in specified populations, and the application of this study to the control of health problems" (p. 42).

Historically, the term *epidemiology* originated from the study of **epidemics** (rapid rises in disease occurrence beyond the expected norm) of infectious diseases such as yellow fever, cholera, and bubonic plague. Contemporary epidemiology focuses on a broad spectrum of health problems including communicable and chronic diseases, injury control, nutrition, and violence (Friedman, 1987).

The use of epidemiological methods dates back to the 5th century B.C. Hippocrates, a Greek physician and the father of modern medicine, was the first to use observation and data collection to describe infectious diseases such as tetanus and mumps. Epidemiological methods were used to investigate and conquer such epidemics as the bubonic plague, which killed 25 million Europeans in the Middle Ages. Into the 17th and 18th centuries, vital record collection and analysis became important tools in determining the impact of the great epidemics on communities by examining age distribution and seasonal changes in the number of deaths. John Graunt (1620–1674) is credited with the first analysis of birth and death records, published in *Natural and Political Observations Made upon the Bills of Mortality,* as cited in Hennekens and Buring (1987). During a time when bubonic plague caused deaths to outnumber births, his report contributed to the understanding of the pattern of this disease in the London population.

John Snow (1813–1858) wrote about his epidemiological investigation of the London cholera epidemic in *On the Mode of Communication of Cholera,* as cited in Hennekens and Buring (1987). His important work is considered the first application of epidemiological methods. Snow investigated an outbreak of cholera in London and linked the cause of the epidemic to a contaminated water supply. He used observational methods, neighborhood interviews, and analysis of death records according to geographic location to show that death rates were higher in a community whose water source was supplied by one particular water company.

In the southern United States, a Public Health Service physician named John Goldberger (1874–1927) conducted a famous epidemiological investigation on **pellagra,** a deficiency disease causing gastrointestinal, mucosal, neurological, and mental symptoms. Using methods established by John Snow, Goldberger determined the cause of pellagra to be dietary rather than infectious, as was previously believed. The epidemiological methods used were observing those with and without the disease and interviewing local residents about environmental conditions and dietary habits.

Prior to the discovery of disease-producing microorganisms, many diseases were attributed to poverty, overcrowding, and poor environmental conditions and occurrences. Contemporary epidemiology mirrors the technological advances of the past century and the changes in life expectancy. During the past century, life expectancy in the United States has increased by nearly 60%. In 1900, life expectancy was 47 years [U.S. Department of Health and Human Services (USDHHS), 1990]. In 1998, life expectancy was 77 years (USDHHS, 2000). Evolutionary changes of an aging population linked with the cure and control of many communicable diseases has resulted in the modern epidemics of chronic diseases such as heart disease, cancer, and stroke. Table 14-1 illustrates this evolutionary shift in the leading causes of death in the United States from 1900 to 1998 (when adjusted for age). Applying epidemiology to the study of chronic diseases such as cancer as opposed to that of communicable diseases has required the development of more complex research methods because of the long induction period between exposure to a disease-causing agent and appearance of signs of the disease.

REFLECTIVE THINKING

Assessing Your Community

- Can you call to mind a particular disease, health concern, or injury that affects your community?
- Can you describe the population in the community that is most affected by this particular problem?
- What factors may be contributing to the problem?

BASIC CONCEPTS IN THE EPIDEMIOLOGICAL APPROACH

The epidemiological approach is an application of the scientific method and assumes that health, disease, and injury do not occur randomly. The historical development of epidemiological methods illustrates the necessity of investigating a health problem before everything is known about the disease etiology. For example, prior to the discovery of the microorganism responsible for cholera, John Snow used epidemiological methods to show that a contaminated water source was causing a cholera outbreak in London. Similarly, community health nurses working in health districts and neighborhoods may employ epidemiological methods to investigate health, social, and environmental problems. This section

TABLE 14-1 Ten Leading Causes of Death in the United States, 1900 and 1998, All Ages

1900	1998
Pneumonia/influenza	Heart diseases
Tuberculosis	Cancer
Heart diseases	Stroke
Stroke	Chronic obstructive pulmonary disease
Diarrhea/enteritis	
Nephritis	Accidents
Cancer	Pneumonia/influenza
Injuries	Diabetes
Diphtheria	Suicide
Other	Nephritis, nephrotic syndrome and nephrosis
	Chronic liver disease and cirrhosis

From National Center for Health Statistics. *(1999). Ten leading causes of death in the United States. [On-line]. Available: www.cdc.gov/nchs.*

REFLECTIVE THINKING

Causes of Death

- As a community health nurse, what resource would you use to find data about the leading causes of death in your community?
- What are the leading age-specific causes of death in your community?

provides an overview of several key concepts framing the foundation and historical development of epidemiology.

Epidemiological Triad: Agent, Host, and Environment

One of the functions of the epidemiological approach to the study of disease is to determine the etiology, or cause, of the disease or risk factor. Although most of the concepts inherent in the science of epidemiology evolved from the study of infectious diseases, these concepts can be applied to noninfectious diseases and conditions as well (Lilienfeld & Stolley, 1994). The concepts of epidemiology can also be applied to the study of injuries and, more recently, have been applied to the study of health and wellness. In order to study the etiology or

causality of a health problem, the epidemiologist systematically views three multifactorial elements: agent, host, and environment.

Agent

The **agent** is a toxic substance, microorganism, or environmental factor, such as radiation or a lifestyle, that must be present (or absent) for the problem to occur. Analytic epidemiology seeks to link the agent to the disease or condition in order to determine causality. In other words, the epidemiologist must examine factors that influence the probability of contact between, for example, an infectious agent and a susceptible person or population, known as a host. To illustrate the concept of an agent linked to the development of a disease or risk factor, consider the relationship between asbestos exposure or smoking and the development of lung cancer or the relationship between type A behavior and heart disease. According to Lilienfeld and Stolley (1994), disease agents and etiologic factors can be classified into four categories: nutritive elements, chemical agents, physical agents, and infectious agents.

Nutritive elements can be described as excesses or deficiencies within a host, such as vitamin or protein deficiencies. Cholesterol is one example of a nutritive element that can be viewed as an agent of disease, in this case, hyperlipidemia. **Chemical agents** include poisons and allergens. Examples of poisons include pharmaceuticals taken in excess, carbon monoxide, and caustic substances such as lye. Allergens are agents such as ragweed and poison oak and may also include medications or foods. **Physical agents** include radiation, excessive sun exposure, and mechanical agents. Because mechanical agents may be more difficult to conceptualize than other physical agents, two examples are presented here to clarify this concept.

In the 1950s, when jet aircraft were in the initial stages of development and usage, many of the pilots being trained to fly the new airplanes were found to have hearing loss in some decibel ranges. Upon investigation, it was determined that the high-pitched sounds emitted by the jet engines damaged the ear and caused permanent hearing loss in certain decibel ranges. Since that discovery, pilots and others working around jet aircraft have been required to wear protective ear coverings to block out damaging sounds.

More recently, with the advent of computer technology and the widespread use of computers in the office and home, many people have developed a type of carpal tunnel syndrome. In computer users, this condition has been traced to the position in which the hands are held for long periods of time when working at a computer. Consequently, those who use the computer for many hours a day are now advised to change hand positions often and to take periodic breaks from their work at the computer.

Infectious agents of disease include metazoa, such as hookworm; protozoa, including those causing malaria and toxoplasmosis; bacteria, associated with syphilis, tuberculosis, and other diseases; fungi; and viruses. An example of an infectious agent is one that causes foodborne illness such as salmonellosis; the illness is caused by the bacterial contamination of certain (usually uncooked or undercooked) foods, which are ingested by a susceptible host.

Host

The **host** is the person or population on which the agent acts. Before the host population is examined, the persons composing a population must be looked at individually. In this way, the epidemiologist or community health nurse can determine those factors that individuals possess that might be factors linked to a particular disease or disability. In examining the individual host, the epidemiologist must look at demographic characteristics including age, gender, ethnicity, socioeconomic status, marital status, nutritional and immune status, genetic or familial factors, occupation, physiological or psychological state, preexisting conditions or disease, and lifestyle. Each of these characteristics will have an impact on the development of disease or other conditions as well as on the general health or wellness of the individual host. Although the host is, technically, always an individual, epidemiology is a science that examines the presence of disease or risk factors in populations over time. Thus, epidemiologists examine a group or population of hosts in which a particular agent or risk factor is present. To draw conclusions about disease, injury, or wellness in a population without closely examining individual host characteristics for common factors can lead to misinterpretation of data and, in turn, false conclusions.

Through scientific investigation, we have become increasingly aware of the role played by genetic factors in the development of disease. Sickle cell anemia and hemophilia are two examples of genetically transferred disease. Age is also an important factor; whereas some diseases appear to primarily strike young people, others develop with the aging process. Gender must also be considered, in that some diseases or conditions are more common among women or among men. For example, although cases of breast cancer are occasionally seen in men, this disease primarily affects women. Some diseases are more common in one ethnic group than in another. The higher rate of sickle cell anemia among African Americans is an example of an ethnically related factor. The psychological or physiological state of the host must also be considered. Pregnancy, obesity, and high blood pressure are among the many physiological states that may place the individual at risk for disease, disability, or injury. Stress, one of many psychological factors, is now recognized as an important factor in the development of some diseases and conditions. Preexisting disease and immunocompetence are also key factors affecting susceptibility and resistance to disease. The development of opportunistic infections such as tuberculosis or toxoplasmosis among persons with AIDS is an example of poor host resistance. Risk factors for disease are increasingly being attributed to lifestyle factors: Amount and type of exercise, elements of diet, including fat and alcohol intake, and smoking habits, among others, are now seen as key risk factors in the development of certain diseases and conditions. Marital status may also be an indicator of the probability of developing a particular disease or of life expectancy. People who are married or partnered, for example, may have a longer life expectancy.

Environment

The third concept inherent in the epidemiological triad is **environment.** The environment comprises those factors outside of the host that are associated with the development of disease, disorder, or injury. Elements of environment that must be considered when linking agent and host include geographic factors (climate, latitude, and altitude), occupational hazards, and personal and secular trends (changes in lifestyle patterns or environmental risks over years or decades, such as sewage treatment or availability of immunizations).

The interaction of host and environmental factors is very important in tracing the etiology of disease and other conditions. Whether being examined by the epidemiologist or the community health nurse, the importance of individual host characteristics, or factors, cannot be overemphasized.

With regard to the impact of environmental factors (those outside of the host) on disease development, physical environment is important in that certain diseases are more prevalent in a particular climate or geographic location or even at certain times of the year. Malaria, for example, is a disease that is rare in the United States but indigenous to many parts of Africa. Biological factors are those related to density of populations, sources of food and water, and the presence of disease agents in the area being studied. Whether the host lives in an urban or rural setting may be a factor related to disease development. For instance, people living and working close together in cities may be more susceptible to influenza outbreaks than are their counterparts in rural areas. The occupation of the host must be carefully examined for exposure to pathogens. Historically, one can recall the discovery of the prevalence of lung disease among miners. More recently, researchers have examined the relationship between agricultural pesticide use and disease development among farm workers as well as between silicate exposure and asbestosis.

The significance of the epidemiological triad should thus be evident. Equally significant is the interrelationship among the three parts of the triad. For example, occupation is viewed as a characteristic of the host, but where the host works constitutes an environment. Further, the occupation of the host in a particular environment can cause exposure to chemical or mechanical agents. Likewise, socioeconomic status (a host factor) can affect the nutritional state and the ability to obtain adequate and safe housing (an environmental factor). For instance, the media have reported numerous cases of lead poisoning among children who have been exposed to old lead-based paint (an agent) on walls in pre-1950 tenements or on older cribs. Furthermore, disease vectors (agents), including rats, cockroaches, and fleas, may also be rampant in substandard conditions. See Figure 14-1 for an illustration of the epidemiological triad.

Many of the host and environmental factors thus far mentioned constitute distinct areas of scientific study, such as genetics, microbiology, geriatrics, pediatrics, and sociology, to name a few. The task of the epidemiologist is to attempt to examine and integrate pertinent elements from many different disciplines in order to assemble the data needed to analyze a particular disease or condition and trace its etiology (Lilienfeld & Stolley, 1994). The same process may be used by community health nurses in identifying factors related to disease, disability, or injury among their clients.

It is important to understand the concepts of agent, host, and environment in that they are basic to the science of epidemiology. These three factors and their parts must be considered whenever and wherever the epidemiologist seeks to determine the etiology of a disease, whether the goal is eradication of the disease or the development of preventive measures.

The goal of epidemiology therefore is to understand the causal factors that interact to increase the risk of dis-

---

✳ DECISION MAKING

Lead Poisoning

As a community health nurse, you have determined that several of your youngest clients, who live in urban older housing, are exhibiting symptoms of lead poisoning.

◆ What host factors might predispose the children to this condition?

◆ How might you determine the agent involved?

◆ What environmental factors might you suspect that could be related to the condition, and what steps might you advise the parents to take to correct those factors?

---

ease or injury in order to prevent the initiation of the disease process or injury. However, causal relationships are complex. The term *web of causation* has been used to depict causal factors that contribute to the disease process or injury. Diez-Roux (1998) recommended a paradigm that considers multiple levels of factors that affect and contribute to disease. This paradigm expands epidemiological studies to broader contexts such as neighborhood characteristics and downward to the genetic/molecular level.

The Natural History of a Disease

One goal of epidemiology is the eradication or prevention of health problems. A logical first step for the epidemiologist, then, is to understand the natural history of the disease in question. The **natural history of a disease** can be defined as the unaltered course that a disease would take without any intervention such as therapy or lifestyle changes. One primary application of epidemiology is to study the natural history of a disease in order to develop therapeutic interventions or prevention strategies. The natural history of a disease can be understood by viewing the concept as a continuum, with exposure to the agent suspected of causing the disease or condition at one end, through the development of signs and symptoms of illness in a progression of severity, to the ultimate outcome of the disease, whether that be disability or death, at the other end (see Figure 14-2).

The most common analytic study design used to determine the natural history of a disease is the cohort study, which will be discussed in detail later in this chapter. Understanding the natural history of disease is of vital importance to epidemiologists and others who seek to discover the etiology of disease, design strategic therapeutic interventions, and develop preventive or screening measures in order to alter the outcome of a particular

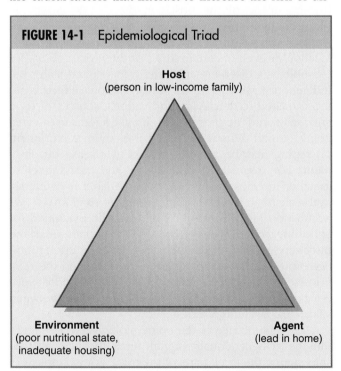

FIGURE 14-1 Epidemiological Triad

Host
(person in low-income family)

Environment
(poor nutritional state, inadequate housing)

Agent
(lead in home)

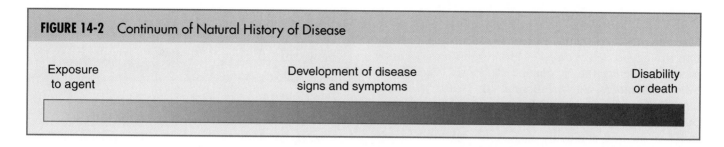

FIGURE 14-2 Continuum of Natural History of Disease

Exposure to agent

Development of disease signs and symptoms

Disability or death

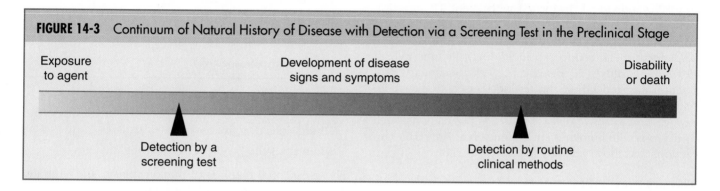

FIGURE 14-3 Continuum of Natural History of Disease with Detection via a Screening Test in the Preclinical Stage

Exposure to agent

Development of disease signs and symptoms

Disability or death

Detection by a screening test

Detection by routine clinical methods

disease process or condition. Community health nurses also use the concept of the natural history of disease in client education, when informing clients about their diseases or conditions and encouraging behavior or lifestyle modification as a means of altering the course of the disease or condition in question.

Figure 14-3 illustrates the natural history of a disease continuum with incorporation of detection via a screening test in the preclinical stage.

The usefulness of screening tests to detect early disease depends on available and effective treatments at the time of detection. Additionally, the possibility of a **false-negative test** (test that is negative when the individual actually has the disease of interest) and a **false-positive test** (test result that is positive when the individual does not have the disease of interest) should be minimal; that is, the test should have sufficient **sensitivity** (the probability of a positive result for an individual who has the disease) and sufficient **specificity** (the probability of a negative result for an individual who does not have the disease).

Concept of Prevention

Prevention is another key concept to epidemiology. Epidemiologists seek to identify characteristics that cause or predict a disease or condition. This identification of potential risk factors may result in prevention of disease when intervention strategies can be established. Measures that delay the onset of a disease or prevent it altogether are called preventive. The three **levels of prevention** are called primary, secondary, and tertiary.

A taxonomy of the three levels of prevention reflects the continuum of the natural history of a disease. Primary

prevention strategies or interventions foster health promotion and wellness before a disease or symptoms develop (Green, 1996). Secondary prevention activities target early diagnosis, treatment, and detection of disease to prevent disability. Tertiary prevention strategies and activities focus on limiting disability once disease develops. Community health prevention strategies include health education for health promotion, public health measures, legal or regulatory sanctions for health protection, and health services for screening and preventive care.

Primary Prevention

Primary prevention typically involves several key strategies: health education, regulatory strategies, and health care services. These strategies are used in many disease prevention programs. Health education programs targeting populations at risk for cancer, for example, include antismoking campaigns, fiber-rich diet promotion to reduce colon cancer, and promotion of sunscreen use to prevent harmful sun overexposure. Regulatory strategies that limit carcinogens in the environment and alert the public to potential hazards have been employed in such states as California to promote cancer prevention. Cigarette taxes constitute another example of regulatory strategy, specifically with regard to the primary prevention of lung cancer. Immunization is an example of preventive health care services, constituting an important component in the primary prevention of childhood infectious diseases. Vaccination against hepatitis B to prevent liver cancer is another example of primary preventive health care.

Secondary Prevention

Screening tests constitute a common secondary prevention strategy to detect disease before symptoms occur or would be detectable by routine diagnosis (Greenberg, Daniels, Flanders, Eley, & Boring, III, 1996). Screening tests should provide for early treatment and enhanced outcome. One such example is the Mantoux skin test, a standard method of identifying persons with tuberculosis (TB) infection when placed, read, and interpreted properly. The individual diagnosed with latent TB infection benefits from treatment to prevent disease onset. A complete and properly taken course of treatment for latent TB infection can reduce an individual's lifetime risk of developing active TB disease by 90%. Secondary prevention targeted tuberculin testing is used to detect infected individuals and provide treatment to prevent progression to active disease to at-risk populations, such as persons with human immunodeficiency virus (HIV) infections and those recently infected with TB.

Tertiary Prevention

Tertiary prevention strategies seek to reduce complications and limit disability once disease develops. Tertiary care is the major focus of the health care industry. As the natural history of a disease continuum progresses to disease development, treatment of disease and rehabilitation are the primary activities.

TYPES OF EPIDEMIOLOGICAL STUDIES

As mentioned earlier, the purpose of the epidemiological approach is to study the distribution and determinants of health problems in groups or populations. Epidemiological methods of study may also be used by nurse researchers. The community health nurse must therefore become familiar with both epidemiological literature and clinical nursing research in order to integrate both into practice. This section provides an overview of two major approaches to epidemiological study designs.

Table 14-2 summarizes the types of epidemiological studies.

Observational Studies

Observational studies are nonexperimental in nature. They primarily describe, compare, and explain disease, disorder, or injury occurrence in a population. There are two general categories of observational studies: descriptive and analytic.

Descriptive Studies

Descriptive epidemiological studies contribute to the investigation and understanding of a health problem by asking the following questions:

TABLE 14-2 Types of Epidemiological Studies

OBSERVATIONAL STUDIES	INTERVENTION STUDIES
Descriptive	
Correlational	Prevention trials
Cross-sectional/survey	Therapeutic trials
Case reports and case series	
Analytic	
Case-control study (retrospective)	
Cohort study (prospective)	

Who has the problem *(person)?*

Where does the problem occur *(place)?*

When does the problem occur *(time)?*

These essential features of person, place, and time are the necessary elements of descriptive studies. Data such as sex, age, occupation, ethnicity, marital status, and socioeconomic status may be factors in who gets a particular health problem. Where a person lives or works provides information regarding the place where the disease or injury is occurring. Timing of a disease, such as seasonal occurrence or epidemic outbreak, is important in determining when a disease may occur. For example, descriptive studies were invaluable in initially understanding and identifying the presence of acquired immunodeficiency syndrome (AIDS) among young homosexual males in the United States in the early 1980s. Three types of descriptive studies—correlational studies, cross-sectional surveys, and case reports and case series—are useful in examining the factors of person, place, and time.

A **correlational study** is useful when the community health nurse investigator wants to compare neighborhoods and examine a particular disease in relationship to a potential risk factor. Epidemiological measures are assessed on a group rather than an individual basis. For example, if a community health nurse notices a number of children with leukemia in the health district and suspects a contributing environmental contaminant in the area, a correlational study could be initiated to compare leukemia rates among children of a health district in a neighboring town. This statistical comparison may or may not confirm higher leukemia rates in the nurse's health district. The information is specific only to the population groups under study in the geographic areas. Correlational studies are used in the initial assessment phase of investigating potential exposures (risk factors) of diseases.

The second type of descriptive study design, the **cross-sectional survey,** also may constitute the initial assessment phase of a more in-depth study. The cross-sectional survey could be used to assess a health problem such as TB infection among homeless persons, for example. By using a representative group (cross section) of individuals, such as those residing in a particular shelter, to represent the homeless population of a community, a survey using TB skin testing could be performed. This type of study occurs at only one point in time but can be helpful in associating disease prevalence and possible causes.

Case reports and case series constitute the third type of descriptive study design. Case reports detail histories of individuals or groups with unusual health problems and are significant in the identification of potential new diseases. For example, some of the first known cases of AIDS were described in the medical literature as case reports. A case series is a compilation of case reports.

Analytic Studies

Analytic studies go beyond describing the occurrence of health problems in a population by comparing groups of individuals in order to study associations and causal relationships. The purpose of **analytic epidemiological studies** is to search for causes of disease occurrence.

The first type of observational analytic investigation is the **case-control study.** In this look-back study design, also known as a **retrospective study,** groups of individuals are assembled after a disease has occurred. The epidemiologist compares groups with similar characteristics to examine risk factors associated with a disease occurrence. The structure of the case-control study requires that two study groups be assembled by the epidemiologist. One group of individuals who have a specifically defined disease (the cases) is compared with another group of individuals who do not have the disease (the controls). Members of both groups may share certain characteristics such as age and sex. Both groups are then studied using questionnaires, interviews, or testing in order to determine possible exposures or characteristics that may be attributable to the disease under study. Most notable among etiologic associations discovered via the case-control study design are the relationships between viral illness among young children, aspirin use, and Reye's syndrome and the relationship between toxic shock syndrome and tampon use.

The second type of observational analytic investigation is the **cohort study,** or **prospective study.** In this study design, the epidemiologist assembles a group of individuals who are free of the disease under study (the cohort) and follows the group into the future to determine etiologic factors contributing to disease development. This type of epidemiological study is one of the most effective methods to show potential causes of a disease. The best-known cohort study in the United States is the Framingham, Massachusetts study, which began in the 1950s. Framingham was chosen as the site for this study because it exhibited a number of characteristics that would allow the investigators to follow the study population for a number of years: a stable population; a wide range of occupations; one hospital, which was utilized by the majority of the population; and annually updated population lists (Hennekens & Buring, 1987). In this study, investigators identified and examined a cohort of 5127 Framingham men and women, each 30–50 years in age and free of coronary heart disease. Data were assembled on demographic characteristics, medical history, cigarette smoking, and several clinical and laboratory parameters. Members of the cohort have been followed and reexamined at regular intervals since the initial information was collected (between 1950 and 1952). Epidemiologists are studying these individuals to determine potential risk and predictive factors contributing to the development of coronary heart disease. Findings from this cohort study have contributed significantly to the understanding of the causal relationship between smoking, high blood pressure, high serum lipids, and heart disease. The study has added significantly to the body of knowledge on cardiovascular diseases. The Framingham Heart Study is considered a classic in the annals of epidemiology, both in describing the natural history of a disease and in determining the etiologic factors in the development of a particular disease.

Another example of an ongoing cohort study is the Nurses' Health Study, which began in 1976, with funding from the National Institutes of Health (NIH). Nurses' Health Study II was established in 1989 with funding from NIH also. The major motivation for developing the Nurses' Health Study II was to select a study population younger than the original Nurses' Health Study cohort. Both studies use biannual questionnaires to collect information on reproductive factors, lifestyle practices, and diet in relation to the occurrence of breast cancer, heart disease, and other major illnesses in women (*Nurses' Health Study Newsletter,* 2000).

Both case-control and cohort studies have limitations in the final analysis of the study results. In the case-control study, the epidemiologist selects individuals who already have a disease; thus, this method is potentially susceptible to selection and observation bias. **Bias** is an error in study design that results in incorrect conclusions regarding the association between potential risk factors and disease occurrence. The cohort study design is less prone to bias because individuals are selected and observed before disease occurrence. Experimental, or intervention, studies greatly reduce the role of bias by randomly assigning individuals to study groups.

Intervention Studies

Intervention studies are experimental in nature and require the epidemiologist to alter the behavior of the individuals participating in the study rather than merely observe the behaviors. Also known as randomized controlled clinical trials, intervention studies can best demonstrate the relationship between cause and effect. The structure of the study design requires a group of individuals (the study population) and a treatment or intervention to be tested. Individuals are randomly assigned to either the experimental (treatment) group or the control (no-treatment) group. Members of the experimental group receive the treatment or intervention, and members of the control group receive no intervention. Providing the study is conducted properly, comparison analysis of the two groups following the treatment or intervention may provide epidemiological evidence of a cause-and-effect relationship. Pharmaceuticals approved for therapeutic use are frequently tested using this study design.

There are two types of intervention studies: prevention trials and therapeutic trials. **Prevention trials** use experimental methodology to test measures or interventions among individuals and groups to prevent disease in a healthy population. Common examples of prevention trials are vaccine field testing and fluoridation of community water supplies to prevent tooth decay. **Therapeutic trials** are usually conducted among individuals who are identified to be at risk of a certain disease or who already have symptoms of the disease being studied. The intervention given to the experimental group may be a drug, behavior change, or surgical intervention, for example, a new medication for hypertension. The control group may receive the current usual care or no intervention. Both the experimental and control groups are followed up for a specified time in order to determine the effects of the intervention.

EPIDEMIOLOGICAL MEASUREMENT

As discussed earlier, epidemiology focuses on describing the presence and distribution of a disease or other health-related condition in a population and identifying associations between that disease or health-related condition and possible causative factors. In order to accomplish either of these objectives, the frequency of disease must be measured. Such measurement allows comparison of disease occurrence between groups. Within a given population, groups that exhibit a particular exposure or characteristic can be compared, as can groups that either do not exhibit the condition of interest or have not been exposed to the disease of interest. In this way, the epidemiologist may gain information useful in determining disease etiology or developing preventive measures.

Measures of Disease Frequency

Several techniques are used to measure disease frequency. The most basic measure of **disease frequency** is a simple count of those individuals who have the dis-

ease of interest. Such a count is of limited use to epidemiologists, however. In order to successfully determine the distribution and probable etiology of disease in a population or geographic area, the epidemiologist must know the size of the population of which affected individuals were a part (e.g., a city) and the time period during which information on the presence of the disease was obtained. Knowing the base population and the time period for data collection permits the comparison of disease frequencies among two or more groups of people or populations. To illustrate this concept, consider the following hypothetical scenario:

> City A reports 56 cases of tuberculosis, while city B reports 35 cases. With only this information, the county public health officer would assume that city A had a larger outbreak of TB and therefore required more financial resources and public health nurses to combat the spread of the disease. However, if city A has a population of 75,000 and city B has a population of 15,000, it can be seen that city B actually has the more severe problem with the disease. If a time element is factored in—for example city A's cases are reported for a period covering one year, and city B's cases occurred during a six-month period—the picture becomes even clearer. Resources should be deployed to city B, where the situation is much more serious.

Prevalence and Incidence Rates

The most commonly used measures of disease frequency are the prevalence rate and incidence rate. The **prevalence rate** is defined as the proportion (percentage) of the population that has the disease or condition at a given time. **Point prevalence** refers to the total number of persons with a disease at a specific point in time. The **incidence rate** is defined as the rate of change from the nondiseased state to the diseased state among persons at risk and reflects new cases of the disease or condition in a specified time period (Hennekens & Buring, 1987). Rates are special forms of proportions that include a time specification. All rates have a numerator and a denominator. The numerator is the number of events (disease incidents) or conditions of interest, and the denominator is the number of people in the population from which the numerator (affected individuals) was derived.

Other common measurements of disease frequency with which the student should be familiar are morbidity and mortality rates, special types of incidence or prevalence rates. The **morbidity rate** is the incidence of nonfatal cases of disease in the total population at risk during a specified point in time. The usefulness of the **attack rate** is illustrated by the following situation:

> A number of patrons of a local restaurant presented in local emergency rooms on Mother's Day evening

RESEARCH FOCUS

The Long-Term Effects of a Cardiovascular Disease Prevention Trial: The Stanford Five-City Project

Study Problem/Purpose

This study examined the long-term effects of a community-based health education intervention trial to reduce the risk of cardiovascular disease. During the last 40 years, epidemiological studies have established that hypertension, cigarette use, obesity, elevated plasma cholesterol, and sedentary lifestyle are related to the pathogenesis of cardiovascular diseases. It is important to conduct community-based education programs as a public health measure.

Methods

Two treatment cities in California (those who had received a community-based health program) and two control cities were selected to participate in this study. Persons 12–74 years of age who resided in randomly selected households in the four cities were eligible to participate. The initial study (one city) of the intervention trial, with results published in 1990, was designed to test whether a comprehensive program of community organization and health education produced favorable changes in cardiovascular disease risk factors, morbidity, and mortality. This current study (four cities) was conducted as a follow-up, population-based, cross-sectional survey, three years following the conclusion of the main health education intervention.

Findings

Blood pressure improvements observed in all cities from baseline to the end of the intervention were maintained during the follow-up in those cities who received the treatment but not in the control cities. Cholesterol levels continued to decline in all cities during follow-up. Smoking rates leveled out or increased slightly in the treatment cities and continued to decline in the control cities but did not yield statistically significant net differences. Both coronary heart disease and all-cause mortality risk scores were maintained or continued to improve in the treatment cities while leveling out or increasing in the control cities.

Implications

These findings suggest that community-based cardiovascular education programs can have sustained effects. However, the modest net differences in risk factors point to the need for new designs and interventions. The use of smaller, more frequent surveys, interventions of shorter duration, longitudinal follow-up of high-risk cohort samples, and evaluation of qualitative parameters at various levels are needed. The Stanford Five-City Project is one of the most comprehensive cardiovascular disease risk reduction studies conducted in the United States and the first to conduct a long-term follow-up of the main intervention effects (the community-based education programs).

Source: From Winkleby, M. A., Taylor, C. B., Jatulis, D., & Fortmann, S. P. (1996). The long-term effects of a cardiovascular disease prevention trial: The Stanford five-city project. American Journal of Public Health, 86 (12), 1773–1779.

with complaints of nausea, vomiting, abdominal pain, and diarrhea. Investigation by the local health department revealed that all of those who were taken ill had eaten brunch at the restaurant. After interviewing all Mother's Day patrons, it was determined that of those attending the brunch, nearly all became ill (attack rate) following the ingestion of certain food items. The source of the outbreak was traced back to poor refrigeration and lack of stringent sanitary measures among staff preparing those particular foods. Public health measures were instituted to prevent further illness.

The **mortality** (death) **rate** can reflect both incidence and prevalence. The **case fatality rate** refers to

deaths from a specific disease. The general formulas used to calculate the mortality and case fatality rates are found in Figure 14-4 along with the other rates discussed.

Vital Statistics

More specific rates are used by scientists, including epidemiologists, when examining incidence or prevalence in special populations. These are major public health rates, also known as vital statistics. **Vital statistics** are the result of systematic registration of vital events such as births, deaths, and health events. The statistical reports generated from the assembled data have many uses. For example, birth and death statistics are used to calculate estimated life expectancy, and health and disease statistics are used to

FIGURE 14-4 Equation Used in Computing Prevalence, Incidence, Morbidity, and Mortality Rates

prevalence rate *(P)* = $\dfrac{\text{number of cases (new and old) existing at a given point in time}}{\text{size of the population at a given point in time}}$

incidence rate *(I)* = $\dfrac{\text{number of new cases of disease at a given point in time}}{\text{population at risk of becoming new cases at the same point in time}}$

morbidity rate = $\dfrac{\text{new nonfatal cases of disease}}{\text{total population at risk}}$

attack rate = $\dfrac{\text{number of people ill in the time period}}{\text{total number of people at risk in the time period}}$

mortality rate = $\dfrac{\text{number of deaths from a disease (or all causes)}}{\text{total population}}$

case fatality rate = $\dfrac{\text{number of deaths from a disease}}{\text{number of cases of the disease}}$

identify changes in leading causes of death over time. The **cause-specific death rate** is the number of deaths due to a given cause each year.

The **maternal mortality rate** reflects the deaths of mothers at the time of birth or shortly thereafter. Equations used in computing vital statistics can be found in Figure 14-5.

Sources of data for these measures are many and varied and include birth and death certificates; census figures (for populations); disease registries; the Centers for Disease Control and Prevention (for notifiable diseases); various national surveys such as the National Health Interview Survey; hospitals (discharge records); insurance providers; exposure or trauma registries; and tumor registries. Also useful to the investigator are employment statistics and air and water quality statistics. The Internet is a newer but valuable source for data on vital statistics.

The measures calculated from information compiled by these various sources allow epidemiologists and public health practitioners to construct a picture of the state of the nation's health. In this way, we can learn which diseases are the leading causes of death in various age groups or in other populations and in the nation as a whole. We can also learn which diseases or conditions are most prevalent in given populations and which are geographically widespread. This information guides scientists (including nurse researchers and investigators), policymakers, and others engaged in research or the development of new treatment modalities. For example, decisions can be made regarding priorities for the allotment of financial and personnel resources and the development of treatment or preventive measures.

The information provided by the various public health measures discussed here also provides a historical record of diseases in the population. For example, according to the U.S. Public Health Service, the two leading causes of death in 1900 were pneumonia/influenza and tuberculosis, whereas heart disease and cancer were the leading causes of death in 1998. Such data provide information about the results of lifestyle changes, treatments developed for disease (including pharmaceuticals), and similar variables. Such information could only be surmised had these vital records not been kept.

Measures of Association

Thus, measures of disease frequency are a basis for comparing populations. Such comparisons are valuable to epidemiologists investigating the relationships (associations) between disease agent, host, and environment as discussed earlier in the chapter. In epidemiology, **measures of association** are defined as those statistical measures used to investigate the degree of dependence between two or more events or variables. Events can be classified as statistically associated when they occur more frequently together than could be accounted for by chance alone. Statistical association does not always imply causality, however. For example, when a factor and disease are associated only because both are related to some underlying cause, a noncausal statistical association exists. To illustrate this concept, consider an association found between yellow fingers and lung cancer. In other words, many people who developed lung cancer exhibited the phenomenon of yellow fingers. We can be reasonably certain, however, that yellow stains on the ring and middle fingers do not cause lung cancer. Rather, the underlying cause of these stains is smoking, and many heavy smokers do develop lung cancer. The association between yellow fingers and lung cancer would therefore be labeled noncausal.

Two of the most frequently used measures of association in epidemiology are relative risk and attributable risk. These measures indicate the degree of increased likelihood that one group as compared with another group will develop a disease or condition, or the degree of higher dis-

FIGURE 14-5 Equations Used in Computing Vital Statistics

<u>Rates Whose Denominators Are the Total Population</u>

crude birth rate $= \dfrac{\text{number of live births}}{\text{total mid-year population}} \times 1{,}000$

crude death rate $= \dfrac{\text{number of deaths during the year}}{\text{total mid-year population}} \times 1{,}000$

age-specific death rate $= \dfrac{\text{number of deaths in a given age group in a year}}{\text{average mid-year population in the age group}} \times 1{,}000$

cause-specific death rate $= \dfrac{\text{number of deaths due to a given cause in a year}}{\text{total mid-year population}} \times 100{,}000$

<u>Rates and Ratios Whose Denominators Are Live Births</u>

infant mortality (death) rate $= \dfrac{\text{number of infant deaths in one year (under 1 year of age)}}{\text{number of live births in the same year}} \times 1{,}000$

neonatal mortality (death) rate $= \dfrac{\text{number of newborn deaths (under 28 days of age)}}{\text{number of live births in the same year}} \times 1{,}000$

fetal death ratio $= \dfrac{\text{number of fetal deaths in one year (20 + weeks)}}{\text{number of live births in the same year}} \times 1{,}000$

maternal mortality rate $= \dfrac{\text{number of maternal deaths in one year (from complications)}}{\text{number of live births in the same year}} \times 100{,}000$

<u>Rates Whose Denominators Are Live Births Plus Fetal Deaths</u>

fetal death rate $= \dfrac{\text{number of fetal deaths in one year}}{\text{number of live births plus fetal deaths in one year}} \times 1{,}000$

perinatal mortality rate $= \dfrac{\text{number of fetal deaths (under 7 days)}}{\text{number of live births plus fetal deaths in one year}} \times 1{,}000$

ease frequency in one population as compared with another. The concept of **risk** refers to the probability that a disease or a condition will develop in a given time period.

Relative Risk

Although epidemiologists widely use several relative measures, only the most common are discussed here. Relative measures indicate the likelihood of an exposed group's developing a disease *relative* to those who are not exposed. The rate ratio (RR), also called the **relative risk** or the risk ratio, is the ratio between the rates in the exposed and unexposed groups. Cohort studies such as the Framingham Heart Study, discussed previously, are the source of data for relative-risk determination:

$$RR = (I_e / I_u)$$

where I_e represents the *incidence* rate among the *exposed*, and I_u represents the *incidence* rate among the *unexposed*.

Attributable Risk

Attributable risk provides information about the effect of the exposure or the increased risk of disease in those exposed as compared with those who are unexposed.

This measure expresses the number of cases of disease attributable to the exposure of interest. It is useful as a measure of the impact of a particular exposure on public health. Attributable risk is expressed as follows:

$$AR = (I_e - I_u)$$

An allied measure is **attributable risk percentage (AR%),** which is defined as the proportion of the disease of interest in the population being investigated that could be prevented by eliminating the exposure. This is a measure of the impact of an exposure on public health, assuming that the association is one of cause and effect. Attributable risk percentage (also called rate difference or risk difference) is expressed by the following formula:

$$AR\% = \frac{I_e - I_u}{I_e}$$

Measures of association are calculated with the aid of a two-by-two table, also called a four fold table or a contingency table (see Figure 14-6).

The relative risk or risk ratio is also utilized by epidemiologists to judge whether a valid observed association is likely to be causal. A relative risk value of 1.0 indicates that incidence rates of disease in exposed and

Out
of the Box

New Jersey Information Systems

In the late 1980s, the hospitals and the state health department in New Jersey each wanted a reliable perinatal database, although admittedly for different reasons. To support epidemiological analyses, the health department wanted the capacity to monitor and record prenatal and birth events electronically. Hospitals wanted to be able to submit paperwork electronically, and to have more prenatal and medical information about pregnant women before they presented in labor at the emergency room. The state hospital association wanted a more accurate research database in order to analyze epidemiological trends, assess risk in different hospital markets, and obtain reliable data for negotiations with insurers. Since it seemed that a single information system might work for all the parties, the state's Director of Maternal and Child Health convened an advisory group of state personnel and hospital representatives.

The innovative group struggled with the competing interests. The group's product was an electronic birth certificate that would provide the state health department with aggregate statewide data to support surveillance, vital registries, and epidemiological investigations. Each hospital could customize the birth certificate to meet its own needs. Within two years of its implementation, all the hospitals in the state were voluntarily registering their births electronically, and the comprehensive birth data were being used to populate the immunization database. Similar electronic ventures emerged in New Jersey throughout the 1990s—an interactive immunization registry, a laboratory reporting system for multidrug-resistant pathogens, and an environmental emergency notification system, among others. As the technology blossomed, these autonomous projects were joined into a single overarching electronic network that supports a variety of medical and public health objectives. The goals of all these projects are similar—to simplify the reporting of key events; to create reliable databases that can provide usable information for clinical, epidemiological, and policy-planning purposes; and to provide meaningful feedback to providers that will help guide clinical decision making and support more effective medical practice. ■

✳ DECISION MAKING

Teenage Pregnancy and Birth Rates

◆ What are the pregnancy and birth rates among teenagers in your community? What percentage of infants born to teenage mothers in your community exhibit low birthweight or other neonatal problems?

◆ What resources exist in your community to advise or assist pregnant teens?

◆ Where would you look for information on teen pregnancies and births in your community?

ment of disease. In other words, if an individual or host is exposed to the agent or risk factor, he or she has a greater likelihood of developing the disease under study. Conversely, a relative risk value of less than 1.0 indicates that the individual with that factor is less likely to develop the disease or other event under study. Use of the two-by-two table is illustrated in Figure 14-7.

Odds Ratio

The last relative association measure to be discussed here is the exposure odds ratio, which is calculated when incidence rates are unavailable. The **odds ratio (OR)** for a population approximates the relative risk (RR) when the specific risk of disease for both the exposed and unexposed groups is very low. The odds ratio is expressed by the following formula:

$$OR = \frac{a/c}{b/d} = \frac{ad}{bc}$$

A two-by-two table can be used to determine this measure.

Information used to calculate the odds ratio is collected via a case-control study, discussed earlier in this

nonexposed populations are the same and that, therefore, no association exists between the variable, or risk factor, being studied and the development of the disease of interest. A relative risk value greater than 1.0 indicates that a positive association does exist between the exposure to the risk factor being examined and the develop-

FIGURE 14-6 Two-by-Two Table

	(D) Disease	(D̄) No disease	
Exposed (E)	a	b	a + b
Unexposed (Ē)	c	d	c + d

Using a two-by-two table, relative risk (risk ratio) would be calculated in the following manner:

$$RR = (I_e/I_u) = \frac{a/a+b}{c/c+d} =$$

$$l_e = \frac{\text{those exposed who develop disease}}{\text{those exposed with disease} + \text{those exposed with no disease}}$$

$$l_u = \frac{\text{those unexposed who develop disease}}{\text{those unexposed with disease} + \text{those exposed with no disease}}$$

FIGURE 14-7 Calculating Relative Risk Using the Two-by-Two Table

Data for 37,840 live births in an urban county for one year, by birth weight

Outcome at One Year

	Dead	Alive	Total
≤2,500 g	530 (a)	4,340 (b)	4,870
>2,500 g	333 (c)	32,637 (d)	32,970
	863	36,977	37,840

The relative risk of mortality at one year associated with low birth weight is calculated in the following manner:

$$RR = (I_e/I_u) = \frac{a/a+b}{c/c+d} = \frac{530}{4,870} \text{ divided by } \frac{333}{32,970} = 10.78$$

Stated in words, the relative risk that babies born at 2,500 g or less had a death rate at one year of 10.78 times that of babies born over 2,500 g.

FIGURE 14-8 Calculating Odds Ratio Using the Two-by-Two Table

Researchers reported on a case-control study of the relationship between pancreatic cancer and various lifestyle habits, including coffee drinking. Of 902 cases with pancreatic cancer, 347 reported drinking one or more cups of coffee per day. Eighty-eight of the 108 controls reported drinking no coffee per day (Hennekens & Buring, 1987).

	(D) Disease	(D̄) No disease	
Risk factor: coffee drinking	347 (a)	20 (b)	a + b 367
absent	555 (c)	88 (d)	c + d 643
	a + c = 902	b + d = 108	1,010

$$OR = \frac{a/c}{b/d} = \frac{ad}{bc} = \frac{347 \times 88}{555 \times 20} = \frac{30,536}{11,100} = 2.75$$

Stated in words, people who drank one or more cups of coffee per day exhibited odds of having pancreatic cancer 2.75 greater than those of people who drank no coffee.

✳ DECISION MAKING

Disease and Risk Factors

◆ What are the incidence and prevalence of breast cancer in your community?

◆ Is Lyme disease present in your state?

◆ If so, identify any risk factors associated with the presence of this tick-borne disease in your community.

chapter. Because the disease status of the two populations being investigated is already known, case-control studies can be conducted with fewer subjects than is possible in cohort studies. The case-control study is particularly useful in the development of knowledge about a particular disease and its possible causative factors and is frequently used to test hypotheses about the etiology of a disease. In the case-control study, the control group must be carefully selected and must be comparable in demographic characteristics to the case group in order for the results to be valid, that is, to have scientific merit. In other words, the control group must, as nearly as possible, mirror the case group except that they do not have the disease or event of interest. Several sources of controls are commonly utilized in the development of a case-control study. These sources

FIGURE 14-9 Measures of Association

$$\text{relative risk} = \frac{\text{incidence rate among the exposed } (I_e)}{\text{incidence rate among the unexposed } (I_u)}$$

$$\text{attributable risk} = \text{incidence rate among the exposed} \\ (I_e) - \text{incidence rate among the} \\ \text{unexposed } (I_u)$$

$$\text{attributable risk \%} = \frac{I_e - I_u}{I_e}$$

$$\text{odds ratio} = \frac{a/c}{b/d} = \frac{ad}{bc} \text{ (using two-by-two table)}$$

include hospitals, the general (but similar) population, or special groups such as friends, relatives, or neighbors of the cases. The analysis of the case-control study involves comparing cases and controls with reference to the frequency of the exposure or characteristic that is being investigated as a possible etiologic, or causative, factor. This comparison is effected by estimating the relative risk as computed by the odds ratio. A case-control study often precedes a cohort study as an important initial attempt in identifying the risk factors for a particular disease or event. Figure 14-8 illustrates the use of a two-by-two table to calculate the odds ratio in a case-control study. Figure 14-9 summarizes the measures of association.

Perspectives...

INSIGHTS OF A COMMUNITY HEALTH NURSE RESEARCHER

As a nurse researcher, I have recently participated in two projects that have made a strong impression on me. I coordinated a study on immigrant adolescent acculturation and analyzed data collected in a teen clinic in an effort to understand the demographics of the population served as well as reasons for which they visit the clinic. Working with young health educators in these settings, as they seek to educate their peers around healthier behaviors, is both illuminating and inspiring. These health educators, just out of their teens, are often survivors of high-risk behaviors themselves, as well as being members of the target population. This fact alone makes them potent peer educators.

While teen birth rates have dropped significantly in the United States over the last decade, there remain areas and populations in which teen pregnancy remains a problem. In one northern California county, adolescent pregnancies and birth rates among young Latinas, particularly recent immigrants, continue to concern health providers. Intake information at one teen clinic revealed a number of reasons these young women become pregnant. Cultural norms included adolescent motherhood, the pairing of young girls with older men, and the concept that a young man's virility and masculinity are proven by the pregnancy of his partner. At the same time they struggle with acculturation—they desire to become Americanized but retain strong familial and cultural ties to the customs of their country of origin.

In an effort to change some of the cultural and gender biases of young men and bring about a behavior change that might eventually translate into fewer teen pregnancies in the county, this teen clinic has implemented a program to reach young men and train them as peer health educators. Topics covered in their training include the male role in pregnancy and sexually transmitted disease prevention, relationship building, setting academic goals, violence prevention, and alcohol and other substance use and misuse. This fledgling program, funded by the state Office of Family Planning, is a good example of a public and private partnership working to impact the public health problem of teen pregnancy. Although too soon for formal outcome results to be described, some positive outcomes have already been noted. For many of the young men participating in the program, self-esteem has risen as the teens have interacted with other young people and adults in community events and conferences. Workshops conducted by the peer health educators have been well-attended and highly praised. A new awareness of their own health needs has brought many of the participants to the teen clinic for the first time for HIV/sexually transmitted disease testing and health screening. The number of young men seen in the teen clinic increased a substantial 60% in the first six months of 2000 over the same period in 1999. Some of the increase is attributed to the peer education of the young men of the Male Involvement Program.

Building healthy communities and impacting health of individuals and populations often require innovative ideas attacking a health problem on numerous levels.

—Lindsey King Phillips, RN, MS

USING THE EPIDEMIOLOGICAL APPROACH IN COMMUNITY HEALTH NURSING

Disease and Health Status Surveillance

Epidemiological measurement and analysis allow community health nursing researchers to measure health status and disease occurrence in populations. Health status indicators are used to provide a snapshot of the major diseases, disabilities, and injuries in a community for use in establishing health priorities and plans and evaluating programs. **Surveillance** of disease occurrence yields epidemiological intelligence data by providing a systematic count of disease frequency. These data, in turn, can be used to estimate the magnitude of health problems in the community, detect epidemics, understand the natural history of a disease, or detect potential emerging infectious disease threats (Teutsch, Churchill, & Elliott, 1994). Timely surveillance information, then, is key to the public health approach to prevention of diseases and injuries.

As practitioners, educators, and health planners, community health nurses must have fundamental knowledge of and access to population-based disease and health status surveillance data. Such data may be obtained from a variety of sources such as government agencies or may be directly collected by the community health nurse who conducted, for example, a neighborhood needs assessment. State and local public health jurisdictions collect and analyze the immunization rates of school-aged children in most communities. Audits of immunization records may reveal demographic features of the children. This information may, in turn, lead to the identification of barriers to vaccination or of poor access to health care.

Computerized health information systems and registries facilitate the use of medical information in a timely manner. Governmental agencies also publish data on the Internet. Common sources of routinely collected data in the United States include the following:

Centers for Disease Control and Prevention (CDC)

National Center for Health Statistics (NCHS)

Health Care Financing Administration (HCFA)

Bureau of the Census

Agency for Health Care Planning and Research (AHCPR)

National Institutes of Health (NIH)

The Search for Etiology

The community health nurse is an instrumental link in the search for and detection of potential health problems or hazards in a health district. Using the epidemiological approach, the community health nurse can identify connections between community demographics or environmental characteristics and disease occurrence. In a given health district, for example, children with elevated serum lead levels may be treated and returned to the same lead-contaminated environment unless the community health nurse determines the source of exposure. The community health nurse would use the epidemiological approach and knowledge of abatement resources in order to eradicate the lead source.

Casefinding

Another use of the epidemiological approach in community health nursing is casefinding to identify individuals whose health status is at risk. A traditional method of casefinding, contact tracing, aims to identify individuals who may be infected from exposure to a particular disease (e.g., chlamydia) in order to evaluate for infection, provide appropriate treatment, and quickly interrupt disease transmission. Community health nurses implementing this investigational approach apply techniques of surveillance and risk identification to their knowledge of the causative organism, mode of transmission, and communicable period.

Determining the Health Status of a Population

The community health nurse may be the first clinician to detect threats to health, or unhealthy behaviors, in a population. Observing a number of clients presenting with similar complaints or symptoms in a neighborhood clinic, for example, can alert the community health nurse to the presence of a disease or high-risk behavior in a population. Once the diagnosis is formulated that a particular problem exists, the community health nurse works with clinicians to determine how widespread the problem may be. Questionnaires, telephone surveys, and outreach through community health fairs or other public venues like shopping malls may be employed. Understanding the demographics of the target population is essential. Cultural and language needs should also be identified to insure the thorough assessment of the population and their full participation in the gathering of data.

Evaluating Care

Using epidemiological measures to assess health status and disease occurrence, determine the etiology of a particular health condition, and design a treatment or prevention modality are important processes in the care of client populations. Equally important is the thorough evaluation of all aspects of client care. Whether the community health nurse is reviewing an individual client's treatment plan and results or looking at interventions and

COMMUNITY NURSING VIEW

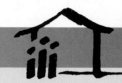

One day during the winter of 1981, seven Laotian refugees who recently came to the United States ate mushrooms from the same batch, picked at a local park that same day. The next day six of the seven were admitted to a small community hospital with symptoms of nausea, vomiting, diarrhea, dehydration, and elevated liver enzyme tests. Although the onset time of the symptoms varied within the group, most experienced gastrointestinal distress within 8 hours. Three of the seven individuals were monitored for liver, kidney, and circulatory complications for 24 hours in the intensive care unit. All seven individuals were discharged without complications within seven days.

Samplings of the remaining mushrooms collected by the hospitalized group were sent to a local university for identification. These mushrooms were identified as belonging to a poisonous genus, *Amanita*.

With help from a Laotian-speaking community outreach worker, the community health nurse interviewed several members of the group. These individuals stated that foraging of wild mushrooms was customary in their homeland and that they therefore continued to forage mushrooms following their arrival in the United States. They further reported that in Laos, a simple boiling method was used to determine whether mushrooms were poisonous or harmless. In Laos, when poisonous mushrooms are boiled with rice, they turn the rice red. Because the locally gathered batch did not turn the rice red, the mushrooms were ingested. The community health nurse determined that

several steps needed to be taken to prevent further poisoning from wild mushrooms. The nurse knew that foraging wild mushrooms was not unique to Laotians or Southeast Asian groups.

Nursing Considerations

Assessment

◆ What data including cultural factors would the nurse need to collect to assess the problem of mushroom poisoning?

Diagnosis

◆ What diagnosis might be made given the data included in the case scenario?

Outcome Identification

◆ What outcomes might be formulated specific to a community approach to mushroom poisoning?

Planning/Interventions

◆ What community notification and educational strategy might the nurse develop and implement to deal with the problem of mushroom poisoning?

Evaluation

◆ How would the community health nurse evaluate the effectiveness of the community intervention?

---

outcomes for an entire target population, evaluation is critical. Among the questions that must be asked and answered are:

- Was the program implementation or medical treatment successful?
- Were the objectives achieved?
- Has the client or target population adapted a healthier lifestyle or minimized risky behavior?
- Is the client or target population satisfied with the outcome?
- Were treatments or programs implemented in a culturally competent manner?

The answers to these questions will help determine the design and implementation of future programs.

Applying the PRECEDE-PROCEED Model

Community health nurses are frequently involved in planning and implementing new health programs or are asked to identify the health needs of their communities. For example, legislation may mandate that local services be implemented for an identified vulnerable population such as pregnant teens or homeless youth. Changes in national immigration policy may result in an influx of refugees requiring specialized health screening. The PRECEDE-PROCEED model uses deductive reasoning in applying an epidemiological approach to community health planning. Developed by Green and Kreuter (1991), the **PRECEDE-PROCEED model** is a health promotion planning framework consisting of two components: a diagnostic component called PRECEDE and a developmental component called PROCEED. PRECEDE was conceptualized by the authors as an acronym for *p*redisposing, *r*einforcing, and *e*nabling *c*onstructs in *e*ducational *d*iagnosis and *e*valuation. PROCEED is an acronym for *p*olicy, *r*egulatory, and *o*rganizational *c*onstructs in *e*ducational and *e*nvironmental *d*evelopment. The model can be used at the primary (hygiene and health enhancement), secondary (early-detection), or tertiary (therapeutic) stage of prevention or treatment and may be viewed as an intervention whose purpose is to "short-circuit illness or enhance quality of life through change or development of health-related behavior and conditions of living" (Green & Kreuter, 1991, p. 22). Green and Kreuter believe that the PRECEDE framework takes into account the multiple factors that shape health status, thereby assisting the user in developing a subset of those factors as targets for intervention and in generating objectives and evaluation criteria. PRECEDE-PROCEED includes a series of phases in the planning, implementation, and evaluation process. Six phases of the model are considered basic; phases 7, 8, and 9 are seen as extensions, depending on the evaluation needs of the health planners. The phases defined by Green and Kreuter (1991) are presented in an abridged format here:

Phase 1. Assessment of needs or problems of the target population. The population concerned should be involved in the process.

Phase 2. Identification of the specific health goals or problems that may contribute to the needs or problems identified in phase 1. Health problems are ranked, and the problem most deserving of scarce resources is targeted.

Phase 3. Identification of specific health-related behavioral and environmental factors (risk factors) that are linked to the targeted problem.

Phase 4. Classification of factors that have direct impact on the target behavior and environment into one of three categories: predisposing factors (knowledge, attitudes, beliefs, values, and perceptions that facilitate or hinder motivation for change), enabling factors (skills, resources, or barriers that help or hinder desired behavioral or environmental changes), and reinforcing factors (rewards and feedback received by the learner following adoption of the behavior).

Phase 5. Assessment of organizational and administrative capabilities and resources for the development and implementation of a program.

Phase 6. Implementation of the program.

Phase 7. Evaluation of the process, which includes examining the program implemented by determining whether the program has met the requirements outlined in each of the previous steps.

Phase 8. Impact evaluation. Examined are the goals of the implemented program and whether the actions implemented affected the problem being addressed by the model.

Phase 9. Outcome evaluation. The results of the implemented program are examined to determine whether the program accomplished the goals for which it was designed.

The uniqueness of the PRECEDE-PROCEED framework allows the community health nurse to determine population needs prior to a program's implementation. Because evaluation methods are established in the planning phase, the achievement of program objectives can be measured throughout the program's phases. The model also was specifically developed with the community rather than the individual in mind, making it particularly useful to community health nurses. See Chapter 16 for more information about the PRECEDE-PROCEED model.

KEY CONCEPTS

◆ Epidemiology is an applied, population-based science embracing the related community health sciences of ecology and demography and focusing on the distribution and determinants of diseases or conditions.

◆ A basic understanding of the epidemiological approach provides the community health nurse with necessary language and methodology to understand, describe, and analyze health problems of communities.

◆ Epidemiology methods are used to investigate the natural history of a disease, to search for disease causes (etiology) or risk factors, to conduct disease surveillance, and to test new treatments.

◆ Concepts basic to the epidemiological approach are that health problems in a population do not occur randomly; that causes are interactions between agent, host, and the surrounding environment; and that the natural history of a health condition provides fundamental information on how to intervene or prevent that condition from occurring.

◆ Observational or nonexperimental epidemiological study designs are used when little is known about a disease, when a disease occurrence is rare, and to make associations or comparisons between those with and those without a disease. Intervention studies or experimental methods are used to compare therapeutic or preventive treatments.

◆ Epidemiological measurements typically encountered by the community health nurse are measures of disease frequency expressed as rates and measures of association (ratios and percentages).

◆ The epidemiological approach is particularly useful to the community health nurse because the focus is population based and the approach provides tools to collect, describe, analyze, and evaluate information about a community.

▨ RESOURCES

American College of Epidemiology: www.acepidemiology.org
American Public Health Association: www.apha.org
Association for Professionals in Infection Control and Epidemiology (APIC): www.apic.org
Centers for Disease Control and Prevention: www.cdc.gov

Centers for Disease Control and Prevention Epidemiology Program Office: www.cdc.gov/epo
Center for Epidemiology and Policy: http://www.med.jhu.edu/cep/
International Epidemiology Foundation: www.epifoundation.org
Journal of Epidemiology and Community Health: http://www.bmjpg.com
National Center for Health Statistics: www.cdc.gov/nchs
National Institutes of Health: www.nih.gov
National Institutes of Health, Division of Cancer Epidemiology and Genetics (DCEG): www.dceg.cancer.gov
Nurses' Health Study: www.channing.harvard.edu/nhs
Surveillance, Epidemiology and End Results (SEER) Program of the National Cancer Institute: www.seer.cancer.gov
U.S. Bureau of the Census: www.census.gov
World Health Organization Global Programme on Evidence for Health Policy: www.who.int/whosis

Chapter

15

ASSESSING THE COMMUNITY

Aida Sahud, DrPH, MSN, RN

MAKING THE CONNECTION

A healthy city is one that is continually creating and improving those physical and social environments—expanding those community resources which enable people to mutually support each other in performing all the functions of life and in developing to their maximum potential.

—Hancock & Duhl, 1985, p. 29

COMPETENCIES

Upon completion of this chapter, the reader should be able to:

- Describe the various ways that communities are defined.
- Examine the concept of community as a holograph.
- Discuss the influence of values on need and explain the various types of need.
- Describe in detail the participation of community members in community assessment.
- Outline the steps in conducting a community assessment.
- Discuss the sources of information about communities.
- Explain the various tools used in community assessment.
- Discuss ways to determine appropriate responses to an identified need.
- Outline the process of setting priorities for action.

KEY TERMS

aggregate	expressed need
community	felt need
community assessment	gentrification
community competence	NIMBYism
community of interest	normative need
community participation	project team
comparative need	social support
	steering committee
	windshield survey

In Chapter 1, a number of definitions of community health nursing and the scope of community health nursing practice were presented. A common theme, however, pervaded all these definitions: The focus of community health nursing is the promotion and maintenance of health of whole populations or communities. This responsibility is ongoing, underpinning the daily practice of community health nurses. If they are to effectively promote the health of the communities they serve, community health nurses must have the knowledge and skills to effectively assess community needs and resources. This chapter explores some key issues in community assessment, including the importance of community participation in community assessment, the stages of the community assessment process, and a number of tools and methods useful in the collection of information required for community assessment.

A POPULATION OR COMMUNITY FOCUS

Since the development of Health for All by the Year 2000, countries around the world have been attempting to implement the principles outlined in the Alma-Ata Declaration [World Health Organization (WHO), 1978] and the Ottawa Charter for Health Promotion (WHO, 1986). National policies have been established to implement Health for All in many countries, and international and national health professional associations have committed themselves to the principles of social justice, equity, and community participation.

Through the International Council of Nurses and various national nursing and public health associations, community health nurses have made a formal commitment to improve the health of the world population. This commitment, like the declarations from which it arose, is based on the recognition that health is determined largely by the social, economic, and political environments in which people live and that effective solutions to health problems must therefore address social, economic, and political issues.

Community assessment is an extremely important component of community health nursing practice. Without adequate assessment, nurses may identify a problem and a corresponding solution before having explored the situation in sufficient depth to fully understand it (Rorden & McLennan, 1992). Comprehensive community assessment not only identifies problems but also addresses the nature of those health problems. Because of the primary role that health assessment plays in promoting the health of communities, community assessment has been identified as one of the three core functions of public health [Institute of Medicine (IOM), 1988].

The four major enabling goals cited in the updated Health for All by the Year 2010 "Briefs" which are based in public health theory include promoting healthy behaviors, protecting health, achieving access to quality health care and strengthening community prevention (*Development of Healthy People 2010 Objectives,* 2000). Subsequently, the advanced-practice nurse is prepared to treat the community as a client. In order to do a thorough needs assessment, she or he will need to consider the political, economic, and social aspects of the community in question. Additionally, just as the community health nurse gathers data on individuals and families for relevant nursing interventions, the advanced-practice nurse will do likewise with a focus on the identified community. The outcome of the data analysis will provide information for future program planning.

Community assessment is not achieved simply by assessing the health of individuals within a community.

Community health nurses must also assess the health of the community itself; identify the characteristics, resources, and needs of the community; and work with community members on those issues that arise, addressing not only individual behavior but also applicable environmental variables. Working to change individual behavior when the environment in which those individuals live has a greater bearing on health results in "blaming the victim" (Ryan, 1976).

Focusing on the community as a whole requires a population focus and the recognition of the community as client (Anderson & McFarlane, 1988; Kuehnert 1995). In order to understand the full implications of such an approach, we must first consider the meaning of the terms *community* and *healthy community* and how need is conceptualized.

DEFINING THE COMMUNITY

The term **community** has been used in a myriad of ways, ranging from the very specific to the quite broad and general. In 1955, Hillery identified 94 different definitions of the term (Rissel, 1996); many more have been developed since. Some authors suggest that the result has been a confusing array of definitions (Rorden & McLennan, 1992). Given its central place in the discussion and analysis of communal life, however, *community* as a term cannot be avoided. An examination of the term and of the common dimensions among its various definitions constitutes an important preface to a discussion of community assessment.

Many of the broader definitions of the term refer to *community* as simply a large group of people or "community as population" (Hawe, 1994, p. 200). It is commonly understood that a community and aggregate differ in definition. An **aggregate** is the identification of a group of individuals with a common concern. The sense of community holds that there are many dimensions which bring people together in order to interact with one another (Caretto, McCormick, 1991). According to these definitions, then, communities are little more than large numbers of individuals.

Such definitions have some similarities to geographic definitions of community, wherein communities are seen as groups of people living in particular places, with locality central to their definition as communities. Definitions of community as populations and geographic areas are those that have generally been used by health planners in their assessment and planning work (Rissel, 1996): "The underlying premise of Healthy People 2010 is that the health of the individual is almost inseparable from the health of the larger community and that the health of every community in every state and territory determines the overall health status of the nation" (*Healthy People 2010*, 2000).

In addition to some of the prior stated definitions of community, Shields and Lindsey (1998) have identified the following variables which need to be considered when defining the "community": context and resource, community as client, and relational and political aspects.

Context and Resource

Community health nurses (CHNs) have placed emphasis on the community and environment in which their clients live. These elements have been perceived as inseparable. Presently, it has been suggested that community be recognized as a resource. This subtle movement is to perceive resource as a contrast to illness (Shields & Lindsey, 1998). When discussing community health nursing, it is encumbent upon us as CHNs to seek the strengths within the individual, family, and community. It is a common practice for CHNs and other health professionals to be hypervigilant to what is not healthful or productive for a family or a community. The suggestion taken here by Shields and Lindsey is to distance oneself and begin to focus and highlight what the family and/or community is doing right. It takes a certain awareness to make this shift of thought. It is a valuable practice since it creates a foundation for future interventions and planning.

Community as Client

This is when the CHN can view the community as a whole entity. It includes individuals and families plus the broader view of the community in respect to health promotion, prevention of disease, sanitation, epidemics, and immunization programs.

Political and Relational Aspects of Community

Community is more than just a place, it is about people's relationships—"about how we are a people; how you are as a person, it is about the 'how' of everyday life. Just as mind, body and spirit are inseparable, so are the individual and community. Thus the relational aspects of community encompass people's relational experiences as well as a relational way of being" (Shields & Lindsey, 1998, p. 26).

The relational way of being extends to and includes power relations in the community. Aspects of gender, class, and social division must be taken into account when perceiving a community. Concerns of drug abuse, poverty, and violence need to be recognized as major public health issues which require that the CHN reach out and influence the sociopolitical powers in order to enhance social change (Shields & Lindsey, 1998).

Davis (2000) has reconceptualized the notion of community by stating that "holographic theory demonstrates that it is possible to create processes in which the whole can be encoded in all the parts, so each part represents the whole. While there is diversity, the essence of holography becomes its wholeness whereby unity forms a whole of knowing" (p. 296). She elaborates even further by stating that "placing parts and whole in context opens the door to help us realize that the dimensions of community and their moral struggles are contextual and complex and do not lend themselves to easy answers" (p. 298). Davis further suggests that the emphasis on community consciousness and humanistic values has not been satisfactorily integrated into community health practice. Her recommendation is to offer the holographic model as a means to look at and understand communities in a new way (p. 294).

The CHN must first ask what is meant by holographic theory? The nurse must also consider how this can be applied to a community assessment. The word *hologram* is derived from the Greek words *holos,* meaning "whole or complete," and *gram,* meaning "message." A hologram has often been described as a very complex lens. It can be, for example, a laser beam which forms and bends the light so that the image of the original object is perceived differently, i.e., other interrelated patterns may appear which would not appear with a single beam of light from the sun or a lamp.

If a hologram is broken or cut up, each small portion contains all the information about the whole object. In this case, if the CHN were to consider the eight integrated and relational patterns identified in Figure 15-1, it would be important to consider that all eight patterns would appear from various sources when doing a community assessment.

An example of this might be a large university located within a moderate-sized urban community. The values and awareness of the university community will have permeated the larger community in which it exists. Equally as important is that community issues will have been fodder for the educational system to digest and integrate into the curriculum. Holding this in mind, it might be assumed that similar values, social justice issues, and levels of sophistication, just to mention a few, will be shared by the population at large. Despite the variation in socioeconomic groups and, more specifically, educational levels, there is a collective consciousness that prevails.

Even in a community crisis, the members of the community, irrespective of income, will share a common understanding of their rights. If there is an outbreak of a communicable disease and a death of a child, the said community will organize itself. It will seek out information and educate itself about the disease. The members of the community will expect to be treated fairly.

The CHN working within a structured system, such as the Public Health Department, will need to look through her holographic lenses in order to assess the whole community.

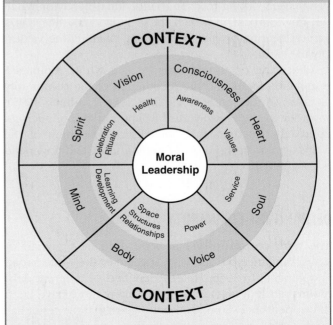

FIGURE 15-1 The Holographic Community. This figure demonstrates that the holographic community embodies a living being of community which lives within each of us

From "Holographic Community: Reconceptualizing the Meaning of Community in an Era of Health Care Reforms," by R. Davis, 2001, *Nursing Outlook, 48*(6), pp. 294–301. Reprinted with permission.

Figure 15-1 demonstrates that the holographic community embodies a "living being" of community which lives within each of us. Eight integrated, relational patterns are set in context. These dimensions are (Davis, 2000):

- The consciousness of community—awareness
- The heart of community—values
- The soul of community—service
- The voice of community—power
- The body of community—space, structure, relationships
- The mind of community—learning, development
- The spirit of community—celebration, ritual
- The vision of community—health

Another visionary, Koerner (2001) recognizes that in this new millennium the global aspect of community must be addressed. She states, "By making the planet our client, we move toward global nursing action. What we do in our country has great implications for the rest of the world." We are in a position to take up leadership in our communities which will provide a model for others. Furthermore, when, "community is our client we will allow some of the issues that foster disease: poverty, safety, clean water and homelessness" to enter into our scope of practice (p. 22).

In their classic work of 1981, Bryson and Mowbray discuss the fact that community programs have not always been well planned. One example that they draw upon is the problem which has continued to emerge since the legislation of deinstitutionalization. This refers to those who were discharged from state mental health facilities and moved into the community. Although the idea was cogent, those with mental illness were transitioned into communities without adequate resources of planning. As a result, what has emerged is an almost insurmountable problem in most urban communities. Displaced individuals often find themselves wandering "lost" through unfamiliar neighborhoods. Brady and Brady (2000) refer to this problem.

They describe a woman with mental health problems walking down the street, having a profound conversation with herself. She is unkempt and uncared for and living in an adult home sponsored by the government for those who are mentally disabled. She was among the first cohort of people with mental health problems released from a state hospital and returned to the "community named the Rockaways" with a myriad of holotropic drugs to assist her in her living situation.

The concept of housing for patients who before would have been placed in a state psychiatric facility is elaborated further by Brady and Brady (2000), who describe the evolution of the housing situation for clients with mental health problems.

Since the change in policy about housing the mentally ill, patients were discharged from psychiatric facilities to single-room occupancies (SROs). These consisted of rooms in older, urban buildings with low rents. The single room may have had a basin with running water, a shared bathroom down the hall, and no cooking facilities. Many discharged patients managed to place their meager belongings in the room along with a hot plate to heat up a can of food or boil water for instant coffee or tea.

As neighborhoods changed and **gentrification** occurred, many of the old tenement-type buildings were replaced by new, unaffordable, condominiums and hotels, leaving this marginal population without housing.

The state of New York created a mental health program whereby the clients were able to live in adult houses in a district called the Rockaways. The problem was that the current residents in the community felt that their property values would decrease if the mentally ill were housed there. Furthermore, there was the problem of **NIMBYism** (Not in My Back Yard). This is a psychological reaction predicated on fear of what someone with a mental illness might do to harm others in the neighborhoods. As a result, hoards of middle-class families left

the Rockaways neighborhood for other "unspoiled" communities. In the Rockaways, the mentally ill continue to maintain themselves without organized community support.

The problem of NIMBYism is more likely to occur when the neighborhood is not in coalition with those making the decisions. Brady and Brady (2000) reiterate that policies and well-rounded statements for review must be presented in community open forums. This allows the residents to have an opportunity to address their concerns. It also allows them to have their myths and stereotypes about the mentally ill dispelled and to participate in the planning process.

Because CHNs typically work in particular geographic areas, it is reasonable to expect that the majority of communities or populations with whom they work will be geographically based. Community health nurses may also work with communities having shared interests and a common sense of belonging as well as with **communities of interest,** groups of people who share beliefs, values, or interests in a particular issue (Clark, 1973) but whose membership may or may not be restricted to the particular geographic area.

Because communities are not homogeneous but experience varying degrees of consensus and conflict, community health nurses may also find themselves working with a number of communities of interest having dissimilar—or even conflicting—needs. For example, one group of people may be working to preserve parkland within a community, while another group may be urging the development of this land for public housing for low-income earners. Community health nurses may also find themselves working with a community whose values are in opposition to those of community health nursing, for example, a group creating racial disharmony. Minkler (1994) warns us that

> while we do need to work closely with communities, to respect their capacities and rights to self-determination, we must at the same time strive to live up to our own ethical standards and those of our profession in not letting blind faith in the community prevent us from seeing and acting on the paramount need for social justice. (p. 529)

Similarly, CHNs may find themselves working with populations or groups who may or may not recognize a sense of common purpose or belonging. For example, a number of elderly people may be living alone and experiencing social isolation within a particular community. These people may seem to the community health nurse to be a community of interest, but they may have no awareness of their shared experiences or needs. Just as the complexity in defining community is reflected in community health nursing practice, so is it reflected in the community assessment process.

DEFINING HEALTHY COMMUNITY

The goal of community health nursing practice—and, hence, the ultimate goal of community assessment—is to promote community health. This raises the questions "What is a healthy community?" and "How will we know when we've attained one?"

Most definitions of health focus solely on individuals, a legacy of the power of the medical model. Given what is known about the influence of the social, economic, and political environments on individual health, being able to define a healthy community may be an important first step in making a significant difference in the population's health.

The public health model recognized by nurses identifies the "determinants of health and the effects of: behavior, biology, environment and the health care system on the health status of individuals and communities" (Association of State and Territorial Directors of Nursing, 2000, p. 1).

Shields and Lindsey (1998) revisit the WHO's definition of health within the context of primary health care and health promotion. They state, "Health promotion as defined in the Ottawa Charter (1986) is the process of enabling people to increase control over, and to improve their health" (p. 24). In order to reach a full state of physical, mental, and social well-being, "an individual or group must be able to identify and to realize aspirations, to satisfy needs, and to change or cope with the environment. Health is, therefore, seen as a resource of everyday life, not the objective of living. According to the Charter, health is a positive concept emphasizing social and personal resources, as well as physical capacities" (p. 24).

It is true that the basic level of learning about a community or another country is to inquire about the infant mortality and morbidity indices and to determine the ma-

jor causes of death. From the wisdom of the previous authors, it is clear that these statistics are the skeleton upon which to consider the broader scope of possibilities.

In an interview with Ilona Kickbusch, who has been Director of Lifestyles and Health for the European Regional Office of the World Health Organization, Flower (1994) discusses the use of a series of indices from the Healthy Cities Project which are used to measure the health of a city. She includes the fascinating things done by cities. An example of this is the development of a new city policy based on findings from the health needs identified in different neighborhoods in Copenhagen. Flower states, "the whole new city health policy, focused on improving social support networks. It moved away from the classic notions of dealing with behaviors such as smoking, drinking and unhealthy diet. The city has defined as a major part of the health problem that people feel lonely, neglected and useless" (p. 52).

Kickbusch incorporates the notion that local government and the grass-roots population must be involved in the process of identifying health needs of the population of the specific city in question.

In order for CHNs and other public health professionals to engage in community work, the Association of State and Territorial Directors of Nursing (2000) recommends three functions which satisfy the government role in health and are linked by continuous evaluation (see Figure 15-2):

- Assessment—encompasses all the activities involved in the concept of community diagnosis, such as surveillance, identifying needs, analyzing the causes of problems, collecting and interpreting data, case finding, monitoring and forecasting trends, research, and evaluation of outcomes.

- Policy Development occurs as the result of interactions among many public and private organizations and individuals. It is the process by which decisions about problems are made, goals and the proper means for reaching them are chosen, conflicting views about solutions are handled and resources are allocated.

- Assurance provides services necessary to reach agreed-upon goals by encouraging private sector action, by requiring it, or by providing services directly. The assurance function in public health involves stimulating the implementation of legislative mandates as well as maintaining statutory responsibilities. (Association of State and Territorial Directors of Nursing, 2000, pp. 9–10)

Community Competence and Community Capacity

Some of the parameters put in place by the Association of State and Territorial Directors of Nursing (2000) remind us that for community competency we must consider the partnerships and expected outcomes set forth

---

REFLECTIVE THINKING

Communities and Communities of Interest

Consider an area where you plan to conduct a community assessment.

- To what communities and communities of interest do members of this area belong?
- Can you identify areas of conflict between any of the communities and communities of interest that you have identified?
- Consider what steps you could take to deal with conflict between competing communities of interest.
- What values would guide your decisions?

FIGURE 15-2 ASTDN Public Health Nursing Practice Model

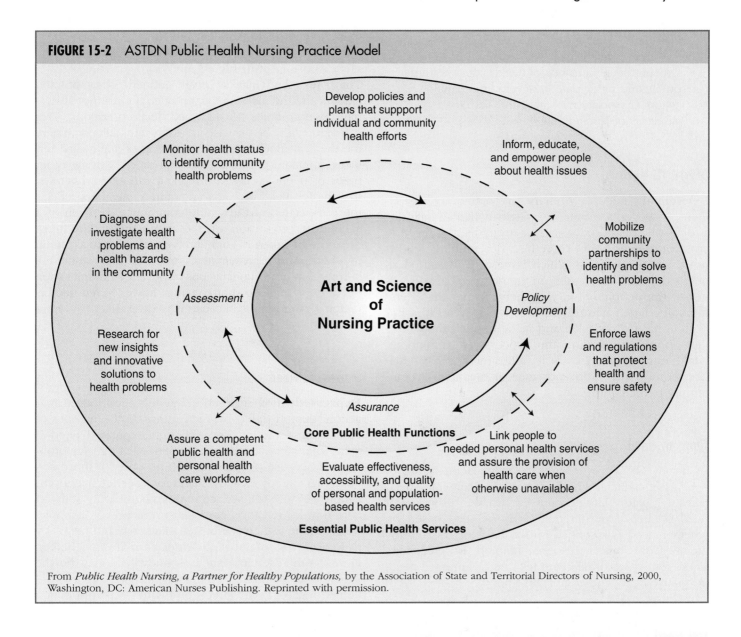

Develop policies and plans that suppport individual and community health efforts

Monitor health status to identify community health problems

Inform, educate, and empower people about health issues

Diagnose and investigate health problems and health hazards in the community

Assessment

Art and Science of Nursing Practice

Policy Development

Mobilize community partnerships to identify and solve health problems

Research for new insights and innovative solutions to health problems

Enforce laws and regulations that protect health and ensure safety

Assurance

Core Public Health Functions

Assure a competent public health and personal health care workforce

Evaluate effectiveness, accessibility, and quality of personal and population-based health services

Link people to needed personal health services and assure the provision of health care when otherwise unavailable

Essential Public Health Services

From *Public Health Nursing, a Partner for Healthy Populations,* by the Association of State and Territorial Directors of Nursing, 2000, Washington, DC: American Nurses Publishing. Reprinted with permission.

by community leaders, including health practitioners. **Community competency** means that the parts making up the whole meet the needs of the inhabitants of that community. (See Chapter 20.) The caliber of the health practitioners is critical since it is their mission to provide information to members of the community and to act as a catalyst for action which will lead to the improvement or protection of health.

Highlights for improving health or protection in a community require that public health practitioners mobilize partnerships. Once the partnerships have been mobilized, public health nurses need to do the following:

- Interact regularly with many providers and services within each community.

- Convene groups and providers who share common concerns and interests in special populations.

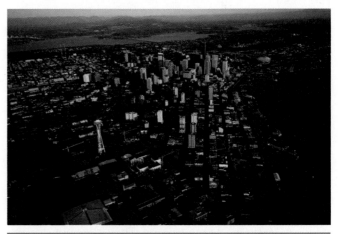

Community health nurses tend to work within geographic boundaries with either the entire community or particular communities of interest.

- Provide leadership to prioritize community problems and develop interventions.
- Explain the significance of health issues to the public and participate in developing plans of action. (Association of State and Territorial Directors of Nursing, 2000, p. 14)

DEFINING NEED

Determining need is primary to community assessment; however, a community assessment also includes a focus on community assets or strengths. Because the concept of need is not value free, determining need is not a simple process. Which issues are identified as needs depends very much on the perspective and values of the people identifying them. Rather than deny the value-laden nature of needs assessment, it is important to acknowledge and make explicit the values that should be driving the process. In community health nursing practice, these values include social justice, equity, and the importance of meaningful community participation.

Types of Need

Bradshaw (1972) recognized the value-laden nature of need assessment, and his framework for examining need takes this nature into account. Bradshaw's taxonomy of need outlines four different types of need based on whether need is identified on the basis of community-member opinion, professional opinion, or precedent. These four types of need are felt need, expressed need, normative need, and comparative need.

Felt Need

Felt need is described as that which people say they need. For example, community members may tell staff at a community health center that they need more antenatal care services within the area. Felt need is important because it reflects that which the people themselves identify as their problems. By itself, however, felt need is unlikely to be comprehensive for a number of reasons. First, people may say that they need only those things that they believe are within the realm of possibility for them; they may not be able to identify those needs of which they are unaware or those needs that they believe will not be met. Second, people may identify only those needs that they believe the person who is conducting the needs assessment wants to hear. They may not, for example, describe anything other than medical needs to a

CHN if they do not understand the broad population-level role of the nurse and, instead, believe that the nurse's role is primarily the provision of clinical care. Third, felt need may be easily influenced by opinion leaders and the mass media, and people may not always have opportunities for informed decision making. This can particularly be the case in health care delivery, where the medical model and the provision of acute-care services dominate public debate. Fourth, as with the other types of need discussed further, it cannot be assumed that the felt need of a few community members reflects the perspective of the whole community, or even of a significant proportion of the community. Care must therefore be taken in community assessment to ascertain the views of a representative sample of the community before coming to conclusions about a community's felt need. Despite these shortcomings, however, felt need is extremely important because it is determined by community members.

Expressed Need

Expressed need is described as felt need turned into action, demonstrated by such things as the number of names on a waiting list. Although expressed need is somewhat more concrete than felt need, it remains problematic because people can sign up only for those services that already exist. Demand for a service may occur simply because the service represents the only solution currently offered for a particular problem. For example, long waiting lists to see obstetricians may not necessarily indicate a shortage of obstetricians in the area. Rather, lack of other services such as midwifery may be the problem or community members may be highly concerned regarding the effects of environmental pollution

---

✳ DECISION MAKING

Needs

A local community group of nonsmokers has asked that a smoking cessation class be added to services already offered at a local clinic. They state that a neighboring community clinic offers one such class.

◆ Which type of need is expressed in their initial request to you?

◆ Given this type of need, what must you consider before making any decision regarding the request?

on the developing fetus, causing many people to visit existing services for additional checkups. Thus, although these problems may manifest as long obstetric waiting lists, more obstetricians may not be the best solution. Also, people tend to sign up on more than one waiting list. For example, people waiting for a nursing home placement may sign up on the waiting list of every nursing home in the area, although they will eventually accept only one place. Thus, adding together the numbers of names on waiting lists may yield an inaccurate picture of need.

Normative Need

Normative need is need determined by experts on the basis of professional analysis. For example, dietitians may determine the recommended daily allowance of protein or fat. Although normative need is the type of need most often regarded as objective and unbiased, it is not without its problems. Professional judgment is based on values in the same way as is felt need, a fact reflected in the way that professional judgment changes over time. Changing beliefs about acceptable cholesterol levels constitute just one example (Becker, 1986). Professional judgment is also often influenced by political agendas, which may make professionals more or less willing or able to publicly present their opinions.

Comparative Need

Comparative need is need determined by comparing the resources or services of one group or area with those of another similar group or area. For example, a given area may be designated as needing more public housing because it has less than do other areas of a similar size and demography. The main shortcomings of this type of need are related to the assumptions on which it is based: that similarity exists between the areas and the response

to the need in the area of comparison was the most appropriate response to the problem, neither of which may be true.

As the preceding discussion illustrates, there are strengths and weaknesses inherent in each of the types of need outlined by Bradshaw (1972): No one type presents a complete picture. When considered together, however, the various types of need provide a much more comprehensive picture than that provided by assessing need via only one method. The responsibility of CHNs lies in critically examining the types of need present in any situation and ensuring that both professionals' and community members' perspectives are included in the process of identifying need.

COMMUNITY PARTICIPATION IN COMMUNITY ASSESSMENT

The WHO, through its Health for All by the Year 2000 program, has identified the importance of active **community participation** at all stages in the assessment, planning, delivery, and evaluation of health services. This sentiment has been echoed at the national level by the American Public Health Association (1991). Attainment of effective community participation is by no means a simple process, however. As is the case with the concept of community, *community participation* must be defined and those kinds of participation likely to be meaningful and effective identified.

REFLECTIVE THINKING

What Type of Need?

- Identify an issue that has been described as a need in your local area.
- Which types of need are present: felt need, expressed need, normative need, and/or comparative need?

REFLECTIVE THINKING

Community Participation

Based on dimensions of community competence, imagine yourself involved in a community project.

- How would you go about encouraging participation from the community?
- What interventions would you make to bridge the gap between those in the community who are isolated and those who are not?
- What would be the most effective means of communication?

TABLE 15-1 Dimensions of Community Competence

DIMENSION	DEFINITION
Commitment	The community members' willingness to invest time and energy into maintenance of the community. Results from community members' realization of the influence that community members have in their own lives, awareness of their own significant role in the community, and recognition that participation in community life yields positive results.
Self-other awareness and clarity of situational definitions	The extent to which components of the community understand their own identity and interests and the ways in which these interests relate to those of other groups within the community.
Articulateness	The ability of groups within the community to articulate their positions and interests and the relationship between their interests and those of other groups within the community.
Communication	The ability of the community to establish common meanings and to effectively send and listen to messages. Effective use of various channels of communication.
Conflict containment and accommodation	The recognition of conflict in a community and the presence of procedures to ensure that conflict is accommodated in such a way that communication channels remain open.
Participation	Members of the community contributing to defining and implementing goals and projects.
Management of relations with the larger society	Understanding and adapting to the larger social system. Effectively using resources that the larger social system offers.
Machinery for facilitating participant interaction and decision making	The presence of procedures and structures for involving community members in decision making.

From "Community Organizing for Health Promotion in the Rural South: An Exploration of Community Competence (Community Interventions)," by A. Denham, S. C. Quinn, and D. Gamble, 1998, Family and Community Health, *21, pp. 1–21. Reprinted with permission of Aspen.*

Community organization is a strategy used to promote health, overcome a problem, or meet a need in the community. Oftentimes, history and social and environmental roots will be incorporated into a discussion so that the people gain a clearer understanding of the issue at hand. Crucial to this process is the participation, commitment, and control of the community members (Denham, Quinn, & Gamble, 1998). The community members working in concert are helped to identify their collective goals and ways of meeting them.

Tables 15-1 and 15-2 identify the eight dimensions implemented by Denham et al. (1998) when they participated in a research study in rural North Carolina. They interviewed 11 community members of different genders and racial backgrounds in order to explore community competence.

In addition to the eight dimensions identified in Tables 15-1 and 15-2, members of the community added the concept of **social support.** This was defined by Eng and Parker (1994) as when "community members know and care about neighbors and show willingness to lend a hand in cognitive, instrumental and emotional support" (p. 210).

APPROACHES TO COMMUNITY ASSESSMENT AND PROGRAM DEVELOPMENT

As mentioned in the previous section, building relationships within the community is a critical part of the community assessment process. The consensus process encourages the involvement of community leaders in developing goals, outcome and process objectives, and plans to meet the objectives. A number of models have been developed and used to develop an effective partnership with community members and to facilitate community participation. These models include the Assessment Protocol for Excellence in Public Health, the Planned Approach to Community Health, and Healthy Cities (Alexander, 2001).

The Assessment Protocol for Excellence in Public Health (APEX/PH) was developed in the United States and designed to facilitate the process of improving public health. The APEX/PH model provides a process for local health departments to assess their capacity to build stronger partnerships with their communities, involve community representatives in identifying their health problems and priorities, and develop a community plan for improving the ability of the health department to

TABLE 15-2 How Community Organization Enhances Community Competence

DIMENSION	MECHANISM
Commitment	• Involving participants in the day-to-day work of the organization through volunteer work or tangible contributions and recognizing them for their efforts. • Creating a sense of community ownership over activities of organization, maintaining community control. • Creating conditions in which people can experience successes. • Soliciting broad-based participation. • Avoiding assumptions about people's level of commitment.
Self-other awareness and clarity of situational definitions	• Bringing individuals together so that they can begin to realize common experiences, interests, and goals. • Raising awareness of the way the power structure operates within a community.
Articulateness	• Creating a sense of community or a supportive, safe environment in which individuals can begin to practice articulating their concerns. • Creating situations for people to feel successful with public speaking. • Creating public forums for community members to express their views. • One-on-one work between individual community members and organizers helping to build confidence.
Communication	• Increasing personal contact between individuals. • Bringing isolated individuals and different cultural groups together so that they get to know each other. Opening new channels of communication. • Sponsoring structured workshops on specific communication skills.
Conflict containment and accommodation	• Establishing a clear goal or mission as a framework for resolving conflicts. • Clarifying issues in order to separate conflicts from personalities or personal animosities.
Participation	• Including all groups or points of view in organizing efforts so that no one feels excluded. • Engaging a broad cross section of the community in defining issues. • Letting community members set the pace for action, especially in high-risk situations. • Highlighting how issues affect people personally.
Management of relations with the larger society	• Attending local government meetings regularly. • Inviting public officials to meet with community members on the community's own terms. • Taking community members to new settings and building confidence by increasing their experience with the larger society. • Providing training in how "the system" works, where to go to deal with issues.
Machinery for facilitating participant interaction and decision making	• Community- or constituent-controlled boards and committees. • Conducting surveys and polls. • Organizing community meetings. • Training in participatory decision making and group process. • Maintaining a high level of informal communication between decision makers and constituents.
Social support	• Bringing people with common needs in contact with each other to facilitate the formation of informal support networks or support groups.
Leadership	• Sharing leadership in order to nurture new leaders. • Including a broad group of individuals in leadership activities. • Identifying individuals with leadership talents or experience and creating an opportunity for them to use their skills. • Providing structured leadership development activities. • Supporting new, inexperienced leaders.

From "Community Organizing for Health Promotion in the Rural South: An Exploration of Community Competence (Community Interventions)," by A. Denham, S. C. Quinn, & D. Gamble, 1998, Family and Community Health, 21, pp. 1–21. Reprinted with permission of Aspen.

meet community health needs identified in the assessment process.

The Planned Approach to Community Health (PATCH) was developed by the Centers for Disease Control and Prevention (CDC) in the United States as a means to plan, deliver, and assess the progress of community-based health promotion programs. The PATCH program is basically a system—a working partnership among the CDC, state health agencies, and the community. There are five general phases in the process (Kreuter, 1984): (1) mobilizing the community by establishing a core of representatives at the local level, (2) collecting and organizing data reflecting local community opinion and health-related variables, (3) choosing health priorities, (4) designing interventions, and (5) evaluating results.

The Healthy Cities model, a demonstration project developed initially in the European office of the WHO, is a model that emerged from the Alma-Ata Declaration and the Health for All strategy. Two key principles of the Health for All by the Year 2000 initiative—multisectoral collaboration and public participation—constitute a central focus of the Healthy Cities model. Although originating in Europe, the Healthy Cities model has been applied in cities and communities throughout the world.

As discussed in Chapters 1 and 5, the Healthy Cities model focuses on the need to reorient medical services and health care systems toward primary health care. The model emphasizes the importance of public involvement in the creation of partnerships between the public, private, and voluntary sectors. The concept of health promotion is central to this model.

THE COMMUNITY ASSESSMENT PROCESS

Having examined some of the main concepts relevant to community assessment, we can now review the community assessment process itself. A number of terms are used to describe this process, including community assessment, community profiling, and community analysis. These terms may also be defined in varying ways. This chapter uses the term **community assessment,** defined as the process of critically examining the characteristics, resources, assets, and needs of a community, in collaboration with that community, in order to develop strategies to improve the health and quality of life of the community (Alexander, 2001).

An example of how the community assessment tool is not an end in itself but the beginning of a process that addresses the community's actual needs is demonstrated by Barry, Doherty, Hope, Sixsmith, and Kelleher in Ireland (2000). While gathering data for their study of "a community needs assessment for rural mental health," they recognized the need to do an assessment in two major stages.

The collected data from a controlled sample ($n = 2500$) was used to determine the group's attention to health and safety practices. They were also interested in data related to attitudes and barriers undertaken for health-promoting actions. In addition, they met with two focus groups of farming organization representatives. Pertinent information which surfaced from these meetings included hazards to safety and health—specifically chemical, machine, and lifestyle practices with concerns about mental health promotion.

The findings from the focus groups revealed concern about rural isolation, depression, and suicide. These findings were congruent with a recent study of the National Task Force on Suicide in Ireland (Department of Health, 1998) which detailed a trend of suicide rates among men between the ages of 15 and 24.

The second stage, predicated on the findings of the first stage, led the researchers to do a data collection from four randomly selected farming communities. The purpose was an "in-depth study of the attitudes, perceptions and current practices of rural residents concerning mental health and safety issues" (p. 293).

The needs assessment study was designed to gain an understanding of how mental health issues are interpreted and dealt with in the context of rural community life (Barry et al., 2000): "Community perceptions and beliefs are considered to play a key role in informing the objectives, content and medium of community intervention strategies" (Barry, 1998, in Barry et al, 2000, p. 293).

Identification of Available Resources

Early in the process, it is necessary to ascertain the time and money available to conduct the community assessment. In this way, the size of the project can be made to correspond to the available resources. The skills and time required of the team involved in the assessment must also be established. Proper review of resources will also help ensure that adequate resources are allocated to address the issues identified in the community assessment. There is little point in expending resources to complete a community assessment if there are neither sufficient resources nor commitment to respond to the needs that arise (Rissel, 1991).

If other community agencies are interested in the community assessment, they may be willing to contribute some resources to the project, particularly if their needs are also addressed. This could constitute a very efficient use of both agency and community resources.

Establishment of Project Team and Steering Committee

Having established why and with what resources the assessment is being conducted, it is then important to establish the project team and steering committee. Com-

REFLECTIVE THINKING

Community Assessment Team Members

What do you think would be the advantages and disadvantages of having insiders conduct a community assessment? Of having outsiders conduct the assessment?

FIGURE 15-3 Organizing the Planning Effort

- Choose a convenient, comfortable, accessible location and agree upon a time to meet.

- Use the initial meetings to build relationships among group members, set a positive tone, and clarify expectations.

- Build in a group process to ensure that your Working Group understands the vision, the planning process, the NEST model, and their roles in making it happen.

- Take the first steps to organize the planning phase by the second or third meeting. By this point, you may be able to:

   Elect a chairperson
   Identify committee goals
   Make a tentative timeline for achieving them
   Identify necessary planning resources

- Establish subcommittees or other structures for getting the work done.

- Develop a way to measure progress.

- Work on making meetings productive.

- Establish ground rules for attendance and participation.

- Use meeting agendas and minutes.

- Create a friendly environment.

- Choose a decision-making style.

   Consensus
   Majority vote

- Create meetings that are fun and involve all of the group members.

From *The Heart of the Community: NEST: A Working Model of Community-Based Long Term Care for Elders,* by C. Mendieta, 1999, San Francisco: Neighborhood Elders Support Team, U.S. Agency on Aging Award #90-AM-2054. Reprinted with permission.

---

munity assessments are rarely completed by a single person; rather, they are best conducted by a group of people with complementary skills.

The **project team** is the group of people who will conduct the community assessment. The team must include a number of people with varying expertise, such that, together, the team has a broad range of skills. It may be made up of outside experts employed specifically for the assessment or employees of local agencies allocated to the project.

The **steering committee** is a group of people from outside the project team who oversee the project, providing outside advice and ensuring that the project achieves its goals. The steering committee typically comprises members of three groups: community health professionals from the area in question, representatives from other organizations that are able to respond to the findings of the community assessment, and representative community members (SCHRU, 1991).

The steering committee is a valuable source of expertise, direction, and support for those conducting the community assessment. This committee also ensures a link between community and project team (necessary if the assessment is to include a community perspective) and plays an important role in formulating recommendations for action on the basis of the community assessment. The steering committee should be of manageable size to facilitate problem solving and decision making; between 6 and 12 people is usually considered workable [Southern Community Health Research Unit (SCHRU) 1991].

The steering committee takes on particular importance when the project team is composed of people who are outsiders. If an outside body is commissioned to perform as the project team on a community assessment, the lack of insider knowledge on the part of team members may cause them to miss or misinterpret important information about the community's history or values. They will also be unaware of any contentious issues about which community members are not speaking. Having community insiders on the steering committee helps compensate for such difficulties (see Figure 15-3).

An example of the project planning process that was used in conducting a community assessment was a project in the Bernal Heights District of San Francisco, California. This was a project that addressed the provision of care to a group of low income elderly. The elderly in this community wanted to remain in their homes as long as possible. Keeping this in mind, a grass-roots group which started the project in 1993 expanded in the late 1990s, with the advent of the Neighborhood Elder Support Team (NEST).

In a community project, a core group often called the "Project Group," participates in the needs assessment. The initial steps of gathering data and sharing meetings to involve the community were initiated with the Bernal Heights Group. A core group of workers called the "Peer Care Coordinators" was established. They were considered "the eyes and ears of NEST in the neighborhood"

(Mendieta, 1999, p. 18). This working group "is willing to commit enough time and resources to actively participate in the creation of the program, not just give advice or ratify decisions" (p. 22). To be most effective, "The Working Group should be made of individuals who understand the culture of the neighborhood and the role of elders" (p. 22).

Other people in the neighborhood concerned with the welfare of their elderly neighbors were called the "gatekeepers." A grocer identified as a "gatekeeper" notices when a customer who usually shops weekly is no longer coming around or a neighbor, another "gatekeeper," notices when an elderly neighbor appears confused when walking his dog.

Through flyers, community meetings, word of mouth, and the media, the people in the community became aware of the services being offered by the NEST program. It is important to note that apart from the willingness of the community to participate, geographical parameters such as mountains, hills, and a few major boulevards within this community aid the members to perceive Bernal Heights as a separate entity within the larger context of the city of San Francisco.

Referrals from neighbors, volunteers, shopkeepers, social groups, and health professionals are made to the Bernal Heights Community Center which houses the NEST program. Peer care coordinators who live in the community and whose average age is 70 are involved, along with volunteers and nursing students who followup by making home visits to an identified client.

Although Mendieta specifically refers to the NEST project, the principles of community organization apply to any group implementing a community project. Mendieta (1999) highlights the fact that the working group will bring community resources into the planning process: "They are a source of both support and leadership. The importance of the commitment, energy, drive, and expertise Working Group members bring to the planning effort cannot be overestimated" (p. 22).

Development of Research Plan and Time Frame

Developing a plan for the entire community assessment process at the beginning will enable the team to keep more or less on schedule. Changing circumstances may, however, require some flexibility in the plan. Outlining a clear time frame at this point will also ensure that all members of the project team and steering committee are aware of the time commitment expected of them (SCHRU, 1991).

Collection and Analysis of Information Already Available

Regardless of the number of potential new resources available for the assessment, it is advisable not to rein-

vent the wheel. Nor can one ignore that which has already been learned about the particular issues being addressed. It is thus wise to collect information that is already available. A literature review to identify ways whereby similar issues have been dealt with elsewhere is invaluable. It is also important to identify the information about the area that is available from secondary sources, information previously collected by local, state, and federal governmental bodies. Such information may take the form of epidemiological and demographic data about the area, policy documents developed at the national or state level, and the like. These are discussed in more detail later.

Any community assessments previously conducted in the area should also be examined. Some such assessments may have examined one particular group of the community rather than the community as a whole. Analysis of the information obtained from the various sources will help the team identify the need for further information.

Completion of Community Research

Having developed an overview of the characteristics of the community and having examined any previously collected information about the community's needs, the next step is to plan ways to collect additional data that are needed. Such data are likely to include needs identified by local community members and other health and social welfare personnel, as well as information related to community history and values. Techniques such as surveys, interviews, and group discussions are particularly useful in data collection. The various methods are discussed in further detail later in this chapter.

Analysis of Results

Once the data collection process is complete, analysis of the results is necessary. This is a crucial stage of the process and includes analysis of both community resources and needs. In needs analysis, it is important to express the need as a problem, rather than a potential solution to the problem. For example, it might be said that there is a need for more dentists in a community. This, however, describes a solution to the problem rather than the problem itself. The problem may be better described as long waiting lists to see dentists. More dentists in the community might then be identified as one of a number of potential solutions to the problem. Making explicit this difference between problems (needs) and solutions may alert the project team and steering committee to a number of possible causes and solutions to each need identified. During the analysis of results, it is important to be mindful of the original purpose of the assessment and to link the analysis back to that purpose.

Another important aspect of the analysis process is to look beyond the immediate issue identified to any underlying problems. Time should be spent critically analyzing any underlying causes of each problem. Analyzing the data in this way increases the likelihood of identifying, and, later, addressing the root causes of issues affecting the health of the community. It may also facilitate the identification of a common basis for a number of seemingly unrelated issues and, thus, a comprehensive response. For example, in exploring the issues facing the Fitzroy Community Health Centre in Melbourne, Australia, staff identified poverty as the underlying cause of a number of these issues (McBride, 1988). Having done so, they were then in a position to identify strategies to address this problem directly, rather than by continuing to react separately to multiple results of poverty.

Reporting Back to the Community

Reporting the findings of the community assessment to members of the community is a vital part of the community assessment process. Community members "own" the information collected in a needs survey as much as do the team members involved in collecting it. Effort should thus be made to ensure that the information collected is returned to the community (Mendieta, 1999).

Reporting back to the community is much more than a formality; doing so provides an opportunity for verification of the findings and identification of any potential problem areas prior to final publication (Barton, Smith, Brown, & Supples, 1993). For these reasons, it is recommended that a penultimate draft be presented to the community for response, rather than simply presenting the final report as a *fait accompli* (Russell, Gregory, Wotton, Mordoch, & Counts, 1996). Any important omissions or areas of contention can then be identified and acted on.

Results can be presented in both verbal and written forms. A combination of approaches is most likely to ensure effective dissemination of the results. Reports must be written clearly to ensure accessibility to a wide range of community members. Some examples of ways to report the findings of the assessment to the community are as follows:

- A brief, widely distributed, user-friendly report
- Public meetings
- Press releases
- Displays in well-frequented areas such as shopping centers
- Presentations to local government and community groups

In addition to fulfilling the moral obligations of the project team, reporting back to the community enables other agencies to act on needs identified and allows community members to lobby for further action if the issues identified so warrant. Conclusions and recommendations from the community assessment direct both the community and health agencies toward appropriate action (Mendieta, 1999).

Setting Priorities for Action

Once the needs assessment is complete and the issues requiring attention are identified, identification of priorities for action is the next important step. This is a point at which the differing values of steering committee members may become apparent, and the perspectives of community members on the steering committee become particularly important (Kang, 1995).

Ruffing-Rahal (1987) identifies consistent contrasts between priorities identified by community members and those identified by health professionals. The danger lies in deciding whose priorities take precedence. Labonte (1994) highlights a PATCH project wherein community members' priorities were ignored because they did not match those identified by a risk factor survey. This is a point at which the full implications of a partnership approach become apparent.

Determining priorities for action is a complex process that must begin with a confirmation of those values that will guide the process. Decision making may be guided by the principles of social justice and equity, which drive primary health care and the new public health movement, as well as by the values implicit in an agency's mission statement and philosophy. A series of questions, such as those listed, may help guide decision making:

- What types of need are present? Do community members consider these to be needs?
- How many people are affected?
- What will be the consequences if these needs are not met?
- Are there critical needs that should be met before other needs are addressed?
- Is it possible to address these needs?
- Do the needs coincide with governmental policies or the department's mission statement?
- Are resources (funds, staff) available? (Wass, 1994, based on Gilmore, Campbell, and Becker, 1989)

The process for determining priorities must also ensure that everyone has an equal opportunity to participate and to influence any decisions. Group rules that recognize everyone's right to speak are important, as are voting processes that allow everyone an equal vote. One process that has been used quite successfully is the nominal group process. This process is discussed in the section on community assessment tools.

FIGURE 15-4 The Ottawa Charter for Health Promotion's Five Levels of Action

- Build healthy public policy.
- Create supportive environments.
- Strengthen community action.
- Develop personal skills.
- Reorient the health system.

From *Ottawa Charter for Health Promotion,* by the World Health Organization, Health and Welfare Canada, Canadian Public Health Association, 1986, Copenhagen, Denmark: FADL Publishers. Copyright by WHO. Used with permission of Oxford University Press.

FIGURE 15-5 The Steps of Brainstorming

1. Present the issue to the group.
2. Invite the group to suggest solutions to the issue.
3. Encourage group members to be creative and to not judge the value of an idea before suggesting it.
4. Write down all suggestions without comment or criticism.
5. Continue the process until all ideas are exhausted.
6. When no more suggestions are forthcoming, analyze the responses.

If the brainstorming process is used to identify appropriate responses to a health issue, the next step involves discussing each suggestion to identify its merits and shortcomings. Suggestions may then be scaled according to their usefulness.

Adapted with permission from *Promoting Health: A Practical Guide,* by L. Ewles and I. Simnett, 1992, London: Scutari Press. Copyright 1996 by Bailliere Tindall, London.

Determination of Responses to the Needs Identified

Once the community needs have been identified, it is necessary to determine ways to best address those needs. Once again, it is important that community members be actively involved in this process. This is a point at which the contributions of community members may be vital, because understanding the issues from their perspective may highlight particular approaches that are either likely or unlikely to be successful. As is true at earlier stages of the community assessment, one of the first steps in this process is to ensure clarity regarding actual needs so that appropriate responses to those needs may be generated.

The Ottawa Charter for Health Promotion (WHO, 1986) provides a useful framework around which responses to needs can be identified. The five levels of action listed by this charter identify a broad range of activities at both the environmental and the individual levels, serving as another reminder that change at the individual level may not necessarily be the most appropriate response to identified needs. A comprehensive response is likely to include action on a number of these five levels, listed in Figure 15-4.

Discussion and idea-generating processes are important at this stage to enable the group to identify a range of innovative and comprehensive responses to the identified needs. One such process is brainstorming. The brainstorming process can prove quite useful for a committee or group trying to decide ways to best address identified problems. The value of the brainstorming process lies in the fact that it provides a forum wherein creativity is encouraged and judgment of ideas is suspended, enabling the development of hitherto unthought of solutions. Brainstorming has been used successfully in a variety of scenarios and may be a valuable tool in developing creative ideas. The steps of brainstorming are listed in Figure 15-5.

Planning and Implementation

Once a strategy or set of strategies to address identified problems has been developed, the next step is to plan the ways that these strategies will be implemented. This

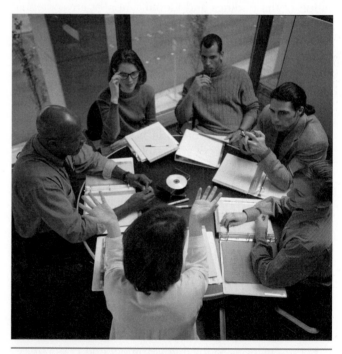

Creative ideas often stem from brainstorming. Present an issue to a group of classmates and then have a group brainstorming session to suggest solutions. Photo courtesy of PhotoDisc.

does not mean that the assessment phase is entirely over; rather, the process must remain flexible and sensitive to changing circumstances and the needs of the community throughout the planning and implementing phases. Certainly, though, a large component of the assessment phase is over, and attention can be focused more fully on the very different set of skills required in effective planning, implementation, and evaluation (examined in Chapter 16).

DOCUMENTING A COMMUNITY ASSESSMENT

Returning to the Bernal Heights NEST program, the following groups have been noted to enhance greater collaboration within the community: senior service organizations, elementary schools, nursing and medical schools, the Department of Public Health, fire department, and funders (Mendieta, 1999, p. 14).

Mendieta (1999) emphasizes that the transition period between planning and implementation can be very intense. Even though the core program has been identified and thoroughly studied, regardless of how organized the group is, some things are likely to change or will need to be changed. These changes often happen quickly and can create stress among the staff. An example (Mendieta, 1999, Chapter 3) was when the staff recognized that although they had sufficient help in organizing the volunteers, providing peer counselors for case management, and creating a senior center, they did not have enough volunteer staff to attend to the administrative duties.

Mendieta (1999) states that the "many hats syndrome" is common in the nonprofit world. NEST staff quickly experienced this pitfall. In addition to providing direct services and performing administrative duties, NEST's small staff was trying to do it all. They were conducting "all levels of outreach, creating program documents and filing systems, greeting the public, answering phones, cleaning the office and running frequent errands" (pp. 38–39).

When a new organization finds itself short staffed, it is common that the staff becomes overwhelmed and the quality of its performance decreases.

Another cautionary note relative to a new program is to have an evaluation design in place before opening the doors. Benefits of ongoing program evaluation include:

- An opportunity to touch bases with your vision and purpose
- Providing important feedback on effectiveness of services
- Validating the work that has been accomplished
- Ensuring staff accountability (Mendieta, 1999, p. 39)

Having an evaluation plan in place is crucial in terms of gathering pertinent data. This is relevant for future planning, grant writing, and general record keeping to provide a means of comparison over time (p. 41).

COMMUNITY ASSESSMENT TOOLS

There are a number of valuable tools for use in collecting the information required in a community assessment. The kind of information obtainable through these tools varies considerably. Some tools facilitate the collection of quantitative data, whereas others provide qualitative data. It is important to note that no one method is likely to provide the full range of information needed in a community assessment. Rather, the kind of information provided by these methods is likely to be complementary; thus, use of multiple methods is warranted. As a general rule, quantitative methods facilitate a description of the extent of social phenomena, whereas qualitative methods facilitate the exploration of the underlying rationale of attitudes and behaviors (Chu, 1994). If the community assessment is to move beyond describing an area to *understanding* that area and its related issues of concern, some in-depth, qualitative methods must be used. In this way, the issues raised and their contributing factors can be explored (Baum, 1995). Regardless of the tools ultimately chosen, it is important to have people with expertise in the available assessment methods on either the project team or the steering committee.

The following summary of the various tools and methods constitutes an introduction to this topic. Some of the methods involve the analysis of information already collected, whereas others involve the collection of new information. Examination of information already collected is referred to as secondary data analysis. Applicable data include epidemiological and demographic information, national or regional policy documents, and previously conducted needs surveys. Methods that involve the collection of new information, or primary data, include participant observation, surveys, key-informant interviews, group techniques, and community forums. Figure 15-6 illustrates the various tools used in community assessment.

Demographic and Epidemiological Data

Demographic and epidemiological data can provide a great deal of useful information about a community. Demographic information includes the age, gender, and ethnicity compositions of the community. Other social and economic indicators, such as employment levels, levels of home ownership, and population rates, are also valuable. Epidemiological data identify the rates of morbidity and

FIGURE 15-6 Community Assessment Tools

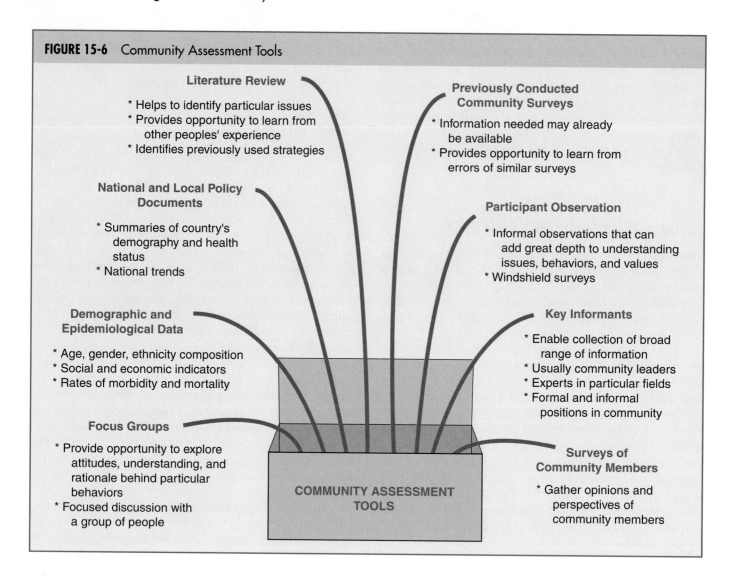

Literature Review

* Helps to identify particular issues
* Provides opportunity to learn from other peoples' experience
* Identifies previously used strategies

National and Local Policy Documents

* Summaries of country's demography and health status
* National trends

Demographic and Epidemiological Data

* Age, gender, ethnicity composition
* Social and economic indicators
* Rates of morbidity and mortality

Focus Groups

* Provide opportunity to explore attitudes, understanding, and rationale behind particular behaviors
* Focused discussion with a group of people

Previously Conducted Community Surveys

* Information needed may already be available
* Provides opportunity to learn from errors of similar surveys

Participant Observation

* Informal observations that can add great depth to understanding issues, behaviors, and values
* Windshield surveys

Key Informants

* Enable collection of broad range of information
* Usually community leaders
* Experts in particular fields
* Formal and informal positions in community

Surveys of Community Members

* Gather opinions and perspectives of community members

COMMUNITY ASSESSMENT TOOLS

mortality in the population, for identification of leading causes of death and diseases within population subgroups and local communities. In addition, epidemiological information now includes data related to injuries (Murray & Lopez, 1996).

In the 1980s there was growing recognition of the limitations of epidemiological data, particularly since the major indicators used to assess population health status were mortality indices (Brown, 1985). Rather than describing the health of the population, epidemiological data focused on mortality data. Given the WHO's definition of health as being more than the absence of disease, this has been a shortcoming. Billings and Cowley (1995) further point out that mortality data can be misleading. This is particularly true when rates are relatively low, because the rates say nothing about the state of the majority of the population who remain alive (Patrick, 1986). Morbidity data have also been criticized because it cannot be assumed that incidence rates equate with need for services (Billings & Cowley, 1995; Stalker, 1993).

In addition to the above statistical limitations, there are others as well, ones that reduce their practical value to policymakers (Murray & Lopez, 1996). First, even the mortality data may be fragmented and partial, even not available in some countries. Second, estimates of the numbers killed or affected by certain conditions or diseases may be exaggerated beyond their demographically plausible limits. Third, traditional health statistics do not provide policymakers with sufficient indicators to compare the relative cost-effectiveness of different interventions. Because of these problems with the use of traditional population health status indices, primarily mortality rates, the WHO, the World Bank, and the Harvard School of Public Health worked to address these problems with their landmark study, *The Global Burden of Disease and Injury*. Further discussion of this study is included in Chapter 3.

Additional concerns about epidemiological data have also emerged in conjunction with the growing awareness of environmental health issues. Epidemiological data that

Perspectives...

INSIGHTS OF A COMMUNITY HEALTH NURSE

As a community health nurse, you never know exactly where you will find yourself or what you will do if you are asked to carry out a community assessment. It can, by definition, be a community of geographical location or one of common interest. My experience was in the Western Highlands of Guatemala, where I was assigned to six villages. My primary purpose was to give "charlas," talks on various health topics. Some of them included rehydration therapy, nutritional resources, hygiene, sanitizing water/vegetables, cooking with a protein substitute, dental hygiene education, women's reproductive health, and discussions about hypertension. The members of the six villages were poor farmers struggling to feed their families and to maintain a shelter.

When doing an assessment, one of the most critical features is to collect as much data about the community as possible. Some of the concerns in my communities included a high infant mortality rate (with estimates of 60/1000), poor prenatal care, and deficiencies in nutrition for pregnant women and small children. Another public health issue was the death of children due to gastrointestinal illness and dehydration. Often, the parents needed to be educated about the signs and symptoms of dehydration and how, with home remedies, they could rehydrate the child.

A study done in Guatemala by public health professionals demonstrated that 95% of families always had salt and sugar available along with some lemons. The majority of families had access to potable water. Upon advisement, the mothers would boil the water for 15–20 minutes using firewood.

Sugar, salt, and lemon (for flavor enhancement) are necessary for the rehydration remedy recommended by the WHO.

During some of the charlas, the women would place eight teaspoons of sugar and one teaspoon of salt in a small plastic bag. We would first prepare the rehydration remedy so that everyone could taste it. Then we would all share in counting out the spoonfuls until each woman had a little bag to carry home. I suggested that they keep the bag of ingredients and the recipe, done in drawings (for those who couldn't read), in the kitchen hanging on a wall.

I worked closely with the home educator (Clara) and two agriculturists, Arturo and Paco, who had worked in these communities for approximately 10 years.

Arturo and Paco taught the men how to rotate crops in a way that did not overuse the minerals and nutrients of the earth. They were dedicated to teaching them how to use measures other than pesticides for their crops. Paco taught the women how to grow small trees for the purpose of reforestation. Clara did the same work that I was requested to do. She also provided information and applications about how women could start small businesses. Selling snacks at the school house was one possibility. She taught them how to extract Eucalyptus oil from the trees for assisting in respiratory problems.

From the information already provided in this short piece, you, as a community health nurse, can already identify some of the health and environmental problems of these communities.

Using powers of observation and asking questions of the housewives, the farmers, the home educator, and agriculturists are other ways to collect data from the community. Other resources include other health professionals, doctors, nurses, and religious people who serve the communities.

Asking key informants for help and capitalizing on the rapport that they had already built with the community members helped me to gain entry into the communities. Every time that I went to a village with Clara, Arturo, and Paco, they graciously introduced me as a Peace Corps volunteer and a community health nurse. I then could explain that I was there to help them with any project they wished to do.

The project was discussed with the village and the "felt" need was identified as having personnel nearby to provide minimal health care. The nearest hospital or public health clinic was at least 45 minutes away from the villages. The community members really didn't have much money, if any, to pay for services. Lack of transportation was another barrier.

It was decided, with the help of Clara, Arturo, and Paco, that each village would select two representatives for a month's training to become health promoters. The people in the village agreed that each community would select one man and one woman. The criteria for the candidates were that (1) they had to be motivated to help their communities, (2) they needed to be respected by the community so their

(continues)

Perspectives...

friends and neighbors would come to them for minimal health care, (3) they had to be able to read and write even if it was at the primary grade level, (4) the person could be of any age. It took six months before the villages came to a consensus about the candidates.

The youngest participant in the project was a mature 13-year-old girl who was highly motivated to learn and help her village. She was accepted by the other participants as well as her village. The eldest person was in her sixties. She also was respected by the community.

Keeping within the cultural norms, the course was developed with "icebreakers" so as to have some *conocomiento* (getting to know each other). We provided appropriate food snacks at midmorning and midafternoon. Little open tacos with carrots, beets, and cheese along with a rice drink were their favorites. Breaks originally scheduled for 15 minutes were changed to at least a half hour because the longer break seemed to work better for the group. Active participation and interactive learning were the main principles used in the course. The students were very highly motivated to learn everything they could. They took their new role very seriously. It was a question of wanting to learn and being proud to be representing their villages. They earnestly wanted to be as prepared as possible.

The success of this project was due to collaboration between the grass-roots communities, the Guatemalan official agencies (i.e., Public Health and Digesa—the Agricultural Department), and the Peace Corps. The early planning meetings drew about 20 people. As we reached our goal of starting the program, the responsibility and planning depended on three people: the public health representative, the rural nurse, and myself.

With our dedication and steadfastness and the support of the community, we certified 12 health promoters. We held a graduation celebration, bringing in the Guatemalan flag and playing the national anthem for the participants who successfully completed the course. The formality of the graduation was congruent with the formality of the culture. The period of time from the project's inception until the student graduation was two years.

In terms of evaluation and the sustainability of the project, I had the opportunity of visiting the health promoters two years after graduation. Ten of the 12 were still providing service to their respective communities. The two who weren't had either moved away or had found full-time employment elsewhere. The Guatemalan public health professional was still training community health promoters and the program was thriving.

—Aida Sahud, DrPH, MSN, RN

focus on those health problems involving a simple cause-and-effect relationship and no delay in the onset of symptoms may be of limited use (Auer, 1988; Brennan, 1992). There are many situations in which long time frames and complex interrelationships result in the suffering of many people before epidemiological evidence of the problems is identified (Wass, 1994). Even given all of the various shortcomings, however, epidemiological data, used and recommended for use in the *Global Burden of Disease and Injury* study, remain a key source of information for community assessment purposes.

Barton et al. (1993) warn that secondary data such as demographic and epidemiological information is often not available for the exact area being assessed. In fact, community boundaries rarely correspond to census tracts. In such situations, inferences may need to be drawn about the community in question on the basis of information gathered for larger statistical areas. Local information gathered via discussion with local key informants can then be used to determine whether the issues

reflected in the broader data are true for the local community (Barton et al., 1993).

Because it constitutes part of the public record, demographic and epidemiological information should be relatively easy to access in industrialized nations. In addition to being available directly from the governmental bodies that collect it, this information also may be obtained from the regional health department or public health offices. This may not be the case, however, in the developing nations of the world, where information may be difficult to obtain.

National and Local Policy Documents

National policy or strategy documents, such as *Healthy People 2000* in the United States (U.S. Department of Health and Human Services, 1991), *Achieving Health for All: A Framework for Health Promotion* in Canada (Epp, 1986), and *Health for All Australians* in Australia (Health Targets and Implementation Committee, 1988), may provide useful summaries of a country's demography and evidence of health problems. As national documents, they may also contribute to the decision to address a particular health issue. It must be remembered, however, that these documents are political in nature and that issues may therefore be exaggerated or downplayed depending on current political agendas. Also, as political documents, the extent to which they reflect felt need depends on the extent to which meaningful participation processes were incorporated into the policymaking process. If such participation processes are largely nonexistent, the documents are likely to reflect only normative or comparative needs.

The other important point to note about national documents is that they reflect national trends, which may or may not accurately reflect the local picture. Different localities clearly have different needs; and if local needs do not reflect national needs, national policy documents may be of limited use.

Literature Review

Reviewing current literature can help identify the particular issues facing people in certain situations and can highlight typical or potential needs (McKenzie & Jurs, 1993). A literature review may afford the project team insight garnered from the work of others. In this way, the team can build on, rather than unnecessarily repeat, previous work.

A literature review will also uncover strategies used by others in addressing particular needs. Such information proves very useful when it comes time to plan appropriate responses to the needs identified in the assessment process.

Previously Conducted Community Surveys

Any previously conducted community surveys constitute useful sources of information about a community for three central reasons. First, the local information needed may have already been collected by others, minimizing duplication of effort and the unnecessary use of resources. Second, through either critical examination of any corresponding reports or discussion with those who conducted previous surveys, it is possible to learn from any errors made in those surveys. Third, all necessary information may already be available, and no further community research may be needed, although this is seldom the case.

Participant Observation

Community health nurses are in an excellent position to learn about community beliefs, values, and issues through observation, having many opportunities to observe and listen to people during the daily interactions of community health nursing practice. Such opportunities occur both when working directly with individual clients and

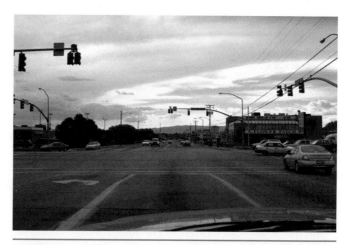

From the car, the nurse can observe communities in action.

groups and when living and moving among the community. This process of observation can be cultivated by taking every opportunity to listen and to take notice of occurrences (Twelvetrees, 1987). For those community health nurses who are not members of the communities with which they work, this may require making a conscious effort to participate in some of the everyday activities of the community: for example, attending local shows, walking through the various parts of the community, or shopping as the locals do. This type of informal observation can greatly enhance understanding of issues, behaviors, and values in a community and becomes particularly important when working with people who are unable or unwilling to articulate their views (Bowling, 1992).

Developing networks with a wide range of individuals and groups as part of daily practice can also help increase awareness of emerging health concerns (Peckham & Spanton, 1994). Indeed, Eng, Salmon, and Mullan (1992) urge health care professionals to be active members of their communities, while being careful not to take over from community members in local leadership roles.

The term **windshield survey** describes the process of observing a community by driving a car or riding public transportation through that community. Windshield surveys enable the observation of such things as housing quality, recreation facilities, the movement of people throughout the area at varying times of the day, areas of congregation in the streets, and the atmosphere of different areas of town (Shuster & Goeppinger, 1996). All such observations contribute to understanding the area and what it is like to live there.

Key Informants

Interviewing key informants is one relatively efficient way to collect a broad range of information about a community. Key informants are people who, by virtue of

Out
of the Box

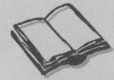

A Grass-Roots Community Project Serving Women in Oakland, California

A community need was identified which was to provide integrative health measures to a group of low-income women in Oakland, California, with cancer. It was clear from the target population that many women had been struggling with various forms of cancer. The majority had been receiving treatment from both medical and nursing professionals. In many cases, they had expressed a desire to try some complementary measures in their treatment but could not afford to pay for them. Many women were identified as low income when they first came to this integrative care clinic. Many others had become low income after they had undergone medical treatment such as radiation and/or chemotherapy and were too weak to work. Oftentimes, the illness itself robbed them of their energy and their financial resources, making it impossible for them to work full time and to pay for the services they wished to have.

The efforts of a group of community organizers, professional women and representatives of public health, joined together and developed a vision for the women with cancer to be able to receive a number of different complementary treatment modalities:

acupuncture, Eastern and Western herbal remedies for symptom control, massage/therapeutic touch, and visualization/relaxation sessions. In addition to these modalities, the clinic provides organic vegetables and other foodstuffs, such as bread for the clients.

The clinic has trained a number of community volunteers to provide the above-mentioned services gratis to the clients. The commitment of each volunteer is to create an atmosphere of "community," a sense of belonging, along with providing specific treatment modalities to the client. Each person volunteers for at least a day a month and makes a minimum of a year's commitment. The herbs and foods are donated through the collaboration of other organizations in the community.

The administrative officers are constantly attending to the organization and efficient running of the clinic. In addition, they are committed to writing grants to maintain the offering of services to the women in the community. This occurs within the context of quality assurance.

It is within the purview of the community health nurse to identify a community need and find a way of organizing groups within the community to manifest needed services. Models such as the integrative care clinic identified have come about by having a vision and a dedicated group of women to organize and provide services. ∎

---

their positions in the community as community leaders or experts in a particular field, are able to identify problems and issues affecting that community. Key informants may hold formal or informal positions in the community; it is important to include both types of key informants because their perspectives may vary greatly. For example, the viewpoint of the mayor may differ substantially from that of the leader of a local self-help group. At the same time, however, the perspectives of key informants may differ from that of the general community. Thus, interviewing key informants is never assumed to be equivalent to interviewing community members not in leadership positions.

There are three main groups of key informants (Ong, Humphries, Annett, & Ritkin, 1991):

1. People who are in key positions in the community because of their professions, such as health professionals, social workers, and police

2. People who are leaders within the community, such as leaders of self-help groups or volunteer organizations and counselors

3. People who are centrally placed because of their social roles in the community, such as corner shopkeepers or postal workers

Because they typically have lived in the area for some time, key informants may be able to tell you a great deal about the community, including the historical and cultural base, the major problems, and the experience of living there. There are some important points to note, however, about the use of key informants. First, key informants must be chosen carefully to ensure that those chosen have a good understanding of the community and that their perspective is likely to be a representative one. Second, key informants should not be used in isolation at the expense of talking to the actual people affected by the issue or problem at hand (Gilmore et al.,

1989). Doing so introduces the risks that assumptions about community members will be accepted as fact and that vested interests will unduly influence the results.

Because they facilitate exploration and discussion of issues as they arise, semistructured interviews are commonly used in ascertaining the views of key informants. Although it is possible to use a survey approach with key informants, doing so is unlikely to yield the same depth of material.

Surveys of Community Members

If a community assessment is to take account of felt need, soliciting the opinions and perspectives of community members is vital. Surveys may be used both to ask residents about unmet needs and to evaluate existing services. Surveys may also be used to collect direct information about people's health experiences, attitudes, and behaviors.

A number of different survey methods may be used in community assessment, the most common being face-to-face interviews, telephone surveys, and self-administered questionnaires (Hawe, Degeling, & Hall, 1990). These three forms of information collection are compared in Table 15-3. Which one is used depends on the type of information that must be collected. Information regarding issues that can be clearly and simply expressed may be obtained via a self-administered questionnaire, whereas information regarding issues that require sub-

stantial thought and exploration might be best obtained via interviews (Hawe et al., 1990). Similarly, it may be possible to examine some issues via the use of a set of structured questions, whereas a less structured approach in the form of either semistructured or unstructured interviews may be more suitable for exploring other issues.

The type of information sought is not the only variable to be considered, however. Cultural differences may play an important part. For example, interviews may be the most appropriate method when working with members of an ethnic group having a strong oral culture. Similarly, asking direct questions may be considered rude in some cultures. In such a circumstance, a general discussion may be more appropriate, even if the issues of concern seem straightforward to the professionals involved in the community assessment.

If survey findings are to be generalized to the community, the sample chosen for the survey must be randomly selected to ensure representation of the population in question. Furthermore, the data collection instrument must be valid and reliable (McKenzie & Jurs, 1993). Involving people with expertise in the development of the survey instrument and survey plan is vital.

The Nottingham Health Profile, used in both Britain and Australia, represents a useful example of a questionnaire for collecting information on health experiences and perceived health status. Such information complements information received from analysis of service use

TABLE 15-3   A Comparison of Three Models of Data Collection

	SELF-ADMINISTERED QUESTIONNAIRES	TELEPHONE SURVEYS	FACE-TO-FACE INTERVIEWS
Cost	Cheapest method per respondent	Low to medium cost per respondent	Most expensive method per respondent
Coverage	Can reach a widely scattered sample	Can reach a widely scattered sample, but only those with phones	Depends on personal contact
Response rate	Lowest, especially with groups of low socioeconomic status	Medium response rate	Highest response rate
Standardization	Standardized	Standardization depends on the interviewer	Standardization depends on the interviewer
Privacy for asking sensitive questions	Good, least likely to cause embarrassment	Some "anonymity" for giving replies	May be difficult
Probing	Does not permit clarification; misunderstanding will go undetected	Allows for probing, reduces misunderstanding and missing answers	Allows for probing, reduces misunderstanding and missing answers
Literacy	Requires literacy	Not restricted by literacy, but language skills important	Not restricted by literacy, but language skills still important
Observation	No observation possible	Listening to respondent	Listening to and watching respondent

From Evaluating Health Promotion, *by P. Hawe, D. Degeling, and J. Hall, 1990, Sydney, Australia: MacLennan & Petty. Copyright 1996 by MacLennan and Petty, Sydney. Reprinted with permission.*

and is of particular value because of the likely correlation between perceived health status, health attitudes, and health behavior. The fact that such self-reported information may be more valuable than morbidity and mortality figures in predicting service use means that this profile could be invaluable in community assessments (Baum & Cooke, 1989). Furthermore, because it retains a social health perspective and can be used to demonstrate the influence of socioeconomic status on health, the Nottingham profile, unlike many other behavioral surveys, precludes the risk of blaming the victim.

Focus Groups

When groups of people hold discussions regarding a specific area of interest to the community assessment, the groups are known as focus groups. Focus groups provide opportunities to explore attitudes, understandings, and the rationales behind particular behaviors or attitudes among groups of people (Hawe et al., 1990) and can be of value in developing a greater understanding of the needs of groups who may have been largely neglected by the health system (Stevens, 1996). They also provide researchers with opportunities to listen to a group of people explore an issue of concern.

A typical focus group is limited in number to 8–12 people to facilitate in-depth discussion and participation by all group members (McKenzie & Jurs, 1993). Focus groups are conducted in an informal atmosphere. The researcher acts as facilitator, guiding the group through a semistructured interview schedule related to the topic of interest. Because focus groups are designed to uncover the range of opinions and feelings on various aspects of the topic, the questions used are open ended, and freedom of expression is encouraged (Murphy, Cockburn, & Murphy, 1992). The facilitator remains relatively unobtrusive and does not disrupt the flow of discussion, thereby enabling group participants to explore the issues and respond to each other's comments without external judgment (Hawe et al., 1990; Stevens, 1996). Focus group discussions are taped so that they can be analyzed after the event (Murphy et al., 1992).

Within the relative safety of such a group, participants may feel comfortable expressing views that they may not be willing to share individually. Also, group members are able to build on each other's comments and come to conclusions that they may not have considered outside of the group context (Stevens, 1996). For these reasons, focus groups can be of great value in community assessment.

Focus groups are most effective when group members are relatively homogeneous. People invited to participate in a focus group may share certain characteristics such as age group, gender, cultural background, education, or socioeconomic status (Stevens, 1996). Within the boundaries of their shared characteristics, however, people may be chosen to reflect a variety of different attitudes toward the topic at hand in order to facilitate discussion and identify important issues. If the people in a focus group were to be too similar, there might be little for them to discuss; conversely, if focus group members were to not share certain assumptions or history, productive discussion may be impossible (Hawe et al., 1990).

Focus groups may be useful at various points during the community assessment process—from exploring the rationale behind a particular high-risk behavior to developing action plans to address community problems from the perspective of those people affected by the problems. For example, a group of young people might be invited together to discuss the issues of mental health or youth unemployment. Through a discussion of the youths' experiences, researchers might reap a deeper understanding of the underlying dynamics of these experiences. The focus group might then be asked to explore possible solutions to the identified problems. Brainstorming, discussed earlier, may be a valuable technique in such a situation.

Focus groups constitute a very useful way of exploring in some depth the perspectives of people who may not normally have a voice but whose inclusion in the assessment process is important. It is important to note, however, that although focus group participants are chosen because they are typical of their particular subgroup, they are not a representative sample. This means that the outcomes of focus groups cannot be generalized to the entire community (McKenzie & Jurs, 1993).

Community Forum

A public meeting or series of public meetings can provide a valuable opportunity to assess the range of public

---

✳ DECISION MAKING

Planning an Elder Center

A group of elder adults (ages 65 and over) says that their community needs a center where the elder members of the community can meet and socialize. It is determined that a needs assessment will be done.

◆ Outline a plan to begin a needs assessment process that you would recommend to the steering committee and project team.

◆ Include a list of the tools that could be used to identify who would be members of your project team and your steering committee. Incorporate the stages of the community assessment process.

RESEARCH FOCUS

Dimensions of Participation and Leadership: Implications for Community-Based Health Promotion for Youth

Study Problem/Purpose

For researchers and practitioners to gain a better understanding of coalition building in three major communities as it relates to community health promotion for youth.

Methods

The Houston-Harris County Community Partnership project was funded by the Center for Substance Abuse Prevention (CSAP) from 1991 to 1996. As part of an evaluation scheme to examine ecological changes in each intervention community, information was gathered and summarized in case studies. Interviews with staff, community members, and agency representatives were conducted. Participatory observation occurred at all committee and subcommittee meetings, and school district and police statistics were collected for each community. Additionally, two surveys assessing individual change variables were conducted. The qualitative and observational evaluation data findings from these case studies are presented to explore the three dimensions outlined below.

Findings

The three communities addressed in the study were Alianza, Brighton, and Centro. Dimensions for each community were scope; indigenous, skilled leadership; and formality of relationships: (1) Scope is the level at which community problems will be addressed; (2) indigenous, skilled leadership is the willingness and ability of the community to identify indigenous, skilled leadership; and (3) formality of relationships is looked upon within the group. The three cases studies were analyzed according to all three dimensions.

Of the three communities, two were able to enhance options for youth to stay healthy. These coalitions were clear about their scope of activities and the formality of their relationships. The Alianza community quickly nominated a community outreach worker to serve as a paid leader. It ultimately realized substantial community change. Brighton experienced difficulty in identifying a skilled leader for the outreach position, and as a result they organized themselves at a slower pace with fewer positive results realized. Centro encountered difficulties in all three dimensions and was unprepared to collaborate in a meaningful way. Hostile interactions with the nonindigenous community outreach worker and with each other created an unfavorable environment for all three dimensions.

Some of the other benefits that emerged, particularly from the Alianza community, included numerous youth and school-based programs, more involvement of Hispanic parents in the schools, and an emphasis on diverse role models among school personnel. Students were also cited as having reconnected to their roots of origin with pride rather than shame as "a wet-backs." Art, in the form of a student-produced mural, raised cultural awareness among the student group.

Implications

Practitioners must take time to identify a clear scope of activities and be selective about working with communities able to identify local leadership. Some communities may not be ready to clarify their scope or identify leadership; therefore, practitioners should not force their engagement but implement strategies to facilitate their awareness and motivation for action while working with communities that are ready for implementation.

Source: Reininger, B., Dinh-Zarr, T., Sinicrope, P. S., & Martin, D. W. (1999). Dimensions of participation and leadership: Implications for community-based health promotion for youth. Family and Community Health, 22(2), 72–82.

---

opinion on an issue or to identify a number of possible solutions to an issue. Unlike a focus group, a community forum can be conducted with a large number of people. In fact, community forums are advertised widely to encourage maximum community participation. Because some people are more likely to be able to attend or to publicly express their view, however, a community fo-

rum is unlikely to be representative of a community. The purpose of the community forum should be made clear beforehand and again at the outset of the forum so that participants do not expect that issues discussed will necessarily be acted on by health professionals in the manners identified at the forum. This is particularly important because certain people or groups may attempt to dominate

RESEARCH FOCUS

The Effects of Community Policies to Reduce Youth Access to Tobacco

Study Problem/Purpose

This study tested the hypothesis that adoption and implementation of local policies regarding youth access to tobacco can affect adolescent smoking.

Methods

A randomized community trial was conducted in 14 Minnesota communities. Seven intervention communities participated in a 32-month community-organizing effort to mobilize citizens and activate the community. The goals were to change ordinances and merchant policies and practices and enforce practices to reduce youth access to tobacco. Outcome measures were derived from surveys of students before and after the intervention and from tobacco purchase attempt in all retail outlets in the communities. Data analyses used mixed-model regression to account for the clustering within communities and to adjust for covariates.

Findings

Each intervention community passed a comprehensive youth access ordinance. Intervention communities showed less pronounced increases in adolescent daily smoking relative to control communities. Tobacco purchase success declined somewhat more in intervention than control communities during the study period, but this difference was not statistically significant.

Implications

This study provides compelling evidence that policies designed to reduce youth access to tobacco can have a significant effect on adolescent smoking rates.

Source: Forster, J. L., Murray, D. M., Wolfson, M., Blaine, T. M., Wagenaar, A. C., & Hennrikus, D. J. (1998). The effects of community policies to reduce youth access to tobacco. American Journal of Public Health, 88, 1193–1198.

discussion, potentially leaving less articulate people concerned that their views will not be considered. If well advertised beforehand and used for the purposes of information sharing and information gathering, a community forum can be a valuable tool in the community assessment process (Cooney, 1994).

A community forum should be facilitated by one or several people, depending on the size of the group. In addition, someone should take specific responsibility for recording the proceedings of the forum. As taping of large groups is not always successful, taking notes during the forum is recommended.

Nominal Group Process

The nominal group process is a technique that can be used in small-group settings to identify issues or rank priorities. It was designed to overcome the problem of some group members' dominating the discussion and, thus, preventing quieter members from voicing their perspectives. There are a number of steps in the nominal group process.

First, the question at hand is presented to the group members. This question might be related to problems that they see in the local community or to solutions to particular problems already identified. Group members are asked to work individually on this question for approximately 10–15 minutes.

Next, using a round-robin technique so that all group members participate equally, group members are each asked to contribute an answer. This process is continued until all responses are listed on a board; no critiquing or discussion is allowed. Each response is then allocated a number. The meaning of each response is then clarified with the group, allowing participants to explain their rationale when necessary.

Participants are next asked to "vote" on the priority of the identified problems or issues. Each participant is asked to rank, say, the top five issues or responses. Participants allocate from five points (for the issue to which they assign the highest priority) down to one point (for the issue to which they assign the lowest priority). Finally, points allocated by all participants are collected and collated. The problem or issue with the largest number of points is accorded top priority, and so forth, down to those issues with no points being accorded the lowest priority (Green & Kreuter, 1991; Van de Ven & Delbecq, 1972).

In this way, the nominal group process allows everyone to vote anonymously and equally. Findings are therefore much more likely to be representative of the group than are the findings of a focus group or community forum, where particular individuals may dominate. For these reasons, the nominal group process can be useful in setting priorities.

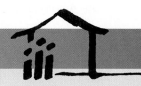

COMMUNITY NURSING VIEW

A community health nurse working in a low-income urban area has been asked to participate on a steering committee working to develop an after-school program for approximately 200 students whose parents are unable to pick them up until 5:30 P.M. The school day ends at 2:50 P.M. The goal of the program is to keep "latch key" children off the streets and out of trouble.

Several months earlier, an accidental shooting occurred in the home of one of the children who attended this school. The incident occurred when two 12-year-old boys were home alone playing with a rifle. One of the boys accidentally shot and severely injured the other. Since this incident, latch key children have been the focus of articles in the local newspaper.

The idea for the program came from the mayor of the city. If successful, the program will be a model for other schools in the region. The steering committee has been meeting for several months, holding three meetings to date. The only nurses on the committee will be the community health nurse and a school nurse.

Nursing Considerations

Assessment

◆ Who else might be on the steering committee? Why?

◆ Who might be on the project team? Why?

◆ What questions should be asked about the type of data to be collected?

◆ What type of data should be collected?

◆ Which needs assessment tools might be used to collect the data?

◆ What questions must be answered to ensure appropriate planning?

Diagnosis

◆ What nursing diagnosis might be formulated specific to the accident?

Outcome Identification

◆ The goal of the program is to keep the children off the streets. What other positive outcomes could be realized if this program is successful?

◆ What is the benefit to the community?

◆ What is the benefit to the children and the families?

Planning/Interventions

◆ Who should be involved in the planning with regard to the where, when, who, and how of program development?

◆ What factors should be considered when planning this program?

◆ How would costs play a part in the planning?

◆ Given that this is a low-income urban community, who might cover the costs of this program?

◆ Where could the steering committee look for funds?

Evaluation

◆ If the program is shown to have low enrollment, what might be the sources of the problem? How might these sources be identified?

◆ What might be suggested as the next course of action if the program were to be deemed unsuccessful?

◆ What might be suggested if the program were to be deemed successful?

◆ What process could this steering committee use to select its evaluation methods?

◆ What indicators could the steering committee use to evaluate program effectiveness?

◆ What process might the steering committee use to evaluate its own effectiveness in program planning and development?

KEY CONCEPTS

◆ Three dimensions that are important to consider when defining community health are status, structure, and process.

◆ The population focus of community health nursing requires an understanding of the purpose and process of comprehensive community assessment.

◆ Holographic Theory may be used to define community as a whole, with numerous processes, in which the parts are encoded in the whole and the whole within each part.

◆ Community assessment is part of a complex process of identifying and responding to problems, needs, and issues affecting populations.

◆ The different types of needs that must be considered when conducting a needs assessment include felt need, expressed need, normative need, and comparative need.

◆ Comprehensive community assessment considers the needs of a community, its assets, and the resources available to perform the assessment.

◆ Community members and health professionals bring different, but complementary, perspectives to the identification of community health needs and assets. Thus, community members must be involved in the identification of health needs and assets as well as the planning of programs to address those needs.

◆ The purpose of the assessment must be clearly defined and the available resources for conducting the assessment identified to ensure that adequate resources are allocated to complete the assessment.

◆ A research plan and time frame must be developed and agreed on by the project team and the steering committee members.

◆ A community assessment should include the collection and analysis of data currently available in addition to the collection and analysis of new data.

◆ A variety of information sources and methods of obtaining data are available to and valuable in community assessment, including demographic and epidemiological data, national and local policy documents, previously conducted surveys, literature reviews, participant observation, windshield surveys, key informants, surveys of community members, focus groups, community forums, and the nominal group process.

◆ The results of the community assessment must be communicated to the community either orally, in written form, or in both ways.

◆ The plan to address the identified needs must be developed with input from community members.

◆ Community assessment is the beginning of a process to respond to community health problems and needs; it is not an end in itself.

RESOURCES

Community development: Promoting health through empowerment and participation: http://www.hc-sc.gc.ca/hppb

Community health assessments: http://www.hcwp.org

Practical holography: http://www.holo.com/holo/book/book1.html

Public health assessment: http://www.atsdr.cdc.gov/HAC/PHA/sharon/sha_toc.html

Tobacco use control: An example of community health improvement in action: http://www.allina.com/Allina_Journal/Winter1997/roski.html

Using performance monitoring to improve community health: Conceptual framework and community experience: http://www.nap.edu/html/concept/#inter

Welcome to Darebin Community Health: http://www.darebinch.com.au

PROGRAM PLANNING, IMPLEMENTATION, AND EVALUATION

Claire Budgen, RN, BSN, MSN, PhD
Gail Cameron, RN, BSN, MN

Go to the people
Live among them
Start with what they know
Build on what they have
But of the best leaders
When their task is accomplished
Their work is done
The people all remark
We have done it ourselves

—Author unknown

COMPETENCIES

Upon completion of this chapter, the reader should be able to:

- Explain the programming processes of planning, implementation, and evaluation.

- Discuss ways that the Health for All movement, with its strategies of primary health care and health promotion, is changing community nurses' work with programs and people.

- Describe the ways that societal trends, health care reform, and definitions of health affect programs.

- Examine program issues through the different lenses of caring, phenomenological, feminist, and critical social theories.

- Identify the ways that multilevel change theories may be used to guide programming.

- Differentiate among types of community organizing: community development, social planning, and social action.

- Critique programming models for their usefulness in various community situations.

KEY TERMS

community organization

cost analysis of health programs

formative evaluation

outcome evaluation

process evaluation

program

program evaluation

program implementation

program planning

programming

programming models

structural evaluation

summative evaluation

Community health nurses use programs to improve the health of communities. The intent of this chapter is to provide nurses with background enough to undertake the work of planning, implementing, and evaluating community health programs. Nurses are being challenged to work with programs in new ways, in response to the global Health for All movement, with its accompanying strategies of primary health care, health promotion, and population health (World Health Organization [WHO], 1978, 1986, 1997). Use of primary health care and health promotion principles, in combination with principles of programming, means that from the viewpoint of the community, priority health issues are

dealt with effectively, resources are well used, and the community is strengthened.

Community nurses have derived basic programming principles from nursing, health, business, education, and social science theories as well as from their nursing practice. The term "program" has various meanings. **Program** is most simply defined as a collection of activities intended to produce particular results (Dignan & Carr, 1992, p. 5). In community health programs, activities focus directly on health issues or on health determinants, and the desired result, ultimately, is improved health of the community.

When people talk about a "program," they sometimes speak only about the activities that appear most directly connected to health improvements and not about the less visible but foundational interactive work. For example, a prenatal education program might be thought of as a package of educational material on topics deemed relevant for prenatal health. In actuality, the program may include activities such as connecting with parents-to-be using multiple outreach strategies, meeting with participants in settings close to where they live, ensuring that participants have the opportunity to discuss their health interests, and adjusting educational topics in the program to focus on what participants see as most important. Thus the prenatal program may be somewhat different each time it takes place, although the same basic educational package is used and the same goal is met, that is, to have people better prepared for birth and a new baby.

To assist the reader to gain a comprehensive understanding of what is included in a successful community health program, the term **programming** is used to encompass the whole sequence of processes to be undertaken which together produce the program and the desired results. Thus, programming is process oriented. The extent to which these processes can be detailed ahead of time varies with the nature of the program, as is evident in the example of the prenatal program.

Community health nurses most often have conceptualized programming processes similarly to the nursing process, that is, framed as assessment, planning, implementation, and evaluation. These terms are used commonly in programming work across disciplines. However, a word of caution is needed. When programs are based on primary health care and health promotion principles, nurses work to enable communities to increase their control over and to improve their health; thus communities need to be full participants in programming processes. Full participation creates empowerment; what full participation should comprise must be decided within the context of the program. Many health care practitioners (and associated bureaucracies) are only minimally familiar with a participatory, partnership model of care and have limited knowledge about how to share control (Eisler, 2000). Also, the "health care system as expert" model has predominated to such an extent that many community members are not experienced at taking control and making decisions in partnership with health care practitioners. However, there is evidence that both community members and health care practitioners can learn and benefit from using a partnership model (Clarke & Mass, 1998).

In the past, program planning, implementation, and evaluation activities frequently were based on the premise that communities were the recipients of programs rather than partners in programming. There is value now in considering other ways of thinking about programming to ensure that conceptual space is created for processes that are truly enabling for the community (i.e., create opportunity for community control). For example, Sheilds and Lindsey (1998) recommend that community nurses interested in health promotion move away from nursing process language and use a framework based on the work of Freire (1970, 1993) that comprises listening and critical reflection, participatory dialogue, pattern and theme recognition, envisioning action, action, and reflection on action.

Similar ideas and language are appearing in the literature of other disciplines as community health practitioners and researchers develop new knowledge about how best to influence and support change through programs (McKenzie & Smeltzer, 2001). Regardless of the programming framework a nurse prefers, knowledge of a variety of frameworks is helpful because community nurses work with people from diverse programming backgrounds and may need to bridge differences. What is most significant to the success of programs is the quality of the working relationships among people and the health focus of their actions.

In this chapter, current thinking about community health programming is brought forward, in particular lessons from the Health for All movement of the past two decades. The framework of program planning, implementation, and evaluation will be used, informed by principles of health promotion and primary health care. **Program planning** is defined as the process of exploring the community situation, deciding on a more desirable situation, and designing actions to create the desirable situation. **Program implementation** is carrying out the designed actions. **Program evaluation** is defined as both an ongoing process of reflecting on plans, actions, and results, so that programs can be improved along the way, and, at the conclusion of the program, assessing the results or outcomes, the community situation "now," and what might be done next. Then planning begins again; programming thus is cyclical. In concise terms, programming involves analyzing the situation, setting goals, taking action, and evaluating the results. Throughout these processes, community nurses and community members are advised to work in partnership.

Successful programming does not take place in isolation from the situation or setting within which it occurs. In this chapter, health programming is considered in the context of health care reform and societal trends. Also, primary health care, health promotion, and common definitions of health are examined in relation to the practicalities of programming. Some of the theories, models, and "how to's" of program planning, implementation, and evaluation are explored. Because change is inherent in programming, the use of change theories is also discussed. The intent of this chapter is to provide nurses with background enough to reasonably undertake the work of community health programming.

HEALTH PROGRAMMING IN CONTEXT

Thoughtful consideration of the context within which a health program will be developed and implemented contributes directly to program success. Local contexts are nested with regional, national, and international contexts. Although contexts vary considerably, important factors and trends relevant to health usually can be identified if the nurse is open minded, observant, and questioning and works in partnership with the community.

Health Care Reform and Societal Trends

Health care reform issues and societal trends are macro-level contextual factors that must be considered in programming. Societal trends include increasing global interconnection, environmental degradation, and shifting demographics, increasing technology, and changing health issues; one response has been the restructuring of health care organizations. Organizations generally are under strong pressure to change in order to survive in rapidly changing local and global environments.

Health care systems, under pressure "to do more with less" or "to do better with the same" are using industrial and corporate models to guide reform. Of greatest concern in health care are appropriateness of care, quality, accessibility, equity, and costs. Business theories can provide useful ideas for the administration of health care. Nurses must be aware, however, that business theories generally are based on principles of market justice that may conflict with the social justice orientation of nursing and the Health for All movement. A business orientation may cause programmers to be "insufficiently appreciative of the human dimension" (Hammer, as cited in Pratt, 1997, p. 81).

The values underlying reform approaches and program decisions must be openly examined so that profit or short-term cost savings do not take precedence over people and long-term costs. For example, in the health maintenance organization initiative in the United States, *prevention for profit* has many times taken precedence over *prevention to improve the health of the population;* the original goal of increasing access to prevention services has been overshadowed by excessive profit taking.

People and governments have difficulty thinking in the long term and for the whole population. For example, after years of beneficial experience with a not-for-profit national health care service (with some private for-profit components), Canadians are experiencing pressures to move to a more privatized and "for-profit" system of care. The claim is that this move would increase efficiency and contain costs. Long-term evidence from the United States and other countries does not support the claim (Armstrong, Bourgeault, Choiniere, MyKhalovskiy, & White, 2000; Canadian Public Health Association, 2000; Evans, Barer, & Marmor, 1994). When health care for a country is examined in totality, long-term economic and health benefits for the whole population result when appropriate health care is accessible for all at a reasonable cost to the community and country (Fuller, 1998; Federal, Provincial and Territorial Advisory Committee on Population Health, 1999; Labonte, 1998; WHO, 1998).

To achieve the Health for All goal, programmers must consider health program appropriateness, accessibility, and quality of outcomes for communities in relation to human and material costs for both the short and the long term. Nurses working in community programming are well positioned to participate in reform; to anticipate and observe the impact of various strategies; to ask and to assist communities to ask critical questions; and, through the inclusion of political-action strategies in programs, to influence the direction of system changes and resource use. In the past, nurses might not have considered this sociopolitical type of work as part of programming; but nurses are accountable to the public, and if health care system issues are a priority for the community, their inclusion in programming is appropriate (see Chapters 4, 5, and 18).

Health problems also are changing. Epidemiological data in the United States and Canada reveal high mortality and morbidity related to social, economic, political, and physical environmental conditions (e.g., substance misuse, accidents, violence, abuse, suicide, homelessness, occupational and environmental hazards, and inadequate nutrition and activity) and also to chronic disease (e.g., cardiovascular disease, cancer, HIV/AIDS, diabetes) [Federal, Provincial and Territorial Advisory Committee on Population Health, 1999; U.S. Department of Health and Human Services (USDHSS), 2000]. To a large extent, these conditions and diseases are preventable. New communicable diseases "only a plane ride away" are being reported along with drug-resistant strains of old diseases such as malaria and tuberculosis. Needed are effective prevention programs at the socie-

tal, community, and individual levels (see Figure 16-1). Research on prevention programs has increased significantly. Studies rich in information about different programs can be found via health care database searches. Appropriate allocation of health care resources to prevention programs, in comparison with treatment services, has not yet occurred in most countries. Nurses involved in programming may need to search for resources to support preventive programs. National coalitions and associations are sources of support for prevention program information, funding, and other resources (see Appendix A).

Dramatically changing technologies have created an unprecedented flow of information and a multitude of new health programs. Technologies have "done wonders" but have also engendered ethical, legal, social, and economic dilemmas, as well as iatragenic health effects (Armstrong et al., 2000). Nurses should anticipate encountering these dilemmas and effects in their work in programming and also should explore technology-based opportunities. Careful programming in partnership with communities helps ensure that the technologies used are acceptable, appropriate, and affordable.

Demographic data in the United States and Canada indicate an increasing proportion of elderly people, increasing cultural and racial diversity, a steepening socioeconomic gradient (increasing poverty and wealth and a widening gap between), increasing numbers of children living in poverty, and changes in the profile of families and communities (Federal, Provincial and Territorial Advisory Committee on Population Health, 1999; USDHSS, 2000; Provincial Health Officer, 2000) (see also

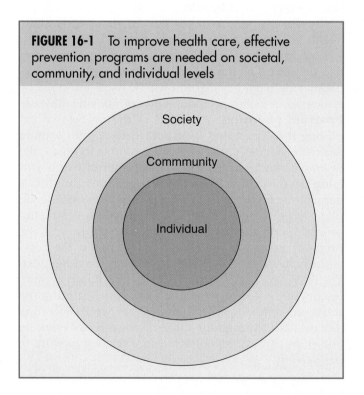

FIGURE 16-1 To improve health care, effective prevention programs are needed on societal, community, and individual levels

Chapter 3). Increasing global population, political problems, and wars put pressure on countries to accept immigrants and to share resources. Equitable creation, conservation, and distribution of resources are challenges for all levels of government and for nurses involved in programming. Distribution of wealth in countries is strongly correlated with health. Where there are wide gaps between rich and poor, health is negatively affected, with particularly devastating effects on the life-long health and development of children and, thus, of nations (Keating & Hertzman, 1999).

Racial, socioeconomic, and other prejudices are impediments to equity that nurses must be prepared to counteract or circumvent in programming. Smith (1997) encourages community health nurses to mobilize resources through the development of both local and global partnerships rather than focusing on scarcity of resources. Resources can be created, used, counted, and distributed in many different ways. A broad definition of resources includes ecological, social, economic, and human "capital" (Hancock, 1999).

Societal trends are significant to health programming because they are linked with the health of communities and with the types of programs that would be most helpful. Certain groups are at greater risk, and the health-related circumstances of these groups need careful consideration for the benefit of the whole community. Also, programs must be designed differently for different subpopulations or aggregates within communities. Nurses who consider the ways that health care system changes and societal trends are affecting communities and subpopulations can use this knowledge to avoid pitfalls, realize opportunities, and improve programming success. Opportunities for nurses to make positive contributions through programming have never been greater. See Figure 16-2.

Definitions of Health for Programs

In programming, nurses will encounter three common approaches to health: medical, behavioral, and socioenvironmental. A fourth approach, ecological, is receiving renewed attention. Health and health-related issues are defined differently within each approach, and each is associated with different types of programming. The concept of programming "upstream," that is, at the origin of problems, is of special interest. Nurses must consider the definition(s) of health being used in a program to ensure maximal usefulness for the community.

Medical, Behavioral, and Socioenvironmental Approaches to Health Programs

The medical approach focuses on disease and disability (Labonte, 1993, pp. 27–32). Health programs using this approach tend to be practitioner managed and focus on detection, treatment, and reduction of risk factors. In preventive practice (public health in the United States and Canada), although the program is delivered to the individual, the intent is improvement in the population's health (e.g., hearing and vision screening of young children and immunization programs). A high percentage of the population must therefore be reached. The irradication of smallpox through massive immunization programs is an example of the successful application of the medical approach in the global population.

In the behavioral approach, health is defined as physical functional ability and healthy lifestyle behavior.

FIGURE 16-2 Stories of Justice as Told by Fish

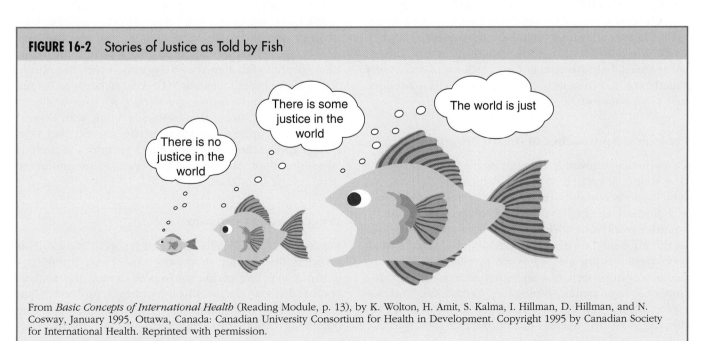

From *Basic Concepts of International Health* (Reading Module, p. 13), by K. Wolton, H. Amit, S. Kalma, I. Hillman, D. Hillman, and N. Cosway, January 1995, Ottawa, Canada: Canadian University Consortium for Health in Development. Copyright 1995 by Canadian Society for International Health. Reprinted with permission.

Behavioral programs thus focus on the reduction of risky behavior and the promotion of healthy lifestyles. Such programs may be supported by public policy such as "no smoking" and seat belt legislation. Again, the underlying intent is to improve the health of the population. With the behavioral approach, practitioners and communities may negotiate strategies to improve individual health behavior and lifestyle.

The socioenvironmental approach encompasses social wellness, being connected to others, having a meaningful life, and being in control. Socioenvironmental programs are intended to improve social and environmental conditions that support health and to reduce both psychosocial risk factors (e.g., isolation, low self-esteem, and low perceived power) and socioenvironmental risk conditions (e.g., poverty, dangerous environments, consumerism, and inadequate education). With this approach, communities are likely to determine the issues, goals, and strategies; practitioners then assist communities to plan and implement programs. Examples are family caregivers, support networks, and media watch programs to detect and change media messages that are hazardous to health. The health interest in social and environmental conditions includes an interest in collective community lifestyles (Frohlich & Potvin, 1999).

Each of the three approaches has appropriate and inappropriate applications; a collaborative rather than competitive view is helpful overall. Community health nurses may want to use a single approach or a combination of approaches within a given program, depending on the situation. Familiarity with each approach and a critical view regarding the most appropriate approaches for given situations are strengths nurses can develop and bring to community health programming. Health care practitioners tend to use the single approach with which they are most familiar; community health nurses who understand all three approaches can work effectively with a wide variety of others and, in some cases, help diverse groups work more effectively together (e.g., physicians, psychologists, social workers, and city planners).

Ecological Approaches to Health Programs

Of particular relevance to community health programs is a fourth approach to health which is not new but which has become more visible as concerns about environmental issues have moved to the top of health agendas worldwide (WHO, 1998). Ecological models of health are based on ecosystem theory; the world and all its dimensions are viewed as interconnected. Thus, an ecological approach encompasses aspects of all three previous approaches: biological, behavioral, and socioenvironmental. Ecological theory contributes a cautionary note to nurses that programs need to be considered for their potential effects on systems and people other than those immediately involved and later in time. For example, an immunization or infant rehydration program may save the lives of children, but unless the children have enough to eat, death and disability are simply delayed.

Ecological models used in combination with Health for All strategies direct all sectors of society to put health on their agendas and to recognize their accountability for the health consequences of all their decisions (WHO, 1986). This has been termed "health imperialism," but no one denies that this supports Health for All interests. Although nurses might give priority to the health of humans and others might see the health of the natural environment or of the economy as the priority, ecological models suggest that a long-term view needs to be taken that includes their interconnectedness for the well-being of both the planet and people. To this end, Minkler (1999) suggests a balanced rather than dichotomized view of individual and social responsibility and reminds us that, literally, "we are all in this (with this planet) together" (p. 135).

Hancock (1993) and Hancock, Labonte, and Edwards (1999) have put forward several ecological models. For community-level programs, two models are of interest. The human development model emphasizes connections between health and environmental and economic well-being, with a particular focus on viability, equity, and sustainability. The health and community ecosystem model adds community interests such as liveability, adequate prosperity, and conviviality (see Figure 16-3). This latter model emerged from Healthy Cities/Communities program work within the Health for All movement. Methods for evaluating programs guided by ecological models are being developed and tested (see Table 16-4 later in this chapter). Ecological models invite the practitioner to look holistically at the situation, enabling more effective programming. However, all approaches have limitations. Ecological models have been associated with the phrase "complexity breeds despair" (Green, Richard, & Potvin, 1996). Fortunately, nurses are known for their ability to deal with complexity; they routinely work with diverse people in complex community environments. Also, ecological approaches can guide small programs as well as large; therefore, the nurse who is new to programming need not be intimidated.

Programming Upstream

Regardless of the health approach favored, consensus is growing that health programs must focus more "upstream," meaning taking into consideration the societal context that manufactures health or health problems (Butterfield, 1990; Steingraber, 1997) (see Chapter 11). The community health nurse might, for example, examine de-

FIGURE 16-3 Two Ecological Models for Community Health

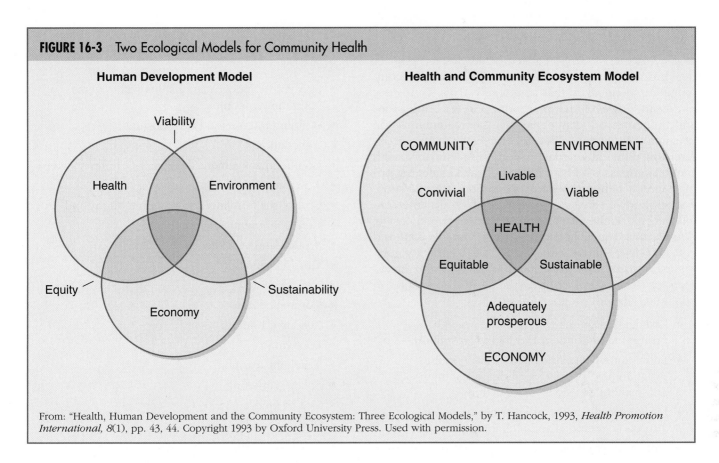

From: "Health, Human Development and the Community Ecosystem: Three Ecological Models," by T. Hancock, 1993, *Health Promotion International, 8*(1), pp. 43, 44. Copyright 1993 by Oxford University Press. Used with permission.

mographic and epidemiological data about smoking and raise questions regarding the reasons that smoking predominated among the more established and affluent male members of society until its health hazards were recognized. Other questions that might be raised include why it now predominates among those with fewer social and economic resources, including young people, particularly young females (Provincial Health Officer, 2000; Provincial Health Officer, 1996). In a community where increasing numbers of young people are starting to smoke, an upstream approach would guide the nurse to consider the context within which individual smoking behavior is created and maintained. A smoking prevention program in the local community might include assisting young people and other groups:

Furthest upstream:
- To analyze information relevant to youth from regional, national, and international smoking reduction groups
- To gain skills at coalition building and lobbying to further curtail tobacco production, marketing, and use
- In countries where tobacco companies are paying governments for tobacco-related health costs, to lobby governments to ensure that a substantial

portion of "tobacco payback" funds are used for the protection and strengthening of youth

Upstream:
- To critique local market and social forces related to youth smoking
- To lobby local merchants to reduce marketing of tobacco to young people
- To develop environments for young people that support nonsmoking (consider social and physical environment)

Still upstream (prevention for young people at the individual lifestyle level):
- To develop a peer health education network around nonsmoking
- To develop personal skills around not starting to smoke

Downstream:
- To quit smoking

Furthest downstream:
- For tobacco-related health problems, to develop a self-care support group for those with lung problems

PRIMARY HEALTH CARE PRINCIPLES FOR PROGRAMS

As a component of an integrated health system, primary health care focuses on the main health issues of a community as defined by that community. This focus does not mean, however, that practitioners never bring issues and programs to a community (e.g., new immunization programs). Primary health care, done well, may look different in different regions or countries. Primary health care encompasses a broad range of health strategies; primary are health promotion, prevention, rehabilitation, and supportive services. Curative services are an essential but not dominant component. This comprehensive, non-discipline-specific model should not be confused with selective primary care models such as primary nursing and primary care medicine (McMurray, 1999). Enactment of Health for All/primary health care principles in community health programs means:

- Essential programs with increased health promotion and illness and injury prevention
- Full community participation throughout the programming process, including defining issues and making decisions about actions
- Use of socially acceptable, appropriate, and affordable methods and technology
- Universal, equitable access to programs close to where people live, work, play, and study
- Collaboration among all sectors (community, health, environment, social, political, economic, business, education, religion, private and public organizations, government) (WHO, 1986; Stewart, 2000)

On the basis of primary health care principles, nurses involved in community programming must be prepared to work with a wide cross section of people in ways that support meaningful participation. For both nurses and community members, knowledge and skills are useful in the areas of:

- Forming working relationships with diverse community people
- Building intersectoral relationships
- Negotiation
- Conflict management/dealing with different views
- Advocacy
- Consensus building/finding common ground
- Coalition and alliance building
- Written and verbal communication
- Group facilitation
- Networking
- Committee work
- Resource finding
- Lobbying
- Teaching/learning
- Social marketing
- Use of media
- Proposal and report writing
- Political action
- Budgeting

Although the list may seem intimidating, community nurses and community members already will have developed many of these capacities in other settings and will be able to assist one another (Buresh & Gordon, 2000). The reader also is referred to the extensive multidisciplinary literature available on these topics (nursing, social work, political science, community psychology, business, and education).

In primary health care, participation does not mean placing unreasonable expectations on community people. Participation does mean that community people are

---

✳ DECISION MAKING

Which Health Approach to Use?

In the region where you work, several cases of active tuberculosis and two deaths from untreated tuberculosis have been identified. Neighborhoods in the region are diverse (e.g., some very poor, others affluent). You have been asked to help plan new programs to deal with the problem.

- ◆ What do the various health approaches offer in this situation?
- ◆ Which approach(es) would you recommend using? Why?

✳ DECISION MAKING

Is Primary Health Care Achievable?

In the region where you work, families with members experiencing cancer must travel for treatment to a city 250 miles away. Costs to families are high in terms of both dollars and disruption to work, school, and support networks.

- ◆ Using primary health care principles, what possibilities do you see for improving this situation?

fully informed, make decisions, use their own expertise, and have the opportunity to develop new capacities, including knowledge and skills. Practitioners have expertise and power that they use on behalf of the community (e.g., interpreting epidemiological data, providing current health information, teaching group facilitation skills, and connecting with resources). According to primary health care, the views of community people must always have priority consideration in programs (Shediac-Rizkallah & Bone, 1998). Further, the views of those external to the community must be considered in relation to the views of those in the community. Programming is a mutual process. This is not to idealize the notion of community or participation. However, programming will not be helpful if nurses do not ground their work in the community.

Health Promotion Principles for Programs

Health promotion, health protection, and disease prevention, although closely related and sometimes overlapping in the realm of application in programs, can be differentiated theoretically (see Chapter 10). Prevention programs are geared toward eliminating the negative, that is, preventing the occurrence of disease and disability. *Health protection* implies changing physical and social environments to improve health; changes in legislation and regulation are components.

Health promotion is framed positively; that is, enhancing health and well-being. Conceptualized by WHO (1986) as a process that enables people to take control of and improve their health, health promotion has been defined by some practitioners as a way of "being" rather than of "doing." The focus is on the way a practitioner relates with others rather than the type of program. Hartrick (2001) describes health promotion as a relational process of mutual engagement that strengthens capacities that are already there. Labonte (1999) gives an example where "health promoters use their 'professional' powers (status, access to material resources) transformatively, making them available to community members to increase their own power" (p. 368). In the example, health promoters assisted community members to make and eventually maintain on their own a relationship with a housing authority official. The result was permission (previously denied) for a community garden that the community members were able to sustain, partially through the ongoing mutual relationship with the housing authority and partially through their increased ability to mobilize resources. The notion of skill building is enriched when thought of in terms of power. When guided by the WHO definition, health promotion programs and health-promoting practices have a distinctly political and socially critical dimension. The politics of enabling others to increase control implies that the "others" will experience an increase in power to act on their own behalf.

Health promotion programs have tended to focus on individual lifestyle change; there is a shift to programming that includes change in collective community lifestyles and environmental conditions. In the 21st century, Labonte (1999), who has worked in health promotion around the world, predicts:

> Health promotion will be challenged to act on two concerns that underpinned public health activism a century ago: social justice (reducing inequalities in wealth and power) and healthy environments (increasing sustainable social and economic practices). (p. 365)

The Jakarta Declaration on Health Promotion into the 21st century (WHO, 1997; see also Chapter 11) reinforces the need for social responsibility and strong environmental action, investment for health development, infrastructure for health promotion, partnerships, and programs that increase community capacity and empower the individual.

Population health, an approach receiving renewed attention in the Health for All movement, is intended to assist countries to deal more effectively with the social, economic, political, and physical environmental conditions that are determinants of health. Some governments are shifting their interests from health promotion to population health. Although population health is criticized by some as being too epidemiological in focus and not sufficiently activist, if the data truly are used to shape government policy, health improvements will occur. However, because the status quo is challenged when power is directed toward changing inequities that negatively affect health, governments often find appropriate policy change difficult. In community programs, nurses will find both health promotion and population health strategies useful (see Hamilton and Bhatti's combined population health promotion model; Figure 16-10 on p. 390).

Theorists and activists in health promotion caution about professional practitioners' inclination to take over processes intended to strengthen others; governments and organizations tend to do the same (Baum & Sanders, 1995). It is tempting to take over control when one believes one knows that which is best in a given situation. The result is another form of "power over," implying social control and maintenance of inequities, rather than the intended "power with," implying social change and transformation to a more equitable state. Social control has contributed significantly to community health, for example, through health-focused regulatory actions of governments to prevent environmental degradation and protect workers' health. Eng, Salmon, and Mullan (1992) have identified different models of intervention for social change and social control (see Table 16-1). Social change must be more emphasized if the Health for All goal is to be reached.

TABLE 16-1 Comparison of Social Change and Social Control Models of Intervention

SOCIAL CHANGE	SOCIAL CONTROL
• Social analysis	• Epidemiological/demographic analysis
• Focus on strengths	• Focus on weaknesses
• Goal is health outcome and increased community competence	• Goal is health outcome
• Organized around human categories	• Organized around disease
• Asks "What are people's motives?"	• Asks "How can we motivate people?"

From "Community Empowerment: The Critical Base for Primary Care," by E. Eng, M. E. Salmon, and F. Mullan, 1992, Family Community Health, 15*(1), p. 5. Copyright 1992 by Aspen Publishers, Inc. Reprinted with permission.*

EMPOWERMENT AND PARTNERSHIP

Central to health promotion are the concepts of empowerment and partnership. The concept of empowerment has multiple meanings. As both a process and an outcome, it was considered to be an abstract concept difficult to create through programs. However, there now is evidence that empowerment can be supported relatively easily and that the gains in health outcomes for individuals and communities are significant (Butler & Marquis, 1998; Clarke & Mass, 1998; Skelton, 1994; Perlmutter & Cnaan, 2001; Wallerstein, 1992).

Empowerment can be simply defined as gaining power. Most appealing is the notion that power can be created through transformative interactions among people: the power of possibility, the power of affirmation, the power of new ideas, and the power of self-created knowledge (Freire, 1970, 1993; Chinn, 2001). Rissel (1994) argues that this win-win form of empowerment occurs only in the psychological realm and that when material resources are involved, empowerment means win-lose, hence the struggle to maintain the status quo by those who benefit materially from it. Others see this win-lose conceptualization as learned, unhealthy for communities, and subject to change (McKnight & Kretzmann, 1992). McKnight and others have been involved in many programs where communities have successfully reconceptualized power relations and capacities and created important improvements in health for communities (McKnight, 2001).

In health care, the implications are that empowered individuals and communities will make positive use of the power they gain; that is, they will be able to think critically, act in their own best interests, create more equitable access to resources, develop their own resourcefulness, work well with others, and respect their own and others' diversity. Obviously, certain values, knowledge, and skills are components. A further implication is that empowerment is associated with improved health and a reduced need for health care services (Frank, 1995). Community empowerment is associated with the concept of community competence, the ability of the community to function effectively as a unit of problem solving (Ross, 1955, as cited in Minkler, 1990, p. 268). These idealized views of empowerment have been tested and critiqued as practitioners have attempted to shape health programming in ways that support others' empowerment. Sustainability of empowerment has proven to be more of a challenge than initial community empowerment, not surprising when communities are embedded within oppressive social and environmental conditions (Shediac-Rizkallah & Bone, 1998). Labonte (1993) derived from his varied community practice an empowerment pathway from personal care (individual development), to small-group development (mutual support), to community organizing (around issues), to coalition building/advocacy, to collective social and political action. Some practitioners contend that nurses should focus only on personal care and small-group development; however, nurses have learned that "the personal is political" (Chinn, 2001) and that good personal care may require movement to other actions along the pathway.

Concern has been expressed that empowerment and health promotion theory may be used by some as insincere rhetoric to disguise a shifting of the burden, as opposed to the profit, of health care to someone else (e.g., from government to citizens or from health care practitioners to families). Bringing the idea of empowerment into health programming suggests that nurses must tend to their own empowerment as well as to the empowerment of others. Nurses have been observed at some times to be the recipients of disempowering behavior, at other times, the perpetrators (Roberts, 1983). Although this finding is not surprising in a world where disempowering acts are prevalent, it does not need to continue. Nurses need to think about how they are positioned and how they position themselves in power relations (Bassett-Smith, 2001). Nurses have been challenged to value their knowledge and closeness with people and to become more comfortable and visible in using their considerable strengths to improve health and the inequities and power imbalances that affect health (Buresh & Gordon, 2000). Health care administrators and policymakers, to meet their legal accountabilities to the public, have been challenged to ensure that nurses have authority and voice to fully participate in systems (Fletcher, 2001). These challenges can be met, at least partially, through more critically reflective practice in community health programming (Johns, 1999).

Empowerment, partnership, and participation are linked in the nursing literature with relational ethics and advocacy. Schroeder and Gadow (2000) suggest:

> When community is defined as partner, univocal decisions are not valid, for all views become legitimate influences in decision making. In an advocacy approach, practitioners become free to engage with a community as a particular partner rather than an abstract aggregate and to act on the belief that true expertise resides in the community itself. (p. 86)

Nurses and others alike contribute their voices, knowledge, and skills. Nurses have expertise in health care; community members have expertise in their own lives and communities and their own health. Nurses may have particular difficulty working in partnership with and respecting the expertise of community members whose cultural backgrounds are different from the nurses' own. Nurses may be uncomfortable with visible differences, and also with invisible differences, because, like an iceberg, much that is influential in culture is not visible and accidentally can be bumped into. At the beginning of programming work, nurses can talk with community members about the fact that lack of familiarity with one another's cultural perspectives may create discomfort and misunderstanding at times and that open dialogue is helpful. This means establishing a commitment from everyone to voice openly questions and discomforts and to listen carefully to each other. Bishop's (1994) concept of "becoming an ally" may be helpful in enabling nurses and diverse community members to find common ground, that is, a place upon which they can build their work together. Relational caring and phenomenological theories also are useful in this endeavor. A cultural interpreter may be helpful, that is, someone who understands the cultures and can translate, just as with languages.

Another concept linked with empowerment and participation in the literature is human agency, that is, the human capacity to decide, to act, and to direct one's life (Tang & Anderson, 1999). Human agency is supported when nurses work in equal partnership "with" others rather than "doing things to" or "for" others. In the familiar "doing to/for" style, the nurse as "expert" may simply decide that which must be done and do it, or the nurse may act under the direction of another "expert" such as an organization without being aware of constraining human agency. Nurses also have agency, of course, and may experience diminished agency. Becom-

ing aware of the ways in which programming activities, as well as surrounding societal structures, may decrease agency, is a process that requires considerable critical reflection because much is taken for granted in the ways we work and live. Nurses support agency in programming when they reflect on their work and strive to work in partnership with others as coearner/teachers, co–decision makers, and coactors.

This partnership style is applicable to all nursing relationships: that is, with individuals, communities, colleagues, other practitioners, agencies, and government. Working in partnership does not mean that nurses do not act at times without the full participation of the community, e.g., in crisis or emergency situations when quick action is required, such as during a sudden outbreak of a communicable disease or a disaster. At these times, human agency may be viewed as threatened by external forces, and the nurse acts as an advocate for the community, "doing for" only in essential ways and only for as long as needed.

THEORETICAL LENSES

Theories enable community nurses to use already developed ideas to guide and strengthen their work with programs. Theories provide nurses with different lenses through which to see situations; each lens provides a different view and understanding. Models are visual representations of theories. The adage about not needing to "reinvent the wheel" applies here, as do the ideas of "improving the wheel" (theory) through testing it in practice and "altering the wheel" to suit different situations (i.e., creating new theory from practice). Bateson (1990) speaks about the value of improvisation and reflection as one lives, works, participates, and observes. As theories are the science of programming, improvisation and reflection are the art.

Meta-Theories

> If you have come to help me, you are wasting your time. But if you have come because your liberation is bound with mine, then let us begin. (Lily Walker, an Australian aboriginal woman, as cited in Labonte, 1993, p. 35)

Meta-theories provide broad descriptions and explanations of general happenings in the world. Of particular interest in nursing at this time are caring, phenomenological, feminist, and critical social theories. Phenomenological, feminist, and critical social theories are helping nurses understand and transform the underlying ideas and responses that support the social construction of inequities.

Caring

Caring may be defined as the moral imperative to act ethically and justly. Caring theories are explored elsewhere (see Chapter 1); however, relational caring theory will be briefly discussed here because of its specific relevance to programs informed by health promotion principles. Community nurses are commissioned to provide care (programs) in ways that maintain dignity and respect, knowing that the ways will vary for different people (Canadian Nurses Association, 1997). Being respectful of differences is easy to talk about but very challenging to do. Relational caring theory offers new "how-to-do" ideas. In relational practice, the nurse attends to the relationship with different clients by making an open space in the communication where the nurse and clients can cocreate a relational narrative, that is, a story in which they develop shared meaning about experiences and about the work they will do or are doing together, each being an expert and also vulnerable (Gadow, 1996). Using the familiar concept of a story enables nurses and clients to stand back from the situation and also to be creative. Listening, authenticity, respect, clarification of intent, honoring ambiguity and complexity, and imagination comprise caring practice that is informed by a relational ethic (Hartrick, 2000). The relational narrative (story) or shared meaning that is created is ever changing as the nurse and others work together. Relational caring theory is as relevant in community programs as in individual and family care.

Phenomenological Theory

Use of phenomenological theory enables nurses to understand people's lived experience within the context of culture, time, and place. It is the meaning of people's lives as lived by them (Leonard, 1991). For example, urban people who are living in poverty may experience their lives as a daily struggle to find food (from food-banks and garbage cans), find a place to sleep (under a bridge, at a shelter), relieve stress (find a cigarette butt to smoke, a warm place to sit), and avoid danger (gangs, thieves, police).

Phenomenology provides community health nurses a lens through which to understand the world from the viewpoint of clients. The nurse asks clients to speak of their experiences, listens carefully, and avoids translating the story into nurse language or jumping in with interpretations. The nurse may learn that the idea of impoverishment as avoidable may not be part of the lived experience of poverty. What choices can be seen when a person is struggling to get through the day, frequently encountering rejection and hostility? From this place of understanding, meaningful work with clients can begin. Thus, that which is sometimes called "the apathy of the poor" can be reconceptualized into the need to create possibilities.

The experience of being listened to and understood is a powerful one that validates and strengthens clients (Attridge, Budgen, Hilton, McDavid, Molzah, & Purkis, 1997). Most practitioners would say they routinely work this way, but clients would disagree. Although it is challenging to work in this way when pressures of busy schedules and agency policies impinge, doing so is essential. Using phenomenological theory in programming can help the nurse understand the experiences of the different people who comprise a community and a programming team. Effective action is based on understanding (Covey, Merrill, & Merrill, 1997).

Feminist Theory

Feminist theories provide a lens through which socially constructed inequities based on gender and power relations can be seen and challenged (Bent, 1993). For example, when poverty is examined as a gendered situation, research reveals that poverty is not equally distributed among males and females and that the causal patterns as well as the impacts and the responses of others such as social organizations are different. Gendered beliefs are embedded in the operation of social, educational (including family), political, and legal institutions around the world. Many gendered practices are harmful to a particular gender, such as the practice in some countries of males eating before females, leaving females inadequately nourished and at risk, especially during childbearing. Although feminist theories are intended to create knowledge to improve women's lives, these theories also enable a more critical look at men's lives. For example, of concern in North America is the gendered circumstance of suicide where young men take their lives at a rate substantially higher than young women; one must ask, is there something in our privileging of males that is harmful to their health?

Bateson (1990) points out that certain gendered knowledge is health promoting and may be helpful to the other gender. For example, women's greater experience with balancing multiple commitments and handling discontinuities and diversities (as a result of their family and work roles) makes them a source of knowledge about interdependence and flexibility. Often, there is value in critical examination from the perspective of each gender. For example, Bateson notes:

> Many women raised in male dominated cultures have to struggle against the impulse to sacrifice their health for the health of the other. But many men raised in the same traditions have to struggle against pervasive imageries in which their own health or growth is a victory achieved at the expense of the other. (p. 240)

Programming based on gender-sensitive research can take into account the different experiences of males and females, and more helpful programs can be designed (Van Norstrand, 1993). Feminism challenges community health nurses to:

- Question the influences of gender in a given situation (in combination with other categorizations such as culture, age, size, sexual orientation, ability, and the like)
- Determine whether the influences are benefiting or harming the health of the various people involved
- Support beneficial and reduce harmful influences

Critical Social Theory

Critical social theory is a lens that focuses on the transformation of existing social orders with the intent of changing power relations and social positioning to promote greater freedom, equality, and social justice. Social orders determine the distribution of wealth and work, including that work which does not count (e.g., housework); access to resources such as education, health care, and law enforcement; and media images about various groups, including religious, ethnic, family, age, and the like (Habermas, as cited in Stevens, 1989). There is no one critical social theory. Rather, from systematic social critique by those who are in oppressed positions, critical theories are developed relevant to their specific position (e.g., from experience with racism, poverty, environmental destruction, homophobia, or gender bias) (Kendall, 1992).

The domination and privileges of one group over another often are assumed to be natural or "just the way it is." For example, the work of one health care discipline may be taken for granted to be more important than the work of another; the existence of poverty may be viewed as a natural phenomenon or the result of an inadequate work ethic; the superior socioeconomic status of one race or class over another may be assumed to be the result of natural superiority; and the protest that industry cannot switch to environmentally safe production methods without shattering the local, national, or global economy may be viewed as a basic truth. Historical and cultural comparisons can help uncover the roots and development of dominant social constructions.

Use of a critical social theory lens invites the nurse to ask questions (Bassett-Smith, 2001):

- *To expose existing social formations:* Whose voice is heard? Not heard? Is my voice heard? What is frustrating or contradictory in my position?
- *To raise questions about those interests that are served and not served by these social formations:* Who benefits? Who does not benefit?
- *To explore the way social formations are produced and reproduced:* What is actually taught in families? In schools? In health care agencies?

REFLECTIVE THINKING

Theoretical Lenses

Think about a community that has significance for you. Imagine looking at your community through the different lenses of caring, phenomenological, feminist, and critical social theories.
- What do you see with each?
- Are there similarities in the views? Differences?

- *To create images of new possibilities:* What would "better" look like?
- *To identify actions through which transformation can be achieved:* What must happen to create "better"?

Dialogue (mutual interaction) and consciousness raising are part of critical theorizing. The social critique does not end at the point of blaming the oppressor or the oppressed but at the place of challenging and changing the rules that support the undesirable imbalance in power. Use of critical social theory is an optimistic act that enables nurses and communities to see the established order of society as only one way the world can be constructed and to appreciate and use the power they have to transform their worlds for the better (Hagedorn, 1995; Bassett-Smith, 2001).

Caring, phenomenological, feminist, and critical social theories can assist community health nurses to achieve Health for All goals in their programming work. These theories offer explanations about how meaningful connections can be made with people having diverse characteristics, how people experience the world, and how people hold different truths and ideas about that which is desirable and that which is possible. Further, use of these theories can raise awareness about barriers to health and can facilitate health-promoting action.

Change Theories

Other theories useful in programming are change theories. Programs always have some level of change as a goal: individual, family, group, organization, community, societal. Programs often are directed at more than one level of change. For example, a program aimed at assisting teenage mothers and fathers may include change at the individual level to increase the mothers' and fathers' relational and parenting knowledge and skills; change at the family and group levels to build mutual support and problem solving; and change at the organizational, community, and societal levels to provide employment and housing that enable teenage parents to care for their children while completing school, participating in neighborhood support networks, and working for pay via flexible arrangements with employers and social agencies. Community, organizational, and societal change is connected to public policy and politics (see Chapter 18). Change theories are interspersed throughout this text. Of particular interest in this chapter are change that is emancipatory or empowering, and change at the community level.

Transtheoretical and Relapse Prevention Models of Change

The nurse will encounter many programs aimed toward individual change, often as components of larger community change programs. Many programs involve education (see Chapter 10). Two extensively used individual change theories, transtheoretical (Prochaska, Johnson, & Lee, 1998) and relapse prevention (Marlatt & George, 1998), derive from social learning and cognitive theories (see Figures 16-4 and 16-5). Learning is viewed as occurring when individuals interact with others, and challenges arise when individuals work to change behavior patterns that have been constructed and maintained through social interaction.

In the transtheoretical change model, the individual moves from not thinking about change in the near future, to seriously thinking about change (in the next six months), to actively planning changes, to overtly making changes and taking steps to maintain changes and avoid relapse (McKenzie & Smeltzer, 2001). Relapse is common, but the opportunity is there for another change effort, hence the spiral diagram. Individuals can identify where they are at in the model, and strategies to assist them can be designed accordingly. (For a plain-language handbook see Prochaska, Norcross, & Diclemente, 1996.)

According to the relapse prevention model, because relapse is common in health behavior change, the programmer needs to prepare individuals for the possibility of relapse and teach them how to avoid relapse and, in case of relapse, how to get back on track without guilt or giving up. Possible global self-control strategies are identified in the circles of the model, in correspondence with specific experiences of the individual, identified in rectangles. Use of the model is intended to improve personal knowledge and skills so that individuals are prepared to cope well with typical experiences as they try to develop healthier behaviors. Therefore, global strategies need to be translated into specific strategies for individuals. Role playing, relaxation and imaging techniques, contracts, and reminder cards have been used to help individuals develop personally relevant self-control strategies. Those individuals who have made changes are often very helpful in assisting others to change (ripple effect).

The transtheoretical and relapse prevention models both involve critical awareness and skill building at each stage and are cyclical. Individuals may move through the stages several times before their lifestyle patterns are as they want them to be. The use of these theories can be empowering when a program incorporates a critique of societal influences along with the strengthening of individual competence as long as individuals are neither pressured nor blamed.

Diffusion Theory

Diffusion theory provides a useful lens through which to view group, organizational, and population change. The theory explains the way that information and

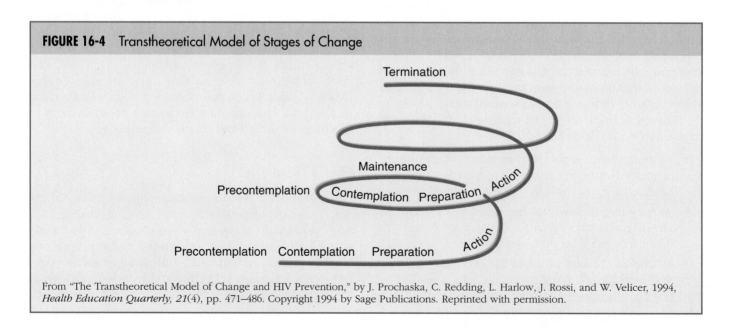

FIGURE 16-4 Transtheoretical Model of Stages of Change

Termination

Maintenance

Precontemplation Contemplation Preparation Action

Precontemplation Contemplation Preparation Action

From "The Transtheoretical Model of Change and HIV Prevention," by J. Prochaska, C. Redding, L. Harlow, J. Rossi, and W. Velicer, 1994, *Health Education Quarterly, 21*(4), pp. 471–486. Copyright 1994 by Sage Publications. Reprinted with permission.

FIGURE 16-5 Relapse Prevention Model

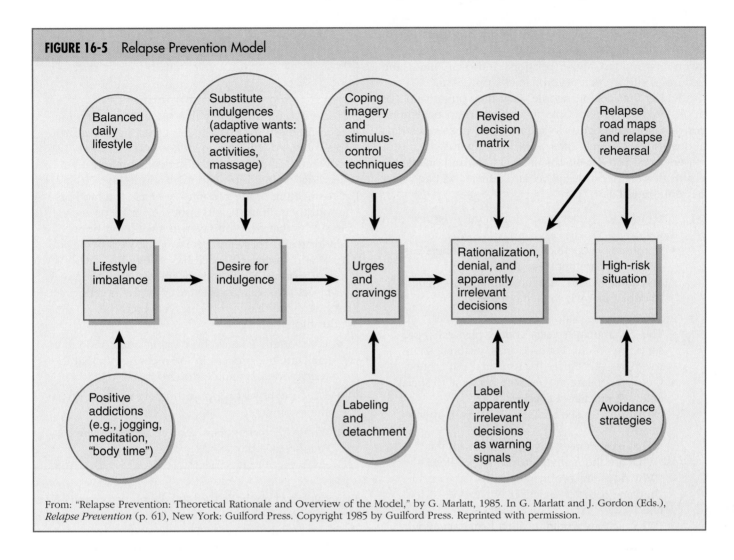

From: "Relapse Prevention: Theoretical Rationale and Overview of the Model," by G. Marlatt, 1985. In G. Marlatt and J. Gordon (Eds.), *Relapse Prevention* (p. 61), New York: Guilford Press. Copyright 1985 by Guilford Press. Reprinted with permission.

change spread through populations unevenly. According to diffusion theory, systematic processes (awareness, interest, trial, and adoption) are engaged in sequentially by different segments of the population (Rogers, 1998). Change is seen as progressing in a bell-shaped curve from innovators (risk takers), to early adopters (respected opinion leaders), to early majority adopters (deliberators), to late majority adopters (responders to the norm), to laggards (marginalized people or cynics). Diffusion processes are enhanced when people are aware of the advantages of the change, are provided opportunities to explore the compatibility of new and current practices, are supported in adopting change, and are offered opportunities for trial and modification (Rogers, 1998).

Implications for programmers are that different approaches must be used to reach (i.e., establish meaning for) different segments of the population at different times. For example, according to the theory, innovators respond best to cognitive approaches, early majority adopters to motivational approaches, and late majority adopters and laggards to reducing perceived barriers. The approaches must be timed so that each of the vari-

ous segments in the population is introduced at the right time to that which is most meaningful to them. Diffusion theory can be used to guide programming aimed at multiple levels of change (e.g., adoption of healthier eating habits by high school students, or a "healthier eating" program in a school food service, or a Heart Smart nutritional program in restaurants across a region). Use of diffusion theory is compatible with Health for All programs when the focus is on social change rather than control.

Freire's Theory of Freeing

To support emancipatory change and empowerment, Freire (1970/1993), a Brazilian educator, developed a methodology of problem-posing dialogue (termed by some a theory of "freeing") intended to help people uncover the root causes of problems, see possibilities for transformative actions, and act to change social inequities rather than adapting. Practitioners around the world have found Freire's methods highly effective for helping people who are stuck in complex, disadvantaged, and marginalized situations become effective in improving their health and health-related situations. The underpinnings of critical social theory are apparent in Freire's use of "conscientisation," that is, bringing to awareness hidden power relations and overcoming the culture of silence that accompanies oppression.

Rather than telling people what they ought to do or think, Freire invites people to engage in an egalitarian conversation (dialogue) to identify and pose questions about issues. Communities work from their own values, experiences, and definitions of situations, and practitioners work to support the process. Freire's approach may be represented as:

1. Listening to understand community issues and themes:
   - Community identifies issues; practitioners ask: "What is important to you?"
   - Practitioners learn/use the community language to depict that which is important.

2. Problem-posing dialogue:
   - The community selects codes (physical representations of the issue—stories, pictures, songs, role plays—that place the issue in social context).
   - Question posing moves from personal to social analysis; practitioners ask:
     "What do you see and feel? What is happening here?"
     "What experiences have you had with this?"
     "What are the many parts of this problem?"
     "Why does this problem exist?"
     "Imagine a better situation. What does it look like?"
     "What actions would create a better situation?"

3. Action and reflection:
   - Community tests out their ideas for action in the world.
   - Community reflects on their action.
   - Action and reflection become a deepening spiral over time as the community works to change complex, embedded problems. (Wallerstein & Bernstein, 1988)

Community Organization

Community organization, a multifaceted theoretical approach to promoting change at the community level, incorporates many of the concepts of interest to nurses. Community organizing has a long history, originating in situations where adverse social conditions prompted the formation of coalitions to create systemwide change. Lillian Wald's work in the late 1800s with the settlement house population of New York provides one example of the way that community nurses can use community organization to dramatically improve the health of a community.

Community organization was the original term coined by social workers to represent the collection of

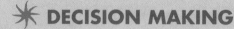

✳ DECISION MAKING

Top-Down and Grass-Roots Processes

You work for an agency that offers a program for teen mothers. You have been given an educational plan with corresponding videos and handouts covering topics such as baby development, feeding, crying, birth control, and the like. At the first meeting of the program, you ask the mothers about their interests and issues. Your focus is on ensuring that everyone gets to speak and be understood. The teens talk about always being "on call" and having no social life. They also speak of being worried about money and whether they will ever get off social assistance. After the meeting, you realized that you had not covered the educational plan.

- Using Freire's ideas, how might you continue to facilitate the process in the meetings so that the teens' priorities guide the group?
- How might you support the development of their competence?
- How will you explain your choices to your employer/supervisor?

principles and methods for influencing community-level change (Drevdahl, 1995); *community organizing* now is the term commonly used. The classic typology of community organizing includes three methods: social planning, social action, and community development (previously called locality development) (Rothman & Tropman, 1987, as cited in Minkler, 1990). Incorporated, in varying degrees in these methods are the concepts of participation (people working together), relevance (starting where people are), and empowerment (increasing community choice and competence). Each model is associated with different change strategies and roles for health care practitioners (see Table 16-2).

Social planning is the most "top-down" of the models. In this model, much of the planning work is carried out by practitioners. Issues may be identified by the practitioner rather than (or, sometimes, in addition to) the community. The process is one of rational problem solving based on empirical data and expert technical assistance. Social planning is a familiar model in public health programs based on a population-focused, epidemiological problem-solving approach. Many programs offered by community nurses are based on a social planning model. For example, in well-baby programs topics and activities may be largely predetermined by practitioners, who gather and analyze data about babies, health and parenting and design interventions accordingly. The

TABLE 16-2 Community Organization Models

	COMMUNITY DEVELOPMENT	SOCIAL PLANNING	SOCIAL ACTION
Categories of community action	Self-help; community capacity and integration (process goals)	Problem solving with regard to substantive community problems (task goals)	Shifting of power relationships and resources; basic institutional change (task or process goals)
Practitioner roles	Enabler, catalyst, facilitator, teacher	Fact gatherer and analyst, program implementer	Activist, advocate, negotiator
Change strategies	Building community connection and caretaking	Planned change, social marketing, health education	Political action, lobbying, confrontation
Primary definer of issues and actions	Community (practitioner input)	Practitioner (community input)	Community (practitioner input)

From "Models of Community Organization & Macro Practice: Their Mixing and Phasing," by J. Rothman and J. Tropman, as cited in "Improving Health through Community Organization," by M. Minkler, 1990, in K. Glanz, F. M. Lewis, and B. K. Rimer (Eds.), Health Behavior and Health Education *(pp. 264–265), San Francisco: Jossey Bass. Copyright 1987 by Itasca County Historical Society. Adapted by permission of Jossey-Bass, a subsidiary of John Wiley & Sons, Inc.*

process whereby community nurses advocate for babies (child protection) while maintaining caring, empowering relationships with parents (parenting support) has been described as a "figurative dance" and "exquisitely complex" (Zerwekh, 1992, pp. 102, 104).

Community development and social action models are more grass roots, or "bottom up"; in other words, the community identifies the issues, is fully involved in decision making throughout all processes, and most often determines the processes. Practitioners may teach community people needed skills so that they can act on their own behalf. Community development is intended to bring people together to solve community problems and build community competence, consensus, and a sense of community. Social action is the most political of the models, with the intent of action being inequity correction, institutional change, and power redistribution.

In using community organization, Drevdahl (1995) cautions:

When professionals initiate a program they may think, "How can I get you (the community members) to participate in what I want to achieve?" This reasoning is antithetical to community organization tenets when the objective is to examine relationships of power and create opportunities for community change. (p. 16)

Community nurses are using community organization models and meeting with impressive successes (English, 2000) as well as some frustrations (Chalmers & Bramadat, 1996). Employing agencies and program funders sometimes want greater up-front specification of program goals, timelines, and quantifiable results than is possible with minimally prestructured models of pro-

gramming, such as community development and social action. Also, the targets for change under the social action model may be either the agency (or government) that employs the nurse or powerful organizations in the community (e.g., a factory polluting or a gang terrorizing a neighborhood). These situations may create conflict and in some cases result in sanctions against involvement. Other confounding factors may arise from the need for confidentiality versus the open information sharing inherent in participatory processes and from the nurse's personal desire for control or discomfort with conflict. Despite these challenges, community organizing has become an important approach to promote community health.

In programming practice, community organization models often are blended to address the multiple factors influencing the health of a community. Of importance is that nurses use these models, as well as other models and theories, on the basis of thoughtful judgment regarding that which would be most helpful to the community. Although nurses may feel passionately about a particular model or theory, being dogmatic is not useful.

Community Organization in Action: Planned Approaches to Community Health and Healthy Cities/Communities

Two examples of community organizing associated with the Health for All movement are the Planned Approach to Community Health (PATCH) and Healthy Cities/Communities programs. The PATCH programs are sponsored by the Centers for Disease Control and Prevention (CDC) in the United States to promote partnerships among the CDC, local communities, and state and local health agencies to plan, implement, and maintain local health promotion programs (Goodman, Steckler, Hoover, & Schwartz, 1993). The PATCH programs use a social planning approach that incorporates some features of community development: PATCH includes:

- Communities develop advisory committees with representatives from agencies and the public.

- The CDC provides training and technical assistance so that the advisory committee can conduct structured interviews with identified community leaders and assess needs using an established behavioral risk survey (oriented to major chronic diseases).

- The committee collects and analyzes data, decides priority health issues and designs, and implements interventions to improve health in these areas.

Many PATCH programs have been implemented and evaluated throughout the United States. From an evaluation of 27 programs (Steckler, Orville, Eng, & Dawson, 1992), findings indicated increased awareness of health issues, implementation of new programs, and improved communication among agencies and public participants. Not surprising, but of concern, was the additional finding that the risk survey was too complex for the community partners to deal with, and it directed attention to predetermined health problems, which were not necessarily of primary interest to the community. The evaluators further concluded that funding and technical support were insufficient throughout to fully support program goals. Overall, participants expressed enthusiasm for PATCH but noted difficulty in maintaining the considerable commitment required.

Challenges with PATCH are being addressed. Green and Kreuter (1993) suggest that technical tasks be done by professionals. Tensions such as those that arose around the use of the predetermined risk survey are common with social planning approaches. Local people are most keen to participate when issues have personal meaning for them (community development), whereas health professionals may be assigned responsibility for preventing and controlling the most prevalent population health problems as determined by epidemiological data (social planning). Green and Kreuter question, "Is it necessary for us to create an integrated model that intertwines these two divergent approaches through all aspects of the planning and implementation process?" (p. 221). Green & Kreuter's (1999) recent work indicates that they are "intertwining" social planning and community development based on results of extensive field research (see PRECEDE-PROCEED section).

In operation worldwide are WHO-inspired Healthy Cities/Communities programs (English, 2000; see also www.amulet.nbca/designinghealthycities). These programs are based on community development and so-cial action models. Related successes have been credited to the wide general appeal of the concept and the use of strategies that promote intersectoral collaboration, local participation, shared vision, and community ownership. Program foci and processes are determined by the participants.

The Healthy Cities/Communities initiative has stimulated a diverse range of programs that are meaningful to specific communities. The programs generally focus on reducing risk conditions (e.g., making public parks safer and developing community walks and bicycle paths for all ages). Difficulties arise when funders from the health sector want to see measurable reductions in disease risk factors (which the programs are not immediately geared toward) and measurable improvements in health (although tools for measuring "broadly defined" health are not well developed). Funders from sectors other than health have other interests that must be addressed. Programmers may not be able to bridge the gap between that which the program can realistically affect and that which funders recognize as worthy.

Another challenge for Healthy Cities/Communities programs is that social action naturally gives rise to conflict between competing interests of the powerful and less powerful (e.g., developers' wanting land rezoned for building versus parents' wanting a park for youth recreation). In addition, local issues often are affected by external forces such as national policies or multinational corporations (Labonte, 1998). Because the vision of Healthy Cities/Communities programs has public appeal, those who do not want a particular change may stall and use diversionary tactics rather than being open about the conflict and thus risking political fallout. Skillful negotiation, early conflict recognition, and open conflict management have proved essential in most community organizing efforts (Bless, Murphy, & Vinson, 1995). Sustaining Healthy Cities/Communities programs takes considerable energy and political savvy; nevertheless, the concept continues to inspire commitment. The Canadian Forum on Health (Ritchie, 1997) and *Healthy People 2010* (USDHHS, 2000) document the gains made through community social action and Healthy Cities/Communities programs and continue to recommend community action as a national health strategy.

PROGRAMMING THEORIES AND PRACTICALITIES

With context appreciation and an array of potentially helpful theories providing the background, the nurse is well prepared to bring programming into the foreground. Nurses may use their knowledge of context and theories to assist with both the substantive content and organizational process requirements of programming

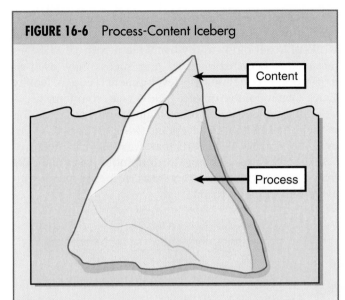

FIGURE 16-6 Process-Content Iceberg

Content

Process

From *Basic Concepts of International Health* (Reading Module, p. 13), by K. Wolton, H. Amit, S. Kalma, I. Hillman, D. Hillman, and N. Cosway, January 1995, Ottawa, Canada: Canadian University Consortium for Health in Development. Copyright 1995 by Canadian Society for International Health. Reprinted with permission.

(i.e., the focus of the program and the way the program will operate). (See Figure 16-6.) Community health programs vary from being relatively simple and narrowly focused, such as a heart health program for local firefighters, to being highly complex and broadly focused, such as a Healthy Cities program. When a program is broadly focused and comprises many different components, the term *project* rather than *program* may be used; however, basic programming ideas continue to be applicable. The content or focus of a program may appear to be "the program," but nurses have learned that the processes through which the program is realized comprise the majority of the work.

Use of Language

The language appropriate for nurses to use in programming varies depending on the participants. When a nurse is submitting a proposal to get funding support for a program from a level of government, the language used will be different from that used by a nurse working with a group of laypeople to create an action plan that everyone can follow. The nurse must therefore be "multilingual" within English (or other languages). Adjustment of language to suit the situation and participants supports primary health care and health promotion principles and enables participation throughout programming by all stakeholders (those who are likely to be affected by the

program in some way). Stakeholder participation and partnership increase the likelihood that the program will create the desired health outcomes, including increased community competence.

Deciding about Participation

Decisions about participation should be based on the community situation, the theories being used, and stakeholder preferences. To support partnership throughout the processes, planning and advisory groups of some type with representatives from all stakeholder groups may be formed, or the style may be more loosely structured (Bracht, 1990). Organizational support structures and styles of operating often change during programming to facilitate progress toward the desired results and, also, because participation may change over time.

Envisioning the Process

Programming processes of planning, implementation, and evaluation are most easily described in a linear sequential format. In practice, however, these processes overlap and must be revisited often during the time span of a program. Community assessment, sometimes called community analysis, may be viewed as either a part of planning or a separate process occurring prior to planning. Evaluation, in particular, must be integrated throughout. To be done well, the processes of planning, implementation, and evaluation, like most things, require practice, particularly given the constantly changing nature of people, settings, and resources (McKenzie & Smeltzer, 2001). Nurses should anticipate ambiguity and remember that reflection and improvisation will contribute to clarity and direction.

Programming Models

Programming models are representations of approaches to programming that offer explanations of the processes involved. To provide guidance throughout programming processes, communities and nurses together may either create their own model or choose to use an already tested programming or planning model. Sometimes a model is recommended by a funding agency. Numerous choices are available in the literature. Because all models are based on values and assumptions, the nurse should ensure that the chosen model is either consistent with Health for All ideas or can be adequately adapted. Several models are described next. Following these descriptions is a section on some practicalities of programming useful with all models.

Healthy Communities: The Process

Grass-roots community development is the focus of the Healthy Communities: The Process model (British Columbia Ministry of Health, 1989). This model is useful when diverse community people come together to work on health issues; a brief manual is written in language intended to be clear to people lacking community organizing experience. The phases of the model are entry, needs assessment, planning, doing, and renewal. The circular movement through the phases and the main tasks to be accomplished during each phase are depicted in Figure 16-7. Near the completion of each phase, a pause

is recommended so that the community group can reflect on "Did we get the job done? Where are we now? What worked? What didn't and why? What next?" (p. 11). This model has been extensively and successfully used in grass-roots community development and Healthy Cities/Communities projects. Now that community development is becoming more familiar in health care, the model is gaining more acceptance with funders and with evaluators who use participatory research methods. Nurses may want to change the terminology in the model from "needs" to "issues or interests" to better match with a strength-oriented focus.

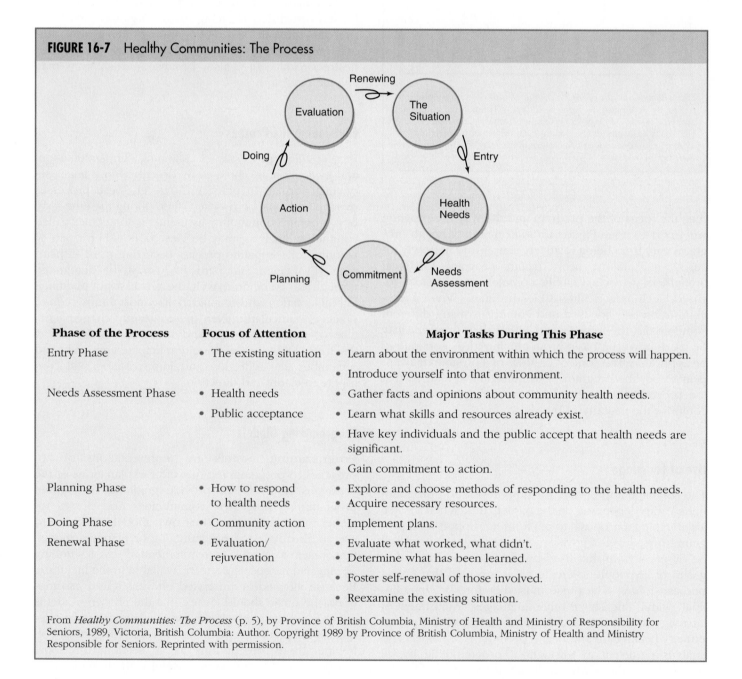

FIGURE 16-7 Healthy Communities: The Process

Phase of the Process	Focus of Attention	Major Tasks During This Phase
Entry Phase	• The existing situation	• Learn about the environment within which the process will happen.
		• Introduce yourself into that environment.
Needs Assessment Phase	• Health needs	• Gather facts and opinions about community health needs.
	• Public acceptance	• Learn what skills and resources already exist.
		• Have key individuals and the public accept that health needs are significant.
		• Gain commitment to action.
Planning Phase	• How to respond to health needs	• Explore and choose methods of responding to the health needs.
		• Acquire necessary resources.
Doing Phase	• Community action	• Implement plans.
Renewal Phase	• Evaluation/ rejuvenation	• Evaluate what worked, what didn't.
		• Determine what has been learned.
		• Foster self-renewal of those involved.
		• Reexamine the existing situation.

From *Healthy Communities: The Process* (p. 5), by Province of British Columbia, Ministry of Health and Ministry of Responsibility for Seniors, 1989, Victoria, British Columbia: Author. Copyright 1989 by Province of British Columbia, Ministry of Health and Ministry Responsible for Seniors. Reprinted with permission.

FIGURE 16-8 Guiding Principles for Health Promotion Organization

- Planning must be based on a historical understanding of the community. Conditions that inhibit or facilitate interventions must be assessed.

- Because the issue or problem is usually one of multiple (rather than single) causality, a comprehensive effort using multiple interventions is required.

- It is important to focus on community context and to work primarily through existing structures and values.

- Active community participation, not mere token representation, is desired.

- For the project to be effective, intersectoral components of the community must work together to address the problem in a comprehensive effort.

- The focus must be on both long-term and short-term problem solving if the change is to endure beyond the project's demonstration period.

- Finally, and most important, the community must share responsibility for the problem and for its solution.

From "Community Organization Principles in Health Promotion: A Five Stage Model," by N. Bracht and L. Kingsbury, 1990, in N. Bracht (Ed.), *Health Promotion at the Community Level* (p. 74), Newbury Park, CA: Sage Publications. Copyright 1990 by Sage Publications. Reprinted with permission.

FIGURE 16-9 Model of Community Organization Stages

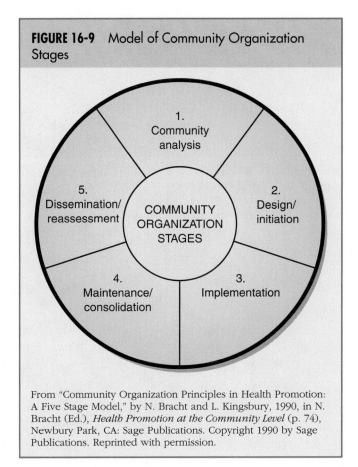

From "Community Organization Principles in Health Promotion: A Five Stage Model," by N. Bracht and L. Kingsbury, 1990, in N. Bracht (Ed.), *Health Promotion at the Community Level* (p. 74), Newbury Park, CA: Sage Publications. Copyright 1990 by Sage Publications. Reprinted with permission.

Health Promotion at the Community Level

Bracht and Kingsbury's (1990) model for health promotion at the community level is well grounded in community organization theory (see Figure 16-8). Although this model is similar to Healthy Communities: The Process, the language is intended for practitioners. The model has effectively guided extensive as well as small community programs. The five phases of the model are community analysis, design initiation, implementation, maintenance/ consolidation, and dissemination/reassessment (see Figure 16-9).

Population Health Promotion Model

The broad planning model referred to as population health promotion combines the main ideas that have emerged from health promotion and population health theory and practice over the past two decades (Hamilton & Bhatti, 1996) (see Figure 16-10). The model guides program content decisions; that is, it answers the questions "On what should we take action?" "How should we take action?" and "With whom should we act?" (p. 6). The model is appealing because of its integration of Health for All concepts and strategies. Depicted in the cubic-style model are health determinants, health promotion

strategies, and levels at which action can be taken (WHO, 1986). A short manual gives multiple examples of ways the model can be used to create a program, starting from a health determinant, health concern, specific population, or at-risk group (see Figure 16-11). Some community health providers have redesigned the population health promotion model by converting the cube into a North American native medicine wheel style (nesting circles) and adding gender and culture as health determinants (Health & Community Services, 1998). Manuals and a colorful mobile model are available to aid planning.

Diagrammatic Models: Logic Models and Conceptual Maps

If a program is defined as a collection of activities designed to produce particular results, it is reasonable that diagramming that which is envisioned would be helpful to those involved. Diagrammatic models show via graphic designs how program components are related to produce desired results (i.e., values/interests, goals, program activities, results). The exercise of creating the diagrams (e.g., logic models, conceptual maps) brings people together to think through on paper the relationships among goals, program activities, and predicted outcomes. The values,

FIGURE 16-10 Population Health Promotion Model

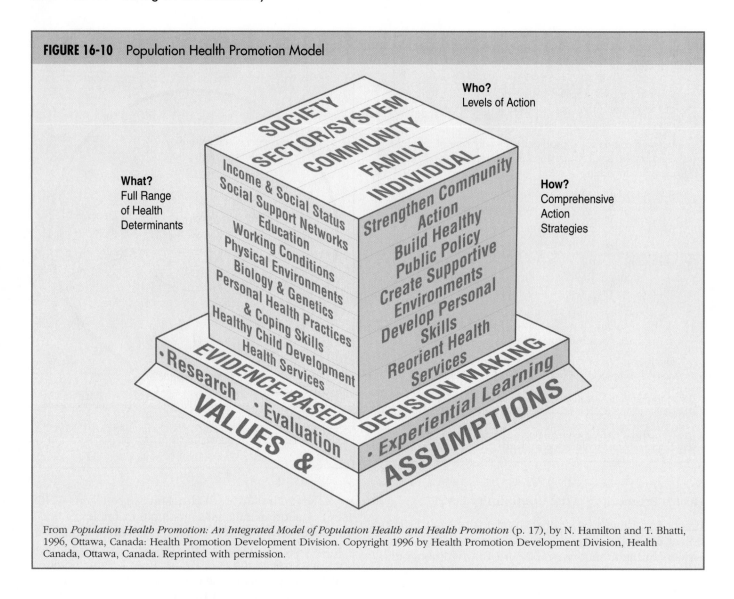

From *Population Health Promotion: An Integrated Model of Population Health and Health Promotion* (p. 17), by N. Hamilton and T. Bhatti, 1996, Ottawa, Canada: Health Promotion Development Division. Copyright 1996 by Health Promotion Development Division, Health Canada, Ottawa, Canada. Reprinted with permission.

assumptions, and hypotheses shaping the program can thus be made more visible. Choices can then be made about those things that should and should not be included (program content).

Logic models derive from systems theory and use formal language and symbols; conceptual maps use plain language and symbols or pictures. The underlying intent of both is to depict that which is occurring in sequence. Three examples of logic models are provided: modeling, a logic chart (Wong-Reiger & David, 1995) and a program outcome model (United Way, 1996). The reader is cautioned that terminology varies and must be clarified for each type of logic model. For example, results occurring close to a program may be called outputs, impacts, or short-term outcomes, while results occurring further from the program may be called intermediate or long-term impacts or outcomes. The sequential logic, rather than the language, is of prime importance.

Modeling was originally developed for educational programs (Borich & Jemelka, 1982). A series of sketches are used to diagram inputs (basic requirements for the program to work), activities (events intended to produce change), modifiers (factors that affect program activities and, thus, influence outcomes for better or worse), and outcomes (the changes following from program activities) (see Figure 16-12). Modifiers, as factors that support or constrain a particular change, must be tended to during programming.

Wong-Reiger and David (1995) use different shaped symbols to indicate program activities, service delivery (the tasks to create the activities), immediate results, and ultimate results (as long term as can be reasonably attributed to the activities and also measured) (see Figure 16-12). When creating the diagram, they suggest working backward, from the long-term desired outcomes, to in-

FIGURE 16-11   Using the Population Health Promotion Model

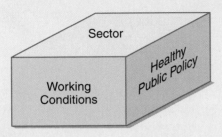

Sector

Healthy Public Policy

Working Conditions

Focus on the Determinants of Health

For example, industry can examine the effects of emerging technologies on working conditions and can adopt health-enhancing options.

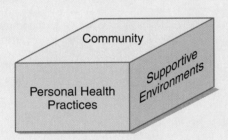

Community

Supportive Environments

Personal Health Practices

Focus on a Specific Health Concern

For example, schools and workplaces can make nutritious foods available in their cafeterias.

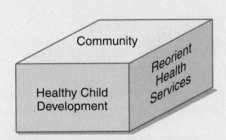

Community

Reorient Health Services

Healthy Child Development

Focus on Group at Risk

For example, community clinics can make appropriate primary care services accessible to young families.

FIGURE 16-12   Modeling: A Group Support Program

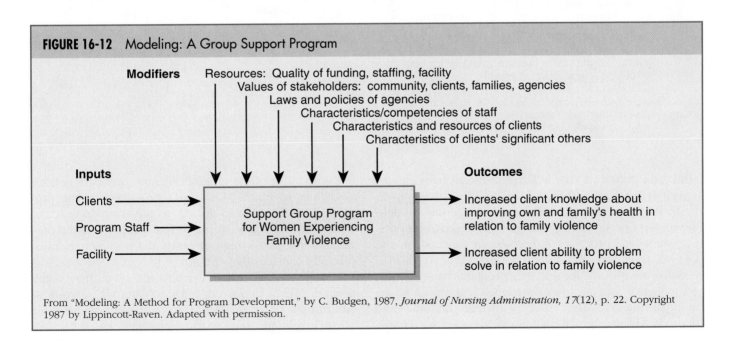

Modifiers   Resources: Quality of funding, staffing, facility
Values of stakeholders: community, clients, families, agencies
Laws and policies of agencies
Characteristics/competencies of staff
Characteristics and resources of clients
Characteristics of clients' significant others

Inputs

Clients

Program Staff

Facility

Support Group Program for Women Experiencing Family Violence

Outcomes

Increased client knowledge about improving own and family's health in relation to family violence

Increased client ability to problem solve in relation to family violence

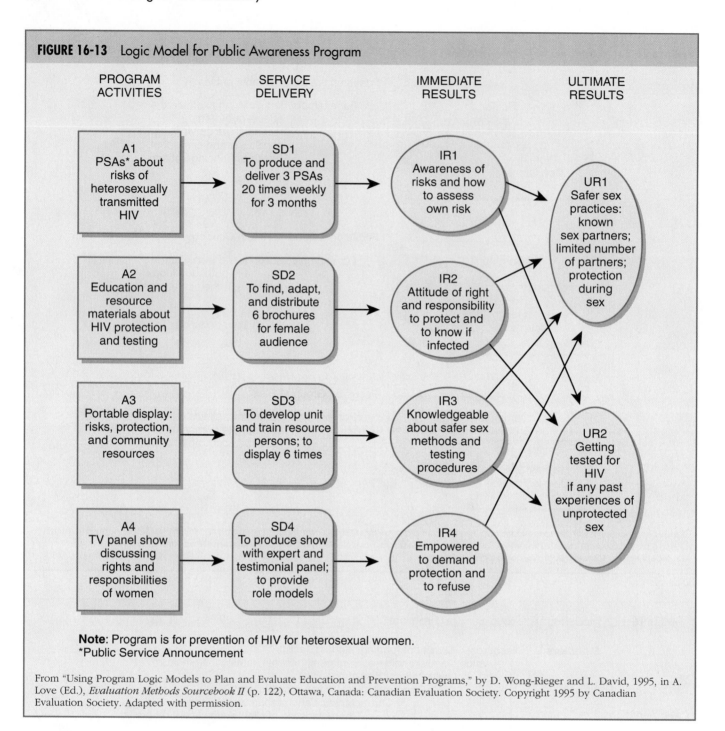

FIGURE 16-13 Logic Model for Public Awareness Program

PROGRAM ACTIVITIES | SERVICE DELIVERY | IMMEDIATE RESULTS | ULTIMATE RESULTS

A1 PSAs* about risks of heterosexually transmitted HIV

SD1 To produce and deliver 3 PSAs 20 times weekly for 3 months

IR1 Awareness of risks and how to assess own risk

UR1 Safer sex practices: known sex partners; limited number of partners; protection during sex

A2 Education and resource materials about HIV protection and testing

SD2 To find, adapt, and distribute 6 brochures for female audience

IR2 Attitude of right and responsibility to protect and to know if infected

A3 Portable display: risks, protection, and community resources

SD3 To develop unit and train resource persons; to display 6 times

IR3 Knowledgeable about safer sex methods and testing procedures

UR2 Getting tested for HIV if any past experiences of unprotected sex

A4 TV panel show discussing rights and responsibilities of women

SD4 To produce show with expert and testimonial panel; to provide role models

IR4 Empowered to demand protection and to refuse

Note: Program is for prevention of HIV for heterosexual women.
*Public Service Announcement

From "Using Program Logic Models to Plan and Evaluate Education and Prevention Programs," by D. Wong-Rieger and L. David, 1995, in A. Love (Ed.), *Evaluation Methods Sourcebook II* (p. 122), Ottawa, Canada: Canadian Evaluation Society. Copyright 1995 by Canadian Evaluation Society. Adapted with permission.

termediate outcomes that indicate progress, to program activities (see Figure 16-13).

In the United Way (1996) program outcome model, the results of program activities are categorized as outputs (i.e., immediate products of the program) and outcomes (i.e., initial, intermediate, and long term) (Figure 16-14). As outcomes become longer term, programs have less direct influence. Also, outputs sometimes are considered to be initial outcomes (e.g., number of free condoms distributed). There is no "right" categorization; what is important is the sequential logic.

Regardless of the type of diagram, there are general guidelines to follow. Outcomes produced by the program should be related directly to the situation (i.e., the issues, values, needs, or goals) that gave rise to the program. When predicting outcomes, the programmer must carefully consider the strength of program activities; it is tempting for the novice to expect too much from small programs (e.g., to prevent teen smoking via a two-hour educational program). After program components have been identified, the relationships among them are mapped; in instances where relationships are not sound,

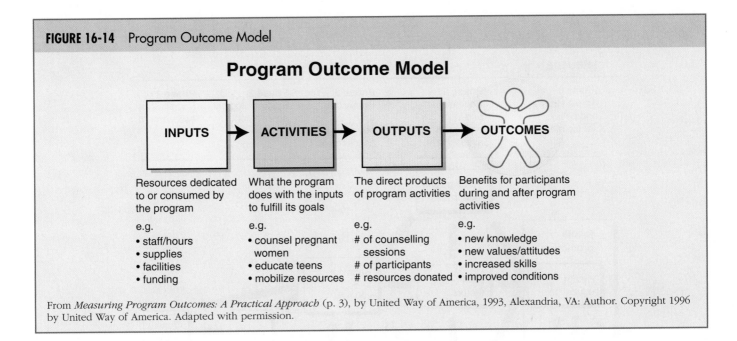

FIGURE 16-14 Program Outcome Model

From *Measuring Program Outcomes: A Practical Approach* (p. 3), by United Way of America, 1993, Alexandria, VA: Author. Copyright 1996 by United Way of America. Adapted with permission.

changes in components are made. Also, gaps or extensive overlaps between desired outcomes and activities are eliminated.

Use of diagrammatic models can expedite understanding of the program by funders and others. The language can be adjusted to suit the audience. Several diagrams may be drawn for a program, starting with general program components and moving to greater specificity as needed. Funders may appreciate diagrams at the most general level; practitioners and others may prefer more specific diagrams. For example, at the level of interest for funders and administrators, a large program to deal with families experiencing male violence to female partners may include:

- (Activities) education, access to shelter and protection; (goals) to decrease health problems and reduce health care costs

Practitioners working directly in the community with families need more specificity. For example, in the situation of male violence to female partners, a program might include:

- (Activity) support groups for women and children; (goals) to increase knowledge and protective skills

- (Activity) support groups for men; (goals) to increase relational skills and decrease violent behavior

- (Activity) coalition work with public and private organizations; (goal) to increase shelter facilities for women and children

- (Activity) alliance building with police; (goals) to increase protection for women and children and containment of men.

Although the primary intent of diagrammatic models is to make clear the connections between values, goals, program activities, and outcomes, other relevant program dimensions may be included for practical purposes. For example, specific resource requirements may be noted (e.g., 20 hours of nursing, space for group meetings, 60 handouts), and the power, or "dose," of activities may be shown (e.g., two-hour support group once a week for six weeks). Program costs are then easy to estimate, and, if the evaluation shows that the outcomes are positive but not to the extent desired, a power increase may be recommended (e.g., extending the support group to 12 weeks or making it ongoing).

Diagrams such as logic models and conceptual maps may be created in many forms for planning purposes, updated later as programming progresses, and used finally to guide evaluation. Cartoonlike sketches are sometimes helpful in depicting the human experiences represented within the diagrams. Of importance is not the form of the diagrams per se, but that the diagrams visually depict that which is planned, is happening, or has happened. Constructing diagrams in conjunction with community participants promotes clarity, shared vision, and ownership.

Precede-Proceed

The PRECEDE-PROCEED model (Green & Kreuter, 1999) is a comprehensive educational and ecological framework for health promotion programming that has been used in a myriad of ways to guide the planning, implementation, and evaluation of numerous large and small health programs (see Figure 16-15). The long-term use of the model has permitted testing and refinement. Although

FIGURE 16-15 PRECEDE-PROCEED Model for Health Promotion Planning and Evaluation

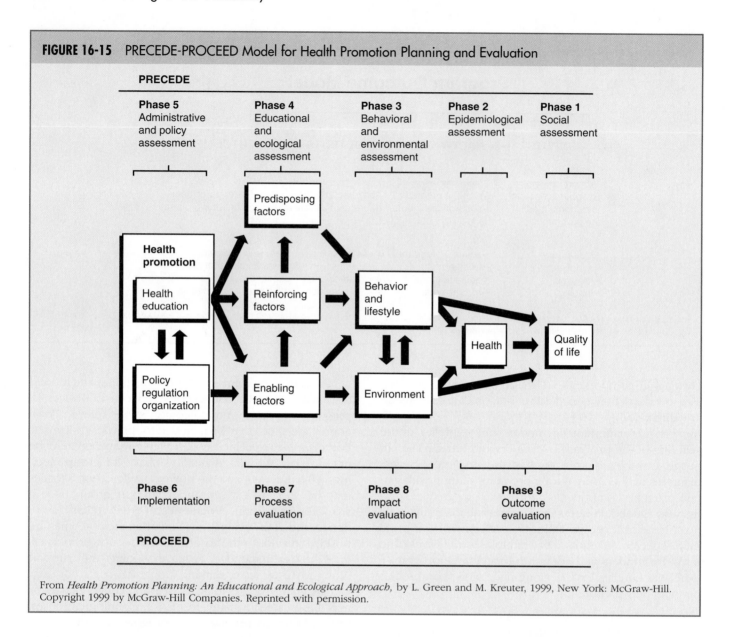

From *Health Promotion Planning: An Educational and Ecological Approach,* by L. Green and M. Kreuter, 1999, New York: McGraw-Hill. Copyright 1999 by McGraw-Hill Companies. Reprinted with permission.

the model has a strong social planning orientation, more recently, some community development principles have been incorporated. For example, the term *diagnosis* has been replaced by the term *assessment,* because people using the model in field work linked diagnosis with "problems only" and no identification of strengths. As well, there now is a stronger message about ensuring that the program is meaningful from the viewpoint of the community through more full community participation.

PRECEDE-PROCEED is an acronym for the components of the model. PATCH programs were based on PRECEDE, and the results led to the development of PROCEED. In the model, social, epidemiological, behavioral, environmental, educational, ecological, policy, and administrative dimensions are assessed, and multilevel strategies are designed to improve health status and quality of life. Subjective quality of life is placed ahead of objective health status. Similar to logic models, the user may

start by identifying desired outcomes (i.e., phases 8 and 9) (ideally with the community), then identifying possible causes and finally interventions. Also, if the approach is community development, phase 2 may be omitted. An example of model use follows.

- Phase 1. Social Assessment: Involve the target population in a self-study to identify their needs and aspirations in relation to their quality of life.
  Program: College students were interviewed and then surveyed about their health interests. Concerns were expressed about unplanned pregnancy and sexually transmitted diseases (STDs).

- Phase 2. Epidemiological Assessment: Use epidemiological data to enable identification and ranking of health goals or problems that might contribute to the quality-of-life issues.

Program: Sexually active students reported lack of condom use. STD and pregnancy rates in national data were similar to those reported by students in the self-study (relates to *Healthy People 2010* objectives 7-3—Health, risk behavior information for college and university students— and 25-11—Responsible adolescent sexual behavior).

- Phase 3. Behavioral and Environmental Assessment: Identify and rank health-related behavioral risk factors and environmental risk conditions related to the goals/problems.

  Program: Risk factors and conditions were embarrassment, cost, accessibility, trusting partner, and partner refusal.

- Phase 4. Educational and Ecological Assessment: In relation to the goals/problems, identify factors that have potential to influence behavior or environment, and categorize factors as predisposing (knowledge, attitudes, values, beliefs, perceptions of individuals that can be altered through direct communication), enabling (skills, resources, or barriers controlled largely by societal forces and systems that make possible a change in behavior or environment), or reinforcing (feedback and rewards given to support changes made).

  Program: Predisposing factors were relationship skills, sexual health knowledge, and skills in condom use. Enabling factors were readily available condoms at low cost. Feedback and rewards were social support and college credit for involvement in peer education program.

- Phase 5. Administrative and Policy Assessment: Determine capabilities and resources available to develop and implement program.

  Program: Campus health and health department willing to collaborate and to provide funds, teaching time, educational material, and condoms for two years. College administration agreed to support the program (e.g., physical plant staff assistance).

- Phase 6. Implementation: Based on resources, select methods and strategies of interventions and implement.

  Program: Students, nurses, and faculty developed and implemented peer educational strategies for relationship skill building and sexual health knowledge, including condom skills. Faculty arranged credit for students involved. Condom machines ($0.25 per condom) were put in all washrooms.

- Phases 7, 8, 9. Process, Impact, and Outcome Evaluation: Respectively evaluate the implementation of the program, the immediate results, and the longer term results in terms of changes in quality of life for the target population (see section on evaluation for details on these types of evaluation).

  Program: Numerous issues arose in the implementation (e.g., maintenance of condom machines). Throughout implementation, opportunities to evaluate program activities were provided and activities were adjusted accordingly. At the end of two years, students were again interviewed and surveyed. Results were used to determine whether the program should be continued, changed, or stopped.

The depth developed in each phase of the model depends upon resources as well as goals. Although the model is conceptually complex, many practitioners have found it practical when they are dealing with multilevel community change. An advantage is that the model is well recognized by government agencies and funders and is available via computer program EMPOWER from Jones and Bartlett Publishers (www.jbpub.com). For more information about the model and its relationship to epidemiology, see Chapter 14.

More About Programming Practicalities

Whether a specific programming model or a more ad hoc approach is used, the nurse will benefit from additional organizational skills and knowledge about ways to actualize programs. The subsequent several sections focus on the practicalities of planning, implementation, and evaluation, with Health for All theory providing an underlay (see Table 16-3).

Program Planning

Program planning is the process of exploring the situation, deciding on a more desirable situation, and designing actions to create the desirable situation. Again, it is important to remember that in actual situations these processes are intertwined and, depending on the situation, the community and nurse may start with an issue, goal, idea for action, or assessment and work in a circular fashion to complete the picture. For example, a community group or agency may ask the nurse for assistance to decrease violence (goal), implement a heart health program (action), or assess the community to identify health issues and community capacities (community analysis and issues identification).

The nurse who is new to programming may be impatient to proceed to the "action" and do something about that which from the nurse's point of view is an obvious health problem or issue. But planning is action and should not be considered simply as a prelude to . . . action, although it does play a vital role in this respect. Not only does it have its own (intervention) implications, it is a process that continues through all

TABLE 16-3 Program Planning, Implementation, and Evaluation: Questions to Ask

PROGRAM PLANNING	PROGRAM IMPLEMENTATION	PROGRAM EVALUATION
Analyzing the Community What is the situation?	How can we ensure we do "good" and "no harm"? How can we keep things on track? How can we deal with the unexpected?	Was the program carried out as planned? What has changed as a result of the program? Were the results worth the effort? What is the situation now?
Identifying Issues What is important? Whose views have been heard? Whose views have not been heard? What issue is most important at this time? What are the parts of the issue? Why does the issue exist?		
Clarifying Goals What would be a more desirable situation? What do we want to happen?		
Designing Actions What should be done to create the more desirable situation? What resources are needed, and where can they be obtained? Who can do what?		

action phases, making a total programme more purposeful, giving it a greater direction, increasing its amenability to control, and yielding a clearer vision of its effectiveness. (Steuart, 1959/1993, p. S22)

An analogy can be made between planning a health program and creating an architectural design for a building. The more carefully the architects consult with the people for whom the building is being constructed, the greater the likelihood that the building will be satisfactory to those people. The more clearly specified the vision of that which is wanted, the more likely the vision's realization. Although it is impossible to anticipate and plan ahead for everything, the more thoroughly the components are detailed and possible pitfalls are anticipated, the greater the chance that the actual building process will proceed smoothly and the building will meet the needs of the clients. Also, the more the architects attend to the physical and social environments where the building is to be located, the more likely the building will be compatible with the environment, appreciated by the neighbors, and viewed as an overall positive addition to the neighborhood. It is much the same with program planning.

To carry the analogy a bit further, if a social planning approach were to be used, the architects might bring one or several building plans for consideration, oversee the project, and provide expert assistance; the people for whom the building is being constructed might, in turn, suggest alterations and provide information about preferred choices throughout. In a community development approach, the architects might work to assist the people to plan and build the building themselves and provide assistance as needed and as negotiated. In a social action approach, the architects might join with the people in lobbying to get resources and to change zoning in a neighborhood so that the desired and needed building can be constructed in the location where it is most needed.

Community Analysis

What is the situation?

Community analysis or assessment, that is, exploring the community situation, for programming purposes may be done in a comprehensive, largely "up-front" way or in more targeted or ongoing ways as people come together to plan and more information is needed. Assessment frameworks are developed from particular perspectives. Assessment consistent with Health for All strategies focuses on community competence as much as (or more than) needs. And, of course, the community and the nurse work in partnership to determine ways and times to best accomplish assessments. McKnight and Kretzmann (1992) describe ways to map community capacity so that communities can be built "from the inside out," thereby increasing community competence rather than community dependence on outside services.

In the United States, the Assessment Protocol for Excellence in Public Health (APEX/PH) tool was developed by local health departments in response to the recommendation that all departments regularly and systematically evaluate community needs; the Protocol for Assessing Community Excellence in Environmental Health (PACE-EH) is an additional tool for assessing community perceptions and environmental conditions (by the National Association of County & City Health Officials) (McKenzie & Smeltzer, 2001). APEX-PH and, more recently, PACE-EH have been used to collect communitywide data that can provide valuable information for community health programs. Similar data sources are available in many countries. Chapter 15 includes a comprehensive discussion of community assessment.

Identifying Issues

What is important?

Whose views have been heard?

Whose views have not been heard?

What issue is most important at this time?

What are the parts of the issue?

Why does the issue exist?

Issues of interest or concern must be identified. Freire's problem-posing dialogue can be helpful for doing so, especially if the participants are struggling to identify the determinants of an issue. When a more desirable situation is envisioned, action plans (community development and social action language) or intervention strategies (social planning language) can then be developed to change the current situation.

Planning should not proceed unless there is strong consensus within the community that the issue in question is a priority. Because communities often are not homogeneous, achieving a shared view may take time. Nurses sometimes are sent to a community to address an issue or problem that has been identified outside the community; for example, a nurse working for a public health service may be asked to develop an immunization program or a wellness program for teens. Dialogue around any such issue must occur to foster community ownership of the issue and the solutions. Often, a nurse or agency issue is intertwined with an issue of priority to the community. After the community connects with an issue, the community and nurse can proceed to work together. If the community does not connect with an externally identified issue, the nurse must either drop or delay that issue and instead address the priorities of the community. Why should the community become involved with something that is not important to them?

Information-generating strategies that nurses can use in assisting a community to clarify and rank issues include community forums, focus groups, nominal group processes, Delphi techniques, key informant interviews, and surveys (see Chapter 15). These strategies also can be used to uncover community views on program goals and preferred actions to achieve those goals. There is no one right way to use these strategies.

Nominal Group Process

Nominal group process can be particularly helpful when consensus decisions must be made at a community meeting by people who have varying levels of skill at expressing themselves in groups. One way of using nominal group process is to ask the group to brainstorm by having each person contribute an idea (possibly in round-robin style) until everyone has exhausted all their ideas. During brainstorming, the group is encouraged not to censor any ideas but, rather, to bring forward as many ideas as possible. All ideas are written down (e.g., on chalkboards or large paper fastened to the wall). After brainstorming, time is taken for people to clarify (but not debate) the proposed ideas. Everyone is then invited to vote for the ideas that they think are priorities (or best action strategies). Voting can be achieved by giving everyone a marker or a predetermined number of stickers and asking them to mark ideas as they walk around the room during a refreshment break. The priority ideas are then discussed, and plans are developed. Remaining ideas are recorded for possible consideration another time (Delbecq, 1983).

Delphi Technique

The Delphi technique is a multistep survey method that is useful for identifying issues of importance and achieving consensus when it is not practical for people to meet face to face. Advantages are that input is obtained via regular or electronic mail and everyone is given equal chances for input without undue influence from other participants. A limitation is that participants must be comfortable with reading and writing and prompt about returning mail. Participants receive initial questions, data are analyzed, results (issues identified and rankings) and any new questions arising are returned to participants for further comment, and so on, until adequate information and consensus are obtained. Sometimes a planning group generates the first list of issues; other times, one or two broad questions are asked: for example, What are the most important health issues in your community? Why do these issues exist? Following the Delphi, program planning proceeds around the top ranked issues. Three survey rounds are average; occasionally more rounds are needed (Dignan & Carr, 1992).

Fostering Participation

The people who are hardest to reach are sometimes neglected in the planning phase. These people, who often do not come to events such as community forums, may be the most marginalized or at risk—and may be the people whom the program is most intended to benefit. Bracht (1990) argues that it is the practitioner who finds it "hard to hear" rather than the client who is "hard to reach" (p. 256). Whatever must be done to make early, meaningful connections with these people should be done. Much time has been wasted planning programs for people who have not participated in the process, with program failure a common result. Skelton (1994) speaks of empowerment in terms of the power of voice and exit: that is, being heard and leaving or not participating. From this point of view, nonparticipation may be seen as positive for the participants and as requiring a change in the nurse's approach. If the planning phase is not appropriately welcoming for people, why should they later be receptive to intervention strategies?

A method of fostering participation (and voice) among seniors was incorporated in one community development project, in which one of the authors (Cameron) participated. A steering committee with a balance of seniors and practitioners was formed. Community forums were held in settings frequented by seniors. Those who came to community forums were invited to join a networking process whereby they designed questions, practiced interviewing, and then went into the community to interview other seniors. Through snowball sampling, interviewees suggested additional names of people who had not participated (e.g., house-bound seniors). The interviewers were paid as research assistants from a government grant. Opportunities for empowerment and increased community competence among seniors are apparent in this method, and, not surprisingly, meaningful information was gained about seniors' views and wishes (goals).

Clarifying Goals

What would be a more desirable situation?

What do we want to happen?

Communities sometimes express their goals broadly. For example, the community may want children to grow up healthier. In this case, further exploration is required to identify factors that are influencing the situation (e.g., poor food or a lack of safe places to play and learn). Sometimes called targeted assessment, this more specific exploration ensures that action strategies can be sensitively designed to achieve desired results. Action strategies are different depending on the determinants. Goals are general statements about that which is desired (e.g.,

to improve the health of children). More specific and detailed subgoals (termed objectives in social planning language) can provide better direction for the action plan (e.g., to provide adequate daily nutrition for all children). Although familiarity with this more formal programming language is a necessity, the nurse must not use such language in a way that obscures meaning for those involved. Program goals and objectives become the intended results (see the discussion on diagrammatic models).

Program subgoals, or objectives, may be devised for all factors that influence an issue, thereby interconnecting the subgoals with the achievement of the overall goals. For example, for the goal to improve children's health, subgoals or objectives might be, for all community children, to provide adequate daily nutrition and exercise, to immunize against common communicable diseases, to create equitable access to education, and to provide a safe environment at home and school. Priorities can then be established relative to importance and resource availability. In doing so, it is helpful to consider both significance and likelihood of achieving success. The first objective may be to identify and mobilize resources. When possible, objectives are phrased to specify the desired results, those persons being targeted, and the time frame; for example, in community X, immunize for influenza 90% of adults 65 years and older by December 1. This degree of specificity is not always possible (e.g., when activities are not easily quantified) and also may not always be helpful (e.g., early in programming or in certain community development programs). After goals and objectives are established to the degree of specificity appropriate, alternative strategies for achieving them are considered and, finally, actions are selected for implementation.

For U.S. nurses, the national goals and objectives outlined in *Healthy People 2010* documents are very helpful, because they target specific priority needs of the U.S. population, as identified by a cross section of practitioners and interested citizens (USDHSS, 2000). For example, Objective 24-6 is to increase the proportion of persons with asthma who receive formal patient education, including information about community and self-help resources, as an essential part of the management of their conditions (target 30%, baseline 8.4%, in 1999). In Canada, health goals have been identified nationally and provincially, but objectives often are not specified numerically (Provincial Health Officer, 2000). Although national goals and objectives tend to be oriented to a social planning model, community development approaches may be integrated to increase community control. For example, in one of the poorest and underserved neighborhoods in Canada, nurses joined with neighborhood people for an immunization and harm reduction blitz (e.g., condoms, needle exchange, health information) that reached 8500 people in five weeks

(Munroe, 2000). Entry to the inner neighborhood was guided by neighborhood volunteers working side by side with nurses; immunizations were given in bars and food lines and on the street. Neighborhood people assisted with records and supply management. The program would not have been successful without the guidance and assistance of the neighborhood people; both health agency and neighborhood participants were so pleased that another blitz has been planned.

To use the *Healthy People 2010* objectives (USDHSS, 2000) in a community development process, the community might evaluate how well they meet national or state objectives, decide the significance of the objectives for them, and use gaps as starting points for action. Communities also could be encouraged to think about health care in a different way via introduction to the primary health care model. *Healthy People 2010* describes many programs across the United States that are helping the country move toward Health for All goals. Nurses in other countries also may find the *Healthy People 2010* documents useful because of their comprehensiveness and specificity.

In programming, keeping information organized is an important task. A chart with columns or a diagrammatic model can be used to keep track of goals, objectives, corresponding actions, and desired outcomes. The formality of the documentation will vary depending on the complexity of the program and those who will be using the chart. For example, handwritten lists or diagrams using plain terms may be appropriate for one program (e.g., a community development program for homeless children who live on the streets), whereas typewritten documents using practitioner/bureaucratic language may be appropriate for another program (e.g., a citywide program for sexually transmitted disease prevention).

Designing Actions

What should be done to create the more desirable situation?

What resources are needed, and where can they be obtained?

Who can do what?

Many choices confront nurses and communities as they decide which actions or intervention strategies will be used to achieve the desired results. Programs may include, for example, health education, environmental change, health assessment, immunization, risk screening, illness management, political action, regulatory activities, advocacy, and the like. Each of the change theories and programming models is associated with (but not limited to) particular action strategies. For example, health education and social marketing (e.g., public awareness campaigns) are associated with social planning; these strategies are used in nationwide school and media initiatives in the United States and Canada to stop drinking and driving. Social action commonly uses lobbying strategies such as letter writing and telephone campaigns to change policy, laws, and regulations. Community development uses strategies such as community forums where critical dialogue is supported.

Questions regarding appropriate strategies must be considered simultaneously with questions about resources, including people and time. This tends to be an iterative (back-and-forth) process involving consideration of those strategies that would likely achieve the desired results, the resources that would be required, and the likelihood of getting those resources. Adjustments are made until all three aspects are in reasonable accord. The use of diagrammatic models can be helpful in this process.

Many kinds of action strategies can be created, and imagination is an essential ingredient. Actions may be targeted to change any relevant health determinants. When nurses and their community partners find themselves at a loss to answer the question "What can be done to improve this situation?" use of the theories discussed earlier may generate possibilities. Community pressures and problems—and the efforts to improve them—are seldom completely unique to any one setting. Valuable ideas may be garnered by investigating the approaches being used elsewhere. Searching the literature is one strategy for making such connections; networking via word of mouth, the Internet (Nicoll, 2001), and the telephone is another strategy.

Resources, Budgets, and Feasibility

Resources should be sought both within and outside the community. Capacities within the community may be thought of as resources and, to promote community self-reliance, should be considered before looking for resources outside the community (McKnight & Kretzmann, 1992). For example, a community kitchen program to help teen parents may be well served by having experienced older people or students from a cooking school take turns teaching, rather than bringing in outside assistance. Possible sources of support both within and outside of the community include businesses, social and professional clubs, volunteers, community institutions, and agencies such as churches, schools, colleges, hospitals, and mental health and social services. People will create and mobilize resources and take on a multitude of tasks to achieve goals that are meaningful to them. And, of course, the skills and time the nurse will commit to the program must be counted.

Programs involving volunteers of all sorts are becoming popular as a way to contain costs and, hopefully, support community empowerment (Hutchison & Quartaro, 1995). This is an example where the art of programming is important. To help justify the use of their valuable energy toward a given program, volunteers must benefit from their involvement in some way. The community health nurse can ask volunteers to think about those things that they would find beneficial. For example, in the neighborhood blitz described earlier, volunteers were provided with lunch and honorarium.

To be feasible, a program must have adequate resources. Resource needs can be determined by noting the resources required next to each action strategy. Expenses can then be listed next to the resources, and a budget can be prepared. A budget lists expenses (costs for the resources required) and expected income (available funds or donations) and income sources (see Table 16-4). Resource documents must be updated on an ongoing basis; the complexity of such documentation varies with the nature of the program. Resource documents guide the distribution and tracking of program resources and are also useful when applying for resources (e.g., for funding from an agency) and when compiling program reports (see Figures 16-16 and 16-17).

Managing Tasks and Time

Program planning must be linked with time estimates and task specification. Preliminary time frames are developed on the basis of any fixed time requirements. For example, if students are involved, note when the students must have their work completed; if elders need immunizations prior to flu season, note when the immunizations should be finished; or if an agency has provided funding for a project, note when a final report is expected. From fixed time requirements, the nurse and community can work backward to the present; if there are no time requirements, working forward from the present is possible.

Time and task management tools may be used during all phases of programming and are especially helpful when a number of people are working on different aspects of the program. All tools can be modified, for example in terms of the language used. A simple tool can be created by expanding diagrammatic models or the previously described chart that lists goals, objectives, and action strategies. Timelines indicate tasks or activities that must be done and by whom and when. Making an optimistic and an alternative timeline (if things take longer)

TABLE 16-4 Community Health: Indicator Categories

A: Determinants

Sustainability
  Energy use
  Water consumption
  Renewable resource consumption
  Waste production and reduction
  Local production
  Land use
  Ecosystem health

Viability
  Air quality
  Water quality
  Toxics production and use
  Soil contamination
  Food chain contamination

Livability
  Housing
  Density
  Community safety and security
  Transportation
  Walkability
  Green/open space
  Smoke-free space
  Noise pollution

Conviviality
  Family safety and security
  Sense of neighborhood
  Social support networks
  Charitable donations
  Public services
  Demographics

Equity
  Economic disparity
  Housing affordability
  Discrimination and exclusion
  Access to power

Prosperity
  A diverse economy
  Local control
  Employment/unemployment
  Quality of employment
  Traditional economic indicators

B: Processes

Education
  Early childhood development
  Education/school quality
  Adult literacy
  Lifelong learning

Governance
  Voluntarism/associational life
  Citizen action
  Human and civil rights
  Voter turnout
  Perception of government leaders
    and services
  Healthy public policy

C: Health Status

Quality of life
  Well-being
  Life satisfaction
  Happiness

Mastery/self-esteem/coherence

Health-promoting behaviors

Disability/morbidity
  Stress/anxiety
  Other morbidity/disability measures
  Health utility index

Mortality
  Overall mortality rate
  Infant mortality rate
  Suicide rate

From "Indicators That Count! Measuring Population Health at the Community Level," by T. Hancock, R. Labonte, and R. Edwards, 1999, Canadian Journal of Public Health, 90 (Suppl. 1), p. S24. Copyright 1999 by Canadian Public Health Association. Reprinted with permission.

Note: *The indicators were developed for the Health and Community Ecosystem Model, Figure 16-3.*

FIGURE 16-16 Gantt Chart and Budget for Public Awareness Program

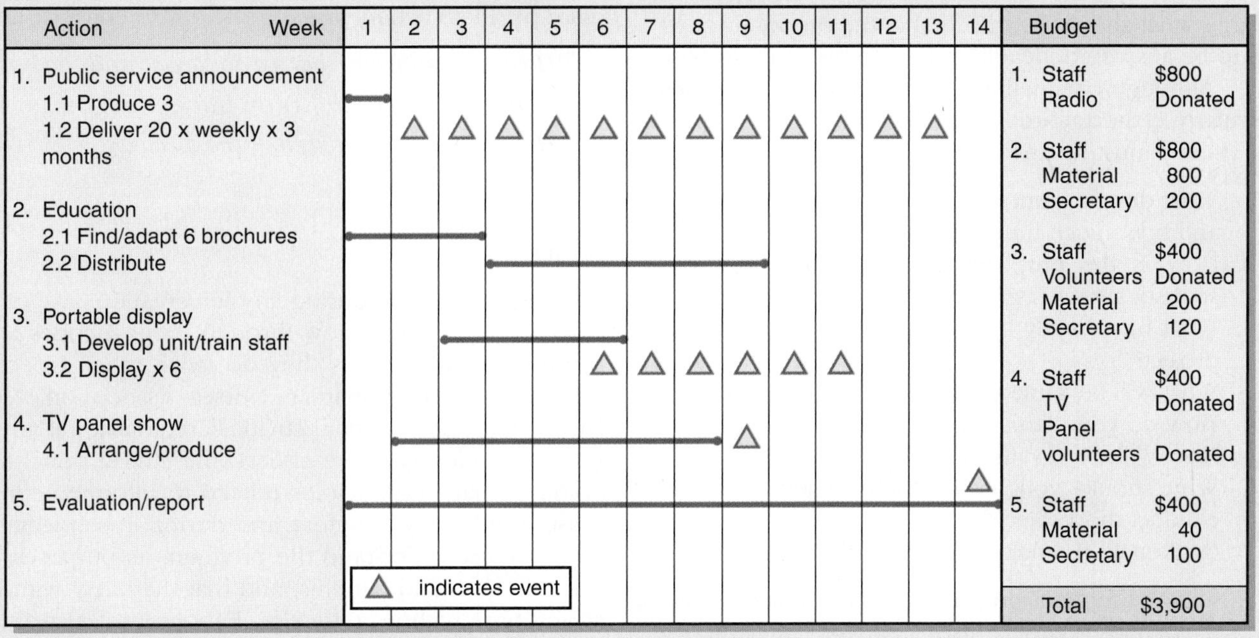
Action
Week
1
2
3
4
5
6
7
8
9
10
11
12
13
14
Budget
1. Public service announcement
1.1 Produce 3
1.2 Deliver 20 x weekly x 3 months
2. Education
2.1 Find/adapt 6 brochures
2.2 Distribute
3. Portable display
3.1 Develop unit/train staff
3.2 Display x 6
4. TV panel show
4.1 Arrange/produce
5. Evaluation/report
indicates event
1. Staff $800
Radio Donated
2. Staff $800
Material 800
Secretary 200
3. Staff $400
Volunteers Donated
Material 200
Secretary 120
4. Staff $400
TV Donated
Panel volunteers Donated
5. Staff $400
Material 40
Secretary 100
Total $3,900

FIGURE 16-17 Sample Budget

Income/Resources

Funding	______	
Grants	______	
Donations	______	
	Subtotal	$______

Expenses

Staff	______	
Supplies	______	
Equipment	______	
Space	______	
	Subtotal	$______
	Balance(+/−)	$______

may be wise. As with all aspects of programming, flexibility is needed in combination with goal directedness.

A commonly used time and task management tool is a Gantt chart, which has the tasks to be completed listed on the vertical axis and the time periods (days, weeks, months) marked on the horizontal axis (Hale, Arnold, & Travis, 1994). Dots indicate the start and completion points for each task, and the connecting line provides a visual indicator of the time period estimated (see Figure 16-16). Gantt charts now are available in work management computer software programs.

Grant Writing

To get adequate resources for a program, nurses may need to submit a proposal to an agency or foundation that grants funds for health programs. Sometimes nurses submit proposals to their own employing agency. A grant proposal is simply a written request for money (and occasionally for other resources). Writing a grant proposal is a systematic, step-by-step process (McKenzie & Smeltzer, 2001, p. 226):

- Locate grant money.
- Find out how to apply for it.
- Write a request, i.e., proposal.

A source must be found that grants funds for the kind of program the nurse is undertaking. For example, a community service group, such as Kiwanis, may focus on helping children and be willing to fund a program to improve youth health in a community, or a cancer society will fund a smoking prevention program. Local, state or provincial, and national sources may also have funds available (see Appendix A for an inventory of U.S., Canadian, and other national sources). Also, funding agencies may send out requests for proposals; nurses need to watch for these and be prepared to work in a short time frame.

After a potential funding source is located, it is a good idea to contact the funding agency to discuss whether the nurse's program idea "fits well" with agency interests and to clarify what should be included in the proposal (questions to be answered, deadlines for submissions, and format). Although guidelines vary among agencies, particularly in the amount of detail required, certain questions usually must be answered:

1. What do you want to do, how much will it cost, and how much time will it take?
2. How is the proposed project related to the sponsor's interests?
3. What has already been done in the area of the project?
4. What will be gained if this project is carried out?
5. How do you plan to do it?
6. How will the results be evaluated?
7. Why should you, rather than someone else, conduct this project?
(McKenzie & Smeltzer, 2001, p. 228)

In writing the grant proposal, the wise nurse follows agency guidelines precisely, uses language familiar to the agency, and makes use of any work already completed (e.g., a Gantt chart developed with a community). Accuracy, clarity, and appearance (grammar and spelling) are important because the reviewer must make a judgment based on what is visible and competition for funds usually is keen (similar to a job application). Helpful strategies for improving the quality of a proposal are to ask others (respected colleagues or persons familiar with the agency) to critique your proposal prior to submission and also to review a proposal that was previously funded by the agency.

Documenting Programs

Record keeping should be accurate and designed specifically to support programming processes and program activities. Program documentation is comparable to record keeping for individual clients in agencies, although community participants may maintain the records themselves, and records may be kept open to all participants. Record keeping can serve to promote participation. Both quantitative data (objective measures such as dates of meetings and numbers of participants) and qualitative data (verbal descriptions, journals, pictures, and case stories) can be used to document processes and program activities.

Keeping a simple journal can assist the nurse in tracking actions and the nurse's critical reflection on processes and events. Documentation can save time and prevent conflict by recording previous decisions, meeting attendees, and discussions among attendees. Documentation is also a rich source of data for program evaluation because it serves as a record of those things that actually occurred. Accuracy and usefulness are improved when documents are compiled promptly.

Program Implementation

Program implementation is the process of putting the program plan into action. Some questions to consider are:

How can we ensure that we do "good" and "no harm"?

How can we keep things on track?

How can we deal with the unexpected?

Ethics

Of special interest during implementation are ethical considerations and follow-through. Ethical codes apply in programming just as they do in all other aspects of nursing practice (Canadian Nurses Association, 1997). Nurses must ensure that activities are adjusted if anyone is experiencing negative effects (the ethical principle of doing no harm). Principles related to informed consent must be adhered to before and during implementation. People must understand the program, its purposes, any possible risks and benefits, and that they may withdraw at any time without difficulty. People must also understand confidentiality and negligence (failure of a person to act in a reasonable manner given the accepted standards of conduct for persons with the same qualifications and background). Safety issues must be considered throughout; for example, people who work in high-crime neighborhoods must take precautions such as traveling in pairs and during daylight hours, and meetings must be held in locations offering safe and easy access.

Follow-Through and Dealing with the Unexpected

The implementation of a program may be time limited (e.g., a six-week healthy lifestyles program or a six-month letter-writing campaign) or may occur over a long period and in a more intermittent manner (e.g., a community development project that takes place over a period of many months). Structured social planning or social action interventions may be piloted, phased in over time, or implemented in totality (McKenzie & Smeltzer, 2001). Tasks, time, and resources must be carefully monitored during implementation (e.g., staying within budget).

Just as they did in earlier processes, the concepts of partnership and participation apply during the implementation process (e.g., getting people together regularly to refresh their sense of purpose and humor). All involved should be invited to use their observation skills to ensure that actions are implemented as planned or adjusted as necessary to keep the actions moving toward the desired result.

With community work, the follow-through process is sometimes like trying to keep an eye on a ball when the ball is moving in an unpredictable pattern and the playing field is full of hills and gullies. Continue to listen, negotiate, and deal promptly with differences and conflicts. If the program must continue after the nurse's involvement has ceased, community follow-through and its long-term implications should be incorporated into planning to ensure program continuity after the nurse leaves (Shediac-Rizkallah & Bone, 1998).

Program Evaluation

Was the program carried out as planned?

What has changed as a result of the program?

Were the results worth the effort?

What is the situation now?

What should be done next?

Program evaluation is a process to assess the performance of a program (Dignan & Carr, 1992, p. 143). Health care programs commonly are evaluated in terms of three dimensions (Mullet, 1995):

- Responsiveness: how well the program dealt with the issues which gave rise to the program

- Effectiveness: the extent to which desired outcomes were achieved

- Efficiency: whether as much as possible was achieved, with the least use of resources

Evaluation of these dimensions is rarely straightforward.

A systematic sequence of activities is performed to complete an evaluation: choosing questions to be answered, creating an evaluation plan or design, deciding the kinds of data needed to answer the questions and ways of obtaining these data, collecting and analyzing the data, and interpreting the results. There is no set of fixed rules to apply; rather, evaluation approaches must be flexible to permit answering of the most important questions (Dignan & Carr, 1992). Nurses must remember that different questions are important to different stakeholder groups. Use of basic research principles (including ethics) will ensure both rigor and relevance. Method selection from quantitative (empirical analytic), qualitative (interpretive), and participatory action (critical) research traditions facilitates appropriate evaluation of any program. The selection of specific methods should be based on the nature of the evaluation questions.

The extent of evaluation possible is largely determined by resource availability. An allocation of 10% of the program budget for evaluation is recommended (WHO European Working Group, 1998). Resource considerations must include appropriate expertise to design and conduct the evaluation. If people working directly with the program do not have the necessary expertise, they should find an external consultant who does. University faculty and private consultants usually can be found. Practitioners and community people are sometimes reluctant to designate resources for evaluation, preferring instead to see the resources used to enhance the program. In response, the nurse-programmer might ask the question "Why would you want to do more until you know the effectiveness of what you are already doing?"

Evaluation Types

Evaluation may be formative, occurring throughout all programming processes, or summative, occurring at an end point. **Formative evaluation** provides information to those planning and implementing the program "along the way" and permits improvements to the program while activities are in progress. **Summative evaluation** provides retrospective information about the performance of the program up to the point when the evaluation was completed. Summative evaluation is more likely to be used to make decisions about whether the program should continue and, if so, with what changes. According to Pirie (1990), it is important to inform program stakeholders that evaluation results are not the only factor in such decisions; for example, budget cuts and political pressures may result in the termination of a successful program.

Evaluation is frequently conceptualized in terms of process, structure, impact, and outcomes. Donabedian (1996) developed this now classic framework to study the quality of medical care. *Process* is the term used to describe all the activities undertaken to produce change. **Process evaluation** answers the question "Was the program implemented as planned?" If not, what was altered and why?" The evaluator will want to know, so that implementation issues can be understood. Programs are rarely implemented exactly as planned. For example, a program activity may be altered based on formative evaluation, such as changes in a parenting program based on participants' midterm feedback.

Structure is the term used for all the resources required to support the program process. **Structural evaluation** is the assessment of resources used in the

---

✳ DECISION MAKING

Disaster Planning: What Applies?

You have been invited to join a committee to design a disaster plan for a small town.

◆ Drawing on your community health programming knowledge, what ideas, principles, and processes do you think might prove useful in this different programming context?

◆ What ideas would likely not prove useful or would need modification?

program. Data about structures (sometimes called maps) are used to help determine costs. Process and structural evaluations provide an essential underlay for outcome evaluation because the interpretation of program outcomes rests on an understanding of the program as it occurred. The program could erroneously be judged as unsuccessful when, in fact, it was not fully implemented.

Outcomes are the results of the program. **Outcome evaluation** is the determination of program results at different points in time. The terms *outcome* and *impacts* are sometimes used interchangeably and sometimes to reflect time differences. Immediate and short-term outcomes are assessed close to the program to determine whether the results were the effects intended (e.g., on completion of a smoking cessation program, the number of participants who quit smoking). In the longer term, outcomes are assessed to determine whether changes further from the program, occurred as intended (e.g., one year later, the number of participants who were not smoking). Long-term outcome evaluation requires resources for longitudinal tracking. Sensitive indicators of impacts and outcomes are selected on the basis of the following questions:

What changes are reasonable to expect?

What would indicate that the program resulted in changes?

What would permit discovery of unexpected changes?

Sensitive indicators identify the information that would reveal the changes being created by program activities. Indicators might be, for example, safety, behavior, quality of life, health-related policies, participation, individual health status, population health status, use of

✳ DECISION MAKING

Sensitive Indicators

You are a resource person for a self-help support group for people experiencing chronic pain. Group members are helping each other manage pain by sharing ideas and encouragement. At the group's request, you have invited different health care practitioners (e.g., Therapeutic Touch, massage, medical, physiotherapy) to share their approaches. Group members also are working to change the regional government's compensation policy, which restricts benefits for persons who experience chronic pain following on-the-job injuries.

◆ What indicators might be sensitive to and reflect changes resulting from the group activities?

resources, and the like. Satisfaction of stakeholders may or may not be a good indicator of program success (e.g., parents of teens may not be satisfied about condom machines in school washrooms, but the program may help prevent disease and unwanted pregnancy). (See Table 16-4 for indicators developed for an ecological community health model.)

Evaluation As Comparison

Evaluation is a process ultimately intended to determine the worth of something, presumably in comparison with some norm or standard of "goodness." In program evaluation, comparison may be made with:

- A similar program (e.g., comparing one nursing center with another);
- A different program (e.g., comparing weight gains of infants going home on an early maternity discharge program with weight gains of infants who are kept longer in the hospital);
- Established norms (e.g., comparing condom use by local teens with condom use by teens as reflected in national data);
- Established practice and outcome standards (e.g., best practices, benchmarks);
- Pre- and postprogram assessments (e.g., nutritional patterns of college students before and after the lowering of cafeteria prices for healthy foods);
- The same program over time (e.g., utilization statistics, historical record keeping, and periodic inventories that permit comparison with previous performance) (Green & Kreuter, 1999).

Quality assurance and quality improvement are well known evaluation approaches based on comparisons with established practice and outcome standards and changes over time within the same program (see Chapter 17). Appropriate comparisons can be difficult to make with many community programs because of the complexity of situations (e.g., transient community members); comparisons also can be challenging with new innovative programs (Hilton, Budgen, Molzahn, & Attridge, 2001). When comparisons cannot be made in a straightforward way, creativity is helpful (e.g., the nurse may consider that which would likely have happened to the people or in the community if the program had not been implemented and provide evidence to substantiate the answer).

Another evaluation approach based on comparison is the tracer method (Kaluzney & Veney, 1999). A health problem is traced through the community or population and comparisons are made with population subgroups and variables such as socioeconomic conditions, gender, age, health care access, and the like. The method is analogous to the use of radiopaque tracers in biomedical care which indicate the health of organs and glands. The tracing of smoking behavior through a population is described in the section on "upstream" programming. The picture of the problem revealed in the tracing can provide information about causative factors and, also, the effectiveness of health care programs that are implemented to reduce the problem.

Health Promotion Evaluation

According to the WHO European Working Group, evaluation of health promotion programs should be participatory; use multiple methods; focus on capacity building of individuals, communities, organizations, and governments; and be appropriate to the complexity (WHO, 1998, p. v). Participatory evaluation approaches increase the likelihood that results will be directly useful in creating community change. Both process and outcome evaluations are recommended. Considerable progress has been made in the development of participatory methods, and these methods are becoming more accepted by funders (Butler & Marquis, 1998; Labonte, Feather, & Hills, 1999; Lindsey, Sheilds, & Stajduhar, 1999; Smith, 1998).

Data Sources and Collection Methods

After the type of evaluation and overall evaluation questions have been decided, the next step is selection of data sources and data collection methods. Data already collected for purposes of assessment, planning, and implementation should be used for evaluation whenever possible. For example, assessment data may have been gathered about community health status during program planning; after program implementation, these same kinds of data may be gathered and a before-and-after comparison performed.

Data sources usually are people and documents; collection methods include interviews, focus groups, observations, and surveys. Standardized tools may be used or tools may be created specifically for the program. As appreciation increases for clients' rights, abilities, and responsibilities, the subjective perspectives of program participants are becoming more valued by programmers and funders. Nurses must ensure that the participants' experiences with the program are understood as fully as possible from their perspectives. This has been an ongoing struggle in evaluation (e.g., in quality assurance programs) that is only now being addressed through use of critical and interpretive (qualitative) inquiry methods.

All program documentation has potential for use in evaluation (e.g., records of meetings and group sessions, letters, media coverage, pictures). Nurses are encouraged to use innovative as well as traditional data sources and collection methods.

Evaluation Models

As much as is possible, evaluations must be designed to answer questions pertinent to each of the stakeholder groups, for example practitioners, various groups of community people, agencies, and funding bodies. Each group will likely be interested in different aspects of the evaluation; dissemination of findings to these groups may therefore require the preparation of separate reports and recommendations. Funders generally want quantified information derived from measurements of risk factor and risk condition reduction or improvements in health. In some situations, providing such information is not feasible; in other instances, that which is important to health cannot be quantifiably measured. Because funders deal primarily in these terms, however, the nurse must find a way to translate the effects of the program into terms meaningful to funders (or others).

Numerous models for program evaluation exist. Diagrammatic models developed earlier in the process may be used to guide evaluation. Two evaluation frameworks that are useful in the current health care context are those of Pirie and Mullett. Pirie (1990) designed a series of questions to ensure that evaluation information would be directly useful "to people and their programs" (p. 201). The questions as outlined below have been altered to reflect a partnership, health-promoting style of relating.

- *Questions for the planning stage:*
  Why should this program be developed?
  Are the resources appropriate?

- *Questions for the program implementation stage:*
  Is the program being implemented as planned?
  Is the program reaching the people/organizations intended?
  Who is the program failing to reach and why?
  What are participants' views about the program?
  Are participants satisfied with their experience?

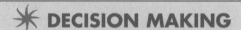

☀ DECISION MAKING

Evaluation

A community agency funding a public awareness program for HIV prevention in heterosexual women has asked you for advice about the evaluation (see Figures 16-13 and 16-16 for program activities, desired results, evaluation budget, and timeline).

◆ Given the limited evaluation budget and short timeline, which types of evaluation would you recommend?

◆ What comparisons might be made?

◆ What data sources and collection methods might be used?

FIGURE 16-18 Program Performance Evaluation Framework

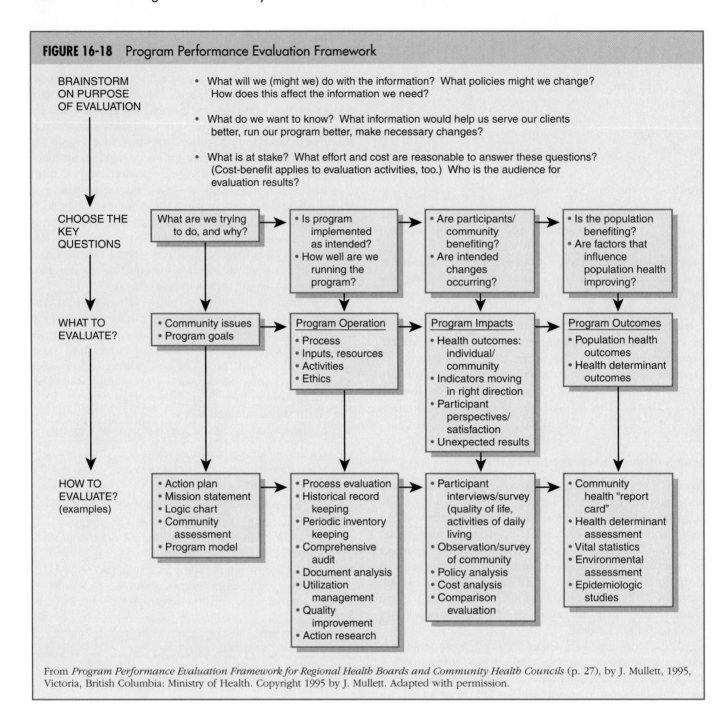

From *Program Performance Evaluation Framework for Regional Health Boards and Community Health Councils* (p. 27), by J. Mullett, 1995, Victoria, British Columbia: Ministry of Health. Copyright 1995 by J. Mullett. Adapted with permission.

- *Questions about program outcomes:*
  What, if anything, is changing as a result of the program?
  Is the program having the effects it was designed to have?

Based on these general questions, nurses and their community partners can design specific evaluation questions relevant to their programs or these general questions may be used "as is" in interviews and surveys. This framework can be used to guide summative evaluation by altering the tense of questions.

A framework developed by Mullett (1995) for British Columbia's health care reform effort is intended to be a user-friendly evaluation guide for a broad range of health programs and stakeholders (see Figure 16-18). This

RESEARCH FOCUS

Effectiveness of Community-Directed Diabetes Prevention and Control in a Rural Aboriginal Population

Study Problem/Purpose

The increasing prevalence of non–insulin-dependent diabetes mellitus (NIDDM) in native Canadian populations is having profoundly negative health impacts. The strongest risk factors for NIDDM are lifestyle related, including obesity, physical inactivity, and inappropriate diet. Lifestyle is shaped by the cultural, health, social, educational, and economic environment of the community. In response to the problem, a community-based diabetes prevention and control project of 24 months duration was initiated. General aims of the project were to modify risk factors, encourage meaningful community participation, develop culturally relevant interventions, and enable the community to assume responsibility upon completion of the project. The project was federally funded (NHRDP-Canada).

Methods

The study combined community development, participatory action research approaches, and quasi-experimental design. An intervention community and two control communities were chosen so that comparisons could be made. Sites were semirural Okanagan First Nations communities. The intervention community had a population of 707, high-risk cohort $n = 62$; the two control communities, 659 total population, high-risk cohort $n = 43$. The research team included six native tribe members from the study community, one native nurse, a diabetes nurse specialist, two nursing faculty members, and a doctoral student. An advisory team of eight community members worked with the research team. Nursing students worked as research assistants.

A seven-month preintervention included training of workers and interaction with the communities to achieve mutual understanding of the situation. Measurements of physiological, anthropometric, and behavioral variables among established diabetics and persons at familial risk were taken prior to and at two points after the 16-month intervention. Program implementation consisted of socioenvironmental and behavioral inter-ventions designed by the community and research team together. Interventions stressed individual and community strengths and capabilities to deal with diabetes. Interventions comprised numerous communitywide, group, and individual activities combining exercise, education, nutrition, smoking cessation, and social interaction activities. An array of people with special knowledge and skills participated in health activities (community members of all ages, tribal council, media, diabetic/heart/cancer associations, grocery stores, health practitioners, etc.). Over the duration of the study, quantitative and qualitative data were collected via minimally structured interviews, lifestyle surveys, blood tests, blood pressure readings, anthropometric measures, and observation.

Findings

Prior to the interventions the communities had limited knowledge about healthy lifestyles and diabetes. This was also true of those members with diabetes. Following the interventions knowledge increased; health-promoting activities were designed and people participated; outside resource people were invited into the community for the first time; the tribal council hired a full-time recreation coordinator; and several activities have continued after the project. One continuing activity is a walking event in remembrance of a beloved native research team member who was killed near the end of the study; the walk has been held yearly. Approximately 200 people (20% of community) have participated each time.

Community members reported that they are developing a sense of community cohesiveness and of possibilities and that internal community conflict is decreasing. These data were provided during open interviews, rather than via questionnaires. Although efforts were made to adapt the questionnaires to the cultural perspective of the community, participants reported "hating" filling out the questionnaires. Among high-risk cohorts, although individuals reported that their lives were "getting better" and that they were hopeful for the future, individual behavior and physiological status did not improve.

(continues)

Implications

The project was not successful in reducing risk factors in the high-risk cohort. The project was successful at helping the community increase competence, mobilize resources, and begin to change their social and political environments in directions supportive of healthy lifestyles. The change theories on which the study was based suggest that environmental and lifestyle changes take considerable time, especially with populations who have been severely marginalized. The project likely was too short. Also, interventions must be powerful enough to create the desired changes. Because the interventions were largely carried out by community people who were themselves learning about diabetes and modification of environments and lifestyles, the interventions may not have been strong enough. The researchers concluded that replication of the study over a longer period and with increased intervention strength and measurement tools more appropriate to the people and the community is warranted.

Source: Daniel, M., Green, L., Marion, S., Gamble, D., Herbert, C., Hertzman, C., & Sheps, S. (1999). Effectiveness of community-directed diabetes prevention and control in a rural aboriginal population in British Columbia, Canada. Social Science and Medicine, 48, 815–832.

framework is comprehensive and must be tailored to fit the program. In particular, the "How to Evaluate" examples are primarily geared toward social planning and must be significantly modified to be appropriate for community development, social action, and small programs.

Cost Analysis

In this era of health care reform and associated concerns regarding cost control, evaluation is linked with accountability to the public to ensure that health improvements are worth the funds spent. **Cost analysis of health programs** is the evaluation of the costs of a program in relation to health outcomes. There are many ways to examine costs, for example (McKenzie & Smeltzer, 2001; Rossi & Freeman, 1999):

- Cost accounting: comparison of the projected and actual costs of a program
- Cost effectiveness: comparison with another program, cost per effects or outcomes achieved (e.g., costs and outcomes of two programs to decrease falls in the elderly)
- Cost benefit: comparison of benefits (in dollars) of different programs with program costs (e.g., with falls prevention programs, calculate the costs in ratio to the benefits or outcomes, such as dollar value of no injury versus fractures)

Because all that is important to health is not readily measurable or easily converted into monetary terms (e.g., palliation, community competence, environmental change, quality of life), new approaches to cost analysis are needed. Values and needs that gave rise to a program, short- and long-term health outcomes, and human and material costs must be considered. The use of a case study is often helpful to illustrate the human dimension along with material costs. With large programs, community health nurses are advised to seek the assistance of a consultant; with small programs, nurses can analyze the resource and budget information in combination with the process, structure, and outcome evaluation data.

Cost analysis is sometimes simple; at other times, it is complex. For example, the cost analysis for a home intravenous drug therapy program may simply compare the costs of home care with the costs of hospital care. In contrast, the cost analysis for a community cardiovascular disease prevention program may require 20 years of follow-up. When more immediate information is needed with regard to programs such as the latter, the nurse can make comparisons with other similar programs for which cost analysis has already been performed. With prevention program cost analysis, a bit of a conceptual leap must often be made when comparing the cost of prevention with the cost of disease. *Healthy People 2010* (USDHSS, 2000) provides information about the costs of treatment for common diseases and injuries in the United States. Costs for a prevention program can be compared with the costs of treatment. For example, a campus health program (along with other factors, no doubt) was associated with a 30% reported increase in condom use by students (Budgen & Bates, 1996). Condoms are highly effective (but not foolproof) in reducing the transmission

Perspectives...

INSIGHTS OF STUDENT NURSES

Based on the observation that pregnant women often were not well prepared for hospital delivery or for early discharge, our plan was to develop an antenatal clinic. In a BSN health promotion course, we learned the importance of clients identifying their own needs and of the input of other health care providers. We therefore conducted interviews and a survey of clients, public health nurses, hospital maternity nurses, and physicians. Results revealed that there were already a number of programs in place. Our question then became, "Why aren't clients using them?" Further investigation indicated the need for integration of hospital and community resources and for consistent information for clients, especially about breastfeeding. We thus changed our plan to focus on the following:

- Improve continuity of care (reduce the need for multiple visits)
- Identify at-risk clients early (those with particular needs)
- Increase access to prenatal classes and other educational opportunities
- Streamline hospital admission
- Decrease the amount of paperwork
- Provide consistent breastfeeding information postpartum

We developed a working committee that included a public health nurse who works with pregnant teens, the planned maternity care coordinator (who liaises between hospital and public health nurses), a family physician, an obstetrical nurse (who also was pregnant), an obstetrical unit clerk, and the obstetrical and pediatric clinical coordinators. We also obtained additional input from clients, midwives, obstetrical nurses, obstetricians, and the college prenatal educator.

Many viewpoints were presented, and it was challenging to obtain consensus on the way to achieve the client's needs while meeting regional, community, and hospital philosophies and fiscal responsibilities. As discussions and meetings were held, actions were gradually agreed on, and progress was made.

- Approval was given by administration for a preadmission clinic for clients at 28–30 weeks of gestation. The focus is client-identified educational needs, risk identification and referral, completion of hospital forms, admission and discharge planning, and a tour of the obstetrical unit.
- To improve prenatal education, support for clients to attend prenatal classes is offered at the clinic (e.g., funding), as is information about prenatal videos available at the public library and video stores.
- To streamline information and reduce paperwork, care mapping has been developed with the help of interested hospital nurses and implemented. The form replaced three other forms, and the information obtained is faxed to public health nurses to improve continuity of postpartum follow-up.
- A breastfeeding workshop was held for public health nurses, hospital nurses, and lactation consultants. Nurses were encouraged to identify their learning needs, and client feedback about inconsistencies in teaching was incorporated. Nurses were given paid time from work to attend.

Implementation of the preadmission clinic is the joint responsibility of hospital and public health nurses. Depending on client demand, a clinic will be held one afternoon per week and one Saturday per month. Public health nurses, hospital nurses, and prenatal educators interested in working at the clinic are mentored by the obstetrical coordinator.

Evaluation of the clinic will include surveys of clients, nurses, and physicians to obtain quantitative and qualitative information about their positive and negative experiences. For comparison purposes, length-of-stay statistics were gathered prior to and following the implementation of the clinic.

During the year-long programming process to streamline and improve maternity care, we learned the importance of letting go of our own ideas. Obtaining input from all involved shaped and helped with the acceptance of change. In acknowledging and respecting diverse views and working together, we were able to achieve the consensus necessary to make the program a reality. Support and encouragement for each other as agents of this change are assisting us to maintain the momentum to follow through on the work.

—Maureen Spinks, RN, BSN student
Jean Jacobsen, RN, BSN student
Lisa Porter, RN, BSN student

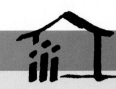

COMMUNITY NURSING VIEW

A nurse has been asked to develop a program for teens at a local high school. The nurse has been told that teachers are concerned about "bullying" on the school grounds, parents are worried about conflict among students from different cultural backgrounds, and the school principal would like help to improve support for students with serious medical problems.

Nursing Considerations

Planning/Implementation

- Given the preliminary information available about the high school, what overall *approaches to health* might be most helpful for this high school community?

- What *theories and models* might be useful initially? Later?

- *Who* should be included in the initial work? *What* are the urgent and longer term issues?

- *How* should the nurse deal with the fact that three issues have been raised?

- How might the nurse and community find out more about the current situation and issues of importance? (*diagnosis*)

- What would be a better situation? (*identification of goals/outcomes*)

- How can the desired situation be created? (*action strategies*)

- What are the resource requirements and availability? (*feasibility*)

- Among the many possible actions that could be undertaken, how would the nurse determine those that are best?

- What *ethical issues* might be anticipated?

- What forms of *documentation* might be useful?

Evaluation

- What would indicate that programming work was helping the community?

- What *types* of evaluation would be appropriate?

- The nurse will be able to work with the school intensively for a year but then will need to decrease involvement. What might be done to assist the high school to continue on with the program after the nurse's involvement has decreased or ceased?

---

of sexually transmitted disease. Cost estimates in the literature indicate that health care for one person with HIV/AIDS dramatically exceeded the annual costs of the health program. Cost estimates in the literature also were found for chlamydia, a less costly but more prevalent sexually transmitted disease among young people. The conclusion was thus drawn that the program was worth the cost.

Cost analysis, like other components of programming, becomes easier with practice. The community health nurse who adds the skills of cost analysis to programming will be well equipped.

In conclusion, throughout planning, implementation, and evaluation, Health for All goals can be achieved through programs when nurses understand the context, use theory thoughtfully, and work with communities in partnership (see Figure 16-19). The community health nurse can be a significant force in the Health for All initiative. See Out of the Box for an example of program planning and evaluation in action.

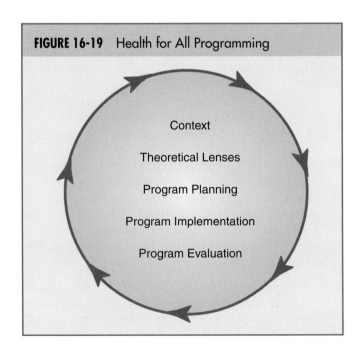

FIGURE 16-19   Health for All Programming

Context

Theoretical Lenses

Program Planning

Program Implementation

Program Evaluation

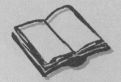

Out
of the Box

Passing the Baton: Long-Term Programming to Create a Healthy Campus Community

When creating community change, a challenge can be the long-term nature of the endeavor. At a Canadian University College campus, successful programming around smoking has been created by "passing the baton" from one group of students to another. In 1998, nursing students, as a course project, assisted with the design and conduct of a campus health survey. Results indicated that students were concerned about smoking at building entrances (in-door smoking had been banned). Nursing students in the following semester conducted additional research about people's opinions and smoking behavior on campus and about smoking policy at other North American institutions. In another course, students used the research results collectively to develop a position paper that they presented to the university Board of Governors. The students requested that outdoor designated smoking areas be developed, away from building entrances, and that the smoking policy be updated. The three-point intent of the request was to (a) decrease exposure to second-hand smoke, (b) promote healthy lifestyles by decreasing the visibility of smoking, and (c) reduce litter from cigarette butts.

The Board asked the president of the University College to deal with the issue; the president delegated the request to Administration, Physical Plant and Campus Health. The resulting coalition (Working Group on Designated Outdoor Smoking Areas) has worked three years using various programming strategies to change smoking on campus, while simultaneously dealing with the politics which arise from different views (e.g., rights of individuals versus the community, rights of smokers versus nonsmokers, defeat of provincial legislation on workplace smoking). Dealing with differences and finding common ground have meant slow progress. For example, the update of campus smoking policy did not have enough support to occur initially; however, health education and peer support strategies by Campus Health were supported. In some instances progress temporarily

went backward, for example, the stoppage of tobacco sales at a University College vendor was followed by a student association approval for installation of a cigarette machine in the nearby student-managed pub.

Administration and Physical Plant initially took action to demarcate outdoor smoking areas away from building entrances and, one year later, used Safer Campus grant funds to build "garden-type" gazebos for smoking. Physical Plant has maintained the gazebos and "friendly" signage at all entrances (e.g., "Out of consideration for others, please smoke only in gazebos").

Implementation of the "smoking" gazebos has required a continuing process of community development, political action, health education, social marketing, and evaluation research. The involvement of students from semester to semester keeps the project progressing. Campus Health nurses have worked to maintain partnerships with student associations and students (nursing, international, and others). Students have conducted further surveys on utilization issues as course projects, and, also, students have been hired as wellness assistants to work on Butt Busters health education campaigns. The Butt Busters campaign originated with Home Support students as part of their community course work. The campaign has involved multiple posters (student designed) and "walk about" distribution of rewards (and encouragement) for gazebo use. Rewards have been donated (e.g., parking passes, food vouchers). Smoking at building entrances has decreased and butt litter has been reduced, but not to the extent desired; therefore programming continues.

Research findings have been used to improve the gazebos (e.g., addition of garbage cans) and to raise campus community consciousness. Campus Health nurses obtained grant funds from a Health Region Tobacco Reduction program, enabling the development of smoking cessation and reduction programs. Students and Campus Health nurses have written articles for the student newspaper; and the occupational health and safety officer recently has agreed to assist

(continues)

Out
of the Box (continued)

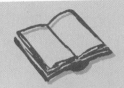

in reaching faculty and staff, e.g., through the news journal.

Most recently, a newly hired senior administrator has offered to take an updated smoking policy through the necessary approval steps, and a policy has been developed by the occupational health officer with input from the Working Group. Policy implementation is planned for 2002; health education, gazebo use, and smoking cessation will continue to be supported by Campus Health in partnership with students.

This project illustrates the strength of human resistance to change and the power of human persistence and patience in creating a healthier community. Success requires programming that is flexible and evolutionary, taking into account the interests of all people and keeping the goal in focus. ■

—*Rebecca Aaron, RN, BSN*
Colleen Aitken, RN, BSN

KEY CONCEPTS

◆ Health programming work includes the processes of planning, implementing, and evaluating programs for the purpose of improving health.

◆ The WHO's primary health care and health promotion strategies are of special interest to nurses as they create programs that contribute to the goal of Health for All.

◆ Dramatic, multilevel change (societal, community, individual, and environmental) is required for the achievement of Health for All.

◆ Community empowerment, community competence, partnership, intersectoral collaboration, and a broad definition of health are fundamental concepts in Health for All programs.

◆ Successful health programs take into account the societal and health care reform context.

◆ Community health nurses use caring, phenomenological, feminist, critical social, and multilevel change theories to assist their work with people and programs.

◆ Community organization, a multilevel change theory comprising community development, social planning, and political action, provides useful guidance for many Health for All programs.

◆ The science of programming is the theoretical knowledge that community nurses use; the art is the way nurses work with communities.

RESOURCES

Association of State and Territorial Health Officials: www.astho.org
Canadian Nurses Association: www.cna-nurses.ca
Center for Cross Cultural Health: www.crosshealth.com
Community Toolbox, University of Kansas: www.ctb.ku.edu
Cross-cultural health care programs: www.xculture.org
Diversity intervention to improve health programs: www.diversityrx.org
Evaluation, Australia: www.aes.asn.au
Evaluation, Canada: www.evaluationcanada.ca
Evaluation, United Kingdom: www.evaluation.org.uk
Evaluation, U.S.A.: www.eval.org
Grants Net: www.os.dhhs.gov/grantsnet
Grantsmanship Center: www.tgci.com
Health Canada (and Statistics Canada): www.hc-sc.gc.ca
Health Communication Network: www.hc-sc.gc.ca/hppb/socialmarketing
Health Promotion Institute, University of British Columbia: www.ihpr.ubc.ca
Society for Public Health Education: www.sophe.org
Specific prevention program areas and grants: www.cancer.org; www.cancer.ca; www.diabetes.org; www.americanheart.org; www.lungusa.org
Wellness Councils of America and Canada: www.welcoa.org

QUALITY MANAGEMENT

Sue A. Thomas, EdD, RN

MAKING THE CONNECTION

Chapter 16 Program Planning, Implementation, and Evaluation

The performance of a health care organization is in direct proportion to its planned, organized, systematic commitment to excellence.

—Ellie Green, 1997, p. 257

COMPETENCIES

Upon completion of this chapter, the reader should be able to:

- Discuss the meaning of quality within the context of health care.
- Examine the historical development of the focus on quality care in health services.
- Discuss the role of organizations in health care quality.
- Explain quality assurance (QA)/quality improvement (QI) as dimensions of quality management.
- Discuss total quality management (TQM)/continuous quality improvement (CQI) as a management philosophy.
- Discuss the use of evaluative models in quality assurance program development.
- Examine approaches for implementing CQI.
- Describe the use of TQM/CQI in community/public health settings.
- Discuss the implications of quality management for community health nurses.

KEY TERMS

performance
 improvement

performance
 measurement

quality assurance/
 quality improvement

total quality
 management/
 continuous quality
 improvement

Rising health care costs, questions about effective interventions, and the need for efficient delivery of health care services have resulted in the focus on quality measurement, management, and improvement. Professional organizations, consumers, government agencies, academic centers, and research laboratories are concerned with the highest quality outcomes for the lowest cost (Young, 1998). The emphasis on quality, cost-effective outcomes addresses the need to use outcome information to measure and demonstrate the effectiveness of health care practices.

Community health nurses and other health professionals have a vested interest in health care quality. Because of their concern about quality services, objective and systematic evaluation of health care quality is a priority, coupled with ongoing quality improvement.

This chapter will explore the concept of quality, the historical development of quality in health care, the meaning of quality assurance and improvement, the use of evaluative models in quality management, and the implications of quality management in community health nursing.

DEFINING QUALITY IN HEALTH CARE

Health professionals and clients alike are concerned with defining quality of care. Quality of care may have different meanings for health professionals and clients (Lynn & McMillen, 1999). Health professionals evaluate quality based on clinical outcomes, cost, access to services, functional status, staff mix, client satisfaction, and other measures.

Historically, there has been less attention given to client's views of quality care. Oermann and Templin (2000), however, conducted a study with 239 clients and found that high-quality nursing care was defined as nurses who were caring, concerned, and competent. In addition, communicating effectively with clients and providing them with information about their health problems were viewed as important indicators of quality care. These findings were also similar in a research study with veterans who were receiving care in an ambulatory setting (Oermann, Weglarz, & Templin, 1999).

Defining quality in health care is evolving. There is no one universal definition of quality, however, that is applicable across the health care system (Katz & Green, 1997). Initially, technical aspects of client care were the primary focus in definitions of quality in health care. The National Association of Quality Assurance Professions defined quality as levels of excellence demonstrated and documented in the process of client care based on available knowledge and achievable at a given organization (Lutz, 1994).

The Joint Commission on Accreditation of Health Care Organizations (JCAHO) defined quality as "the degree to which patient care services increase the probability of desired outcomes and reduce the probability of undesired outcomes given the current state of knowledge" (Katz & Green, 1997, p. 8). The JCAHO identified 10 indicators that determine the quality of care: appropriateness, availability, continuity, effectiveness, efficacy, efficiency, respect and caring, safety, and timeliness.

Quality has also been defined as continuous striving for excellence and a conformance to guidelines or specifications (Davis, 1994). The Institute of Medicine (IOM) defined quality health care as "the extent to which health care services . . . have a net benefit. . . . That benefit is expected to reflect . . . client satisfaction and well being, broad health status and quality of life outcomes, and the processes of client-provider interaction and decision-making" (Lohr, 1990, p. 4).

REFLECTIVE THINKING

REFLECTIVE THINKING

Perceptions of Quality

- What does quality in health care mean to you?
- Why is it important to examine the meaning of quality in health care from both health professional and client perspectives?
- How would you examine the meaning of quality care from the client's perspective?

It can be seen that there are different definitions of quality in health care, depending on the context. Donabedian (1990) suggests that no one all-embracing definition will be sufficient because there are different dimensions—the meaning of quality from the health professional perspective, which focuses on the possibility of benefit and harm to health; the clients' expectations of benefits and/or harm and other outcomes; and the social definition, which focuses on the cost of care, the benefit/harm continuum, and the distribution of care as valued by the population.

It is important to mention that terms used in health care quality management are those that were initially used in business—terms such as quality assurance (QA), quality improvement (QI), total quality management (TQM), and total quality improvement (TQI). Health care, as a major American industry, examined the quality strategies used by other businesses to foster excellence as well as economic efficiency (Katz & Green, 1997).

Quality assurance/quality improvement refers to the process that ensures certain standards of excellence are being met in the delivery of care (Lalonde, 1988). Quality assurance is concerned with the accountability of the provider to deliver quality care (Davis, 1994). Quality improvement refers to the process of attaining a higher level of performance or quality that is superior to previous levels and the actual attainment of that quality level (JCAHO, 1994).

In the late 1980s, the JCAHO noted that even though quality could not be ensured, quality could be measured and then subsequently improved. In order to measure quality, key indicators of the quality of a service would need to be identified. The indicators would be monitored and the quality of the outcomes measured. Outcomes refer to the results, or consequences, of care or lack of care.

Therefore, to improve the quality of the outcomes, those key processes that led to the outcomes would need to be identified. Improvement efforts would then focus on the processes with the intent that the quality of the outcomes would be improved as well. Thus, quality improvement became a critical concept in quality management (Katz & Green, 1997).

Total quality management/continuous quality improvement refers to a management philosophy that emphasizes the processes and principles that focus on continual improvement (McLaughlin & Kaluzny, 1994). Further discussion of this philosophy will be included later in this chapter.

One of the major business experts who has had a significant influence in health care quality management is W. Edwards Deming. Deming identified 14 points that addressed the development of quality and its continual improvement (Walton, 1986). Deming's focus on continual improvement is based on the belief that it is necessary in order to develop more efficient systems that will result in higher quality at lower cost. Thus, continual improvement is a major theme today in the various definitions of quality. Further discussion of Deming's influence will also be presented later in this chapter.

HISTORICAL DEVELOPMENT OF QUALITY IN HEALTH CARE

The focus on quality of care is not new. It has traditionally been an issue in health care delivery. In nursing, for example, in the 1860s Florence Nightingale worked to improve hospital care through the development of a method to collect and report hospital statistics (Wold, 2000). Subsequent to Nightingale's pioneering efforts in setting standards for care, a greater emphasis was placed on licensing accreditation and evaluation in nursing programs in the early 1900s in the United States.

Initially the major focus was on quality assurance, with the emphasis focused on developing standards of care. In community health nursing, the Standards for Community Health Nursing Practice were submitted to the American Nursing Division members in 1973 and were revised in 1986 and 1999.

In 1972 the Joint Commission on Accreditation of Hospitals (JCAH), for example, specified the standards for care in writing, with evaluation of care based on the standards required. The quality of care expected was made explicit by the written standards that directed the way the service was to be provided and the results that were expected from the care provided. Standards therefore defined quality.

In 1976, The National Association for Healthcare Quality was founded in the United States (NAHQ, 2001). It has become the nation's leading organization for health care quality professionals with the goal of promoting the "continuous improvement of quality in healthcare by providing educational and development opportunities for professionals at all management levels and within all health care settings" (NAHQ, 2001). NAHQ works to improve the quality of health care through professional education information exchange, certification, and assistance on current professional standards of performance. It includes members across the health care continuum and professional disciplines.

In the mid-1980s JCAH became the Joint Commission on Accreditation of Health Care Organizations (JCAHO) and began focusing on quality control for hospitals and home health nursing. JCAHO reported that quality could be improved. Since the 1980s continuous quality improvement has become a primary issue for all health care professionals.

In community health nursing specifically, frameworks and guidelines for community health/public health nursing practice have been developed by both the American Nurses Association (ANA) (1982) and the American Public Health Association (APHA) (1996). In 1978, the Association of Community Health Nursing Educators (ACHNE) was established. One of its concerns was the quality of nursing education. In 1991 and 1993, three reports were published by ACHNE which identified curriculum content required to prepare community health nursing students for practice in the United States (ACHNE, 1991a, b, 1993).

More recently, the Quad Council in 1997 (ANA, APHA Public Health Nursing Section, ACHNE, and the Association for State and Territorial Directors of Nursing) examined the scopes and standards of public health and community-based nursing practice. The focus on obtaining quality health outcomes for populations served was critical in this process.

INTERNATIONAL DEVELOPMENT OF ORGANIZATIONS FOR QUALITY HEALTH CARE

Effective leadership in the delivery of quality health care is not only a national concern but an international one as well. It is necessary therefore to discuss international organizations that focus on quality to enhance our knowledge of reciprocal and synergetic collaborations.

In 1985, a group of health professionals met in Udine, northern Italy, to discuss quality assurance issues in health care. From this group of professionals, it was determined

---

REFLECTIVE THINKING

Perspectives of Quality Care

- Why is it important to develop a knowledge of historical perspectives in health care quality?
- What do you think the major focus should be in delivering quality health care? Why?

---

that an international society should be formed. The organization is the International Society for Quality in Health Care (ISQua, 2001). The purpose of ISQua is to provide an opportunity for individuals and institutions to share expertise via an international multidisciplinary forum. The objectives of this international society are (ISQua, 2001, p. 1):

1. To promote quality improvement on a continual basis in health care internationally

2. To focus on the methodologies needed to facilitate quality in health care and to develop programs and activities related to these

3. To organize scientific meetings of the society and to encourage the organization of such meetings on both a global and a regional basis

4. To publish the *International Journal for Quality in Health Care* and other relevant publications

5. To promote external evaluation of health care, including the provision of an internationally agreed-on method of assessment of health care standards and also for an internationally agreed-on method of accreditation for health care accreditation organizations

6. To promote research and education in quality improvement in health care, with particular regard to cost effectiveness, cost benefit and cost utility analysis, clinical epidemiology, and measures of quality of life and consumer satisfaction

7. To maintain relationships with relevant organizations concerned with assuring quality improvement and optimal standards in health care

ISQua's first international conference was held in Paris, France, in 1986. Since then there have been yearly conferences. ISQua's conferences have provided a valuable forum for exchanging information and sharing ideas and updates on practice from countries throughout the world (ISQua, 2001). The current ISQua's secretariat was established in Australia in 1995 and is located in Melbourne. It is supported by members, with leading quality health care providers and agencies from over 60 countries.

Another major organization that represents a network of national societies dedicated to quality improvement in health care at national/international levels is the European Society for Quality Healthcare (ESQH), based in Limerick, Ireland. ESQH was founded in 1998 by a group of presidents and former presidents of national organizations for quality health care in Europe under the auspices of ISQua (ESQH, 2001).

The purpose of ESQH is to achieve its aims through collaborative action within the network and in association with other European health-related organizations. The aims of ESQH are (ESQH, 2001):

- To support quality improvement in health care in Europe
- To strengthen the integration of European national societies' knowledge and experience

- To provide a contact and influencing agency with other health-related organizations in Europe and around the world

To accomplish its goals, information sharing on quality health care occurs in spring and fall workshops each year. In addition to the ESQH workshops, there are a number of projects that address quality improvement. One of the projects is the focus on further development of a European Clearing House on Health Outcomes and Evidence-based Medicine. There are also projects that address the development of a pan-European Information Technology system delivering information to the public, professionals, and other health authorities (ESQH, 2001).

It is important, as stated earlier, that community health nurses have a knowledge not only of quality improvement actions in their own communities and own nations but internationally as well. We can learn from each other, share knowledge and experiences in quality health care through collaborative networking at all levels. It is critical that we do so.

QUALITY ASSURANCE/QUALITY IMPROVEMENT

An examination of the concepts of QA/QI in health care is important in terms of the influence of industrial experts such as Phillip B. Crosby, Joseph M. Juran, and W. Edwards Deming. Various approaches to ensure quality care have emerged since the 1950s based on the work of these business experts (Katz & Green, 1997).

Approaches to Quality Assurance/Quality Improvement

A discussion of the specific approaches to QA/QI is necessary. Crosby (1979) identified 14 steps that addressed his beliefs. Crosby's work was based on these steps and his belief that quality is achieved through compliance with defined specifications or standards.

Juran (1988) proposed three approaches to quality: quality planning, quality control, and quality improvement. Quality planning refers to determining who the clients are, assessment of the clients' needs, and the service that addresses the needs and developing processes to address the needs. Quality control focuses on the evaluation of the performance of the service in order to assess the difference between actual performance and goals. Quality improvement establishes an infrastructure with project teams designed to carry out improvement projects.

W. Edwards Deming (1986) is well known for his work with the Japanese after World War II. His management philosophy and techniques became the standard in Japan, with his influence highly recognized. Deming strongly emphasized the development of quality and its continual improvement. Deming's focus on continual improvement is evident today in definitions of quality in business as well as in health care.

Deming identified 14 points as guidelines for addressing quality improvement (Deming, 1986, p. 23):

1. Create and publish to all employees a statement of the aims and purposes of the company or other organization. The management must demonstrate constantly their commitment to this statement.
2. Learn the new philosophy, top management and everybody.
3. Understand the purpose of inspections, for improvement of processes and reduction of cost.
4. End the practice of awarding business on the basis of price tag alone.
5. Improve constantly and forever the system of production and service.
6. Institute training.
7. Teach and institute leadership.
8. Drive out fear. Create trust. Create a climate of innovation.
9. Optimize toward the aims and purposes of the company the efforts of teams, groups, staff areas.
10. Eliminate exhortations for the work force.
11a. Eliminate numerical quotes for production. Instead, learn and institute methods for improvement.
11b. Eliminate management by objectives. Instead, learn the capabilities of processes and how to improve them.
12. Remove barriers that rob people of pride of workmanship.
13. Encourage education and self-improvement for everyone.
14. Take action to accomplish the transformation.

Total Quality Management (TQM)/Continuous Quality Improvement (CQI) Processes

Total quality management/continuous quality improvement are terms that refer to a management philosophy that has been used successfully in the industrial sector initially, more recently in health care. TQM/CQI refers to a focus on the processes that address the goal of continuously improving those processes. It focuses on problem prevention and continuous improvement. This management philosophy is thus process driven and focuses on teamwork, leadership, empowerment of employees, individual responsibility, and continuous system improvement of processes in order to improve quality outcomes (Berwick, 1989). It seeks to eliminate errors in process before negative outcomes occur, instead of waiting until after the negative outcomes to correct professional performance.

The major characteristics of TQM/CQI include the following (McLaughlin & Kaluzny, 1994, p. 4):

1. Empowers clinicians and managers to analyze and improve processes
2. Adopts a norm whereby client and provider preferences are the primary determinants of quality
3. Develops a multidisciplinary approach that moves beyond traditional department and professional lines
4. Provides the motivation for a rational data-based collaborative approach to process analysis and improvement

TQM/CQI uses QA/QI methods and tools. However, it does not use only these methods. Traditional QA/QI methods address primarily the adherence to professional standards required by external accrediting agencies. They focus primarily on problem detection and improvement—a focus on deficiencies. The primary goal of QA approaches is to monitor the process and outcomes of client care for the purpose of problem identification, intervention, and data collection regarding interactions between the client and health professional.

TQM/CQI focuses on problem prevention and continuous improvement as referred to previously. Evidence of a continual improvement of all processes of service, practice, and governance is what is expected now by health care organizations, regardless of negative occurrences (Katz & Green, 1997).

DEVELOPING A QA/CQI PROGRAM

The purpose of developing a QA/CQI program is to promote the continuous improvement of quality in health care. The primary objective is to assure quality outcomes for clients.

Developing a well-organized quality management system in health care is the key to achieving quality. It is important therefore to understand various approaches

---

✳ DECISION MAKING

QA/CQI Program Development

You have been asked to participate in developing a QA/CQI program.

◆ What steps do you think should be taken initially to begin the process?

---

used in program development. There are three important approaches associated with a quality management system: performance knowledge, quality measurement, and performance improvement (Katz & Green, 1997). A well-developed quality management system includes each of these approaches. To omit one reduces the ability of the organization to affect its performance level of care. The approaches are identified in this discussion as separate items. However, in actual practice they blend together.

Performance Knowledge

Before any quality-of-care performance measurements can occur, there are important steps that must be addressed:

1. Identification of the clients and scope of services provided
2. Identification and prioritization of major service functions and processes
3. Dissemination of existing federal, state, and professional standards that address structure, process, and outcomes and development of performance standards that are organization specific

It is critical that all staff are provided with information regarding the role of standards in achieving performance targets and the importance of complying with written standards and expectations.

Performance Measurement

Performance measurement refers to the use of indicators that enable health care organizations to measure outcomes as a function of individual and organizational performance. Indicators provide a critical method for examining outcomes and/or key processes. The term indicator refers to a particular type of measurement—a performance measure. It is a valid and reliable outcome measure related to one or more performance dimensions (Katz & Green, 1997). Currently there are worldwide trends toward the measurement of processes and outcomes which focus on performance improvement in health care. Initiatives in many countries have introduced clinical and other performance indicators. ISQua has instituted an international indicators initiative. The first meeting in Budapest in 1998, hosted by ISQua, on es-

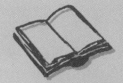

Out of the Box

Evaluating Quality Care

A health-promoting organization was founded in 1997 in San Diego, California. The purpose of this organization was to reduce the recidivism of women released from jail. The rise in the incarceration rate of women in the United States (the majority of whom are mothers) is a major public health and social problem. In order to assess the problem, Welcome Home Ministries was founded in 1997 by Carmen Warner-Robins, MSN, RN, MAT, FAAN, a jail chaplain and nurse who currently serves as the executive director. Warner-Robins' passion was to serve women and promote healing in the women's lives.

Based on an evaluation of outcomes following the release of women from jail in southern California, it was found that when many women were released they had only the clothes on their backs, few belongings, and nowhere to turn except to their old networks. Based on these findings, the Welcome Home Ministries was developed in order to create a caring community and healthy future for the formerly incarcerated women. The mission of the program is to create a faith-based support system for women in their transition from incarceration to productive citizenship. A variety of services are offered: (1) provision of clothing, food, toiletries, and a reintegration network; (2) weekly support and prayer groups and worship fellowship; (3) as-

sistance in networking for housing, jobs, and rehabilitation programs; and (4) provision for activities that improve self-esteem.

In order to evaluate the quality of Welcome Home Ministries, a participatory action research project was conducted with 21 formerly incarcerated women and 5 community volunteers who participated in a systematic planning process to determine priorities, develop action teams, and evaluate program effectiveness. This action research project was presented at the International Caring Conference in Scotland in June 2001. The conference was sponsored by the International Association for Human Caring and the University of Stirling, Department of Nursing and Midwifery, attesting to the international recognition of this program.

The results of the action research project pointed to the success of the program. Of the 226 women who have participated or are currently participating in Welcome Home Ministries, only 7 were known to have returned to jail. The involvement of formerly incarcerated women to assist women newly released from jail indicated that caring communities can make a difference with this highly vulnerable population. One of the women who received assistance from Welcome Home Ministries stated, "Welcome Home has given me unconditional love and support. My sisters have shown me that there is hope in every one of our lives." ∎

---

tablishing an international framework of performance indicators in health care resulted in the agreement to continue dialogue about an international approach to indicators. Since 1998, an international steering group of ISQua members who are experts in the indicators area has been appointed to work on this endeavor. At the Buenos Aires 2001 ISQua Conference, designated events focused on the indicator initiative (ISQua, 2001). This international effort thus highlights the importance of community health nurses developing knowledge about performance measurement.

Performance Improvement

The **performance improvement** approach focuses on a continuous effort to strive to improve the service delivered through a process of action planning. A number of steps are included in the process (Katz & Green, 1997):

1. Organizing a process improvement team
2. Developing and implementing an improvement action plan
3. Assessing and documenting improvement
4. Communicating the results of the outcome

A performance improvement plan requires a proactive approach, collaboration, and creativity. It fosters the exchange and development of ideas and solutions and is an essential process for the entire organization.

Use of Evaluative Models in QA Programs

Evaluating quality in health care, and nursing in particular, has become a priority given the effects of health care costs on accessibility, the consumer demand for improved quality care, and the increase in nurses' involvement in health agency policy formation. It is important therefore to examine the evaluative models that are used in QA programs.

One of the most widely used frameworks for evaluation of health care programs is Donabedian's (1981, 1985, 1990) model, which addresses three major components for evaluating quality:

1. Structure—refers to evaluating the characteristics of a health care setting, such as facilities, equipment, client mix, qualifications of health care providers

2. Process—refers to evaluating activities as they relate to expectations and standards of health care professionals in client care management

3. Outcome—refers to the result or consequence of the health care (or lack of care) provided, such as change in the client's status following intervention and the effect of the intervention on how the client functions

Donabedian's model can be used in developing a QA program. One of the major reasons for the use of this model is the focus on outcomes. Outcomes are the key to evaluation of health care providers and agencies by accrediting bodies, Medicare and Medicaid, and insurance companies. Across the United States, managed-care organizations, large employer groups, and other health care organizations are using outcomes measurement tools to measure and evaluate the results of health care. Outcomes measurement is defined as the systematic observation, at a point in time, of outcomes indicators. An outcomes indicator measures such things as performance of functions, processes, and outcomes over time (Maloney & Chaiken, 1999).

There are various types of outcome measures in health care. These include physical/clinical (mortality and morbidity), economic (cost/benefit), and humanistic (quality of life) measurements. An examination of the development of outcomes measurement tools over the past two decades indicates that the definition of

RESEARCH FOCUS

Implementing a Caring Model to Improve Patient Satisfaction

Study Problem/Purpose

The purpose of the study was to evaluate the effect of implementing a caring model on client satisfaction. Client satisfaction has become an important outcome indicator to measure the quality of care. Acknowledging the importance of nurse caring behaviors and the impact on client satisfaction is recognized as an important measure of organizational effectiveness.

Methods

This study used a descriptive design to evaluate the difference in client satisfaction before and after implementing a caring model. (Eight nurse-client satisfaction attributes were incorporated into the caring model.) A survey instrument was used to measure client satisfaction. The impact of the caring model implementation on client satisfaction was compared six months preintervention to six months postintervention, with the study conducted in a 48-bed acute-care community hospital that was part of a multihospital corporation. An analysis of variance and leverage analysis were used to analyze the results of caring behaviors on client satisfaction.

Findings

The results of the study provided evidence that nurse caring behaviors significantly influenced the client satisfaction responses. Assessment of the eight nurse-client satisfaction attributes indicated that clients valued effective nurse caring behaviors. The greatest magnitude of change occurred in the three months immediately following the implementation of the caring model. Findings at six months postintervention suggested a positive trend for improved client satisfaction. However, the change was less, pointing to a need for ongoing education related to the importance of caring behaviors.

Implications

Nurses' caring behaviors can influence client satisfaction. However, to sustain the influence of the behaviors on client satisfaction, ongoing educational experiences for nurses are necessary. Caring behaviors must become an integral part of the organizational philosophy and culture. Nurses' socialization to a caring philosophy is essential in all nursing practice arenas.

Source: Dingman, S. K., Williams, M., Fosbinder, D., & Warnick, M. (1999). Implementing a caring model to improve patient satisfaction. Journal of Nursing Administration, 29(12), 30–37.

outcomes has expanded and now includes results of significance to clients, such as clients' assessment of their own health and evaluation of the quality of care received.

The major goals of outcomes measurement and management is to utilize the data collection to improve the quality of care in the future. Quality improvement strategies can be developed and implemented with the hopes of future improvement.

The conducting of outcome studies in nursing, for example, provides the information that health care organizations can use to determine which nursing therapeutic interventions offer the best clinical, humanistic, and cost-effective outcomes as well as validate the outcomes of their care. The ability to identify health status changes as a result of nursing care provides data that demonstrate nursing's contribution to health care delivery. What must be kept in mind, however, is that there are many uncontrolled factors that have an effect on health status.

THE USE OF QA/CQI IN COMMUNITY AND PUBLIC HEALTH SETTINGS

Monitoring the quality of service provided to clients in community/public health agencies is required. Systematic evaluation of care is thus a priority within the practice of community/public health nursing. The increasing involvement of nurses in program management and the required monitoring and improvement of the quality of care point out the importance of nurses having the knowledge to participate in this endeavor.

Guidelines such as *Healthy People 2010* provide a prioritized identification of targeted health objectives for the United States, coupled with current health statistics about health promotion and disease prevention. *Healthy People 2010* identifies specific targets with recommended performance goals. The Community Health Improvement Process (CHIP) proposed by the IOM in its report "Improving Health in the Community: A Role for Performance Monitoring" (Durch, Bailey, & Stotto, 1997) is another model that describes how private health care organizations and public health agencies can work together at a community level to monitor performance in order to improve the public's health. Monitoring the health of communities would be a private-public collaborative project, which would reduce the fragmentation that exists in the health care system.

Participating in the planning, implementation, and evaluation of a model QA/CQI program in health care agencies requires that nurses have an understanding of the various approaches used to monitor the quality of care. Traditional approaches used to protect the public include the assurance of a level of competency among health professionals, such as credentialing, accreditation, and certification. Additional approaches utilize methods

that incorporate other evaluation strategies. As discussed previously, evaluation of structure, process, and outcomes is necessary in a model QA/CQI program.

Structure

In public health and other community settings, the evaluation of structure is not a new concept. Evaluation of structure is a major method for evaluating quality of care. Structure refers to the philosophy and objectives of the agency that serve to identify the standards.

The philosophy is a written statement about the health agency's beliefs about excellence in service, practice, and leadership (Katz & Green, 1997). Values are identified which refer to beliefs such as caring, justice, and accountability—beliefs about how caring, justice, and accountability for example guide the agency's and nurses' ethical decision making. Values provide a basis for organizational caring actions. When objectives are formulated, resources such as facilities, equipment, and personnel are identified.

Process

Evaluation of process standards is important and is another major method for appraisal of the quality of care given by health professionals, such as public health nurses. Process standards outline how the knowledge and skills of nurses are operationalized. Written process standards refer, for example, to standards of care such as the ANA standards for nursing practice, agency procedures, practice guidelines, and documentation. Process standards translate the agency's values into actions and those processes for which the agency will be required to address.

Outcomes

The increased emphasis on outcomes research, measurement, and management in community/public health agencies, not only in the United States but other countries as well, requires that community health nurses are knowledgeable about this method. The evaluation of outcome standards, or the results of nursing care, for example, through enactment and completion of a process is difficult.

Evaluation of outcome standards requires evaluating the methodology used to collect and analyze the health-related data, the methodology used to systematically analyze which interventions are most effective in terms of outcomes and cost, and how the outcome measures used meet the tests of reliability, validity, and reproducibility (Figure 17-1).

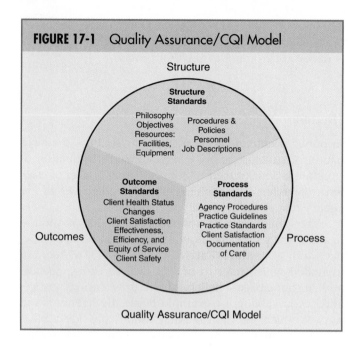

FIGURE 17-1 Quality Assurance/CQI Model

Structure

Structure Standards

Philosophy
Objectives
Resources:
Facilities,
Equipment

Procedures &
Policies
Personnel
Job Descriptions

Outcome Standards

Client Health Status Changes
Client Satisfaction
Effectiveness,
Efficiency, and
Equity of Service
Client Safety

Process Standards

Agency Procedures
Practice Guidelines
Practice Standards
Client Satisfaction
Documentation
of Care

Outcomes

Process

Quality Assurance/CQI Model

Evaluation, Communication, and Action

The interpretation of the evaluation of structure, process and outcome standards in an agency is a critical part of the process. The identification and communication of strengths and weaknesses between the quality care standards of the agency or program and the practice of the nurses or other health care professionals are necessary. A formal report should be written and discussed with designated staff and administration members.

Evaluative judgment requires critical thinking. It involves making judgments about the quality of care provided by the agency. The judgments made about the quality of care must be communicated to both administration and staff. Identification of necessary changes to improve the quality of care and possible ongoing courses of action to improve the quality should include both staff and administration.

After the possible courses of action are considered, taking definitive action to improve the quality of care must occur to ensure that the CQI model is operational. The critical aspect in this process is that QI is continual and that regular feedback is provided to staff.

QUALITY MANAGEMENT IN COMMUNITY HEALTH NURSING

Improving the health of communities is a national and global challenge. Community health nurses are in a very important position to continue to participate in health status improvement of our populations. Community and public health nurses have used strategies such as community assessments, case management, targeted population interventions, and other healing modalities across the health care continuum for many years. Lillian Wald,

Perspectives...

INSIGHTS OF A NURSING CONSULTANT

Serving as a consultant to program managers in a local public health department highlighted the critical importance of examining the processes and methods related to quality management. Working with program managers to develop quality assurance and continuous quality improvement plans for each program was an experience that attested to the necessity for addressing the importance of quality management in the education of community/public health nurses.

The assessment of quality in the delivery of community health nursing services is not new. However, the emphasis on developing a systematic ongoing process for quality improvement is at the forefront today. The imperative for delivering high-quality care to all members of our community requires a commitment to developing strategies and action plans to improve care.

Action plans that address the monitoring of quality care and performance improvement underpin the work of the health care team across the entire continuum of care. Action plans that describe the monitoring of quality improvements in community/public health nursing services on an ongoing basis are examples of caring in action. Monitoring service effectiveness, responsiveness to clients, timelines in the provision of services, efficiency, and equity provides the opportunity to evaluate our practice, to manifest caring about the populations we serve. Taking the time to reflect on our practice and promote quality in health care at local, national, and international levels is a commitment to excellence.

—Sue A. Thomas, EdD, RN

for example, utilized these strategies over a century ago, as did other nursing leaders such as Mary Breckinridge, in order to improve the public's health.

Because of increased demands for quality care at this time in our history, community health nurses, as well as other health professionals, are required to systematically evaluate the quality of their care. Developing a well-designed quality management system is critical—one that addresses QA and CQI.

It is important that nurses participate in organizations that provide a forum for engaging in dialogue about quality in health care, organizations such as the National

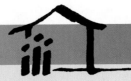

COMMUNITY NURSING VIEW

Susan, the new program director of an interfaith agency's nursing center designed to provide services to the homeless/near homeless, is responsible for monitoring the quality of service provided to the clients who use the nursing center. She is beginning the initial phase of reviewing the current QA/QI system.

The nursing center provides health services to the identified high-risk population; it is staffed by nurse practitioners, RN volunteers, and student PHNs. Nursing services, based on the philosophy of caring practice, provides basic health services, health screening and referral, and case management. The nursing center focuses on health promotion, disease prevention, and healing. It is a well-recognized nursing service, one that is valued by the community.

Nursing Considerations

Assessment

◆ In order to prepare for the QA/QI system review, what initial steps should Susan take?

◆ What critical information does Susan need in order to begin the QA/QI review?

◆ What evaluative data should Susan review that address the structure and process of care given? That address evaluation of care?

Diagnosis

◆ Given the nature of the review process, what possible problems might be anticipated?

Outcome Identification

◆ Why is it important for Susan to determine how health outcome is defined by the program?

◆ What are the different outcome measures that Susan would need to consider?

Planning/Interventions

◆ Who should Susan plan to include in the QA/QI system review process? Why?

◆ How might Susan communicate the results of the review and to whom?

Evaluation

◆ What process might Susan implement to evaluate the effectiveness of the QA/QI system review?

Organization for Healthcare Quality and the International Society for Quality in Health Care. Recognition and knowledge of other organizational efforts to improve quality care, such as the European Society for Quality in Healthcare, are also necessary. It is through our various forums for multidisciplinary dialogue that we as a nation, and we as nurses, can contribute to the promotion of quality improvement on a continual basis in community/public health settings.

KEY CONCEPTS

◆ Community health nurses have a vested interest in quality health care and ongoing quality improvement.

◆ There are different definitions of quality in health care, depending on the context.

◆ The concepts of quality assurance and quality improvement were originally conceived by business experts.

◆ There are international organizations that focus on the importance of promoting quality health care.

◆ Various approaches to ensure quality care have emerged based on the work of P. Crosby, J. Juran, and W. Edwards Deming.

◆ Quality assurance/quality improvement programs are required in public health agencies that use federal and state funds.

◆ Total quality management and continuous quality improvement are terms that refer to a management philosophy used in health care.

◆ Continuous quality improvement in health care is a major focus in quality management.

◆ Developing a well-organized quality management system in health care is the key to achieving quality.

◆ One of the most widely used frameworks for evaluating the quality of care in health care organizations is Donabedian's model, which focuses on structure, process, and outcome.

◆ Systematic evaluation of nursing care is a priority in the practice of community/public health nursing.

◆ Participating in the planning, implementation, and evaluation of a QA/CQI program requires that community health nurses have a knowledge of the various approaches used to monitor quality of care.

◆ By learning about quality in health care through national and international multidisciplinary organizations that focus on quality practice and performance improvement, community health nurses can participate in promoting research in

quality improvement and assure that there are optimal standards in health care.

 RESOURCES

International Society for Quality in Health Care: http://www.isqua.org.au

European Association for Health Care Quality: http://www.esqh.net/index.html

National Association for Health Care Quality: http://www.nahq.org

POWER, POLITICS, AND PUBLIC POLICY

Cynthia O'Neill Conger, PhD, RN

MAKING THE CONNECTION

*Genuine politics—politics worthy of the
name, and the only politics I am willing to
devote myself to—is simply a matter of
serving those around us: serving the
community, and serving those who will come
after us.*

—*Havel, 1992*

COMPETENCIES

Upon completion of this chapter, the reader should be able to:

- Discuss the concept of caring applied at the community level.
- Describe the concept of power, including the varied power bases.
- Explain the differences in the terms *politics* and *policy*.
- Discuss how a bill becomes a law in the United States.
- Discuss the differences between collective values and traditional values and how they affect policy development.
- Discuss the American Nurses Association (ANA) grass-roots political nurse network.
- Discuss issues that will enhance nursing's political base.
- Describe specific political action strategies and how they can affect health policy.
- Identify several resources for participating in political activism.
- List and describe several nursing organizations involved in public policy formation.

KEY TERMS

amended	lobby
author	policy
coalition	political
collective	action/political
health care policy	activism
healthy public policy	politics
house of origin	power
incrementalism	sponsor
killed	testimony
	veto

Politics is about communities: the local, state, national, and international communities. The profession of nursing has had an interesting past in regard to political involvement and is now recognizing its unique contributions for the future.

It is important to revisit the efforts made by the nursing profession and some of its political pioneers. Early leaders in nursing, including Florence Nightingale and Lillian Wald, modeled political activism as an important role in nursing. Despite the involvement of these early leaders, widespread political involvement by nurses has not been realized. There are many reasons, including gender issues, the socialization process, and the obstacles that can be inherent in power, the political process, and the development of health policy. However, during the past two decades there has been a heightened awareness among nurses about the political process, political activism, and the building of nursing's political base.

This chapter will explore the above concepts and political processes. The chapter will focus on health policy development and how the community health nurse can be involved in shaping nursing practice and public policy by employing strategies of political activism. This chapter concludes with an overview of sources of information and organizations involved in health policy formation.

CARING AND THE POLITICAL ACTIVIST— HISTORICAL PERSPECTIVES

It is no accident that the founder of public health nursing in the United States was also an avid political activist. From the very inception of the Henry Street Settlement, Lillian Wald recognized the link between politics and the economic and social needs of the public. Like Florence Nightingale many years earlier, Wald astutely realized the connection between poor social, environmental, and economic living conditions and the poor health of the people living in those conditions. Like Nightingale, Wald conceptualized nursing not as a profession whose mission was limited to offering comfort and care in specified health care institutions but as one that encompassed the whole of people's lives. She chose to practice her nursing skills in the community and opened the Henry Street Settlement in one of the poorest neighborhoods of Manhattan to improve not just individuals' health but the health of the community as well.

Though the initial purpose of the Henry Street Settlement was to serve as a clinic for neighborhood residents, it gradually developed into a political power base for Wald's many social and political activities. Combining a fierce sense of justice with a social conscience, Wald quickly attracted like-minded women to the Settlement. Among the members of her inner circle was Lavinia Dock, a nurse, feminist, educator, and union organizer. Adelaide Nutting was an innovator in nursing education at Columbia Teachers College as well as a suffragette. Lina Rogers Struthers became the head of the first public school nursing service. Together, these women shared and supported each others' ideas and activities for social improvement. Included among the many political issues Lillian Wald participated in were the sanitation and health care problems in New York City's tenements, worker conditions, labor unions, children's rights and health issues, racial justice, and feminism and the suffrage movement.

Lillian Wald developed both a public and a private self that allowed her to accomplish major social reforms. "Through her public self she connected her caring with activism by initiating practice and policy changes via administrative and organizational skills, persuasiveness, coalitions, delivering testimony and political power" (Backer, 1993, p. 128). Wald conceptualized the community health nurse as a health professional who both witnesses and seeks to improve the health, economic, and social conditions of those people with whom she works. This conceptualization is the foundation supporting nursing activism in the policy arena.

Caring beyond the Individual and Family

Although the history of nursing nationally and internationally is connected to population-focused care and social justice, medical advances changed the face of health care. Cure of illness became possible rather than merely symptomatic care, and nursing changed focus from populations and prevention of disease to individuals and cure. This narrowing focus resulted in social and political withdrawal. The once well-deserved reputation of nursing as a social change force faded into history (Conger & Johnson, 2000).

Many people continue to see nursing as a hands-on, one-to-one activity. The nurse is assumed to be the bedside practitioner, the one health care professional who is accessible and constantly available for the client. Community health nursing, with its emphasis on groups of people, known as aggregates, that are at risk for health problems, as well as its focus on entire communities, has long been seen as different from other nursing specialty arenas that focus on sick individuals in hospitals or clinics. This broader focus often requires a mental leap by nursing students as they are introduced to the concepts of aggregate nursing and population-focused practice. Similarly, the political activists among nurses are seen not as "real nurses," who by definition would remain at the bedside, but rather as people who have somehow lost touch with the basics of health care and health care recipients. However, actions by the American Nurses Association (ANA) in recent years serve to discount this notion. Nursing has evolved into a more sophisticated political player (Lescavage, 1995). The ANA has assumed a more proactive stance in the health policy arena. In 1980, the ANA spearheaded the notion of nurses as social advocates and activists through publication of the *Social Policy Statement* (ANA, 1980) delineating the reasons and approaches for nursing involvement in social issues. *Nursing's Agenda for Health Care Reform* (ANA, 1991) outlined nursing's solution to the health care crisis. Demonstrating that the *Agenda for Health Care Reform* and the *Social Policy Statement* could move from words into action, the ANA took a very visible stance in

the health care reform debates that occurred in Washington, D.C., during 1992 and 1993 (Conger & Johnson, 2000). Following these debates, the *Social Policy Statement* was updated (ANA, 1995). And the first nursing journal related to nursing and health policy, *Nursing Policy Forum,* was begun. Unfortunately, the journal was short-lived, but, in the year 2000, *Policy, Politics, and Nursing Practice* took its place. Yet recent studies and news events reflect a gradual awareness by consumers about the linkages between a community's social and economic conditions and its health status. Consider recent news articles citing the concern about tuberculosis rates and its prevalence in homeless and immigrant populations (Fielding & Ulene, 2000; Kelly, 2000; Roberts, 2000). Consider the increasing American obsession with violent crime and teenage gangs, often associated with poor urban neighborhoods (Constantino, 2000; Hopkins, 2000). Recall the poorly defined political campaign for "family values" in the 2000 presidential race, which attempted to link single-parent households to a variety of social ills including high rates of teen pregnancies. Yet few of these sensationalistic news stories examined and unraveled the many interlinked causes that contribute to the problems reported (Blyth & Evans, 2000; Ruben, 2000; Simon, 2000).

Clearly, the community health nurse is one of the few health professionals who directly observes many of the sources or causes of preventable health problems. The community health nurse visits the homes of families lacking the resources to adequately feed and clothe themselves. The community health nurse often participates in community clinics and identifies children who have never had a visit with a primary care provider for routine health maintenance. The community health nurse may be the first to notice a number of similar cases of illness within the community and to identify environmental or toxic hazards affecting a community's health. Backer (1993) stated:

> Nurses today face social conditions similar to those confronted by Wald and her colleagues. These issues include inadequate or lack of health care for many Americans, as well as their lack of housing, employment, and education, and the threat of infectious diseases. (p. 128)

The community health nurse may be the first to realize the presence or scope of health problems affecting large segments of the population, and this most certainly is a mandate to action for the caring professional.

Earlier in this textbook, the reader was exposed to the elements of caring applied to communities. Community health nurses demonstrate caring for populations by recognizing and accepting the multiple elements that make a community the place that it is: a place where people work, play, and live together. The nurse supports the growth and empowerment of communities as they seek new ways to improve their health status. But often problems that affect a community's well-being arise not from within the community but from outside the community. Economic, social, environmental, and cultural factors may directly influence a community, and yet decisions about these factors may be occurring miles away from the community of concern. Often, decisions are made at the county, state, or federal level that directly affect communities. Off-shore oil drilling, lumber and land use regulations, hazardous materials disposal—all these are issues that are not only subject to heated national debate but also hold the potential for affecting the small communities to which they are adjacent. These issues, so clearly related to health, will be decided at the political and policymaking levels.

As the industrialized nations move forward, we are witnessing the end of the Industrial Revolution, which began at the start of the 20th century. We are seeing the beginning of a new world whose economy depends less on labor and production and more on the gathering and exchange of information. The rapidly escalating use of computers and the international exchange of information and data have led some people to call this the Information Age. Health care has been revolutionized as well by this explosion of information exchange. And at the center of the changing health care arena will be nurses, representing the largest number of health care workers. At a time when many see this new paradigm of health care delivery as computer and information based, it is important that nurses ensure that the human, caring aspects of health care be incorporated as well into the new system. Nurses need to become political players in health care reform. Not only do nurses need to be prepared to debate the issues; they need to step forward and define the health care issues in the 21st century.

CONCEPTS OF POWER, POLICY, AND POLITICS

The concepts of power, policy, and politics are important for the nurse to understand. Power has traditionally been viewed by many nurses as a negative concept. The discussion of the many dimensions of power and the various power bases will provide nurses with another way of viewing and applying the concept in their practice setting. The concepts of policy and politics are also often associated with negative images such as smoke-filled rooms, bribes, and payoffs, to mention only a few. Both terms are value laden and thus can be perceived as ethical or nonethical depending upon the situation. A detailed discussion of all three concepts—power, policy, and politics—will provide the student with a framework for the rest of this chapter.

Power

Power is defined as the ability to influence others, the ability to do or act, and achievement of the desired result. Nurses have not been socialized to the concept of

---

REFLECTIVE THINKING

Communities

- What types of communities do you know that are currently feeling threatened by pending governmental regulations?
- Why would communities dependent on only one main industry (such as tourism, lumber, coal mining) be most vulnerable to policy changes?
- How would the loss of a major industry affect the health status of a community?

---

power. To many, the concept carries with it a negative connotation. Many nurses view themselves as powerless, and, often, the public also perceives nurses as powerless. There are several reasons, most having to do with gender: (1) Nursing is a female-dominated profession; (2) power is related to the male gender; (3) power is not "feminine"; (4) the majority of nurses still work in male-dominated organizations (hospitals) with powerful males (physicians); and (5) the profession is perceived as altruistic rather than power based.

Even though nurses are the largest professional group in the health care industry, they still have not fully appreciated their potential and used the power they could attain. As one nurse who participated in a political internship program stated, "The internship experience reemphasized to me the importance of one strong nursing voice. One in 44 female voters in America is a nurse. Though nurses are an extremely large segment of the population, they have not yet learned to harness the political power of their numbers" (Chaffee, 1996, p. 22).

In order to change the concept of power from negative to positive, we must remember that power is multidimensional and that there are many sources or bases of power. Understanding those facts can help in the analysis of the dynamics of power in specific situations. The more bases of power one incorporates, the more powerful she or he will become.

A typology of power bases has been established by various authorities (Mason, Talbott, & Leavitt, 1993, p. 120):

1. Coercive power is rooted in real or perceived fear of one person by another.
2. Reward power affects behavior as one person perceives the potential for rewards or favors by honoring the wishes of a powerful person.
3. Legitimate power derives from an organizational position or title rather than from a personal quality.

4. Expert power comes from knowledge, special talents, and skills; it is person power as contrasted with position power.

5. Referent power is apparent when a subordinate identifies with and follows the direction of a leader whom the subordinate admires and believes in.

6. Information power results when one individual has (or is perceived to have) special information that another individual desires.

7. Connection power is accorded to those who are thought to have a privileged connection with powerful individuals or organizations.

Policy

Policy is the governmental practice that guides and directs action in all spheres of social interaction such as national defense policy, environmental policy, economic policy, and health care policy. **Health care policy** is action taken by government to direct decisions and actions to safeguard and promote the health of the public and provide for health care services. "Policy encompasses the choices that a society, segment of society, or organization makes regarding its goals and priorities and how it will allocate its resources" (Mason et al., 1993, p. 5).

In the early stages of policy formation, the direction may not be completely clear, as in the current profusion of health care reform measures being proposed in various countries worldwide. Eventually, however, a number of measures that have been proposed, debated, and approved will coalesce to show a picture of governmental purpose and direction. Though many people may speak of policy as if it were a plan or a single decision, governments often express one intent while enacting policy with differing or even opposite effect from the stated goal. It is important for nurses to distinguish between stated values or spoken goals and the actual direction dictated by public policy, for it is that actual direction rather than the stated values that will affect our lives.

Who determines policy? Although elected officials propose and participate in the development of policies, the public, including nurses, has a role in shaping public policy. Milio (1981), in her classic text, *Promoting Health through Public Policy,* writes about the importance of nursing's becoming involved and participating in shaping health policy. Nurses at all levels—at the bedside, in administration, and in the community—are affected on a daily basis by public policy. Individual nurses can influence policy decisions at all governmental levels. Organized nursing's unified efforts, such as those outlined in *Nursing's Agenda for Health Care Reform* (Tri-Council for Nursing, 1991) is a good example of a **collective,** or group pursuing an agreed-upon goal, action or set of actions, and a **coalition,** which is a temporary alliance of diverse members who come together for joint action in support of a defined goal. It is impor-

tant that nurses be proactive in the earliest stages of policy development so that they can exert nursing's influence early in the political process.

Although it might seem ideal to develop an idea and be able to enact it into law quickly, our government is structured to allow input from a variety of persons at many stages of policy development. It is these many opinions, and the resulting modifications to legislation or policy being developed, that determine what the final law looks like. Although this system of weighing various opinions, making compromises and modifications, eliminating controversial pieces of legislation, pressuring influential groups, and courting or opposing political parties can seem frustrating to some outside observers, many find it fascinating and exciting. The formation of policy involves the use of the political process.

Politics

Politics means "influencing." "It is defined as a process by which one influences the decisions of others and exerts control over situations and events. It is a means to an end" (Mason et al., 1993, p. 6). Frequently, politics is associated with conflicting values, and multiple interest groups compete for scarce resources. Being involved in politics and developing actions and strategies to influence the political process is known as **political action** or **political activism.**

Mason et al. (1993) have advanced four spheres of political action: "Politics and policy are usually associated with government, but there are three other spheres for nurses' political action: the workplace, professional organizations, and the community" (p. 10). The community encompasses all three spheres of influence, which are an integral part of the community:

> The community is a social unit with a variety of special interest groups, community activities, health and social problems, and numerous resources for solving those problems. The community can be a neighborhood, or it can be international connections that will characterize the world into the twenty-first century. (p. 10)

Nurses can effect change in all four spheres of political influence. The four spheres are interconnected and overlapping, and nurses' involvement in one sphere will affect the other spheres (Mason et al., 1993). See Figure 18-1.

How has nursing evolved as a body politic—that is, as the political arm of nursing? Cohen, Mason, Korner, Leavitt, Pulcini, and Sochalski (1996) have advanced a framework that conceptualizes the political development of the nursing profession. They identify four stages of development to "analyze previous accomplishments and plan future actions that will enhance the political involvement of nursing as it seeks to improve the health care delivery system" (p. 259).

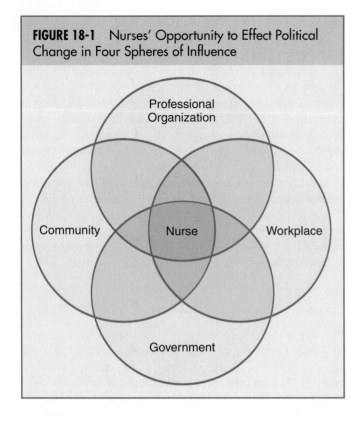

FIGURE 18-1 Nurses' Opportunity to Effect Political Change in Four Spheres of Influence

The fourth and final stage in the profession's political development has not been realized and is termed "leading the way." Cohen et al. (1996) state:

> In this stage nurses become the initiators of crucial health policy ideas and innovations. Reaching this stage will require that nursing seek out, develop, and support its visionaries and risk-takers. The further the professional development, the more the public will benefit from nursing's expertise and advocacy. (pp. 263–264)

Now, during the period of reorganization of health care delivery in the United States and other countries, is a crucial time in transition toward stage 4. Pursuit of stage 4 can be enhanced in the following ways (Cohen et al., 1996):

- Build coalitions and constituencies.
- Enhance leadership development.
- Mobilize nurses to run for office.
- Integrate health policy into curricula.
- Develop public media expertise.
- Increase sophistication in policy analysis and related research.

Because community health nursing focuses on the health of population groups, it is, by definition, political in nature. Community health nurses need to be advocates for aggregates with special needs and special concerns or problems. To be an advocate for special populations includes using a variety of political strategies and becoming sophisticated players in the political system.

POLITICAL PROCESSES: HOW LEGISLATION IS MADE

An important initial step in becoming a political activist is to have a basic grasp of the political system, to understand how laws are made, and to examine the finer points of the political process in a particular community, state, or nation. When nurses take time to study how laws and political decisions are made, they realize where they can effectively influence those decisions as health care professionals.

Think about some issues involving health that should be addressed in a community. Has there been a communicable disease outbreak recently in the community, and how would the community treat or prevent future outbreaks of this disease? Is there anything nurses can do to improve the health of children or to decrease the incidence of domestic violence? What can be done to facilitate healthier lifestyles for a particular population? Almost any health issue can be influenced by well-crafted legislation. Many health problems are negatively affected by legislation that either gives inadequate consideration to all the ramifications of the law (perhaps by not involving enough health care experts such as nurses)

The first stage of nurses' political activism, which began in the 1970s, sought to promote political awareness of nurses. At this time, the first of many books and articles were published that emphasized the importance of nurses' becoming politically active to advance the profession. The need for a power base among nurses was emphasized by the ANA, the primary professional nursing association in the United States. These efforts began the identification of ways nurses could become involved in politics (Cohen et al., 1996).

The second stage highlighted the activities that enhance the profession's identity as a special interest in the political arena and began to develop its own sense of uniqueness. This stage was "characterized by a new sense of identity emanating from the development of nursing coalitions and the building of nursing's political base" (Cohen et al., 1996, p. 261). During this stage in the 1980s, the ANA's political activities expanded and a grass-roots political network was developed and grew rapidly. There was a sudden increase in specialty organizations, many of which became politically active.

The third stage in the political development of the nursing profession, occurring in the 1990s, was marked by "political sophistication." The major achievements during this stage were (1) the development of Nursing's Agenda for Health Care Reform, discussed later in this chapter; (2) the appointment of nurses to federal panels and agencies; and (3) increasing savvy shown by nurses in areas such as election strategies and public relations techniques (Cohen et al., 1996).

or is altered by people with differing economic or political motives.

The Legislative Process

The U.S. government has three levels of governance: federal, state, and local. Local government may include counties, cities, or different specified districts such as school districts, hospital districts, or other special-interest areas. Local politics may differ radically from one city or county to another. Major decisions may be made by city councils or county supervisors.

Federal and state governments are similar to each other. They both have three main branches: legislative, executive, and judicial.

The executive and legislative branches are intended to be open and accessible to the people and are able to be influenced by citizens in order to make laws that serve everyone equally. However, the way in which citizens may wield their influence differs for each branch.

The Legislative Branch

The legislative branch is the law-making body of government. On the federal level, the legislative branch, Congress, is made up of two bodies: the U.S. Senate and the U.S. House of Representatives.

A single bill may be considered by several different committees. Once it has been passed by the committee(s), it is returned to the **house of origin.** The house of origin is the governing body of which the bill's **author,** the legislator who submits the bill, is a member (i.e., either the House or the Senate). The bill is presented in its **amended** (i.e., including any changes made to the printed bill) form for a full vote by all the members of the house of origin. The members vote, and the bill is either passed or defeated, or **killed.** Once a bill has passed through its house of origin, it is then sent to the other house and the process is repeated. It may go through committees and then be voted upon by the full membership of that house. Only after a bill has been passed by both houses of the legislature is it sent to the executive branch of government and signed into law or vetoed by the chief of the executive branch. On the federal level this is the president, and on the state level it is the state's governor. See Figure 18-2.

There are many ways that nurses can influence the legislative process. At the state level, nurses may serve as the **sponsor** of a bill: that is, the originator of the idea for the bill. An individual nurse may contact her or his representative to meet and suggest an idea, or, more commonly the state nurses association will propose an idea to a legislator. The legislator who first introduces a bill to the legislature is then known as the bill's author. Once the bill is introduced, nurses may augment its progress by garnering support for the bill from lobbyist groups within the state. Many health care groups actively follow and **lobby** (take actions to influence legislators to take a certain position on prospective bills or issues) a number of bills as they progress through the legislative process. Several health-related associations may align with each other in order to stimulate legislators to pass legislation that may benefit them all.

Joining with special-interest groups to lobby politicians is one of the most effective means of supporting legislation because legislators recognize that such groups represent large numbers of potential voters. Seeking the support of influential groups is the business of politicians. Politicians want to serve and please the people who voted them into office because these constituents represent future votes the next time they run for office.

Aside from joining lobbying groups, nurses have a unique and perhaps more powerful lever for influencing health legislation: their experience within the health care system. Every nurse who has held a job in nursing has seen the health care system in action and the effect it has on clients. Each nurse has a story to tell. Often a story well-told will influence a politician to support or oppose a piece of legislation. Providing **testimony,** or evidence in support of a bill, at legislative committee hearings, keeping track of pieces of legislation, and calling or writing a legislator may have a significant impact on a proposed bill. In order to track and affect legislation at key times in the life of a bill, interested parties must contact committees and key players at the appropriate state and federal levels. Figure 18-2 depicts the typical progress of a bill at the federal level. The left side of the figure indicates points in the process at which community health nurses might become involved and influence legislation.

The Executive Branch

The executive branch of government is responsible for carrying out the laws passed by the legislative branch. At the federal level, the chief executive is the president of

---

REFLECTIVE THINKING

Community Political Structure

- How is your local city or county structured?
- Who are the major decision makers in your city or county?
- Who are the official (i.e., elected or appointed) leaders in your community? Who are the unofficial leaders? Consider church, cultural, and business leaders and the roles they play in your town.
- Who do you know who has participated in local or state politics?

FIGURE 18-2 How a Bill Becomes a Law at the Federal Level in the United States

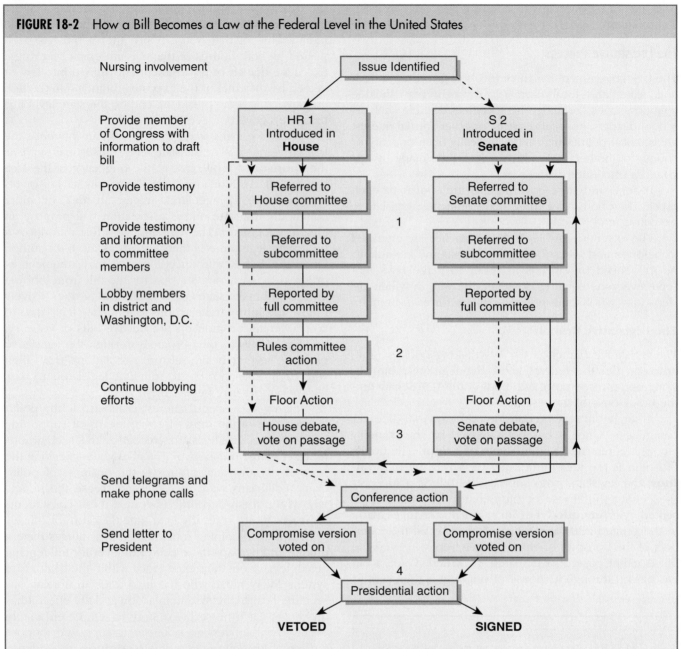

¹A bill goes to full committee first, then to special subcommittees for hearings, debate, revisions, and approval. The same process occurs when it goes to full committee. It either dies in committee or proceeds to the next step.

²Only the House has a Rules Committee to set the "rule" for floor action and conditions for debate and amendments. In the Senate, the leadership schedules action.

³The bill is debated, amended, and passed or defeated. If passed, it goes to the other chamber and follows the same path. If the two chambers pass a similar bill, both versions go to conference.

⁴The President may sign the bill into law, allow it to become law without his signature, or veto it and return it to Congress. To override the veto, both houses must approve the bill by a 2/3 majority vote.

From *Policy and Politics for Nurses: Action and Change in the Workplace, Government, Organization and Community* (3rd ed.), by D. J. Mason, S. W. Talbott, and J. K. Leavitt, (Eds.), 1998, Philadelphia, PA: W. B. Saunders. Reprinted with permission.

the United States. At the state level it is the state's governor. Among the responsibilities of the executive branch are signing bills passed by the legislative branch and making them into laws. The chief executive has the power to **veto,** or reject, bills passed by the legislature.

If the legislative branch wishes to override an executive veto, a second vote on the bill is taken in both houses and a two-thirds vote is required to effect an override.

At the federal level, another responsibility of the executive branch includes appointing persons to key positions such as cabinet members, ambassadors, and federal judges. Nursing organizations can support the appointment of persons with knowledge of health care issues to key posts. Kristine Gebbie, a nurse and former Secretary of Health in the state of Washington, was appointed to chair the President's AIDS Commission by President Clinton in 1993. Other executive duties include making treaties with other nations and, most important, reporting on the state of the nation to the legislative branch. The president makes a yearly State of the Union address to Congress in January.

At the state level, many of the laws passed by the legislature are then sent to regulatory agencies that transform the laws into enforceable regulations. The regulatory agencies are considered to be part of the executive branch, and the directors of these powerful agencies are appointed by the governor.

Nurses should feel comfortable writing or calling either the White House or their state governor's office to offer comments on pending legislation or upcoming appointments. Comments by citizens are tallied by staff, and opinion trends can significantly affect executive decisions. In addition, a brief well-told anecdote of some personal encounter that illustrates an opinion may be utilized by a leader to make a point in a political debate.

The Judicial Branch

The third branch of government is the judicial branch. This branch is the court system of the federal government. The judicial branch is divided into three levels: federal district court, appellate courts, and the Supreme Court. Most federal cases originate in district courts, whose decisions may be appealed to the appellate courts and, finally, the Supreme Court of the United States. The judicial branch is responsible for interpreting federal law, and it has the power to resolve disputes over the Constitution that might arise from the legislative and executive branches.

Regulation

Regulations are intended to promote individual accountability for actions and to protect the public health and welfare. Regulations specify how policies are to be realized; they fill out the details of new or amended laws.

At the federal level, proposed regulations are published in the *Federal Register,* after which concerned parties may comment on the proposed regulations and suggest changes. Community health nurses can have input into regulations that affect their professional practice as well as legislation that shapes public health policy.

PARTICIPATION IN HEALTH POLICY FORMATION

Whereas the concept of politics may seem overwhelmingly broad and intimidating to many Americans, the concept of public policy is even less clearly delineated. What is public policy, and how does it affect us? Why would a

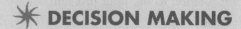

✳ DECISION MAKING

Political Influence

A federal bill related to early intervention for pregnant women is at the committee level. As a community health nurse you are aware of how important the passage of this bill would be to your practice.

◆ What could you and other community health nurses do to influence this legislation?

person in a caring profession, whose expertise involves working with people around health issues, be interested in policy? If you find yourself asking these questions, consider the following effects of policies today:

- Both prescription and nonprescription drugs in the United States are tightly regulated by the Food and Drug Administration. Yet tobacco containing nicotine, one of the most harmful drugs known to humans, remains unregulated. As noted in Chapter 3, tobacco is the major cause of premature death and disability worldwide.

- Statistics indicate a strong link between the number of handguns in a given society and the number of gunshot-related injuries and deaths. Yet the U.S. government has yet to ban personal weapons.

- Attempts to hold down Medicare costs in this country in the early 1980s caused the initiation of measures limiting days in the hospital for the elderly. Yet, health care professionals have increasingly warned of the increased potential of incomplete recovery for persons released prematurely to their homes.

All of these issues represent different aspects of public policy. Clearly, they are connected to the health of the people in communities where community health nurses work. Nurses are in a unique position to address many health problems that can be modified by public policy. Because community health nurses share common goals with clients and because they recognize that individuals are embedded in family and community systems, they are prepared to play a vital role in policy and population-based efforts to enhance care. In the next sections, public policy and specific strategies nurses can use to help shape it will be explored in more depth.

What is Healthy Public Policy?

Successful problem solving requires finding the right solution to the right problem. We fail more often because we solve the wrong problem than because we get the wrong solution to the right problem. (Ack-off, 1974, p. 1)

Doctoral programs exist that prepare professionals in policy analysis and development of good policy, so a full discussion of how to develop healthy public policy is beyond the scope of this chapter. However, that said, it is important for the novice in public policy to understand why and how a public policy is a good one.

Health problems brought to public attention, whether to a local, state, or federal government or to an organization with a health mission, are those that have not been solved at the private level. Problem types include needs, values, or opportunities for improvement. Problems emerge into the public arena because of their nature, scope, and/or severity. What on the surface appears as a relatively simple, straightforward issue or problem may have a number of definitions and implications that are not readily apparent? Every stakeholder in the issue may have a different definition. For example, when California produced legislation that allowed refusal of medical care to undocumented individuals, the health care delivery system interpreted this as a way to reduce unrecoverable costs for care. However, for some in the Hispanic community, the problem was defined as discrimination. Why does this occur? It occurs because the policy analysts, policymakers, and other stakeholders hold competing assumptions about human nature, values, government, and opportunities for social change (Dunn, 1994). The complexity of the problem of child health in developing countries demonstrates this point. For years the approach to solving the problem was getting public health (vaccinations and sanitation) and illness care services into the area. When dramatic results were not realized, other factors were examined. It was discovered that family health was related to the education level of the women. As women became more educated, family health improved. Thus, in many developing countries, improvement in health is directly related to societal and values change.

Therefore, **healthy public policy** is policy which has been developed through the process of problem definition with the input of stakeholders and from various perspectives. Alternative solutions to the problem have been analyzed in depth as to actual, potential, and unforeseen outcomes as well as examined for impacts on stakeholders. It is important to note here not only does this happen at the governmental level but also that it is required of organizations that set health policy such as the World Health Organization (WHO).

One healthy approach to policy development globally is the Healthy Cities movement. It strives to impact health by involving the people of the community in identifying assets and needs and mobilizing action at the grass-roots level within the community to solve their own problems through projects aimed at influencing the physical and social environments in which the people live and work. The outcome of this is often policy at the local or national level. Healthy Cities is an innovative grass-roots approach to health promotion and disease prevention. Originating in Europe in 1986, Healthy Cities has been a successful model to ensure that the local community is involved and participates in the treatment of its health problems.

Mission of the Healthy Communities Program

In the United States, the National Civic League (NCL), a private, nonprofit organization, championed the Healthy Cities model. The notion of Healthy Cities was redefined to Healthy Communities to reflect the notion that communities exist within cities and change often occurs at levels smaller than the city designation. However, a city may be defined as a community. The Healthy Communities Program is based on the principle that challenges faced by communities are so complex that new ways to describe and solve them are needed. In the past, decision makers tended to view community problems through a microscope, in isolation of each other, and, therefore, addressed them externally one at a time. The Healthy Communities Program allows a wide-angle view of a community's strengths and problems, exploring the relationships that exist between them, and finding deeper solutions that can ripple through many problems. This broader approach suggests not only a fresh definition of community issues but also a new manner in which citizens, government, not-for-profits, and the private sector must work together. This concept can be practiced in community work through the application of the following principles (www.ncl.org/NCL/hci.htm#Principles):

- A broad definition of health that goes beyond the absence of disease to address the root-cause problems in communities and includes economy, education, parks and recreation, arts, mental health, community spirit, and unity

- A collaborative, consensus-based approach to problem solving that involves a diverse group of citizens from the community

- An assets-based approach to problem solving that defines people and relationships by their skills and abilities rather than by their needs and deficits

- Addressing challenges at the systems level in the community rather than doing another short-term, low-impact project

- Creating a shared vision for the future that captures a community's hopes and dreams and guides their collaborative work in the community

The Healthy Communities Program was developed by the NCL as an initiative to carry out work based on the principle that citizens need to be involved in the operation of their community in a strong way. The program assists in community development to empower communities to identify their own assets and needs and develops political power. The Paso Del Norte Initiative in El Paso, Texas, is one example. In 1997 the Paso del Norte Health Foundation committed a total of

$2.5 million over a three-year period for the Healthy Paso del Norte Initiative. The NCL trainers and facilitators worked for six months with nine border communities to assist them in the development of their Healthy Communities process and imparted to them the skills and tools necessary to follow through. These communities have each developed regional health councils that have identified priorities and developed action plans and strategies for improving their quality of life (www.ncl.org/NCL/hci.htm#Principles).

Both the Healthy Cities and Healthy Communities models have been successfully used at the local, state, national, and international levels. Local health departments and community health nurses can serve as advocates, facilitators, and catalysts to develop communities toward the solution of their own problems. In other words, they are part of the team in the communities in which they have roles as professionals. Another focus for political activity for nurses centers on the *Healthy People 2010* objectives.

Healthy People 2010 Objectives— Guide for Healthy Public Policy

Healthy People 2010 provides an excellent foundation for the development of healthy public policy at the workplace, local, state, and national levels. See Figure 18-3. Embedded within each objective is a policy issue. For example, Objective 1-1 relates to improving the nation's proportion of persons with health insurance.

FIGURE 18-3 *Healthy People 2010* Objectives Related to Policy—a Sample

1-1. Increase the proportion of persons with health insurance.

1-2. (Developmental) increase the proportion of insured persons with coverage for clinical preventive services.

1-4. Increase the proportion of persons who have a specific source of ongoing care.

1-5. Increase the proportion of persons with a usual primary care provider.

1-6. Reduce the proportion of families that experience difficulties or delays in obtaining health care or do not receive needed care for one or more family members.

1-7. (Developmental) increase the proportion of schools of medicine, schools of nursing, and other health professional training schools whose basic curriculum for health care providers includes the core competencies in health promotion and disease prevention.

1-8. In the health professions, allied and associated health profession fields, and the nursing field, increase the proportion of all degrees awarded to members of underrepresented racial and ethnic groups.

From *Healthy People 2010, Understanding and Improving Health*, by U.S. Department of Health and Human Services, 2000, Washington, DC: U.S. Government Printing Office.

Policy Formation

Occasionally, ambitious proposals seem to radically change the course of a country's public policies. In the United States, for example, much of the criticism of President Clinton revolved around his overly ambitious attempts to make major policy changes. His proposals for health care reform and for reform of the criminal justice system via a major crime bill were at odds with the current direction of policies in those areas. Rarely has a president tackled a major restructuring of national policy; however, historians can quickly cite the few instances. One example is the New Deal by President Franklin Roosevelt during the 1930s. The New Deal was a term applied to a number of economic and social measures initiated to bolster the national economy and productivity. Social Security was one government program that emerged as part of the New Deal. Other examples are President Johnson's Medicare and President Clinton's welfare reform.

Although it is easier to visualize public policy by imagining the larger sweeping reforms mentioned above, most public policy is in fact created in small, individual steps. Individual laws, enacted piece by piece, relating to a common concept such as welfare, health access, or education come together to form a direction that is, if not mutually decided upon, at least silently con-

doned. This approach is called **incrementalism.** The policy environment around a problem is altered in small increments rather than in a rational approach, which redefines the entire policy environment for an issue.

Policy, then, is rarely developed with a broad vision in sweeping reforms. It is an incremental process in which pieces are added and refined as policymakers see fit. The ultimate goal of nursing involvement in politics is not to become overly concerned with the political process but rather to use that process as a tool to influence public policy.

In policy formation, there is often a conflict in values. When nurses begin a study of public policy, and specifically health policy, it is necessary to examine the values of the society that has developed the policies. MacPherson's (1987) article examining health care policy and values lists three areas in which U.S. culture differs significantly from nursing values. The opposing values include individualism versus collectivism, competition versus cooperation, and inequality versus equality. She points out that the fierce individualism that has created self-reliant heroes like explorers and cowboys also has undermined the capacity of Americans for commitment to one another. It is natural, then, in a country such as the United States, which stresses individualism, pursuit

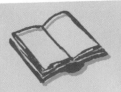

Out
of the Box

In 1999, an important action plan was formed which enhanced the Healthy Cities/Communities movement in the U.S. A national network of community and organizational leaders was created called the Coalition for Healthier Cities and Communities (CHCC). The CHCC brings together more than 1000 local, state, and national organizations, collaborative partnerships, and citizens to assist in creating healthier communities.

Instead of operating as a membership organization from a centralized location, the CHCC acts as a clearinghouse for leaders and communities who choose to use the services. Thirty states are represented by network liaisons to the CHCC and support state and local Healthy Communities initiatives by providing education and policy assistance.

The CHCC plays an important role in shaping private sector and public policy in their efforts to enhance the Healthy Communities initiatives in action planning. This coalition (www.healthycommunities.org) is becoming a critical base from which to further build a policy agenda that addresses the improvement of the economic, social, and physical well-being of people and communities. The coalition provides a valuable learning base through the availability of case studies, success stories, best-practices information, educational materials, training programs, "outcomes" research, and various other datasets. ■

of self-interest, and competitiveness, that health care policies tend to promote structured inequalities (p. 3).

Traditional U.S. ideals of individualism and the free market are in conflict with nursing values and especially with the work and concepts inherent in community health nursing. Community health nurses work to promote a collective identity among the aggregates they work with in order to empower the community to resolve health-related problems. They see the strength of communities as residing in an increasing ability to plan and work together toward common goals. Cooperation and collaboration rather than competition yield a strong base from which to identify and deal with community problems.

Emerging values emphasizing collectivist or community-oriented solutions are challenging traditional values. Col-

lective orientation emphasizes society's responsibility to solve social problems. Debates regarding collective versus individual rights have been increasing in U.S. politics; examples include struggles to enact legislation on the wearing of seatbelts, use of motorcycle helmets, gun control, and health care reforms (Weis, 1995):

> Americans will not be able to solve the problems of the health care system unless the country shifts priorities and biases away from an individual-centered view of health and human welfare toward a more community-centered approach. (p. 26)

Collectivism strives for collaborative efforts or partnerships throughout society.

Nursing and the Political Network

There are over 2.6 million registered nurses in the United States. One in 44 registered voters in the country is a registered nurse (ANA, www.nursingworld.org/centenn/cent1990.htm, May 2, 2001). Nurses make up one of the largest voting blocks in the nation and individually, through our votes, can have a great impact on policy at the state and national levels. In addition to individual efforts, nursing professional organizations impact policy.

Although some specialty groups follow legislation pertinent to their particular group, the vehicle for collective action or political action is nursing's primary professional organization in various nations throughout the world. Worldwide, the major international organization is the International Council of Nurses (ICN), discussed previously in Chapter 5. In the United States, for example, the ANA is the major organization. The ANA has a long history and has been the major voice for nursing at the federal level. The ANA began in the early part of the century and formed a special committee on legislation in 1923. "Throughout its history, ANA has demonstrated its commitment to the delivery of quality, cost-effective health care services to the public by fostering high standards of nursing practice and by lobbying the U.S. Congress on health issues affecting the public" (Mason et al., 1993, p. 582).

In 1951, ANA opened its Washington, D.C., office in order to have access to legislators and to lobby Congress on issues important to the nursing profession. In 1992, the ANA launched an effective "Nursing on the Move Campaign." The ANA moved its entire headquarters from Kansas City to Washington, D.C., Capitol Hill, to be more visible to policymakers in Congress. The primary departments involved in legislative activities at ANA headquarters are Government Relations, American Nurses Association Political Action Committee (ANA-PAC), and Political Education, hub of the political network grass-roots program.

The Government Relations Department at ANA headquarters includes a cadre of lobbyists and political staff who ensure that nursing is visible and active during key policy debates. The primary purpose of the Government Relations Department is to lobby and network with legislators. This department is concerned with a myriad of issues and concerns about which lobbyists and staff must become knowledgeable and gain expertise in order to move key and important legislation for nursing and health care.

In 1971, a small group of nurses in New York State organized the "political arm of ANA." The name of the group was Nurses for Political Action (NPA). "A political action committee increases member participation, empowers its members to play a greater role in the development of public policy, raises money to contribute to candidates running for political office and better positions the profession in the legislative arena" (ANA, 1996, p. 5).

In 1974, under the auspices of the ANA, the political action arm became Nurses' Coalition for Action in Politics (N-CAP). Its focus was on education, stimulating participation, and political education of nurses as well as nonpartisan fund raising. In 1986, N-CAP was renamed the ANA-PAC.

By 1994, ANA-PAC ranked the third largest health care political action committee in the United States, surpassed only by the American Medical Association (AMA) and the American Dental Association (ADA). Owing to thousands of nurses who contributed to ANA-PAC, it became the fastest-growing PAC association from the 1991–1992 election cycle to the 1993–1994 election cycle. During the 105th Congress, the ANA-PAC lobbied for nursing legislation in Congress. The 105th Congress enacted legislation to provide direct Medicare reimbursement to all nurse practitioners and clinical nurse specialists; the Community Nursing Organization demonstration project was reauthorized; and there were significant increases in funding for the Nurse Education Act programs and the National Institute of Nursing Research. In addition, all three nurses who ran for reelection to the House of Representatives in the 2000 campaign were successful. ANA-PAC also endorsed 252 candidates for federal office in the 1998 general election (204 Democrats and 47 Republicans) who, as demonstrated by their campaigns or voting history, were friendly toward nursing and public health issues. An extraordinary 88% of those endorsed candidates were elected to the 106th Congress. This success rate is the best in ANA-PAC's 26-year history. For the third consecutive election cycle, ANA-PAC raised more than $1 million from nurses across the country to support candidates and issues (ANA, www.nursingworld.org/gova/federal/anapac/gpacfaq.htm, May 2, 2001).

The development of nursing as a special interest included the growth of ANA's political activities. In 1981, the ANA established its political nurse network. The ANA legislative network is coordinated by the ANA's Department of Political Education in Washington, D.C. The goal of this legislative network is to have a grass-roots structure of nurses established in every one of the 435 congressional districts in the United States. District activities are coordinated under the leadership of a nurse residing in that particular district, who assumes the role and title of Congressional District Coordinator, or CDC. This nurse acts as a liaison between Washington and her or his district. In the late 1980s, the ANA legislative network also established Senate coordinators (SCs), accomplishing the ANA's goal to have one nurse as primary contact to all senators and congresspersons across the nation. The ANA's political network proliferated across the United States and enabled nurses to organize within their congressional districts and states, thereby increasing their visibility, access to legislators, and influence in the political process.

Congressional district coordinators and Senate coordinators work with the ANA's political and legislative departments to keep abreast of issues and serve as the ANA's link educating nurses on the political issues and process and educating members of Congress on nursing's issues. These nurses gather information on the local "political scene" for ANA and ANA-PAC, work on the campaigns of ANA-PAC–endorsed candidates, provide information on federal legislation, and encourage nurses to lobby. As the CDC for the First Congressional District of California, this writer can attest to the influence this network has on nursing's political machine.

In 1993, during the health care reform debate, the ANA coordinated an action team, Nurses Strategic Action Team (N-STAT). This grass-roots program established communication links and mobilized nurses to respond quickly to congressional decisions in order to influence the health care reform debate. The former CDCs and SCs, which were established in the early 1980s, became known as the N-STAT Leadership Team during the period of the Clinton administration's health care reform debates during the 1990s. The N-STAT Team continued to establish effective working relationships with their senators and representatives in Congress through political and grass-roots activities. The other arm of N-STAT is the Rapid Response Team. The Rapid Response Team is basically a communication network; its members provide thousands of voices speaking to public policymakers on nursing and public health issues. Nurses may become members of the team if they belong to their state nurses association (SNA). "The heart of nursing's power on Capitol Hill lies in the participation of thousands of nurses at the grass-roots level; as that participation increases, so will the voice and victories of nursing in the legislative arena" (ANA, 1996, p. 4).

Recognizing and Prioritizing the Issues

One unique purpose of the ANA and SNAs is to shape public policy about health care to be consonant with the goals of nurses, nursing, and the public health. The ANA establishes policies and goals for the profession that form the basis for nursing's contribution to the advancement of health care policy.

These goals serve as the foundation for a variety of ANA program activities. One of these activities is the ANA's legislative and political effort. The ANA seeks enactment and implementation of legislation that will benefit the health and welfare of the nation's citizens. It also participates in the election of candidates to public office who are knowledgeable about and supportive of the profession's policies.

In addition to political and legislative activities, the ANA is involved in other nursing activities and health care issues such as access to quality health care services, financing of health care, funding for nursing education and nursing research, human rights, and the economic and general welfare of nurses.

As indicated above, the ANA has many categories for prioritizing its political efforts. In the formulation of health policy, it is important to identify the issues and prioritize them. In this section, nursing issues on a national and international level will be identified and issues that will enhance the political development of nursing will be explored.

On the national level, the following list of nursing issues is by no means exhaustive. However, it will provide the reader with an overview of current nursing concerns. It is important to remember that policy formation is often a lengthy process; an issue may carry over for several sessions of Congress before legislation is passed.

ANA nursing issues are as follows:

- Health care reform: the next step
- Medicaid reform and Medicare restructuring with prescription drug benefits
- Community nursing organizations (CNOs)
- Workforce and quality issues
- Patient safety
- Long-term care

One issue previously included on this list was reimbursement for advanced practice nurses. As mentioned earlier, ANA lobbying efforts during the 105th Congress resulted in legislation supporting reimbursement.

It is important to identify that ANA priorities incorporate legislation supporting the health of the public as well as legislation specific to nursing as a profession. Nurses will be seen as self-serving if their policy and political activity focus solely on maintaining or expanding the profession. This has been an issue in state legislatures to a greater degree than Congress. If SNAs actively and regularly lobby for policies related to the health and well-being of the public, policymakers will tend not to view their activities toward professional policies as self-serving (Conger & Johnson, 2000).

There are specific issues that will enhance the political development of nursing. These issues cannot be prioritized because it is important to remember that (1) the stages of nursing's political development are not time bound; (2) depending on the issues, there may be movement back and forth among stages; and (3) the events that categorize each stage of nursing's political development are ongoing and are not intended to end or be replaced by those of other stages (Cohen et al., 1996).

Some of the issues that will enhance nursing's body politic are:

- **Development of nursing as a special interest**
  The development of nursing as a special interest has not been a hasty process. It was necessary to grow as a profession—to move schools of nursing into academia, develop nursing's unique theory base, and increase research in nursing. The profession strived to develop its own identity. Attainment of nursing as a special interest will always be advantageous to nursing as well as the public. In the later stages of political development, nursing can advocate for groups in society or a community to improve the well-being of others.

- **Continued growth of the Political Action Committee for Nurses**
  The ANA-PAC was discussed in depth previously. Suffice it to say, the PAC must continue to grow financially to maintain its position as a major political force impacting elections and legislation. Representing the largest group of health care workers, the voice of nurses must be heard by decision makers at least as strongly as physicians, health care organizations, and pharmaceutical and medical supply companies. This takes not only money but also commitment by nurses to be involved in grass-roots efforts at the local level by contacting local legislators to support or reject legislation; working to elect officials supportive of the public's health and nursing as a profession; and working with local leadership, boards of health, and bureaucracies to impact policies and programs.

- **Building coalitions**
  The formation of nursing coalitions in the legislative arena is very important for nursing. One powerful coalition, the Tri-Council of Nursing—consisting of the ANA, American Association of Colleges of Nursing (AACN), National League for Nursing (NLN), and American Organization of Nurse Executives (AONE)—was very significant in the development of a plan for nursing's agenda for health care reform. There are three reasons to enter into coalitions: to "borrow" power, to build a base of support, and to prevent another group from challenging a plan (Mason et al., 1993, p. 169). Perhaps all of those reasons were influential in the success of the agenda.

The ability to forge coalitions and compromises symbolized a new level of maturity for the profession. Coalitions are not limited to coalitions of nursing organizations. Much strength comes from coalitions of a broad range of organizations with interest in a special policy. For example, the nursing coalition of the Utah Nurses Association, school nurses, and colleges of nursing sought support from the Utah Educational Association, Utah Medical Association, and the Parent Teacher Association (PTA) in support of school nursing legislation, which would increase the ratio of nurses to students in schools. Legislators are more responsive to broad-based support by involved interest groups. In the future, the profession will need to build coalitions beyond nursing for broad health policy concerns. "Nursing will have to form political and economic coalitions, not only with consumer groups, but with the other economic and political players in ways which will associate nurses with these groups" (Porter-O'Grady, 1994, p. 36).

- **Fostering nurse appointments and campaigns**
Appointments of nurses to federal panels and agencies, ranging from the Prospective Payment Assessment Commission to the Agency for Health Care Policy and Research (AHCPR), have increased over the years. Also, there has been a proliferation of nurses elected or appointed to positions at the federal and state levels of government. By 1996, 71 nurses held elected positions in state legislatures, and many more were members of legislative staffs in Congress or state governments. In the future, the profession needs to mobilize nurses for campaigns to promote the election of nurses to public offices. Until nurses can be more a part of the legislative arena, it will be difficult to influence "healthy policy."

- **Increasing research and policy analysis**
Congress established the National Center for Nursing Research in 1985, which Congress upgraded to the National Institute of Nursing Research in 1993. In the last several decades, nursing research has grown immensely, but policy research has not. Research on nursing's political socialization is still in its infancy. "Actual policy studies in nursing have minimally increased since Milio's (1981) comprehensive literature review in nursing and no nursing policy analysis research has been done by nurses" (Hall-Long, 1995, p. 27). In the future, nursing needs to increase research related to nursing's political socialization, education, and participation. In addition, "nursing needs to develop sophistication in conducting policy analysis, policy research, and nursing

research with policy implications" (Cohen et al., 1996, p. 265).

- **Increasing education in relation to policy formation and participation**
During the first stage of nursing's political development, the importance of including health policy in nursing curricula was recognized. This importance was espoused by nursing leaders in the mid-1980s and into the 1990s. "Nurses must incorporate a political component into their professional role identity. A political thread must be woven through the nursing curricula" (Brown, 1996, p. 3).

In her article "Community Health Learning Experiences and Political Activism: A Model for Baccalaureate Curriculum Revolution Content," Williams (1993) suggested that political activism content, theory, and practice be a part of community health nursing curricula. She stated that with their "emphasis on public health programs and services, legislative influences on health care, and health policy issues, community health nursing content and practice are the logical areas of the baccalaureate curriculum for political activism education" (p. 353). However, Conger and Johnson (2000) suggested that assigning policy and political activism content to the community health nursing course alone tends to compartmentalize policy and political activism as a process related to community health nursing alone rather than as a process integral to all nursing practice arenas. They suggest that policy content should be a thread throughout the curriculum with exemplars appropriate to the practice arena of concern. For example, bicycle helmet safety or gun safety would be appropriate considerations for the pediatric nursing course and motorcycle helmet policy should be an issue for a critical care nursing course. Both Williams (1993) and Conger and Johnson (2000) agree that nursing faculty should be involved in political issues and activities so that they can serve as role models and mentors for students. Students are constantly hearing about and are interested in health-related political issues: health care reform, America's aging population, motorcycle safety, and right-to-life and living-will concerns, to mention just a few.

In its 2000 document *Essentials of Baccalaureate Nursing Education for Entry Level Community Health Nursing Practice,* the Association of Community Health Nurse Educators (ACHNE) recommended that the theoretical content of baccalaureate programs should include health policy and political and legislative concepts and processes including nursing's role in affecting policy (ACHNE, 2000). Both the American

Association of Colleges of Nursing (AACN) *Essentials of Baccalaureate Education for Professional Nursing Practice* (1998) and the ANA *Scope and Standards of Public Health Nursing Practice* (1999) recommend inclusion of policy and the political process content in the baccalaureate curriculum and public health nursing practice. Unfortunately, although these documents bow to the concept, implementation has not been widely accomplished.

In the future, nursing educators can make sure that political content is included at the baccalaureate level. To hasten this action, The Commission on Collegiate Nursing Education (CCNE) and the NLN Council of Baccalaureate and Higher Degree Programs in Nursing, the two programs ensuring quality nursing education, could include the requirement of political action content as one of the criteria for the accreditation of baccalaureate programs in nursing.

- **Reaffirm nursing's agenda for health care reform**
  Nursing's Agenda for Health Care Reform (Tri-Council for Nursing, 1991) was a milestone for the profession in terms of consensus building and collaboration among organizations. For the first time, the entire profession had a document that depicted the values that nursing stands for in terms of health policy and quality client care. This document enhances the ability of nurses to represent themselves to legislators and others during deliberations of health care reform (Cohen et al., 1996). The development of the agenda reflected a new level of maturity for the nursing profession. In the future, there must be a reaffirmation of nursing's agenda for health care reform and a commitment to be diligent in all efforts to create meaningful reform.

- **Participation in health care reform and health care delivery**
  Evaluating the effectiveness of the nation's health care system continued at a rapid rate during the 1990s. The issues are complex and have profound implications for nursing in an evolving health care delivery system. To date, there have been many problems in health care reform because of the current "erosion" of care. In the future, there will be reorganization of health care delivery and new opportunities for true health care reform. "Nursing offers just what the American health consumer hopes for. This is the time to take the lead and aggressively persevere in negotiating a truly reformed and effective health-based system" (Porter-O'Grady, 1994, p. 38).

There is a fit between the values of the community health nurse and the values of the community. The more the profession pursues its political development and participates in policy making, the more the public will benefit from nursing expertise and the advocacy that nurses can provide on behalf of the public.

Nursing's Role in Shaping Health Policy

Nurses are becoming more political in their workplace and community and on state, national, and international levels. In the workplace, collective bargaining unions are becoming prevalent. Nurses participating in such unions must know the political structure of an organization and the negotiating process. The SNAs and the ANA in the United States have legislative networks in place. Nurses in increasing numbers are participating and taking leadership in these networks. Knowledge of politics and political action is needed if nurses are to participate in decisions about the health care system of which they are so essential a part.

Community health nurses need to be politically active in the community because of shared values and because of the pervasive role the government has on health care. The local level delivers direct services to combat risk factors for disease and injury and seeks to improve

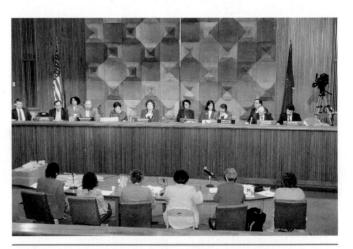

Nurses Making a Presentation before a State Legislature. Photo courtesy of the New York State Nurses Association.

✳ DECISION MAKING

The Future

Nursing has come a long way in its political development. What particular ideas or strategies would be important to enhance nursing's future development?

health levels through government-funded clinics and other programs. Community health nurses need to educate policymakers regarding the needs of the public. Policymakers rarely have backgrounds related to health and may be unaware of health issues or lack understanding of the implications for the health of the public. Policymakers at all levels need input from nurses.

Communicating with legislators or other policymakers is necessary for effective political action. Communicating with a legislator may be accomplished by writing letters, telephoning, attending meetings, and participating in events featuring legislators. The use of e-mail is questionable. While computers are available to most legislators, use of the computers varies greatly. Some legislators are computer literate and others refuse to use them. Some categorize the use of e-mail at the same level as mass mailings of the same content. You must know the preference of your legislator if you choose this method of contact.

Each of the above methods is effective in a particular situation. Constituent letters, if well written, can be a powerful vehicle for ensuring that multiple voices are heard. Use of the telephone in contacting your legislator can save time; also, it often provides a more direct and rapid means of delivering your message. Scheduled meetings with legislators in their district or legislative offices are an important activity for nurse leaders. As the role of the state and federal legislature in determining health issues continues to escalate, personal communication with individual legislators becomes increasingly important. Visits by nurses as health care professionals provide for face-to-face dialogue on pertinent health issues and allow for personalization of an organizational relationship with the legislator and the legislator's staff. Finally, attending candidate campaign events is very important. Endorsing candidates and contributing to (and/or working in) their campaigns ensure our influence as nurses with elected officials. Refer to Table 18-1 and Figures 18-4, 18-5, and 18-6 for specific guidelines on communicating with legislators and other policymakers.

To help shape health policy, one must know and use the strategies of political action. Communicating with a policymaker is only one example of political action; there are many other strategies nurses can learn and use to affect health policy. Many of these strategies were discussed in the previous section as the issues pertinent to nursing's political development were explored. Political action strategies may be categorized into levels of sophistication from the least to the most sophisticated: basic political participation, political awareness, political activism, and political sophistication. These levels and strategies are summarized in Table 18-2. By reviewing this table, the nurse should be able to recognize her or his personal level of sophistication. This table will also provide the nurse with information about how she or he can use additional political action strategies in order to reach a new level of sophistication.

It is important for community health nurses to focus on health policy issues that concern the public, because nursing values can improve the health and health care of people. Emerging values may remain on a collision course with dominant or traditional value systems in our country. Nursing's long-held belief in a more collective approach to health care should continually be voiced. Nurses can help shape the values debate to seek support for increased access to quality, cost-effective health care

---

TABLE 18-1 Writing to Your Legislator

DO	DO NOT
1. Use plain or personal stationery when you write as an individual. If you are writing as the representative of a group, use the organization's stationery. If using e-mail, be sure to identify yourself and/or organization in the beginning of the correspondence.	1. Make threats or personal attacks.
2. Identify the bill with which you are concerned, using title and number when possible.	2. Berate your legislator. If you disagree with him or her, give reasons for your position.
3. If you belong to an association that evaluates legislation, know its position. You have maximum impact when you back up your association's position.	3. Overstate or exaggerate your position.
4. Be concise and factual.	4. Use xeroxed copies of letters, printed postal cards, or form letters.
5. Let the legislator know how the particular measure will affect his or her district.	5. Write only letters of criticism.
6. Include enough pertinent facts and reasons to substantiate your position.	

From Political Action Handbook for Nurses, *by L. Freed, 1996, Santa Rosa, CA: Professor Publishing.*

FIGURE 18-4 Telephoning Your Legislator

Preparation

1. Decide the purpose of your call, and list the points you wish to make in the course of the telephone conversation.
2. Know the number of the bill you want to discuss, its author, its general purpose and contents.
3. If possible, find out when and where the next action is scheduled on that bill.
4. If you are representing an organization, know approximately how many organization members live or work in the legislator's district.
5. Make sure you understand and can explain simply your rationale for support of or position on the legislation.

Suggestions for Conversation

1. Make the reason for your call clear at the beginning of the conversation.
2. State your name and what county you work in, the association position you hold (if any), and the legislative district in which you live (if applicable).

3. If you are calling about a bill and the legislator is not available, ask to speak to a legislative aide.
4. Ask for the appointment secretary or personal secretary if you are calling to make an appointment with the legislator.
5. As briefly as possible, state the state nurses association's position on the bill or issue and clearly stress the local support of that position.
6. Try to determine the position held by the legislator on the bill or issue.
7. If you spoke with a legislative staff person, make a note of the name.
8. Thank the legislator or legislative staff person for his or her time and assistance.
9. Make a brief report, verbally or in writing, to the state nurses association legislative chairperson or other appropriate person.

From *Political Action Handbook for Nurses,* by L. Freed, 1996, Santa Rosa, CA: Professor Publishing.

FIGURE 18-5 Meeting with Your Legislator

Contacting the District Office

1. Contact the district office during legislative recess or make arrangements to visit your state capital or Washington, D.C.
2. Write or call in advance for an appointment.
3. Make your appointment for a specific time period; usually half an hour to an hour in length is appropriate.
4. If the meeting is going to focus on a specific legislative topic, let the legislator's staff know this at the time the meeting is arranged.
5. When a legislator is not available, make an appointment with the legislator's staff person.

Preparing for the Meeting

1. Select a small group of knowledgeable nurses to attend meetings.
2. Meet as a group in advance of the meeting with the legislator to:
   a. Determine the primary goal of the meeting.
   b. Identify which issues or legislation need to be discussed to meet that goal.

c. Review the rationale for positions on issues or legislation.
d. Determine the roles and responsibilities of individual members for the conduct of the meeting.

During the Meeting

1. Be prepared to be brief and speak to the point.
2. Stick to the topic(s) you planned to discuss.
3. Supply a fact sheet or other information on the topic or issue being addressed.
4. Leave on time unless the legislator clearly wishes to continue.
5. Thank the legislator (or staff person) for his or her time.

After the Meeting

1. Take time to debrief and to summarize impressions of the meeting and the legislator's positions.
2. Write a brief summary of the meeting and forward it to the legislative chairperson of the state nursing association.
3. Discuss and plan strategy for follow-up.

From *Political Action Handbook for Nurses,* by L. Freed, 1996, Santa Rosa, CA: Professor Publishing.

FIGURE 18-6 Reasons for Participating in Events Featuring Legislation

1. To get better acquainted with legislators.
2. To listen to legislators' concerns.
3. To question legislators about issues and bills in your state capital and Washington.
4. To make a statement to your legislators about the viewpoint of your state nursing association.
5. To showcase your clout as an organization.

From *Political Action Handbook for Nurses,* by L. Freed, 1996, Santa Rosa, CA: Professor Publishing.

TABLE 18-2 Levels of Political Sophistication and Political Action Strategies

LEVEL	POLITICAL ACTION STRATEGIES
Basic	• Voting
	• Reading newspapers, magazines, and journals
	• Understanding the political process
Political awareness	• Learning about politics, policy, and PACs
	• Lobbying: writing a legislator, telephoning a legislator
	• Participating in a grass-roots political network—local or state level
	• Participating in voter registration programs
	• Campaigning
	• Supporting nursing organizations
Political activism	• Lobbying: meeting with a legislator, participating in events featuring legislators
	• Participating in a grass-roots political nurse network–federal level
	• Leading a grass-roots political nurse network
	• Participating in coalition building
	• Participating in campaigns
	• Contributing to PACs
	• Electioneering
	• Attending conferences and workshops and completing internships related to policymaking
	• Supporting nursing organizations and lobbying for their interests
	• Presenting testimony—local level
	• Participating in community partnerships
Political sophistication	• Forming coalitions
	• Presenting testimony—state or federal level
	• Becoming appointed to federal panels or agencies
	• Conducting public policy research
	• Running for public office

Contributed by L. Freed.

for all Americans. "Nurses are in a unique position to take the heartbeat of their clients and translate it into caring health policy. The time is now for us to capture our legislators' attention and make our concerns known" (Jennings, 1995).

AFTER A BILL BECOMES LAW

Take the opportunity to read a bill that has become a public law. You will notice that most policies, which become law, are written in general terms. There are few if any specific instructions as to how to implement the law. The role of the *legislative branch* of government is to determine the "shoulds" or "oughts" related to issues. Laws are usually written in broad terms to provide flexibility and adaptability over time (Loquist, 1999). Determining the way the

law will be implemented in detail is the role of the *executive branch* of government. The law is assigned to the appropriate department in the executive branch. For example, health-related law would be assigned to the Department of Health and Human Services. Here rules and regulations for implementation of the law are established. It is important for nurses to realize that their work is not done once a bill becomes a law. Rules and regulations have a major impact on the direction a law or program developed to implement the law takes. Nurses have an opportunity to influence the nature of rules and regulations that define program implementation.

Oftentimes laws are challenged in the *judicial branch* of government through the courts system. The role of the Supreme Court of the United States is to determine whether or not a law brought before it is consistent with the intent of the U.S. Constitution. An example of this you may be familiar with is laws related to abortion. *Roe vs. Wade* was a case which challenged the federal law against women's free choice for abortion. In 1973, the Supreme Court, through the *Roe vs. Wade* case, determined that the law preventing abortion was unconstitutional. This case, in effect, overturned a law established through the legislative process. Periodically through the years this decision has been challenged in the Supreme Court but has always been upheld. A number of states have tried to limit women's rights for abortion, but through the courts, these state laws have been overturned.

Oftentimes legislation passed at the federal level opens the door for state legislatures to determine if a particular program is of interest for them. The Children's Health Insurance Program (CHIP) is one example of this. The intent of the program and federal money were made available to states that were interested in enacting legislation and developing their programs as they saw fit to mesh with the rest of their health care financing philosophy and approach. This is a common practice. States frequently develop more specific rules and regulations than the program at the federal level and, in turn, will pass the program down to the local level for implementation. Of course, each level is accountable to the level above it. For example, the Women, Infants, and Children's (WIC) Program is implemented at the local level. How it is implemented varies according to the values and needs of the local community. In some, the program is centralized into one office; in others it is totally decentralized. In some it is located in the local health departments; in others it is carried out by a private, nonprofit organization.

SOURCES OF INFORMATION

There are many sources of information and resources for nurses who are interested and wish to participate in political activism. The most important first step in the decision to take a political stance and attempt to influence the political process is to become an informed student of politics. To become informed, one must read, listen, and watch. Local newspapers, magazines, and even professional journals are filled with reports of policy decisions. Radio and television news reports are both excellent sources of information and a gauge of public opinion.

When an issue or a piece of legislation is of particular interest or concern, be sure to know the topic well. The nurse should become knowledgeable about the issue or bill so that when it is debated he or she will be able to answer any questions that may be posed by lawmakers, voters, or others. Nurses should study the political process to ensure they can anticipate the paths the legislation or politician needs to travel. Nurses should form coalitions with organizations that are similarly interested in the issue and should identify the point in the

political process where they are most likely to have the most influence; this point will depend on the resources, alliances, and strategies developed. With persistence, political activism can be the most rewarding way of demonstrating community health nursing's strength in caring for the people community health nurses serve.

The following sections include selected resource information. This list is not exhaustive. Refer to Appendix B for more resources.

Books

Policy and Politics for Nurses: Action and Change in the Workplace, Government, Organization and Community, 3rd ed., by Mason, Talbott, and Leavitt (1998), is an excellent book suitable for a reference in nursing and politics. *Health Policy and Politics: A Nurses Guide* (Milstead, 1999) covers a broad range of policy and political strategies, decision points, activities, and outcomes. It is an outstanding book for a nurse who is interested in becoming a change agent for health.

Healthy People 2010 by the U.S. Department of Health and Human Services (2000) includes the current U.S. health priorities for disease treatment and prevention and serves as a logical starting point for nurse activists. Familiarity with the *Healthy People 2010* priority areas provides both a priority list for nurses and an insight into the discrepancies between the country's stated agenda and the actual actions taken on that agenda. Accessing the Internet for updates on *Healthy People 2010* is also important. *Healthy People in Healthy Communities* (U.S. Department of Health and Human Services, 2001) is a planning guide for building community coalitions, creating vision and partnerships, and measuring results toward improving the health of a community. An examination of similar initiatives in other countries will enhance nursing's knowledge of global actions to improve health.

Magazines and Newsletters

The American Nurse is the official publication of the ANA. This monthly news magazine is distributed to state nurses associations and ANA members and includes invaluable information on policy issues and political action.

Capitol Update is the legislative newsletter for nurses. This bimonthly newsletter is compiled by the Departments of Federal Government Relations and Political and Grassroots Programs at ANA Headquarters, Washington, D.C. Each issue usually includes "Legislative Update," "In the Agencies," "Political Update," and announcements. This newsletter is a must for the political activist.

Policy, Politics, and Nursing Practice is a quarterly nursing journal published by Sage. Its scope is broader than policy and politics alone, including articles related to health services research and political initiatives at both

Perspectives... ✳

INSIGHTS OF A NURSING ACTIVIST

While many health care issues are decided by Congress and state legislatures, local government officials often have the power to impact the health of a community and should not be overlooked. County and city officials frequently control funding for health departments, mental health programs, and substance-abuse treatment programs. Many larger community problems often encompass health care issues. It is important for nurses to be familiar with their local elected officials and understand the role they play in health care decisions. As an advocate for the health care needs of women and children in my community, I learned the importance of understanding the organization and power structures of local government.

In 1992, I was part of a group of concerned citizens in Utah County, Utah, who came together to develop a better way to respond when a child made an allegation of sexual abuse. One of the issues we faced was how to provide specialized medical examinations for children at a cost the community could afford. We wanted to create a system for the investigation and prosecution of child abuse that put the needs of the child and family first. At that time when a child made a disclosure of sexual abuse he or she was taken to multiple agencies for repeated examinations and interviews. Advocates for community change wanted to create a model center that would encourage a multidisciplinary approach and take the trauma out of investigating and prosecuting child sexual abuse. In conjunction with two other communities, we developed the concept of the Children's Justice Center.

The Children's Justice Center is a "homelike" facility where professionals are brought to the child to provide interviews, examinations, and support to both the child and family. Prior to the development of the Children's Justice Center there was only one place in Utah where a child could receive a medical examination from a health care provider with specialized training in sexual abuse. We believed that the children of our community would be best served if we could provide a nurse practitioner with specialized training in sexual abuse examinations at the Children's Justice Center.

To achieve this change in our community, we needed the support of our county commission and the county attorney. The county commission funded the health department, which would be the local health care entity to provide financial support and supervision for the nurse practitioner. The county attorney is the person responsible for prosecution of child abuse in Utah County. His support was needed in order for the nurse to be able to testify as an expert witness in child abuse cases.

The county attorney did not want to use nurses as expert witnesses in child abuse cases. He believed that juries preferred to hear medical testimony from a physician. We gathered data from other communities and other prosecutors who worked with nurses as expert witnesses. After several presentations to the Utah County Commission, we were able to convince the commissioners that our program would be the best option for the children of Utah County. Eight years later our program has become a model for the state of Utah. Last year the legislature funded a team of nurse practitioners to perform examinations throughout the state.

—Susan Chasson, RN, MSN, JD

the national and international levels. It is an excellent resource for current nursing involvement in the policy arena.

Specialty Organizations

Many specialty nursing organizations such as the American Association of Critical Care Nurses (AACN), the Association of Women's Health, Obstetrical, and Neonatal Nurses (AWHONN), and the Association of Operating Room Nurses (AORN), to name just a few, are active in politics and distribute legislative newsletters. Nurses who

belong to a specialty organization and wish to increase their political involvement should request specific newsletters from their organization.

Political Internships

Nurse in Washington Internship (NIWI) is an internship program sponsored by the National Federation for Specialty Nursing Organizations (NFSNO). This program is for nurses who wish to develop legislative knowledge and skills of political activism. This annual intensive four-day program educates nurses throughout the United

States about the policy process in the nation's capital. Since its inception in 1985, many nurses have developed the ability to become participants in nursing political activities. Mary Wakefield, nurse and Chief Staff to U.S. Senator Kent Conrad (D-ND), stated, "There is a direct link between what happens in D.C. and how we practice, what we teach, and what we research" (Chaffee, 1996, p. 21).

The Robert Woods Johnson Health Policy Foundation (RWJF) established the Robert Woods Johnson Health Policy Fellowship Program (HPFP) in 1973. The HPFP provides the opportunity for nurses to be active participants in health policy development at the national level. To date, 151 fellows, 8% of whom are nurses, have participated. RWJF has expended more than $13 million in support of the program.

As stated in the 1998 program brochure, "The HPFP is designed to develop the capacity of outstanding midcareer health professionals in academic and community-based settings to assume leadership roles in health policy and management." This career development program provides opportunities for midcareer professionals to gain an understanding of the health policy process and to contribute to the formulation of new policies and programs. Today, the program aims to enrich the substance of the health policy debate at both the federal and state levels.

Six fellows, primarily with academic backgrounds, are selected to participate in the program each year. The fellows arrive in Washington in September and begin a 12-week orientation period during which they are introduced to key officials and staff from both the legislative and executive branches. Today, most fellows choose to work in one Congressional office (either House or Senate) for the duration of their fellowship; however, they are free to choose up to two placements in either congressional offices or the executive branch. The program has always been bipartisan, with fellows serving in the offices of both Republicans and Democrats. During their assignments, fellows draft legislation, perform background research, organize and staff hearings, brief members of Congress on particular issues prior to committee and floor votes, respond to constituent requests, and represent their offices at conferences. After completion of the program, fellows have used the experience to play a more active role in health policy–related activities at their home institutions and/or in their home states, and particularly in their local professional societies and affiliations (www.rwjf.org/health/fellowse.htm, May 14, 2001).

ORGANIZATIONS INVOLVED IN POLITICS AND POLICY

Nursing and health care organizations provide an opportunity for nurses to influence health and public policy through collective action. Perhaps one of the best examples of collective action in the United States was Nursing's Agenda for Health Care Reform, a policy statement on national health care. More than 60 organizations supported the agenda. Many nursing organizations have recognized the importance of political action for their members. And some specialty nursing organizations have enhanced their specialty by intense political involvement. It is also important for nurses to be active participants in multidisciplinary organizations such as the American Public Health Association (APHA), because their participation can lead to coalition building. Representation in multidisciplinary groups strengthens political efforts.

These nursing organizations have been involved in politics and political activism longer than other nursing organizations: ANA, SNAs, NLN, and the Tri-Council for Nursing. By the mid-1980s, owing to the growth of specialty groups, there was also a proliferation of specialty organizations.

The ANA began in the early part of the century and formed a Special Committee on Legislation in 1923. The departments that have to do with politics and policy are:

Government Relations—lobbies legislators and follows legislation in Congress

ANA-PAC—a powerful political action committee

Political Grassroots Program—a political grass-roots network for nurses

The SNAs determine preferred state policy and lobby on most issues of concern to nursing. They also have their own PACs. Each state has an affiliated association with the ANA.

The NLN was formed in the early 1950s and has joined with the ANA on many issues of concern to nursing. This organization is one arm of the Tri-Council for Nursing, which developed Nursing's Agenda for Health Care Reform. Although the focus of the League is on nursing education and the accreditation of schools of nursing, the NLN has participated in policy and political debates at all levels of government.

The Tri-Council for Nursing originated in 1981 and is composed of the ANA, NLN, AACN, and the American Organization of Nurse Executives (AONE). (AONE joined the alliance in 1985 without any change in the title.) Its purpose is to facilitate coordination and communication on key professional issues and to promote federal legislation of mutual concern. The alliance has played a major role in advancing the profession and the nation's health in the policy arena (Hall-Long, 1995).

The National Federation for Specialty Nursing Organizations (NFSNO) is "a loosely structured alliance of large and small nursing specialty organizations whose purpose is to coordinate efforts of practice, education, and other areas of mutual concern among nursing organizations" (Hall-Long, 1995, p. 26).

RESEARCH FOCUS

Impact of a Children's Health Insurance Program by Age

Study Problem/Purpose

The State Children's Health Insurance program (SCHIP), commonly known as CHIP, was created by the Balanced Budget Act of 1997. This act gave states that passed legislation for a CHIP a portion of $24 million over a five-year period to provide health insurance to children who do not qualify for other public programs yet whose parents cannot afford to purchase private insurance.

The purpose of this research study was to examine variables related to lack of health insurance before health insurance was obtained compared with these same variables one year after the children had been on one of two publicly funded low-cost health insurance programs, including CHIP. Indicator variables were: regular source of care, use of specific services, unmet need or delay in obtaining services, and childhood activities limited by parents because of lack of health insurance. Three research questions were asked: (1) Before enrollment in the health insurance program, were there any differences in indicator variables across age groups? (2) After being enrolled in the program for one year, was there any improvement in indicator variables? (3) After being enrolled in the health insurance program, was the magnitude of differences in indicators across age groups the same or different?

Methods

The study was conducted among a sample of 887 families randomly selected from 5864 uninsured children enrolling in one of two CHIP-related programs during 1995 in western Pennsylvania. A parent was interviewed within 2 weeks of acceptance into one of two programs relating to indicator variables prior to acceptance into the health insurance program. The families were interviewed again at 6 months and 12 months following acceptance. Interviews consisted of demographic information, fixed response questions, and open-ended questions and reflected the care of all children in the family. A group of children who were enrolled during 1996 served as a comparison group. Children were divided into four groups: 0–5 years, 6–10 years, 11–14 years, and 15–19 years.

Findings

Findings from this study indicated that there were significant differences in most indicator variables across age groups before enrollment. After one year of enrollment, there was significant improvement in most indicators within each age group and for the total group. After one year, the differences across age groups had decreased markedly and in some cases disappeared (p. 1057). After examining the comparison group, researchers concluded that the change could not be attributed to an improvement in the health care delivery system since the levels of indicator variables were similar to those of the study children.

Implications

The findings of this study indicate a pattern of poor health care, as reflected by indicator variables, especially for older children. Lack of access to the health care system for all age groups of children greatly reduced the exposure to health promotion, disease prevention, and early intervention for health problems, especially with the adolescent age groups. For adolescents, this reflected lost opportunities related to substance abuse and pregnancy. The findings of the study also indicated that when low-cost insurance is available, families seek health care.

Source: Keane, D. R., Lave, J. R., Ricci, E. M., & LaVallee, C. P. (1999). The impact of a children's health insurance program by age. Pediatrics, 104(5), 1051–1058.

The National Organization Liaison Forum (NOLF) was formulated in the early 1980s. It is a diverse forum within the ANA made up of a coalition of nursing organizations. Its purpose is to "provide a unified approach to national policy issues and nursing interests" (Hall-Long, 1995, p. 26).

The AACN Certification Corporation certifies critical care nurses and promotes critical care nursing practice that contributes to desired client outcomes through the CCRN certification program in adult, pediatric, and neonatal critical care nursing. This corporation is a separate affiliate of the AACN, the world's largest specialty nursing organization. In an article titled "AACN Perspective, Redefining Nursing in the Midst of Health Care Reform," Caterinicchio (1995) states, "Nurses are constants in every phase of health care delivery—and reform.

Through a shared and mutual commitment to promote a health care system driven by the needs of patients and their families, nurses have the power to set the tone for change across the entire nation" (p. 9).

The AONE is an association dedicated to advancing the practice of nurses who facilitate, design, and manage care. The organization focuses on resources that promote education, advocacy, research, information sharing, networking, and career advancement opportunities. Since 1994, the AONE has strengthened its linkages between the national organization and the Organization of Nurse Executives (ONE) at the state and local levels. It strengthened its linkages because the AONE recognized that both leadership and policy development begin at the local level, where real health care reform is taking shape (Swan, 1995).

The American Academy of Nurse Practitioners (AANP) is an organization that includes all nurse practitioner specialties. Its purposes are to promote high standards of health care delivered by nurse practitioners and to act as a forum to enhance the identity and continuity of nurse practitioners at a national and international level. The organization actively promotes health policy through its governmental affairs activities in Washington, D.C. Participating in the development of health policy has become an important part of the role of the nurse practitioner (Towers, 1995).

The American Association of Occupational Health Nurses (AAOHN) is the national professional association for registered nurses who provide on-the-job health care for the nation's workers. As the largest group of providers of health care at the worksite, occupational health nurses are key players in directing public policy. After many years of working with the Occupational Safety and Health Administration (OSHA), in 1993 the OSHA of Occupational Health Nursing was established. In an article about AAOHN, Livsey (1995) states, "In today's work environment, it is imperative that nurses take a proactive position in influencing health policy at national, state, and local levels" (p. 14).

There are other specialty nursing organizations involved in politics. Some have their own lobbyists on Capitol Hill; others do not. It is important to remember not to work alone on a policy or issue and thus fragment nursing. The more one specialty organization can work with other organizations to form coalitions, the more influence the profession will have on legislators and other policymakers. The following is only a partial listing of other specialty nursing organizations involved in the policy arena:

- American Nephrology Nurses' Association
- Association of Operating Room Nurses
- Organization for Obstetric, Gynecologic and Neonatal Nurses (NAACOG)
- Oncology Nursing Society

Another national organization is the American Public Health Association (APHA), which was founded in 1882 and represents approximately 50,000 public health workers. It is a multidisciplinary organization representing varied health professionals and health organizations. The APHA has numerous special-interest sections, including a Public Health Nursing Section. The association is nationally and internationally recognized for its expertise and leadership in public health. The APHA frequently provides testimony to Congress and is involved with both public policy and regulatory issues. The APHA is a member of the World Federation of Public Health Associations and serves as that organization's secretariat.

The Agency for Health Care Policy and Research (AHCPR) is one of eight agencies of the U.S. Public Health Service. This agency was established by Congress in 1990 and is the nation's focal point of health services research. The AHCPR seeks answers to some of the most pressing health concerns facing the population and serves as a bridge between researchers, clinicians, and policymakers. Participation by nurses from all backgrounds is welcomed and encouraged by the agency (Bavier, 1995).

INTERNATIONAL HEALTH ISSUES

Global health policy needs to be considered at two levels. The first level is international policy, with direct involvement of the United States that impacts the health of U.S. residents specifically. These policies, such as the North American Free Trade Agreement (NAFTA), may not be directed at health issues but impact health on a daily basis. The second level is policies of other countries that have potential impact on the health of the people of the United States. The third level is comprised of international policies, for which the United States is an indirect participant, through agencies such as the World Health Organization or World Bank, which primarily impact the health of other nations.

U.S. International Policy Directly Affecting United States

Not only do local, state, and national policies affect the health of the population of the United States, so does U.S. international policy. Consider the fierce political battles waged over NAFTA, which opened trading between the United States, Mexico, and Canada on January 1, 1994. The numerous health consequences of this international policy could not have been foreseen. One impact is reflected by the dramatic increase in tractor-trailer truck traffic on the major north-south freeways leading into Mexico. The 900-mile corridor of Interstate 35 between the Texas-Oklahoma border and Mexico alone carries 32% of the NAFTA-related tractor-trailer truck traffic. The tractor-trailer traffic through Dallas/Fort Worth and Austin nearly doubled between 1992 and 1996 (personal communication, Gabriela Garcia, Texas Department of Transportation, May 1, 2001). The resulting number of deaths and injuries involving tractor-trailer trucks increased by 23% between 1993 and 1999 on the Texas freeways (Personal Communication, Tom Vinger, Texas Department of Public Safety, May 1, 2001).

Secondary effects of this increased truck load include noise pollution and air pollution. In 1994 there was only one bridge between Laredo, Texas, and Nuevo Laredo, the Mexican city across the Rio Grande River from Laredo. A new international bridge opened September 2000 to ease traffic congestion on the old bridge and to move traffic out of Laredo. The result was a significant drop in carbon monoxide levels at the old bridge. Figure 18-7 shows the actual reduction in carbon monoxide for the three months following the bridge opening compared with the same three months from the year before.

One can only imagine the effects of the new free-trade agreement signed during the 2001 Summit of the Americas held in Quebec. The accord, signed by leaders of 34 countries in North, Central, and South America, would open borders to free trade beginning December 2005 (Deans, 2001).

Another impact of NAFTA is the daily migration of workers across the Texas-Mexico border and its relation to health insurance coverage. In the 2001 legislative session, Texas considered House Bill 2498 and Senate Bill 1826, which would allow health maintenance organizations (HMOs) in Texas to contract services provided by an HMO delivery network located in the United Mexican States. In this way, workers living within 62 miles of the border on the Texas side, workers crossing from Mexico to work in Texas, and those living in Mexico working for U.S. companies located in Mexico could seek covered health care in Mexico rather than crossing the border for health care. As of May 15, 2001, this legislation had passed favorably out of the House; substitute legislation passed favorably out of Senate committee but is stalled

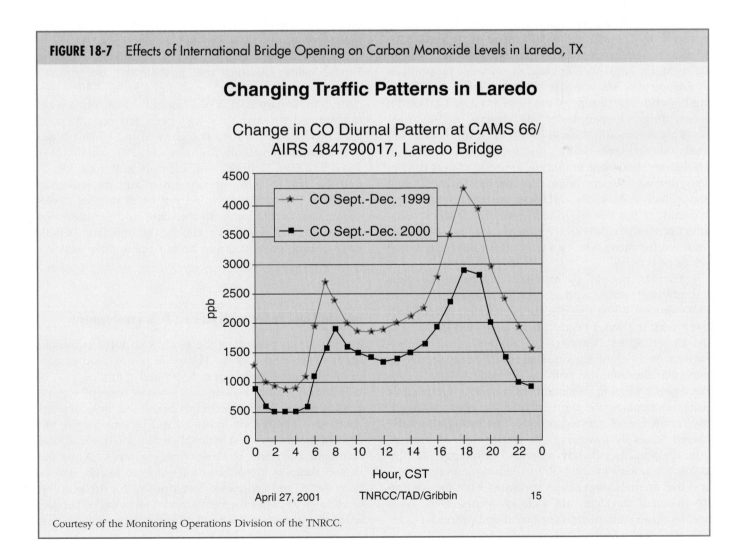

FIGURE 18-7 Effects of International Bridge Opening on Carbon Monoxide Levels in Laredo, TX

Courtesy of the Monitoring Operations Division of the TNRCC.

on the floor of the Senate. This would be the first legislation of its kind providing reimbursement for regular health care provided by non-U.S. health care providers covered by U.S. health care plans. In the past, health insurers have allowed foreign health care if it were related to a travel emergency. When passed, this legislation will open the door to a number of other efforts of this type.

Public policies that mandate withholding medical services from immigrants are affecting western and southern border states in the United States and have a major impact on the health of populations in many near-border towns in California, Arizona, and Texas. Some health care programs continue to provide services to undocumented immigrants despite the policy.

International Policies Indirectly Affecting the United States

In the not-so-recent past, the United States had little need to be concerned about health policy in other countries affecting the health of North Americans. For the most part, the oceans provided effective barriers preventing most health problems from entering North America. It is not so now. The availability and speed of air travel have all but erased borders between continents. U.S. chain stores and restaurants are found in epidemic proportions in Europe and Asia; diseases found in Europe and Asia are threats to the people of the United States. Two health issues are good examples of this concern.

Foot and mouth disease (FMD) in cloven-hoofed animals (sheep, goats, cattle, and swine) is occurring in epidemic proportions in Europe, especially Great Britain. This disease has not been documented in the United States since 1929. While FMD does not infect humans, an epidemic of this disease in the United States will directly affect economics and dietary patterns, resulting in poorer nutrition for those who can least afford increases in the prices of protein.

Animals, people, or materials that bring the virus into physical contact with susceptible animals can spread FMD viruses. While this disease is prevalent throughout the world, the water borders have protected Britain and the United States. Not so today, although there are numerous methods of transmission for this disease, two in particular illustrate the point to be made by this example: People wearing contaminated clothes or footwear or using contaminated equipment pass the virus to susceptible animals and infected products are brought into the United States by travelers (U.S. Department of Agriculture, www.aphis.usda.gov/oa/pubs/brofmd.pdf, May 14, 2001). Therefore, in addition to a ban on imported meat and live animals, prevention measures have focused on international travelers and include treatment of shoes and baggage examination for prohibited products.

A second example of current interest is bovine spongiform encephalopathy (BSE), commonly referred to as mad cow disease. Since it was identified in the mid-1980s in Britain, mad cow disease has resulted in the slaughter of millions of cattle—and the deaths of 10–15 people per year from the related brain-wasting disease which is a variant of Creutzfeldt-Jakob disease (vCJD), first identified in 1994. BSE appears to have originated from scrapie, an endemic spongiform encephalopathy of sheep and goats that has been recognized in Europe since the mid-18th century. It has since spread to most sheep-breeding countries and is widespread in Britain, where until 1988 the rendered carcasses of livestock (including sheep) were fed to ruminants and other animals as a protein-rich nutritional supplement (www.aphis.usda.gov/oa/bse, May 15, 2001).

The United States has instituted prevention measures since 1997. Food and Drug Administration (FDA) regulations have prohibited such feed from going to ruminants in the United States because scientists believe the disease spreads when cows eat remains of potentially infected animals. In addition, importation of European cattle has been banned. Herds of cattle imported from Europe around the time of the outbreak have been quarantined and euthanized (www.aphis.usda.gov/oa/bse, May 15, 2001).

As with HMD, BSE is a public health issue for the United States. Although laws prohibit the use of ruminant byproducts in feed, mistakes can and have occurred. In January 2001, a number of cattle in Texas were quarantined for fear they had been fed contaminated feed produced by a feed company in the United States (www.latelinenews.com/ll/english/1042591.shtml, May 15, 2001). Had authorities or scientists in Europe identified the risk of transmission earlier and implemented laws, the United States would not be at risk for development of an outbreak. In this case and in numerous others, the U.S. population can be the unwilling beneficiary of problems occurring because of another nation's poor policy judgment.

International Policy with Indirect U.S. Involvement

Seventy-seven percent of the world's population lives in nonindustrialized nations. These are poor countries economically and depend upon developed countries for economic and health assistance. However, except for the eradication of vaccine preventable disease, little benefits have been realized by industrialized nations for the billions of dollars invested in health, educational, social, and economic programs in developing countries. While the United States is involved in international health, education, social, and economic development for the purpose of altruism to better the health and well-being of people, at least as important are political and policy ramifications.

The primary U.S. agency involved in international health is the United States Agency for International Development (USAID). USAID's history has a long history dating back to the Marshall Plan reconstruction of Europe after World War II and the Truman administration's Point Four Program. Since 1961, when President Kennedy signed the Foreign Assistance Act and created USAID by executive order, USAID has been the principal U.S. agency providing assistance to countries recovering from disaster, trying to escape poverty, and engaging in democratic reforms (www.usaid.gov/about, May 15, 2001).

Andrew Natsios, the program administrator for USAID, testified before the Senate Appropriations Committee Subcommittee on Foreign Operations on May 8, 2001. In his testimony he stated (Natsios, www.usaid.gov/press/spe_test/testimony/2001/ty010508.html, May 15, 2001):

> Foreign assistance is sometimes the most appropriate tool, when diplomacy is not enough or military force imprudent. In general, foreign assistance works hand-in-hand with other foreign policy tools. Foreign assistance implements peace agreements arranged by diplomats and often enforced by the military; foreign assistance supports peacekeeping efforts by building economic and political opportunity; foreign assistance helps developing and transition nations move toward democratic systems and market economies; foreign assistance helps nations prepare for participation in the global trading system and become better markets for U.S. exports. All of these activities help build a more peaceful, stable, and prosperous world—which is very much in the interest of the United States.

USAID has identified four pillars that will "cut through all programs of the agency and improve the Agency's effectiveness as a key foreign policy instrument of the [Bush] Administration. The pillars will coordinate and focus Agency resources and capabilities to address globalization and conflict" (Natsios, www.usaid.gov/press/spe_test/testimony/2001/ty010508.html, May 15, 2001). These pillars are economic growth and agriculture, global health, conflict prevention and developmental relief, and the global development alliance that reflects a public/private partnership internationally.

Other U.S. organizations that play a less political role in international health include the APHA, the Red Cross, and the Centers for Disease Control and Prevention (CDC). The first two depend upon volunteers and are nonprofit organizations. The CDC has been described elsewhere related to national initiatives. International efforts of the CDC focus on toxic substances and disease, epidemiology, chronic disease prevention and health promotion, environmental health, health statistics, HIV/AIDS, sexually transmitted diseases, tuberculosis, infectious disease, injury prevention, immunizations, and occupational health and safety.

International Health Organizations

The WHO, Pan American Health Organization, and United Nation's Children's Fund (UNICEF) are organizations actively involved in improving health and promoting policies toward this end. They have been described in detail in Chapter 5.

The World Bank is another agency that influences health policy internationally. It provides approximately $16 billion in loans to over 100 developing countries and supports 457 health-related initiatives. Many World Bank–financed health projects emphasize the prevention, control, and treatment of specific conditions such as malaria, diarrhea, measles, and HIV/AIDS through strengthened primary health services. For example, it worked with the government of India and donors to finance a 1993 leprosy project that improved outreach to poor communities and promoted more effective treatment and service packages. The number of registered leprosy cases dropped from 1.7 million in 1992 to 0.5 million in 1996. More recently, the World Bank has become increasingly active in health sector reform projects undertaken in partnership with governments. While issues vary from country to country, the guiding principles of this work are to ensure equity, access, quality, consumer satisfaction, and efficiency in the financing and provision of health services, while controlling the growth in expenditures for health in line with economic growth (www.wbln0018.worldbank.org/HDNet/HDdocs.nsf, May 15, 2001).

An important role of the World Bank is to help governments of countries with which it works. The objectives toward this goal are based on the view that building efficient and accountable public sector institutions is mandatory if sustainable development is to be maintained. A lesson learned from East Asia (and to some extent Russia) is that good policies are not enough, that the World Bank cannot afford to look the other way when a country is plagued by deeply dysfunctional public institutions that limit accountability and set perverse rules of the game. Anticorruption strategies include developing coalitions of government, civil society, nongovernmental organizations, and others within a country. Coalitions have proven to sustain reform but also can strengthen and sustain political will to act against corruption (www1.worldbank.org/publicsector, May 15, 2001). The World Bank, in control of the purse strings to aid developing countries, has a great deal of power to affect political change and impact health policy internationally.

International Nursing Organizations

The International Council of Nurses (ICN) was formed by a group of British nurses at the turn of the century. It is composed of over 90 nursing associations (only one from each country may belong). The ANA is the member from the United States. The organization provides a medium through which national nursing associations share their common interests and goals and work together to influence policy supporting and improving the health of the people of their nations.

LAWS THAT AFFECT COMMUNITY HEALTH NURSING PRACTICE

Laws at multiple levels affect community health nurses. Laws relating to the public's health specifically and to the social and economic environments define and limit the services community health nurses can provide by defining the limits of their practice as well as resources available to their clients: individuals, families, aggregates, and communities. Laws related to nursing practice define the professional boundaries of community health nursing practice. In addition, laws defining malpractice and negligence apply to community health nursing as well as hospital-based nursing practice.

The legislature of a state or Congress enacts *statutory law*. The focus of this chapter has been primarily on how nurses can influence statutory law. At the local level, city councils and other forms of local government institute *ordinances;* county boards of health can institute *health ordinances*.

The rules and regulations developed by the executive branch are called *administrative law*. While this type of law does not go through a system similar to the legislative process, it does become open for public comment. At the federal level, rules and regulations proposed are published in the *Federal Register* and public hearings are set for comments about the proposals. Rules and regulations may be changed after this public input. This is an excellent time for nurses and nursing organizations to collaborate with others interested in impacting the direction of the rules and regulations. At state and local levels, notice of public hearings are posted in newspapers and widely advertised in newsletters and mailings to organizations with special interest in the issue or program.

Law developed as a result of court decision is called *judicial* or *common law*. An example is *Roe vs. Wade* and the abortion issue discussed earlier. Judges should be impartial and, therefore, it is not appropriate for individuals or groups to lobby them. However, judges do reflect the values of the society of which they are part. For example, a decision made by a judge in a rural area of Alabama may not be the same as one in New York.

Advocacy and social justice are two guiding principles of community health nursing practice. As such, we have the professional responsibility to work to change laws, established at any level, that negatively impact the health of our clients as well as negatively impact our nursing practice.

Professional Laws

Not only are rules and regulations developed for laws and programs that impact our clients, rules and regulations are developed that define the practice of community health nursing. Community health nurses, as all registered nurses, are required to take the NCLEX licensing examination. Some states such as California require a registered nurse to qualify for a Public/Community Health Nursing Certificate, issued by the state, that reflects educational preparation in the area to practice as a public/community health nurse.

In 1998 Utah was the first state to adopt into law the concept of the mutual recognition of nursing licenses, as proposed by the National Council of State Boards of Nursing. This arrangement has many positive results. It will reduce the cost for individuals to maintain licensure in more than one state, facilitate career moves, and make it easier for nurses to cross state lines temporarily to assist with disasters. For health care employers, it will expand their ability to quickly fill positions from a larger pool of nurses licensed to practice in the state. For regulators, there should be a reduction in the number of licenses issued, thus reducing costs; and since a person will only have one license, it should improve the ability to track and take action against those few nurses who are involved in improper activity, thus improving client safety (www.ncsbn.org/files/mutual/9814utahnews.asp, May 14, 2001). As of August 1, 2001, 13 states have enacted legislation to become a member in the Multi-State Compact. These states are Utah, Texas, Arkansas, Delaware, Iowa, Maryland, Nebraska, North Carolina, South Dakota, North Dakota, Wisconsin, Idaho, and Mississippi (personal communication, Texas Board of Nurse Examiners, May 14, 2001).

Specific laws and standards relating to safe and professional nursing practice are applicable in community health nursing just as in all other locations and practice specialties. See Table 18-3 for a sample of recent laws affecting community health nursing. This includes practicing within the scope of the law as set by your State Board of Nursing. It is imperative that you review agency policies as well as your Nurse Practice Act to determine the requirements and limits of practice as they apply to your level of licensure and practice arena. In a court of law, your practice decision in question will be examined as it relates to agency policy, your Nurse Practice Act, and acceptable standards of practice as defined by the ANA. Copies of the Standards of Practice for your practice arena can be ordered through the ANA web site.

TABLE 18-3 Sample of Recent Laws Affecting Community Health Nursing Practice

LAW	MAJOR IMPACT
Omnibus Budget Reconciliation Act of 1981 (PL 9735), Block Grants for Social Services	Consolidated categorical grants for specific populations into block grants, which shifted power to the states allowing states to develop more individualized programs reflective of unique needs.
	Four grants focused on programs and services in the areas of preventive health services, substance abuse and mental health, maternal and child health, and community health centers.
	This major change in funding allocations impacted the structure of health departments and changed many of the programs they provided.
Omnibus Budget Reconciliation Act Expansions of 1985, 1986, and 1989	**1985:** Required employers to provide group medical coverage for laid-off workers and their dependents for up to 36 months (COBRA) and added hospice benefits for Medicaid patients.
	1986: Began the era of prospective payments for illness care focusing on hospital services.
	1989: Fee schedules for physicians were regulated to encourage less high-tech care.
	This bill and its expansions were the first efforts to expand insurance coverage to impact the rising numbers of uninsured in the country and to bring down the cost of illness care.
The Health Objectives Planning Act (PL101-582), 1990, 1991	**1990:** Supported *Healthy People 2000* and provided funding to help improve the public's health.
	1991: Funding for health promotion and disease prevention was added.
	1992: Changed the name of the Centers for Disease Control to the Centers for Disease Control and Prevention (CDCP), which indicated a change in focus from disease to prevention initiatives.
	All of these increased the focus on and visibility of community/public health efforts aimed at promoting health and preventing disease to reduce the burden of high illness care costs.
Personal Responsibility and Work Opportunity Reconciliation Act (PL 104-193), 1996	Known as Welfare Reform Act, this law limited the lifetime limit of Welfare benefits to 5 years and changed the name of Aid to Families with Dependent Children (AFDC) to Temporary Assistance to Needy Families (TANF). Some states have limited benefits to less than 5 years.
	This program has the potential to impact the health and well-being of low-income families by further increasing the numbers subsisting under the federal poverty income levels.
Health Centers Consolidation Act (PL 104-299), 1996	Consolidated funding for homeless programs, migrant health, and community health centers.
	This resulted in more freedom in the development of programs to serve underserved populations. This law also supports funding for rural health centers serving underserved populations.
Health Insurance Portability Act (PL 104-191), 1996	Required group health plans to limit time that preexisting conditions would not be covered to 12 months. Time insured under a former plan must be credited to the 12 months limit if there was no break in coverage.
	This impacted the status of chronically ill children and adults who previously were often refused coverage under group plans, thereby reducing the number of people seeking help for health care through the public sector.

COMMUNITY NURSING VIEW

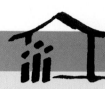

David Olds et al. (1997) conducted a study of prenatal and home visitation by nurses. The study found that early childhood visitation resulted in positive outcomes. The number of subsequent pregnancies was reduced, and child abuse and neglect were reduced. This study has impacted the practice of community health nursing by providing evidence for the outcomes of nursing home visitation related to primary prevention. This highly acclaimed and tested model improves the social functioning of low-income first-time mothers and their babies. To date, there have been two randomized clinical trials: one in Elmira, New York, and the other in Memphis, Tennessee. Other replication sites are in place, and there are plans to expand to 20 replication sites across the nation. The trials produced the following results:

♦ 25% reduction in cigarette smoking during pregnancy among women who smoked cigarettes at entering the program

♦ 80% reduction in rates of child maltreatment among at-risk families from birth through child's second birthday

♦ 56% reduction in the rates of children's health care encounters for injuries and ingestions, from birth through child's second birthday

♦ 43% reduction in subsequent pregnancy among low-income, unmarried women by first child's birthday

♦ 83% increase in the rates of mother's labor force participation by first child's fourth birthday

In 1997, an Assembly bill was presented in the California legislature that provides for a home visitation program for low-income mothers to aid in the prevention of maternal and child health problems and to improve outcomes of mothers and children.

Nursing Considerations

Assessment

♦ This piece of legislation is very important for community public health nurses; what initial data would be important to collect in order to effectively lobby for the bill?

♦ What data would be necessary to begin planning and intervention strategies?

♦ Which body of your state legislature would be the best choice for introduction of the bill? Why?

♦ Who would you choose to sponsor your bill?

♦ How much will this program cost the taxpayers? Will the costs for the program outweigh the cost currently outlaid to not have the program?

Diagnosis

♦ How would you state a community diagnosis for this situation?

Outcome Identification

♦ What are the expected outcomes of this legislation?

Planning/Interventions

♦ This legislation is at the committee level. According to knowledge about how a bill becomes law, how should the community health nurse proceed?

♦ What other information is needed?

♦ What should the community public health nurse specifically do to affect this piece of legislation?

♦ What strategies are necessary to "track," or follow, this legislation?

♦ How can the community public health nurse involve other nurses to influence this piece of legislation?

Evaluation

♦ How might the community public health nurse have developed a stronger power base to influence this legislation?

KEY CONCEPTS

♦ Early community public health nurses were involved in influencing health-related policy decisions. However, only in the last two decades has nursing become visible in the political arena.

♦ The community health nurse is one of the few health professionals to realize the scope of health problems affecting large segments of the population; this knowledge is a mandate to action for the caring professional.

♦ By learning the various power bases, the nurse can understand and use power in a positive and productive way.

♦ Policy represents the actions of a government and develops incrementally over time.

◆ Politics is associated with conflicting values, and often multiple interest groups compete for scarce resources.

◆ Four stages of political development in the nursing profession have been identified in order to analyze previous accomplishments and plan future actions.

◆ Local politics may differ radically from one city or county to another; federal and state governments are similar to each other.

◆ The private sector, including nurses, can influence legislation in many ways, especially through influencing the process of writing regulations.

◆ The community health nurse should use the political process as a tool to influence health care policy.

◆ Nursing values, although different from the public's traditional values, are useful for focusing the policy debate on issues of human rights, individual worth, and caring.

◆ Nursing's political network encompasses the professional associations with their myriad activities including lobbying, electioneering, and grass-roots political action.

◆ In the international community, nursing's basic problems and issues are very similar to national issues.

◆ Community health nurses need to be politically active in the community because of community and professional shared values and because of the pervasive role the government has on the impact of health care.

◆ Major strategies for political action include lobbying, electioneering, coalition building, and participating in political networks.

◆ Nurses can access a variety of specialty organizations with expertise in political activism to ensure that nursing's voice is heard at all levels of government.

◆ The primary goal of the World Health Organization is to attain the highest possible level of health for all people.

◆ International policy affects the United States even though the United States may not have had direct involvement in establishing the policy.

◆ Supporting international health policy and programs is important for political reasons.

◆ Laws that affect community public health nursing practice are laws which impact public health resources, services, and programs as well as laws, rules, regulations, and standards focused on nursing itself.

RESOURCES

American Nurses Association: http://www.nursingworld.org
American Public Health Association: http://www.apha.org
American Red Cross: http://www.redcross.org
Center for Health and Public Service Research: http://www.nyu.edu/wagner/chpsr
Coalition for Healthier Cities and Communities in the U.S.: http://www.healthycommunities.org
Federal Register: http://www.access.gpo.gov
Healthy People 2010: http://www.health.gov/healthypeople
International Council of Nurses: http://www.icn.ch
International Healthy Cities Foundation: http://www.healthycommunities.org/international_healthycities.html
Journal of Health Affairs: http://www.healthaffairs.org
National Civic League: http://www.ncl.org
National Council of State Boards of Nursing: http://www.ncsbn.org
Pan American Health Care Organization: http://www.paho.org
Robert Wood Johnson Foundation: http://www.rwjf.org
United Nations: http://www.un.org/english
United States Agency for International Development: http://www.usaid.gov
United States Congress: http://www.access.gpo.gov/congress
World Health Organization: http://www.who.int/home-page
World Bank: http://www.worldbank.org
World Federation of Public Health Associations: http://www.wfpha.org

VARIED ROLES OF COMMUNITY HEALTH NURSING

Diane Stafanson, RN, MSN, NP

Your behavior influences others through a ripple effect. A ripple effect works because everyone influences everyone else. Powerful people are powerful influences.

If your life works, you influence your family.

If your family works, your family influences the community.

If your community works, your community influences the nation.

If your nation works, your nation influences the world.

If your world works, the ripple effect spreads throughout the cosmos.

. . . All growth spreads outward from a fertile and potent nucleus. You are a nucleus.

—Heider, 1985, p. 107

COMPETENCIES

Upon completion of this chapter, the reader should be able to:

- Discuss possible effects on the nurse when making a role transition from an acute-care practice to community-based practice.
- Compare and contrast the multiple role functions (clinician, advocate, collaborator, consultant, counselor, educator, researcher) of the community health nurse.
- Analyze the significance of nurse actions in the role of case manager for the client maneuvering through a complex health care system.
- Compare and contrast the roles of community health nurse generalist and community health nurse specialist.

KEY TERMS

advanced-practice
  nurses

advocacy

aggregates

biometrics

case management

clinical specialist

collaborate

community health
  nurse generalist

community health
  nurse specialist

consultant

coordination

counseling

demography

multidisciplinary team

reference group

role ambiguity

role conflict

role incompetence

role modeling

role overload

role rehearsal

role strain

role transition

self-care

self-determination

The history of community health nursing in the United States reflects a practice of nursing focused on caring for people with the greatest needs. The earlier commitment of community health nursing is reflected today as community health nurses continue to strive to promote the health of individuals and families and the communities of which they are a part. The health needs of society and consumer demand are bringing about a significant increase in community-focused services. Although the practice settings are varied, the basic concepts of health, health promotion, and disease prevention and an appreciation of cultural di-

versity are needed. Nursing assessment and intervention are being directed toward the needs of **aggregates** (groups of people with similar needs) as well as individuals. Society's changing demands require that today's community health nurse function in a variety of roles and practice settings.

ROLE TRANSITION

Nursing students as part of the educational experience are required to undertake new roles as they move through the required clinical rotations. These learning experiences can produce **role strain,** which Leddy and Peppe (1998) describe as "a subjective sense of distress when role related stress is related to one or more of the following areas:

Role conflict: the existence of clear but competing or incompatible expectations

Role ambiguity: the degree to which role expectations are unclear

Role overload: perceived inadequacy of time to achieve quantity or quality of exceptions

Role incompetence: perception of inadequate skills, knowledge or ability to satisfactorily meet role expectations (p. 80)

The transition from the acute-care setting to the community requires a structured program to assist the new community health nurse in acquiring the knowledge and skills necessary to fulfill a new role. This eases **role transition** and fosters role socialization. When transitioning to a new role, a nurse must learn new role behaviors, review previously learned material, and mediate any conflicts between the different role expectations. The nurse must internalize the values of the new role, adopt the appropriate behaviors, and identify significant role models. Role socialization is enhanced by observation of others in the role (**role modeling**), internal preparation and overt practice of new role behaviors (**role rehearsal**), and participation in planned group activities with others involved in role transition (i.e., a **reference group**). The nurse manager along with other health care professionals, the **multidisciplinary team,** are critical factors in the success of the nurse's development in a new role. The new community health nurse must recognize the broader scope of practice, embrace the autonomous nature of the practice, and communicate needs to those who may be of help during the role transition.

MAJOR ROLE FUNCTIONS

Community health nurses must demonstrate a caring and comprehensive client-centered practice in performing multiple role functions regardless of the employment setting. These role functions include:

- Advocate
- Collaborator
- Consultant
- Counselor
- Educator
- Researcher
- Case manager
- Clinician

The nurse who implements these roles demonstrates a caring and comprehensive client-centered nursing practice (see Figure 19-1).

Advocate

The caring practice of community health nursing is dependent on an understanding of the roles that community health nurses play in working with individuals, families, and communities. Figure 19-1 illustrates the varied roles of the community health nurses. **Advocacy** as it is directed toward individuals, families, and communities implies caring and the nurse's willingness to be supportive. This process of advocacy protects the rights of

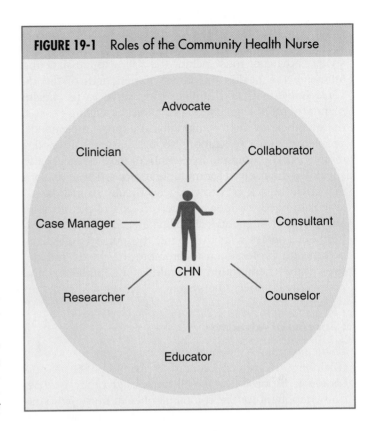

FIGURE 19-1 Roles of the Community Health Nurse

Perspectives...

ROLE TRANSITIONS

A stressful time for Registered Nurses in the RN to BSN program where I served as faculty becomes very evident the first night of the Family and Community Health Nursing class. Comments and concerns arose in several areas, from "you mean that I have to go into someone's home" to "I am a CCU nurse, I don't remember much about pregnancy or child development" to "I never plan to leave my hospital, so why do I need to take this class?" The clinical experiences take place in an urban area and the nurses live mostly in suburban areas or in a higher income area within the urban setting, and so questions of safety frequently occur. These comments and concerns are valid, and I certainly appreciate that many will not choose to become public health nurses, although some will shift to other community-based practices in nursing. My goal as both lecturer and a clinical instructor is to change the way that they look at their clients in the hospital. By this I mean for them to begin to think of clients as members of a family living in a community which may or may not have the resources to ensure the support that may be needed by the client and the family. The

clinical experience is so structured that they visit clients throughout the life span and develop more skills in health promotion and disease prevention activities for the whole family, not just the identified client. As part of this experience, they begin to build their knowledge of community resources—e.g., Women, Infant, and Children (WIC), sources of free food and meals to senior day care centers. As the class and clinical experiences develop, the nurses become more aware of the complexities of the health and welfare system and the need to become politically involved in the life of the community.

For community health nurses, identifying the strengths of families and communities, the knowledge and skills gained from home visiting, collaboration with multiple agencies in the community, and the increased awareness of their role in ensuring a system that meets the basic needs of clients are all relevant to their practice as professional nurses regardless of the employment arena they choose.

—Diane M. Stafanson, RN, MSN, NP(c)

others and validates and encourages the client's right to self-determination. For community health nurses, the style of advocacy must include the ability to translate and articulate the health and illness experiences of the diverse individuals and families they serve to the health planners and policymakers. They must be willing to assist the members of their community to express their needs, problems, and expectations to the appropriate policy members. The community members may be unable to speak for themselves for multiple reasons. These reasons may include lack of knowledge; difficulty or inability to articulate needs or ideas; perceived lack of power; fear; and physical or mental disability. Because of close and frequent contact with the client, the nurse is often the best health professional to promote the needs and desires of the client within the realm of a complicated and potentially cumbersome system.

Concepts of Advocacy

Client advocacy is essential to the nurse-client relationship (Klainberg, Holzemer, Leonard, & Arnold, 1998). A professional responsibility for all nurses, advocacy is especially important for the community health nurse, who has a broad exposure to social situations, is closely tied to the family and community, and has a philosophical basis for advocating for the group (Kosik, 1972). Public health philosophy supports the appropriate use of social programs, fosters decision making within the family or community network, and promotes **self-care** (health care performed by the client) and **self-determination** (the right to make one's own choices) by the individual or group.

Advocacy has been described as encompassing both simple and complex actions. Advocacy is perhaps simplest when it involves actions of loving and caring for others. This premise of caring is supported by Mayeroff (1971), who in his classic reference describes caring actions that may precisely apply to the role of the nurse advocate:

> When I care for an adult, . . . I try to avoid making decisions for him. I help him make his own decisions by providing information, suggesting alternatives and pointing out possible consequences, but all along I realize that they are his decisions to make and not my own. If I made his decisions for him, I would be condescending to him and treating him as a child; and by denying his need to take responsibility for his own life, I would be denying him as a person. (p. 34)

Advocating for the client, family, and the community provides an opportunity to demonstrate a caring concern on the part of the community health nurse. The process of advocacy is one of mutuality and self-determination.

The nurse must know the health care system, the law, and the unique characteristics of the client. The advocate must know how to use the system to achieve the desired outcomes while still promoting client self-determination. Advocacy is essential for the provision of ethical health interventions.

As an advocate, the nurse informs the client of available services, supports the client's requests, and assists with the receiving process. Being a true advocate requires a willingness on the part of the nurse to fully invest in the client-nurse relationship. Advocacy is time consuming and demands a client-focused approach. The nurse must in one sense be a risk taker, being willing to intervene on behalf of the client to ensure that the system does not prevent access to necessary services to which the client is entitled.

Characteristics of an Advocate

Characteristics of an advocate include the ability to relate to clients and co-workers. The willingness to cope with pressure and manage stress is essential. As an advocate, the community health nurse must be self-motivated, tenacious, and flexible and possess outstanding communication skills. The advocate values the humane and just treatment of others and demonstrates cultural sensitivity with clients, families, and the members of the multidisciplinary team and the community at large.

Goals of Advocacy

The goal of client advocacy is twofold: client independence and system improvement. In making the client more independent, the nurse encourages the client to be an active participant in individual health care. The client must remain at the center of the care process and feel supported in decisions. To this end, the nurse expands

---

✳ DECISION MAKING

Client Advocacy

Nurses often interact with clients whose values and beliefs differ from their own. It is important to identify ways that your own values and beliefs affect your interactions with clients. How might you respond to the following situations?

◆ Your belief system supports abstinence as the only acceptable contraceptive practice. You are a school nurse and are approached by a teenaged girl who is sexually active and desires information and access to condoms and the birth control pill.

◆ You believe that people must have their basic safety and security needs satisfied in order to progress to independence. You are the case manager for several families whose income is significantly below the poverty level. The families live in substandard housing, and their apartments are vermin infested. How might you advocate for these families? To what community groups would you address your concerns?

the client's understanding of those services that can be expected from the system, the reasons those services are needed, and the ways that those services might be obtained. In all actions of advocacy, the nurse fosters both client and system acceptance of client participation. The system must support active participation by clients and social groups in health care decisions that affect them. Active decision making ensures the client's progress toward self-care, the desired outcome of advocacy interventions (Powell, 1996).

The second goal of advocacy is to improve the system to make it more sensitive and relevant to the needs of the individual or group (Powell, 1996). The community health nurse "uses tools of public health policy development and advocacy for needed policy changes to improve the health of communities" (Kuehnert, 1991, p. 5). This is accomplished by implementing such actions as assessing client/community needs, planning appropriate programs, developing policies, implementing change, evaluating outcomes, and remaining committed to the process until change is accepted.

Advocacy Interventions

Advocacy interventions are implemented on multiple levels. Advocacy occurs with individuals, families, communities, and social systems (Flarey, 1995). The community health nurse is active at each of these levels during the course of professional practice. At times, the focus may be on one level more than on another. The needs of different clients, groups, or social situations require varied time and energy commitments from the advocate. The nurse must be sensitive to difficulties the client may encounter and must develop the ability to identify potential barriers to the well-being of the client at each level. The nurse must also be sensitive to the barriers which limit effective community advocacy and intervention. Often there is a conflict of the public health priorities among the policymakers at all levels of government (local, state, and federal). The impact of categorical funding is often the compartmentalization of the scope of the work, thus increasing and complicating the caseloads for community health nurses and diminishing response to the community.

For example, an unmarried teen mother may not be able to negotiate the health system to apply for Medicaid coverage, thereby restricting access to health care for herself and her infant. The community health nurse can advocate for the teen mother by implementing interventions that reduce barriers to the services.

Some advocacy changes may be possible only at the community level. Larger social issues, for example, may be addressed at the level of public policy development. Such larger social issues may include, but are not limited to, poverty, homelessness, unemployment, gender issues, violence, and illiteracy. The nurse advocating at the public policy level needs expertise in skills of problem solving, negotiation, conflict resolution, and change processes (Kuehnert, 1991; Spradley & Allender, 1996).

The political arena provides access to the legislative system, an established vehicle for social progress. Involvement in the political process challenges all of the abilities of the nurse in the advocate role.

An example would be a community health nurse who sits on the board of directors of a women's crisis shelter. In this example, the nurse is aware that recent legislation and new state guidelines mandate that an increase in shelter services be provided. However, no increase in state funding has been appropriated to support the newly mandated services. The community health nurse takes the problem to the county commission to petition for county funding as a yearly budget item. Such funding would ensure a state source of income for the women's shelter, allow for an increase in services to cover the state mandate, and generate local commitment to women's needs in the county.

Consumers of health care demand that they be participants in the decisions affecting their health care at both the individual and group levels. The Society for Healthcare Consumer Advocacy identifies the following values for individual health care consumers:

Dignity of the consumer shall never be compromised.

The right to control one's own decisions shall be respected.

Caring and compassion are as important as technology.

Education and information are vital to informed health care decision making.

The Society affirms that the values and ethics of health care advocates are the foundation of professional practice, and that collaboration with other health care professionals is essential [American Hospital Association (AHA), 2000]. It is the responsibility of the advocate to foster this participation. As the consumer becomes more involved, the advocate must become better prepared in order to impart the necessary knowledge and power to the consumer. The nurse must develop expertise in political processes, client-focused care, community and social issues, and the acquisition of health care resources in order to empower the client in self-management.

Collaborator

To **collaborate** means to work with others toward a common goal. It is a process of joint decision making in an atmosphere of mutual respect and cooperation. Collaboration should always be the mode of interaction between the community health nurse and the client and is an equally important nursing role when the nurse functions as part of a team. Whether collaborating with an individual, a family, an agency, or as part of a team, the community health nurse is involved in joint decision making regarding the most appropriate action to be taken to resolve problems (Clark, 1999).

Perspectives...

COMMUNITY HEALTH NURSE AS HEALTH CARE LIAISON

In my various roles as a nurse working in a community, I have often found myself functioning as a liaison between the medical and nonmedical facets affecting people's lives. For example, as a community mental health nurse, I worked with a social worker to screen every person in my catchment area who was referred for admission to the state psychiatric hospital. We did screenings in hospitals, homes, board and care facilities, and facilities for the elderly. I shared information about physiology, medications, and similar aspects of medical situations with my co-worker, and she helped me navigate the social service system. I found that it was never safe to assume that because a client was in a hospital or under the care of a physician that all possible physiological sources of the symptoms had been ruled out. I often found that physicians were unaware that long-term doses of even mild tranquilizers or other medications can build to toxic levels in an elderly person and cause confusion and other symptoms of brain dysfunction. Even something as routine as a chest x-ray to rule out lung infection was sometimes not done when psychiatric symptoms were noted.

As director of a psychiatric day treatment center, I found many clients who had not seen a family physician or had dental care for years. As a nurse, I was often the only professional who was thinking about care of the whole person.

While working with mentally ill clients, I routinely trained operators of board and care facilities. Part of that training included information about the physical health of their boarders who were our clients and who usually had no families or other advocates for their well-being.

As a Peace Corps volunteer in a Muslim country in the mid 1990s, I had easy access to all hospitals when I said I was a nurse. I was able to observe how students were being taught, summarize my findings, and participate in decision making for professional education programs. I could also interpret the findings for those involved in teaching English to medical school students and to Peace Corps staff.

In my role as a VISTA volunteer, I worked with a small staff of child development specialists. When there was an opportunity to hire a new person to manage a program which provided support to parents of newborns, I suggested that we look for a nurse for this position. At first, this suggestion was not considered helpful, until I explained all the things a nurse could do in this position. I think my being a nurse in a community development role helped convince them to hire a nurse. They did—and they are glad now.

—Joan Heron, RN, PhD

Concepts of Collaboration

Nurses in all settings work as members of a team. In acute-care settings, team members are generally other health care professionals. In community health settings, the nurse is part of a truly multidisciplinary team that includes not only other health care workers but also members from community organizations, social service agencies, judicial systems, political entities, schools, religious organizations, volunteer networks, and other non-health-related professions. The complex demands of clients and populations in many community health settings require a multidisciplinary approach in order to promote optimal outcomes. All members of this multidisciplinary team work together to bring about optimal health and well-being for the client, whether that client be an individual, family, group, or community. The ANA (1999) Scope and Standards of Practice clearly articulate the importance of collaboration with multidisciplinary team members. As described in the ANA's *Standards for Community Health Nursing* (1999), "community health nursing practice requires planning

and sharing with others in the community to promote health for the community, family, and individual. Through the collaborative process, the special abilities of others are used to communicate, plan, solve problems, and evaluate services" (p. 14).

Successful collaboration requires that the multidisciplinary team develop a common purpose, communicate to effectively coordinate efforts, and recognize the unique and complementary skills possessed by each team member. Each team member brings special abilities and expertise to the collaborative process. With strong support and active participation of all members, "the team communicates, plans, anticipates and solves problems, and evaluates services" (ANA, 1987, p. 4).

Although they do share some similarities, collaboration and coordination are inherently different. **Coordination** is the efficient management of services without gaps or overlaps. The nurse as coordinator may or may not consult with others in carrying out that which is essentially a management function. Collaboration, on the other hand, involves joint decision making between two or more people (Clark, 1999).

Characteristics of a Collaborator

Effective collaboration requires skills in communication and problem solving. The nurse must be able to communicate effectively with the client, family, group, or team. With other team members, the nurse shares client needs and possible interventions to bring about the resolution of problems. With the client, the nurse engages in joint problem solving to identify needs and evaluate alternative solutions. Together, all members of the team, including the client, select an appropriate alternative. Collaboration continues as solutions are implemented and evaluated. Collaboration does not work when each team member designs and provides a program from a particular area of expertise and then "coordinates" by informing others of the plan. To be successful, collaboration must be a joint effort on the part of the client and all team members to identify mutual goals and acceptable means for meeting those goals (Clark, 1999).

The community health nurse as team member must develop assertive communication skills and be able to describe the nurse's unique contribution to the health team as an equal partner. The nurse as collaborator works with individuals from other disciplines, service providers, political entities, and community agencies to establish effective networks to expedite client services. This networking may require continual redefinition and development. Political astuteness and maturity on the part of the nurse will assist in overcoming the turf issues, financial constraints, and competition that combine to make collaboration a complex and involved process. Although collaboration is a relatively new role for nurses, they must actively promote the collaborative process to secure the delivery of high-quality services to the client. Collaboration succeeds when there are feelings of mutual respect and collegiality among all members of the team (ANA, 1998).

Consultant

Every community health nurse is a **consultant.** Each time a nurse gives information or assists a client in choosing between alternative actions, the nurse is using consulting skills. Consultants help clients understand their problems and assist them in making wise decisions. Consultants are catalysts, persons who bring about change or changes. From a perspective of expertise, the nurse consultant promotes decision making and change by providing information and alternatives. Consultation as a skill is part of almost every professional activity that involves problem solving. The nurse also acts as consultant when helping a client improve specific skills or make more effective plans. See Table 19-1 for a comparison of consulting, counseling, and educating roles.

Components of Consultation

The consultant has traditionally been viewed as an expert, or someone with specialized skills and knowledge, who is able to propose solutions for identified problems. The consultant is expected to be a resource, someone who can provide information that will assist the client to make decisions based on alternatives. The consultant may be viewed as a change agent who uses process consultation to bring about change in a given situation. In process consultation, the consultant helps the client perceive, understand, and act on events that occur in the client's environment. A consultant can be seen as a trained teacher and an expert in a particular specialty. The successful consultant must be able to motivate others and be able to get things done even when not in direct charge of the people concerned (Shi & Singh, 1998).

In nursing consultation, there are generally three types of clients: the individual client, the group client, and the community or secondary group (see Figure 19-2). The individual client may be a patient, family member, fellow nurse, or other professional. The group client is

TABLE 19-1 Comparison of Counseling, Consulting, and Educating

COUNSELING GOAL	CONSULTING GOAL	EDUCATION GOAL
Decisive action is taken.	Decisive action is taken.	Present facts.
		No decisive action is taken.
Example	**Example**	**Example**
Explore methods of cessation and help client decide best course of action.	Set goals and objectives to stop smoking (obtain nicotine gum; begin program within two days of obtaining nicotine gum; complete prescribed regimen; monitor adherence to regimen; monitor nonsmoking for a period after regimen has been completed).	Present dangers of smoking. Present cessation techniques.

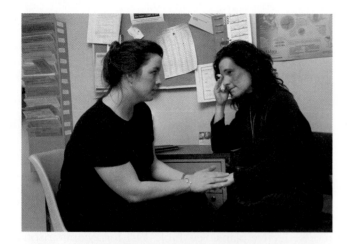

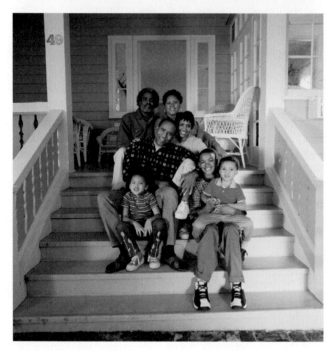

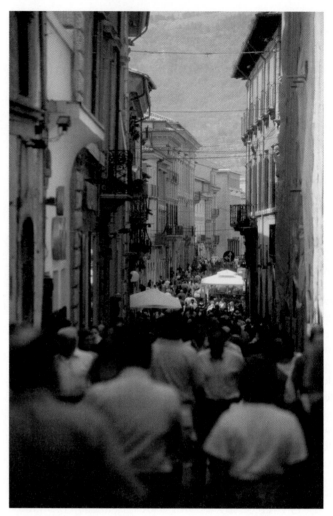

FIGURE 19-2   Types of Clients Encountered in Nursing Consultation: a. Individual Client, b. Group Client, c. Community Group

usually a small cohesive unit or primary group of 10 or fewer people. Examples of such groups include families, unit staff nurses, or other nurse groups. The community or secondary group is a larger, more diverse and complex social system. This community group is more impersonal; examples include community organizations, large health care agencies, schools, governmental agencies, and foundations.

The nurse consultant fulfills multiple roles. In addition to specific consulting duties, the nurse will likely be expected to fill one or more of the following roles: leader, expert, coordinator, resource person, clinical specialist, teacher, and researcher. As leader, the nurse consultant assists and directs others toward a desired goal. The quality of leadership is key in determining the suc-

cess or failure of a consultant. In a consulting arrangement, the nurse must develop informal power based on interpersonal relationships and expert knowledge. As expert, the nurse has unique skills to bring to a particular problem. The client must believe that the consultant has pertinent information, skill, or ability that can help. As coordinator, the nurse plans, organizes, supports, energizes, and inspires. The nurse is able to manage conflict and to synchronize events to produce minimum conflict and maximum collaboration. As resource person, the nurse consultant brings knowledge and assistance in the wise use of resources. The nurse provides information about resources so the client can make informed choices from a variety of alternatives. As clinical specialist, the nurse consultant provides a unique service by bringing specialized knowledge, skill, and experience to the situation. As teacher, the consultant helps the client actively learn new information, skills, and abilities. As researcher, the nurse consultant is involved in fact finding. This is a key function of the consultant, whether in developing a database, assessing and diagnosing client problems, or producing a formal research proposal. The consultant is researching, whether by simply listening or by conducting a complex formal survey.

Many nurses may initially be uncomfortable functioning in the role of consultant because it differs from the traditional role of "doing for" the client and, instead, consists of helping others gain the expertise and ability to do for themselves. A consultant remains relatively distant from the problem at hand, giving advice but not personally investing in the outcome. Indeed, a consultant must be willing to stand by without directly controlling anything. Although there to influence and give advice, the consultant generally does not have the authority or position power to implement change. The optimal relationship is one in which the consultant shares knowledge and expertise in a collaborative relationship. The client allows the consultant to take the lead in exploring a problem, and the consultant respects the client's right to make the final decision. It may be a challenge for the consultant to balance the supportive role with the objectivity and distance that must be maintained for credibility to be enhanced.

Counselor

Counseling at its most basic level is the process of helping clients choose appropriate solutions to their problems. Clients generally seek counseling when they are unable to make decisions about health or personal concerns. Counseling involves exploration of feelings and attitudes on the part of the client and is directed toward helping the client develop self-understanding. The community health nurse has an important role as counselor. Clients may, e.g., want to explore concerns regarding the "right birth control method" for them or seek guidance about their parenting skills and/or explore their feelings about caring for an elderly, ill family member. For a review regarding counseling theories and techniques, refer to Chapter 10.

Educator

Community health nursing has embraced the responsibility of educating individuals, families, and communities since the days of the Henry Street Settlement. Health education is considered one of the major functions of the community nurse and is deemed an essential nursing responsibility regardless of the setting where the nurse is employed. Education is a necessary role function for the promotion of health and welfare of individuals and societies. Education is one of the avenues via which the nurse enables the client to make informed decisions regarding personal, family, or community health practices and lifestyle choices. Although educating the individual is considered important, the majority of education implemented by the community health nurse is directed toward aggregates rather than the individual and focuses on health promotion, health maintenance, and disease prevention with the goal of not only imparting information but also helping to change behaviors. (Spearmann, Daugherty, & Reign, 2000).

Examples of educating aggregate groups in the community include classes on managing hypertension, physical fitness, preparing for labor and delivery, and classes to teens on preventing sexually transmitted infections. Chapter 10 explores educational theories and the nurses' role.

Characteristics of a Nurse-Educator

It is important that the nurse-educator view the client as a responsible, thinking individual who has the right to make choices regarding individual health behavior. It is essential for the nurse-educator to assess the knowledge base of the learner and the perceived need for information prior to undertaking teaching (Redman, 2001). With this perspective, the nurse-educator will include the learner in the planning process and will advocate for the learner until the individual can take responsibility. The attitudes, behaviors, and style of the teacher affect learning outcomes (Rankin & Stallings, 1996).

In order to foster success in the learner, the professional nurse-educator must keep several important concepts in mind and must continuously evaluate him- or herself with respect to these concepts. By doing so, the nurse will develop further skill in interpreting the needs of the learners and in adapting the teaching process to best meet those needs.

The role of nurse-educator is challenging yet offers significant rewards. Community health nursing affords boundless opportunities to teach in any setting with any number of individuals. This teaching-learning exchange is vital in developing an informed client who is capable of making health-promoting changes in self, family, and the community. An in-depth discussion of the education process, including teaching methodologies and learning theories, is presented in Chapter 10.

Researcher

The community health nurse participates in the research process at multiple levels. The nurse may be involved in activities such as identifying problem areas; collecting, analyzing, and interpreting data; applying findings; and evaluating, designing, and conducting research. All research efforts are designed to provide a specialized, scientific knowledge base for nursing practice. This foundation enables the nursing profession to anticipate potential health problems of society and to remain accountable for care interventions. This ability, in turn, ensures that nursing interventions remain current and relevant to society's needs. At a minimum, the community health nurse is expected to read current research and apply the findings to practice as a consistent part of professional actions (Burns, Garrett, & Grover, 2000).

Goals of Nursing Research

As researcher, the nurse seeks to discover, investigate, understand, explain, and predict phenomena. The research process comprises specific actions to collect data and synthesize information. The steps of the scientific research process are as follows:

1. Identify the question.
2. Review related literature.
3. Select a conceptual framework or model.
4. Select a research design and methodology.
5. Collect and analyze data.
6. Interpret and discuss results.
7. Identify implications for practice.
8. Communicate findings to others.

These steps ensure that the research process as well as the findings can be reviewed, evaluated, and critiqued by other investigators (LoBiondo-Wood & Haber, 1994).

To manage future health concerns, the researcher will be challenged to answer research questions on issues related to HIV/AIDS, infectious disease, chronic physical and emotional conditions, and injury prevention. The identification and evaluation of public health nursing interventions is an additional area of research in this time of health care scarcity. Social issues including escalating health care costs, disability related to aging, social violence, poor pregnancy outcomes, poverty, homelessness, substance abuse, and other such community-level concerns must also be studied thoroughly (ANA, 1999). Other broad areas for nursing research as outlined by the National Institute of Nursing Research (NINR) are discussed later in this chapter. Participation in research at the community level can range from collecting data to chart auditing and participating in small pilot studies to creating and managing large longitudinal studies. There is a place for community health nurses at all levels and in all settings to be involved in ongoing research.

Characteristics of a Nurse-Researcher

The researcher embodies several characteristics. Among these are a spirit of inquiry, energy, drive, creativity, and perseverance. The investigator must be open minded, analytical, detail oriented, and able to communicate findings.

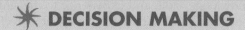

✳ DECISION MAKING

Nursing Research

Research in community health practice is challenging. The variables can be difficult to identify and measure. Consider ways that you might structure your research to answer the following:

◆ How might you measure the "health" or "wellness" of your community?

◆ You have decided to implement a teaching project on stress management to a group of well elders. What criteria might you use to measure the effectiveness of your nursing interventions?

◆ You are a new occupational health nurse at a local plastics factory. What questions might you ask the employees to better understand their need for and interest in health promotion topics?

Even if not involved in the full research process, the nurse must actualize these characteristics in order to critically review and analyze the research of others before applying findings to practice (Spradley, 1996; Shelov, 1994).

To develop new strategies and new tools to meet the changing needs of clients and health care delivery systems, the researcher must prepare to meet research challenges. Shelov (1994) outlines several necessary components for meeting future needs:

• The community health researcher must gather good data. Data must be reliable, valid, reproducible, objective, and sufficiently flexible for application over time.

• The researcher must carefully identify the needs of populations. High-risk population groups must be targeted so that specific and relevant strategies can be developed and implemented. The population group must be involved in the processes of decision making and program and/or policy development in order to increase group interest and commitment to behavior changes.

• The researcher must measure and analyze the outcomes of the specific interventions. Accurate evaluation provides information necessary to modify or restructure future interventions.

• The researcher must accept that technology cannot answer all social and health problems. The greatest research challenges lie in the psyche, behavior, motivations, values, and needs of individuals and populations. These phenomena may be the most difficult to assess through the scientific process as it is now designed.

Research-based solutions to current and future health issues are necessary to enable society to work toward a healthier future. Critical-thinking skills, creativity, flexibility, and tenacity are essential to ensure the success of research-based decision making and practice in community health nursing. The research role of the community health nurse is an essential component in the identification, analysis, and application of strategies that lead to positive health outcomes and promote the self-care of populations. (See Research Focus.)

Case Manager

Coordination of care is difficult in a health care system with many differing public and private programs, services, agencies, and institutions. Because of its complexities, the system frequently breaks down, creating fragmentation of care for the client. Obvious gaps in services, duplication of resources, and difficulty in accessing care are among the manifestations of this breakdown, some of which contribute to escalating health care costs.

RESEARCH FOCUS

Promoting the Health of Adolescent Mothers and Their Babies

Study Problem/Purpose

There is ongoing public concern about adolescent pregnancy and parenting because of its impact on maternal child health and on the social and economic implications of early pregnancy and parenting. Changing federal welfare reform with its emphasis on self-sufficiency presents an additional stressor for the adolescent parent. Community-based interventions to improve the health and social outcomes for disadvantaged adolescent mothers need to be identified and evaluated.

Methods

Pregnant adolescents referred to a county health department were randomly assigned to either an experimental (EIP) group or to a control traditional public health nursing (TPHN) group to evaluate the effects of an early intervention program that uses a public health model on health and social outcomes of adolescent mothers and their children and the quality of the mother-child interaction. The 121 adolescents in the sample were predominantly minority and from impoverished backgrounds. They were followed from pregnancy through six weeks. Intensive and comprehensive visits by public health nurses and preparation for motherhood classes were provided to adolescents in the EIP group.

Nursing intervention for the EIP group utilized a case management approach with approximately 17 home visits on a regular basis during the second and third trimesters through the first year of motherhood. Interventions were directed to the following five areas: health, sexuality and family planning, maternal role, life skills, and social support. During the postpartum period, the interventions included information on family planning, infant care, and well baby health care. For the traditional targeted public health nursing group, one to two home visits were made prenatally with a focus on assessment and counseling related to prenatal care, self-care, preparation for child care, and well baby care.

Findings

The findings were based on medical records data. Other measures included maternal self-reporting of selected behaviors, nurses' interviews, and the Nursing Child Assessment Teaching Scale. Early findings show that both groups had reduced low-birthweight (LBW) and premature infants. Infants in the EIP had significantly fewer total days of birth-related hospitalization and rehospitalization than those in the TPHN group during the first six weeks of life. Adolescents in the EIP had a lower school dropout rate than that of the TPHN group.

Implications

These results reinforce the importance of public health nursing care in terms of prenatal and perinatal outcomes for adolescents. The support of the adolescent pregnant and new mother will help to improve the health and social outcomes for the often-disadvantaged adolescent mother and in the long run will decrease the costly utilization of health and social welfare programs.

Source: Koniak-Griffin, D., Anderson, N. L., Verzemnieka, I., & Brecht, M. L. (2000). A public health nursing early intervention program for adolescent mothers: Outcomes from pregnancy through 6 weeks postpartum. Nursing Research, 49(3), 130–138.

Furthermore, concerns regarding the quality of services rendered are ever present. One response to the problems of our health care system is **case management.** Case management is the application of strategies for coordinating and allocating services for individuals who cannot manage their own care or who cannot negotiate the health care system.

Case management programs have been implemented in every conceivable public and private setting throughout the United States. Case management is seen as an effective method of delivering services to individuals needing assistance maneuvering through the health care system and is especially effective for those with long-term care needs. Those who are physically and emotionally disabled, frail and elderly, chronically ill, nursing home residents, or members of high-risk groups—those who require multiple services and who are involved in the system over a long period of time—are excellent candidates for case-managed services.

The case manager's role is to deliver "cost efficient individualized and coordinated care to patients and clients with chronic illness and disabilities" (Chen et al., 1999, p. 27). Good problem-solving techniques and an ability to perform accurate assessments and to identify variables that effect healing and functioning are essential. It is important to note that the case manager's role is not to control people but to control the care provision process. The community health nurse is in an excellent position to function in the role of case manager because of long-term commitment to the client, a focus on considering the wide range of client needs and matching the client to needed services, experience with the referral network, and professional skills in comprehensive assessment and care planning, implementation, and evaluation (Powell, 1996; Chen, Leahy, McMahon, Mirch, & Devinney, 1999).

Concepts in Case Management

Multiple concepts are inherent in case management. Kane (1990) quotes the *Encyclopedia of Aging* definition of case management as "a service function directed at coordinating existing resources to assure appropriate and continuing care on a case-by-case basis" (p. 2). Case management requires focused and skilled assessment in the planning of services. The process is built on comprehensive functional assessment, identifies measurable outcomes, and incorporates collaboration and networking for the allocation of health services (Chen et al., 1999).

Case management is further identified as a process that coordinates services by implementing an individual service plan developed in response to client needs and problems. This plan addresses the gap between complex client needs, services offered by providers, and increasingly limited health care resources. The overriding goals of case management are to minimize fragmentation of services and maximize individualization of care. The term *caseload* refers to the number of clients being followed by a particular nurse.

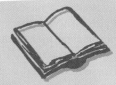

Out of the Box

Case Management in Community Health Nursing

The Prenatal to Three Initiative (Raising Healthy children in San Mateo County, California) established a new, culturally competent, comprehensive health care program for all county Medicaid perinatal families. Begun in 1996, this program is powerful and effective because it engages over 31 diverse health care and community providers in coordinated perinatal case management services, instilling a new care philosophy with creatively integrated services/social support for low-income families. Public health nurses (PHNs) provision of care to this population aggregate of pregnant women and their infants through age 3 enables the development of a relationship-based care that is built on mutual trust. PHNs utilize the "Touchpoints" concepts of physician T. Berry Brazelton to help in developing a connection with the parents, providing anticipatory guidance to parents about predictable times when a baby goes through a growth spurt and the family may experience disorganization, dysfunction, and regression; focusing on the parents' concerns and building on family strengths. PHNs provide education and support to community workers and child care providers in Touchpoint training classes. Case management advocacy has helped families to navigate managed-care procedures, access child care, and receive transportation, translation, and other services. Public health nurses collaborate, refer, and consult with other team members, including community health workers, social workers, nutritionists, substance-abuse counselors, and mental health workers actively engaged in providing support to the families. Outcomes of this collaborative program of service include the following:

- *Reduced abuse/neglect, developmental disabilities, accidents/injuries, and failure to thrive*
- *Less anemia, tooth decay, number of hospitalizations for common illness, and infant deaths*
- *Increased rates of immunization*
- *Improved family functioning and parental satisfaction*

Adapted from Health Plan of San Mateo, Peninsula Partnership, and San Mateo County Health Services Agency, 1999. ■

Managed Care and Case Management

The definition and role of the nurse as case manager are fluid in today's health care system and will continue to evolve. The advent of managed care will affect the community nurse in functional roles and practice settings. Because Medicaid and Medicare populations in the United States are rapidly being moved into mandated managed care programs, implications for the role of community nurses in health departments, clinics, home health agencies, and other organizations using managed-care frameworks are profound. Because they are likely to lose the safety net funding they have received for providing primary care services to Medicaid clients, public health departments will continue to see changes. The number of home health agencies has been significantly decreased nationwide as a result of many factors, including managed-care organizations and Medicare mandates for prior authorization and a restriction of services to the acutely ill population being served and often inadequate financial reimbursement to the home health agencies, making it too difficult for them to meet their own financial obligations. Nurses employed in managed-care organizations will be challenged to incorporate community nursing principles into their practice as they become responsible for applying population-based care to system enrollees in a cost-effective manner. Case management functions may potentiate nurses becoming administrators of client care rather than being caregivers. This shift from a primary care focus will have ramifications for nursing practice, such as increased need for task delegation, increased use of unlicensed assistive personnel, and a blurring of practice boundaries and authority lines.

Functions in Case Management

Case management comprises six major functions that must be present in all case management models. These functions are case finding, assessment, care planning, implementation, monitoring, and reassessment and evaluation (Wolfe, 1998).

Case finding: Case finding is the identification of those individuals from a population who will benefit from case management services. Case finding was founded on the philosophy that not all individuals require case management. Only those individuals who were unable to function at the level necessary to effectively care for themselves or manage independently were considered for case management (Redford, 2001). Appropriate cases were identified through the screening of applicants, information and referral networks, or brief assessments of key dimensions that showed need or eligibility. Case finding has evolved to now include many or all of the enrollees in health maintenance organizations (HMOs) or other managed-care programs. Such programs manage enrollees to the degree necessary

to reduce costs while striving to ensure access to quality care. Enrollees may be grouped with other individuals with similar health needs and be assigned to specific case managers in order to more effectively track concerns and facilitate services. High-risk neonates, the fragile elderly, and those with chronic diseases such as diabetes, hypertension, and asthma are examples of aggregates who benefit from case management (Cohen & Cesta, 1997).

Assessment: Assessment means a full-scale, multidimensional, standardized, functional assessment of the client's needs and resources. Assessed are a comprehensive range of dimensions, including functional abilities, physical health, emotional well-being, social function, environment, current service involvement, and family support. The information obtained from the assessment process provides the case manager with practical and measurable data from which problems are identified and service plans are developed, implemented, and evaluated.

Care planning: Care planning is the core function of the case management process. The case manager takes the data identified via the assessment and, with the client, develops a service plan. This plan incorporates client preferences; specifies the type, amount, and source of services; identifies family roles and responsibilities; and specifies the nature and intensity of the case manager's role. Service planning commits the agency to the client for a specified period of time, makes claim to identified resources and establishes client and provider expectations.

Service planning requires the case manager to have a broad knowledge base, abilities in the analysis and synthesis of information, and skills in client teaching, counseling, and service negotiation. The case manager must be aware of the availability, limitations, and accessibility of service alternatives and must be skilled in the effective integration of these services (Redford, 2001; Chen et al., 1999).

Sometimes the clients' and family's needs are overwhelming and the problems so numerous that one does not know where to begin. In reality, the case manager must indicate that there will be numerous long-term problems that ultimately will be needed to be dealt with. The establishment of short- and long-term goals is helpful (Mullahy, 1998). For example, in working with a pregnant teenage girl, the short-term goals might be focused on her attending prenatal appointments, regularly taking prenatal vitamins, and remaining in school. The long-term goal would focus on a healthy outcome for both the mother and infant.

The use of standardized care plans and critical pathway tools is increasing in the community setting. The data derived from these processes allow agency nurses to better track clients by monitoring their signs and symptoms and contrasting and comparing variances to expected health responses. Tracking client health in this manner allows the nurse to anticipate potential problems and respond quickly to actual problems to minimize untoward health responses. The use of computers to track and compile the data collected from these tools is helpful to the nurse in providing high-quality care.

Implementation: Implementation is when the service plan is enacted. It is challenging to arrange services that adequately and effectively meet the needs and preferences of the client while also keeping costs to a minimum. Costs of services must be factored into decisions regarding the best service alternatives. Both formal and informal, traditional and nontraditional networks and resources are used to enact the service plan (Redford, 2001; Mullahy, 1998).

Monitoring: Monitoring is the function that provides information regarding the appropriateness, adequacy, and effectiveness of the service plan. The case manager monitors the well-being of the client in response to the service plan. Changes in the condition or circumstances of the client are noted. The services received are also evaluated. Services are monitored for timeliness, appropriateness, amount, duration, and effects. Monitoring service providers is important. Each provider is evaluated against specified performance standards. The overall purpose of the monitoring function is to ensure that the service plan is assisting the progress desired for the client. Monitoring requires knowledge of the services requested, an understanding of specific performance standards, attention to service goals, and responsible documentation. Modifications are made to the service plan as necessary (Redford, 2001).

Reassessment and evaluation: Reassessment and evaluation is a formal process that occurs at regularly scheduled intervals. Evaluation also occurs at times of client hospitalization, nursing home admission, illness, family crisis, or other precipitous, triggering events. This function provides for the assessment and evaluation of the total service plan and/or the entire case management process. Data are used to evaluate the effectiveness of the service plan in meeting the identified client goals and outcome objectives. This function provides information regarding the effectiveness of case management as a service-coordinating strategy. The information collected may be used in research investigations targeting client outcomes following case management interventions (Kane, 1990; Redford, 2001).

Characteristics of a Case Manager

The case manager must have a high level of professional competence, including in-depth clinical knowledge, an understanding of the service system, and experience with cost containment strategies. The case manager needs

skills in negotiation, collaboration, and conflict resolution in order to broker for services. Mullahy (1998) identifies what she calls the intangible characteristics of a good case manager. She includes among other qualities a sense of humor, a belief in one's ability to make a difference, approachability, optimism, keenly developed ethical principles, and a commitment to professionalism (p. 420). An appropriate educational background is necessary to better prepare nurses in these areas. An integration of case management content in baccalaureate and master's nursing programs is essential for professional preparation. Continuing-education programs are necessary for nurses who must incorporate case management skills into their careers. Opportunities for nurses as case managers are continuing to expand.

The demand for well-managed and coordinated client services requires a pool of highly qualified and well-educated professionals. Case management is a logical path for community health nurses because of their educational preparation and community experience. Continuing-education programs that update knowledge, skills, and experiences in case management strategies will enhance the nurse's proficiency as a case manager. Legal, ethical, and social obligations must be well understood by the nurse and incorporated into the service delivery plan. As case manager, the nurse, along with other community service providers, is challenged to develop and refine management systems that promote client well-being, that are fair to all (clients, case managers, and service providers), and that cost no more than necessary (Shi & Singh, 1998). Table 19-2 presents examples of the roles of community health nurses.

Clinician

Community health nursing differs from most traditional nursing roles in its focus on the community as client. Personal health services focus on individuals and may include services to help individuals maintain health, recover from illness, or adapt to long-term disabilities. Public health, however, addresses the health of individuals within the broader context of the community. Although community health nursing practice may include nursing care of individuals, families, and groups, the primary responsibility is to the health of the community as a whole (Clark, 1999). Community health nursing promotes the health of the public. The services and programs emphasize health promotion and maintenance and the prevention of disease. The aim of illness prevention and risk reduction is the promotion of optimal health of the total community. Although community health activities may change over time, the goals of community health nursing remain congruent with those of *Healthy People 2010* which are dedicated to the principle that

> regardless of age, gender, race, ethnicity, income, education, geographic location, disability and sex-

TABLE 19-2 Various Roles of the Community Health Nurse

ROLE	EXAMPLE
Advocate	Speak for the needs of the homeless.
Collaborator	Work with a parent, teacher, principal, physician, and social worker to develop a plan to facilitate the successful integration of a child with a disability into a public school setting.
Consultant	Provide assistance to a program coordinator to develop a client satisfaction questionnaire.
Counselor	Assist adult children to explore their feelings about nursing home placement for a parent and discuss other options available to them.
Educator	Teach a prenatal class on nutrition and healthy habits.
Case manager	Coordinate support services for an elderly woman and her husband, who has Alzheimer's disease. Explain Alzheimer's respite services, support groups, nursing home and long-term care facilities. Assist with insurance issues. Assist the woman to obtain transportation as she no longer drives.
Clinician	Provide information to a group of teenagers regarding safe-sex practices. Plan, implement, and evaluate a program to decrease drug use by adolescents.

ual orientation . . . every person across the Nation deserves equal access to comprehensive culturally competent, community based health care systems that are committed to serving the needs of the individual and providing community health. (USDHHS, 2000)

Most nurses with a background in acute care do not have experience with a broad community-based practice perspective. Associate degree and diploma programs in nursing generally do not provide a theoretical background for community health practice. Beginning in the late 1960s, baccalaureate programs in nursing had established curricula to prepare nurses for entry-level positions in public health nursing. With the current trend of relocation of the acute-care work force to community and public health delivery systems, the number of nurses needing to pursue the recommended educational preparation for community health practice is significant (Association of State and Territorial Directors of Nursing, 2000).

The ANA and the Association of Community Health Nursing Educators (ACHNE) recommend that two levels of community health nurses form the core personnel for community health nursing practice: the **community health nurse generalist,** educated at the baccalaureate level, and the **community health nurse specialist,** prepared at the master's or doctoral level. In this model, the focus of baccalaureate-prepared nurses is clinical practice with individuals and families within a community context. The focus of master's-prepared nurses is the health needs of the community, whereas the doctorally prepared nurses focus on health policy and research. This staff may be assisted by clinical nurse specialists from other nursing fields, nurse practitioners, nursing care associates, and ancillary nursing

personnel. Community health nurses also work with and collaborate with other members of a multidisciplinary team.

Community Health Nurse Generalist

The community health nurse generalist functions in the broadest practice role. This role combines nursing, epidemiology, case management, and resource coordination. The generalist provides care in a wide variety of settings to individuals, families, and groups while maintaining an understanding of the values and concepts of population-based practice. The community health nurse generalist participates with the specialist in community-wide assessments and in the planning, implementation, and evaluation of programs and services. The educational preparation and the knowledge and skill of the community health nurse generalist makes for a valuable partnership with the specialist in communitywide services.

Community Health Nurse Specialist

The ANA (1999) identifies the **clinical specialist** in community health nursing (CNS) as having significant expertise in assessing the health of communities. The CNS possesses skills based on knowledge of epidemiology, demographics, biometrics, environmental health, and community structure and organization. The community health CNS engages in research, theory development and testing, and policy development. Beecroft (1997) sees the CNS role as one that builds upon knowledge and expertise in working with systems and is able to develop, market and evaluate programs. The CNS is viewed as a change agent.

The community health nurse specialist may perform all of the functions of the generalist. In addition, the nurse specialist brings expertise in working with families and groups, in formulating health policy, and in assessing communities and has proficiency in carrying out all phases of population-focused programs. The specialist has skills in epidemiology, **demography** (the statistical study of populations, including health, disease, births, and deaths), **biometrics** (the application of statistical methods to biological facts), community development, and management. The community health nurse specialist engages in research, theory development and testing, and health policy development (ANA, 1986).

The advanced-practice clinical specialist in community health nursing is educationally prepared at either the master's or doctoral level as are other advanced practical clinical specialists. Nurse practitioners, nurse midwives, and nurse anesthesiologists play significant roles as **advanced-practice nurses.** Much debate has centered on the similarities and differences in the roles of the CNS and nurse practitioner (NP). Both roles originated in the mid-1960s to meet perceived health care needs. The CNS role was proposed by nurse educators in response to a need to improve client care. The CNS role was envisioned as an avenue for advancement for the talented nurse who wished to remain in direct contact with clients. The CNS would provide expert physical, social, and psychological support to clients; educate clients and families in the management of health problems; consult with nursing staff and other disciplines; and conduct research related to nursing practice outcomes (Gray, 2001).

The CNS is described as an expert practitioner with graduate preparation in a nursing specialty. Subroles of practice include clinical practitioner, educator, researcher, and consultant. The community health CNS would fulfill all of the roles of the community health nurse generalist plus be involved in conducting community assessments, assessing for populations at risk, and developing and implementing population-focused programs (ANA, 1986).

The NP movement evolved in response to a perceived shortage of physicians, particularly generalists willing to meet the needs of underserved populations. This new role was not supported by all nurses. Health professionals of the 1960s divided health care workers into those who cured illness and those who gave care. Nursing was seen as a caring profession, and, whereas CNSs were applauded for expanding that role, NPs were categorized as suspect because their role included both caring and curing. Some experts felt the NP role was a step backward because it threatened the independence of the nursing profession (Gray, 2001).

Many community health nurses have pursued additional education to assume the role of advanced-practice nurse practitioners providing primary care services. Nurse practitioners are prepared to provide a full range of primary health care services. They engage in independent decision making and provide health care to individuals, families, and groups throughout the life span. Nurse practitioners are skilled in assessment and intervention. In many states, their practice includes prescriptive privileges and other treatments commonly viewed as within the domain of medical practice. Nurse practitioners maintain a strong nursing focus by providing anticipatory guidance and counseling about health maintenance and disease prevention. The NP diagnoses actual and potential health problems and, with the client, plans appropriate treatment. Nurse practitioners operate under protocols and consult with and refer to other disciplines.

Despite the differences, there are many similarities in the components of the NP and CNS roles. Teaching and counseling individuals, families, and groups are major responsibilities for both groups. Although the tasks of conducting physical examinations, ordering laboratory tests, and prescribing medications are commonly associated with the NP role, a significant number of CNSs also carry out these activities depending on their legal authority and scope of licensure. Clinical nurse specialists are more likely to be expected to teach staff and run support groups, but many nurse practitioners also perform these functions. Although differences remain in terminology and description of practices, there are many overlapping functions in the two roles, and some nurse educators are now merging these roles (Gray, 2001).

The need for community health nurses prepared at the generalist and specialist levels will increase in the future. To truly function in the clinician role, the nurse must remember that community health nursing is not defined merely by the setting. Community health nursing practice is characterized by its focus on aggregates, the community, and high-risk populations. The beginning community health nurse may face the dilemma of "not seeing the forest for the trees" (individuals versus aggregates). Baccalaureate nursing programs have, in the past, focused on sick individuals. Community health nurses must expand their thinking from individuals to families, high-risk groups, and the entire community. Concurrently, emphasis is shifting from treatment of acute illness to the prevention of illness and promotion and maintenance of health. Community health nurses who do not focus care on the total community are not fulfilling the potential of the role in promoting the health of the community.

The present trend in community health nursing is to bring about the need for more graduate-prepared clinical specialists. Populations most in need of graduate-prepared community health nurses include elders, the homeless, adolescents, the unemployed, and other populations at risk. Health conditions needing specialist services include at-risk pregnancies and low birthweight; HIV and AIDS; Alzheimer's and other chronic diseases of elders; and stress-related injuries and illness. Community health nurses are being employed throughout the community, in health departments, schools, industries, home health, hospice, and multiple other

COMMUNITY NURSING VIEW

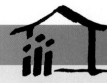

After one month of orientation that included observation of home visits, a new public health nurse working for the health department is excited at the prospect of performing independent home visits. This is her first day doing so.

The nurse's first client today is Sophia, an 18-year-old who has a 2-month-old daughter. Sophia is being followed through the teen parenting program. The program services include assessment for growth and development of the baby; nutritional status of the mother and infant; mother-child relationship; family support system; education regarding parenting, birth control, and nutrition; referrals to support groups; community resources; and educational and child care opportunities.

Sophia recently enrolled in the program, and this is her first experience with a public health nurse. The nurse phoned Sophia prior to the home visit and reviewed her role and the program services. When the nurse arrives at the door, Sophia is sitting on the back porch drinking tea and smoking cigarettes. The baby is lying in a playpen nearby. Sophia tells the nurse that she has been looking forward to the visit. "My friend had a nurse visit her too, and she really thought it was cool. I have been waiting to talk with you about my boyfriend and what I should do—he's a pain, and I'm really upset. He isn't helping me out with the baby. I've asked him and he doesn't want to do anything. What can I do?"

Nursing Considerations

Assessment

◆ How might the nurse establish rapport with Sophia?

◆ What data should be collected regarding Sophia's request for the nurse to help her with the issue regarding her boyfriend?

◆ What additional data should be collected on this first home visit?

Diagnosis

◆ What initial diagnoses might be formulated?

Outcome Identification

◆ What initial outcomes would be formulated specific to Sophia's anxiety related to her boyfriend?

◆ How should the nurse intervene following Sophia's statements about feeling upset?

Planning/Interventions

◆ What critical factors should the nurse include in the planning process?

◆ What would the initial plans be for working with Sophia?

Evaluation

◆ How would you evaluate the outcome of the nurse's interaction with Sophia?

◆ What would you include in the evaluation?

---

settings. Current health care changes hold many possibilities and exciting opportunities for community health nursing as the health care system rediscovers the importance and cost-effectiveness of prevention, and caregivers again teach people ways to be in control of their own health via healthy lifestyles. The objectives of the *Healthy People 2010* initiative serve to outline the numerous ways that the nurse may influence the health of communities. Nurses have a great opportunity to be key players in addressing many of the health care problems facing society.

KEY CONCEPTS

◆ The transition from acute-care practice to community-based practice requires the nurse to broaden professional skills and personal perspective and to view the community as client.

◆ The community health nurse is an advocate for individuals, families, groups, and communities. The nurse is influential in the development of independence and self-determination (self-care) in the client/community.

◆ In implementing health-promoting interventions with clients, the community health nurse fulfills multiple functional roles such as collaborating, consulting, and counseling. The nurse implements the educational process to enhance the client's understanding of beneficial lifestyle and behavioral changes and is committed to the implementation of research-based practice. The nurse participates in the research process to varying degrees.

◆ The community health nurse implements case management strategies to reduce the fragmentation of care that is common for individuals who are unable to negotiate the complexities inherent in the health care system.

◆ There are multiple clinical roles and preparation levels for the community health nurse. Both generalist and specialist skills are necessary to provide interventions to aggregates with varying needs.

◆ The American Nurses Association, National League of Nursing, and National Institute of Nursing Research have outlined recommendations for meeting the challenges of nursing practice in the United States. These recommendations emphasize cooperation between nursing education and clinical delivery systems to prepare nurses for community-based, population-focused, and prevention-oriented practice.

RESOURCES

ADVOCACY

Political action links for nurses: http://www.academic. scranton.edu/facultyu/zalonm1/political

CASE MANAGEMENT

Case management resource guide: http://www.cmrg.com
Bridging acute care and community case management systems: http://www.cde.psu.edu/C&I/CaseManagement

COLLABORATION

Community collaboration: http://www.pmsd. org/academy/page7
Collaboration, conflict, and power: Lessons for case managers: http://www.findarticles.com/cf_0/m0FSP/3_56908980/print

COMMUNITY HEALTH NURSING

Journal of Community Nursing: http://www.jcn.co.uk/home
Community health promotion: Challenges for practice: http://www.harcourt-international.com/catalogue/title
Community health education: Settings, roles, and skills for the 21st century: http://www.opengroup.com/mnbooks/083/ 083420987X
Community-based nursing practice project: http://www. southalabama.edu/nursing/fuld
Advanced practice community health systems nursing: http://www.son.washington.edu/eo/fa_achn.asp

RESEARCH: COMMUNITY HEALTH NURSING

Research & the community: Health, stress, and coping: http://www.umich.edu/~miwh/courses
Improving research utilisation in community nursing: http://www.fons.org/projects
Center for Nursing Research: http://www.nursing.virginia.edu/ centers/research

Diane Stafanson, RN, MSN, NP

MAKING THE CONNECTION

*What would it mean to live in a
city whose people ever changing
each other's despair into hope?
you yourself must change it
what would it feel like to know your country
was changing?
though your life felt arduous
new and unmapped and strange
what would it mean to stand on
the first page of the end of despair?*

—*Adrienne Rich, 1986*

COMPETENCIES

Upon completion of this chapter, the reader should be able to:

- Describe the similarities and differences between home health nursing and community health nursing.
- Discuss the role of the nurse in a public health setting.
- Recount the role of the nurse in providing hospice services to dying clients and their families.
- Describe the role of the school nurse in meeting the broad health needs of students, staff, families, and the community for whom he or she is responsible.
- Examine the role of the occupational and environmental health nurse in implementing cost-effective programs from administrative/management, nurse, and worker perspectives.
- Chronicle the challenges in providing quality nursing services to clients in a correctional setting.
- Define forensic nursing and its processes.
- Examine parish nursing and its historical background.
- Compare and contrast the differing standards of nursing practice as outlined by the American Nurses Association (ANA), the American Association of Occupational Health Nurses (AAOHN), and the National Association of School Nurses (NASN).

KEY TERMS

block nursing

correctional health nursing

employee assistance program (EAP)

environmental health

ergonomics

forensic nursing

home health nursing

hospice

industrial hygiene

occupational/ environmental health nursing

palliative services

parish nursing

school nursing

telehealth

toxicology

Role specialization in nursing is not a new concept. Nurses participating in acute-care settings generally function in a specialized area of client care that best meets their professional area of interest. Community health nurses provide care to aggregates in varied settings utilizing their expertise as generalists and in their roles as clinical nurse specialists and nurse practitioners. As noted in Chapter 2, community-based nursing practice was first established by Lillian Wald and Mary Browser in 1983 to meet the health needs of a community in New York City by establishing what was known as a Settlement House. Community health nursing programs today serve those at risk, for example, a program in Michigan where nurses serve homeless and marginally housed African American women, and in San Francisco, California where runaway teens receive nursing care. Whatever the practice setting community-based nurses need to coordinate and collaborate with hospitals and community agencies to ensure that the needs of their clients are being met and their levels of function are being optimized.

PRACTICE SETTINGS FOR COMMUNITY HEALTH NURSING

Community health nurses provide care to aggregates in multiple settings. Some nurses function as home health or hospice nurses, for example. In each of these capacities, the nurse delivers care in a variety of locations, but generally in the client's home. The nurse's caseload is an aggregate assembled because of individual disability, diagnosis, or need. Other nurses practice in stationary community settings such as public health departments, neighborhood schools, industrial or business environments, or correctional facilities. Caseloads are composed of groups of people within these settings who need interventions for actual or potential health needs. Regardless of the location or setting, the community health nurse provides a comprehensive health program for individuals, families, groups, and communities. In each setting, with all clients, the nurse provides services that emphasize caring, compassion, respect, and dignity.

Public Health Nursing

Previous generations of public health nurses identified the need for community-based programs whereby people who were at risk were connected with community services such as those provided by health departments. Public health nurses were at the forefront of many policy reforms that helped bring family planning, workplace safety, and maternal and child health services to people in need.

Since the inception of public health nursing, public health nurses have made a unique contribution to the health care system. Beginning with Lillian Wald, visiting families in their homes has been central to public health nursing practice, thereby providing nurses with the opportunity to see firsthand the difficulties that individuals and families experience in their homes and communities. In addition to the home-based interventions, public health nurses work in other community-based services such as nursing centers, screening programs, and health education outreach efforts (Clark, 1998).

Today, they continue to contribute significantly to the health of the community. As discussed in Chapter 1, public health nursing, as defined by the American Public Health Association (APHA), Public Health Nursing Section (1996), is "the practice of promoting and protecting the health of populations using knowledge from nursing, social, and public health sciences" (p. 1). The primary focus of public health nursing is to promote health and prevent disease for population groups. Public health nurses may provide care to individuals and families within a population group; however, the focus is on the population, with an emphasis on identifying individuals who may not request care but who have health problems that put them and others in the community at risk.

Role Functions of the Public Health Nurse

Public health nurses work in the neighborhoods and homes of some of the most vulnerable people (ANA, 1999). Their practice includes the assessment and identification of populations who are at risk or high risk for disease, threat of disease, poor recovery, and injury. These populations include the aging population, whose numbers will increase significantly in the near future, children and adults with chronic illness and disabilities, impoverished women and children, homeless and near-homeless persons, families who are dealing with violence in their homes and neighborhoods, those with substance abuse problems, and people threatened by the return of acute and chronic communicable diseases.

Public health nurses are involved in the interdisciplinary activities associated with the core public health functions of assessment, assurance, and policy development. Public health nurses translate knowledge from the health and social sciences to individuals, families, and

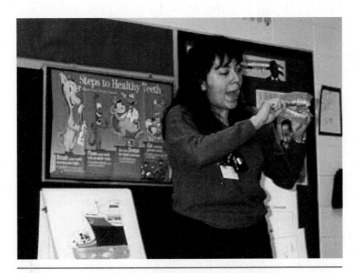

A few of the many places community health nurses can be found working and caring for clients are schools, churches, correctional facilities, and places of business.

population groups through advocacy, targeted interventions, and program development. Public health nurses work to ensure that services are available and accessible. They function as health educators and care managers, working with and through relevant community leaders, interest groups, employers, families, and individuals, and they are involved in social and political actions, all to improve health care access and availability (APHA, 1996; ANA, 1999). See Figure 20-1.

Public health nurses practice in community-based health agencies, particularly health departments in counties throughout the United States. In health departments, public health nurses contribute to the surveillance and monitoring of disease trends within the community. Emerging patterns of diseases that may threaten the public's health are identified, and interventions are planned, implemented, and coordinated. Public health nurses also contribute to the monitoring of environmentally caused illnesses, immunization levels, lead poisoning incidence, infant mortality rates, and communicable disease occurrence in order to identify problems that threaten the public's health. Public health nurses also function in other community-based agencies with varying degrees of public health focus.

FIGURE 20-1   Scope and Standards of Public Health Nursing Practice: Standards of Care

Standard I. Assessment: The public health nurse assesses the health status of populations using data, community resources identification, input from the population, and professional judgment.

Standard II. Diagnosis: The public health nurse participates with other community partners to attach meaning to those data and determine opportunities and needs.

Standard III. Outcomes Identification: The public health nurse participates with other community partners to identify expected outcomes in the populations and their health status.

Standard IV. Planning: The public health nurse promotes and supports the development of programs, policies, and services that provide interventions that improve the health status of populations.

Standard V. Assurance: Action Component of the Nursing Process for Public Health Nursing. The public health nurse assures access and availability of programs, policies, resources, and services to the population.

Standard VI. Evaluation: The public health nurse evaluates the health status of the population.

From *Scope and Standards of Public Health Nursing Practice,* by American Nurses' Association, 1999, Washington, DC: American Nurses Publishing. Reprinted with permission of American Nurses Publishing.

Public health nurses are being challenged to provide care in an environment of budgetary constraints. With the advent of Medicare and Medicaid reimbursement for designated services by public health nurses, case management skills and documentation of outcomes are a necessity. Many public health agencies provide combined public health/home health services, which for some nurses requires an updating of their knowledge and skills needed for home health care.

Home Health Nursing

Home health nursing is a dynamic specialty requiring outstanding knowledge and skill in assessing, intervening, and evaluating nursing actions. Nurses function as case managers and in this role must be able to navigate the market-driven health care system with its restructuring and corporation. Managed care and the new Medicaid prospective system are changing how home health agencies can conduct business (Ayer, 2000). The Department of Health and Human Services defines home health care as "that component of a continuum of comprehensive health care whereby health services are provided to individuals and families in their places of residence for the purpose of promoting, maintaining or restoring health, or of maximizing the level of independence while minimizing the effects of disability and illness, including terminal illness" (Warhole, 1998).

The primary purpose of home health services is to allow clients to remain in their homes to receive health care services that would otherwise be offered only in health care institutions. The home health nurse provides skilled nursing interventions to clients who have acute or intermittent medical conditions or who are terminal. The client must be under the supervision of a physician (Thobaben, 1998). The nurse implements these medical orders as a part of the overall nursing care plan.

Home health nursing is delivered through a variety of agencies and organizations. Home health services have traditionally been provided through visiting nurses' associations and community health agencies. As demand for services increases and opportunities for business emerge, however, hospitals are expanding their services into the home health field, and other private organizations are entering the arena. The inclusion of private, for-profit businesses in home health has affected the delivery of care by community, nonprofit health care agencies. This highly competitive market has made it difficult for many community agencies with limited resources to survive. In California alone, there was a 19% decline in the numbers of home health agencies between 1997 and 1998. [California Association for Health Services at Home (CASAH), 2000]. Significant legislation issued on January 12, 2001, by the Health Care Financing Administration (HCFA) will for the first time allow for a combination of both in-home and telehome care visits which will be reimbursable. For additional information, see Out of the

---

FIGURE 20-2 Scope and Standards of Home Health Nursing Practice

Standard I. Assessment: The home health nurse collects client health data.

Standard II. Diagnosis: The home health nurse analyzes the assessment data in determining diagnosis.

Standard III. Outcome Identification: The home health nurse identifies expected outcomes customized to the client and client's environment.

Standard IV. Planning: The home health nurse develops a plan of care that prescribes interventions to attain expected outcomes.

Standard V. Implementation: The home health nurse implements the interventions identified in the plan of care.

Standard VI. Evaluation: The home health nurse evaluates the client's progress toward attainment of outcomes.

From *Scope and Standards of Public Health Nursing Practice,* by American Nurses' Association, 1999, Washington, DC: American Nurses Publishing. Reprinted with permission of American Nurses Publishing.

Box (CASAH, 2000). See Figure 20-2 for American Nurses Association (ANA) Home Nursing Standards.

Home Health Links to Community Health Nursing

Home health nursing's historical link to community health agencies has forged multiple similarities between these specialties. Social and cultural changes and economic and business trends, however, have led to the development of some significant differences. It is important to distinguish between public health nursing and home health nursing in order to understand performance expectations, to appreciate the common historical origins, and to identify present dichotomies. By clearly distinguishing between the two, one can acknowledge, appreciate, and evaluate the integrity and uniqueness of each specialty. It is also important to recognize the commonalities between the two areas to foster the sharing of information that supports the practice of each. It is vital that the home health nurse have knowledge of public health practices and have the skills to provide a public health/family focus. Likewise, in order to enhance community support of clients who require home health services and the nurses who provide those services, the home health nurse must be aware of the needs of this aggregate. See Figure 20-3 and Table 20-1.

A comprehensive program of care for the home health client requires multidisciplinary expertise over a wide range of services. The home health nurse must be well informed and skilled in the various public health role functions in order to ensure the delivery of comprehensive and effective care to the client and family.

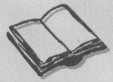

Out of the Box

Significant New Legislation Should Help Home Care Agencies

*The passage of the Medicare, Medicaid, and SCRIP Benefits Improvement and Protection Act of 2000 should help significantly in the financial support to home care agencies and the recipients of their care. Among other benefits is an additional one-year delay in the 15% cut in the home health benefit along with a revision to the home-bound definition which will allow services to those clients who are attending an adult day care program. Significant legislation in January 2001 by the HFCA in response to the legislation discussed above will enable a home health care agency to provide reimbursable **telehealth** phone visits to accomplish and/or enhance client care when an actual "hands-on" visit is not required. This important change will require staff development classes as well as training for family members who are doing the daily care in the use of the technological equipment needed to carry out the monitoring and care of the client. Early evidence shows that use of this technology is reducing the utilization of critical care services and overall cost of care. Clients with pulmonary and cardiac diseases are examples of aggregate populations well served by this new technology (Kelly, 2001; Marks, 2001).* ■

FIGURE 20-3 Similarities between Public Health Nursing and Home Health Nursing Statement of the Scope and Standards of Hospice and Palliative Nursing Practice

Practice environment: Nursing care is provided to clients in their place of residence whether their own residence, a nursing home facility, homeless shelter, etc.

Provision of services: Home health nursing care is frequently offered by official public health nursing agencies.

Nursing goals: Nursing interventions promote the community members', the clients', and the caregivers' active participation in promoting, maintaining, and restoring health to individuals, families, and the community as a whole.

Reimbursement for services: Public health nursing and home health nursing services are reimbursed by Medicaid and Medicare dollars.

From *Statement on the Scope and Standards of Hospice and Palliative Nursing Practice,* by Hospice and Palliative Nurses Association. 2000. Kendall/Hunt Publishing. Adapted with permission of Kendall/Hunt Publishing Company.

Role Functions of the Home Health Nurse

The functions of home health nurse as clinician, educator, and collaborator merit special mention. As clinician, the nurse works with clients throughout the life span as well as along the wellness-illness continuum. The nurse must be creative and adaptable when providing interventions in light of limited resources, in restricted environments, and in practice isolation. The home health nurse is the practitioner who provides critical information regarding client status to the multidisciplinary team. This information is obtained from continuous physical and functional assessment and evaluation of client response to interventions.

As clinician, the nurse is confronted with advancements in health-related technology. Improvements in home intravenous therapy, pain management techniques, portable ventilator management, total parenteral nutrition, computer-assisted documentation, and other intervention tools increase the nurse's need for continuing education. This education may be formal or informal

but must be supported by nursing management to guarantee the delivery of up-to-date, skilled nursing interventions.

As educator, the nurse provides information to promote health for the client and family. The nurse is responsible for implementing teaching/learning strategies to assist the client in adapting to personal circumstances. The nurse and client, in partnership, identify needs, set goals, and develop and implement an educational plan. Interactions characterized by caring and compassion throughout the teaching/learning exchange support the development of trust between the nurse and client.

The nurse collaborates with the multidisciplinary team to create a plan that optimizes client response. This collaboration is required in home health nursing in order to ensure continuity of care. Although members may vary, the team frequently includes a nurse, physician, physical therapist, occupational therapist, speech pathologist, social worker, homemaker/home health aide, and clergy member. Regardless of the composition of the team, it is important to remember that the delivery of comprehensive, skilled nursing care is and will continue to be the predominant component of home health services (ANA, 1999). The home health nurse is responsible for the management and coordination of care. As such, the nurse coordinates client access to multiple community resources. The home health nurse must therefore have a working knowledge of broad community health concepts.

The population in need of home health nursing services continues to grow and will do so in the future. As

TABLE 20-1   Differences between Public Health Nursing and Home Health Nursing

	PUBLIC HEALTH NURSING	HOME HEALTH NURSING
Practice focus	Population	Individual/Family
	Wellness	Illness
	Primary prevention	Secondary, tertiary prevention
Caseload acquisition	Case finding from community at large	Referral by physician or agency
	Self-referral	
	Referral by agency or physician	
Entry into service	Medical diagnosis, risk potential	Medical diagnosis
	Social diagnosis	
Interventions	Continuous	Episodic

it does, there will be increased competition for clients as well as for qualified personnel. Increasingly, health services are being provided by private organizations. Services are expected to expand to include wellness and health promotion activities and high-technology interventions. In order to meet this broad scope of services and to implement the professional standards set forth for home health nursing, registered nurses holding a minimum of a baccalaureate degree in nursing—and whose competencies and skills therefore parallel practice expectations—will be sought after (Josten, Clarke, Oswold, Stoskopf, & Morrow, 1995). Specialization via master's preparation and professional certification are endorsed by professional nursing as means to better prepare the nurse to assist clients and families, enact social policy, and conduct research (ANA, 1999).

Hospice Care

Hospice care is a coordinated program of **palliative services** (which alleviate pain or other symptoms without curing) delivered to terminally ill clients and their families. Interventions provide for the physical, psychological, social, and spiritual care of dying persons and their families (Murray & Zenter, 1997). Hospice emphasizes the caring and comfort aspect of care over the curing aspect via interventions to alleviate symptoms and control pain in the client and provide support and instruction to the family and significant others. Caring and comfort interventions include actions that preserve the humanity and protect the dignity of dying clients and their loved ones. Such interventions take place in a variety of settings, depending on the availability and accessibility of services. To support the restoration of health to the survivors, bereavement interventions continue for loved ones after the death of the client.

Clients are eligible to receive hospice care when it is certified by a physician that the client has fewer than

six months to live and when the client is willing to receive palliative, as opposed to curative, care. Clients are best served by a comprehensive hospice program that "provides centrally coordinated home care, inpatient, acute, and respite care, and bereavement services for the family and others deeply affected by the death of a client" (ANA, 1999, p. 17). Such a program is guided by a multidisciplinary team of professionals who coordinate skilled care through a holistic, dynamic, individualized plan of care that prescribes interventions to attain expected client and family outcomes (Hospice and Palliative Nurses Association [HPNA], 1999). The client and family are integrated into the team and define their rights and responsibilities regarding pain and symptom control, comfort interventions, home emergencies, and identification and use of available resources (ANA, 1999).

Standards of hospice and palliative nursing as "a holistic philosophy of care that is implemented in a variety of care settings and within a matrix of affiliative relationships in collaboration with the patient and family and other members of the interdisciplinary team. The hospice and palliative nurse must be flexible in dealing with the inevitable role blending that often occurs (HPNA [2000] Statement on the Scope and Standards of Hospice and Palliative Nursing Association, p. 3). See Figure 20-4.

The importance of the multidisciplinary team is addressed in the standards. The HPNA (2000) describes hospice practice as conducted within an "affiliative matrix" (p. 2). In such a matrix, the development and maintenance of collaborative relationships within the hospice team are critical. Role blending occurs as the nurse functions as case manager, coordinator of the plan of care, advocate, and educator. Because of the associated clinical expertise and close contact with the client and family, nursing care is recognized as the cornerstone of hospice services (ANA, 1987). In many hospice care agencies, the only paid personnel are the nurse and maybe a social worker.

FIGURE 20-4 Statement of the Scope and Standards of Hospice and Palliative Nursing Practice

Standard I. Assessment: The hospice and palliative nurse collects client and family data.

Standard II. Diagnosis: The hospice and palliative nurse analyzes the assessment data in determining diagnosis.

Standard III. Outcome Identification: The hospice and palliative nurse identifies expected outcomes individualized to the patient and family.

Standard IV. Planning: The hospice and palliative nurse develops a plan of care that prescribes interventions to attain expected outcomes.

Standard V. Evaluation: The hospice and palliative nurse evaluates the patient and family's progress toward attainment of outcomes.

From *Statement on the Scope and Standards of Hospice and Palliative Nursing Practice*, by Hospice and Palliative Nurses Association. 2000. Kendall/Hunt Publishing. Adapted with permission of Kendall/Hunt Publishing Company.

Dimensions of Hospice Care

Healing is an essential concept of caring and underlies hospice philosophy. Healing may be analyzed across physical, psychosocial, and spiritual dimensions (*Nurses Handbook of Alternative and Complementary Care,* 1998). Interventions related to the physical dimension are geared toward supporting restoration to maximum wholeness. In this dimension, the client is assessed for physiological responses to his or her disease process. Interventions related to the physical dimension include pain relief, symptom control, maintenance of skin integrity, energy conservation, and nutrition management. Modalities that enhance client control of these responses may include autogenic training, relaxation techniques, biofeedback, self-hypnosis, and/or Therapeutic Touch.

The psychosocial dimension refers to the emotional, psychological, and social health of the client and family despite loss and grief (Leddy & Pepper, 1998). Related interventions are geared toward optimizing this dimension and include supporting a sense of power and control in the client and family, promoting positive self-concept, alleviating feelings of loneliness and isolation, and fostering the communication of feelings and needs. The hospice nurse strives to assist with the peaceful acceptance of inevitable death by fostering communication and encouraging the life review process. Interventions that promote client control over his or her life may reduce anxiety and generate feelings of harmony for the client and the family.

The spiritual dimension refers to the spiritual, religious, and relationship needs of the client and family (HPNA, 2000). With hospice care, spiritual interventions support the client and family to come to terms with death. Assessment of the spiritual needs of the client and family is the responsibility of the hospice nurse. Interventions include recognizing the spiritual needs of the dying person, assisting the client in meeting those needs, and enhancing a sense of wholeness and closure. The importance of the spiritual dimension in working with the dying cannot be overemphasized. Igoe (1984) states, "The essence of hospice seems to be found in the spiritual dimension" (p. 160). It is critical that the caregiver assure hospice clients that they will be well cared for, surrounded by those they love, and treated with love and respect in their efforts to arrive at spiritual peace (Igoe, 1984).

Types of Hospice Programs

Hospice programs vary in organizational structure and service delivery. Community needs, leadership, funding sources, political influences, and available resources for health care, spiritual care, and social services affect the availability and structure of hospice care. Hospice programs may be owned and operated by public agencies, hospitals, home health agencies, extended-care facilities, or other independent organizations. As with home health services, hospice organizations may be financially structured as nonprofit or for profit. They may serve clients in their homes or in inpatient facilities, be freestanding or part of a larger institution. Regardless of the organizational structure, a hospice program must meet strict criteria to become Medicare certified and receive reimbursement for services rendered.

Hospice programs employ registered nurses as either full-time hospice nurses or home health, hospital, or community staff nurses with varying hospice caseloads. Trained volunteers are critical members of the hospice team and constitute a significant source of support for the client and family. Also provided by hospice programs are physician services, various therapy services, spiritual and bereavement counseling, home health aide services, homemaker services, medical supplies, short-term inpatient care, and other specialized care providers as necessary to achieve the outcomes of the plan of care (HPNA, 2000).

Role Functions of the Hospice Nurse

A high level of professional competence is required to function effectively as a hospice nurse (HPNA, 2000). The hospice nurse must be skilled in all of the functional roles required of the nurse in the community setting and also have a strong background in acute care. Three role functions deserve specific discussion with regard to hospice care. As educator, the hospice nurse supports client and family decision making by providing information specific to the client's situation across the physical, psychosocial, and spiritual dimensions. As consultant, the nurse provides expert knowledge combined with an understanding of the client's needs and strengths to empower the client to make decisions about the dying process. The other members of the multidisciplinary team rely on the nurse's accurate and comprehensive judgment in order to make appropriate decisions regarding care. As advocate, the hospice nurse upholds the desires of the client. In the dying process, clients often become too weak and disadvantaged to defend their wishes. The hospice nurse must practice with a heightened sense of ethics in considering the client's decisions (ANA, 2000; HPNA, 1999).

The nurse is responsible for coordinating the services provided to the dying client and grieving family members (Clark, 1998). Close and frequent interaction with dying clients and their distressed families may deplete the nurse's physical and emotional reserves. The nurse must therefore carefully balance the needs of the client and family with personal limitations. The hospice nurse requires administrative and peer support in order to manage personal needs as they arise. Appropriate interaction with and utilization of all members of the multidisciplinary team will strengthen the support network for the hospice nurse as well as for the client and family.

Hospice nursing involves the delivery of holistic, sympathetic, empathetic, personal care to dying individuals and their families during a critical phase of family life (HPNA, 2000). The provision of such comprehensive client/family care and the autonomous professional practice characteristic of hospice nursing afford the nurse numerous opportunities to develop clinical and leadership skills. The hospice movement is expected to grow rapidly as individuals and families continue to seek a comfortable and humane death with caring professionals who will assist and guide the process without controlling it.

School Nursing

School nursing is a branch of community health nursing that seeks to identify or prevent school health problems and intervenes to remedy or reduce these problems. The school nurse is a licensed, professional nurse; licensure or certification is preferably through an appropriate association. The majority of nurses employed as school nurses are educationally prepared at the baccalaureate level. Their scope of practice and their credentials are frequently overseen and regulated by the individual state board of education and/or the local school districts. In some communities, school nurses are also hired by public health departments who contract with school districts. This alters the role. The role for school nurses today requires functioning as health managers and coordinators of care. The trend is to encourage nurses working in schools to obtain graduate preparation as school nurse practitioners or clinical specialists for school-aged children. The nurse implements primary, secondary, and tertiary prevention strategies to promote optimum wellness in the school-aged client. Prevention interventions target students who have potential health concerns, acute or chronic diseases, handicapping conditions (speech, hearing, visual, and orthopedic impairments), emotional or family problems, mental retardation, or learning disabilities. Other health-related issues that demand attention include accident awareness, tobacco use, chemical abuse, sexual activity, pregnancy, and various types of violence. The school nurse should be familiar with the year 2010 national health objectives in order to provide appropriate screening, monitoring, and services that support meeting these objectives. The school nurse contributes directly to the students' education by implementing prevention strategies that promote the physical, emotional, and social health of students so they are prepared to learn.

School Nursing Service Populations

School nursing takes place in both public and private schools with enrollments ranging from several students to several thousand students. Services are delivered to students and staff across the health care continuum. Nurse competencies must therefore run the spectrum from pediatric and adolescent to general adult health care. Because the school community is a microcosm of our society, a functioning knowledge of public health concepts and occupational health principles is vital to the school nurse. School nursing is considered "community-based and community-focused, with the school community at the center of interest and the recipient of nursing services" (Resnicow & Allenworth, 1996).

School health services have expanded in recent years due to the inclusion of programs for disabled and disadvantaged students, the relatively new phenomenon of children with acute or chronic health problems attending school, the increased numbers and types of communicable diseases, and the incorporation of students in need of specialized treatments. Contemporary school services may also include wellness programs for students and staff. The challenge of keeping students and staff healthy enough to attend school and be in condition for optimal teaching and learning will continue. As such challenges continue and grow, so too will the responsibilities of and opportunities for the school nurse.

REFLECTIVE THINKING

Hospice Care

- How might you provide spiritual support to those with values that differ from your own?
- In what ways do you manage your needs when you are experiencing loss?
- How has your ability to communicate been affected when you are grieving?

As a specialty practice, school nursing has identifiable and measurable standards of practice. Because the school nurse most often works in isolation and is generally evaluated by nonnurse administrators, these standards are an essential foundation of practice. Both the administrator and the nurse must have an in-depth understanding of these standards and be committed to applying them. A summary of these standards is provided in Figure 20-5.

Role Functions of the School Nurse

The National Association of School Nurses (NASN, 1998) outlines three overlapping roles for the school nurse: the generalist clinician role, the primary care role, and the manager and coordinator of care roles. The nurse in the generalist clinician role provides health services, counseling, and health education to students and families. These services are integrated into the school as an important part of the total educational program. This nurse is usually employed by the school, by the school district, or by a local governmental agency such as the health department (Tyrrell & Eyles, 1999).

The generalist clinician is located in the school and provides services during school hours. The nurse is incorporated into the daily functions of the school community. Students, families, faculty, and staff recognize the nurse as being an available professional resource for health concerns. In this role, the nurse is able to identify students, families, and staff at risk (case finding), develop and implement appropriate interventions for identified health needs, and formulate appropriate policies and programs to resolve actual and potential problems. Interpersonal violence and substance use are major contributors to premature death, disability, and social problems among U.S. youth. Homicide is the leading cause of death among 15- to 24-year-olds and the number one cause of death among black and Hispanic youth (Lowrey, Cohen, Modzelesdki, Kann, Collins, & Kolbe, 1999).

The primary care role is carried out by nurse practitioners who practice under physician-approved protocols and standardized procedures. The school nurse practitioner diagnoses and treats health problems and coordinates care with other health professionals. Management of minor acute and chronic illnesses, health education, and environmental health support are provided. Annual health assessment for the well child/adolescent and developmental assessment are included within this primary care role (NASN, 1998). Many of these practitioners have implemented school-based clinics, school-linked services, and collaborative, community-based services. School-based clinics are offered near the families who need them and furnish an accessible location for persons seeking professional health care. The school nurse needs to be aware of changing legislation which impacts the health of school children. The 1997 Child Health Insurance Plan Act is significant in that it helps to provide financial assistance for states to promote the health of low-income children. This legislation is known most commonly as the Healthy Families Program (State of California, 1997). Figure 20-6 offers examples of items to monitor in the school-age client.

As manager, the school nurse is responsible for a variety of actions defined by the NASN. The management role includes program planning for the provision of comprehensive services to clients in the school community. Effective management strategies ensure a continuum of care from the student's home, to community health provider, to school, and back to home (Zanga & Oda, 1987).

FIGURE 20-5 Standards of Professional School Nursing Practice: Standards of Care

Standard I. Assessment: The school nurse collects client data.

Standard II. Diagnoses: The school nurse analyzes the assessment data in determining nursing diagnoses.

Standard III. Outcome Identification: The school nurse identifies expected outcomes individualized to the client.

Standard IV. Planning: The school nurse develops a plan of care/action that specifies interventions to attain expected outcomes.

Standard V. Implementation: The school nurse implements the interventions identified in the plan of care/action.

Standard VI. Evaluation: The school nurse evaluates the client progress toward attainment of outcomes.

From *Standards of Professional School Nursing Practice,* by National Association of School Nurses (NASN), 1998, Scarborough, ME: Author. Reprinted with permission.

FIGURE 20-6 Examples of Items to Monitor in the School-Age Client

Physical health

Emotional health

Health habits (smoking, eating, drug abuse, sexual activity)

Pregnancy

Potential abuse (sexual, emotional, verbal, physical)

Chronic absenteeism

Failing grades

Medicine intake and reactions

Interaction with peers, teachers, and other authority figures

Safety issues

Social concerns (home environment, homelessness, poverty, domestic violence)

✳ DECISION MAKING

School Nursing

As the nurse in an elementary school, you have witnessed an increasing number of students with complex physical and emotional problems being mainstreamed into the classroom. At the same time, money, resources, and services are dwindling.

◆ What school and community resources might you approach for assistance in meeting the needs of these students?

◆ As the school nurse, how would you influence the health of aggregates faced with decisions regarding gang membership? Violence? Drug and alcohol use? Cigarette use? Teen pregnancy?

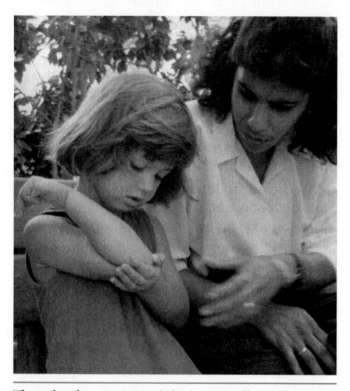

The school nurse treats injuries as well as offering counseling, screening, and other services.

Because the school nurse may coordinate programs on several campuses, carry a large and active caseload, and supervise other school nurses, volunteers, or health aides, management and leadership skills are crucial. The school nurse is in a position to influence health policy formation, to obtain political and parental support for program development, and to secure maximum participation from the community (Tyrell & Eyles, 1999).

An essential management function of the school nurse is to conduct research. The NASN's Standard 9 ad-

dresses the need for school nurses to participate in research or research-related activities to further the knowledge base for school-based health outcomes. Many studies conducted on the school-aged population have been done by professionals other than school nurses. The NASN (1998) challenges nurses within the specialty to conduct studies and promote research-based practice. Data collection and documentation of school health efforts, interventions, and outcomes are beneficial to the development of effective programs. Such information is crucial to the formation of district and/or governmental health policy and to the delineation of the scope of school nursing practice (Tyrell & Eyles, 1999).

The school nurse of today is a valuable resource for students, families, and staff who are continually confronted with a multitude of physical, mental, social, and behavioral issues. The nurse is a competent case finder, clinician, educator, manager, collaborator, and researcher and is available as a health resource for the community served. As the center of school health services, the school nurse supports the education process by promoting the overall health of students and staff.

Occupational/Environmental Health Nursing

According to the American Association of Occupational Health Nurses (AAOHN), **occupational/environmental health nursing** is a specialty practice providing health care services to workers and worker populations (AAOHN, 1999). This practice is an extension of community health nursing and focuses on the promotion, protection, and restoration of workers' health within the context of a safe and healthy work environment. Occupational nursing is a synthesis and application of principles from nursing, medicine, **environmental health** (the study and prevention of environmental problems), **toxicology** (the study of poisons), and epidemiology. It incorporates concepts from safety, **industrial hygiene** (the study of the workplace environment and its relationship to impaired health of workers or community citizens), and **ergonomics** (the study of the relationship between individuals and their work environment) and adopts principles from the social and behavioral sciences. A rapidly changing and evolving practice setting, occupational health is dynamic and fluctuates in response to changing health care, business, economic, political, ecological, social, and cultural demands (AAOHN, 2001).

Goals of Occupational/Environmental Health Nursing

The occupational/environmental health nurse, often the only health care professional in the industrial setting, holds a key position working with management to develop strategies to improve the health of workers. The work of the occupational health nurse benefits the corporation by giving rise to a healthy, involved, and productive work force.

The workplace provides an ideal community for the implementation of health promotion, health protection, and health restoration strategies. Individuals come together in the workplace, representing a cross section of the societal picture of physical, behavioral, cultural, and emotional variables. The workplace environment changes as society transforms. Work-force demographics mirror these societal transformations. The work force is increasing in age, diversity, educational level, skill, and desire to influence changes in work environment (AAOHN Position Statement, 2001). The health and wellness issues that emerge in conjunction with changing demographics are the domain of the occupational health nurse.

Role Responsibilities of the Occupational/ Environmental Health Nurse

The occupational/environmental health nurse has multiple clinical, educational, and administrative responsibilities. Clinical responsibilities include preplacement assessment, annual physical examination, diagnosis and treatment of acute minor illnesses, emergent care, and counseling. Educational obligations consist of identifying teaching/learning needs, developing programs, and evaluating learning outcomes. Administrative duties include performing referral and follow-up, monitoring the worksite, implementing corporate and governmental regulations, communicating worker health needs to corporate management, and various other administrative tasks (Cookfair, 1996). Nursing interventions may be geared toward the individual worker, a group of workers on the same unit, or a population of workers with similar actual or potential needs. Standards of occupational and environmental health nursing can be found in Figure 20-7.

Traditionally, the occupational health nurse has delivered direct care on a one-on-one basis. In this individual orientation, the occupational health nurse is usually located in an office, and the worker approaches the nurse for assistance. Interventions include direct services such as individual assessment, one-on-one counseling, treatment of illness and injury, worker compensation case management, or individual crisis management (Maciag, 1993).

Although individual interventions are important, occupational health nurses must consider alternative ways of providing health services with limited resources. Individual interventions are narrowly focused and expensive in terms of time and resource allocation. With the rising cost of providing individual health care interventions, the occupational health nurse must meet the challenges of containing costs, ensuring quality programming, and targeting services via planning, research, and policy development. A section of the *Healthy People 2010* objectives addresses occupational safety and health challenges. The related objectives guide actions for occupational health

---

FIGURE 20-7   Standards of Occupational and Environmental Health Nursing Practice

Standard I. Assessment: The occupational and environmental health nurse systematically assesses the health status of the individual client or population and the environment.

Standard II. Diagnosis: The occupational and environmental health nurse analyzes assessment data to formulate diagnoses.

Standard III. Outcome Identification: The occupational and environmental health nurse identifies outcomes specific to the client.

Standard IV. Planning: The occupational and environmental health nurse develops a goal-directed plan that is comprehensive and formulates interventions to attain expected outcomes.

Standard V. Implementation: The occupational and environmental health nurse implements interventions to attain desired outcomes identified in the plan.

Standard VI. Evaluation: The occupational and environmental health nurse systematically and continuously evaluates responses to interventions and progress toward the achievement of desired outcomes.

Standard VII. Resource Management: The occupational and environmental health nurse secures and manages the resources that support an occupational health and safety program.

Standard VIII. Professional Development: The occupational and environmental health nurse assumes accountability for professional development to enhance professional growth and maintain competency.

Standard IX. Collaboration: The occupational and environmental health nurse collaborates with employees, management, other health care providers, professionals, and community representatives.

Standard X. Research: The occupational and environmental health nurse uses research findings in practice and contributes to the scientific base in occupational and environmental health nursing to improve practice and advance the profession.

Standard XI. Ethics: The occupational and environmental health nurse uses an ethical framework as a guide for decision making in practice.

From *Competencies and Performance Criteria in Occupational and Environmental Health Nursing*, 1999, American Association of Occupational and Environmental Health Nurses. Reprinted with permission.

---

services. It is the nurse's responsibility to implement cost-effective interventions to achieve these objectives.

The occupational health nurse plays a big role in maintaining the health and safety of employees by assessing the worksite for hazards and potential hazards and reducing risks that could lead to a disaster situation.

The nurse assists in developing written disaster plans appropriate to risks inherent in the worksite. The nurse must be versed in disaster prevention and planning and must be skilled in communicating with company administration, community resources, and at-risk workers. Disaster plans are designed to prevent or minimize injury and death of workers and nearby residents. Additional priorities for planning include development of an effective triage system, interface with community resources (fire, police, emergency, hospital and public health departments), minimizing property damage, and facilitating resumption of business activity. Although the nurse is rarely solely responsible for planning and implementing the disaster plan, as a member of the team, the occupational health nurse may function as clinician. The occupational health nurse also plays a significant role in preventing and reducing workplace violence. On an average, 20 workers die of a work-related injury each week and *1 out of 6 of these fatalities can be attributed to violence in the workplace* (AAOHN, 2001).

Future occupational health nurses will need broad business skills. The nurse analyzes trends, develops programs, contains costs, identifies problems, and proposes solutions to health-related issues. Occupational health services, like other corporate functional areas, exist solely to support the overall goals of the corporation. In addition to the health and welfare of the workers, the corporation is critically concerned about profits, losses, productivity, and future economic health. The occupational health nurse must be committed to supporting the goals of the organization. The nurse attends to the health of workers, realizing that a sick, less-productive work force is expensive to the economic health of the organization (Clark, 1998).

The occupational health nurse is responsible for proposing well-planned and cost-effective health programs to corporate management. Expert skills in data collection, data analysis, and program planning, combined with abilities in persuasive communication, are essential for obtaining corporate support and resources for service needs (Maciag, 1993). The nurse must be familiar with the current and future goals of the corporation to be successful in providing services that complement and support these objectives. Adaptability and flexibility are skills required for the nurse to meet these responsibilities.

The occupational health nurse influences worker health behavior in numerous ways and may be a catalyst for voluntary personal behavioral change on the part of the worker. The nurse may implement strategies such as simple awareness-promoting interventions (e.g., posters, lectures, or demonstrations), information contests, or worksite health and nutrition fairs to educate the work force about healthy lifestyles and behaviors.

More stringent measures that affect worker behavior are by-products of mandatory governmental regulation. Many environmental interventions are the result of governmental policy. The Occupational Safety and Health Administration (OSHA) and the National Institute of Occupational Safety and Health (NIOSH) are federal agencies involved in developing regulations related to occupational health and safety. OSHA is part of the U.S. Department of Labor. It enforces occupational regulations at the federal, regional, and state levels. NIOSH is a division of the Centers for Disease Control and Prevention (CDC), a part of the U.S. Public Health Service. NIOSH is a data collection center that makes recommendations regarding occupational hazards. The increase in regulations to ensure safe work practices, smoke-free environments, and employee-exposure control necessitates that the occupational health nurse be well informed regarding current regulations and be able to understand and apply OSHA and NIOSH regulations. The nurse should be skilled in educating the work force regarding all regulations and be supportive of efforts to comply with them. Figure 20-8 lists items of which the occupational health nurse should be cognizant.

Employee Assistance Programs

Large companies with sufficient resources may finance long-term, in-depth programs designed to affect worker behaviors, beliefs, and attitudes in an effort to improve morale and productivity and reduce health risks and absenteeism. One example is the **employee assistance program (EAP).**

Employee assistance programs may take the form of counseling, chemical rehabilitation, stress management training, or other similar initiatives considered helpful in supporting workers' attempts at maintaining or restoring productivity. The occupational health nurse's involvement in an EAP may be at the referral level, or the nurse may function as coordinator or counselor. Occupational health is currently seeing growth in employee assistance programs. Such programs benefit workers by supporting

---

FIGURE 20-8 Examples of Potential Agents That Occupational Health Nurse Needs to Monitor

Exposure to:

- Pesticides
- Allergens
- Asbestos
- Wood dust
- Cement dust
- Metal dust
- Lead
- Noise
- Repetitive-motion problems
- Safety violations

them in regaining or maintaining productivity and benefit corporations by creating a human-oriented, supportive environment for their workers and by sustaining a productive work force (Thompson, 1989).

Role of the Occupational/Environmental Health Nurse

Multiple factors will determine the role functions, scope of practice, and contributions of the occupational health nurse in the future. Among these factors are the ways that occupational health nurses execute the scope of occupational health practice, are viewed by other nurses and professionals in related fields, perceive themselves in the professional role, organize as a professional group, involve themselves in corporate and/or governmental affairs, and generate scholarly research. The role of the occupational health nurse will also be affected by the types of injuries, illnesses, and issues encountered by the worker of the future. Occupational health nursing is creating a solid and unique framework for practice by fostering research. In a rapidly changing and increasingly complex work environment, research is a vital component for the delivery of appropriate, quality services. Rogers (1989) states that occupational health nursing is a scientific, applied discipline that "has an obligation to seek opportunities to expand the frontiers of occupational health nursing knowledge and to be discontent with the status quo" (p. 497).

The role of the occupational health nurse is diversified and complex. The occupational health nurse is in a position to coordinate a holistic approach in the delivery of health services in the work environmental (AAOHN, 2000). The nurses in the occupational health setting must embody new ways of thinking, demonstrate political astuteness and expertise in communication, demonstrate flexibility and the ability to deal with ambiguity, as well as possess a knowledge of economics and health care delivery. Population-based practice that focuses on outcome measurement, quality assurance, and advocacy will continue to be imperatives for practice in the 21st century.

Research in Occupational/Environmental Health Nursing

Occupational health nurses are encouraged to create opportunities for participating in and conducting research to contribute to the growing body of knowledge (AAOHN, 2001). Occupational nursing research priorities have been identified and targeted, with the AAOHN Board categorizing 11 research priorities into 3 broad areas. The first area of research is related to the effectiveness of occupational health nursing interventions in the following areas:

- Primary health care delivery at the worksite
- Health-promoting nursing interventions

REFLECTIVE THINKING

Occupational Health Nursing

- To what degree should the occupational health nurse be involved in employee assistance programs?
- What about confidentiality? If an employee were considered unstable and a risk to fellow employees would you report this finding to appropriate management/authorities?

- Programs on employee productivity and morale
- Ergonomic strategies to reduce worker injury and/or illness

The second broad area of research targets the strategies for dealing with occupational health issues, including the following:

- Methods for handling complex ethical issues related to workers' health
- Strategies for minimizing work-related health outcomes
- Mechanisms to ensure quality and cost effectiveness of programs
- Factors that influence worker rehabilitation and return to work

The final area of research is related to identifying hazards and reducing risks at the worksite. Areas of interest include the following:

- Occupational hazards of health care workers
- Factors that contribute to behavioral changes and self-care
- Factors that contribute to sustained risk-reduction behavior related to lifestyle choices (Rogers, 1989)

Correctional Health Nursing

Correctional health nursing is a branch of professional nursing that provides nursing services to clients in correctional facilities. Facilities in which individuals are incarcerated include prisons, jails, youth detention/correction centers, adult probation/parole divisions, and other similar restricted settings. Individuals who are perceived to be threats or to owe debts to society are retained in correctional facilities to maintain the public order. Individuals incarcerated in such environments vary from juveniles to aged adults and include both women and men (Moritz, 1982; ANA, 1995).

Challenges in Correctional Nursing

The correctional health nurse functions in a non-health care setting governed by an overriding attention to individual safety and institutional security. The nurse works with men, women, and youth for whom society has little regard and minimal interest in spending scarce public resources on personal health needs. The inmate/client usually does not have a choice regarding the services provided or the practitioner providing those services. Furthermore, the health services provided may be inadequate because of poor resources, outdated equipment, difficulty in accessing the client for assessment and treatment, lack of health or security personnel, or limited opportunity to involve support services and networks (Little, 1981; Peternelj-Taylor & Hufft, 1997). These factors combine to create a stressful, complex, and challenging work setting that demands the nurse be competent in multiple areas. The National Association of Correctional Nursing (NACN) was established in 2000 to provide direction and support to nurses employed in the correctional system. The goal and mission of the NACN is to advance the respect and credibility of our profession. Through the strength and number of our members, NACN is determined to establish correctional nursing as a legitimate and recognized nursing specialty. We shall advance the skills and knowledge of our members through dissemination of information from other correctional health care organizations, while improving upon the core nursing skills unique to correctional nursing through testing and certification (NACN, 2000).

The ANA Position Statement (revised 1988) states its opposition to nurse participation in capital punishment. ANA views nurse participation in executions as contrary to the goals and ethical traditions of the profession.

Scope of Nursing Services in Correctional Settings

Nursing services provided to inmates range from brief ambulatory or emergent care to comprehensive health programs. Clients range from the healthy to the acutely or chronically ill and include individuals who are mentally ill and/or developmentally or physically challenged. The aging population in the correctional setting presents a challenge to those caring for them. Public perception has assumed a strong link between violent behavior and mental illness. The most recent studies have shown this to be untrue. According to the American Psychiatric Association, a "small subgroup of people with severe and persistent illness is at risk of becoming violent" (ANA, 1994). The Department of Justice states that at least 6.4% and possibly as high as 8% have a severe mental disability. It is believed that 90% of persons with current illness are not violent. The correctional nurse has a responsibility to the mentally ill, institutionalized patients to advocate for high-quality and accessible treatment as well as protect this vulnerable prison population who are frequently victims of violence themselves (National Mental Health Association, 1995). Nursing responsibilities to in-

carcerated clients include health education, suicide prevention, communicable disease control, alcohol and drug rehabilitation, somatic therapy, psychosocial counseling, emergency care, and environmental health. The nurse must be educationally and experientially prepared to provide and/or coordinate comprehensive services for clients needing interventions in these areas. As the number of women inmates increases, women's health issues will move to the forefront. Incarcerated women will need obstetric, gynecological, and parenting services and support. The correctional health nurse is committed to the provision of care to all individuals regardless of the nature of their crimes or the duration of their incarcerations (ANA, 1995).

The scope and standards for practice in a correctional facility as outlined by the ANA have been adopted by the American Correctional Health Services Association, an organization open to all correctional health care professionals. The *Scope and Standards of Nursing Practice in Correctional Facilities* (see Figure 20-9) guides professional practice and performance for the correctional health nurse (ANA, 1995). The standards recognize the right of all people to have access to adequate health care.

Case finding is particularly important in the correctional setting. The nurse must be able to assess individuals who, among other things, are at risk for suicide, communicable disease, and alcohol and drug problems. Suicide is a significant cause of death for incarcerated youth. Potential for suicide is especially high for juveniles housed in adult facilities. Identification of at-risk individuals is critical for providing effective interventions to reduce suicidal tendencies and behaviors (Peternelj-Taylor & Hufft, 1997; NACN, 2000).

Crowded facilities, poor hygiene, and sexual activity may contribute to the transmission of communicable disease. Health education coupled with epidemiological

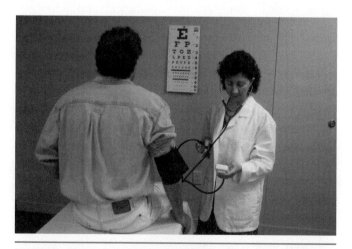

Working in a correctional facility offers many challenges to the nurse; however, rewards can be found in opportunities to function as a group leader, innovator, teacher, planner, and caregiver.

strategies is necessary to reduce new disease cases and lessen the effects of current cases. Chemical abuse is another serious problem for many inmates before, during, and after incarceration. In order to effect change, the nurse must therefore be competent in the areas of case finding, treatment programs and detoxification regimes, individual and group counseling, health education, and client referral (NACN, 2000).

FIGURE 20-9   Standards of Nursing Practice in Correctional Facilities

Standards of Care

Standard I. Assessment: The nurse collects client health data.

Standard II. Diagnosis: The nurse analyzes the assessment data in determining diagnoses.

Standard III. Outcome Identification: The nurse identifies expected outcomes individualized to the client.

Standard IV. Planning: The nurse develops a care plan that prescribes interventions to attain expected outcomes.

Standard V. Implementation: The nurse implements the interventions identified in the care plan.

Standard VI. Evaluation: The nurse evaluates the client's progress toward attainment of outcomes.

Standards of Professional Performance

Standard I. Quality of Care: The nurse systematically evaluates the quality and effectiveness of nursing practice.

Standard II. Performance Appraisal: The nurse evaluates his or her own nursing practice in relation to professional practice standards and relevant statutes and regulations.

Standard III. Education: The nurse acquires and maintains current knowledge in nursing practice.

Standard IV. Collegiality: The nurse contributes to the professional development of peers, colleagues, and others.

Standard V. Ethics: The nurse's decisions and actions on behalf of clients are determined in an ethical manner.

Standard VI. Collaboration: The nurse collaborates with the client, significant others, other criminal justice system personnel, and health care providers in providing client care.

Standard VII. Research: The nurse uses research findings in practice.

Standard VIII. Resource Utilization: The nurse considers factors related to safety, effectiveness, and cost in planning and delivering client care.

From *Scope and Standards of Practice in Correctional Facilities,* by American Nurses' Association, 1995, Washington, DC: American Nurses Publishing. Reprinted with permission of National Association of School Nurses.

Individuals in correctional facilities are isolated from family and other social support systems. This separation can result in significant distress to the individual and the family. Clients and/or family may be sullen, angry, or scared and may therefore be unwilling or unable to communicate needs. Manipulative behaviors and "game playing" are frequent patterns displayed by inmates. These issues demand skilled communication from the nurse in attempting to build rapport and develop a therapeutic relationship with clients. To be successful, the nurse must know ways to respond to and manage these patterns (Peternelj-Taylor & Hufft, 1997). It is important for the nurse to include family and significant others in the plan of care as much as possible. A solid background in communication theory, family theory, and group work is essential to the success of interventions (ANA, 1995).

The scope of practice for the nurse in a correctional setting is limited strictly to the delivery of nursing services. Under no circumstances should the nurse participate in activities linked to security or inmate correction. The nurse does not participate, either directly or indirectly, in surveillance, strip searches, disciplinary decisions, or health-threatening actions such as lethal injections. Rather, the nurse implements all aspects of the nursing process to promote, maintain, or restore the health of the client (ANA, 1995). Figure 20-10 lists several health-related concerns that the correctional health nurse must monitor in the inmate.

Attention to safety is particularly important for the nurse working in a correctional setting. It is imperative that the nurse retain a deep respect for the nature of the environment and be committed to security protocol. The nurse is held to all security regulations that apply to other facility personnel and must maintain a balance between the risks inherent in a controlled environment and the delivery of quality care (ANA, 1995). This balance challenges the nurse's ability to provide nondiscriminatory, nonprejudicial services to inmates within a setting characterized by opposing philosophical orientations: Whereas corrections officers focus on security for both the setting and the inmates and staff, inmates focus on personal survival and hopes for freedom, and nurses and health care staff focus on the health and well-being of the inmates

---

FIGURE 20-10   Examples of Problems the Correctional Health Nurse Needs to Monitor

- Depression
- Communicable diseases
- Rape
- Signs of trauma
- Substance abuse
- Chronic and acute illnesses
- Pregnancy

whom they serve. Given these differing orientations and foci, the potential for conflict is great (Peternelj-Taylor & Hufft, 1997).

Communication strategies that foster rapport and open exchange with correctional personnel (e. g., guards, counselors, and administrators) are critical in order to continue appropriate interventions without breaching safety and security protocol (ANA, 1985; Peternelj-Taylor & Hufft, 1997). Educating each group about the functions and expanded services that can be provided by the nurse will promote the acceptance of the nurse as a capable and valuable member of the facility. In return, the nurse must respect the responsibilities and actions of members of the other groups and function within the standards and scope of practice. Communication efforts that further understanding among groups will lead to collaboration, mutual assistance, and coordination of actions to ensure positive outcomes (Peternelj-Taylor & Hufft, 1997).

Ideally, the nurse in the correctional setting should receive specific orientation, inservice education, and continuing education to support practice in this specialty. The nurse should be minimally prepared with a baccalaureate degree in nursing. Nurse specialists and nurse practitioners with masters preparation are frequently employed in correctional facilities. These nurses function in broad clinical and administrative roles. They participate in and conduct research to further the foundation of correctional health nursing practice (ANA, 1995).

Many issues combine to make nursing in the correctional setting a challenge. The nurse practicing in the correctional setting is often the only health care provider in the facility, a setting that is focused on security needs rather than health needs and that allocates few resources to adequately support nursing interventions. The nurse may have few role models and may receive little or no feedback regarding interventions or practice competency. Furthermore, the nurse has little control in the decision-making processes related to inmate health needs and treatment options. Also, educational programs to obtain training in correctional health practice may be unavailable. Finally, the nurse may perceive a lack of support and feel isolated and misunderstood by peers.

Correctional health nursing also offers many potential rewards, however. Such rewards include opportunities to function as group leader, innovator, teacher, planner, caregiver, counselor, coordinator, and researcher. Furthermore, the opportunity for personal growth via identifying values, studying human behaviors, and contributing to the health and well-being of those who otherwise may not receive such care can generate a sense of personal satisfaction (Peternelj-Taylor & Hufft, 1997). Nursing practice in the correctional setting is, and will continue to be, exciting, stimulating, challenging, and potentially rewarding and enjoyable work.

Forensic Nursing

Today's forensic nurses are also called *the new detectives* as nurses join with other investigators in combating crime and violence. With the ever-increasing violence in this country, there is a definable role for nurses who have special educational preparation in the field of crime-related deaths and injuries. Nurses must be knowledgeable about the legal and custody requirements of the institutionalized client (Lynch, 1999). **Forensic nursing** can be defined as "the application of nursing to law. Forensic nursing addresses the legal, civil, and human rights of victims and perpetrators of violent crime" (Lynch, 1999, p. 28).

Since 1992, facilities accredited by the Joint Commission on Accreditation of Health Care Organizations (JACHO) have had to establish policies and procedures to train staff to identify crime victims and to work with survivors of child, domestic, and other abusive situations. The emergency room nurse is often the first to observe trauma in the clients served. The community health nurse working in the clinical area or in the process of home visiting must be aware of suspected or actual abusive situations such as child abuse and neglect, domestic violence, and elder abuse and be aware of the legal requirements for the nurse who suspects or has actual knowledge of family violence. See Figure 20-11 for standards of forensic nursing practice.

Parish Nursing

Parish nursing is a relatively new adaptation of the older religion-based nursing models of health care delivery. This congregation-based approach to health care delivery was revived during the mid-1980s by Reverend Granger Westberg to better employ the faith and support network of congregations to meet the health promotion and disease prevention needs of members. Grouping individuals by congregation or religious affiliation provides a means of identifying populations by value orientation, spiritual direction, and community and cultural associations. Reverend Westberg considered spiritually motivated registered nurses as ideal practitioners to provide

---

REFLECTIVE THINKING

Treating Clients Incarcerated in a Correctional Facility

How do you feel about providing health care to an individual who has committed murder? A client who has been convicted of sexually abusing a child? A client convicted to selling drugs?

the link between health sciences and human needs (Westberg, 1990). The ANA recognized parish nursing as a specialty in 1997.

Description of Parish Nursing

A parish nurse is a registered nurse who provides holistic nursing services to the members of a faith congregation as a part of the ministerial team. The nurse promotes the health of parishioners and their families by integrating theological, psychological, sociological, and physiological perspectives of health and healing with the beliefs and culture of the congregation (Ryan, 1990). Principles of holistic health and human caring are employed. These nurses work with other practitioners and health care agencies and with the ministerial team to enhance the quality of life for all members of the congregation (Schank, Weis, & Matheus, 1996). Parish nurses do not provide hands-on, invasive treatments; rather, they provide a framework to move individuals and families toward better health states (Solari-Twadell & Westberg, 1991).

Because the parish nurse functions independently and must be proficient in accessing community resources, it is recommended that entry-level parish nurses have baccalaureate degrees and three to five years of nursing experience. Additionally, the parish nurse must be spiritually mature and have the confidence and experience to fulfill multiple roles. Participation in a parish nursing educational program is considered essential for successful practice (Schank et al., 1996). Information about such programs in the United States can be obtained through the National Parish Nurse Resource Center.

The Congregation As a Community Setting

Religious congregations are considered effective settings for addressing the health needs of a population for a variety of reasons. First, religious organizations and congregations are found in virtually every community in every culture. Second, faith congregations have long histories of serving their communities through social activities and educational programming. Third, religions focus

---

FIGURE 20-11 Scope and Standards of Forensic Nursing Practice: Standards of Care

Standard I. Assessment: The forensic nurse shall provide an accurate assessment based on data collected or the physical and/or psychological issues of the client as related to forensic nursing and/or forensic pathology.

Standard II. Diagnosis: The forensic nurse shall analyze the assessment data to determine a diagnosis pertaining to forensic issues in nursing.

Standard III. Outcome Identification: The forensic nurse will identify expected individual outcomes based on the forensic diagnoses of the client.

Standard IV. Planning: The forensic nurse develops a comprehensive plan of action for the forensic client appropriate to forensic interventions to attain expected outcomes.

Standard V. Implementation: The forensic nurse implements a plan of action based on forensic issues derived from assessment data, nursing diagnoses, and medical diagnoses, when applicable, and scientific knowledge.

Standard VI. Evaluation: The forensic nurse evaluates and modifies the plan of action to achieve expected outcomes.

Standard VII. Ethics: The forensic nurse's decisions and actions reflect and are guided by client, personal, and professional ethical considerations.

Standard VIII. Collaboration: The forensic nurse collaborates with the client system, other health ministers, health care providers, and community agencies in promoting client health.

Standard IX. Research: The forensic nurse uses research findings in practice.

Standard X. Resource Utilization: The forensic nurse considers the effectiveness measures of appropriateness, accessibility, acceptability, and affordability of resources in the development and implementation of health promotion programs for clients.

From *Scope and Standards of Forensic Nursing Practice,* by American Nurses' Association, 1997, Washington, DC: American Nurses Publishing. Reprinted with permission of American Nurses Publishing.

✳ DECISION MAKING

Correctional Nursing

All clients, including those who are incarcerated, have basic rights that must be upheld. They have the right to individualized care; the right to act according to their own values, beliefs, and cultural practices; and the right to know about and participate in personal health care decisions (Faris, 1995).

◆ How might you preserve individual cultural practices of incarcerated individuals?

◆ What could you do to encourage clients who may lack fundamental interpersonal and social communication skills to participate in their personal health care decisions?

◆ Examine your personal values regarding the right to live in a safe, free society and your right to be treated with dignity.

◆ How would you assist imprisoned clients to improve their health and quality of life if their values and their behaviors toward others in society were in conflict with your own?

on problems of the human spirit, problems that often are related to the development of and/or response to illness. Fourth, religious communities are rich in traditions of service, support, and volunteerism in humanitarian efforts. Fifth, religions can provide a model of cooperation between science, medicine, and faith communities to better serve populations (Westberg, 1990). Nurses working closely with parishioners can facilitate this desirable cooperation. Finally, faith congregations are one of the few institutions that interact with individuals and families from birth through death (Solari-Twadell & Westberg, 1991). This relationship allows the parish nurse to effectively use a life span approach when managing client and family health needs.

Role Functions of the Parish Nurse

The role of the parish nurse incorporates "whole-person ways of ministering to people who are hurting" (Westberg, 1990, p. 38). Parish nurses can integrate caring principles into practice by focusing on the beliefs and values of the individual and can effectively combine the strengths of humanities and science, medicine and religion, doctors and clergy, and spirituality and health to better client outcomes (Westberg, 1990).

Several functional roles are paramount to the practice of parish nursing. These include counselor, collaborator, case manager, manager, educator, and advocate (ANA, 1998; Miskelly, 1995). As counselor, the parish nurse discusses individual health concerns, refers clients for health interventions, and makes home, hospital, and nursing home visits (Westberg, 1990). In this role, the nurse may empower clients to better express themselves to both health professionals and other members of the ministerial team (Westberg, 1990). As collaborator, the parish nurse serves as a liaison to multiple community resources and services. The nurse may also function as a case manager, assisting clients in navigating the complex health care system (Schank et al., 1996). As manager, the nurse organizes support groups within the congregation and recruits, trains, and supervises volunteers to extend resources throughout the parish community (Holst, 1987; Westberg, 1990). As educator, the parish nurse promotes health through various teaching modalities. The nurse provides seminars, conferences, classes, and other educational activities to raise the health consciousness of the parish community and to "foster an understanding of the relationship between lifestyle, personal habits, attitudes, faith, and well-being" (Holst, 1987, p. 15). The nurse strives to enable individuals to become more active partners in the management of their personal health resources. A nurse working with a congregation can reinforce and validate religion's ancient and contemporary concerns about personal hygiene, health, and well-being (Holst, 1987). As advocate, the nurse attends to the needs of the underserved members of the congregation and fo-

cuses on gaining access to needed services (Schank et al., 1996). See Figure 20-12 for ANA standards of parish nursing.

Models of Parish Nursing Practice

Most parish nursing practice is described as one of four differing models: the institutional/paid model, the congregational/paid model, the institutional/volunteer model, and the congregational/volunteer model. In the institutional/paid model, the nurse is employed by a local hospital, community agency, or long-term care facility that contracts with one or more congregations for nursing services. The employing agency provides the salary, benefits, institutional support, and supervision to the nurse. In the congregational/paid model, the congregation employs the nurse directly, providing salary, benefits, and supervision through the congregation and the ministerial team. In the institutional/volunteer model, the agency and the congregation have a contractual relationship for services and support, and the nurse volunteers his or her time when rendering needed services. The contract, when the services are volunteered, outlines actions and expectations of involved parties to ensure a well-communicated and well-structured program of services. The congregational/volunteer model differs from this in that the contractual relationship is between the nurse-volunteer and the congregation (Solari-Twadell, 1990; ANA, 1998). Models will continue to develop or be modified as the role of the parish nurse is shaped and refined.

Future Development

Parish nursing is a developing specialty area in community health nursing that is making a significant contribution to the advancement of the health of faith communities. Parish nurses enjoy the unique opportunity of discovering the ways that deep spiritual beliefs and religious values affect health by working with individuals and families of faith communities. This increased awareness of beliefs and values in the faith community in turn allows the nurse to effectively support parishioners in improving their health practices. Understanding a faith tradition, using the health ministry, employing the support community, and providing opportunities for service and spiritual growth combine to make parish nursing fascinating, stimulating, and meaningful.

Block Nursing

The early history of public health nursing in London and the United States was the practice of **block nursing.** This practice recognized the need for nursing interventions for vulnerable individuals and families living in the nurse's own neighborhoods. Lillian Wald's immersion in the 19th century to the problems sur-

FIGURE 20-12 Scope and Standards of Parish Nursing Practice

Standard I. Assessment: The parish nurse collects client health data.

Standard II. Diagnoses: The parish nurse analyzes collected data about the client to determine the diagnosis.

Standard III. Outcome Identification: The parish nurse, with the client, identifies expected outcomes specific to the client's desired health outcomes.

Standard IV. Planning: The parish nurse assists the client in developing a plan for health promotion and other interventions that empowers the client to achieve desired health outcomes. The plan identifies the self-care activities to be done by the client, the interdependence with other systems, the interventions to be performed by the parish nurse, and the collaboration with and referral to other health care professionals and providers on the basis of the expected outcomes.

Standard V. Implementation: The parish nurse assists the client in implementing the interventions identified in the health promotion plan.

Standard VI. Evaluation: The parish nurse continually evaluates client responses to interventions in order to determine the progress made toward desired outcomes.

Standards of Professional Performance

Standard I. Quality of Care: The parish nurse systematically participates in evaluation of the quality and effectiveness of his or her parish nursing practice.

Standard II. Performance Appraisal: The parish nurse evaluates his or her own nursing practice in relation to professional standards, relevant others, and regulations.

Standard III. Education: The parish nurse acquires and maintains current knowledge in the nursing practice and health promotion.

Standard IV. Collegiality: The parish nurse contributes to the professional development of peers, colleagues, and other health ministries.

Standard V. Ethics: The parish nurses' decisions and actions reflect and are guided by client, personal, and professional ethical considerations.

Standard VI. Collaboration: The parish nurse collaborates with the client system, other health ministers, health care providers, and community agencies in promoting client health.

Standard VII. Research: The parish nurse uses research findings in practice.

Standard VIII. Resource Utilization: The parish nurse considers the effectiveness measures of appropriateness, accessibility, acceptability, and affordability of resources in the development and implementation of health promotion programs for clients.

From *Scope and Standards of Parish Nursing Practice,* by American Nurses' Association, 1998, Washington, DC: American Nurses Publishing. Reprinted with permission of American Nurses Publishing.

---

rounding lack of care to the vulnerable populations living on the lower east side of New York led to her forming partnerships with those living there to help meet the needs of the people. In todays limited health care delivery system for vulnerable populations, it is necessary to use nurses and well-trained volunteers to provide care to individuals and families living in close proximity to their own home. They can help to provide the social support needed as well as the financial costs. Saint Pauls Minnesota/Ramsey County Health Department developed such a program in the 1980s which today is under the direction of a nonprofit community nursing center. The costs are being met by the Health Care Financing Administration. This program, as well as the NEST Project in San Francisco, California, described in Chapter 15, is an example of block nursing programs which, through the volunteer services of community members, enable seniors to remain safely in their homes (Jamison, 1990; Reinhard et al., 1996; Mendietta, 1999).

FUTURE DIRECTIONS

The future continues to hold exciting and challenging opportunities for community health nursing. The proposed health care reforms of the 1990s are for the most part unrealized, and the unmet health and illness needs of the population remain. The high-cost, complex, and fragmented U.S. health services remain largely unchanged. The professional nurse for this new millennium must continue to serve the traditionally direct clinical concerns of individuals. To be an effective and active partner in promoting health care, the professional nurse must become a committed partner in structuring the political agendas and appropriated strategies that will lead to implementation of policies that will promote health at the community level (Shi & Singh, 1998; Williams, 2000). Wieck (2000) asks the question of where is nursing going as we enter into this new millennium. She sees hospitals that provide mostly care in intensive care units supported largely by technologies and computers. She affirms that most of

RESEARCH FOCUS

Community Assessment: A Church Community and the Parish Nurse

Study Problem/Purpose

The purpose of this study was to conduct a community assessment for the church and newly employed parish nurse. The goals of the community assessment were to determine the health status of parishioners, identify their perceived health needs and perceived barriers to meeting those needs, and assist the church and parish nurse in developing a health program for their faith community.

Methods

A qualitative and quantitative research design was used. Four hundred and twenty-one questionnaires were completed, and six focus groups were held to validate the data. The focus groups were made up of 4–17 members representing diverse groups in the community.

Findings

The identified health needs of this faith community are similar to the goals of *Healthy people 2000* [U.S. Department of Health and Human Services (USDHHS), 1993]. The community perceived themselves to be in good physical health. The two major concerns expressed surrounded the high-risk behaviors of the adolescents and lack of support services for the elderly. The focus group discussions revealed their willingness to support the efforts of a parish nurse and also demonstrated the importance of the spiritual dimension and their belief in the power of prayer in health and well-being.

Implications

These findings affirm the importance of assessing a community as a first step in planning a health program. Each community is unique and will demonstrate the health problems and risk factors and perceived needs of its members. The parish nurse is able to determine goals and objectives and clarify the types of programs and interventions needed.

Source: Swinney, J., Anson-Wonkka, C., Maki, E., & Corneau, J. (2001). Community assessment. A church community and the parish nurse. Public Health Nursing, 18(1), 40–44.

---

health care will be provided and utilized in communities. Wieck indicates that todays criticism for professional nursing is related to the lack of vision and that nursing has not defined where it wants to be in 10–15 years from now. We are too busy just putting out fires day by day. As she looks at a future for professional nursing, Wieck posits that, by 2015, due to nurse-led initiatives:

- Persons will be in unusually good health.
- Every community will have a nursing center with residents being assigned to an advanced-practice nurse.
- Hospitals will be under the direction of critical care advanced-practice nurses who practice in consultation with physicians, pharmacists, and chaplains to manage care.
- Care will be given by nurses with advanced education in computer analysis and therapeutic reasoning.
- Hospice and home health will be provided by professional nurses whose education is based on critical thinking and problem solving.

- Home health and hospice and palliative care nurses will move in or out of the home under the direction of the advanced-practice nurse in the community-based nursing center.
- Nursing will be a university-based program with most nurses being educated at the master's level as advanced-practice nurses.

Wieck's challenges for professional nursing are congruent with those addressed in *Public Health Nursing: A Partner for Healthy Populations* (Association of State and Territorial Directors of Nursing, 2000). Community health nurses need to be educationally prepared at the baccalaureate level with a foundation in public health nursing. This educational preparation enables them to develop competency in the three core functions identified by the Institute of Medicine report on *The Future of Public Health* (IOM, 1998). These core competencies (Assessment, Policy Development, and Assurance) are identified as part of the *Standards of Practice for Public Health Nurses* and are essential skills for nurses working in community-based settings such as correctional institutions, schools, and occupational health. Community-based nursing practice and settings are influenced by

Perspectives...

INSIGHTS OF A COMMUNITY HEALTH NURSING PROFESSOR

Nurses who practice in community settings must have a different skill set from nurses who practice in structured settings such as hospitals or skilled nursing facilities. Community health nurses have to be more independent, more creative, and able to apply knowledge from a broad range of disciplines. We must be flexible to work effectively with a wide variety of clients and staff from other disciplines. We must have excellent communication skills and a sound theoretical grounding in systems theory, family theory, and epidemiology. In addition to a broad generalist knowledge in nursing, I like to focus on three main themes—tolerance of ambiguity, management of complexity, and appreciation of context—to guide the thinking of nursing students in developing practice skills appropriate for community health nursing.

I tell students at the beginning of my rotation that one of the most important attributes of a community health nurse is a tolerance of ambiguity. When we enter the world controlled by the client, as in a home visit, we frequently enter uncharted territory. My major challenge, in teaching community health to BSN students, has been to convince students to "unlearn" the task orientation so carefully cultivated in the hospital settings, while retaining the skill sets needed to provide care to clients. Nursing students frequently measure "nursing worth" by the number of concrete psychomotor skills, such as injection and IV insertion, that they have mastered and may not consider therapeutic communication, for example, as a skill to be mastered. They are anxious to "do to" rather than "be with." They want to see patients, rather than clients. They are used to specific direction, in the form of procedures, policies, and definite time schedules for the completion of tasks. Lacking the protocols that closely define nursing activities in the hospital setting, they frequently assume that nothing important is being offered in this particular clinical rotation. They are uncomfortable with ambiguity and unable to operate independently without "permission." It is my responsibility to teach students how to function in a world where the details may not be neatly compiled in a patient record, complete with medical diagnosis and treatment plans. They must develop a tolerance for ambiguity.

The complexity of clinical decisions made with clients and vulnerable populations in unstructured environments requires a level of clinical decision making different from that of the hospital or clinic nurse. Nursing practice has dependent functions and independent functions. Community health nurses frequently provide those independent nursing functions that are not dependent on physician's orders. They must decide which nursing interventions are most appropriate, based on an assessment of the client, family, environment, and availability of resources. Many of my clinical teaching strategies revolve around managing the tension between the challenge and the frustration for a student with novice skills who is faced with complex situations. Rarely will the community health nursing student work with clients in need of a simple intervention. Most of our clients have multiple needs and lack resources to meet those needs. If students feel they are unable to "make a difference" for those clients, they may lose motivation in the course. In order to prepare students for these situations, I use case studies and small-group work to critically examine problems in a wide variety of clients and situations. I can then guide students through simulated problem-solving scenarios based on the realities that they will encounter in the field.

The context of hospital nursing practice can easily become that of community health nursing practice. Personnel, clients, and visitors operate within the context of the hospital. Consequently, we begin to view our interactions with clients and family through a unidimensional lens. This helps the hospital nurse to become "more efficient" and increases productivity in accomplishing hospital tasks. Nursing in the community cannot be unidimensional. We must understand the context within which the particular client and family relate to each other and to the larger community. An ability to appreciate contextual variations and design nursing interventions accordingly is a skill necessary in expert community health practice.

Understanding tolerance of ambiguity, management of complexity, and appreciation of context can bring a depth and richness to nursing practice in the community. Nurses, whether they are novice or expert, who can think in multidimensional ways using these concepts are needed in community-based settings.

—Marjorie Barter, EdD, RN

Associate Professor, University of San Francisco

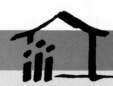

COMMUNITY NURSING VIEW

You have been the school nurse at Bjorn High School for the last two years. The students are mainly children of the local wheat farmers in this Midwestern area. There is a significant increase in the number of pregnant adolescents. Last year over 30% of the graduating senior girls were pregnant and/or mothers of young babies. The faculty has asked that you do "something about this problem." The parents have not expressed any concerns to you about this. The students have been asking you for information on birth control and sexually transmitted infections. You passed their request to the principal and brought it to the attention of the faculty. No plan of action has been forthcoming.

Nursing Considerations

Assessment

♦ What data might the school nurse collect to bring to the parents, students, faculty, and school administration?

♦ How might the school nurse assess the students' knowledge regarding birth control and sexually transmitted infections?

Diagnosis

♦ What initial diagnoses might be formulated?

Outcome Identification:

♦ What initial outcomes would be formulated specific to the data collection?

♦ What outcomes would be identified to measure the students' knowledge regarding birth control and sexually transmitted infections.

Planning/Interventions

♦ Who should the nurse include in the data-gathering process?

♦ What/who should be included in identifying student knowledge?

♦ Who would be the crucial players in the identification and development of the educational interventions?

Evaluation

♦ How would you evaluate the outcome of the data collection?

♦ What would you include in the evaluation of the educational interventions?

---

the proactive role nurses are willing to take. Today's professional nurses are capable of assuming leadership roles in the promotion of programs that optimize health of the aggregate communities which they serve.

KEY CONCEPTS

♦ The public health nurse promotes and protects the health of populations, incorporating knowledge from nursing and the social and public health sciences. The public health nurse uses an interdisciplinary approach associated with the core public health functions of assessment, assurance, and policy development.

♦ The nurse employed in the home health specialty creates a bridge between the acute-care institution and community practice. The home health nurse incorporates a multidisciplinary approach to provide skilled interventions to the client and family. When delivering health services in the home environment, the nurse considers the family as the basic unit of care.

♦ The hospice and palliative care nurse delivers holistic and personal palliative nursing interventions to dying clients and their families. The nurse provides the client and family with skilled interventions, counseling, and emotional support and is considered the cornerstone of hospice services.

♦ The school nurse functions as a total health resource for the students, staff, families, and community with whom he or she interacts. The nurse's overriding objective is to promote optimal health in the school population and, in turn, support the educational process.

♦ The occupational/environmental health nurse safeguards the safety and health of workers through the implementation of interventions derived from numerous other disciplines. The nurse synthesizes principles from these multiple disciplines and blends them with objectives outlined by business and industry to promote a healthy and productive work force.

♦ The nurse practicing in a correctional facility functions as health advocate for incarcerated clients. The nurse ensures that clients have access to quality health services in an atmosphere of dignity and individual worth.

◆ Parish nursing focuses on promoting the health of individuals and families within the context of their values, beliefs, and practices of their faith communities.

◆ The forensic nurse has an important role in investigations aimed at combating crime and violence.

◆ The block nursing model provides a venue in which vulnerable populations and families living within the nurse's own neighborhood obtain needed social support and nursing services.

◆ Standards of community health practice have been outlined by the ANA. These standards have been modified by professional nursing organizations

such as AAOHN and NASN for application to specific community-based nursing specialties. The standards address elements essential to the delivery of quality interventions.

RESOURCES

American Association of Occupational Health Nurses, Inc.: http://aaohn.org
American Nurses Association: http://www.ana.org
American Nurses Foundation: http://www.nursingworld.org/anf
Hospice and Palliative Nurses Association: http://www.hpna.org
International Association of Forensic Nurses: http://www.forensicnurse.org
National Association of School Nurses: http://www.nasn.org
National Mental Health Association: http://www.nmha.org

Unit

V

CARING FOR INDIVIDUALS AND FAMILIES IN THE COMMUNITY

The focus of Unit V is on those processes that are important to caring for individuals and families in the community, including the home visit, the developmental issues needed to be considered, and the understanding of family dynamics.

IN THIS UNIT

Chapter

21

THE HOME VISIT

Janice E. Hitchcock, RN, DNSc

This is the true nature of home—it is the place of Peace; the shelter, not only from all injury, but from all terror, doubt, and division.

—*Ruskin, 1865, p. 606*

COMPETENCIES

Upon completion of this chapter, the reader should be able to:

- Recount advantages and disadvantages of the home visit.
- Describe the process and issues of the home visit.
- Relate the dimensions of assessment in the home setting.
- Explain the use of nurse-client contracting to keep the nursing process goal directed and focused.
- Cite the most common interventions used when providing home care to families.
- Describe telehome health care.
- Explain the community health nurses's focus on health promotion and prevention when working with families in the home.
- Detail issues of termination of the nurse-client relationship.

KEY TERMS

caregiver	partnership
contacting phase	telehome health
contract	termination phase
entry phase	
family strengths	
Outcome and Assessment Information Set (OASIS)	

Nurses make health care visits to the home for many reasons. Public health nurses "are in a unique position because they are the professional group that has the opportunity to visit families in their own homes to detect health concerns and prevent problems before they become serious" (Kristjanson & Chalmers, 1999 p. 365). Home health care providers focus primarily on care of the sick and, in the case of hospice nursing, the dying. Although nurses who visit families in the home sometimes have different objectives, the process of the home visit remains essentially the same.

THE HOME VISIT

The goal of home health—to improve health and the quality of life—has a long history (Hanks & Smith, 1999). Specific activities depend on the needs of the family and on the agency for which the nurse works. Agencies from which nurses make home visits include visiting nurse associations, hospice, public health departments, home health agencies, and school districts. Many hospitals also have home care programs that employ community health nurses to provide follow-up for the hospital's clients.

Advantages

The advantages of home visits over providing care to clients in an agency setting are multiple. When family members can be cared for at home, hospital stays are shortened and overall costs to the family are reduced. From the client's point of view, the client has greater control over the interaction. The nurse is in the client's home and must adhere both to the client's wishes regarding interactions and to the goals of the visit. In many families, for instance, the offer of food or drink to a visitor is a ritual that conveys welcome. A caring way to respond in such a situation is suggested by Wright and Leahey (2000), who recommend a statement such as "Thanks, but maybe we could work first and then have coffee afterward" (p. 218). In this way, work and social boundaries are differentiated without offending the family's sense of hospitality.

Families tend to be more comfortable and, therefore, less anxious in their home environments; thus, they are also more receptive to teaching. Their motivation to learn necessary skills is enhanced because, at home, they have direct experience in the daily management of their health problems. They have identified areas in which they lack knowledge and are inspired to learn how to more effectively care for themselves. Their interest in participating in the health care needs of family members is also increased.

The nurse is able to observe the interplay of factors that influence the client's health status as the process is happening. Specifically, the nurse has more access to infants, children, and other members of family life such as pets, boarders, roommates, and grandparents. The family's social environment and rituals can also be observed (Wright & Leahey, 2000). Through interactions with the family, the nurse comes to understand potential as well as actual health problems and is therefore able to intervene before problems escalate into serious health concerns. The nurse can identify environmental resources and hazards that affect the client's health. Because contact with the family usually occurs over a longer time period than that associated with hospital care, the nurse also has an opportunity to assess the client in activities of daily living and to note health changes. While the mandate of the home health nurse is providing care to the ill client rather than to the family as a whole, the broader family assessment is also important because it affects the health of the individual client.

Disadvantages

Although home visiting provides valuable insights into families and offers interventions unavailable in the hospital, there are disadvantages to be considered. Nurses

TABLE 21-1 Advantages and Disadvantages of Home Visiting

ADVANTAGES	DISADVANTAGES
Costs less than hospitalization.	Nurse's value system and style of practice may not be compatible with providing services in the home.
Affords client greater control over interaction.	More time consuming than care provided in a hospital or clinic setting.
Family more amenable to health education.	No easy access to emergency equipment or consultation.
Nurse can observe factors that influence family health.	Personal safety concerns.
Nurse can observe family interactions.	Cannot work with groups.
Allows for early intervention.	Distractions more difficult to control.
Allows for identification of environmental resources and hazards.	Family resents intrusion into home and/or prefers health care setting.
Allows for assessment of family over longer period of time than is possible during hospitalization.	Potential for caregiver exhaustion.
Facilitates family participation in health care.	
Facilitates family focus and individualized care.	

must weigh whether their value systems and styles of practice are compatible with providing nursing services in the home setting. Nurses with a strong need to control a situation or to be perceived as an authority would have difficulty with ever-changing family circumstances and different lifestyles. Kristjanson and Chalmers (1999) suggest several questions that nurses can ask themselves regarding these issues: "Do [I] hold on to power and control? Do [I] like to be the authority and the expert? Can [I] work in a non-judgmental way with different families?" (p. 369).

Visiting a client at home takes more time than does an appointment in the hospital or clinic setting. Home visiting also negates working with groups of people having similar concerns. Home visiting assumes a greater likelihood that the interview will be interrupted by things such as children needing attention or a visiting neighbor. The home setting offers no immediate access to emergency equipment or to consultation with other disciplines as is available in a medical setting. Furthermore, the client's home may be situated in a neighborhood that is known to be dangerous. In addition to these aforementioned disadvantages, the family caregiver may consider home care a drawback, as well. Providing care to a family member in the home can be exhausting for the **caregiver.** In the family, the caregiver is usually a spouse, parent, or child. It is thus important to assess caregiver needs and arrange for support as needed. (See Chapter 24 for further discussion of caregiver issues.)

Some clients resent the intrusion of the health worker into their homes and prefer the more formal climate of the health care setting. In appropriate situations, however, the home visit offers a dimension of health care that can be provided in no other setting. See Table 21-1 for a summary of advantages and disadvantages of the home visit.

REFLECTIVE THINKING

Advantages and Disadvantages of Home Visiting

Consider your own experiences and expectations of home visiting.

- Do you agree with Table 21-1 regarding the advantages and disadvantages of home visiting?
- For you, do the advantages outweigh the disadvantages, do the disadvantages outweigh the advantages, or do you think they are evenly balanced? Why?

HOME VISIT CONSIDERATIONS

Community health nursing is guided by the nursing process just as is nursing care of individuals. Most family nursing involves working with both individuals in the family and the family as a whole: Individual members may have specific health problems and needs that must be addressed, these problems may have an impact on the family, and the family may have a specific impact on the individual and his or her health. Family decisions regarding the

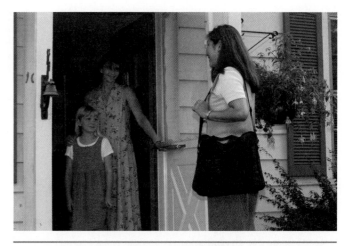

Being perceived with apprehension by the family is commonplace for the nurse conducting an initial home visit. The effective use of social skills to convey caring can ease the family's apprehension.

needs of an ill family member play a large part in the progression of treatment and recovery.

Phases of the Home Visit

Byrd (1995a,b, 1998) developed the concept of home visiting as a process having three phases. The first phase, the **contacting phase,** encompasses the antecedent event (when the nurse becomes aware of an individual or family who is identified as desiring or needing a visit) and the going-to-see phase (when the nurse journeys to the home and gains information about the neighborhood and the family's place in it). The context of the antecedent event may be a voluntary or required request for service because of illness or the identification of a risk for health problems. The nursing strategies for promoting trust ease movement into the second phase, the **entry phase,** which moves from the going-to-see phase to the seeing phase. During this phase the nurse observes and interacts with the family, learning about them and their life situation and planning interventions with their input. These experiences facilitate the **termination phase,** which encompasses the telling phase. The telling phase emphasizes referral and documentation of the situation. During this phase, interventions are evaluated and plans made with the family for future visits. Although most visits provide interventions that support family life, Byrd (1995a) cautions that "the visit may have had nega-

tive consequences such as stigmatizing the family as neglectful or poor" (p. 87). It is important that the nurse consider strategies to minimize these negative outcomes, for instance, by reinforcing **family strengths** (those characteristics that allow a family to manage its life successfully). See Chapter 24 for a more detailed discussion of family strengths.

The first contact with the family is usually via telephone to arrange a time for the home visit. On this initial call, the nurse introduces herself, identifies the purpose of the visit and the agency to which the referral has been made, confirms the client's address, and requests permission to make a home visit at a mutually acceptable time. If the client does not have a telephone, it may be necessary to make an unscheduled visit. After the nurse has met with the family, a neighbor may be identified who can take calls for future contacts. If the family is not home, the nurse should leave a card providing the nurse's name, telephone number, and agency and either asking the client to call to schedule an appointment or indicating a time when the nurse will return. There will be times when the family is consistently unavailable or has moved. Zerwekh (1992) asserts that knowing ways to locate disappearing families is a skill that is foundational to all other work with families in the home: "Effective locating requires community networking, persistence, an extensive map collection, the courage to knock on many doors, and the wisdom to 'sniff out violence' and back away as needed from a threatening household or neighborhood" (Zerwekh, 1997, p. 26). A reasonable effort should be made to effect a successful contact.

In many cases, a health provider, rather than the client, seeks the nurse's services. Under such circumstances, the nurse particularly needs effective social skills

FIGURE 21-1 Visitor Safety Issues

Appearance and Communication

1. Wear a name badge and/or uniform that clearly declares your professional affiliation.

2. Be sure that agency staff know your visiting schedule, including the name, the date, and the time of the visit and your expected return.

3. Let clients know in advance the approximate time of your visit. If you need further directions, ask the client for them rather than stopping to ask someone on the way. If possible, call clients just before the home visit so they can watch for you and come out to greet you.

4. Walk slowly around animals so that you do not frighten them. Ask clients to secure menacing pets before the visit. Never run away from a dog.

5. Do not carry a purse. Before leaving for the visit, lock your purse in the trunk of your car or cover it with a blanket. Keep change for a phone in a shoe or pocket.

6. Use a mobile car phone; however, do not leave it in the car during a visit.

7. If you enter the residence during a domestic dispute, leave and call to make another appointment.

When Traveling By Car

1. Be sure your car is in good working order and has enough gas to get you back to your agency.

2. Provide for the unexpected in winter by keeping a blanket in the car; in the summer, keep a thermos of cool water. It is also prudent to keep a nonperishable snack in the glove compartment.

3. If you have car trouble, do not accept rides from strangers. Turn on emergency flashers and wait for the police, or call for help if you have a mobile car phone.

4. Keep your car locked when parked or driving. If possible, keep windows closed.

5. Stay in your car or leave the area if confronted with a situation that does not feel right.

6. Park in full view of the client's residence. Avoid parking in alleys or deserted side streets. Put a sign in your car that identifies your agency.

7. If safe parking is a question, it may be necessary for your agency to hire a driver to take you to and from the client's residence.

On Foot

1. Keep one arm free and have nursing bag and equipment ready when exiting from the car.

2. Walk directly to the client's residence in a professional, businesslike manner.

3. When passing a group of strangers, cross to the other side of the street, if appropriate.

4. When leaving the client's residence, carry car keys in your hand, holding the pointed ends between your fingers. Doing so renders the keys an effective weapon.

During Visits

1. Use common walkways in buildings; avoid isolated stairs.

2. Always knock on the door before entering a client's residence.

3. If relatives or neighbors become a safety problem, make joint visits, arrange for escort services, schedule visits when they are gone, or close the case.

4. Do not enter a home if firearms are visible; contact supervisor.

5. Do not make a visit if someone at home is on drugs or is abusive.

Other Tips for Safety
Defense Techniques

1. Scream; yell "FIRE!"

2. Kick shins, instep, or groin.

3. Bite, scratch.

4. Blow a whistle attached to your key ring.

5. Use chemical spray.

6. Use your nursing bag as a defense weapon.

7. Arrange a "check-out" phone call.

Nursing Considerations

1. Visit neighborhoods of questionable safety in the morning.

2. Neighborhoods that are extremely unsafe may be ones that cannot be served.

3. In the event of robbery, never resist.

4. Notify your agency for further instructions in the event of any car trouble, auto accident, or other incident when personal safety is in question.

5. Document:

   a. Any threat to personal safety while on duty.

   b. Any animal or human bites (give paperwork to infection control manager).

6. Seek medical attention as needed.

7. Consult with agency manager about notifying appropriate public officials of personal safety violations.

Adapted from "Home Visit Safety," by R. Rice, 1998, *Home Healthcare Nurse, 16,* pp. 241–242, and *Manual of Home Health Nursing Procedures* (pp. 303–304) by R. Rice, 1995, St. Louis: Mosby Yearbook.

to convey caring for the family and to clarify the purpose of the visit with the family. It is important to listen to the family's concerns and to work with them. An authoritative approach is likely to result in a passive or rejecting response (Kristjanson & Chalmers, 1999). Zerwekh (1997) notes that trying to take over in the home is a prescription for alienation and disconnection.

Prior to a subsequent visit, it is important to call and reconfirm the appointment. Families are likely to be distracted by other concerns and may therefore forget a scheduled visit. A brief call will remind them of the nurse's visit and provide the opportunity for the nurse to assess the current status of the client. It is important to remember that priorities and clients' needs change (Monks, 2000).

Safety

When making home visits, the nurse must consider her own safety. Although most home visits do not present a safety risk, some do. There has been an increase in community and interpersonal violence (Fazzone, Barloon, McConnell, & Chitty, 2000). Areas of particular concern are those where gangs are known to exist or those having a high proportion of drug users. Review Figure 21-1 for guidelines to maximize the personal safety of health care professionals working in the community and home settings. (See the accompanying Research Focus for what constitutes unsafe conditions in or near client's home and conditions that impact personal safety of staff.)

Fostering Positive Client Response

When preparing for a subsequent visit, review plans from the previous visit and establish priorities with regard to the problems or issues to be addressed. In consultation with the family, develop objectives at primary, secondary, and tertiary prevention levels and relative to the client's readiness to deal with the issues at hand. Detecting the client's readiness to change is an important competency. Zerwekh (1997) cites three dimensions of timing interventions to foster a positive client response. The first is detecting the right time to initiate an approach: for instance, recognizing that a client needs to tell his or her story before considering possible solutions. The second dimension is the persistence of the nurse in visiting so that she or he will be there when the client is ready. If visits are not consistent, the client has no opportunity to develop enough trust to be willing to discuss true concerns. The third dimension is timing interventions on the basis of future problems and possibilities. This aspect of timing anticipates family needs, such as changes in developmental stages, and allows the nurse to discuss these

expected changes with the family so that they will be prepared for the changes when they occur.

In consultation with the family, the nurse plans both interventions related to the nursing diagnoses and ways to evaluate the outcome of the interventions. It is important to remember that planned assessments and interventions may have to be postponed because of other family needs that take priority during a particular visit (Byrd, 1995a). Because there is usually a specific health problem to be addressed, home care interventions may be prescriptive. In all cases, however, the best results will occur when the family is fully involved in the care and is ready to assist as needed.

Two additional areas that need emphasis have to do with how one conducts oneself in the home and what to do if offered food or gifts. It is important to remember that the nurse is a guest in the home and must treat the client with respect. Be sure to ask permission for any activity. For instance, to examine a medicine cabinet in order to monitor medications, ask the client for permission to do so and explain the reason for doing it. In general, good communication skills provide a framework for working effectively in the home. See Chapter 10 for more information regarding interpersonal communication.

A client may invite the nurse to have coffee and/or other food. In many families, food is used as a way to connect to others. It is important to determine if not accepting a beverage or some food will increase or decrease family acceptance and act accordingly. Clients from some ethnic groups may interpret the decline of the offer for a beverage or food as a rejection.

Some clients will offer gifts or money, especially at termination of visits. While accepting money is never appropriate, a small gift that cements the end of the relationship is acceptable. Be sure to thank the client, acknowledging your appreciation of the gift and confirming that it is a symbol of the end of the relationship. If a client tries to give you something frequently, the best approach is to decline and reaffirm that the relationship is one in which you are there to facilitate the client's progress and is assured without such gifts. It is important to be sure the client knows that gifts are not necessary to assure quality service.

The Nursing Bag

When making a home visit, the nurse comes equipped with a nursing bag. This bag usually contains equipment for basic assessment (sphygmomanometer, stethoscope, thermometer, etc.), medical asepsis (disinfectant, soap, toilettes, etc.), and waste disposal (plastic bags). During the home visit, standard precautions must be observed. Although the principles are the same in any situation,

RESEARCH FOCUS

Personal Safety, Violence, and Home Health

Study Problem/Purpose

This is a qualitative study to investigate anew the personal perception issues related to home health staff safety in a large Midwestern region and its surrounding areas and to address gaps in the existing literature. Research goals were as follows:

1. Serve as a source for understanding the personal safety risk issues facing home care staff in a large Midwestern region and its surrounding areas.
2. Provide an understanding of how perceived threats to personal safety may impact patient care and patient outcomes.
3. Identify strategies for increasing the personal safety of direct care staff.
4. Identify organizational, educational, and procedural issues that impede or enhance staff safety.

Methods

A triangulated qualitative design was used that included focus groups, in-depth individual interviews, critical event narratives, and a participant self-report form. Research questions focused on personal safety risks perceived by staff and administrators, the context and impact of risks on the delivery of home care and patient outcomes, and strategies that decrease safety risks. Risk to personal safety was defined as any perceived or actual threat of loss or injury to a person's physical and/or emotional well-being or possessions.

A purposive sampling was used: 61 participants of whom 56 were women and 5 were men, representing administrators and a mix of direct care staff roles from a total of 13 home health agencies.

Findings

Seven major themes emerged:

1. *Unsafe conditions:* situations that threaten the personal safety of staff within the patient's home or neighborhood in urban, suburban, and rural areas. These situations included:
   - In or near patient's home:
     - (a) Men or adolescents loitering around the patient's home or street
     - (b) A known felon living in the patient's home
     - (c) Verbal, physical, and sexual aggression by patient or by others in the home or community

   - (d) Gangs and gang activity
   - (e) Police raids and drug busts
   - (f) Caught in the crossfire of gunfights
   - (g) Loaded weapons
   - (h) Drive-by shootings
   - (i) Broken glass or debris
   - (j) No phones
   - (k) Poor lighting
   - (l) Poor ventilation
   - (m) "Run-down" homes and broken elevators
   - (n) Rats and hostile dogs
   - Factors pertaining to rural areas:
     - (a) Traveling at night on slick or muddy roads
     - (b) Traveling in remote or isolated areas
     - (c) Loaded weapons in most homes
     - (d) Increase of garage or home-based methamphetamine laboratories
     - (e) Deteriorated homes
     - (f) Increase in domestic violence
2. *Organizational and administrative factors impacting staff safety:*
   - Absence or inaccessibility or written policies and procedures regarding safety
   - Safety policies and procedures not enforced
   - Safety policies and procedures not relevant to home care issues
   - Staff and administrator unfamiliarity with community, neighborhood, and patients
   - Lack or delay of security assistance
   - Cellular phones not provided by agencies for all direct care staff
   - Absence of "call-in" or "check-in" systems
   - Lack or minimal administrative support
   - Staff delay or failure in reporting incidents or verbal, physical, or sexual aggression
   - Staff not always made aware of violent history of patient
3. *Ethical issues:* whether or not to provide care to certain patients in certain areas of the inner city, how much care they should provide, and for how long and whether or not to report observed drug dealing.
4. *Protective factors that kept staff safe:* includes characteristics such as self-confidence, self-reliance, self-motivation, flexibility, "being comfortable with the unknown," and self-assurance about their personal judgment.

(continues)

RESEARCH FOCUS (continued)

5. *Gender, race, age, and experience:*
   - Increased perceived risk in young attractive female staff
   - Male staff expected to take "the most difficult cases" with serious behavior problems
   - Males perceived they got less information about potentially dangerous situations in or near a patient's home than their female partners
   - Male providers not taken seriously by administrators when sexually harassed
   - More threatening for staff of a particular race to go into an area where the majority of people were of a different race
   - Concerns that more experienced staff who feel comfortable become complacent regarding personal safety, which could increase the risk
   - Increased threat of risk when sent to a neighborhood that was not regularly assigned

6. *Education and training:* perceived training about personal safety on the job to not meet their needs. They agreed it was important to have training. Topics of interest included how to handle angry patients, how to avoid power struggles, and how to recognize and protect self against gang and gang activity.

7. *Potential impact on patient care and patient outcomes:* Staff's fears for their personal safety negatively impact patient care to some degree—shorten visits, limit patient education, adjust treatment plans and visit times in response to safety concerns, terminating care.

Implications

All home health agencies need to have ongoing education and training programs specific to home health situations and made available to professional and nonprofessional staff. Comprehensive personal safety policies and procedures relevant to home health care must be developed, implemented, and reviewed with staff several times a year. They must be assessable to all staff, enforced, and evaluated for clinical and cost effectiveness.

Home health agencies need to provide swift and ongoing support critical for a person's recovery from a traumatic or threatening event as well as to provide all level administrators with the essential knowledge, skills, organizational structure, and process to support and guide staff through frightening experiences in the field. Staff must communicate to administrators any incident of threat or harm.

Home health agencies should standardize and centralize a systematic process for collecting and analyzing data regarding all threats to personal safety. They should also have access to information about how threats to staff safety might compromise patient care, especially to the poor, the most vulnerable, and the most in need.

Source: Fazzone, P. A., Barloon, L. F., McGonnell, S. J., & Chitty, J. A. (2000). Personal safety, violence, and home health. Public Health Nursing, 17, 43–52.

✳ DECISION MAKING

Community Awareness

You have been visiting Ms. Alverez for two months. Ms. Alverez has recently returned from the hospital following a stroke that has left her with right-sided weakness. You have helped her to safety-proof her home and adjust to her altered physical condition. When you arrive on your last visit, she has the table set for lunch for the two of you.

◆ How do you respond to her invitation. If you have time to stay? If you do not have time to stay?

◆ What would you do if she offers you a small amount of money as a "tip" to express her appreciation to you for all you have done for her.

some special considerations apply when practicing standard precautions in the home environment. Figure 21-2 outlines information about the proper maintenance of the nursing bag, and Figure 21-3 provides information about maintaining standard precautions in the home.

Health Care Team

The community health nurse works as part of a team of health care providers. The family may have a social worker, rehabilitation therapist (e.g., a physical or speech therapist), or a home health nurse or aide. The nurse must participate in the coordination of health care provided by health personnel. This coordination often includes taking steps to resolve "divergent opinions that occur when different disciplines approach common problems" (Zerwekh, 1991, p. 216). At the same time, the nurse works alone in the home and,

FIGURE 21-2   Bag Technique

1. Maintain an area of the nursing bag as a clean area—reserve for equipment that is directly used on the client. Never enter clean portion of bag without washing hands. Therefore, carry handwashing materials and barriers in another part of the bag.

2. Set the nursing bag on top of fresh newspapers when transporting it in the car.

3. In the client's residence, spread a plastic barrier over cleanest or most convenient work area removed from children and animals. Plastic grocery bags or plastic wastebasket liners make good barriers. Place the bag on the plastic barrier.

4. Never place the bag on the floor; it is considered the dirtiest area.

5. Always carry paper towels and antibacterial liquid soap as well as waterless hand-cleansing solution.

6. Take handwashing items to sink area. Use one paper towel on which to place other items. Use a second and a third towel for washing and drying hands before and after care has been given.

7. After drying hands, use the paper towel to turn the faucet off.

8. Waterless hand-cleansing solution can be used as a substitute for soap and water when there is no water or it is inconvenient to go to the sink.

9. Open nursing bag again and remove items necessary for the visit. If additional equipment or supplies are needed from the bag during the home visit, the handwashing procedure must be repeated.

10. Disinfect all nondisposable equipment that is used to provide care from one client to another with 70% alcohol used with sprayer before returning to the bag. Contaminated equipment or equipment that cannot be cleaned may be transported to the agency in a sealed plastic bag for disinfection. Never place used needles or dirty equipment or dressings in the nursing bag.

11. Do not expose the bag to extreme temperatures or leave it in the car for long periods. Keep in a secure area. If stored in the car, keep it locked in the trunk. If at home, keep it closed and out of the hands of other family members.

12. Clean, disinfect, and restock the nursing bag weekly.

Adapted from *Pocket Guide to Home Health Care,* by K. M. Monks, 2000, Philadelphia: W. B. Saunders, and "Principles of Universal Precautions/Body Substance Isolation," by R. Rice, 1993, *Home Health Nurse, 11*(4), pp. 55–59. Copyright 1993 by Lippincott-Raven Publishers.

FIGURE 21-3   Use of Standard Precautions in the Home Environment

Items to Carry with You

- Sterile (for procedures that require sterile technique), nonsterile (for procedures that may expose staff to the client's blood or other body substances), and utility gloves (to clean up equipment, the work area, or spills)

- One disinfectant that is tuberculocidal and another disinfectant that is effective against human immunodeficiency virus (HIV)

- Product requested by the Environmental Protection Agency with an accepted label that is effective against hepatitis B

- A solution of 5.25% sodium hypochlorite (household bleach) diluted with water to 1:10 (mix fresh daily to maintain effectiveness)

- Masks

- Cardiopulmonary resuscitation (CPR) masks

- Goggles

- Moisture-proof aprons/gowns

- Leak-proof specimen containers

- Sharps containers

- Liquid soap, soap toilettes, dry hand disinfectants (alcohol based)

- Extra clothing stocked in the car in a water-resistant bag

Handwashing

- Wash before and after client contact.

- Wash during client contact if soiled.

- Wash with soap and water immediately after removing gloves (may substitute antiseptic hand cleaner toilettes or other handwashing without water products but wash hands with soap and water as soon as possible).

Use of Gloves

- Wear before contact with nonintact skin, blood, and body substances.

- Change after each procedure.

- After each use, dispose of sterile and nonsterile latex gloves in a leak-resistant waste receptacle such as a plastic trash bag.

- Disinfect and reuse utility gloves. Dispose of and replace when signs of deterioration are apparent.

(continues)

FIGURE 21-3   Use of Standard Precautions in the Home Environment (continued)

Use of Other Protective Equipment As Needed

- Wear disposable gowns or aprons when there is a reasonable expectation of contamination by blood or other body substances. After use, remove and dispose of in a plastic trash bag in the client's residence.

- Wear a face mask whenever there is a reasonable expectation of aerosolization or splattering of blood or other body substances. After use, remove and dispose of in a plastic trash bag in client's residence.

- Wear a face mask and instruct family members to each wear one when caring for a client who needs respiratory isolation. Paste a homemade "STOP" sign outside the client's room to remind family to put on the mask.

- Wear goggles or safety glasses with side shields when there is a reasonable expectation of aerosolization or splattering of blood or other body substances near the nurses's eyes. Clean with soap and water after each use. Discard in plastic trash bag if cracked or heavily contaminated.

- Use disposable CPR masks if required to provide artificial mouth-to-mouth or mouth-to-stoma ventilation.

Sharp Objects and Needles

- Place in a puncture-proof disposable container. A needle must not be bent, sheared, replaced in the sheath or guard, or removed from the syringe after use. Avoid capping needles unless through the use of a mechanical device or a one-handed technique.

- Store sharp's containers on top of the refrigerator in the residence or some other place out of reach of children.

Specimen Collection

- Place blood or other body substances in a leak-proof container and secure in a puncture-proof container during collection, handling, storage, and transport.

- Label the specimen with client's name and identifying data.

- Handle all specimens in a manner to minimize spillage.

- Place containers on the floor of the car during transport.

Exposure Incident

- Use water to irrigate the eye.

- Use soap and water to wash the exposed body part.

- Contact agency for follow-up instructions.

- Document incident.

Adapted from *Handbook of Home Health Nursing* (2nd ed.), by R. Rice, 2000, St. Louis: Mosby.

---

with the family, makes decisions about care appropriate to the family's ever-changing needs. In addition, the nurse often helps the family to connect with other community resources. To help make these connections, the nurse must develop a network of relationships with all sectors of the community.

IMPLEMENTATION OF THE NURSING PROCESS IN THE HOME

It is as important to follow the nursing process in the home setting as in any other setting. Assessment incorporates all family members, both as individuals and as a family unit. Family nursing diagnoses are important in developing appropriate plans and interventions, in collaboration with the family. Evaluation is an ongoing component of the nursing process and is crucial to a timely termination.

Assessment

The nurse's assessment of the family begins before the first home visit. It is important that the nurse review the referral information concerning the client. This informa-

tion provides basic information such as name, age, diagnosis, address, telephone number, insurance coverage, reason for referral, and source of referral. The referral source will vary with each client. A common source is the client's doctor, who recognizes that certain services are needed at home. Because hospital clients are discharged after very short stays, continued teaching and nursing care are often needed after the client returns home.

The first telephone contact is an opportunity to gather data. The nurse should note the client's response to the call. Is the client open to the visit? Does the client remember that a referral had been made? Does the client agree with the reason for the referral or have a different understanding of the reasons that the nurse wants to see him or her? The client's responses and demeanor give the nurse some clues as to the client's perception of the meaning of the home visit.

The purpose of the first home visit is to begin to identify the family's strengths and health needs. It is unreasonable to expect the family assessment to be completed in one visit, or, indeed, in many visits. The first meeting is usually at a time of stress related to the event that precipitated the need for a home visit. The nurse must remember that the family's usual functioning is compromised and that their current behavior may not reflect their usual coping abilities. Objectively assessing families is difficult. It is important to recognize personal bias. The use of assessment tools helps the nurse maintain objectivity. Common assessment tools are interviewing, observation, standardized or unstandardized surveys, questionnaires, or checklists (Thomas, Barnard, & Sumner, 1993). Home health nurses may focus more on client assessment than on family assessment, but both are important regardless of whether the family or the individual is the primary client. The individual and family dynamics discussed in Chapters 24 and 25 provide the information needed to make such assessments.

Interviewing

Community health nurses interview both individuals and families or segments of families: most commonly, committed partners or parent and child. When individuals in families are interviewed, it is important to remember that only one point of view is being represented. Whenever possible, the nurse should make an effort to meet with all family members, either as a group or individually, in order to get an idea of the total family perspective. Although family interviews are more complex than one-on-one interaction, they do elicit data unobtainable in any other way. For instance, the reaction of one family member to another can be observed only in a group interaction.

Before family assessment of any kind is possible, the nurse must establish a trusting relationship with the family. Trust is a critical component of all work with the family (Wright & Leahey, 2000). Initially, family members perceive the nurse as a stranger. Unless they are in extreme stress, family members are unlikely to share their most personal concerns with the nurse. The nurse can expect that initial information obtained may not reflect deeper issues. In addition, cultural factors may cause undeclared stress because family members either do not recognize that they are experiencing stress or do not consider the possibility of getting aid from outside the family to help alleviate the burdens that are causing stress (D'Avanzo, Frye, & Froman, 1994).

As family members become more confident that the nurse is trustworthy, they will reveal more of their real concerns. In addition to their natural reticence to share personal issues and feelings with a stranger, they may have specific reasons to not trust the nurse. If they are taking drugs, are in the country illegally, or have some stigmatizing condition that causes them to fear that their secret will be revealed to a punitive authority, they cannot afford to trust without testing to see whether confidentiality will be maintained. Unless family members come to believe that they can trust the nurse not to report them, they may change residences to avoid further contact. Such an event is undesirable because it prevents them from getting the health care they need.

Observation

Assessment through observation is an ongoing process during each home visit. The nurse can easily observe the condition of the home, the interactions among family members, and the status of the neighborhood and larger community. These observations help the nurse determine the quality of life of the family, identify safety issues, and recognize problems that put the family at risk. See Figure 21-4 for a list of selected observations to make during a home visit.

Other Assessment Tools

Assessment tools help in the organization of family data and provide information to remind the nurse about areas to explore with the family. Family genograms and ecograms, discussed in Chapter 24, can be used to depict the structure of the family. The Wright and Leahey (2000) family assessment model, also discussed in Chapter 24, provides direction for gathering information about the structure, function, and developmental aspects of the family. Murray and Zentner (2001) have developed a family assessment tool that assesses family lifestyle and needs. The assessment tool lists many dimensions of family life that the nurse can observe during the home visit, such as crowding, access to the phone, expression of ideas, and relationship patterns. Other aspects of the tool can be

---

REFLECTIVE THINKING

Home Visit Experience

- Have you ever had a nurse visit your home? If so, what were some of the thoughts and feelings you had about the experience? If you have not had such an encounter, how do you think you would react to such a situation?

- As you think about your own actual or imagined experience with a nurse who is making a health visit to your home, what issues can you identify that would have an impact on your own behavior as a nurse making a home visit?

Perspectives...

INSIGHTS OF A REGISTERED NURSE STORIES INTO LESSONS

I
How to tell my story
    of the stories
    I've been allowed
    to know?
Each with a heroine/hero
each with myth and magic
each sad and true
each strong and full of wonder
    amazing
    I repeat
amazing the lives
    however ordinary
amazing they would tell me
    a stranger
my entré
    is the assumption they make
    about NURSE
I think, I wonder, I worry
will I live up to this?
At times I know
    I don't,
I count on grace.
Lives seem too important to make mistakes
    Yet I learn the human spirit is
        too sturdy
        to crumble completely.
I take their stories in
    absorbing the life so
        that mine is enhanced.
    I'm a robber
but they seem not diminished
    but grateful somehow
    to have a listener.
It's got to be more than that
What about all those theories?
    What about all the postures/
    and definitions?

II
A ninety-year-old professor
    proud and dignified
    took me in and shared the
history of his life
    mostly the good parts
    very few of the bad
        but they were
            there.

The twenty-five year old
    recovered heroin and
    cocaine user
raising a young family
trying in many ways
    beyond herself
to cope with what she had chosen to escape
"It's all still there when
    you come down" she once told me.
Compromising to fit and do the right thing
    in a society that does not
    welcome her
Wanting all the things for her kids
    that others want for theirs,
peacefulness, some joy, a well-received mind
she struggles and her struggles
    make her strong
        a survivor.
A tragic family tale
    of loss and abandonment
    of fear and flight
    of survival
remembered by a child who at seven
    left the only world she
        ever knew
a quiet life on a village farm
    in Cambodia.
Two children for each parent
    to carry
        and one hidden in a womb
        yet to be discovered
But two left behind
    who would surely die
The inconsolable loss sustained
    in an effort that more
        might survive.
The tears in her eyes
    as this
        now eighteen-year-old
        remembers
She rubs her pregnant belly
    just now understanding
    the proportions
        of her mother's loss.
Take it from Helen,
    Life is Hell.

(continues)

Perspectives...

she will engage me and then set
  me to anger and bring me back
    again to an enormous
    attraction.
She could be my aunt Mary
  she's negative enough
and she's rough, Lord the language
  and the volume.
she tells me can't
  but she can
She tells me won't
  but she will
her actions often betray her
an ordinary person
  faced with extraordinary
    circumstances
    her failed marriage of 37 years
    her only daughter's suicide
    her eldest son's death from a boating accident
    her MI
    a stroke at the same time
not familiar or comfortable with
  words like
  grief
  depression
  cope
  mourn
  insight
a woman who always just DID
  now what? and why?
    she asks.
Frustrated and loved by her son John
  who loves and frustrates
    her.
They go round
amazingly they let me see them

love/hate
  one another.

III
So, how about me?
  I am enriched, touched, seized with emotion
    by these experiences
    who wouldn't be?
  I feel a need in
    myself to be less
    guarded
  less in control
the rawness of my nature
  felt
  but rarely shared
what I learned from them.
I thank them all for letting me
  into their lives
they say, "really?"
    doubtful that I
    mean this
    —boy do I mean this.
And hope for us all
    reveals itself to me again
    hope that comes from the
      real lives of
      real people
letting me in
  so briefly
  and so completely
  I look the same
but walk away
  changed.

—Margaret Dodson, RN,
May 3, 1990

---

used to generate questions to ask the family. For instance, the nurse could inquire about the family's knowledge or use of food stamps or about their child-rearing practices. The nurse may use this assessment tool either in whole or in part to obtain needed information about one particular aspect of the family (see Figure 21-5).

An assessment tool available to home health nurses in particular is the **Outcome and Assessment Information Set (OASIS),** a federally mandated requirement for all home health agencies. Its purpose is to measure out-

comes for outcome-based quality improvement; however, it represents a comprehensive assessment for an adult home care client. OASIS has been mandated in all home health agencies since 1999. The data items encompass sociodemographic, environmental, support systems, health status, and functional status attributes of adult (nonmaternity) clients. Selected attributes of health service utilization are also included (Sperling, 1998, 1999).

Many other tools are available for assessing specific aspects of the family, such as the family support scale,

---

FIGURE 21-4 List of Selected Home Visit Observations

Neighborhood

Facilities conveniently available to family (schools, stores, churches, parks, transportation, etc.)

Quality of streets (busy, quiet, well maintained)

People in neighborhood (drug dealers, prostitutes, many or few people, friendly neighbors, children, elders)

Quality of property (well maintained, clutter in yards)

Type, condition, and quantity of animals in the area

Home

Floors and walls: uneven or slippery, loose rugs, cleanliness, heavy articles on top shelves or inadequately hung on walls, unsecured tall book shelves

Walkways and stairways: uneven, broken, or loose sidewalks or paths; absence of or insecure handrails; congested or cluttered hallways or other high-traffic areas; toys or other items in places where people might trip over them; adequacy of night lighting inside and outside

Furniture: hazardous placement of furniture with sharp corners, chairs or stools that are unstable or too low to get into or out of or that provide inadequate support

Bathrooms: presence or absence of grab bars around tubs and toilets, nonslip surfaces in tubs and shower stalls, adequacy of night lighting, need for raised toilet seat or bath chair in tub or shower, presence in medicine cabinet of medications no longer used or out of date

Kitchen: pilot lights in need of repair, inaccessible storage areas, hazardous furniture

Bedrooms: availability of night lights and accessibility of light switches

Electrical: unanchored and/or frayed electrical cords, overloaded outlets or outlets near water, uncovered electrical outlets in places where children can reach them

Fire protection: presence or absence of smoke detectors, fire extinguisher, and fire escape plan; improper storage of combustibles or corrosives; accessibility of emergency telephone numbers

Toxic substances: medications kept beyond date of expiration, improperly labeled cleaning solutions, cleaning materials in unlocked cabinets accessible by children

Communication devices: Note presence of method to call for help such as a telephone or internal intercom in the bedroom and elsewhere (e.g., kitchen) and access to emergency telephone numbers

Medications: Note medications kept beyond date of expiration, adequacy of lighting for medication cabinet or storage, and method of disposal of sharp objects such as needles used for interfections

Family

Children watching TV rather than playing with one another

Parents having similar or different views of a given incident when discussing family health or interpersonal problems

Availability of family members for interviews

Quality and quantity of discipline of children

Family constellation (single parent, three generation, etc.)

From *Fundamentals of Nursing: Concepts, Process, and Practice* (6th ed., p. 142), by B. Kozier, G. Erb, A. J. Berman, and K. Burke, 2000, Upper Saddle River, NJ: Prentice-Hall, Inc. Copyright 2000 by Prentice-Hall. Adapted with permission.

---

which assesses the family's perception of the social support they receive during parenting, the Infant Care Survey; which assesses the mother's comfort with and knowledge of caring for her infant; the Family Hardiness Inventory, which assesses the internal strengths of families in meeting challenges and stress; and the Community Life Skills Scale, which measures the mother's ability to use community and interpersonal resources (Thomas et al., 1993). Janosik (1994) has developed a crisis assessment tool and has suggested questions to raise with family members to facilitate assessment and provide anticipatory guidance (see Figure 21-6).

Use of these tools helps the nurse provide objective, family-centered care through the assessment of family processes, parenting, family coping, health maintenance and management, and home maintenance and management.

Cultural Health Practices

An important component of family assessment is the consideration of cultural health practices. These practices influence all aspects of the nursing process, and understanding them helps the nurse to understand client behavior and to more effectively plan interventions that are consistent with client health beliefs. Selected health practices and cultural assessment tools important to the family are discussed in Chapter 8.

FIGURE 21-5 Family Assessment Tool

Meeting of Physical, Emotional, and Spiritual Needs of Members

Ability to Provide Food and Shelter

- Space management as regards living, sleeping, recreation, privacy
- Crowding if over 1.5 persons per room
- Territoriality or control on the part of each member over lifespace
- Access to laundry, grocery, recreation facilities
- Sanitation, including disposal methods, source of water supply, control of rodents and insects
- Storage and refrigeration
- Available food supply
- Food preparation, including preserving and cooking methods (stove, hotplate, oven)
- Use of food stamps and donated foods as well as eligibility for food stamps
- Education of each member as to food composition, balanced menus, special preparations or diets if required for a specific member

Access to Health Care

- Regularity of health care
- Continuity of caregivers
- Closeness of facility and means of access such as car, bus, cab
- Access to helpful neighbors
- Access to phone

Family Health

- Longevity
- Major or chronic illnesses
- Familial or hereditary illnesses such as rheumatic fever, gout, allergy, tuberculosis, renal disease, diabetes mellitus, cancer, emotional illness, epilepsy, migraine, other nervous disorders, hypertension, blood diseases, obesity, frequent accidents, drug intake, pica
- Emotional or stress-related illnesses
- Pollutants to which members are chronically exposed, such as air, water, soil, noise, or chemicals that are unsafe to health

Neighborhood Pride and Loyalty

Job Access, Energy Output, Shift Changes

Sensitivity, Warmth, Understanding Between Family Members

- Demonstration of emotion
- Enjoyment of sexual relations
  Male: Impotence, premature or retarded ejaculation, hypersexuality

Female: Frigidity (inability to achieve orgasm); enjoyment of sexual relations; feelings of disgust, shame, self-devaluation; fear of injury; painful coitus

Menstrual history, including onset, duration, flow, missed periods and life situation at the time, pain, euphoria, depression, other difficulties

Sharing of Religious Beliefs, Values, Doubts

- Formal membership in church and organizations
- Ethical framework and honesty
- Adaptability, response to reality
- Satisfaction with life
- Self-esteem

Child-Rearing Practices and Discipline

Mutual Responsibility

- Joint parenting
- Mutual respect for decision making
- Means of discipline and consistency

Respect for Individuality

Fostering of Self-Discipline

Attitudes Toward Education, Reading, Scholarly Pursuit

Attitudes Toward Imaginative Play

Attitudes Toward Involvement in Sports

Promotion of Gender Stereotypes

Communication

- Expression of a wide range of emotion and feeling
- Expression of ideas, concepts, beliefs, values, interests
- Openness
- Verbal expression and sensitive listening
- Consensual decision making

Support, Security, Encouragement

- Balance in activity
- Humor
- Dependency and dominance patterns
- Life support groups of each member
- Social relationship of couple: go out together or separately; change since marriage mutually satisfying; effect of sociability patterns on children

Growth-Producing Relationships and Experiences within and outside the Family

- Creative play activities
- Planned growth experiences
- Focus of life and activity of each member
- Friendships

(continues)

FIGURE 21-5 Family Assessment Tool (continued)

Responsible Community Relationships

- Organizations, including involvement, membership, active participation
- Knowledge of and friendship with neighbors

Growing with and through Children

- Hope and plans for children
- Emulation of own parents and its influence on relationship with children
- Relationship patterns: authoritarian, patriarchal, matriarchal

- Necessity to relive (make up for) own childhood through children

Unity, Loyalty and Cooperation

- Positive interacting of members toward each other

Self-Help and Acceptance of Outside Help in Family Crisis

From *Health Promotion Strategies throughout the Life Span* (7th ed., p. 200), by R. B. Murray and J. P. Zentner, 2001, Upper Saddle River, NJ: Prentice-Hall. Copyright 2001 by Prentice-Hall. Adapted with permission.

FIGURE 21-6 Crisis Assessment Tool

Initial Steps

1. Using various sources of information, collect data that indicate the dimensions of the problem.
2. Formulate a dynamic hypothesis concerning the problem and the coping responses of the client.
3. Assess the problem in terms of intrinsic and extrinsic factors and determine a therapeutic approach.
4. Involve the client in problem-solving activities.
5. Negotiate a contract that sets clear, reachable goals.
6. Explain that treatment will be terminated according to the terms of the contract.

General Procedures

1. Obtain demographic data.
2. Define the problem in realistic terms.
3. Assess the mental status of the client(s).
4. Assess the physical status of the client(s).
5. Assess the psychosocial status of the client(s).
6. Assess coping skills of the client(s).

Coping Skills Assessment

1. How does the client deal with anxiety, tension, or depression?
2. Has the client used customary coping methods in the current situation?
3. What were the results of using customary coping methods?
4. Have there been recent life changes that interfered with customary coping methods?
5. Are significant persons contributing to continuation of the problem?

6. Is the client considering suicide or homicide as a way of coping? If so, how? When?
7. Has the client attempted suicide or homicide in the past? Under what conditions?
8. Assess the extent of suicidal or homicidal risk presented by the client. Hospitalization may be necessary as a protective measure.

Planning and Problem Solving

1. Is the present crisis new or a reenactment of similar events that occurred in the past?
2. What alternative methods might have been used to prevent development of the present crisis?
3. What new methods might be used to resolve the present crisis?
4. What supports are available to strengthen new problem-solving methods?

Anticipatory Guidance

1. What sources of stress remain for the client?
2. Using the current repertoire of coping skills, how might the client deal with problematic issues in the future?
3. How might the current repertoire of coping skills be maintained or expanded?
4. Upon termination of the contract for crisis intervention, is further referral or follow-up care necessary?

From E. H. Janosik, *Crisis Counseling: A Contemporary Approach* (2nd ed.), 1994, Boston: Jones & Bartlett. Copyright 1994 by Jones & Bartlett. Reprinted with permission.

Nursing Diagnosis and Planning Care

On the basis of the assessment, the nurse establishes the nursing diagnoses. These diagnoses may be for the entire family or for individuals within the family. In comparison with other community health nurses, home health nurses may assign more circumscribed diagnoses that focus exclusively on the client. Long-term and short-term goals are established in conjunction with the family. Together, expected outcomes that include measurable results within a specific time frame are established. A useful way to confirm these decisions is through the use of a contract.

Contracts

A family **contract** is a critical component of family care that promotes self-care and facilitates a family focus on health needs. Although this type of contract is not legally binding, a pledge of trust and commitment is implicit. The most important component to contracting is the concept of **partnership,** or collaboration: the shared participation and agreement between client and nurse regarding mutual identification of needs and resources, development of a plan, division of responsibilities, time limits, evaluation, and renegotiation (Wright & Leahey, 2000).

Contracting provides the framework for the relationship. It keeps the nursing process goal directed and focused (Wright & Leahey, 2000). The nurse and family must be clear on the responsibilities of each to the relationship, the purpose of the relationship, and any special limitations. For student nurses, one limitation is the

length of time that the nurse will be available to the family. Thus, the time frame, which usually ranges from 4 to 14 weeks, must be made clear, and consideration must be given to the follow-up care that will be provided. In such instances, referral to other community health nurses or to a specific community agency is not unusual. In home health care, a home health nurse is assigned responsibility for the client when the student is no longer available.

The structure of the contract facilitates the termination of the relationship and helps prevent the family from becoming dependent. Because it focuses on the client's unique needs and promotes development of problem-solving skills and autonomy, the process promotes self-esteem in the client. Clients are motivated to do that which is needed to achieve their health goals.

The most common type of contract is an oral contract that is reviewed at each visit. The main consideration is the mutuality of the complete process of client care between nurse and client. Riley (2000) has identified the following elements of a client-nurse contract (p. 51):

- Names of client and nurse
- Purpose of the client-nurse relationship
- Roles of client and nurse
- Responsibilities of client and nurse
- Expectations of client and nurse
- Specific details such as meeting times and structure for confidentiality
- Conditions for termination

A well-developed contract that follows these steps provides distinct direction for nursing intervention. It also provides standards for evaluation because it clearly delineates the expected outcomes (Riley, 2000).

Interventions

In conjunction with the client, nursing intervention begins on the first visit as decisions are made in the planning process about those health needs that should be addressed first and the responsibilities of both the nurse and the client. The timing of the next visit is based on the needs of the client and is mutually agreed on. In home health care, there may be assigned times for nursing visits based on the particular client health problem. A home visit should be planned to last 1/2 to 1 hour. Family members can absorb only a limited amount of information before they are overloaded and unable to take in more. Similarly, the nurse takes in a great deal of information through observation and interview and can easily become overloaded. It is better to arrange a second visit to continue assessment, review that which has been taught, and evaluate progress toward goals rather than trying to accomplish too much at one visit. The home health care nurse usually must accomplish certain activities in relation to the client and may therefore be limited in the amount of time that he or she has available to work with the family. Incorporating the family members in the care of the client, however, allows many opportunities for teaching and for further assessment of family concerns and needs.

Three of the most common interventions are teaching about various health considerations (discussed in Chapter 10), helping families deal with the stress created by health problems, and making referrals for community services.

Family Stress

Some specific considerations related to developing interventions directed toward reducing family stress have to do specifically with parental and caregiver stress. Because parents are usually the family members who determine the ways that the family copes with stress, it is important to address parental anxiety. Although the tendency of the nurse may be to directly protect vulnerable family members such as children or elders, it is equally important to support and educate the caregivers so that they can provide appropriate care to other vulnerable family members. Davis (1998) found that caregivers who were contacted by phone once a week and given the opportunity to problem-solve with the nurse experienced a sense of social support, a reduction in depressive symptoms, and an improvement of life satisfaction in the midst of caregiving. The collaboration of caregiver and nurse, therefore, facilitates the development of strategies that work for the family, decrease stress, and help to improve their quality of life.

Referrals

In making referrals, the important issues to be considered are the three A's: availability, acceptability, and accessibility. Perhaps the most important consideration is the acceptability of the service. If the client is not willing to use the resource, its availability and accessibility are of no consequence. Similarly, no matter how acceptable the service may be to the client, it is of no use if it is inaccessible in terms of available transportation or client eligibility. In some settings, particularly in some rural areas, a service is simply not available, regardless of its acceptability to the client or the client's eligibility.

Promoting Family Strengths

Another intervention is to promote family strengths, thereby allowing family members to focus on their growth-producing dynamics rather than only on their problems. Wright and Leahey (2000) note that commendations to families regarding their strengths are "powerful, effective and enduring therapeutic interventions" (p. 282). While

this intervention is important for all families, it is especially important for vulnerable families. In addition to emphasizing positives, the nurse can also reframe a negative behavior to highlight a positive aspect of the behavior. Alternatives that would facilitate positive behavior can then be considered. For example, if a client does not adhere to the established schedule for taking medications, the deviation can be depicted as an attempt to maintain autonomy rather than as client noncompliance. Emphasizing this positive characteristic supports the client's self-esteem, encouraging the client to reconsider the medication regime and respond in a way that is in his or her best interest.

Communications between Nurses, Clients, the Interdisciplinary Team, and the Home Agency

With the advent of multiple electronic and telecommunication tools, the nurse has many resources with which to communicate with others. The use of cell phones and e-mail is common. For instance, if a client has e-mail, they can contact the nurse if they have a question and the nurse can respond quickly, even if the client is not at home. Most professional contacts have e-mail and can give and receive information quickly. In many agencies, lap-top computers are part of the nurse's equipment. With these, the nurse can document the visit immediately and transmit it to the client's file at the agency. In the near future, other technology will be available that will greatly benefit both providers and recipients of care. (See Out of the Box.)

Telehome Health

Telehome health (THH) or telemedicine is a new adjunct to home visits that is being used in some agencies to reduce home visits (Shaul, 2000). A telecommunication system is installed in the client's home with the

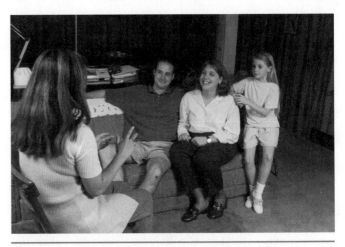

It is important not to overload a family with too much information all at one time.

home base at the agency. The nurse is able to monitor clients and observe and interact with them. For instance, an electronic stethoscope enables the nurse to listen to the client's heart and lungs. It is possible to measure and transmit temperature, weight, blood glucose levels, and pulse oximetry. Benefits are fewer office or home visits, better documentation through the recording and transmitting of still images from the home, and improved confidence in treatment decisions (Hayes, Duffey, Dunbar, Wages, & Holbrook; 1998). With the use of medical sensors and video, nurses can interact with their clients as often as necessary.

Dimmick, Mustaleski, Burgiss, and Welsh (2000) describe a typical nursing consultation via telemedicine as involving

> calling home care patients at a scheduled time once or twice per week, depending on the patient's condition and plan of care. . . . Depending on the patient's hearing capabilities, he or she will either use the speaker-phone or the phone receiver. The telemedicine nurse conducts a televisit appropriate to the plan of care. Both the nurse and the patient can see one another and the camera is movable so that various aspects and views of the patient can be visualized. (p. 126)

The nurse must determine if the client is physically and mentally able to use the equipment and is willing to participate in this type of home visit and if the home environment will accommodate the equipment (Shaul, 2000). Studies have shown that with proper education, most clients do like the telehome visits, particularly if they are supplemented by home visits (Dansky, Bowles, & Palmer, 1999; Shaul, 2000).

Evaluation

Evaluation is an ongoing process that begins prior to each visit. The nurse and family must continually assess the progress of the family toward achievement of expected outcomes and must consider needed modifications to the plan. When goals are achieved, the nurse and client terminate the visits, making sure that the client and family know how to access community resources if needed.

Termination

Termination takes two forms: the ending of each home visit and the final cessation of services. The latter constitutes an important milestone that must be planned well in advance. Termination begins with the first visit. Although the structure of the contract sets the parameters of service, it is important to review with the family that which has been accomplished and to reinforce and support the family's progress. By the time of service cessation, family members will have come to value the nurse's input and will need reassurance that they themselves can make decisions that will positively affect their

health care. The focus on partnership emphasizes this perspective and provides the family with the strength to make independent decisions.

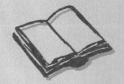

Out
of the Box

New Technologies

The following technologies will be available within the next five years:

1. *Low-cost Internet appliances that are less overwhelming to those who are not particularly computer literate; for instance, e-mail machines are in the early stages of development and soon will be widely available.*

2. *Home monitoring devices for measuring, e.g., blood glucose levels or oxygen tank levels that can be connected to a PC or can automatically dial out will increase reporting accuracy and will be more convenient.*

3. *A "Smart Shirt" will have sensors built into the garment that can transmit vital signs. This sensor will be integrated with computer-based patient record systems.*

4. *Computer devices that are simpler and have larger displays for those with vision deficits are two or three years away.*

5. *Speech recognition used in combination with natural language processing will be useful by the middle of this decade, as will the use of devices with handwriting recognition.*

6. *Video conferencing will be available and will reduce the need for clients to travel.*

7. *Home monitoring via web video cameras will soon be available.*

8. *"Home drug dispensing devices, which would provide monitoring and alert features, including microprocessors in bottle caps to track when bottles are opened," (p. 37) will be available in a few years.*

"Internet and mobile computing, speech recognition, remote monitoring, and personal health records will be some of the most valuable information technologies and applications for the home care and assisted living marketplace during the next five years" (p. 37).

Source: Kleinberg, K. (2001). Technologies to enable home care. Caring 20(1), 36–37. ■

COMMUNITY NURSING VIEW

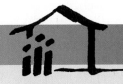

Dan Jewell has been home from the diabetic teaching center for two days. He was diagnosed with adult-onset diabetes two weeks ago. Prior to that time, he had never heard of the disease. His wife, Roberta, attended some classes with him but is still confused about meeting his dietary needs. At the teaching center, Dan learned to give himself insulin injections, but he is very unsure of his technique. Given that he has a friend who has diabetes but who does not have to take insulin, Dan wonders whether he can avoid taking insulin if he is very careful about his diet. His two children, Jerry, 16, and Martha, 13, have been asking questions about diabetes. They are worried about their father's health and also are afraid that they might get the disease. They have read about diabetes and know that it can run in families.

Nursing Considerations

Assessment

◆ What issues do you think must be explored with this family?

◆ Which aspects of care lie in the realm of primary prevention? Secondary prevention?

◆ What assessment tools might be effective with this family.

Diagnosis

◆ What nursing diagnoses are appropriate for this family?

◆ How would you set priorities with regard to the diagnoses?

Outcome Identification

◆ Given the diagnoses you have identified, what outcomes do you expect?

Planning/Interventions

◆ How might you go about developing a contract with this family?

◆ How might you involve the family in contracting to facilitate self-care?

Evaluation

◆ What might you do if an intervention were not working?

◆ How might you know when to terminate with this family?

Sometimes, goals are not completely met because the nurse has to terminate service before the client is ready. For instance, the nurse may have to reallocate time to families who are at higher risk, may take another job, or, in the case of a student, may have completed clinical rotation. In the case of home health, the number of visits is usually prescribed. Whenever possible in such circumstances, the nurse must ensure either a smooth transition to another community health nurse or the provision of an appropriate referral.

A successful termination is one in which both client and nurse feel satisfied that goals have been met or appropriate referrals made. To prepare family members for the last visit, the nurse should spend several weeks working with the family, reviewing client progress, and discussing any remaining issues in order to avoid leaving unfinished business. The nurse should also express and discuss her or his own feelings about ending the relationship. The association of nurse and client typically involves the expression of deep feelings. Disconnecting such a relationship takes much time and effort and should not be performed hastily. Figure 21-7 summarizes the components of the home visit as discussed here and within Byrd's (1995a) framework.

KEY CONCEPTS

◆ The home visit is an important way of providing service to clients. While it has advantages and disadvantages, the home visit offers a dimension of health care that can be provided in no other setting.

◆ The nursing process is carried out in the home setting just as it is in any other setting.

◆ Nursing assessment of the family begins before the first home visit and includes interviewing, observation, use of a variety of assessment tools, and an awareness of cultural health practices.

◆ Contracting promotes self-care and facilitates a family focus on health needs.

◆ Telehome health is a new adjunct to home visits and is used in some agencies to reduce home visits.

◆ The major emphasis of the community health nurse is on primary prevention, including teaching, counseling, and referral to appropriate resources.

◆ Termination is an important part of the home visit.

FIGURE 21-7 Summary of Components of the Home Visit Using Byrd's (1995a) Framework

Contacting Phase Antecedent Event

Client self-refers or agency receives referral from another source.

- Clarify reason for referral.

Phone contact or unscheduled visit with family to arrange home visit.

- Clarify purpose of home visit and who referred family and why.
- Get directions to the family's residence.
- Determine whether any special equipment is needed or is available in the home.

Going-to-See Phase Prepare for Home Visit

Collect information that will be needed about the family.

- Name, address, and phone number
- Map with directions to residence
- Telephone number of agency
- Emergency phone numbers: police, fire, ambulance (in many places, 911 covers all)

Identify any safety precautions that may be needed.

For a first visit, devise a plan for working with the family; for a subsequent visit, review prioritized plans from the previous visit.

Have a list of community resources that may be needed.

Have necessary equipment in nurse's bag and prepare any assessment or permission forms or teaching aids that may be needed.

Leave information with faculty or agency about your planned visit and expected length of stay.

Journey to the Residence

Have adequate gas in your car or adequate money for public transportation.

Observe the neighborhood where the family lives; check for safety, community facilities, people, animals, etc.

Observe the outside of the residence for environmental hazards and general quality of home environment.

Entry Phase (Seeing Phase)

Knock on the door or ring the bell. Stand where you can be seen.

Identify yourself; state your name and agency affiliation.

Ask for the person with whom you made the appointment.

Continue to be alert to your own safety.

Notice who is present and introduce yourself to them.

Allow the family to direct you where to sit. If they do not indicate a preference, ask if you may sit.

On an initial visit, explain the purpose of your agency and the reasons that you have come to their home. On a subsequent visit, review plans made during the previous visit and begin as planned unless the family indicates another priority that takes precedence.

Probable activities during the visit:

- Obtaining signatures on permission forms
- Performing health assessment of client or all family members, as indicated
- Washing hands before and after any direct physical contact
- Providing health education as indicated and written instructions as necessary
- Completing treatments as required
- Reviewing plans of care for the family, assessing for changes, and identifying and problem solving barriers to successful completion
- Identifying health needs of all household members
- Referring family members to appropriate community resources
- Identifying environmental hazards; reviewing concerns and problem solving together with family to find solutions

Conduct all visits in a caring way, providing comfort, support, information, and counseling, as indicated.

Termination Phase (Telling Phase)

Summarize accomplishments of the visit and, with the family, determine that which remains to be completed.

Discuss plans for the next home visit and the work to be completed in the interim by both family and nurse.

Ensure that the family has written documentation of your name, phone number, and agency affiliation.

Discuss referrals with the family and ensure that they have written documentation of the referral agency's name, phone number, and, if available, the name of a specific contact person.

As soon as possible after the visit, document the visit in the format used by your agency. Try to arrange time immediately after the visit to complete the written report.

RESOURCES

Telemedicine Information Exchange: www.tie.telemed.org/homehealth

National Association for Health Care Quality: www.nahg.org
American Health Care Association: www.ahca.org

Chapter

22

CARE OF INFANTS, CHILDREN, AND ADOLESCENTS

Barbara Mandleco, RN, PhD

MAKING THE CONNECTION

I believe that our only national treasure is our children. The one thing that we all have in common is a childhood. This period in our life comes only once, and if someone ruins that, disrupts it, or rapes it, there is no replacement for it.

—Gill, 1995, p. 31

COMPETENCIES

Upon completion of this chapter, the reader should be able to:

- Discuss maternal-child and adolescent health status in the United States.
- Recount developmental theories and conceptual frameworks applicable to infants, children, and adolescents.
- Discuss the relationship between fetal development and the need for prenatal care.
- Cite the respective indicators of infant, child, and adolescent health status.
- Detail the major health risks of infants, toddlers, and school-age populations in the United States.
- Describe the major health risks to adolescents in the United States.
- Discuss nursing's role as it applies to family-centered nursing practice and healthy development during the prenatal period, infancy, childhood, and adolescence.

KEY TERMS

anorexia nervosa	maturation
bulimia nervosa	nonorganic failure to thrive (NFTT)
child abuse	
developmental assessment tools	organic failure to thrive (OFTT)
failure to thrive (FTT)	plumbism
family-centered nursing practice	pregnancy outcomes
growth	pregnancy-induced hypertension (PIH)
health promotion	prenatal risk assessment
human development	
idiopathic failure to thrive (IFTT)	secondhand smoke
	teratogenic effects
infant mortality rate	unintentional injuries
low birthweight (LBW)	very low birthweight

Community health nurses serving families and communities are in unique positions to provide and teach caring behaviors that support healthy development. Child health care focuses on preventing acute and chronic illness while promoting normal growth and development. This chapter focuses on the care and nurturance of children from conception until passage into adulthood and on the roles of community health nurses in serving these populations.

HEALTH STATUS OF CHILDREN IN THE UNITED STATES

Although most children grow up strong and healthy, many others suffer from poverty, abuse, violence, disrespect, hunger, serious injury or chronic illness, family disintegration, inadequate parenting or child care, and limited or no medical insurance. At the Stand for Children Day held on March 12–15, 1997, Miriam Wright Edelman, president of the Children's Defense Fund (CDF) in the United States, introduced the CDF's annual report, *The State of America's Children Yearbook 1997,* by saying:

> If America's children are to grow up educated and productive, they must have a healthy start in life—with the health coverage they need to grow and thrive, healthy communities that allow them to walk safely to school, and the opportunity to learn unimpaired by untreated vision, hearing, and health problems and violence, abuse, and neglect. (Edelman, 1997, p. 1)

Although children are doing better today than when the CDF was established and strides have been made to improve their risks, several issues remain. For example, 1 in 2 children live in a single-parent family at some point in their childhood and 1 in 3 is born to unmarried parents, will be poor at some point in their childhood, and is behind a year or more in school. One child in 5 lives in a family receiving food stamps, and 1 in 6 is born to a mother who did not receive prenatal care during the first three months of pregnancy. One in 8 is born to a teenage mother or never graduates from high school. One in 60 sees parents divorce in any given year, 1 in 138 will die before the first birthday, and 1 in 910 will be killed before turning 20 (CDF, 2000b). Figures 22-1 and 22-2 illustrate the reality for today's American children.

Health Care Coverage of Children

Family income and employment status determine access to health care services and health insurance coverage. Children from low-income and poor families are the least likely to be privately insured because their parents are more likely to be unemployed or employed without health insurance benefits.

Health insurance is important for children to ensure they have a healthy start in life. If they are not insured, they are less likely to do well in school because they do not feel well, see well, or hear well (CDF, 2000b). In 2000, more than 10 million children (one in seven) were uninsured (U.S. Department of Health and Human Services [USDHHS], 2001). The State Children's Health In-

---

FIGURE 22-1 Children's Defense Fund: Key Facts on Youth, 2000

- In 1997, firearms killed 4205 children age 19 and under; of these, 2562 were murdered, 1262 committed suicide, and 306 were victims of accidental shootings.

- In 1997, there were approximately 984,000 confirmed victims of maltreatment (physical abuse, neglect, sexual abuse, medical neglect, psychological abuse, other abuses); three-fourths of the perpetrators of child maltreatment were parents; an additional one-tenth were relatives.

- In 1998, 5.4 million children lived in households headed by a relative other than a parent.

- In 1999, 12.1 million U.S. children (one in six) were poor; 33.1% are African American, 30.3% were Hispanic, 13.5% are Caucasian, and 11.8% were of Asian and Pacific Island descent.

- In 1999, 10.8 million children age 18 and under lacked health coverage; 4.4 million were Caucasian, 3.4 million were African American, and 2.1 million were Hispanic.

- In 1999, an estimated 547,000 children were in foster care; 117,000 of these were waiting for permanent adoptive families.

From *The State of America's Children Yearbook 2000,* by Children's Defense Fund, 2000, Washington, DC: Author. Reprinted with permission.

FIGURE 22-2 Moments in America for Children

Time Frame	Experience
Every 1 second	A public high school student is suspended*
Every 9 seconds	A high school student drops out*
Every 10 seconds	A public school student is corporally punished*
Every 17 seconds	A child is arrested
Every 37 seconds	A baby is born to a mother who is not a high school graduate
Every 56 seconds	A baby is born into poverty
Every 1 minute	A baby is born to a teen mother
Every 2 minutes	A baby is born at low birthweight (less than 5 lbs., 8 oz.)
Every 4 minutes	A baby is born to a mother who had late or no prenatal care; a child is arrested for drug abuse
Every 7 minutes	A child is arrested for a violent crime
Every 10 minutes	A baby is born at very low birthweight (less than 3 lbs., 4 oz.)
Every 19 minutes	A baby dies
Every 41 minutes	A child or youth under 20 dies from an accident
Every 2 hours	A child or youth under 20 is killed by a firearm or is a homicide victim
Every 4 hours	A child or youth under 20 commits suicide
Every 19 hours	A young person under 25 dies from HIV infection

*Based on calculations per school day (180 days; 7 hours/day)

From *The State of America's Children Yearbook 2000,* by Children's Defense Fund, 2000, Washington, DC: Author. Reprinted with permission.

---

surance Program (SCHIP), created under Title XXI of the Social Security Act of 1997, was established as a partnership between the federal and state governments to provide children the health insurance coverage they need. The program is meant to expand health coverage to uninsured children whose families earn too much to qualify for Medicaid but too little to afford private health insurance coverage. Most states provide coverage for children in families at or above 200% of the poverty level ($17,050 for a family of four in 2000) (USDHHS, 2001). The success of the program is measured by the fact that more than 90% of the improvement in children's health insurance coverage between 1998 and 1999 occurred among children in the lower income group (CDF, 2000b).

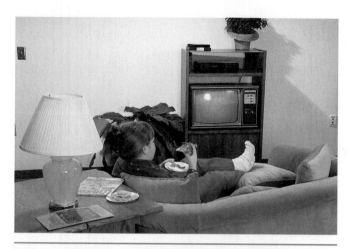

What suggestions might you offer to parents to encourage physical activity on the part of their child?

Immigration Status

Currently one in five children in the United States under the age of 18 (14 million) is either an immigrant or a member of an immigrant family (CDF, 2000a). Immigrant children face many challenges not only related to their health status but also in school because they frequently have difficulty speaking English. The health status of immigrant children is compromised due to intestinal parasites, poor diets, dental problems, anemia, hypertension, orthopedic problems, or other conditions originating in their country of origin (Gavagen & Brodyaga, 1996). They are also at risk because of significant language, cultural, and legal barriers in receiving health care.

THEORETICAL AND APPLIED PRINCIPLES OF CARING

Concepts related to caring, the family, and human development provide the framework for community health nursing practice in the care of individuals and families. The characteristics of an environment that supports health and healing (Chapter 9) also supports normal developmental processes of children. These characteristics—including safety, respect, nurturance, order, and beauty—reflect caring on the part of those responsible for children (Schubert & Lionberger, 1995). When children live in a caring environment, they are more apt to fulfill their potential as adults (see Chapter 9).

Family-Centered Nursing Perspectives

Family-centered nursing practice is based on the perspective that the family is the basic unit of care for its individual members and for the unit as a whole. In addi-

---

※ DECISION MAKING

Family-Centered Nursing Practice in the Community

Imagine that you are a home health nurse who has been referred to an eight-year-old boy with asthma. He is an African American child living in subsidized housing, a government-owned complex for urban poor in a large city. His mother died from asthma six months ago, and he does not want to take his medicine because of his wish to die and be with his mother. He is living with his grandmother and several other family members—adults and children. He receives medical care at a large university medical center. Consider the following questions and determine whether you would interview the child, family members, or health workers in the community.

◆ Who would you interview to gather data and identify problems?

◆ Who would you interview to assess the child's problem?

◆ With whom would you talk in formulating a plan for intervention?

◆ With whom would you communicate in evaluating the intervention outcomes?

---

tion, the family is seen as the basic unit of the community and of society, representing all of human diversity—cultural, racial, ethnic, and socioeconomic. Application of family theory involves consideration of social, economic, political, and cultural factors when conducting health assessments and planning, implementing, and evaluating care of children and families. Although family developmental theory and family functioning are not explored in detail until Chapters 24 and 25, this chapter assumes that the family provides the context for the care of infants, children, and adolescents. Family-centered nursing practice also acknowledges the role of the community, including community agencies and institutions that support and nurture children and their families (Hanson, 2001; Friedman, 1998).

Developmental Processes

The study of **human development** involves the search for principles that address patterned, orderly changes in structure, thought, and behavior over the life span. These changes evolve via an integration of physiological char-

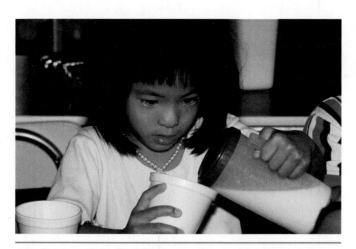

It is imperative that the nurse have a strong background in human development in order to recognize developmental delays and teach developmentally appropriate care.

acteristics; environmental forces; psychological mechanisms such as perception of self, others, and the environment; and acquired coping behaviors (Duvall & Miller, 1984). Developmental processes are influenced by **growth** (increase in body size or changes in body structure and function) and **maturation** (the emergence of genetic potential for changes in physical and mental patterns) (Potts & Mandleco, 2002).

Community health nurses need strong foundational knowledge in human development in order to guide and teach parents and family members to give children developmentally appropriate care. A brief overview of the principles related to developmental theory is presented in Figure 22-3.

The major theories related to childhood and adolescent development are summarized in Table 22-1 (Potts & Mandleco, 2002). The theorists identified in this table cite psychosexual, psychosocial, cognitive, and moral judgment as the areas of concern during the stages of child development. Developmental theories provide tools for understanding child behavior patterns.

The early life of the person is usually divided into periods according to chronological age: the prenatal period (from the moment of conception to birth), infancy (birth–1 year), toddlerhood (1–3 years), preschool (3–6 years), school age (6–12 years), and adolescence (13–20 years). Although somewhat arbitrary, these divisions serve as aids to understanding patterns that apply to most people most of the time (Murray & Zentner, 2001) and thus to understanding normal development.

FIGURE 22-3 Basic Assumptions of Developmental Theory

- Childhood is the foundational period of life; the first five years determine, to a large extent, attitudes, habits, patterns of behavior and thinking, personality traits, and health status.

- Development follows a definable, predictable, and sequential pattern and occurs continually through adulthood, but with individual differences related to the integration of many maturational factors.

- Growth and development are continuous, although a person may appear to stay in one place or regress developmentally.

- Growth is usually accompanied by behavior change, although certain traits may remain with certain adaptations related to maturation..

- Behavior has purpose and is goal directed.

- When one need or goal is met, a person has energy to pursue another need, interest, or goal.

- Critical periods in human development occur as specific organs and other aspects of a person's physical and psychosocial growth are undergoing rapid changes and the capacity for adaptation to stress is weak.

- Mastering developmental tasks of one period is the basis for mastering those of the next developmental period, both physically and emotionally.

- Progressive differentiation of the self from the environment results from increasing self-knowledge and autonomy.

- The developing person simultaneously acquires competencies in four major areas: physical, cognitive, emotional, and social.

- Readiness and motivation are essential to learning. Hunger, fatigue, illness, pain, and lack of emotional feedback or opportunity to explore inhibit readiness and reduce motivation.

- Many factors contribute to the formation of permanent characteristics and traits—genetic inheritance, undetermined prenatal environmental factors, family and society during infancy and childhood, nutrition, physical and emotional environments, and degree of intellectual stimulation in the environment.

- The young child achieves increasing ability to regulate behavior, to think and act in an individual and unique way, and to become more autonomous.

TABLE 22-1 Comparison of Stage Theories of Human Development

AGE PERIOD	FREUD	ERIKSON	PIAGET	KOHLBERG
Infancy (birth–1 year)	**Oral:** receives satisfaction from oral needs being met; attachment to mother important (birth–1 year)	**Trust/Mistrust:** learns world is good and can be trusted as basic needs are met (birth–1½ years)	**Sensorimotor:** *reflexive:* predictable, innate survival reflexes; *primary, secondary, circular reactions:* responds purposefully, repeats satisfying behaviors, develops object permanence, differentiates familiar (birth–12 months)	**Preconventional:** *premoral:* cannot differentiate right from wrong (birth–2 years)
Toddler (1–3 years)	**Anal:** learns to control body functions, especially toileting (1–3 years)	**Trust/Mistrust** (continued) **Autonomy/Shame-Doubt:** learns independent behaviors regarding toileting, bathing, feeding, dressing; exerts self; exercises choices (1½ years–3 years)	**Sensorimotor** (continued) *Tertiary circular reactions:* understands causality; *mental combinations:* simple problem solving, imitation of others. **Preoperational:** *preconceptual:* egocentric thought; mental imagery; increasing language (1–4 years)	**Preconventional** (continued) *Punishment/obedience orientation:* conformity based on fear of punishment (2–3 years)
Preschool (3–6 years)	**Phallic:** learning to control body functions, especially toileting (3–6 years)	**Initiative/Guilt:** goal directed, competitive, exploratory behavior; imaginative play (3–6 years)	**Preoperational** (continued) *Intuitive:* sophisticated language; decreasing egocentric thought; reality-based play (4–7 years)	**Preconventional** (continued) *Instrumental realistic orientation:* conforming behavior based on rewards (4–7 years)
School age (6–12 years)	**Latency:** sexual drives submerged; appropriate gender roles adopted; learning about society (6–12 years)	**Industry/Inferiority:** learns self-worth as gains mastery of psychosocial, physiological, and cognitive skills; becomes society/peer focused (6–12 years)	**Concrete Operations:** understands relationships, classification, conservation, seriation, reversibility; logical reasoning limited; less egocentric thought (7–11 years)	**Conventional:** *interpersonal concordance:* behavior evaluated on intent and other's reactions (7–10 years); *authority/social order maintaining orientation:* obeys out of respect for laws, authority (10–12 years)
Adolescence (12–19 years)	**Genital:** sexual drives submerged; appropriate gender roles adopted; learning about society (12 years and older)	**Identity/Role Confusion:** develops sense of who I am; gains independence from parents; peers important (12–18 years)	**Formal Operations:** capable of systematic, abstract thought (12–older)	**Postconventional:** *social contract/legalistic orientation:* believes laws should further human values and express majority views (12–adolescence); *universal ethical principles orientation:* right/wrong defined on universal, comprehensive, consistent, personal ethical principles. (adolescence–adulthood)

Adapted from Potts, N., & Mandleco, B. (2002). Pediatric nursing: Caring for children and their families. Clifton Park, NY: Delmar Learning.

FETAL DEVELOPMENT AND PRENATAL CARE PRIORITY

Certain events prior to and during the prenatal period are critical to the life of the child. These prenatal influences on development may be identified as normal inherited traits, parental age, prenatal endocrine and metabolic functions, maternal nutrition, **teratogenic effects** (environmental hazards to the fetus), maternal and fetal infections, immunological factors, maternal emotions, and birth defects transmitted by the parents (Murray & Zentner, 2001). The community health nurse may be involved in prevention related to all of these potential or real hazards by assessing, planning, intervening via counseling and/or teaching, and monitoring results. Certain prenatal influences determine risk and priority status for prenatal care.

Prenatal care helps to prevent problems related to childbirth, such as prematurity and **low birthweight (LBW)** (birthweight below 2500 grams). These events affect infant development in vital ways. In fact, a study of more than 4000 children discovered smaller than gestational age infants who may have been malnourished during fetal development had significantly less muscle mass than average gestational age infants. This reduced muscularity could cause delayed motor development in infancy and later in life put them at risk for higher percentage of body fat and impaired glucose tolerance, a prediabetic condition (American Academy of Pediatrics [AAP], 1998).

Given this information, it is easy to see that women who receive prenatal care beginning in the first trimester have more positive **pregnancy outcomes** (health status of mother and infant at birth) than do women who have late or no prenatal care. Lack of prenatal care exacts a high price, both economically and in human terms.

REFLECTIVE THINKING

The High Cost of Prenatal Care

- Imagine that you are a community health nurse in a health center funded by state and federal monies. The budget for public health services is being reviewed, and preventive services are being threatened. You are asked to testify at a hearing and justify prenatal care expenditures in your area. Present your position and your arguments for continuing to provide prenatal services to those who do not have health care insurance and cannot afford private payment.

Prenatal care consists of three basic components: early and continued risk assessment, health promotion, and medical and psychosocial evaluation, care, and follow-up. The **prenatal risk assessment** includes a complete history, a physical examination, laboratory tests, and fetal assessment to determine whether any factors place the pregnancy in jeopardy. **Health promotion** consists of counseling to promote and support healthful behaviors and of prenatal and parenting education. Interventions might address behavior modification related to nutrition; substances to avoid, such as alcohol and other drugs, tobacco, and pesticides; treatment for any existing illness such as diabetes; and referral to community services and resources, both social and financial.

Medically Related Risk Factors

Most women experience pregnancy with few complications to themselves or their infants. For some women, however, pregnancy holds serious risks. These risks may be related to maternal age (adolescents and women over age 35), preexisting medical conditions, socioeconomic status that contributes to poor general health and lack of access to care, or the pregnancy itself. These women are at greatest need of early intervention and continued assessment during pregnancy.

Diabetes Mellitus

During normal pregnancy, endocrine and metabolic adjustments, especially those related to the pituitary, adrenal cortex, and thyroid, occur and affect the developing fetus (Pillitteri, 1999). Related conditions such as diabetes mellitus may exist prior to pregnancy or may develop during pregnancy (gestational diabetes). Either form of diabetes can jeopardize the health of mother and baby if proper diet, exercise, and insulin levels are not maintained. Infants of diabetic mothers (IDM) tend to be large (9 lb or more), and deliveries are often complicated by hypoglycemia, hyperbilirubinemia, and respiratory distress. The community health nurse can help clients avoid these problems by providing continued screening, education, and counseling during pregnancy.

Reproductive History

A woman's reproductive history often helps identify potential risks of pregnancy and can be categorized according to obstetrical history, medical history, and current obstetrical status (Pillitteri, 1999). Specifically, mothers are considered at risk if they have had a pregnancy within the last year, in the past have delivered a low-birthweight infant, had a previous multiple pregnancy, have a history of cardiac, metabolic, or renal disease, had inadequate prenatal care, are over- or underweight, or have any reproductive abnormality (Pillitteri, 1999).

Maternal Infections

Infections during pregnancy can have a major impact on maternal and infant health. Cytomegalovirus (CMV), HIV, syphilis, *Chlamydia trachomatis,* gonorrhea, herpes simplex, rubella, rubeola, mumps, smallpox, viral hepatitis, and toxoplasmosis are among those infections that can have detrimental effects on pregnancy outcomes. The community health nurse has a key role in the screening, counseling, immunization, and/or treatment related to these infections and, thus, in reducing the associated risks to both mother and fetus (Murray & Zentner, 2001).

Pregnancy-Induced Hypertension

Formerly called toxemia, pregnancy-induced hypertension can lead to organ damage in and even death of the mother and impaired development of the fetus. **Pregnancy-induced hypertension (PIH)** is a multisystem disorder characterized by hypertension, proteinuria, and edema. Unless treated, PIH can lead to preeclampsia in the third trimester. Pregnancy-induced hypertension occurs more commonly in primiparas older than 40 or younger than 20 years of age and in women who have had five or more pregnancies or are from a low socioeconomic background. It is also seen more frequently in women who have an underlying disease (diabetes, cardiac disease, essential hypertension), are not Caucasian, have had previous multiple births, or have poor calcium or magnesium intake (Pillitteri, 1999). Women with preeclampsia require weekly monitoring and may need to be hospitalized for closer observation.

Fetal and Maternal Abnormalities

Poor pregnancy outcomes can also be caused by malposition, early separation of the placenta, or other placental abnormalities. The position and size of the fetus and the condition of the cervix are variables to consider when assessing for possible complications in delivery.

Psychosocial Factors and Health Behavior

Psychosocial risk factors include socioeconomic status, psychological factors, and unhealthy lifestyle. Low socioeconomic status is linked directly with poor health, including increased maternal and infant morbidity and mortality. Crowded, often unsafe and unsanitary living conditions, inadequate nutrition, and limited access to health care all have negative effects on the expectant family. Psychological factors that may affect both the mother's understanding of and attitude about her pregnancy and the mother's health-seeking and parenting behaviors include high stress levels, low self-esteem, emotional instability, and domestic violence.

Maternal Stress

Current research indicates that the fetus is affected by maternal stress, although the effects of maternal elation, fear, and anxiety on the behavior and other developmental aspects of the baby are poorly understood (Murray & Zentner, 2001). Folklore has long indicated a link between maternal stress and infant health, but research in this area is quite recent.

Maternal Nutrition

Maternal nutrition is an extremely important variable in fetal health and prevention of complications. Approximately 60 nutrients are known to influence fetal health, and a lack of these nutrients may depress appetite, encourage disease, and retard growth and development, including causing mental retardation (Murray & Zentner, 2001).

Cigarette Smoking

Nicotine is an environmental hazard for the developing fetus and has been associated with premature birth, low birthweight, delayed mental and physical development, and spontaneous abortion (Murray & Zentner, 2001). The

---

✴ DECISION MAKING

Prenatal Nutritional Care

You have been referred to the home of a 20-year-old Caucasian woman who is three months pregnant by her boyfriend. The boyfriend comes around from time to time, but the woman does not know where he goes or what he does at other times. She has a sister living in a neighboring town, but they do not see each other because neither of them has transportation. She works part time at a fast-food restaurant down the street. She receives slightly above minimum wage and is barely able to pay her rent. She gets some food at the restaurant, and her boyfriend buys a few groceries when he is around. She says she is okay because she really does not feel like eating that much. You must make a care plan and decide the immediate focus of attention. Should you:

◆ Provide nutritional counseling and teaching?

◆ Refer her to available resources in the community for food stamps and services?

◆ Ask to include the father of the baby in the planning?

◆ Give her materials and teach her about prenatal growth and development?

Prioritize your selections and provide a rationale.

more the woman smokes, the greater the risk of harm to the fetus. Thus, smoking cessation programs take on new importance during pregnancy. Because **secondhand smoke** (passive smoking) is also known to be harmful to the developing fetus, the pregnant woman should also avoid situations where others are smoking.

Substance Abuse

Pregnant women should avoid alcohol during pregnancy in order to prevent fetal alcohol syndrome, a cluster of permanent birth defects that include mental retardation, delayed motor function, low birthweight, and craniofacial abnormalities. Use of opiates and other psychoactive drugs during pregnancy can lead to addiction in the infant and poor parenting behaviors in the mother. Many drugs used by prescription for medicinal purposes also create environmental hazards for the fetus and should be evaluated carefully for their potential for causing developmental problems (Murray & Zentner, 2001).

Environmental Hazards

Environmental hazards including radiation, chemical waste, contaminated water, heavy metals such as lead and mercury, some food additives, and various pollutants have teratogenic effects, adversely affecting the genetic structure of the fetus and causing developmental abnormalities (Murray & Zentner, 2001). (See Chapter 9 for a discussion of the role of the community health nurse in relation to environmental health issues.)

INDICATORS OF INFANT AND CHILD HEALTH STATUS

Community health nurses play an important role in the prevention of infant mortality and morbidity. By assessing and counseling pregnant women and referring them to perinatal resources for care and education, community health nurses help ensure positive pregnancy outcomes. By monitoring and referring infants to pediatric care, these nurses help improve the health of children. Because they serve as assessment tools for program planning of primary, secondary, and tertiary prevention services, various statistical indicators of child health in the community aggregate of concern are watched carefully. These indicators include the infant mortality rate of the aggregate and both individual and aggregate assessment related to the incidence of low-birthweight infants, nutritional health status, and immunization status.

Infant Mortality Rate

The **infant mortality rate** is the number of infant deaths during the first year of life per 1000 live births. This rate is used as a measure of community and national health status. Compared with other developed countries, the United States ranked 25th in the world in terms of infant

mortality (National Center for Health Statistics [NCHS], 1999). In 1997, the infant mortality rate in the United States reached a record low of 7.2 per 1000 live births (USDHHS, 2000a). This rate is higher among communities of color and among the poor, however. The differences are believed to be related more to socioeconomic status than to ethnicity. The goal of *Healthy People 2010* is to reduce the infant mortality rate to no more than 7 per 1000 live births (USDHHS, 2000a).

Low Birthweight and Child Health

Because they are more likely to die during the first year of life, premature infants and those having low birthweights contribute significantly to infant mortality and morbidity. They are also at risk for long-term health problems such as cerebral palsy, mental retardation, developmental delays, learning disabilities, attention-deficit disorder, and/or sensory deficits (Potts & Mandleco, 2002).

Low-birthweight and **very low birthweight** (less than 1500 grams) survival rates have increased recently as a result of medical and technological advances in respiratory medicine. In 1998, approximately 7.6% of all babies in the United States had low birthweight, and 1.4% had very low birthweight. The incidence of low birthweight is nearly twice as high among African Americans: Approximately 13% of African American infants had low birthweight, and 3.1% had very low birthweight (USDHHS, 2000a). The *Healthy People 2010* goal is to reduce the incidence of low birthweight by 28%, to no more than 5 per 1000 (USDHHS, 2000a).

NUTRITIONAL NEEDS AND CHILD/ADOLESCENT HEALTH

Nutritional status is a very important aspect of nursing assessment in the care of infants, children, and adolescents. Needs change as the child grows, but the need for good nutrition remains constant. Nutrition is the key to maximizing child health and development. Beginning with the preconceptional period, sound dietary habits are important in establishing lifelong health patterns. Nutrition is influenced by socioeconomic, cultural, racial, and ethnic factors, as well as by individual and family food preferences. All of these factors must be considered when assessing child and family nutritional status.

Assessing a child's nutritional status involves obtaining a 24-hour dietary recall, taking comprehensive histories, and measuring height and weight. In adolescents, it is important to evaluate lifestyle and food preferences. The community health nurse may refer the client and family for nutritional and medical follow-up; counsel and educate about nutritional requirements related to specific stages of child development; and screen for nutritional disorders such as failure to thrive, lactose intolerance, obesity, anorexia, bulimia, hypertension, and cardiovascular disease. Table 22-2 summarizes physical signs of health and malnutrition.

TABLE 22-2 Physical Signs of Health and Malnutrition

	HEALTHY	MALNOURISHED
Hair	Shiny; firm in the scalp	Dull, brittle, dry, loose; falls out
Eyes	Bright, clear-pink membranes; adjust easily to darkness	Pale membranes; spots; redness; adjust slowly to darkness
Teeth/gums	No pain or cavities; gums firm; teeth bright	Missing, discolored, decayed teeth; gums bleed easily and are swollen and spongy
Face	Good complexion	Off-color, scaly, flaky, cracked skin
Glands	No lumps	Swollen at front of neck and cheeks
Tongue	Red, bumpy, rough	Sore, smooth, purplish, swollen
Skin	Smooth, firm, good color	Dry, rough, spotty; "sandpaper" feel or sores; lack of fat under skin
Nails	Firm, pink	Spoon shaped; brittle; ridged
Behavior	Alert, attentive, cheerful	Irritable, apathetic, inattentive, hyperactive
Internal systems	Heart rate, heart rhythm, and blood pressure normal; normal digestive function; reflex and psychological development normal	Heart rate, heart rhythm, or blood pressure abnormal; liver and spleen enlarged; abnormal digestion; mental irritability, confusion; burning tingling of hands and feet; loss of balance and coordination
Muscles/bones	Good muscle tone and posture; straight long bones	"Wasted" appearance of muscles; swollen bumps on skull or ends of bones; small bumps on ribs; bowed legs or knock-knees

Note: The physical signs noted here are consistent with but not diagnostic of malnutrition.
From Understanding Nutrition *(7th ed.), by E. N. Whitney and S. R. Rolfes, 1996, St. Paul, MN: West. Reprinted with permission of Wadsworth Publishing Co.*

Infant Nutrition

The first year of life is characterized by rapid growth and development, with the birthweight typically doubling in the first six months and tripling by the end of the first year (Potts & Mandleco, 2002). Such rapid growth requires increased protein and calories. Breast milk serves as the ideal source of nutrients and energy for the first four to six months. When the mother chooses not to breastfeed, commercial formulas constitute a reasonable alternative. Breast milk also contains important antibodies against infections that enter through the gastrointestinal tract. Breastfed infants have fewer infections and allergic reactions than do formula-fed infants. Breastfeeding offers many other advantages including promotion of maternal-infant attachment, more rapid involution of the uterus and return to prepregnancy weight, and lower cost. If the mother's own nutritional status is compromised, however, her ability to produce milk with the appropriate nutritional content may be impaired. Women who consume alcohol, caffeine, nicotine, or psychotherapeutic drugs must be informed that those substances are transmitted in breast milk.

The addition of semisolid foods to the infant's diet at four to six months of age and of finger foods in the lat-

ter part of the first year provides the nutrients essential to growth, oral, and fine motor development (Table 22-3). Healthy full-term infants who are fed on demand tend to regulate their intake appropriately for growth and development and establish their own feeding schedules (Potts & Mandleco, 2002).

Although total energy requirements (kilocalories per day) increase during the first year, energy requirements

TABLE 22-3 Guide for Introduction of Solids

AGE	FOOD	FREQUENCY
4–6 months	Cereal	Twice a day
6–8 months	Vegetables	Once a day
	Fruits	Twice a day
	Juices	Between meals
8–10 months	Meats	Once a day
10 months	Egg yolks	Once a day
9–12 months	Finger foods	At least daily

From Potts, N. & Mandleco, B. (2002). Pediatric nursing: Caring for children and their families. Clifton Park, NY: Delmar Learning.

per unit of body weight decline in response to changes in growth rate. The recommended energy intake drops from 120 to 100 kcal/kg by the first year of age (Potts & Mandleco, 2002).

The most common nutritional problem in infants is iron deficiency anemia. Others are colic, diarrhea, allergies, cow's milk protein-induced intestinal injury, regurgitation, nursing bottle-mouth syndrome, constipation, and burns to the mouth because of formula that is too warm (Lutz & Przytulski, 1997; Stanfield, 1997). Most of these situations can be treated by supplements, varying the diet (amount and type) and parent education (Potts & Mandleco, 2002).

Infant Nutritional Problems

The infant may suffer nutritional deficits because of the presence of socioeconomic risk factors such as low income, low educational level of the parent, and poor food supply. Infants may also be affected by the behavioral choices of the parent, especially health knowledge and lifestyle choices. Biological risk factors such as prematurity or low birthweight put the infant, with immature immune and gastrointestinal systems, at higher risk. When infants demonstrate a loss of weight, delay in development, signs of malnourishment, or failure to thrive (FTT), the root of the problem may be a nutritional deficit. The nutrition of an infant is essential to survival. In the home setting, the nurse, family, and neighbors have the opportunity to make observations that are critical to the survival of the infant. Identification of any of the above problems requires intervention.

The cause of a nutritional deficit may vary from a single reason such as a lack of income in the family to a cluster of causes as in the case of, for example, a low-income, first-time, teen parent who is abusing substances. The community health nurse working with infants needs to have a working knowledge of normal growth and development. Working with that framework, the nurse has the opportunity to intervene in a variety of ways. The more common nursing interventions are parent education about infant nutrition, encouragement of parent participation in parenting classes, and postnatal home visits.

Toddler and Preschooler Nutrition

From infancy to toddlerhood, the appetite decreases. The toddler requires small portions of food, particularly nutritious finger foods. Table 22-4 summarizes a recommended food pattern for adequate toddler and preschooler nutrition.

The preschooler continues to require small portions of food; however, a greater variety of food sources may be required. It is essential that parents offer a wide variety of food sources to promote adequate development throughout this phase. Parents also must set a good example by eating an appropriate diet themselves.

Nutrition of School-Age Children

School-age children grow more slowly than do infants and toddlers, and they eat less in proportion to their size. By the time children reach school age, their eating patterns are generally established. Because snacking is common, especially after school, nutritious snacks are important. To meet the needs of children from low-income families, many school lunch programs have been expanded to include breakfast.

Food choices of school-age children are heavily influenced by their peers. Although school-age children

---

TABLE 22-4 Food Plan for Preschool and School-Age Children Based on the Food Guide Pyramid

FOOD GROUP	NUMBER OF SERVINGS	APPROXIMATE SERVING SIZE*			
		AGE 1–2	AGE 3–4	AGE 5–6	AGE 7–12
Milk, yogurt, and cheese	3	½–¾ cup or 1 oz	¾ cup or 1½ oz	1 cup or 2 oz	1 cup or 2 oz
Meat, poultry, fish, dry beans, eggs, and nuts	2 or more	1 oz or 1–2 tbsp	1½ oz or 3–4 tbsp	1½ oz or ½ cup	2 oz or ½ cup
Vegetables	3 or more	1–2 tbsp	3–4 tbsp	½ cup	½ cup
Fruits	2 or more	1–2 tbsp or ½ cup juice	3–4 tbsp or ½ cup juice	½ cup or ½ cup juice	½ cup or ½ cup juice
Bread, cereal, rice, and pasta	6 or more	½ slice or ½ cup	1 slice or ½ cup	1 slice or ¾ cup	1 slice or ¾ cup

From Townsend, C., and Roth, R. (2000). Nutrition and Diet Therapy. *Albany, NY: Delmar.*

*Use as a starting point. Increase serving size as energy yields dictate, but maintain variety in the diet by making sure all food groups are still appropriately represented.

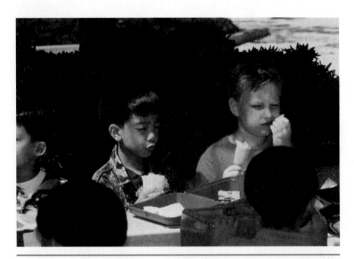

Children base their food preferences on what tastes good rather than on nutritional value. Many of children's favorite foods contain too much salt.

FIGURE 22-4 Facts about the School Lunch Program (NSLP)

1. Established in 1946

2. Federally assisted meal program

3. Provides nutritionally balanced, low-cost or free lunches

4. Serves more than 96,000 public and nonprofit private schools and residential child care institutions

5. Children from families with incomes at or below 130% of the poverty level are eligible for free meals; those between 130% and 185% of poverty level charged no more than 40 cents

From *School Lunch Program Fact Sheet*. [On-line]. Available: http://www.fns.usda.gov/cnd/lunch/about/lunch.

gradually increase the amount of food they eat, the range of foods they accept may be small. Sugar contributes approximately one-fourth of the calories in the average school-age child's diet. Milk, sweetened soft drinks, fruits, fruit juice, and desserts also contribute a great many calories.

Childhood Nutritional Problems

Children are at greatest risk for nutritional deficits because of socioeconomic risk factors, particularly poverty. According to Food Research and Action Center (FRAC, 1998), 59% of all children under age 6 living in a single-parent female-headed household live in poverty. Poor children are typically affected by a cluster of risk factors such as limited food supply, limited food access, parental factors of limited education, unhealthy lifestyle choices, lack of health information and access, and their own poor school performance.

Poor nutritional status is more prevalent in lower socioeconomic groups because of the limited amount and variety of food available. Children with poor nutritional status are frequently hungry. Children who are hungry suffer from unwanted weight loss, fatigue, headaches, increased school absences, poor school performance, and increased illnesses. They frequently have a low intake of iron, zinc, and protein. These children suffer from anemia, which increases their risk for infections and chronic illnesses. In fact, children who are hungry suffer two to four times more health problems than children who are not hungry (FRAC, 1998, p. 4), including slowed growth and development, stunting of height, and decreased protein intake. See Figure 22-4 for information on school lunch programs.

As for infants, the definitive screening criteria for children for nutritional problems are growth and development and maintenance of weight. School-age children have the added screening criterion of school performance. Being underweight or overweight can place a child

at risk for a nutritional or health problem. According to Bronner (1996), obesity can put a child at risk for atherosclerosis, non-insulin-dependent diabetes (NIDDM), hypertension (HTN), and gallbladder disease in adult years. It is estimated that 14% of children are obese. Obesity will be discussed in the section on middle adulthood.

Adolescent Nutrition

Adolescence is a time of rapid physical growth as muscle mass, weight, and height increase. These physical changes mean increased requirements related to nutritional needs, especially calories, proteins, and minerals (calcium, zinc, and iron). Calcium is needed to meet skeletal growth requirements, prevent fractures, and help prevent osteoporosis later (Committee on Nutrition, 1999). Zinc is necessary for final body growth and sexual maturation. Iron intake should be increased to meet normally expanding blood volume need and the increase in lean body mass and to replace iron lost through menstruation. Iron requirements increase to as much as 2.2 mg/day and are associated with the size and timing of the growth spurt, sexual maturation, and menses (Beard, 2000). Males will need more calories than females, especially if they are involved in athletics. Typically female requirements are around 2000 calories per day; males will need from 2500 to 3000 calories per day. Protein needs also increase. Recommended allowances for females range from 44 to 46 grams per day and for males from 45 to 59 grams per day (Committee on Dietary Allowances, 1989).

Adolescents always seem hungry but often do not eat appropriate, well-balanced meals. Instead, they prefer snack foods that are easy to prepare, faddish, and often full of empty calories. Adolescent food habits are influenced by concerns of their body image, peer pressure, emotional problems, busy schedules, or unsupervised meal preparation/purchase. It is not uncommon for teenagers to also often skip meals (breakfast being the most common), eat fast foods, or frequently snack. Therefore, nurses can help parents and adolescents improve their nutrition by explaining the importance of a good diet and encouraging adolescents to be involved in meal planning. Parents also need to realize that adolescents' need for freedom, independence, and peer acceptance may be reflected in their eating habits. If nutritious foods and snacks are available (milk, cheese, yogurt, fruits, vegetables, juices), adolescents are allowed to regularly be responsible for preparing family meals, and food preferences (hamburgers, pizza, burritos) are integrated into meal plans, conflicts around nutritional concerns may decrease. Adolescents and their parents also need to be aware of the recommended dietary allowances and know which foods are high in calcium (milk and milk products), iron (green vegetables, meats), and zinc (milk, meat, fish, eggs). Adolescents should also receive information about nutritious snacks and fast foods available in restaurants (salads, pasta, grilled meats, vegetables, fruits).

All health screening visits for adolescents need to include height and weight measurements as well as questions about eating habits, including dieting, changes in weight, meal patterns, and consumption of empty-calorie, high-fat, high-salt foods. Nutritional evaluations should also include information regarding the family cultural preferences related to food, whether or not there are psychological or psychosocial problems present that affect eating, and whether or not nutritional requirements are understood or being met.

At least three issues related to nutrition may surface during the nutritional assessment: obesity, anorexia nervosa, and bulimia nervosa. Obesity is one of the most serious health problems facing today's children/adolescents. The 1999 Youth Risk Behavior Surveillance (Centers for Disease Control and Prevention [CDC], 2000a) reports 6.8% of Caucasian females and 11.5% of Caucasian males are overweight, whereas 12.8% of African American females and 9.7% of Hispanic females are overweight, and 11.1% of African American males and 15% of Hispanic males are overweight. The rate of obesity is increasing (Birch & Fisher, 1998), and children/adolescents of obese parents are at greater risk of developing obesity than children/adolescents whose parents are thin.

Body mass index (BMI) is the most appropriate indicator of obesity in adolescence because it is precise, readily available in many settings, and reflects weight status based on height and weight rather than on skin fold thickness or measures of adiposity (Cole, 1991). Today, a BMI at the 95th percentile is used to define an adolescent as being overweight (Himes & Dietz, 1994; Troiano, Flegal, Kuczmarski, Campbell, & Johnson, 1995). However, adolescents between the 85th and 95th percentile are considered at risk of becoming overweight (Himes & Dietz, 1994) and should be involved in intervention programs.

Obesity, a complex disease with genetic, behavioral, environmental, and metabolic determinants (Birch & Fisher, 1998; Rosenbaum & Leibel, 1998), occurs when there is an imbalance between energy expenditure and intake. Even though genetics influences energy balance, one's environment also contributes to the situation since the genetic composition of the population changes slower than the rate of obesity (Rosenbaum & Leibel, 1998). Genes and the environment, however, are related because parents usually provide not only a child's genetics but also the child's environment.

Three major environmental factors are thought to be related to genetics and contribute to rising obesity rates: (1) declining amounts of work-related and spontaneous physical activity, (2) increases in the consumption of energy-dense, high-fat foods (Hill & Trowbridge, 1998), and (3) the home environment itself (Strauss & Knight, 1999).

Children today are more sedentary when compared to children a generation ago. In fact, today, about 25% of children do not participate in any regular physical activity, girls participate less than boys, and as one gets older, physical activity actually decreases (USDHHS, 1997). One reason for this decline in physical activity may be that mandatory physical education classes are decreasing in schools as children get older, perhaps due to budget cuts, and television, computer games/use, and video games are popular with young people (Berkey et al., 2000).

Second, children are also consuming diets promoting obesity (high fat, low in fruits/vegetables and complex carbohydrates). High-fat foods tend to be palatable, less satiating, higher in total energy, and of smaller volume, leading to overconsumption (Berkey et al., 2000; Birch & Fisher, 1998; Troiano & Flegal, 1998). In addition, fruits, vegetables, and complex carbohydrates may not be popular with children/adolescents.

Finally, factors related to the home environment promote obesity in children and adolescents. These factors are parental obesity (more often maternal than paternal), low family income, lower levels of cognitive stimulation in the home, and parental occupation. Parental obesity is an important risk factor because of child-parent modeling and genetics. In fact, children from families where one parent is obese have a 40% risk of being obese as an adult. They have an 80% risk of being obese as an adult if both parents are obese (Behrman & Kliegman, 1998). Low family income may be related to obesity because of less healthy eating patterns, decreased activity, and an environment that provides high-fat foods and few fruits and vegetables (Kennedy & Powell, 1997). Lower levels of cognitive development may be related to obesity in children/adolescents because children raised in stimulating and interactive home environments may engage in less sedentary activities (television, video games) and more regular physical activity. Parental occupation is a factor if a parent's education is not used in the occupation or if the occupation is nonprofessional. All these factors are important independent of other socioeconomic factors, including race and caregiver marital status or education (Strauss & Knight, 1999).

Obesity in adolescence may also be connected to not being able or wanting to master the psychosocial and psychosexual tasks of adolescence. Overeating compensates as a regression tactic for self-satisfaction or as a coping mechanism for stress. The resulting obesity becomes yet another obstacle to overcome in achieving developmental milestones. Obesity can ward off pressures associated with puberty and societal expectations and, as long as an adolescent is obese, can repress emotional maturation. For some, obesity can be the reason for their disappointments and eating a method of coping that keeps them connected to their family. This dependence on food and family also interferes with the developmental tasks of separation and individuation. In addition, obesity can interfere with sexuality issues; excess weight protects the adolescent from unwanted sexual advances or attention. Obesity may also represent a way to bring embarrassment and shame to others (parents, family), a way of becoming larger than a person not liked (peer), or aggression directed at the self. It is not unusual for obese adolescents to dislike their own physical appearance, express admiration for thin people, and judge others in terms of their own weight. Psychological counseling as well as nutritional and activity counseling may help adolescents develop more mature methods of coping if their obesity is connected to psychosocial/psychosexual issues.

Childhood and adolescent obesity is a concern today because obese children and adolescents often become obese adults who are at increased risk for diabetes and other chronic diseases or cardiovascular problems. However, it is not uncommon for overweight or obese children and adolescents to also experience psychosocial and physiological effects related to their weight before reaching adulthood. Psychosocial effects include discrimination by others, low self-esteem that persists into adulthood, poor body image, social isolation, depression, and feelings of rejection. Adults may also have inappropriate behavioral expectations for obese and overweight adolescents because often they are early maturers and thought to be older than their chronological age (Behrman & Kliegman, 1998; Dietz, 1998; Hill & Trowbridge, 1998). The obese adolescent's sense of identity can also be affected by derogatory comments made by others, leading to guilt, shame, and consequent overeating, which results in more weight gain, more derogatory comments, and even more poor self-esteem, etc. The physiological effects of obesity during adolescence are listed in Table 22-5.

Categories of intervention for adolescent obesity include adolescent education regarding (1) decreasing time in sedentary activities, (2) increasing time in physical or recreational activity, and parent/adolescent education regarding (3) activity (active caregivers tend to encourage activity in their children) and (4) providing a nutritionally balanced, low-energy diet that is reduced in fat and increased in complex carbohydrates and contains fiber. These intervention categories can be implemented in the school, community, or home. Since the school, community, and home are connected, interventions should consider these sites concurrently.

TABLE 22-5 Obesity Effects: Adolescence	
SYSTEM	**EFFECT**
Cardiovascular	Hypertension, cardiac hypertrophy
Central nervous system	Pseudotumor cerebri
Metabolic	Type 2 diabetes, insulin resistance, hyperlipidemia, increased concentration of liver enzymes
Orthopedic	Blount disease, slipped epiphysis, advanced bone age, increased height
Psychosocial	Isolation, poor self-image, peer rejection, teasing
Reproductive	Early menarche, polycystic ovary disease
Respiratory	Sleep apnea, Pickwickian syndrome

From Potts, N., and Mandleco, B. (2002). Pediatric nursing: Caring for children and their families. Clifton Park, NY: Delmar Learning.

Schools could provide physical activity opportunities by revising or reconsidering current policies and programs regarding physical education classes (Hill & Trowbridge, 1998). Such interventions can provide not only the immediate effects of activity but also sustained effects by encouraging life-long patterns which do not focus exclusively on team-oriented sports and include moderately intense activities (Troiano & Flegal, 1998). School lunch programs could also provide reduced-fat options that contain fiber and have increased complex carbohydrates. Nutrition and diet classes specifically tailored to young people would also be important school offerings.

Communities could interact with school programs to provide opportunities for children and adolescents to be physically active after school and in the summer by providing youth soccer, baseball, basketball, volleyball, and football (Hill & Trowbridge, 1998). Community organizations and agencies concerned about health promotion could provide nutrition and exercise programs at convenient times and locations for busy adolescents and their families.

Families can receive education regarding activity, nutrition, and the role the family plays in prevention. Decreasing television time is important to emphasize because it is a sedentary activity related to weight gain. In fact, children who watch four or more hours of television have greater body fat and BMI than those who watch less (Anderson, Crespo, Bartlett, Cheskin, & Pratt, 1998). In addition, the largest share of advertisements during children's television programming is for food products (Williams, Achterberg, & Sylvester, 1995), most of which tend to be high in simple sugars (cereals) and fat, salt, and sugar (snack foods). Children tend to request foods advertised on television, thereby supporting the premise that repeated exposure fosters preferences (Birch & Fisher, 1998). Parents should be cautioned about the poor nutritional benefits of many foods advertised on television, limit the time children and adolescents engage in sedentary activities, and encourage physical activity.

In addition, parents need to foster healthy eating behaviors in their children and adolescents by making nutritious foods available and accessible that are low in fat and contain complex carbohydrates and fiber. Dietary management should consist of about a 30% calorie decrease in comparison to previous calorie intake by modifying meal patterns and portion size and reducing fat and total calories. Restrictive diets that are very low calorie or protein-modified fast food diets require close supervision and supplementation with vitamins, calcium, potassium, and magnesium. Caloric restriction, however, is not very successful with adolescents; teens like fast, easy results, and weight loss via calorie restriction may take time. Since eating is an important part of adolescent socialization, restricting certain foods or limiting calorie intake may affect interaction with peers (Murray & Zentner, 2001).

Altering food preferences is also important (Domel, Thomson, Davis, Baranowski, Leonard, & Baranowski, 1996). Food preferences are established by providing early exposure to healthy foods, which can influence decisions children and adolescents later make about food consumption; they tend to choose foods they have experienced and therefore prefer. Caregivers also need to be aware of how they interact with their children in the eating context or use food as a reward.

Stringent controls or power struggles in relation to determining what, when, and how much children eat provide few chances for self-control; can encourage preferences for high-fat, energy-dense foods; disrupt children's energy intake; and limit a child's acceptance of various foods (Birch & Fisher, 1998). Feeding practices that encourage or restrict certain food consumption may also decrease the child's ability to pay attention to internal signals of satiety and hunger as a way to adjust intake. In addition, controlling parenting styles can also impede the child's ability to develop self-regulatory behavior, especially when caregivers have problems regulating their own behavior, children demonstrate problems in self-regulation, and caregivers perceive their children to be at risk for developing problematic behavior (Johnson & Birch, 1994). Instead, they should promote behaviors that include moderation and limit consumption of dietary fat and sugar. Parents may also need to change their own nutrition and activity programs (Hill & Trowbridge, 1998) and food preferences if they want to change their child's behaviors on a long-term basis. Figure 22-5 provides suggestions on ways to help overweight and obese adolescents lose weight.

Mechanical methods of weight loss which are frequently advertised in popular magazines are other options

---

FIGURE 22-5 Helping Adolescents with Their Weight

1. Avoid purchasing empty calorie foods; remove empty calorie snack foods from home

2. Ask self before eating, "am I hungry?"

3. Make dining pleasurable

4. Eat only at mealtimes and at the table; avoid empty calorie snacks, reduce dietary intake at least 500 calories daily to lose 1 pound a week

5. Serve individual portions on smaller plates; avoid second helpings

6. Eat slowly by cutting food into small mouthfuls and putting eating utensils down between bites

7. Keep a food diary; examine for empty calories and to see if eating traditional food groups

8. Participate in regular exercise (walking, bicycle riding, swimming, etc)

9. Maintain attractive appearance and proper posture

10. Avoid using food as a reward

11. Praise, feel proud of small weight losses

From Potts, N., and Mandleco, B. (2002). *Pediatric nursing: Caring for children and their families*. Clifton Park, NY: Delmar Learning.

---

which can be used alone or in combination with diet and exercise programs. These methods include steam baths, sauna suits, spot reducers, and special exercise outfits. However, they offer only short-term weight loss. Use of appetite-suppressant drugs, a final treatment option, are typically reserved for adolescents who are severely obese. This treatment option should be managed by a physician or nurse practitioner. On a final note, it is uncommon for weight reduction plans to be successful with adolescents, even though many are used. A more realistic alternative goal for those who have difficulty losing weight and keeping it off may just be to not gain any additional weight.

Eating Disorders

Eating disorders are a complex combination of physical behaviors and psychological beliefs (Potts & Mandleco, 2002). Some experts believe that eating disorders occur because food is the only thing the teen can control in life (Waller, 1998). The disorders are believed to originate from a distorted self-image in which teens see themselves as overweight when in reality they are not (Potts & Mandleco, 2002). Eating disorders have a progressive nature. Usually the changes observed by friends, family, neighbors, or teachers indicate when the disorder becomes a health threat to the teen.

A teen is at greater risk of developing eating disorders in a setting where great emphasis is placed on appearance or weight. Teens involved in certain sports such as figure skating, ballet, gymnastics, or wrestling or teens in modeling are at risk. Use of amphetamines or cocaine to lose weight may increase the risk of an eating disorder. The three most common eating disorders in teens are anorexia nervosa, bulimia, and binge eating.

Anorexia Nervosa

The term **anorexia nervosa** denotes an abnormal fear of becoming obese, a distorted self-image, a persistent aversion to food, and a loss of 25% of normal body weight in a relatively short period of time. The course of anorexia is variable, and the mortality rate ranges from 3% to 10%. Some clients, however, recover completely after the initial episode, while others continue to gain and lose weight. A third group develops chronic disease, and of this group, 5% commit suicide (Steiner, 1998). The emotional, behavioral, and physical characteristics of anorexia are given in Table 22-6.

TABLE 22-6 Characteristics of Anorexia and Bulimia

TYPE	ANOREXIA NERVOSA	BULIMIA NERVOSA
Physical	• Amenorrhea • Lowered body temperature • Lowered potassium and chloride levels if vomiting • Thinning hair • Dry, flaking skin • Lowered pulse rate and blood pressure • Constipation • Insomnia • Lanugo (growth of downy body hair) • Dental caries and periodontal disease if person is vomiting • Broken, split fingernails and toenails • Significantly below ideal body weight (IBW)	• Chronic sinusitis • Swollen and infected glands in the neck and under the jaw • Chronically puffy skin under the eyes and ruptured blood vessels in the cheeks and face • Deterioration of dental enamel due to stomach acids • Gastritis, stomach ulcers, kidney damage, edema • Electrolyte imbalances • Low body weight
Behavioral	• Unusual eating habits: starving, bingeing, purging, food hoarding, and ritualized eating • Preoccupation with meal planning, shopping, and cooking for the entire family while not eating • Hyperactivity and excessive exercise • Chronic or excessive use of laxatives, diuretics, diet pills	• Isolation due to abnormal eating habits and affect • Excessive exercise and other ritualized behaviors • Chronic or excessive use of laxatives, diuretics, diet pills, and emetics • Extreme split between public self (competent, cohesive) and private self (chaotic, unhappy)
Emotional	• Low sense of self-worth: inferiority about IQ, personality, and appearance • Distorted thinking: "If I can't control my environment, at least I can control my body" • Low sense of self-control • High achievement from driven compulsive behaviors • Denial of hunger and delusions about food ingested • Isolation contributing to depression • Outward compliance toward others, alternating with temper tantrums	• Appears more independent and professionally successful than persons having anorexia, who act dependent and tend to be withdrawn • Extremely vulnerable to rejection, especially with men • More outgoing, socially adept, and sexually involved in relationships • Unrealistically high standards of performance and appearance and inability to relax or to savor experiences • More prone to serious personality disorders • Fear of loss of control and of getting fat • Dependence on others for self-esteem and validation

Bulimia Nervosa

Bulimia means "ox hunger." The word *nervosa* was added to the name because, as in anorexia, the person has a nervous fear of gaining weight. **Bulimia nervosa** is also called binge-purge syndrome. It is characterized by episodes of excessive food intake followed by periods of fasting and self-induced vomiting or laxative abuse. The physical characteristics are not as obvious as those of anorexia. It is less likely to be fatal than anorexia because the person is getting some nutrition. The lifetime prevalence of bulimia among women range from 1.1% to 4.2% (American Psychiatric Association, 2000). The emotional, behavioral, and physical characteristics of a person with bulimia are given in Table 22-6.

Binge Eating

Binge eating, or compulsive overeating, is habitual eating to excess due to an irresistible irrational impulse. It begins most commonly in the teen years. Overindulgence occurs at all social levels and is an increasing health risk. Binge episodes become an eating disorder when the eating is (1) more rapid than normal, (2) done until uncomfortably full, (3) done when the person is not hungry yet eats large amounts, (4) done alone because of the embarrassment of the volume consumed, and (5) the cause of feeling disgusted with oneself, depressed, or very guilty about eating (Edelstein, 1989). Recovery begins with meeting another recovered or recovering binge eater or with intervention by family, nurse, or physician. The nurse can play a pivotal role in facilitating this process.

The Community Health Nurse's Role in Identifying and Treating an Eating Disorder

Eating disorders can be identified by the community health nurse. The nurse, especially the school nurse, may be involved in community screening for eating disorders. The home health nurse may be involved in monitoring home nutrition of a client. An appropriate referral to a physician, treatment center, or psychiatric treatment center can be initiated by the community health nurse. The nurse can provide information to the family or client to facilitate the referral process. Eating disorders are typically treated over a long period of time by an interdisciplinary team. The treatment of eating disorders is not just a matter of education but a long process of uncovering the cause and building new coping skills for the client and family.

A good recovery program should evaluate the client's physical condition, nutritional habits, psychological problems and strengths, social situation, family relations, and school or work performance. Individual counseling provides a safe environment to express feelings that have been hidden. Group therapy helps develop new coping skills, socialization, and healthy interests. Family counseling helps educate and support the family to assist in the recovery process. Overeaters Anonymous is a resource for restoration of healthy eating habits modeled after the 12-step program of Alcoholics Anonymous.

Immunization Status

Immunization provides immunity, the ability to destroy a pathogen either actively or passively. Active immunity is produced as a result of the invasion of a pathogen: for example, the varicella zoster virus that causes chicken pox. The virus may invade through accidental transmission from one child to another or may be injected as a vaccine. Either way, active antibodies are developed and may last throughout the person's life span. Passive immunity, which occurs as a result of maternal transmission of antibodies across the placenta to the fetus, is temporary, lasting only several months.

Lack of knowledge and lack of access to care have resulted in increasing numbers of children not being vaccinated. The community health nurse has a major role in screening for infectious diseases, determining immunization status, and educating parents and caregivers about the need for routine immunizations, specific vaccines, and the side effects of same. The immunization schedule developed by the CDC (2001) is summarized in Figure 22-6.

Dental Health

Primary dentition begins when the first tooth erupts, usually at 6 months of age (normal range 4–12 months) and should be complete by 24–36 months of age. Late tooth eruption is usually not a cause for concern if the child is growing and developing normally. Permanent dentition

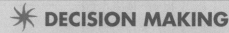

☀ DECISION MAKING

Serving Aggregates of Children in the Community

In your capacity as the community health nurse at a local clinic, you discover that only 10% of the infants enrolled in the clinic have been immunized.

◆ What key decisions must be made by clinic administration and staff in order to address the problem?

◆ What steps should be taken to address this problem?

◆ What other aspects of the data must be considered before any action can be taken?

◆ What clinic and community strategies might be needed?

◆ What role might community health nurses play in addressing the problem?

FIGURE 22-6 Recommended Childhood Immunization Schedule, United States, January–December 2001

Recommended Childhood Immunization Schedule
United States, 2002

Age → Vaccine ↓	Birth	1 mo	2 mo	4 mo	6 mo	12 mo	15 mo	18 mo	24 mos	4-6 yrs	11-12 yrs	13-18 yrs
Hepatitis B[1]	Hep B #1 only if mother HBsAg (−)		Hep B #2		Hep B #3						Hep B Series	
Diphtheria, Tetanus, Pertussis[2]			DTaP	DTaP	DTaP		DTaP	DTaP		DTaP	Td	
Haemophilus influensae Type b[3]			Hib	Hib	Hib	Hib						
Inactivated Polio[4]			IPV	IPV		IPV				IPV		
Measles, Mumps, Rubella[5]						MMR#1				MMR#2		MMR#2
Varicella[6]						Varicella				Varicella		
Pneumococcal[7]			PCV	PCV	PCV	PCV			PCV	PCV	PCV	
Hepatitis A[8]									Hepatitis A series			
Influenza[9]						Influenza (yearly)						

range of recommended ages *catch-up vaccination* *preadolescent assessment*

Vaccines below this line are for selected populations

This schedule indicates the recommended ages for routine administration of currently licensed childhood vaccines, as of December 1, 2001, for children through age 18 years. Any dose not given at the recommended age should be given at any subsequent visit when indicated and feasible. ▨ Indicates age groups that warrant special effort to administer those vaccines not previously given. Additional vaccines may be licensed and recommended during the year. Licensed combination vaccines may be used whenever any components of the combination are indicated and the vaccine's other components are not contraindicated. Providers should consult the manufacturer's package inserts for detailed recommendations.

1. **Hepatitis B vaccine (Hep B).** All infants should receive the first dose of hepatitis B vaccine soon after birth and before hospital discharge; the first dose may also be given by age 2 months if the infant's mother is HBsAg-negative. Only monovalent hepatitis B vaccine can be used for the birth dose. Monovalent or combination vaccine containing Hep B may be used to complete the series; four doses of vaccine may be administered if combination vaccine is used. The second dose should be given at least 4 weeks after the first dose, except for Hib-containing vaccine which cannot be administered before age 6 weeks. The third dose should be given at least 16 weeks after the first dose and at least 8 weeks after the second dose. The last dose in the vaccination series (third or fourth dose) should not be administered before age 6 months.

Infants born to HBsAg-positive mothers should receive hepatitis B vaccine and 0.5 mL hepatitis B immune globulin (HBIG) within 12 hours of birth at separate sites. The second dose is recommended at age 1–2 months and the vaccination series should be completed (third or fourth dose) at age 6 months.

Infants born to mothers whose HBsAg status is unknown should receive the first dose of the hepatitis B vaccine series within 12 hours of birth. Maternal blood should be drawn at the time of delivery to determine the mother's HBsAg status; if the HBsAg test is positive, the infant should receive HBIG as soon as possible (no later than age 1 week).

2. **Diphtheria and tetanus toxoids and acellular pertussis vaccine (DTaP).** The fourth dose of DTaP may be administered as early as age 12 months, provided 6 months have elapsed since the third dose and the child is unlikely to return at age 15–18 months. **Tetanus and diphtheria toxoids (Td)** is recommended at age 11–12 years if at least 5 years have elapsed since the last dose of tetanus and diphtheria toxoid-containing vaccine. Subsequent routine Td boosters are recommended every 10 years.

3. **Haemophilus influenzae type b (Hib) conjugate vaccine.** Three Hib conjugate vaccines are licensed for infant use. If PRP-OMP (PedvaxHIB® or ComVax® [Merck]) is administered at ages 2 and 4 months, a dose at 6 months is not required. DTaP/Hib combination products should not be used for primary immunization in infants at ages 2, 4 or 6 months, but can be used as boosters following any Hib vaccine.

4. **Inactivated polio vaccine (IPV).** An all-IPV schedule is recommended for routine childhood polio vaccination in the United States. All children should receive four doses of IPV at ages 2 months, 4 months, 6–18 months, and 4–6 years.

5. **Measles, mumps, and rubella vaccine (MMR).** The second dose of MMR is recommended routinely at age 4–6 years but may be administered during any visit, provided at least 4 weeks have elapsed since the first dose and that both doses are administered beginning at or after age 12 months. Those who have not previously received the second dose should complete the schedule by the 11–12 year old visit.

6. **Varicella vaccine.** Varicella vaccine is recommended at any visit at or after age 12 months for susceptible children, i.e., those who lack a reliable history of chickenpox. Susceptible persons aged ≥ 13 years should receive two doses, given at least 4 weeks apart.

7. **Pneumococcal vaccine.** The heptavalent **pneumococcal conjugate vaccine (PCV)** is recommended for all children age 2–23 months. It is also recommended for certain children age 24–59 months. Pneumococcal polysaccharide vaccine (PPV) is recommended in addition to PCV for certain high-risk groups. See *MMWR* 2000;49(RR-9); 1–35.

8. **Hepatitis A vaccine.** Hepatitis A vaccine is recommended for use in selected states and regions, and for certain high-risk groups; consult your local public health authority. See *MMWR* 1999;48(RR-12); 1–37.

9. **Influenza vaccine.** Influenza vaccine is recommended annually for children age ≥ 6 months with certain risk factors (including but not limited to asthma, cardiac disease, sickle cell disease, HIV, diabetes; see *MMWR* 2001;50(RR-4);1–44), and can be administered to all others wishing to obtain immunity. Children aged ≤ 12 years should receive vaccine in a dosage appropriate for their age (0.25 mL if age 6–35 months or 0.5 mL if aged ≥ 3 years). Children aged ≤ 8 years who are receiving influenza vaccine for the first time should receive two doses separated by at least 4 weeks.

For additional information about vaccines, vaccine supply, and contraindications for immunization, please visit the National Immunization Program Website at or call the National Immunization Hotline at 800-232-2522 (English) or 800-232-0233 (Spanish).

Approved by the Advisor Committee on Immunization Practices (*www.cdc.gov*), **the American Academy of Pediatrics** (*www.aap.org*), **and the American Academy of Family Physicians** (*www.aafp.org*).

From Centers for Disease Control and Prevention, Jan. 2001.

usually begins at 10–12 years of age. The American Academy of Pediatric Dentistry recommends all children have their first visit to the dentist by 12–18 months of age, and teaching parents about oral hygiene should begin during the infant's first year of life. During infancy, parents should wipe the teeth and gums with a damp wash cloth after feedings and introduce a soft tooth brush, moistened with water, after several teeth have erupted. Toothpaste can be introduced between 2 and 3 years of age, but parents should be cautioned to use only a small amount (pea-sized) to minimize ingestion of fluoride. Flossing can also be started when the child is 2–3 years of age. Parents should supervise or brush the child's teeth until the child is 8–10 years of age since children do not have the motor coordination to be effective before then (Grover, 2000).

Since fluoride is an effective prophylactic agent in preventing dental caries, the AAP recommends supplementation be started at 6 months of age and continued until the child is 16 years of age. Fluoride supplementation is based on the amount of fluoride in the drinking water, and the daily therapeutic dosage is 0.05–0.07 mg/kg/day (Grover, 2000).

Dental problems during childhood and adolescence include malocclusion, gingivitis, and dental trauma. Malocclusion occurs due to dental crowding or mandibular/facial bone growth changes. Usually, braces are needed to redirect facial/mandibular growth and correct tooth positioning. Gingivitis, the inflammation and consequent breakdown of the gingival epithelium, may be the result of ineffective cleaning, high-sugar/simple carbohydrate diets, or increased hormonal activity. The gums may bleed easily and appear swollen and pale. Treatment involves brushing the teeth at least two times a day by using a soft-bristled brush and fluoride toothpaste, flossing daily, eating a well-balanced diet, and regular dental visits (American Dental Association, 2001).

Dental trauma, more common in males, often accompanies sports injuries and involves fractured or avulsed teeth, lacerations of the oral mucosa or gums, or jaw fracture. If tooth avulsion (tooth knocked out of socket) occurs, it may be reimplanted successfully if treatment is begun within 30 minutes. If the tooth cannot be repositioned in the socket, it should be placed in a container of milk rather than being cleaned, and the adolescent taken immediately to the dentist. All cases of dental trauma

TABLE 22-7 Types of Alternative Child Care		
TYPES	**ADVANTAGES**	**DISADVANTAGES**
Center-based care	• Group care for two or more children • Located usually in a home, school, church, or building designed for group care • Center types include nursery school, preschool, parent cooperative • Licensed by local or state agencies • Staff usually trained in child care and development • Structured program of activities for children usually available • Reliable hours of operation	• Regulations vary from area to area • May be placed on a waiting list for admission • Greater adult-child ratio • Care may not be individualized
Family child care	• Small group care • Good adult-child ratio • Located in provider's home • Special arrangements easier to make	• Usually includes provider's children • Licensing by local or state agencies usually not required • Provider(s) may not be trained in child care and development • Hours of operation may not be reliable
In-home care	• Home care provided by sitter or nanny • Provides individualized care • Easier to meet special needs, (i.e. physical, mental, emotional problem) • Provider may do light home task • Do not have to transport child	• Provider may not be trained in child care and development • May infringe on family privacy • Dependent on provider's reliability

From Potts, N., and Mandleco, B. (2002). Pediatric nursing: Caring for children and their families. *Clifton Park, NY: Delmar Learning.*

TABLE 22-8 Choosing Child Care

Does child care provider?

Appear warm and friendly	Accept and respect your family's cultural values
Seem calm and gentle	Seem to enjoy cuddling infants
Seem easy to talk with	Meet infant physical needs
Seem to like themselves and the job	Provide infant stimulation
Treat each child as special	Provide dependable and consistent care
Understand children's stages of development	Provide consistency between home and child care
Encourage good health habits	Seem to have time for all infants
Have previous experience and trained staff	

Does the child care setting have?

Up-to-date license or registration certificate	Fire extinguishers
A clean and comfortable look	Smoke detectors
Enough room to allow children to move freely and safely	Covered radiators and protected heaters
Appropriate staff-child ratio	Strong screens or bars on windows above first floor
Late pick-up policy	Nutritious meals and snacks
Places where children can be alone	A separate place to care for sick children
Child-proofed environment	A first-aid kit
Enough heat and light	Safe gates at top and bottom of stairs
Enough furnishings for all children	A clean and safe place to change diapers, sanitized after each use
Furnishings that are safe and in good repair	Cribs with firm mattresses
Enough clean bathrooms	Separate linen for each crib
Fire safety plan and adequate exits	

Are there opportunities for the child to?

Play quietly and actively	Learn to get along, share, and respect themselves and others
Play alone	Learn about their own and others' cultures
Follow a schedule that meets young children's needs	Crawl and explore safely
Learn new developmental skills	

From Potts, N., and Mandleco, B. (2002). Pediatric nursing: Caring for children and their families. *Clifton Park, NY: Delmar Learning.*

should be treated as an emergency and a dentist seen as soon as possible (Potts & Mandleco, 2002).

Alternative Child Care

Parents are often challenged to find quality alternative care when faced with having to leave their infant or young child with another person. Quality child care, care that is responsive and developmentally appropriate for young children, provides an environment where the child is safe, nurtured, and challenged to learn. Parents must become informed consumers when searching for such care, and the nurse should keep them informed about issues such as availability, affordability, and qual-

ity. Prior to any investigation into alternative child care, it is important for the parent to be realistic about challenges they will face, think carefully about the situation, learn to adapt to leaving their child, set priorities based on family values, and keep communication channels open with the provider (Potts & Mandleco, 2002).

Once the initial ground work has been laid, the next question becomes how to select alternative child care. Table 22-7 provides information on the various types of child care providers available, with advantages and disadvantages of each. Table 22-8 provides guidelines for choosing quality child care.

While searching for quality child care, parents may inquire about the long-term effect on development. Even though this is an area needing further study, research has shown quality child care does not seem to have any persistent effect on child development (Scarr, 1998). In fact, most studies report better school achievement, greater social competence, and fewer behavior problems in children who experience quality child care (Bolger & Scarr, 1995). The child benefitting the most from child care comes from a socioeconomically disadvantaged environment. Quality care may, in fact, provide learning opportunities and social and emotional experiences not available for these children at home (Scarr, 1998).

Family Cultural Health Practices

Community health nurses working with immigrant populations must provide care within the cultural context of ethnic customs and belief systems related to health, nutrition, and parenting. Language difficulties and socioeconomic barriers may create additional stresses on the family system, particularly on the children. Because it may determine health care resources available, immigration status is an important aspect of child and family assessment. See Chapters 8, 24, and 25 for discussions of transcultural family-centered nursing.

Schools

Schools and academic achievement are important in shaping the developing child and adolescent. This is because most children and adolescents attend primary and secondary school and spend an average of 180 days per year in school. In fact, during most of the year, more than a third of waking hours every week is spent in school or school-related activities. In addition, children and adolescents remain in school for more years now than they did in the past because many continue their education or stay in school since they do not have to drop out to support their family. Academic achievement is important because it often reflects not only how well the individual accomplishes long- and short-term goals but also the feelings of success one has in one's own as well as society's eyes. To be effective, schools and curricula should be based on principles of learning and development and provide a climate that encourages exploring knowledge.

Schools can have positive or negative effects on children and adolescents. Often, a student's experience varies according to their parent and family context, peer group, the size of the school, the extracurricular activities they participate in, and the academic track they are on. For some, school is a stabilizing, friendly force that encourages cognitive development, establishes a climate for social interaction, and provides an environment encouraging task completion. School also allows contact with peers and teachers, testing of new ideas, and validating thoughts. Activities and opportunities at school

can provide safe, acceptable outlets for energy and foster development. Schools also can help break barriers related to ethnicity, social class, race, and gender and provide opportunities to participate with others on common goals or engage in in-depth pursuit of an interest. For others, however, school can be a source of stress where threats to safety and self-esteem and constant change occur (Potts & Mandleco, 2002).

MAJOR CHILD HEALTH PROBLEMS

The health of today's infants and children is threatened by many factors that did not exist 50 years ago: HIV/AIDS, gun violence, drug trafficking in schools and neighborhoods, and increasing levels of environmental contamination. Other major health problems are related to parental behaviors, such as smoking, abuse of alcohol or other drugs (see Chapter 31), and family violence (see Chapter 30). Socioeconomic conditions such as poverty and homelessness (see Chapters 32 and 33) further jeopardize children's physical and emotional health.

Some of the major problems for which infants and children are at risk are discussed in this section. Children of all ages are at risk for most of these problems; however, developmental stage determines to a large extent both the response of the child and clues to appropriate intervention. The nurse most often works with the parent(s) to solve child health problems.

Failure to Thrive

When an infant falls below the third percentile for both weight and height on standard growth charts, the condition is termed **failure to thrive (FTT)** (Potts & Mandleco, 2002). There are three general categories of failure to thrive based on causation: organic, nonorganic, and idiopathic. **Organic failure to thrive (OFTT)** is caused by physical health problems such as cardiac defects or infections. **Nonorganic failure to thrive (NFTT)** is usually due to psychosocial factors such as inadequate parenting skills or lack of emotional attachment to the child. **Idiopathic failure to thrive (IFTT)** is unexplained by the usual organic and nonorganic causes and may also be classified as NFTT (Potts & Mandleco, 2002).

Failure to thrive and children at risk for this condition must be identified early to prevent serious long-term problems. If the infant is temperamental, irritable, or at high risk for medical problems at birth, the parent(s) may physically or emotionally detach from the infant, leading to psychological abuse and neglect.

Growth and development tools help the nurse assess the physical status of the child, and observation of the parent-child relationship provides clues to emotional health. By providing emotional support to the parent(s) and by teaching about child development, parenting, and child care, the nurse can prevent parental detachment from the child and help provide a healthy environment for normal infant growth and development.

Cigarette Smoking

Many studies have shown that direct and indirect exposure to tobacco smoke has deleterious effects on health, particularly during pregnancy and childhood. Environmental exposure to tobacco smoke (ETS) is associated with increased rates of respiratory disease, reduced lung growth in children, increased rates of lung cancer, and exacerbation of asthma in children.

The screening of children whose parents smoke should focus special attention on respiratory complications. Health education of parents must emphasize the direct and indirect effects of smoking, especially during pregnancy. Referral to smoking cessation programs and other resources helps protect the health of both children and parents.

Educational and support programs for parents who want to stop smoking are an important aspect of child and family health care. See Chapter 10 for teaching and learning theories, teaching strategies, and health counseling that can help people change behaviors destructive to the health status of themselves and their children.

Unintentional Injuries and Child Health

Unintentional injuries, or accidents, are the leading causes of morbidity and mortality in children ages 14 and under. Children are primarily at risk of death from unintentional injury related to motor vehicle and bicycle-related accidents (as occupants and pedestrians), drowning, fire and burns, suffocation, poisoning, choking, falls, and unintentional shootings (Potts & Mandleco, 2002). Injury rates vary with a child's age, gender, race, and socioeconomic status. Younger children, males, minorities, and poor children suffer disproportionately. Causes and consequences of injuries vary with age and developmental level, reflecting differences in children's cognitive, perceptual, and motor and language abilities as well as in their environments and exposures to hazards. The National SAFE KIDS Campaign was launched in 1988. Since that time, unintentional injury–related childhood mortality has decreased in several areas (see Figure 22-7). The National Center for Injury Prevention and Control (1997) has identified a particular demographic pattern for childhood injuries to aid providers in assessing for risk factors.

Community health nurses play an important role in injury prevention by providing both educational programs for families and communities and screening programs to assess environmental and related medical risk factors. Children at different phases of development are

---

FIGURE 22-7 Trends in Unintentional Injury

There has been a 46% decline in the unintentional injury-related death rate among children 14 years and under over the last 20 years as a result of widespread education, improved safety devices, and better engineering.

Over the past two decades, residential fire–related deaths have declined 55%, and there has been a 60% decline in the death rate from bicycle-traffic injuries among children.

Even though vehicles are used more today and the miles traveled by automobile have increased, over the past 18 years, there has been a 10% decline in motor vehicle occupant-related deaths.

This decline in unintentional injuries may be due to the efforts of the National SAFE KIDS Campaign, which promotes educational and legislative programs meeting its goals of preventing unintentional childhood injury by conducting public outreach programs, stimulating grassroots activities, and working to make injury prevention a priority of public policy. The result of their efforts have been greater use of bicycle helmets, smoke detectors, child safety seats and seat belts.

Courtesy of the National SAFE KIDS Campaign. [On-line]. Available: www.safekids.org.

---

at risk for different injuries, but a child who is developmentally delayed may be at greater risk for accidental injury than another child of the same age (see Chapter 28).

Lead Poisoning

One of the most common pediatric health problems in the United States, lead poisoning, or **plumbism,** was addressed briefly in Chapter 9 as a major environmental issue affecting children. Plumbism occurs in both urban and rural areas and is found most often among toddlers and preschool children. Lead poisoning is likely most prevalent among young children because they engage in the most hand-to-mouth activity; live closer to the floor, where the air holds more lead-containing dust and dirt particles; and have the most rapidly developing nervous systems, which in itself makes them more vulnerable to the effects of lead (www.aap.org/family).

The most common sources of lead ingested by children are dust and soil contaminated with lead from paint that flaked or chalked with age or that was disturbed during home maintenance and renovation. Other sources are "take home" exposures related to parental occupations and hobbies, water, and food (www.aap.org/family). Older buildings still contain lead-based paint, which has not been used in residential structures since the 1950s. Lead poisoning can also occur as a result of environmental contamination by gasoline or industrial waste.

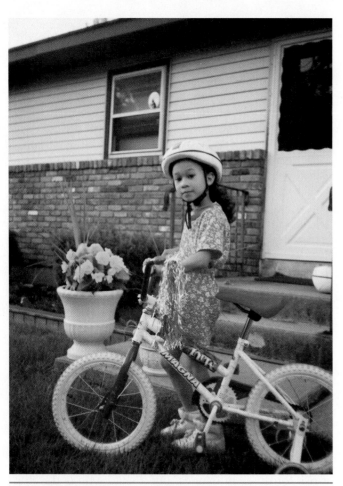

The use of equipment such as safety helmets helps protect children from injury. What other measures can nurses implement and promote to help children protect themselves from harm?

Elevated lead levels interfere with the ability of red blood cells to metabolize iron, resulting in anemia and possible damage to the brain, liver, and other organs. Even low levels of lead exposure, determined by blood levels, can result in mental retardation and behavioral problems (Institute of Medicine, 1995). Symptom severity ranges from no symptoms to a decrease in play activity, lethargy, anorexia, sporadic vomiting, intermittent abdominal pain, and constipation to loss of acquired skills, hyperactivity, bizarre behavior, seizures, and coma. Lead encephalopathy is almost always associated with a blood lead level exceeding 100 μg/dL but occasionally has been found in conjunction with a level as low as 70 μg/dL.

Even though there has been a decline in the average blood lead levels (BLLs) among the population, children continue to be exposed to lead, and it is still a major environmental health problem that could harm their health and impair their ability to learn (CDC, 2000c). Based on data from Phase II of the 1991–1994 National Health and Nutrition Survey (NHANES) III, the CDC estimated that

890,000 children (4.4%) between 1 and 5 years of age had elevated BLLs, above 10 μg/dL (CDC, 1997). The BLL rate was 5.9% among children aged one to two years and 3.5% among children aged three to five years. Children between one and five years were more likely to have elevated BLLs if they were of non-Hispanic, African American heritage, were poor, or lived in older housing. In addition, 21.9% of non-Hispanic African American children and 13% of Mexican American children living in housing built before 1946 had higher BLLs than non-Hispanic Caucasian children (5.6%) living in similar housing (CDC, 2000c).

Due to these figures, in 1997 the CDC changed its national blood lead screening recommendations to an approach that was state based (CDC, 2000c). The CDC also recommended screening children receiving Medicaid for lead unless "reliable, representative blood lead data that demonstrate the absence of lead exposure among this population" exists. Specifically, the recommendations to health care providers were to screen BLLs of all children between one and two years of age enrolled in Medicaid, refer children identified as having elevated BLLs to environmental and public health services, and provide medical management that is appropriate if the blood levels were elevated (CDC, 2000c). Other priority groups for lead screening are found in Figure 22-8.

A critical aspect of treatment for lead poisoning of any degree is to drastically reduce the child's exposure to lead. Interventions may include removing the child from the environment, removing the lead source, and using chelating therapy in cases of lead levels greater than 30 μg/100 mL. Other important nursing interventions include ongoing advocacy for any needed environmental modifications, follow-up for children with lead levels greater than 10 μg/dL, and education focusing on the risk of lead poisoning in the home.

FIGURE 22-8 Priority Groups for Lead Screening

- Children ages 6 to 72 months who live in or are frequent visitors to deteriorated housing built before 1960.

- Children ages 6 to 72 months who are siblings, housemates, or playmates of children with known lead poisoning.

- Children ages 6 to 72 months whose parents or other household members participate in lead-related occupations or hobbies.

- Children ages 6 to 72 months who live near active lead smelters, battery recycling plants, or other industries likely to result in atmospheric lead release.

From *Summary of 1991 Report: Preventing Lead Poisoning in Young Children* (p. 7), by Centers for Disease Control and Prevention, 1994, Washington, DC: Author.

According to the CDC (1994), primary prevention has always been the goal of childhood lead poisoning prevention programs, yet most programs focus exclusively on secondary prevention, that is, dealing with children who have already been poisoned. Programs must shift their emphasis to primary prevention and efforts directed toward identification and remediation of environmental sources of lead. "The purpose of community-level intervention is to identify and respond to sources, not cases, of lead poisoning" (p. 20).

Poverty

As of 1994, 22% of American children lived in families with cash incomes below the poverty threshold, and they are doing less well than their counterparts of three decades ago. Children under six are especially at higher risk because their parents are younger and receive lower wages than they did in the past. Changes that have occurred in poverty are that, today, it is concentrated in inner city neighborhoods with reduced accessibility to jobs, high-quality public and private services (child care, schools, parks, community centers), and informal social supports. For children in poverty, there also is more exposure to serious environmental stressors such as street violence, homelessness, illegal drugs, and negative role models. Deep poverty (50% below poverty threshold) is also more difficult to escape and more chronic in nature. Sluggish economic growth, significant loss of low-skill, high-wage jobs, erosion of government aid, and increases in the number of children living with single mothers (teen and never married) have contributed to poverty in America. Although most children living in poverty are of European descent, the rates of poverty among Latinos, Native American, and African Americans is two to three times higher than in non-Latino Caucasian children (Brooks-Gunn & Duncan, 1997; McLloyd, 1998). (See Chapter 32.)

Poverty affects child outcomes in at least two ways. First, a child's poverty status at three years of age predicts the child's IQ at age five, and persistent poverty has more adverse effects on a child's cognitive functioning than transitory poverty. In addition, children from lower socioeconomic status perform less well than nonpoor children and middle-class children on test scores, grade retention, course failures, placement in special education, high school graduation rates, high school drop-out rates, and the completed numbers of years of schooling. School achievement also declines with the time spent in poverty, and the chance a child will be retained in a grade or placed in special education increases 2%–3% for every year the child lives in poverty. In fact, long-term poverty is associated with deficits in verbal, mathematical, and reading skills that are two to three times greater than those associated with current poverty status. Poverty also affects a child depending on when during the child's life poverty is experienced; poverty during the first five years of life will affect the completed years of schooling more than if poverty occurs during middle childhood and adolescence (Brooks-Gunn & Duncan, 1997; McLloyd, 1998).

Second, there is a higher prevalence of emotional and behavioral problems (externalizing, internalizing) among poor and low socioeconomic status children and adolescents than among children from families where there is higher income. Externalizing behavior problems seen include disobedience, fighting, difficulty getting along with others, and impulsivity, which become more prevalent the longer the children live in poverty. Internalizing behavior problems seen include anxiety, sadness-depression, and dependency (Brooks-Gunn & Duncan, 1997; McLloyd, 1998).

Child Abuse

Child abuse, the willful infliction of physical injury or mental anguish on a child (see Chapter 30), is a major child health problem in the United States. Child abuse may be categorized as physical, emotional, sexual, or a combination of the three. Child abuse is increasing at all levels of U.S. society. Because they often see clients in the home, community health nurses are in an ideal position to detect abuse and neglect and to counsel and educate parents who are at risk for these behaviors.

Nurses and other health professionals are legally required to report suspected child abuse, both physical and sexual. Those who fail to do so are subject to possible fine or licensure loss. Many health care institutions and community-based agencies have specific procedures and guidelines for identifying and reporting child abuse. Community health nurses must be aware of such protocols. Abused children may suffer disproportionately from

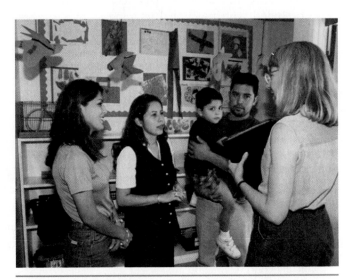

Cultural sensitivity and good communication skills will assist community health nurses in working with children and their families to help prevent child abuse and to protect the children in their care.

anger, noncompliance, low self-esteem, depression, and guilt. In addition, as adults they may abuse their own children or may have poor parenting skills.

Attention-Deficit/Hyperactivity Disorder

Attention deficit/hyperactivity disorder (ADHD) is a clinical diagnosis applied to persistent hyperactivity or inattention and impulsivity that occur more severely and frequently than in other children of a similar developmental level. According to the *Diagnostic and Statistical Manual of Mental Disorders* (APA, 1994), the three diagnostic subtypes of ADHD are (1) hyperactive-impulsive, (2) inattentive, and (3) a combination of subtypes 1 and 2 (most common). Typically, the symptoms appear before the child is seven years old, persist for at least six months before diagnosis is made, and interfere with functioning at home and school (Borowsky, 2000). Difficulties are often school related or academic, but social relations with peers and family members can also occur if the child has mood swings or aggressive behaviors. Many individuals with ADHD have the most difficulties with organizing, preparing, and inhibiting responses (Mercugliano, 1999). Other symptoms, in addition to having a low tolerance for frustration, appear in Table 22-9. Diagnosis is based on data derived from parents, teachers, and the child.

Although the etiology of ADHD is unknown, genetic factors, neurological factors, and dietary ingredients have all been implicated. For example, first-degree relatives have a 25% risk of having similar problems and symptoms of clients with frontal lobe disorders are similar (inattention, hyperactivity, impulsivity). Imaging studies demonstrate brain differences in children with ADHD: right anterior white matter, cerebellar volumes, and anterior corpus callosum are decreased, and there is less brain symmetry. In addition, pharmacological manipulation combined with functional imaging studies suggest decreased energy utilization and blood flow in the striatum and prefrontal cortex (Paule et al. 2000).

The most effective pharmacological treatment (psychostimulants) alters dopamine and catecholamine metabolism. Although aspartame, sugar, and food coloring and additives may cause behavioral problems and hyperactivity in some children, well-controlled studies have demonstrated food additives and sugar have no adverse effects on children's cognitive functioning or behavior even though some caregivers believe certain foods negatively affect their child's behavior (Borowsky, 2000).

Treatment includes behavior management, educational interventions, pharmacotherapy, and biofeedback as well as family education. Behavior management includes reducing family stress, assisting the child follow rules, complete tasks and improve self control, and providing positive feedback for the child's good behavior. Other techniques include clearly defining acceptable/unacceptable behaviors and the accompanying rewards/punishments and periodically varying penalties and rewards to maintain the child's interest. Educational interventions include special education or resource placement (if appropriate) for part of the school day where the setting is smaller and more focused. In addition, providing a nurturing classroom environment where the child will not be embarrassed and their self-esteem will be fostered is important. Finally, closer supervision of the ADHD child in unstructured school areas (cafeteria, playground, halls) is also helpful since they often clash with peers and are easily provoked into misbehavior.

In the short term, pharmacotherapy may result in lower activity levels, longer attention spans, and better impulse control. The most commonly prescribed psychostimulants are ritalin, dexedrine, and cylert. These drugs cause increases in dopamine and norephinephrine, leading to stimulation of the central nervous system (CNS) inhibitory system. Doses are monitored carefully for side effects (tics, hypersensitivity) and adjusted until the response desired is obtained. If psychostimulants are ineffective or produce adverse side effects, clonidine or antidepressants (tofranil, norpramin, pamelor) may be used. Alpha-2 adrenergic agonists can reduce impulsivity and hyperactivity, but lithium, benzodiazepines, antihistaminic sedatives, and buspirone can be detrimental (Popper, 2000). Longer term effects (school achievement, improved social adjustment) are more difficult to obtain by using medications.

TABLE 22-9 Symptoms of ADHD

INATTENTIVE	HYPERACTIVE	IMPULSIVE
Fails to pay attention to details	Fidgetiness	Poor impulse control
Makes careless mistakes	Difficulty remaining seated	Difficulty waiting for turn
Easily distracted	Difficulty playing quietly	Frequently answers questions too soon
Difficulty concentrating on tasks until completed	Feels restless	Interrupts others
Difficulty following directions		
Difficulty organizing		

Biofeedback, a time- and labor-intensive method whereby selective EEG waves are observed and selectively suppressed, has been used with older children. However, it is not currently available for all children. Family education should provide information about the disorder, treatment, and side effects of medications, address concerns, and emphasize family and child strengths. Since many parents feel guilty and confused about the diagnosis, they should be reminded they are not at fault for their child's situation and encouraged to seek ADHD support groups (Borowsky, 2000).

Fifty percent of ADHD children exhibit symptoms into adulthood, including antisocial and criminal behavior, alcohol and drug abuse, anxiety, job changes, and interpersonal difficulties. They also complete less schooling, continue suffering from social skills deficits and poor self-esteem, and hold lower ranking occupations (Mannuzza & Klein, 2000; Young, 2000). However, many have good outcomes and lead productive fulfilling lives.

Effects of Television/Media on Children/Adolescents

Media in America contribute to more adverse health outcomes than to prosocial or positive outcomes. This is especially true in relation to violence, guns, sex, and drugs. For example, cross-sectional, naturalistic, and longitudinal studies as well as several meta-analyses suggest there is a relationship between media violence, real-life aggression, and acceptance of aggressive attitude. Those exposed to violence on television and the media tend to be more likely to commit violent acts. In addition, guns are glamorized in the media; 26% of violent acts committed on the media use guns. Research also suggests adolescents exposed to greater amounts of alcohol or tobacco advertising are more likely to use/intend to use those products when compared to those adolescents who are not exposed to those products. One-third of teens who smoke could link their smoking to tobacco promotional activities. Alcohol advertising in the media stimulates favorable predispositions, greater problem drinking, and higher consumption by young people (Strasburger & Donnerstein, 1999). Figure 22-9 lists the effects of television and media on adolescents.

Parents need to monitor or control the media programming their teens watch and remove the television sets from teens' bedrooms. Specifically, this means limiting all media use to no more than 1–2 hours per day, coviewing television with their children and adolescents, and monitoring their child/adolescent's use of the media (Strasburger & Donnerstein, 1999).

Internet Safety

Although the Internet is an extremely helpful method of expanding a child and family's knowledge about the world, some cautions need to be mentioned so the experiences are safe, enjoyable, and productive. Two im-

FIGURE 22-9 Effect of Television/Media on Children/Adolescents

1. 2–3 hours/day mean less physical activity, reading, interaction with friends

2. 10,000 acts of violence viewed/year; 26% involve use of guns

3. 15,000 sexual references, innuendoes, jokes per year; < 170 deal with abstinence, birth control, pregnancy, STD's

4. 70% of content from prime time dramatic programs contains references to alcohol, tobacco, illicit drugs; over 50% of movies contain references to tobacco/smoking; for every "just say no" public service announcement, 25–50 beer and wine advertisements will be viewed.

From Potts, N. and Mandleco, B. (2002). *Pediatric nursing: Caring for children and their families.* Clifton Park, NY: Delmar Learning.

portant topics related to Internet safety are interacting with others and limiting access to inappropriate content. Often people met on-line are not who they say they are, and the information provided is not always private. Therefore, children and families should be taught to never give out personal information (name, address, age, ethnic background, income, school attended) or information about their friends over the Internet. In addition, they should be cautioned against meeting someone face to face who was originally met on-line, using inappropriate language, or responding to messages that make them feel uncomfortable. Offensive, obscene, violent, pornographic, hate-filled, or racist material is also available on the Internet. Although all but child pornography is legal, guidelines can help families avoid these materials. First, children should understand the kind of sites that are approved by parents, what sites are off limits, and how much time they can spend on a site. In addition, parents should be encouraged to explore the Internet with their children and pay particular attention to games downloaded or copied. Software can also be installed on computers that filter out or block offensive sites. Children should also be shown how to use and evaluate information found on the Internet since not all on-line information is accurate and encouraged to visit noncommercial or other sites that do not sell products specifically to children. Family-friendly Internet sites are listed in the resources at the end of this chapter.

Parenting Education

Parenting in and of itself is difficult enough, but coupled with multiple health problems, financial difficulties, and lack of education, parenting becomes an extraordinary challenge. Parenting education and skill building can have long-lasting positive effects on child and family health. Basic parenting education covers parenting roles, child development (infancy through adulthood), health promotion, nutrition, behavior modification, and stress management.

Through careful screening and assessment, the community health nurse identifies parents or caregivers in need of improved parenting skills and helps them gain access to parenting education resources. The nurse also works to reinforce positive parenting behaviors and monitors the development of parenting skills.

Parents often abuse their children in attempts to teach and discipline simply because they know no other way of approaching these tasks. Figure 22-10 offers some suggestions for positive approaches to the disciplining of children.

FIGURE 22-10 Positive Discipline Guidelines

- Misbehaving children are "discouraged children" who have mistaken ideas about ways to achieve their primary goal—to belong. Their mistaken ideas lead them to misbehavior. We cannot be effective unless we address the mistaken beliefs rather than just the misbehavior.

- Use encouragement to help children feel that they "belong" so that the motivation for misbehaving is eliminated. Celebrate each step in the direction of improvement rather than focusing on mistakes.

- A great way to help encourage children is to spend special time "being with them." Many teachers have noticed a dramatic change in "problem" children after spending five minutes simply sharing those things that they both like to do for fun.

- When tucking children into bed, ask them to share with you their "saddest time" and their "happiest time" of the day. Then share yours with them. You will be surprised what you learn.

- Have family meetings or class meetings to solve problems via cooperation and mutual respect. This is the key to creating a loving, respectful atmosphere while helping children develop self-discipline, responsibility, cooperation, and problem-solving skills.

- Give children meaningful jobs. In the name of expediency, many parents and teachers do things that children could do for themselves and for one another. Children feel that they belong when they know they can make a real contribution.

- Decide together those jobs that must be done. Put them all in a jar and let each child draw out a few each week; that way, no one is stuck with the same jobs all the time. Teachers can invite children to help them make class rules and list these rules on a chart titled "We decided." Children feel ownership, motivation, and enthusiasm when they are included in decisions.

- Take time for training. Make sure children understand what "clean the kitchen" means to you; to them, it may mean simply putting the dishes in the sink. Parents and teachers may ask, "What is your understanding of what is expected?"

- Punishment may "work" if all you are interested in is stopping misbehavior for the moment. Sometimes, we must beware of what works in the present when the long-range results are negative resentment, rebellion, revenge, or retreat.

- Teach and model mutual respect. One way is to be kind and firm at the same time: kind to show respect for the child, and firm to show respect for yourself and "the needs of the situation." This is difficult during conflict, so use the next guideline whenever you can.

- Proper timing will improve your effectiveness tenfold. It does not "work" to deal with a problem at the time of conflict: Emotions get in the way. Teach children about cooling-off periods. You (or the child) can go to a separate room and do something to make yourself feel better and then work on the problem via mutual respect.

- Abandon the crazy idea that in order to make children do better, you must first make them feel worse. Do you feel like doing better when you feel humiliated? This suggests a whole new approach to "time out." Tell children in advance that we all need time out sometimes when we are misbehaving, so when they are asked to go to their room or to a time-out area they can do something to make themselves feel better. "When you are ready, come back and we will work together on solutions."

- Use logical consequences when appropriate. Follow the Three Rs of Logical Consequences: ensure that consequences are (1) *related*, (2) *respectful*, and (3) *reasonable*.

- During family or class meetings, allow children to help decide on logical consequences for not keeping their agreements. (Remember not to use the word *punishment*, which does not foster long-range "good" results.)

- Teach children that mistakes are wonderful opportunities to learn. A great way to do so is to model this yourself by using the Three Rs of Recovery after you have made a mistake: (1) *Recognize* your mistake with good feelings, (2) *reconcile* by being willing to say "I'm sorry, I didn't like the way I handled that," and (3) *resolve* by focusing on solutions rather than blame.

- Ensure that the message of love and respect gets through. Start with "I care about you. I am concerned about this situation. Will you work with me on a solution?"

- Have fun! Bring joy into homes and classrooms.

MAJOR ADOLESCENT HEALTH PROBLEMS

Beginning with the junior high school years, the adolescent period is characterized by dramatic physiological and psychosocial changes. Rapid body growth, changes in body appearance, and surging hormones create an often unpredictable mixture difficult for parents and children alike. Adolescents make a shift from family orientation to peer group orientation, seeking both independence from parents and opportunities to broaden their social horizons. This period is marked by an increasing sense of personal identity and progress in defining social roles, value systems, and life goals. Because adolescents tend to live in the present and with little thought of future consequences, risk-taking behaviors also increase during adolescence, particularly among males. Driving fast and/or under the influence of alcohol, experimenting with controlled substances, and engaging in unprotected sex are examples of potentially fatal risks that adolescents take.

Adolescence in late 20th-century America has become a minefield of problems waiting to explode. Today's adolescent is confronted by an epidemic of sexually transmitted diseases, the most deadly of which is HIV/AIDS, and a world grown increasingly more violent. Family violence, homicide, and suicide rates have skyrocketed in the past 20 years. Teenage pregnancy rates continue to climb, as do the rates of teen suicide. The community health nurse who works with adolescent clients faces a difficult challenge in promoting health and preventing disease and injury in this troubled and troubling population.

The Youth Risk Behavior Surveillance System (YRBSS) monitors priority health risk behaviors among youth and young adults: behaviors that contribute to unintentional and intentional injuries, tobacco use, alcohol and other drug use, sexual behaviors, unhealthy dietary behaviors, and physical inactivity. The YRBSS (CDC, 2000a) reports that nearly three-fourths of all deaths among school-age youth and young adults result from four causes: motor vehicle crashes, other unintentional injuries, homicide, and suicide. A summary report of several national, state, and local surveys cited the following statistics related to health risk behaviors known to increase the likelihood of death: 16.4% of adolescents had rarely or never used a safety belt; 33.1% had ridden with a driver who had consumed alcohol during the 30 days preceding the survey; 50% had consumed alcohol during the 30 days preceding the survey; 26.7% had used marijuana during the 30 days preceding the survey; and 7.8% had attempted suicide during the 12 months preceding the survey. Table 22-10 presents various hazards and developmental characteristics of adolescents as well as appropriate intervention strategies.

Tobacco Abuse

In the fall of 1999, the National Youth Tobacco Survey of approximately 15,000 students in grades 6–12 from 131 public and private schools in the United States discovered that 12.8% of middle school students and 34.8% of high school students used some form of tobacco (cigars, pipes, bidis, kreteks, cigarettes, smokeless tobacco) within one month of the survey (CDC, 2000b). The survey also found that 28.5% of high school students and 9.2% of middle school students currently smoked cigarettes. Most high (91.7%) and middle (87.2%) school students had seen actors smoking on television or in the movies. In addition, more than half of middle and high school students wanted to stop smoking, but only 40% of middle school and 10% of high school students reported they were taught ways to avoid tobacco as part of their school curriculum (CDC, 2000b).

Violence

The second leading cause of death for ages 15–19 and the third leading cause of death for adolescents ages 10–14 is homicide, most due to handgun use (American Academy of Pediatrics Committee on Injury and Poison Prevention, 2000; Webster, Gainer, & Champion, 1995). The homicide rate for black teens is eight times higher than for whites of the same age (Danielson, 1998). Adolescents are also impacted by violence while in school. For example, over 5% of students felt too unsafe to go to school and 6.9% said they carried a gun, knife, or club onto school property at least once in the month preceding the survey (CDC, 2000b). Between 1985 and 1995, the number of students reporting violent crimes at school rose 23.5% (Sniffen, 1998), and recently the arrest rates for rape, homicide, aggravated assault, and robbery during adolescence has increased. Even though most gang-related problems occur in large cities, gang conflict is also seen in smaller cities.

The cause of violent crime committed by young people today has been traced to individual, family, community, and social circumstances. Violent delinquency tends to be more common in working-class than middle-class teens and is associated with depression, drug abuse, lower church attendance, and hopelessness (DuRant, Treiber, Goodman, & Woods, 1996).

Prevention programs targeted to stem the tide of teen violence need to involve nurses, caregivers, schools, and other community agencies. Intervention efforts directed

---

REFLECTIVE THINKING

Violence in the Home

- How do you feel when a child who lives in a home where there is risk for violence asks for your help? Do you want to get involved? Why or why not?

TABLE 22-10 Injury Prevention: Adolescents

HAZARD	DEVELOPMENTAL CHARACTERISTICS	NURSING IMPLICATIONS
Firearms	• Independent, believe are invulnerable • Take unnecessary risks • Need peer approval • Physically active • Responsible for self/others • Curious • Overestimates abilities, stamina, physical development	• Do not carry or use a weapon to deal with conflict resolution • Follow firearm safety rules
Motor vehicles		• Enroll in drivers' education courses • Wear seatbelts (driver/passengers) • Follow traffic rules/speed limit • Do not drink and drive
Poisoning		• Be aware of dangers of drug/alcohol use
Sports		
• Contact sports		• Wear protective gear, including padding/helmets/clothing when participating in contact sports or riding bicycles, all-terrain vehicles, motorcycles; skateboards • Proper use of sports equipment
• Exercise programs		• Assess exercise/fitness programs for safety and ability
• Outdoor activities		• Integrate safety information about outdoor activities (hiking, camping, fishing, back-packing, etc.) into behavior
Water		• Avoid drinking alcohol when boating or swimming
• Craft		
• Swimming		• Learn how to swim • Follow rules regarding water safety

From Potts, N., and Mandleco, B. (2002). Pediatric nursing: Caring for children and their families. *Clifton Park, NY: Delmar Learning.*

toward creating prosocial environments in the home and school may help prevent and reduce aggressive and violent behavior as well.

NURSING ALERT ‹‹‹‹‹‹

Violence

When working with youths who are victims of violence, ask about the victim's relationship to the perpetrator, circumstances surrounding the event, use of alcohol/drugs, predisposing risk factors (violence in the family, unemployment, truancy), and intentions regarding seeking revenge (Danielson, 1998).

Drug Abuse

Illicit drug use is reported by 15.9% of adolescents 12–17 years of age. More than 47% of American high school students have tried marijuana; 26% use the drug monthly. Eight percent of high school students have tried cocaine at least once; 2% have tried heroin or other injected drugs and 16% have inhaled or sniffed intoxicating substances, and over 30% of adolescents have been offered, sold, or given an illegal drug at school (CDC, 2000b). Often adolescents abuse drugs because of curiosity, availability, rebellion, peer pressure, exhilaration, unhappiness at home, the need to overcome feelings of loneliness or insecurity, to be more accepted, to imitate family and friends, to escape, and as an attempt to be mature and sophisticated (Dworetzky, 1995; Kafka & London, 1991; Turner & Helms, 1995).

Nurses, family members, teachers, and community leaders suspecting drug abuse may observe irrational behavior, preoccupation with the occult, decreased quality of schoolwork, irresponsibleness, changes in personality, friends, activities, or appearance, difficulty communicating, rebelliousness, mental or physiological deterioration, unexplainable loss of money or the appearance of new possessions (clothes, CDs, stereo equipment), and actual drug paraphernalia or drugs, including marijuana.

Alcoholism/Alcohol Abuse

Alcoholism and alcohol abuse in adolescence are increasing. Almost 81% of high school students nationally have tried alcohol; 50% reported drinking alcohol at least once over the preceding month of being surveyed; 31.5% report consuming five or more drinks at least once over the past month (CDC, 2000b). Forty-one percent of adolescents report using alcohol and 10%–20% of adolescents are problem drinkers. It is not uncommon for drinking patterns to begin in the eighth grade (Escobedo, Chorba, & Waxweiler, 1995). Often, adolescent behavior relative to alcohol consumption is associated with parental behavior, especially if they are alcoholic or have a drinking problem, peer pressure, or because it makes them feel more mature and is a common social custom. Many adolescents who do drink use it as a mind-altering device since it allows participation in risk-taking activities they might otherwise avoid.

There are numerous hazards of alcohol ingestion. Some may be seen in adolescents, including hepatitis, pancreatitis, gastritis, neuritis, cirrhosis, ulcers of the gastrointestinal tract, impotence, esophageal varices and cancer, cerebellar degeneration, delirium tremens, or birth defects (Murray & Zentner, 2001).

Parents and nurses working with adolescents who abuse alcohol or other mind-altering drugs and their family members need to avoid lectures and judgments. It would be much better to educate adolescents about the detrimental effects of alcohol by describing people who have experienced the effects of excessive alcohol intake. Clarifying values and behaviors relative to leading a healthy lifestyle are also important topics for discussion.

Dryfoos (1998) suggests common characteristics of those who are in jeopardy of not making a successful transition into adulthood because they engage in risky behaviors during adolescence, including violence or substance abuse:

RESEARCH FOCUS

Risky Behaviors

Study Problem/Purpose

To investigate the relationship between risky behaviors (tobacco use, alcohol use, sexual intercourse, poor school performance) and three components of the current and future-oriented self-concept [popular (well liked), deviant (engaging in problem behaviors), conventional (engaging in culturally sanctioned behavior)].

Methods

One-hundred and sixty adolescents from a working class suburban junior high school completed questionnaires measuring their involvement in the identified risky behaviors (tobacco use, alcohol use, sexual intercourse), their current self-concept, and their future-oriented self-concept during the winter of eighth and ninth grades. Grade point averages were obtained from school records.

Findings

There were high correlations between the four risky behaviors, and the prevalence of these risky behaviors increased from eighth grade to ninth grade. Involvement in risky behaviors during eighth grade predicted current and future-oriented deviant self-concept scores in ninth grade. Current popular self-concept scores in eighth grade predicted risky behaviors in ninth grade.

Implications

It is important to realize that how adolescents feel about themselves (self-concept) may be part of the reason they engage in risky behaviors. In addition, when adolescents engage in these risky behaviors early, they have a greater chance of becoming enduring parts of their behavior later. Intervention efforts should be directed toward not only changing one's self-concept so it is more positive but also limiting engagement in risky behaviors.

Source: Stein, K., Roeser, R., & Markus, H. (1998). Self-schemas and possible selves as predictors and outcomes of risky behaviors in adolescents. *Nursing Research, 47*(2), 96–106.

- Early acting out; the earlier a child starts, the longer it will continue and may become more serious as the person gets older.

- The absence of nurturing parents; it is not the number but the quality of parenting that counts; may start early but is a red flag if continues into adolescence.

- Evidence of abuse: creates vulnerability to many negative outcomes.

- Disengagement from school: failing, left behind, or those who have already dropped out.

- Those who are easily influenced by peers: especially apparent in those youth who lack family and school support; tend to conform to peer norms or peer culture instead of societal norms.

- Depression: may be related to stress, abuse, family problems, neighborhood violence, detachment from school.

- Residing in disadvantaged neighborhoods: higher incidence of violence, drug abuse, sexually transmitted diseases (STDs), poverty; less resources such as churches, community police and centers, viable businesses.

- No exposure to the world of work: they do not know anyone in the labor force; lack role models who are employed or have prepared for a career.

Sexual Activity

Half of high school students have engaged in sexual intercourse, and 8.3% experience intercourse before they turn 13 years of age (CDC, 2000b). In fact, 56% of female and 73% of male adolescents report sexual intercourse before turning 18. First intercourse for females occurs at an average age of 17 years for females and at an average age of 16 for males. Nineteen percent of sexually active high school students report having had four or more partners (American Academy of Pediatrics Committee on Adolescence, 2000).

Reasons adolescents use for becoming sexually active may include to feel grownup, enhance self-esteem, experiment, be accepted by friends, have someone to care about, love, and be close to, gain control over one's life, seek revenge, and prove they are "normal" (American Academy of Pediatrics Committee on Adolescence, 2000; Murray & Zentner, 2001). Since few adolescents have the ego strength or decision-making skills to counter peer pressure, they may become sexually active against the wishes of their families and some health care providers.

Predictors of early sexual activity include lack of attentive/nurturing parents, early pubertal development, poverty, history of sexual abuse, cultural and family patterns, poor school performance, lack of school/career goals, and dropping out of school. Factors associated with delay in initiating intercourse include regular atten-

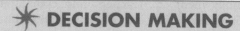

DECISION MAKING

Adolescent Developmental Needs and Pregnancy

You are a community health nurse working at a school-based community clinic serving families of children and adolescents. A 15-year-old Mexican American girl named Maria has been referred for follow-up after treatment for herpes. The referral indicates that she is sexually active and refuses contraception. Upon interview, Maria states that she wants a baby to love and to love her. Although she has a family, Maria states that she feels alone and is therefore trying to get pregnant. One of her former classmates brought her six-month-old baby to a football game, prompting Maria to decide that she wanted a baby.

◆ What developmental needs are involved in this situation?

◆ How might you proceed with a plan of care for Maria and her family?

dance at worship services, stable home environment, and higher family income (American Academy of Pediatrics Committee on Adolescence, 2000).

Sexually active young people participate in behaviors which put themselves at risk for sexually transmitted diseases and pregnancy because they frequently have multiple partners or do not use condoms or other forms of contraception. Refer to Chapter 26 for more information on STDs.

Human Immunodeficiency Virus and Acquired Immunodeficiency Syndrome

Of the 36.1 million people estimated to be living with HIV/AIDS today, 1.4 million are under 15 years of age (CDC, 2001). In addition, 3% of males and 7% of females living in the United States with AIDS were between 13 and 24 when they were initially diagnosed. In adolescents between 13 and 19 years of age, more than half were female, whereas in 20- to 24-year-olds, most (78%) were males (CDC, 2000d). Thirty-four percent of males with AIDS currently between 13 and 19 years of age and 62% of young adults between 20 and 24 years of age were exposed by having sex with other men. In addition, 34% of adolescents acquired their infection because the blood products they received in treating their hemophilia were not heat treated. Almost half the adolescents and young adult women living with AIDS through 1999 were exposed because of heterosexual transmission. Even though only 15% of the adolescent population in America is African American, 60% of AIDS cases reported in

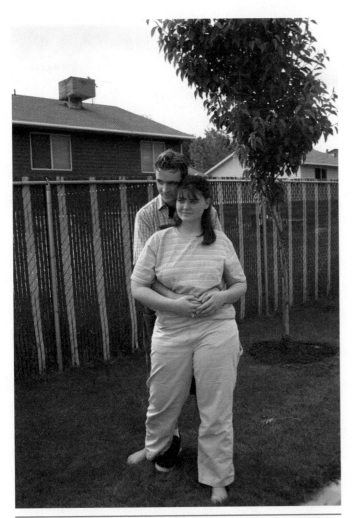

Educating adolescents about sexually transmitted diseases is critical. How might you handle this sensitive issue?

1999 among 13- to 19-years-olds were of this race. Hispanics account for 20% of all reported AIDS cases and 24% of reported adolescent cases even though they comprise only 14% of the population (CDC, 2000e).

Adolescents need to understand the social, medical, psychological, and legal consequences of learning whether they are HIV negative or positive. Community health nurses who offer pretest counseling for adolescents must assess the client's developmental stage and individualize the counseling to the client's developmental needs. For example, the adolescent may be in denial, using magical thinking, or feeling invulnerable. Because some states require specialized training for HIV pretest counseling, it is important to contact the local or state health department about protocols and policies.

Teenagers who are HIV positive provide many legal and ethical challenges. Consent for HIV testing and treatment, limited access to clinical trials, and disclosure of HIV status are all legal issues that confront infected teens, their parents, and health care providers. Laws vary from state to state. Laws related to confidentiality of medical information may not extend to minors, depending on whether the condition presents imminent danger to the young person or others. Treatment may or may not require parental involvement.

Care of the HIV-positive teen involves comprehensive social and medical histories, physical examination, and laboratory tests. The nurse also must follow up with the adolescent who is HIV positive concerning signs and symptoms of HIV-related diseases, types of immunizations given, laboratory values, contraceptive practices, liver function, anemia, and medication regimens. The nurse also must be aware of community resources and agency policies targeting this population.

To help control the spread of HIV/AIDS, community health nurses must understand adolescent development and potential barriers to care. Nurses can participate in community health fairs and school health programs offering HIV/AIDS education that targets teens. Lewis, Battisich, and Schaps (1990) suggest that an effective school-based prevention program should be:

- Clearly derived from theories that recognize the multidimensionality of risk behaviors
- Directed at influencing the general social milieu of the school, not as a separate entity but as an integral part of school life
- Focused on promoting positive influences on social development rather than counteracting negative social norms
- Comprehensive and long lasting, because socialization is a continuous process
- Incorporated into the overall mission of the school to produce a widespread and enduring effect
- Implemented early enough to precede the emergence of problem behavior, because it is harder to change established attitudes and behaviors than to prevent their initial formation
- Monitored and evaluated carefully to ensure that implementation reflects planning

Teens themselves are asking for better AIDS education—straight answers about AIDS and ways to protect themselves. The National Youth Summit on HIV Prevention held in 1995 brought teens together with federal health officials and politicians to discuss preventive measures. Politicians admitted that adults find it difficult to talk about intercourse, much less AIDS.

Adolescent Pregnancy

Most pregnancies occur in those 18–19 years old. Fifty-one percent of teen pregnancies end in a live birth, 35% are aborted, and 14% are miscarriages or still births (American Academy of Pediatrics Committee on Adolescence, 2000). Although birth rates to women under 20 have declined since the 1970s, the United States continues to have one of the highest teenage pregnancy rates among developed countries (Hewell & Andrews, 1996; Ventura, Peters, Martin, & Maurer, 1997). African American teen pregnancy rates are higher than rates in Caucasians and continue to increase (Murray & Zentner, 2001). Most teenage mothers are unmarried. The resulting unplanned pregnancy affects not only the mother and child but also the child's father and their respective families because adolescents are often not socially, emotionally, educationally, economically, or physically ready for pregnancy or parenthood.

Several factors influencing the incidence of adolescent pregnancy have been identified related to individual, family/friend, and society. Individual factors include self-destructive/self-hate feelings and behaviors, egocentrism, low self esteem, loneliness, recent loss, early maturation, independence from family, lack of responsibility, plea for attention, personal fable, self-punishment, and need to prove one's womanhood. Family/friend factors include having a close relative who has experienced an adolescent pregnancy, conflictual mother/father-daughter relationships, sexually permissive peer group, inadequate communication, history of sexual abuse/incest, few girl friends, an older boyfriend, lack of religious affiliation, substance abuse by family or friends, and fulfilling parent prophecy when parents suggest their son or daughter will become pregnant if they do not change their behavior. Societal factors include implied acceptance of intercourse outside marriage, a variety of adult behavioral values, media pressure, inadequate access to contraception, and the availability of public assistance for single young mothers (American Academy of Pediatrics Committee on Adolescence, 2000; Clemen-Stone, Eigsti, & McGuire, 1998; Dworetzky, 1995).

There are risks associated with adolescent pregnancies—medical and psychological. Medical risks include low birthweight (more than double the rate for adults) and neonatal death (almost three times as high as in adults). The mortality rate for the mother is twice as high as for adult pregnant women. Other problems include poor maternal weight gain, pregnancy-induced hypertension, STDs, anemia, and prematurity. Psychological complications include persistent poverty, separation from the child's father, repeat pregnancy, divorce, school interruption, and limited vocational opportunities (American Academy of Pediatrics Committee on Adolescence, 2000).

Improved methods of contraception and the increased amount of sex education courses in the schools reach only a small percentage of adolescents. Not all students who are sexually active attend or have courses readily available, and those adolescents who do participate in the courses may not integrate this information into their behavior because they do not see pregnancy as a concern for themselves or their partners. Therefore, during routine interactions and/or health assessments, nurses should assess the adolescent's knowledge and understanding about intercourse, contraception, and repro-

---

REFLECTIVE THINKING

Adolescent Pregnancy

- What are your feelings regarding adolescents giving up their baby for adoption? What circumstances in your past have shaped your opinion?

---

duction before screening or providing necessary information and support. This includes assessing their understanding and accurate interpretation of risks regarding being sexually active and then discussing sexual responsibility, including abstinence, how STDs are transmitted, and possible consequences of infection and pregnancy. Adolescents who are sexually active should also receive information about the potential outcomes of their behavior, including ways to reduce their risk of becoming pregnant or infected with STDs or AIDS by limiting the number of sexual partners, using appropriate birth control methods, and consistently using condoms. When adolescents with STDs are identified, they should receive appropriate counseling and medical care. When pregnant adolescents are identified, comprehensive prenatal care is essential to reduce maternal and neonatal complications. Pregnant adolescents should also receive information relative to available options. Teens who keep their infants need help becoming effective, secure, and comfortable parents. Information about normal infant growth, development, and care should be provided in an accepting, nurturing environment.

Suicide

The number of adolescents committing suicide has increased dramatically over the last few decades. Now, suicide is the third leading cause of death during adolescence (15–19 years) and the fourth leading killer of younger adolescents (American Academy of Pediatrics Committee on Adolescence, 2000). Over 19% of high schoolers nationally have considered suicide; 8.3% have attempted suicide, and 2.6% required medical attention after a suicide attempt (CDC, 2000b). Sixty-three percent of adolescent suicides in 1997 were committed with a firearm; 91% of suicide attempts involving a firearm are fatal, whereas only 23% of adolescents using a drug overdosage die (American Academy of Pediatrics Committee on Adolescence, 2000).

Frequently, suicide is reported as an accidental death. Even though suicide affects adolescents from all races and socioeconomic groups, some groups have higher rates than others: African American females have the lowest rate; Native American males have the highest rates. Gay and bisexual adolescents have rates of attempting suicide three times higher than other adolescents (American Academy of Pediatrics Committee on Adolescence, 2000). Females are three times as likely to attempt suicide, whereas males are three times as likely to succeed in their attempts.

Stresses related to psychosocial, psychosexual, or physiological issues have been identified as causes for the increasing number of adolescent suicides in the United States (Murray & Zentner, 2001). Often, those adolescents attempting suicide come from families with inconsistent behavioral reinforcement, nonproductive communication patterns, and high levels of conflict/abuse. These youngsters may also feel inadequate or unacceptable, have underlying emotional disturbances, or fail to achieve desired goals. It is not uncommon for seemingly insignificant frustrations and disappointments to precipitate such impulsive acts, which may be committed to increase family and/or friends' attention.

Several warning signs of adolescents who might be at risk for committing suicide have been identified (Conrad, 1991; Fritz & Barbie, 1993). They include but are not limited to experiencing loss due to death or divorce; moving to a different neighborhood, city or state; the appearance of health problems they did not have before; being unable to meet scholastic expectations of teachers, parents, or self; being depressed; changes in eating and sleeping patterns or daily habits; drop in school performance; being lonely or a loner with few friends; truancy; accident proneness; mood swings; increasing alcohol or drug use; feeling rejected, guilty, or hopeless; giving away possessions; withdrawing from people and activities; and writing or talking about death or suicide. Other risk factors are previous suicide attempts, family history of psychiatric disorders, living out of the home, history of physical or sexual abuse, physical ailments, and a recent relationship breakup (American Academy of Pediatrics Committee on Adolescence, 2000).

Suicide prevention programs for teens should be directed at school staff (counselors, school health nurses, teachers), community agency personnel (clergy, police, health care providers, merchants), and students themselves by providing information relative to warning signs, facts, and programs which can enhance self-esteem and social competence. Methods of screening at-risk youth, programs offering peer support, crisis centers, and hotlines as well as restricting the access to handguns, drugs, and other common means of suicide have also been successful. Interventions after a suicide are designed to help prevent or contain suicide clusters and help adolescents cope effectively with feelings of loss they experience with the suicide of a peer.

Nurses working with adolescents need to recognize the seriousness of any of these signs or symptoms, convey concern to the adolescents about those signs, help them feel things will change, listen to and ask about their problems, and refer adolescents with these signs and symptoms to a mental health professional experienced in working with adolescents. Nurse's should not be afraid to ask adolescents directly if they have or are considering suicide, and in fact, the adolescent may be relieved to finally be able to talk about it. It is not uncommon for adolescents unsuccessfully attempting suicide to be merely crying out or asking for help rather than actually wanting to check out or end their life. However, those merely asking for help must be differentiated from those who actually want to end their life because some adolescents attempting suicide later actually succeed. Therefore, follow-up care after gestures is extremely important and crisis intervention for suicide attempts is essential since it can often help the adolescent identify and work through problems, learn alternative ways of coping with stress, and help family and friends be supportive and caring.

NURSING ALERT ‹‹‹‹‹‹

At-Risk for Suicide

- Experiencing loss (death, divorce, move)
- Unable to meet scholastic expectations
- Depression
- Changes in habits
- Drop in performance
- Loneliness
- Truancy
- Accident proneness
- Mood swings
- Increasing alcohol or drug use
- Hopelessness
- Giving away possessions
- Withdrawing
- Writing/talking about death/suicide

Source: Potts, N., and Mandleco, B. (2002). Pediatric nursing: Caring for children and their families. Clifton Park, NY: Delmar Learning.

NURSING ALERT ‹‹‹‹‹‹

Suicide

Take any suicide gesture seriously; convey concern, love, and acceptance; and refer and follow-up to mental health professionals experienced in working with adolescents.

ADOLESCENTS AND FAMILIES

The family is the first and, generally, the most important socializing agent in one's life. Successful socialization is to a large degree a function of the parenting and other familial interactions experienced while growing up. Several changes are likely to impact the type of interactions and quality of relationships adolescents and their parents have with one another. First, adolescents experience physiological changes associated with puberty causing both them and their parents to think and respond differently to one another; parents begin to expect adolescents to act more like adults. While they may not always act more mature, adolescents begin to believe they should be treated more like adults. The cognitive shift to formal operational thinking also impacts young people's relationships with parents. As adolescents are better able to articulate their own concerns when requests are made they disagree with, less compliance may be seen. If parents are not sensitive to adolescents' desires to test their newly found cognitive skills, they are likely to be perceived as defiant. Adolescents also begin answering the question "Who am I?" and exploring attitudes and values they have been taught. This may also increase the level of tension between adolescents and their parents since parents may likely reexperience their own identity, often confronting their own mortality and the notion they are approaching a new stage in their own lives (Potts & Mandleco, 2002).

As young people approach adulthood, they want the opportunity for more autonomy and need to have a sense of self-direction and independence. Parents, however, are often unsure of how to provide their children with opportunities for establishing autonomy. They may even feel threatened by their child's desire for more independence, therefore responding by exerting ever greater amounts of control. The interesting dilemma for adolescents is that, although they are attempting to establish a sense of autonomy and, as a result often act as if they would rather die than be seen with their parents, the unsureness of this period makes the safety found in the parent-child relationship no less important. The task for parents is to recognize the normalcy of their adolescents' needs to push away and begin to explore the world around them, while at the same time recognizing their need to know there is a secure base to return to if their world becomes too unfamiliar or frightening. Indeed, adolescents' attachment to parents is important and has been linked to such characteristics as self-esteem and emotional adjustment (Potts & Mandleco, 2002).

Parent-Adolescent Conflict

As a result of their desire for greater autonomy and their increased level of reasoning and the associated questioning, adolescents are likely to experience greater conflict in their relationships with their parents than children. Most arguments are the "normal, everyday, mundane family matters such as school work, social life and friends, home chores, disobedience, disagreements with siblings, and personal hygiene" (Montemayor, 1983, p. 91). Rarely do they argue about the "hot" topics that are typically identified with adolescence, such as sex, drugs, religion, or politics. This is surprising considering the differences in parent and youth attitudes about these topics. Parents may indirectly attempt to influence their children's behavior regarding these hotter issues through rules and interactions over the more mundane matters families are willing to discuss. For example, parents may be uncomfortable discussing their attitudes and beliefs about adolescent sexuality but will evidence those beliefs through the rules they establish about acceptable clothing, curfews, onset of dating, etc. Montemayor also found most parent-adolescent interactions were peaceful and free of stress. More recently, Barber (1994) found Caucasian, African American, and Hispanic parents and adolescents all disagree about similar issues (e.g., chores and dress). While there were similar proportions of each group reporting chronic (i.e., daily) conflict, substantially lower

---

REFLECTIVE THINKING

Parent-Adolescent Relationships

- Think back to your adolescence. Do you recall ever feeling embarrassed that your parents were with you when you were at the mall or at a dance, even though you may have enjoyed doing things with them when you were around the house? Why do you think you felt uncomfortable? What suggestions would you give an adolescent who is embarrassed to be seen with their parents?

DECISION MAKING

Parent-Adolescent Conflict

Adolescents' attempts for greater autonomy can often result in an escalation in the amount of conflict they have with their parents. As health practitioners, what could you do to help both parents and adolescents understand the normative nature of this experience and what suggestions might you make regarding ways that both could make it a more constructive experience?

levels of conflict were reported by both minority groups when compared to Caucasian families. Barber speculated this may be a function of Caucasians' greater use of an authoritative parenting style, which encourages adolescents to have a greater say in issues relevant to themselves.

Health Promotion

Any adolescent health promotion effort needs to incorporate the adolescents' perspective of what health means and consider their priorities and concerns relative to health and health care services as well as the level of their cognitive development. Often, adolescent concerns related to health are impacted by developmental tasks and crises in the physiological, psychosexual, psychosocial, or cognitive domains since the concerns usually have something to do with their own point of view or context. Many adolescents are reluctant to seek health care because of financial concerns, geographical access, characteristics of the health care provider, or the perceived notion of unavailability of confidential services. Therefore, it is critical providers be respectful and demonstrate openness, competence, honesty, warmth, compassion, and understanding and have the ability to communicate effectively with adolescents and their families.

Several guidelines are also important for nurses to remember when interacting with adolescents. First, the environment should be caring. This means positive relationships are encouraged, individual differences are valued, and strengths and weaknesses acknowledged. Second, nurses need to treat adolescents with dignity and make it a priority to know them as individuals. Third, assessment with the purpose of improving health, describing health-promoting behaviors, and understanding is crucial. Fourth, relationships with families are important to develop and maintain. This means frequent communication between nurses, adolescents, and families and encouraging family participation in many health-issue situations.

Effective nurses also need to know and understand age and maturational level, physiological changes impacting development, and the specific psychosocial needs and developmental changes expected during adolescence. Interactions should always be individualized, and communications need to convey honesty, general concern, and acceptance. Confidentiality and trust can be important issues for adolescents which nurses must acknowledge. Physiological, psychosexual, psychosocial, and cognitive changes normally occurring during this period as well as the many issues and concerns facing adolescents today need discussion and explanation. Any program developed for adolescents, their parents, or both should present information objectively and accurately, and adolescents themselves should be allowed and encouraged to identify and discuss issues and problems they consider important and provide input into planning.

Nurses working effectively with adolescents should demonstrate poise, tolerance, warmth, and empathy. They should always encourage independence and be aware of

hidden adolescent fears or concerns that may be subtly expressed. Nurses also need to be aware of their own biases which may impact interactions or care delivered. Adolescents should be allowed and encouraged to be responsible for as much of their own personal health care as possible and be helped as needed. Finally, adolescents should be assisted in making appropriate decisions impacting their life. If they do not know how to make wise decisions and careful choices, nurses should teach them principles of effective decision making and problem solving.

Nursing care should be provided in settings, sometimes away from parents where the self-conscious adolescent feels welcome and comfortable. Allowing sufficient time and privacy for all interactions is essential, so sensitive topics related to physiological growth, sexuality, personal goals, and concerning behaviors (drug abuse, gang membership, promiscuity) can be discussed in an unhurried and nonjudgmental atmosphere. It is not uncommon for successful interactions to resemble conversations between persons with common interests. The interviewer applies developmental principles, so concrete-thinking younger adolescents understand answers to their specific questions, and older adolescents understand answers to their open-ended and more abstract questions. Confidentiality issues should be discussed early in interactions, since adolescents may confide information to nurses they prefer their parents not know. It is important to make clear early on, however, that some issues may need to be shared with parents, especially when they are younger adolescents still living at home.

Even though adolescence is generally a time of wellness, these young people will seek health care for skin conditions, minor illnesses, school/sports physical, management of chronic illness, high-risk behaviors, and conditions related to sexuality. See Table 22-11.

TABLE 22-11 Five A's of Successful Adolescent Health Promotion

Anticipatory guidance	Establish a trusting relationship before adolescence
Ask	Ask about their behaviors: health enhancing and health compromising
Advise	Advise, even if not asked, about health-promoting behaviors
Assist	Encourage to participate in programs promoting health
Arrange	Arrange follow-up visits or consultations to monitor progress

From Irwin, C. (1993). Topical areas of interest for promoting health: From the perspective of the physician. In S. Millstein, A. Petersen, & E. Nightengale (Eds.), Promoting the health of adolescents: New directions for the twenty-first century (pp. 328-332). New York: Oxford University Press.

IMPLICATIONS FOR COMMUNITY HEALTH NURSING PRACTICE

It is imperative that nurses work in partnership with all segments of society to deal with the problems of aggregates as well as of individuals. Aggregate nursing requires community assessment, planning, and intervention as well as activism and leadership in social and political arenas. Yet, among their variety of roles (see Chapter 19), community health nurses are the major primary health care providers for maternal-child and adolescent care. Careful monitoring and support during these periods of rapid growth and development are essential. During these most vulnerable periods of life, nurses have great opportunities to improve lifelong health. The accompanying perspectives box, written by a public health nurse serving children and families, demonstrates the need for advocacy.

Assessment and Diagnosis

Knowledge of normal growth and development from conception to adulthood is the basis for nursing assessment. Physical examinations, weights and measures, and thorough health histories serve as indicators of health status and give clues to areas of concern. The health history and the child's responses during the examination provide more clues. Close attention is paid to psychosocial factors such as parental expectations of the child, impaired attachment, previous history of abuse or neglect, family violence, and homelessness.

Developmental assessment tools are useful in screening for developmental delays and helping to assess progress. The most common tool used by community health nurses is the Denver II, which screens for delayed gross and fine motor skills, adaptive language, and personal/social skills in children from birth to six years of age. Developmental assessment tools also serve as useful guides for teaching parents those things that a child may be ready to learn but is not yet able to do. A variety of developmental assessment tools are available for infants and preschoolers.

Assessment of family developmental processes and the interrelationship of the child/adolescent and the family is also necessary. Family developmental processes are addressed in Chapters 24 and 25 and provide the context for individual development of the child. A family torn by abusive behavior, alcoholism, drug addiction, or poverty cannot provide an environment where children can reach their developmental potential.

School performance is a crucial aspect of school-age child health and is part of the assessment. If the child is performing poorly academically, further assessment is needed to determine the problem. Testing for vision, hearing, cognitive functioning, and learning disabilities; follow-up medical examinations; and psychological and psychiatric evaluation and testing may be indicated. Poor nutrition and lack of sleep may be overlooked in the search for a cause of poor school performance. Sometimes, children are unable to perform academically and suffer because they are overwhelmed by something that is easily solved.

Assessment of the family-community relationship is also essential because this aspect is critical to the child's growth and development. Family-community relationship determines many factors such as whether the child has health care insurance, transportation services, encouragement and positive support at school, access to churches and other community groups, access to recreational facilities, and the like.

Nursing diagnoses related to child health problems are based on careful, thorough nursing assessment and focus on physical and/or psychosocial factors. Examples of NANDA nursing diagnoses include *Imbalanced nutrition: less* (or more) *than body requirements* and *Risk for impaired parent/infant/child attachment.*

Planning and Intervention

Planning is done with the child, the family, or both. In a situation where a child needs help in learning to use his or her combination lock, for example, planning and intervention could be done with the child alone. More complex matters, however, require total family involvement. There may be a need for teaching or counseling, and the planning for these interventions should be done with the family. There may be a need for referral to community resources or for advocacy on the part of the nurse. In such cases, the family and the nurse together plan that which is to be done and by whom. It is critical that family members be involved in assessment, planning, intervention, and evaluation processes. Other community work may need to be done through social or political action to provide a healthy environment for families and children.

The nursing process is applied in the care of children at all levels of society. First, the nurse can help children within their individual developmental abilities—no more and no less. Second, the nurse can work with the family of the child within the family's developmental ability—by teaching, supporting, or serving as advocate. Third, the nurse can apply the same principles and work with the community to serve the aggregate of children represented by a particular child that happens to be in the caseload.

Evaluation

Evaluation of outcomes for child and adolescent clients must be a part of the planning and the ongoing reassessment. Evaluation of growth is done by weighing and measuring and by keeping track on growth charts. Evaluation of developmental progress is done via use of

Out
of the Box

Insights of a Community Health Nurse Working in Lead Poisoning and Prevention

Nursing practice involves a systems approach in order to develop effective and creative strategies to enhance the health of a particular community. The community health nurse (CHN) works in a multitude of roles that require flexibility and critical systemic thinking skills. Additionally, the role and function of the CHN working with lead-poisoned children, families, and communities require unique skills which include a knowledge base in environmental health and housing. Lead is considered the number one preventable environmental health issue in America today; therefore, it is considered a highly political social justice issue with multiple implications for community outreach strategies. The function of the CHN is the identification, prevention, and case management of lead-poisoned children living in high risk "hot" zones, communities with substandard housing constructed prior to 1950.

The CHN working with this aggregate population must possess essential skills in community building, collaboration, community assessment, and analysis. The level of interventions must be determined by community involvement at various levels. For example, the CHN is a critical player in coordinating and bridging the gap between grassroots community members and housing, environmental, political, and health officials to address substandard housing from a community perspective. The CHN provides critical baseline information and data to these community groups and keeps them informed of additional health indicators affecting a particular community. The nurse is a key player in building and providing "high-risk profiles" of children with multiple health issues such as anemia, low immunization rates, asthma, and dental caries in a particular hot zone. This information is essential for the process of community collaboration in developing effective strategies for children and families affected by lead poisoning.

The most unique factor of working as a CHN with the Alameda County Lead Poisoning Prevention Pro-

gram (ACLPPP) has been the interdisciplinary approach used when a child is identified as being lead poisoned. ACLPPP is the only program in the country that has the health, environmental, and housing components under the same umbrella and management. The program has embraced a comprehensive approach to working with children, families, and communities affected by lead. The CHN's role is to provide a comprehensive systems approach in working with families in order to maximize the potential of the families in our communities. The nurse works closely with the housing and environmental components of the program to ensure that interventions and time frames are being met.

This is an essential process since identifying the source of lead poisoning in the home is the most important factor in preventing further lead exposure and poisoning of children. As parts of the process of working collaboratively within the framework of the program, our CHNs have played a significant role in developing the Case Review Working Committee comprised of housing, environmental, and nursing personnel. The Case Review Working Committee meets bimonthly to review each case, develop action plans, and determine whether a case meets the criteria for enforcement. The property where the poisoned child resides qualifies for enforcement when the property owner refuses to address identified lead hazards in the home. In addition, the committee provides to management status reports and recommendations for any case that requires more aggressive interventions. Needless to say, this process is invaluable in providing quality checks for best practice in the field of lead poisoning.

The primary responsibility of the CHN is to remain as the advocate and liaison between the needs of the children and families affected by lead poisoning while remaining cognizant of additional community concerns and feedback. This responsibility is crucial in order to facilitate the best possible outcomes for children affected and at risk for lead poisoning.

—*Maricela Narvaez-Foster, RN, PHN, MA* ■

Perspectives... ✴

INSIGHTS OF A PUBLIC HEALTH NURSE

I work as a public health nurse for a large county health department serving poor children and their families. One of the most important things I do is serve as an advocate. Advocacy has become even more important recently because families do not know how or are not able to navigate the health care system and need someone who can help with the managed-care process. Because there are so many problems in the changing system, families often need an advocate to help them get needed services. Agents of vendoring services often do not tell clients about available services, and the nurse has to seek out the information for families.

Being an advocate for my clients is so very important. A non-English-speaking family was referred to me because the physician wanted to remove an eight-year-old daughter from the family home. The girl had cystic fibrosis, and failure to thrive had been an issue. The physician was accusing the parents of not giving the child her nighttime feedings containing medication and nutrition. The social worker from Child Protective Services and I made a home visit and found everything in place for the feedings. The mother showed me her equipment and supplies, demonstrated how she gave the feedings, and showed me the records. There was no problem, and the child seemed to be doing very well.

I made an appointment with the mother and child and went with them to see the physician. Everything checked out fine, and the child had gained weight. A resident physician who spoke Spanish saw the child and was very kind to the mother. But the primary physician came into the room after the resident physician had left and continued to insist that the child was not being fed and must be removed from the home. The mother cried all the way home, and I could not comfort her very well because I do not speak Spanish.

I checked out the medical records and talked with people to put the story together. A note posted to the medical record by a physician indicated that the child needed night feeds but that the physician assumed the vendoring agency would not approve because of the cost. As a result, the night feeds had not even been requested! The child had eventually been hospitalized due to weight loss but gained back the weight while in the hospital. Because the child had gained weight during the hospital stay, the physician assumed the child was not getting the night feeds because of negligence on the part of the mother. After the confusion had been cleared up, the physician decided against removing the child from her home, and she is doing well. I am really glad we were there for her and for her family. The language barrier makes things even harder.

I see a lot of children in foster homes who are really suffering. These children *really* need advocates. Because the licensing agencies are not allowed to make unannounced visits to these homes, I have to be their ears and eyes when I make home visits. Probably about half of the foster parents care about the children and are doing a good job. But the other half do not care at all and are just doing foster care for the money: The kids are a commodity. They were probably better off with their biological parents. We need an organization of health care workers just to be advocates for the foster kids in this county.

—Paula, RN, PHN

tools such as the Denver II or other tools considered appropriate for the situation during the first six years of life. School progress is an important evaluative measure during the school-age and adolescent years. Behavior is a strong indicator of the child's well-being and self-esteem.

KEY CONCEPTS

◆ While improving in certain areas because of medical advances, child health in the United States is deteriorating in other areas because of social and environmental health problems such as poverty and violence.

◆ Knowledge of those developmental processes associated with the early years of life provides the foundation for identification of health risk factors and health assessment.

◆ Prenatal care involves careful teaching, guidance, and support of the mother as the fetus experiences this critical period of life.

◆ The aggregate health status of infants and children is determined statistically by keeping records of infant mortality rate, low birthweight, and

COMMUNITY NURSING VIEW

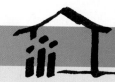

A referral is sent to the public health clinic requesting a public health nursing follow-up visit for a 17-year-old Korean parent of a 2-month-old infant. The teen mother is monolingual and resides with distant relatives.

The community health nurse brings a translator on the home visit. A family assessment is conducted and yields the following information:

◆ Family strengths are that the mother has support from distant relatives; the mother and infant are bonding well; and the mother is highly motivated to learn how to care for the infant.

◆ Areas of concern are that the infant has not gained weight since birth; the infant is breastfeeding only three times per day; the mother has only a sixth-grade education; and the father of the baby is not in the household.

Nursing Considerations

Assessment

◆ How would you obtain the information needed for a family assessment in this situation?

Diagnosis

◆ What nursing diagnoses would be made for the infant? For the mother?

Outcome Identification

◆ What outcomes would be evidenced for the infant? For the mother?

Planning/Interventions

◆ What nursing interventions would be appropriate? Who would you involve in the interventions? What referrals would you make?

Evaluation

◆ How would you monitor and evaluate the results of your interventions?

---

immunization. Growth and development measurements serve as indicators of nutritional need and environmental health needs.

◆ Major health needs of children today are related to family and community environment, challenging community health nurses to address environmental issues in the home and community.

◆ Major health needs of adolescents in the United States are associated with health risk behavior in the areas of sex, violence, and substance abuse.

◆ Community health nurses apply the nursing process using developmental theory as the basis for understanding, as principles are applied to work with individual children, families, communities, and governments.

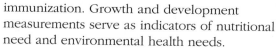 **RESOURCES**

TIPS FOR PARENTS

American Library Association: http://www.ala.org
Family Education Network: http://www.familyeducation.com

50+ Great Sites for Kids and Parents:
    http://www.ala.org/parentspage/greatsites
Franklin Institute Science Museum: http://fi.edu
Library of Congress: http://www.loc.gov
Parents and Children Together Online:
    http://cric.indiana.edu/www/indexfr.html
Parent Soup: http://www.parentsoup.com
Public Broadcasting System: http://www.pbs.org

CHILD AND ADOLESCENT HEALTH

American Academy of Child and Adolescent Psychiatry
    (AACAP): http://www.aacap.org
American Academy of Pediatrics (AAP): http://www.aap.org
American Medical Association Archives of Pediatric and
    Adolescent Medicine: http://archpedi.ama-assn.org.
Planned Parenthood Federation of America, Inc
http://www.plannedparenthood.org
U.S. Public Health Service AIDS Information Hotline
1-800-342-AIDS
CDC guidelines for school and community programs:
    Promoting lifelong physical activity:
    http://www.cdc.gov/nccdphp/dash/guidelines/phactaag.htm

Chapter

23

CARE OF YOUNG, MIDDLE, AND OLDER ADULTS

Deborah Klaas, RN, PhD

MAKING THE CONNECTION

Life's Rainbow
Beginnings are lacquer red
fired hard in the kiln
of hot hope;
Middles, copper yellow
in sunshine,
Sometimes oxidize green
with tears; but
Endings are always indigo
before we step
on the other shore.

—*Banani, 1987, p. 181*

COMPETENCIES

Upon completion of this chapter, the reader should be able to:

- Discuss growth and development theories for the adult years.
- Describe the stages of adult life and tasks to be accomplished in young, middle, and older adulthood.
- Identify the risk factors and conditions most prevalent in each adult stage of life, in terms of emotional, mental, physical, spiritual, and social impact.
- Detail the relationships necessary for healthy existence in each stage of adulthood.
- Describe nursing care as it applies to each stage of development in adult life.

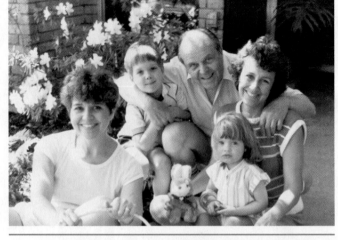

The community health nurse delivers nursing care appropriate to the developmental stage of the client.

KEY TERMS

ageism	male climacteric
ego integrity versus despair	maturity
	menopause
empty nest syndrome	midlife crisis
era	outer (or social) aspect of aging
generation gap	
generativity versus stagnation	presbycusis
	presbyopia
inner aspect of aging	structure building
intimacy versus isolation	transition

The adult years have long been viewed as a stable, nonchanging period of life. Today, however, growth and development are recognized as lifelong processes. The adult years can be as exciting and full of change as are the years from birth through adolescence.

Nurses have always been aware of the developmental stages of the clients to whom they provide care. At all levels of nursing education, a common objective on evaluation forms is related to whether nursing care was appropriate to the developmental stage of the client. The nurse must understand common theories of growth and development in order to determine whether the client is exhibiting behavioral patterns appropriate for the client's given stage of life.

This chapter discusses growth and development of the adult as the basis for assessment, planning, intervention, and evaluation with regard to clients. Just as nursing itself is based on a strong commitment to caring, the nursing process is based on caring (Carpenito, 1999; Anglin, 1994). This chapter begins with a review of some of the growth and development theories for young, middle, and older adults. It examines some of the risk factors and conditions prevalent at each stage of adulthood. The discussion includes consideration of healthy environments as well as healthy relationships with self, partner, family, friends, and neighbors.

THEORIES OF GROWTH AND DEVELOPMENT

Theories about growth and development have been around for many years. Most of them concentrate on those years between infancy and adolescence. One theorist, Daniel Levinson, claims that the study of adult development is just beginning. He has concentrated on the adult years and determined a series of **eras** (periods or stages of development) and **transitions** (periods of approximately five years during which the adult is moving to the next era) through which the adult progresses (Levinson, 1978).

Erik Erikson's theory of development as a series of specific developmental tasks also covers the adult years. His stages of life are related to resolution of crises related in some way to the environment (Erikson, 1963). Tables 23-1 and 23-2 outline developmental stages as envisioned by Levinson and Erikson, respectively.

Because Erikson and Levinson devoted more time to adult development than did other theorists, their theories are more applicable to this chapter. The stages of adult life discussed in this chapter are young adult, ages 20–40

TABLE 23-1   Levinson's Developmental Stages of Adulthood

AGE	SEASON (PHASE)	CHARACTERISTICS
18–20 years	Early adult transition	Seeks independence by separating from family
21–27 years	Entrance into the adult world	Experiments with different careers and lifestyles
28–32 years	Transition	Makes lifestyle adjustments
33–39 years	Settling down	Experiences greater stability
45–65	Pay-off years	Is self-directed and engages in self-evaluation

Adapted from The Seasons of a Man's Life, *by D. Levinson, 1978, New York: Knopf.*

TABLE 23-2   Erikson's Stages of Psychosocial Development

STAGE	AGE	TASK TO BE ACHIEVED	IMPLICATIONS
Trust vs. mistrust	Birth–18 months	To develop a sense of trust in others	Consistent, affectionate care promotes successful mastery.
Autonomy vs. shame and doubt	18 months–3 years	To learn self-control	The child needs support, praise, and encouragement to use newly acquired skills of independence.
			Shaming or insulting the child will lead to unnecessary dependence.
Initiative vs. guilt	3–6 years	To initiate spontaneous activities	Give clear explanations for events and encourage creative activities.
			Threatening punishment or labeling behavior as "bad" leads to development of guilt and fears of doing wrong.
Industry vs. inferiority	6–12 years	To develop necessary social skills	To build confidence, recognize the child's accomplishments.
			Unrealistic expectation or excessively harsh criticism leads to a sense of inadequacy.
Identity vs. role diffusion	12–20 years	To integrate childhood experiences into a personal identity	Help the adolescent make decisions.
			Encourage active participation in home events.
			Assist with planning for the future.
Intimacy vs. isolation	18–25 years	To develop commitments to others and to a life work (career)	Teach the young adult to establish realistic goals.
			Avoid ridiculing romances or job choices.
Generativity vs. stagnation	21–45 years	To establish a family and become productive	Provide emotional support.
			Recognize individual accomplishments and provide appropriate praise.
Integrity vs. despair	45+ years	To view one's life as meaningful and fulfilling	Explore positive aspects of one's life.
			Review contributions made by the individual.

From Childhood and Society *by E. Erikson, 1968, New York: Norton;* Psychiatric and Mental Health Nursing Certification, *by N. Randolph, 1993, Springfield, PA: Springfield.*

years; middle adult, ages 40–65 years; and older adult, age 65 years to death. Because human development is not always a linear process, such arbitrary divisions based on chronological age are not always the best way to view adult development. It must also be kept in mind that with the increasing numbers of older adults, especially adults over 80 years of age, an additional developmental stage of old-old adulthood may be necessary. There have already been further definitions of later maturity as young old (65–74), mid old (75–84), and old old (85 and over) (Murray & Zenter, 2001).

Martha Rogers (1970) noted that human development is the result of the human integrated whole interacting with the totality of the environment. The idea of continuous repatterning of humans and the environment is explicitly depicted by not only growth and development but also the changes resulting from events such as an aging population; short- and long-term effects of limited resources and perhaps excessive resources as well; effects of improved technology/communication; and the current, more transitory nature of families. According to Rogers, individuals age unidirectionally toward greater complexity and organization, a fact supported by research and those working with elderly populations. Community health nurses operationalize Rogers' (1970) assertion that "intervention should be directed toward assisting individuals to mobilize their resources, consciously and unconsciously, so that the man-environment relationship may be strengthened and the integrity of the individual heightened" (p. 134). This theory provides a sound foundation for positively influencing healthy growth and development in the adult at micro- and macrolevels.

DEVELOPMENTAL STAGES AND TASKS OF ADULTHOOD

Like the years of childhood and adolescence, the adult years have definite developmental stages. In recent years, more emphasis has been placed on lowering the death rate among young and middle adults and lowering the number of days of restricted activity among older adults. These objectives are part of the goals of *Healthy People, 2010* (U.S. Department of Health and Human Services [USDHHS], 2000). Policymakers and citizens are looking at each developmental stage and setting priorities for achieving optimal functioning at each level. The nurse, as a member of the health care team, must be familiar with each stage of adult development to promote appropriate healthful behaviors.

Young Adult

The young-adult stage may be the most dramatic of the adult years. These are the years of growing independence and freedom from parental guidance. Often formal education is finished or nearing completion. Some tasks of this life stage include establishing a career, entering into a close relationship and forming a family unit, making friends and taking part in a social group, beginning to take on social responsibilities, perhaps becoming a parent, and, finally, arriving at some philosophical view of life (Bee, 1998). Figure 23-1 lists developmental tasks of young adulthood.

Physical Development

Physically, the young adult is at the peak of efficiency in terms of muscle tone and coordination and has a high energy level. Growth is finished at this stage, and attention must be paid to nutritional needs. If a sedentary lifestyle is adopted, some caloric adjustment is necessary to avoid weight gain. All systems have matured, including the neurological system, which matures at around 30 years

FIGURE 23-1 Developmental Tasks of Young Adulthood

Self

- Acceptance and stabilization of self-concept and body image
- Identifying and resolving conflicts between self and conforming to societal expectations
- Establishing financial and parental independence
- Establishing a satisfying, productive, and economically sound profession
- Establishing a home
- Establishing time and stress management skills
- Formulating a meaningful philosophy of life
- Achieving a more reflective stance about other cultures, mores, and political systems
- Establishing citizenship within the community

Relationships

- Learning to appraise and express love responsibly psychologically as well as physically
- Establishing intimate bonds with partners and/or friends
- Resolving changed relationships within parental family
- Deciding whether to become a parent and carrying out parenting tasks
- Establishing congenial friendships and social groups

Adapted from *Health Promotion Strategies through the Life Span* (7th ed.), by R. B. Murray and J. P. Zentner, 2001, Upper Saddle River, NJ: Prentice-Hall.

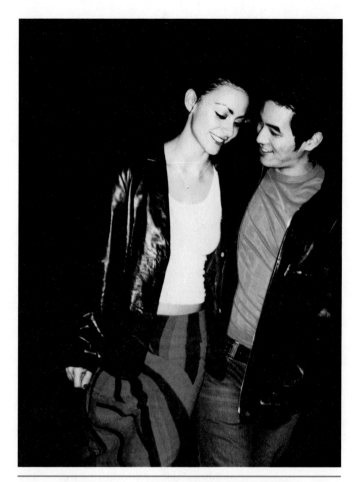

Some of the tasks of young adulthood include establishing a career, beginning to take on social responsibilities, and entering a close relationship.
Courtesy of PhotoDisc.

of age (Murray & Zentner, 2001). Although visual and auditory sensory perceptions are at a peak, the lens of the eye is already losing its elasticity, and close vision is becoming more difficult. Sexual maturity has been achieved, sex drive remains high, and females are well equipped for childbearing, having fully mature female organs.

Cognitive Development

Cognitive functioning of the young adult is more advanced than during adolescence. The young adult uses systematic and sophisticated problem-solving techniques and achieves new levels of creative thought with less egocentrism than is seen in younger individuals. Thinking is more reality based, and mental activities are proficient (Newman & Newman, 1999). Although often formal education is complete at this time, job training, military education, or continuing education are often a part of life. Education is usually directed toward employment, an important part of the young adult's identity. Perform-

ing meaningful, rewarding work produces feelings of worth and accomplishment in the young adult.

Psychosocial Development

Psychosocially, young adulthood is a time of continuing maturation. Erikson (1963) details the crisis as **intimacy versus isolation.** Identity was established in adolescence, and the urge now is to seek love and commitment in a close relationship. To cope with the demands of adult relationships, the individual needs a considerable degree of **maturity.** Developmentally, maturity is a relative state—a state of complete growth or development. Levinson (1986) calls this period **structure building,** when a lifestyle is fashioned. The transition period is one during which the lifestyle is evaluated and modified. This first lifestyle links the individual to adult society, and conflicts may develop when the individual later balances the exploration of new possibilities and options with the need for stability. In the later years of young adulthood, settling down becomes the main issue. Often, the decision to have children is made during this stage, necessitating another adjustment period as new parenting roles are learned and internalized.

Young-Adult Risk Factors

While living in general holds many risks to human life and health, there are risk factors more or less specific to each life stage. These risks can be emotional, mental, physical, spiritual, or social in nature.

From a psychosocial perspective, failure to achieve the developmental task of intimacy results in isolation (Erickson, 1963). Feelings of isolation are linked to risk factors for young adults such as substance use, violence, unsafe sex, and, in some cases, accidents. Specific risks of young adulthood may be more common within certain cultural groups. It is important for community health nurses to recognize these trends without stereotyping clients because they belong to any particular ethnic or cultural group.

Substance Abuse

Young adulthood is a time of major life decisions and life planning. The rigors of career choice, educational opportunities, choice of a mate for life, and decisions about childbearing and childrearing exert considerable stress during this life stage. Rapid, continual advancements in technology and science also contribute to feelings of pressure and inadequacy. A common reaction to the stress of daily life is the use and possibly the eventual abuse of drugs or alcohol. Research indicates that heavy

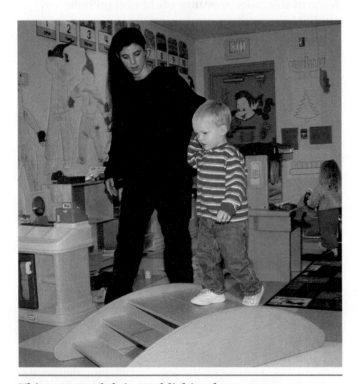

This young adult is establishing her career as a teacher. Establishing a career is an important part of young adulthood.

alcohol use in high school correlates strongly with collegiate polydrug use (Feigelman, Gorman, & Lee, 1998) and that dangers and addictive potential for alcohol and tobacco are seriously underestimated by the same cohort (Donnelly, Hollenbeck, Eadie, Duncan & Eburne, 2000). Alcohol is seen as a means of relaxation and addiction and often not recognized by the drinker until it has seriously interfered in the individual's health and well-being. Cannabis, cocaine, heroin, "ecstasy," and methamphetamine have also become drugs of choice for young adults. Use of these drugs involves significant risks for accidents (Albery, Gossop, & Strang, 1998), high-risk sexual behavior (Bellis, Hale, Bennett, Chaudry, & Kilgoyle, 2000; Klitzman, Pope, & Hudson, 2000; O'Hare, 1999), morbidity, and mortality as well as impairing an individual's resources for achieving appropriate levels of psychosocial development (Haemmerlie, Montgomery, & Crowell, 1999). Recently the Harvard School of Public Health released a study indicating binge drinking occurs in 44% of college students and is associated with significant alcohol-related problems (Wechsler, Lee, Kuo, & Lee, 2000).

The pressures of the young adult years and unresolved past problems can also result in problems with self-esteem and self-image. Low regard for self often accompanies eating disorders. The nurse can identify these inappropriate reactions to stress by conducting a nutritional assessment, a thorough physical examination, and a health history that includes questions about drug, alcohol, and tobacco use.

Suicide

Another reaction to life stress is depression and thoughts of suicide. Suicide is the fifth overall cause of death in young adults in the United States (Murray & Zentner, 2001). The nurse's role in dealing with the risk of suicide in young adults includes both educating the public to the needs of young adults and identifying those at risk. The nurse can also encourage participation in groups as well as express caring concern for the client.

Sexuality

Young adulthood is the time when sexuality reaches its peak. Varieties of sexual patterns are prevalent among young adults, ranging from heterosexuality to bisexuality to homosexuality to masturbation to abstinence (Murray & Zentner, 2001). The individual's reaction to earlier sex education and sexual experience can dictate whether a rewarding sexual relationship is achieved or discomfort and frustration in the sexual role result. Researchers have found that the community can influence how early a person begins having sexual intercourse and whether contraceptive devices are used when sexual activity has begun. If the community offers a variety of opportunities for advancement in education and employment and has formal prohibitions against early sexual behavior and unwed parenthood, a person is less likely to engage in the latter activities. Young women in poor neighborhoods are less motivated to avoid or delay sexual activity than are those in neighborhoods of higher socioeconomic status. Kenney, Reinholtz, and Angelini (1998) found the risk of sexually transmitted disease in women increased with histories of sexual abuse, high-risk behaviors, and sexual precociousness. National Aids Behavioral Surveys found women with risky sexual partners tended to be young, poor, sexually unassertive, and in troubled relationships (Dolcini & Catania, 2000).

Incest or sexual abuse as a child may result in less than optimal adjustment as an adult. Research shows that the common characteristics of adult survivors of incest include a fundamental lack of trust, low self-esteem, and a poor sense of identity (Townsend, 2000). Wingerson (1992) reported 65%–75% of females who abuse drugs or are prostitutes, runaways, or psychiatric outpatients have been victims of childhood incest. Read and Argyle (1999) found a high percentage of paranoid ideation and command hallucinations to kill oneself among adult survivors of incest. When developmental transitions are adversely affected by incest, there are risks of serious psychopathology.

Acquired immunodeficiency syndrome (AIDS) continues to rank highly as a growing cause of morbidity and mortality in the United States despite efforts to educate the general public about high-risk behaviors. Although more males than females in the United States have AIDS, the rate of increase in females is nearly twice that for males (Centers for Disease Control and Prevention [CDC], 2000b). Young adults are at the greatest risk for acquiring this disease. Multiple studies indicate young adults continue to engage in unsafe sex practices, often mitigated by use of substances, and this occurs despite knowledge of HIV and how it is contracted (Cerwonka, Isbell & Hansen, 2000; Skidmore & Hayter, 2000; Kann et al., 2000; Staton et al., 1999). Of great importance to nurses was a study done with young adult nursing students. While they are highly knowledgeable about AIDS transmission, 15%–25% still engaged in high-risk sexual behavior (Zimmer & Thurston, 1998). Although research is ongoing to slow the progress of the disease and develop a vaccine to protect against it, AIDS is at this time a fatal disease. (See Chapter 26 on communicable diseases.) The nurse can evaluate the sexual health of the young adult via a careful, discreet sexual history. The community health nurse is in a unique position to uncover sexual problems through caring interactions and to help the young adult find the necessary therapy.

Reproductive Health Problems

Unwanted pregnancies and sexually transmitted diseases are two major health risks among young adults. The nurse should be involved in providing education about sex and family planning options. Educating clients about primary prevention of pregnancy and making referrals to agencies that are appropriate to the client's beliefs and values are two ways the nurse can help the client. A non-judgmental attitude is vital for community health nurses dealing with sexually active adults. The nurse must be able to disperse factual information about sexually transmitted diseases.

Infertility is a growing concern of young adult couples. As many as 15% of young couples fail to conceive after a year of unprotected intercourse. Investigation into both partners is important because infertility factors are shared equally in men and women (Murray & Zenter, 2001).

Violence

Violence is a major physical risk factor in the young adult stage of life, especially violence of African American against African American. Violence can be self-directed, as discussed earlier, or directed toward others. Nurses can directly address the issue of violence by helping young adults develop healthy parenting techniques and helping young children develop nonviolent conflict resolution skills. See Chapter 30 for further discussion of family violence.

Accidents

According to *Healthy People 2010,* death rates among young adults increase 35% above those of later adolescence. Seventy-four percent occur as the result of external preventable causes such as automobile accidents, homicides, and suicides. Motor vehicle accidents are the leading cause of death for persons aged 20–24. Other accidental injuries include falls, drownings, and poisonings (USDHHS, 2000).

Community health nurses work to prevent injuries in their communities, in homes, schools, workplaces, and wherever there are people. Injury prevention requires acute observation skills in noticing potential safety hazards and collaborative skills in working with others to rectify

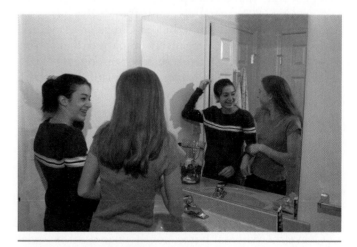

Experiences of childhood and adolescence affect self-esteem and social development throughout adulthood.

unsafe conditions. Safety education is also provided in community settings to promote personal safety.

Cancer

Cancer of the testes and cancer of female reproductive organs occur in young adults. Of concern then is the CDC's (1999) report that 26% of young women engaging in premarital sex do not get screened for cervical cancer. Malignant germ cell tumors of the testes peak in early adult life. Ovarian tumors reach a peak incidence in young adults and testicular cancer is increasing (Henderson, Bernstein & Ross, 1999). Klotz (1999) reported testicular germ cell cancer has increased by 60% over the last 30 years in Ontario, rates that parallel alarming increases in the United States as well. Research strongly implicates environmental pollutants causing hormonal disruption as an underlying factor in the growing rates of testicular cancer (Klotz, 1999). The nurse can teach breast and testicular self-examination and make recommendations for pelvic examination and Pap smears. It is important at this time to educate young adults about early signs of cancer. Even with education, young adults are often oblivious to danger signs and need to be reminded often.

Teaching about life habits that contribute to cancer is part of the nurse's role. Cessation of cigarette smoking for the individual and reduction of parental smoking for children's health are important, as are dietary considerations.

Balancing Multiple Roles

Young adults often find themselves in the position of having to balance a variety of responsibilities such as career advancement, raising children, spousal relationships, and caring for aging parents. The demands of each responsibility in isolation is great but altogether present staggering demands on energy, physical and emotional health, and flexibility. The National Association for Female Executives and Genesis Eldercare conducted a survey among 800 members and found that 89% of responding women reported elder caregiver–associated stress and frustration negatively impacted their lives. They noted the often inadequately supported role of caregiver harmed their careers and relationships with children and significant others (Timon, 2001).

Employment and Housing

Social risk factors are related to the community where the individual lives, which is determined by several factors. Insufficient education or employment opportunities limit choices. The individual remains in an environment that is stifling and without the conditions necessary for successful functioning. In cases in which the individual does not leave the parental home, coresidence restricts social development. Multiple studies have documented the importance of housing to the health and well-being of young adults and families (Cumella, Grattan, & Vostanis,

1998; Fullilove, Green, & Fullilove, 1999). Efforts to move people off welfare rolls have reported some success. However, Cancian and Meyer (2000) noted that only one in four young women who were formerly recipients of welfare work consistently full-time, suggesting employment alone is not a guarantee of economic success.

The community health nurse is involved in the well-being of the young adult and is concerned about public policy involving much more than just physical health. The allocation of funds, the amount spent on prevention, and those persons who make decisions regarding allocation of tax dollars are only a few of the many social issues that are of importance to nurses.

General Factors Contributing to Young-Adult Well-being

Young adults face a variety of challenges as they enter the world of long-term relationships, work, and possibly parenthood. Learning to balance multiple consuming roles is a significant stressor. Community health nurses assess young adults for stress and teach clients nutritional, psychosocial, and physical ways to optimize their health during this potentially draining and turbulent phase of the life span. In addition to providing individual and family care, community health nurses conduct public education classes for younger families regarding healthy means of coping with demands inherent in this age group as well as educate the general and corporate sectors for added social support. Further, they provide a multitude of resources for health-related concerns of members of the young adult cohort.

Middle Adult

Middle adulthood covers approximately the ages of 40–65. This period was once considered old age; but as life expectancy has lengthened, middle age has replaced and pushed old age up into the seventies, eighties, nineties,

---

REFLECTIVE THINKING

Your Own Young Adulthood

Reflect on your own period of young adulthood, keeping in mind the risk factors of substance abuse, suicide, sexuality, violence, and accidents.

- Of these factors, which ones affected you?
- How did these factors shape your life as it is now?
- How will they affect your life in the future?

and beyond. These middle years are the years of stability and structure. Recently the MacArthur Foundation established the Research Network on Successful Midlife Development, the first comprehensive, scientific description of normal midlife in the United States. Research from this project indicates that midlife tends to be a time of emotional, physical, interpersonal, and financial stability. It also found that poor physical fitness and self-destructive habits suggest major national health problems as this cohort moves into old age (John D. and Catherine T. MacArthur Foundation Research Network on Successful Midlife Development, 2001). Figure 23-2 lists developmental tasks of middle adulthood. Middle-aged adults are the stable, mature slice of society responsible for the day-to-day functioning of the world. Most of the power in our society—in politics, business, education, and religion—rests with middle-aged individuals.

Physical Development

Physically, middle age reflects the progression of the aging process. The skin loses its tautness, and wrinkles along with pouches and sagging begin to show on the face and neck. Hair becomes thinner or loses color. Muscle is gradually replaced by adipose deposits, resulting in a thickened midsection and thinner extremities. Decreased bone density and decalcification of bones lead to a change of posture and the beginning of loss of height, especially in the female (Murray & Zentner, 2001). Gradual losses in nerve conduction and muscle function slow movement and impair sensations. Blood vessels are less elastic and lead to cardiovascular disorders and hypertension. **Presbyopia,** or decreased accommodation due to lessened elasticity of the lens of the eye, leads to the necessity for reading or bifocal lenses for close visual acuity. **Presbycusis,** or diminished hearing, begins in middle age, with acuity for high-frequency sounds being first to be lost (Murray & Zentner, 2001).

Changes in body shape in middle adulthood are often compounded by obesity. The prevalence of sedentary lifestyles and unaltered dietary patterns result in overweight adults. People may no longer participate in the regular programs of physical exercise more common in the younger years. At this stage of life it is necessary to reduce caloric intake and adjust the amounts of fat, fiber, protein, and carbohydrates. Also extremely important for cardiovascular health as well as weight maintenance is a program of regular exercise. Due to lack of proper nutrition and resources, hard physical labor and lack of money for age camouflaging and repairing beauty aids, those of lesser socioeconomic status often show signs of aging earlier (Andrews & Boyle, 1999).

FIGURE 23-2 Developmental Tasks of Middle Adulthood

- Maintain a comfortable home.
- Develop financial and emotional security for later years.
- Maintain resilience to changing role, responsibilities, interests, abilities, and shared households.
- Maintain or regain emotional and sexual intimacy.
- Maintain contact with grown children and their families.
- Adapt to departure of child(ren).
- Recommit energy once focused on child care to community life.
- Use competencies to deepen interests and community involvement.
- Meet the needs of elderly parent(s) in a way that is satisfactory to parents and middle-aged children.

Adapted from *Health Promotion Strategies through the Life Span* (7th ed.), by R. B. Murray and J. P. Zentner, 2001, Upper Saddle River, NJ: Prentice-Hall.

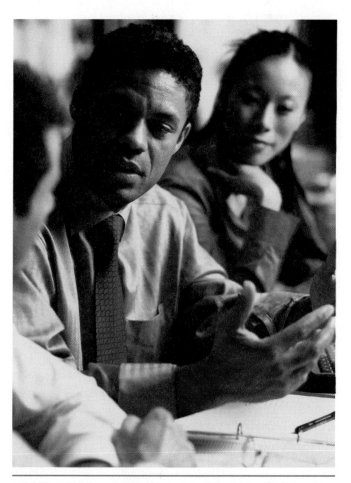

Middle-adulthood developmental tasks include acting as a leader and mentor for less experienced people, whether in the workplace or in the community.
Courtesy of PhotoDisc.

REFLECTIVE THINKING

Physical Signs of Aging

- Which, if any, of the physical signs of middle age do you have?
- What symptoms of aging can you recognize in your parents? In your acquaintances?
- What differences can you identify in the ways that men and women cope with signs of aging?

Cognitive Development

There are no major differences between young and middle-age adults in memory. The ability to learn is unimpaired and often enhanced by experiencially enhanced motivation, flexibility, confidence, and maturity. Problems are viewed from a broader perspective, improving solutions; however, because the middle ager tends to consider more variables, the process may appear slower (Papalia & Olds, 1998). Riegel (1973) characterized mature thinking as being *dialectical* in nature, meaning contradiction and opposing viewpoints are welcomed for intellectual stimulation, deeper understanding, and problem resolution. Creativity is believed to peak during the middle years as the result of an ongoing accumulation of social, contextual, and intuitive intelligence (Papalia & Olds, 1998). In general, middle-aged cognition involves integrating and synthesizing expanding life experiences, actively seeking alternate perspectives and new knowledge, and thoughtful confrontation with self and others.

Psychosocial Development

Psychosocial development during the middle-adult years is typified by self-assessment and introspection. Erikson (1963) defines the developmental task of this life stage as a resolution of the crisis of **generativity versus stagnation.** Individuals have the urge to contribute in some way by providing for others directly or indirectly through altruistic, enterprising, charitable, and service-oriented activities. Actions taken on behalf of others evidence a convergence of personal and societal needs (Murray & Zentner, 2001). Generative middle adults are comfortable with who they are and feel a love of others. Levinson (1978) defines this life stage as beginning with a transition period of reassessment by the middle adult. Various degrees of searching and self-assessment go on before the individual proceeds to making choices and building new structures. According to Erickson (1963), the consequence of not achieving generativity is a sense of stagnation or self-absorption. Behaviors regress to earlier stages of behavior, such as adolescence or younger, and are characterized as immature, or lacking in development.

One final phenomenon in this stage of life is the **empty nest syndrome,** launched by the last child leaving home. This period requires adjustment as the couple learns to live alone as a couple again. Some couples react negatively, discovering that, with the children gone, they have nothing in common. Such couples no longer "know" each other after years of involvement with their children's activities or their relationships have no meaning without the children. For other couples, this is a positive time, and their relationships deepen and become stronger.

Middle-Adult Risk Factors

The middle adult faces many of the same risks as does the young adult. Life stresses continue and, in fact, may actually escalate. The risk of turning to alcohol or drugs to relieve and cope with those stressors remains present.

Midlife Crisis

Unique to this stage of life are several age-related factors. The first of these is the **midlife crisis,** a transition first identified by Carl Jung (1933). At approximately 40 or 50 years of age, the individual begins to lose the sense of purpose and responsibility that has been a part of life. A sense of uselessness and incompletion takes over, resulting in a feeling that some crucial element is missing. Some individuals endure these years of struggle and emerge as stronger, more mature people. Others resist the honest appraisal and examination of life necessary to survive and make drastic career and marital changes in an attempt to bring meaning back into their lives (Murray & Zentner, 2001). The research developed by the Network on Successful Midlife Development (1999) suggests that professional and media reports of midlife, both exaggerated and experienced by those in midlife as less qualitatively and quantitatively. The nurse can be instrumental in assisting the client through this phase of development by using good communication techniques and crisis intervention tactics. Referrals can be made to counseling centers and support groups. The nurse recognizes that this crisis or transition is a part of the development of the middle-adult years and can be used for positive growth and change.

Generation Gap

Another risk factor of the mid-adult years is the conflict between parents and adolescents. Called the **generation gap,** this conflict results from the need for young adults to move out and away from the world their parents have created. This move toward independence involves experimentation and, often, revolt against the parents' world. The parents may respond with resentment and insistence on conformity, and the battle lines are drawn. Again, the community health nurse is in a unique posi-

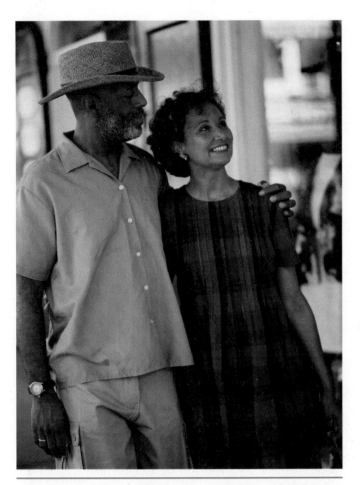

After children have left home, a couple must adjust to being "just a couple" again. Courtesy of PhotoDisc.

tion to assist the client in resolving these difficulties. Recognition of the developmental stage and acceptance of the necessity for tolerance are two strategies that can be used. Humor can also be used to lighten the discussion and to make a point without offending either parent or teenager (Mendenhall, 1999).

Middle-aged adults may find themselves in a position of caring for adolescents and increasingly aging parents and/or living with adult children who have returned home. Although these can be rewarding circumstances, they bring new demands, roles, and commitments (Abaya, 2001). The nurse can assist the adult caregiver to accept the fact that their parents' dependence may be appropriate for their point of life. The nurse can assist the client in recognizing those things that must be done and finding the necessary resources. This sandwich generation, responsible for both children and parents, faces increasing stress as their aged parents decline in ability. The stress on all can be reduced if caregiving situations are regarded as a function of families, not just of individuals (Abaya, 2001). The eventual death of parents can be a relief or another source of stress, depending on how well the middle adult has resolved the child-parent relationship. Again, as in the young-adult years, depression

can be a reaction to the accumulated stresses of middle-adult years. The nurse must be aware of the symptoms of clinical depression, such as changes in appetite and sleep patterns, loss of interest in all activities, fatigue, indecisiveness, or recurrent thoughts of death (American Psychiatric Association [APA], 2000). Suicide is a concern at any age, and care must be taken to recognize the symptoms and help the individual.

Accidents

In middle age accidents are the fourth leading cause of death. The three leading causes of death by accident are (1) automobile collisions, (2) work-related accidents, and (3) falls in the home (Bee, 1998). Fractures and dislocations are the leading cause of injuries occurring at home, during recreational activities, and in the workplace.

Health Problems

No single disease or illness is unique to these years, but health problems do occur. Cardiovascular disease, cancer, pulmonary disease, diabetes, obesity, alcoholism, and glaucoma are major problems of middle adulthood. Cancer ranks as the number one cause of death among people 45–64 years of age. Heart disease is the second leading cause, and cerebrovascular disease ranks third (CDC, 1999). Better maintenance of health is required at this age, and careful assessment must be performed by the nurse to identify potential health problems. The nurse must be aware of health risks particular to certain cultural groups. Hispanics, African Americans (Smelzer & Bare, 2000), and Native Americans (National Diabetes Information Clearinghouse [NDIC], 2001) have higher rates of diabetes than those of Northern European extraction. African Americans have higher rates of hypertension (Smelzer & Bare, 2000), and type A personality traits carry a higher risk for heart attacks and strokes (Murray & Zentner, 2001).

The female climacteric, better known as **menopause,** occurs during the middle-adult years. The associated decline in hormone production produces a wide variety of physical and psychological effects, many of which are undergoing scientific study. Although many women experience no ill effects, menopause is often viewed as a disease treated by estrogen replacement therapy, other hormones, and various medications (Wasaha & Angelopoulos, 1996). The usual symptoms of menopause include hot flashes, vaginal and libido changes, increased risk of osteoporosis and cardiovascular disease, skin changes, and mood alterations. For women who are unwilling to take replacement estrogen and other medications, alternative therapies include exercise, dietary changes, and herbal preparations (Wasaha & Angelopoulos, 1996).

The **male climacteric** usually occurs in the late fifties or early sixties. Less noticeable than menopause, this period may entail some episodes of dizziness, hot flashes, sweating, or headaches. Although males do not lose their reproductive power, sexual hormone production does diminish, and sexual response changes. Some hypertrophy of the prostate gland can begin in these years, resulting in urinary frequency and nocturia (Sheehy, 1995).

Sexuality

Sexual behavior in the middle adult varies between males and females. Males peak in desire in the late teenage years and early twenties, whereas females peak in the late thirties or early forties (Murray & Zentner, 2001). A close, loving relationship, however, is vital in promoting and sustaining a satisfying sexual relationship.

Financial Concerns and Relationship Problems

Major social risk factors of this age include financial concerns, meaningful employment, and relationship problems. Financial concerns often result from rising inflation and cost of living. A job where output is valued over the employee as a person can lead to dissatisfaction and despair. At this time of life, attention becomes focused on the remaining productive work years and whether retirement funds are going to be sufficient to allow a satisfactory lifestyle in the later years.

At this middle stage of life, divorce and all its resultant problems constitute an increasingly common occurrence. Whether the divorce is amicable or acrimonious, major life changes of this type result in stress. If young children are involved, custody questions arise; with older children, there are problems of behavior and supervision. New living arrangements are a source of stress as attempts are made to re-create a stable home and community. Another increasingly common occurrence is the return of adult children (Abaya, 2001). Research is focusing on whether the adult child always benefits or whether the aging parent also is positively affected by the arrangement. Family or cultural beliefs about family structure often dictate the success of alternative living arrangements. The community health nurse can be helpful to all parties in resolving conflicts and helping the individuals work through problems. Communication skills and a sense of humor, again, are valuable tools in helping adults through the risks of middle-adult life.

Older Adult

Late adulthood, from age 65 to death, is more prone to negative stereotyping than is any other life stage. The stereotypes surrounding aging are partly a result of our cultural emphasis on youth and beauty and partly a reflection of our own anxieties about aging and death. The older adult faces the last years of life with few role models, fewer societal definitions, and even fewer directions for dealing with death, the final stage of life. This portion of our population is the most rapidly growing segment,

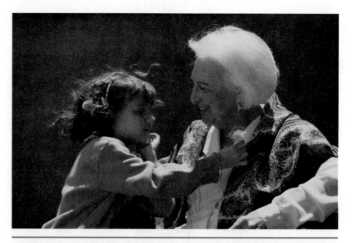

A grandparent can have a very positive influence on grandchildren. In your own life, did you have a grandparent who had a positive effect on you?
Courtesy of PhotoDisc.

and older adults are beginning to be seen as a diverse group with widely differing opinions and needs. The developmental tasks of the older adult include adjusting to physical and health changes; forming new family roles as in-law and grandparent; facing retirement with static or reduced income; associating with own age group; and developing enjoyable and meaningful postretirement activities. Figure 23-3 lists the developmental tasks of the older adult.

Physical Development

Aging does not occur at the same rate for all people. In fact, aging manifests in widely divergent ways in different individuals. Many factors affect the diversity of aging, including heredity, lifetime illness, lifestyle, and stress. Some general characteristics held in common by those aging include gender differences in aging, irregular cel-

> ### REFLECTIVE THINKING
>
> #### Aging and Perception of Aging
>
> - At what age do you think a person is old?
> - Can you identify behaviors in a person over 70 years of age that would make him or her seem much younger?
> - Imagine yourself in your eighties and enjoying a relationship with someone of the opposite sex. How would that relationship be different from a relationship at a younger age?

FIGURE 23-3 Developmental Tasks of the Older Adult

- Recognize and adjust to physical and mental changes in the aging process.
- Adjust to societal views of aging.
- Determine where and how to live remaining years.
- Continue emotional and sexual intimacy with partner.
- Establish a safe and comfortable household to fit changing needs.
- Adjust to retirement income or supplement income with remunerative activities.
- Maintain maximum level of health through health care, diet, physical activity, and satisfying interpersonal relationships.
- Maintain contact with children, grandchildren, and other living relatives.
- Maintain interest in people outside of the family in friendship, social, civic, and political responsibilities.
- Pursue alternate resources for need satisfaction and new interests.
- Adjust and maintain a sense of meaning in life throughout losses of older adulthood.
- Establish a significant philosophy of life and draw on spiritual resources.
- Reassess the self, integrating the past with the present to achieve a sense of coherence.

Adapted from *Health Promotion Strategies through the Life Span* (7th ed.), by R. B. Murray and J. P. Zentner, 2001, Upper Saddle River, NJ: Prentice-Hall.

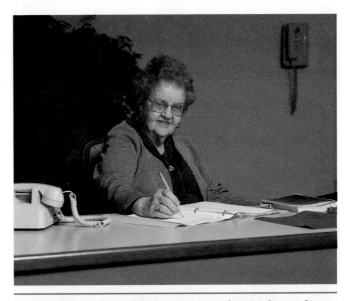

This older adult is able to maintain her independence and self-esteem through volunteer work. Describe the importance of incorporating information such as the ability and desire to make a contribution to society to an older adult's nursing care.

lular aging causing differences among function of organ systems, a cumulative affect of aging traits, and lessening of organ reserves with age (Papalia & Olds, 1998). Often an individual working with an aging person may first notice the most obvious signs of aging—changes in skin, face, hair, and posture (Ebersole & Hess, 1998). It is important to keep in mind that aging does not automatically mean loss of function. The ability of the individual to adapt to physiological aging determines the level of health (Taylor, Lillis, & LeMone, 2001).

Systemic Changes

Internally, or systemically, the signs of aging involve all body parts. The interrelatedness of all organ systems becomes prominent when there is deficiency in one or more. Cardiovascular and respiratory systems are less efficient because of a reduction in strength and adaptability of related organs. Blood vessels harden and react more slowly, causing the heart to work harder and less effectively. The gastrointestinal and urinary systems may also decrease in efficiency, with associated decreased peristalsis and less effective excretion of toxins and wastes from the body. Constipation, a common problem

of the older adult, and urinary frequency reflect these systemic changes of aging (Smelzer & Bare, 2000).

Reduced blood flow to the brain as well as reduced oxygen and glucose use begin at approximately 60 years of age. However, age-related brain atrophy varies widely and is not uniform in all older adults. The structural and physiological changes in the brain do not always manifest as performance disabilities in the elderly (Ebersole & Hess, 1998). Muscle mass and muscle strength diminish in older people, but some of this loss can be counteracted by regular exercise. Bone density is reduced in elderly persons, particularly in females, and bones become more brittle. As the thymus gland ages, it begins to degenerate, reducing circulating lymphocytes. Lymph tissue decreases, leading to a reduction in immune response. Further, there is reduced production and function of T and B cells, which may influence the increased rates of malignancy in this cohort. Rheumatoid arthritis may be caused by increased autoimmune responses (Papalia & Olds, 1998).

Sexuality

Sexuality in the older adult shifts in emphasis from procreation to companionship, intimate communication, and a pleasurable physical relationship (Ebersole & Hess, 1998). Physical changes that influence coitus include decreased vaginal lubrication in the female and a less intense and slower erection in the male. As with most aging changes, there are wide variations, even at a biological level, and many older adults lead full, rich sexual lives. A common problem in Western society is the increasingly large number of older females in proportion to fewer older men. The nurse can address sexuality when doing

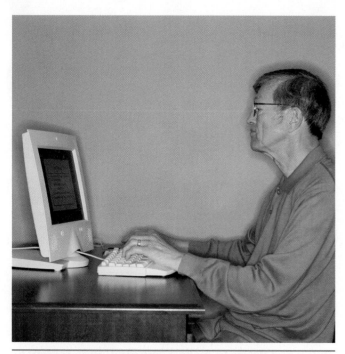

An older adult maintains cognitive skills by remaining mentally active. Courtesy of PhotoDisc.

an assessment and give the older adult the support and advice necessary in this sensitive area.

Sensory Changes

Sensory capacities change in the elderly person. A decrease in neurons accompanying aging may lead to a diminished sense of equilibrium and balance (Papalia & Olds, 1998). Visual acuity declines due to age-related changes in the eye. The lens continues to lose elasticity, becomes cloudy, and admits less light. The pupils become smaller, and the eyelids sag and may interfere with vision. Risks for cataracts, glaucoma, and age-related macular degeneration increase in the aged. Hearing loss continues, with further reduction in hearing of higher frequencies and eventual trouble discerning consonant sounds. Taste and smell sensitivity decline with age, resulting in lessened appetite and enjoyment of food. The skin is less sensitive to touch, and the older adult is less aware of changes in pain and temperature sensation (Murray & Zentner, 2001).

Because these systemic and sensory changes are considered inevitable, some people regard aging and the older adult years as an overwhelming, rapid decline into sickness, incapacity, and death. The older adult takes longer to recover from illness, suffers from a greater number of chronic diseases, and has less resistance to disease. However, the older adult is capable of enduring the changes of aging and functioning very ably. Age-related changes differ greatly in time of onset, and the individual's attitude toward aging often influences the extent to which these changes affect function. Most older adults continue their activities and lifestyles with minimum adjustment to the changes of aging.

Multiple studies have found that exercise is essential to elders' physical and mental health and well-being as well as being a natural retardant of the aging process. The importance of health care professionals promoting exercise among elders was emphasized by McMurdo (1999). She noted that imaginative efforts should be made to help older people identify activities they will enjoy and that often health care professionals are too protective of elders when it comes to exercise.

Many health problems of older adults are improved by exercise. Regular exercise reduces weight and stress, lessens the risks of hypertension and atherosclerosis, and improves glucose metabolism among older adults. Improved physical mobility and balance lead to fewer accidental falls. Last, elderly individuals who exercise are more inclined to change other lifestyle factors related to heart disease, such as high-fat diet and smoking.

Cognitive Development

The cognitive development of the older adult shows a reduction in reaction time but, as with the middle adult, no decline in intellectual function. Again, certain variables affect the measurement of the older person's intellectual functioning: decreased visual and auditory acuity, slowed responses to stimuli, loss of recent memory, and altered motivation, among others (Murray & Zentner, 2001). Cultural differences can also influence measurement of intelligence. For example, because Hispanics are very concerned about hurting someone's feelings, they might respond politely even when they do not understand. Reaction times will often be slower under stress, and many older adults have endured social and environmental losses that cause stress. Other factors that can influence the measurement of cognitive ability in older adults are isolation, level of education and length of time since school attendance, interest, and the conservation of time and energy for other more meaningful tasks (Murray & Zentner, 2001). One important factor to consider when making any judgment about cognitive development in the older adult is the fact that the process of aging is unique to the person. Aging does not occur in the same way in all individuals. This is especially true with regard to mental abilities.

Memory and Memory Loss

One major area of concern in the mental health of the older adult is memory and memory loss (Bee, 1998). The older person who is mentally active and well educated will not show the same problems with memory as will those adults without similar opportunities to use their minds. Research is showing that active participation in education may benefit older people's health (Newman & Newman, 1999). Long-term memory seems to remain intact longer than does short-term memory, possibly because of the frequency of recall of these memories. It is difficult to measure memory in this population because there are so many variables that can affect the measure-

RESEARCH FOCUS

Influence of Companion Animals on the Physical and Psychological Health of Older People: An Analysis of a One-Year Longitudinal Study

Study Problem/Purpose

The purpose of this study was to evaluate the effect of companion animals on the physical and psychological health of older people and to determine if relationships between physical and psychological health and human social networks were modified by a companion animal.

Methods

A random sample of 995 persons aged 65 and over (mean 73 years) participated in a longitudinal study consisting of a telephone interview at the beginning of the study and 1 year later. A battery of tests were administered by phone, assessing social activities, support, well-being, physical and psychological health, pet ownership, and pet attachment.

Findings

Pet owners tended to be younger, married or living with someone, and more physically active. Activities of daily living diminished more rapidly in non–pet owners than in pet owners. However, the direct relationship of owning a pet to psychological well-being was not significant. A complex relationship existed between pet ownership and an older person's well-being.

Implications

Pet ownership may be instrumental in enhancing a person's ability to maintain activities of daily living, thus independence. More investigation is required to determine if a relationship exists between pet ownership and well-being in older adults.

Source: Raina, P., Waltner-Toews, D., Bonnett, B., Woodword, C., & Abernathy, T. (1999). Influence of companion animals on the physical and psychological health of older people: An analysis of a one-year longitudinal study. Journal of the American Geriatrics Society, 47(3), 323–329.

---

ment. Memory changes or alterations in mental functioning usually result from physical or mental disorders often found among elderly people and are generally not a normal part of the aging process.

Psychosocial Development

The psychosocial development of the older adult is an interesting phenomenon. This is a time for assessment of self and life, a time to look back over that which has been achieved and to prepare for the end of life. Erikson describes the task of this stage as **ego integrity versus despair** (Erikson, 1963). Ego integrity means the coming together of all aspects of the past and an acceptance that this life was the only life to be lived. Without this sense of ego integrity, the individual suffers despair, a sense of futility, and the feeling that life was too short and that nothing was accomplished. With despair comes a fear of death, anger at the whole aging process, resentment of younger people, and feelings of inadequacy and worthlessness (Erikson, 1963).

Levinson's (1986) theory of development proposes a transitional period at this stage of life wherein fundamental changes in body and personality lead to fear that the individual has lost all identity and must find a new inner energy with which to survive these last years. The individual in this period has suffered losses, either death of peers, serious illness, or other catastrophes, and is forced to look for new inner strength. In the late years of adulthood, the individual becomes more turned inward, less involved in family and society, and more concerned with inner resources.

Death is considered the final developmental stage and, as such, requires careful preparation. Attitudes toward death have changed over time. In earlier days, dying was an event that took place at home in the company of friends and family. Today, over 70% of deaths in American cities occur in institutions (Murray & Zentner, 2001). This tendency has made death remote and, in some cases, a fearful experience. The hospice movement has begun to affect this picture by providing support for the client and family to face death in the home. The community health nurse is often the person who assists the family and the client to come to terms with the approaching death. It is vital that the nurse, as the principal caregiver, provide support and leadership during this process (Lindeman & McAthie, 1999).

Retirement and Life Review

Two important events in this stage of life are retirement and performing a life review. The way an individual responds to retirement depends largely on the relationship with the job or career. If the work was meaningless, repetitive, and boring, retirement may be a relief and a pleasure. However, many occupations are satisfying and

✳ DECISION MAKING

The Age to Retire

Imagine you are a community health nurse working with the family of a frail 85-year-old woman. She lives with her daughter and her husband. The son-in-law is 68 years old, has a chronic heart problem, and receives a disability stipend. The daughter is 62 years old and has been employed as a bookkeeper at a fruit cannery for many years. She states she has not been feeling well and is finding it difficult to work all day and come home to care for her mother, who is needing more and more help. She says she would like to retire so she could stay at home with her mother but is afraid there will not be enough income to keep their home and maintain their lifestyle.

◆ What factors must be considered in her decision?

◆ How can you assist her in making this decision?

FIGURE 23-4   Important Questions When Considering Retirement Communities

- Do the weather, culture, and recreational activities fit your lifestyle?

- After talking with residents, participating in activities, and eating a meal, can this community offer what you need to live fully and happily?

- Have there been any complaints about this community with any governing, business, or associated agencies?

- What kind of insurance and bonding are carried to protect you if the agency encounters financial difficulty?

- What are the lease termination and refund policies?

- Is the deposit refundable and will interest be applied?

- Are monthly fees variable and, if so, will the agency provide a history of increases?

- What are policies regarding vehicles, parking, and visitors? Are there accommodations so visitors can stay on the premises?

- Have you reviewed all documents you are asked to sign with competent legal assistance?

- Have you taken your time to make your decision, visiting different facilities?

Adapted from *Health Promotion Strategies through the Life Span* (7th ed.), by R. B. Murray and J. P. Zentner, 2001, Upper Saddle River, NJ: Prentice-Hall.

---

fulfilling and carry high status and power. In such an instance, retirement may be devastating. Care should be taken to preplan leisure activities or new careers to perpetuate feelings of self-worth and usefulness. Adjustments in relationships are also necessary, as job-related social opportunities often are no longer available. Marital relationships need time to adjust to this new way of life as previous roles are eliminated and new roles become more clearly defined. Financial conditions must also be considered, especially if retirement brings a reduction in income. Figure 23-4 lists anticipatory actions for the retiring person.

There is no mandatory retirement age in the United States, and most older adults are still highly qualified to perform their jobs. Some people choose to retire in their fifties or sixties. Others choose to retire from one position or career and take on another career at age 60 or 70. Older people often express a need for achievement and challenge. Retirement can be a time of vital aging in which the individual, after a lifetime of work, has the time to pursue interests and hobbies there was no time for previously. Elderhostel (an organization of education and adventure for those over 55) is thriving. Elders are healthier and more active than in years past, moving from work to retirement in numbers previously unseen. In the United States our self-perceptions are often greatly influenced by what we do for a living. Thus, when a person retires, there is an effect on most other roles and relationships. Retirement often means changes in social, emotional, financial, and possibly physical circumstances in the individual's life (Papalia & Olds, 1998).

All of these life changes remind individuals that time is limited and they are approaching the end of their lives. Thus, one last task necessary at this stage of life is life review. Most of one's life's work is accomplished. Butler (1963) described life review as

a naturally occurring, universal mental process characterized by the progressive return to consciousness of past experiences, and, particularly, the resurgence of unresolved conflicts; simultaneously, and normally, these revived experiences and conflicts can be surveyed and reintegrated . . . it is shaped by contemporaneous experiences and its nature and outcome are affected by the life-long unfolding of character. (p. 66)

Acceptance of life facts and the final making of peace with the self are important to the individual in accepting the inevitability of the approaching death.

Facing Death

Dying marks a developmental transition in a person's life. It involves living every day to its fullest as well as preparing for the end of life and the severing of relationships.

Perspectives...

INSIGHTS OF A NURSING STUDENT

"Oh my, this man is 98 years old!" I thought to myself when my first client was assigned to me during my community health rotation. My interest is in maternal/child nursing, my experience is in labor and delivery as a doula. I had limited experience with older clients and now I was assigned one to visit at his home. My concern was not so much in providing care. I knew I was capable of performing physical, functional, and environmental assessments. I knew how to look for potential risk factors in each of these areas and was confident I could perform at an appropriate level. No, this was not my concern. I was concerned that I would be unable to facilitate therapeutic communication with a 98-year-old man. Both of my grandfathers died when I was very young, and I had never had the opportunity to get to know any other elderly gentleman. I was not quite sure if I would be able to be relaxed and supportive with Raymond G., a 98-year-old widowed and retired college professor, as I was capable of being with new mothers and their infant children.

The first lesson I learned about communicating with an older person is to talk slowly. This I discovered during my first phone call to Raymond to set up our first appointment. "I'm sorry, could you repeat what you just said?" was his response to most of my statements during that first phone call. It was a course in patience and enunciation. By the end of the conversation I managed to keep my remarks brief, slow, and loud. As a result we were able to schedule a visit for the following Tuesday in the early afternoon. I spent the next week rereading chapters on working with the elderly in my community health nursing text and outlining my plan for our initial visit.

The days flew by and Tuesday morning arrived. After preconference, I reviewed my initial plan, then called Raymond to confirm our appointment. At the agreed-upon time I walked up the path to his front door. I was able to look through the screen as I walked up the steps, and I saw an elderly gentleman, dressed in khaki pants and a cardigan sweater, sitting in a chair right inside the door. He looked up and smiled, then invited me in. Our visit was short, about 30 minutes, and we spent the time sitting across from each other in chairs he had carefully placed in the living room. I enjoyed hearing about his life, his deceased wife, his grown children, and his fondness for gardening. He explained that he was "eight plus ninety, that's 98" and that he didn't expect to live to see 100, nor did he want to. He introduced me to his companion, Tiffany. "She's a good cat," he said, "she loves to sit with me and never talks back." He and

Tiffany had been together for eight years, and Raymond made it clear that she was quite special to him. Although I didn't want to seem too familiar, I did want to begin a general assessment of the surroundings. I asked Raymond if I could take a look around before I left. He told me to feel free to do so, and I was able to make a first assessment of the home environment before leaving.

I sat in my car for a few minutes reflecting on our visit and was surprised to discover I had really enjoyed visiting with Raymond in his home. Raymond was very easy to talk with, very appreciative of the visit, and had many interesting things to say. I looked forward to getting to know him over the course of the semester. Unfortunately, I was able to visit with Raymond only three times before he suffered a massive MI, which resulted in his death one week later. I had been in touch with Raymond's son, John, and his wife, Sheila, regularly during the course of our relationship, and in the two weeks following Raymond's death we continued to keep in contact. I was able to assist them in finalizing the relationship they had with our student community health group (Raymond had been our client for many years) and even found a new home for Tiffany. This was a great relief for the family, because they were unable to keep her but were devastated at the idea of putting her down.

As I said earlier, my emphasis is in maternal/child health. I have worked with many women and infants during the first few weeks of life, a position I have found to be both invigorating and rewarding. I didn't expect to gain, so soon, the experience of assisting someone through the last days of life, but I know my life was enriched because of it. I know I made Raymond's last week a little more pleasant for him. Both he and his son, John, told me how much my visits meant, and I know Raymond would be pleased that Tiffany has a nice new home. I gave Raymond the gift of caring, but he gave much to me as well.

My life has been enhanced as a result of my short, but meaningful, relationship with Raymond. I have gained valuable insight into the practice of community nursing and into the final stages of life. For Raymond, life had become mundane. He was homebound and had few visitors. Yet he had a mind filled with rich memories and wondrous experiences that he was willing to share with me during our visits. He enjoyed talking about his life and told me more than once that, although it had been a good life, he was ready to "go see my wife." Raymond taught me that the final stage

(continues)

Perspectives...

INSIGHTS OF A NURSING STUDENT (continued)

of life is not to be feared, but embraced. He taught me that it's ok to look back at life and rejoice while preparing for death, that just having someone there to listen who cared about what he had to say was one of life's pleasures. I will always remember fondly my re-

lationship with Raymond, and I promise to be a good companion to Tiffany, who, by the way, is adjusting nicely to life in my home.

—Pamela Rasada
Student Nurse

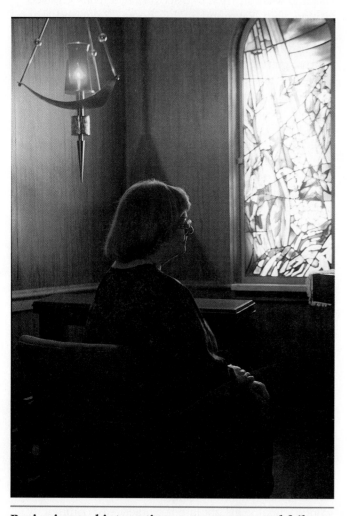

Reviewing and integrating past successes and failures for a sense of wholeness are essential for developing Erikson's developmental stage of integrity.

The community health nurse can assist the client and family in a growth-producing experience until death actually occurs. The client must be assessed for level of knowledge and acceptance and then supported in the process of accepting death. An atmosphere of open honesty and trust is vital during this last stage of life (Lindeman & McAthie, 1999).

REFLECTIVE THINKING

Loneliness and Aging

- Have you ever been alone and unable or unwilling to reach out to others?
- Can you think of ways to help a recently widowed elderly person combat loneliness?
- Do you think financial status has any impact on loneliness? On isolation?

Older-Adult Risk Factors

The risk factors faced by older individuals are many, but most older adults live healthy, productive lives. These individuals, well elders, are growing in number and provide our society with a rich source of experience and wisdom (Papalia & Olds, 1998).

Some of the mental and emotional risk factors at this age are depression, isolation, dementia, and dealing with losses. These include loss of loved ones, loss of job status and prestige, loss of income, loss of independence, and loss of an energetic and resilient body (Lindeman & McAthie, 1999).

Depression

Depression is the most common psychiatric disorder among older adults and is often a reaction to the losses experienced during these years (Varcarolis, 2002). The disease is characterized by intense sadness, hopelessness, pessimism, and low self-regard. Somatic complaints are more common than mood disturbance in elderly persons. Depression rates are very high among the elderly, but depression is not a part of "normal aging." In 1999 the Surgeon General released disturbing information about suicide in the elderly. The highest rates of suicide are in those over 65, with white men over 85 completing the most suicides. Firearms are the weapons used most often to complete suicide in this age group, and attempts are completed far more frequently than in any other age group. Most elderly suicide victims (70%) visited a health care provider within the month preceding their suicide (U.S. Public Health Service, 1999). See Chapter 29 for more information. The nurse needs to follow up on symptoms of depression to determine whether suicidal intentions are present, then find treatment resources.

Loss and Social Support

Isolation can result from physical barriers such as curbs, steps, and the weather or emotional barriers such as fear of crime, depression, and losses such as transportation independence and the death of a spouse and friends. Research indicates there is a broad range of emotional responses to the loss of a spouse, but these responses do not differ significantly between men and women (Quigley & Schatz, 1999). Ostir, Markides, Black, and Goodwin (2000) found emotional well-being evident in a positive affect is different from simply an absence of depression and seems to protect individuals against physical decline in old age. In either case, the older adult is often unable to access appropriate services, act as his own advocate, or coordinate the care he needs (Murray & Zentner, 2001). Although community health nurses can neither reverse the process of aging nor make the associated losses less painful to the older adult, they can listen to the client's complaints, act as a liaison between client and other professionals, and support the client and family in many ways. Because the older adult often relies heavily on family members for assistance, it is important for nurses to work with families as well as individuals. Intergenerational bonds seem to constitute an important factor in the older adult's capacity to survive.

Each stage of growth and development has specific environmental needs above and beyond the common needs of all ages. Chapter 9 explores environment in more detail. Relationships in each developmental stage constitute important aspects of environment.

Because older adulthood is the time when major losses occur, it is vital that older adults have good social support in their personal environments. Family members who love and respect the older individual are important, especially when death and disease have decimated the circle of friends and perhaps taken one's spouse. A better quality of intergenerational interactions usually results in more satisfied elders (Bee, 1998). Often, grandchildren form special relationships with the elderly person and share activities that are very satisfying to both parties (Bee, 1998). Sibling relationships among older adults have not received enough attention, although for many older people, siblings are the only surviving support system (Blasinsky, 1998). Because the older-adult stage of life spans such diverse conditions and abilities, care must be taken to include an array of support systems for all older adults, from the young-old to the old-old.

Community health nurses operate within the environment of the client and must be aware of the importance of the relationships within that environment. They must be aware of all the issues that affect the well-being of clients and must take an interest in social issues, community concerns, and civic matters in addition to health-related issues.

Dementia

Although the majority of older adults experience little or no cognitive impairment, the fear of losing mental capacity is often expressed. Dementia, especially dementia of the Alzheimer's type, is feared most of all. Because this disease often covers a 6- to 20-year course, it has an especially devastating impact on older adults. The community health nurse is often the individual who serves as support and liaison for the family of the Alzheimer's victim. The nurse can act as a resource to the family in locating respite services, home care assistance, and, eventually, long-term care placement options. Education of the elder with Alzheimer's disease should always be accomplished in ways that enhance the person's self-confidence, done with a minimum of environmental distraction in a low-pitched, clear voice and using short, concise, concrete material. Give them plenty of time and help them make associations with prior information. Including a significant other in the lesson will help the client use the information (Murray & Zentner, 2001). See Chapter 27 for more detailed information about chronic conditions.

Sensory Impairment

Sensory impairment is a factor affecting all elderly persons. Visual and auditory problems accompany progressive aging. Blindness and deafness are real risks and require special care to ensure that communication is maintained. Older adults who are hearing impaired have been shown to adapt to the stresses of late life more poorly than those who are not impaired (Stein & Bienenfeld, 1992). Figure 23-5 lists guidelines for helping persons who are blind. Figure 23-6 lists guidelines for communicating with individuals who are hearing impaired.

Reduced pain and temperature sensations can cause safety problems. Older adults need to have more covering on their beds, keep their thermostats higher in the winter, and be aware of ways to prevent hypothermia. Reaction to pain is a warning system, and care must be taken when pain sensation is reduced. Burns or frostbite can occur without warning. Foot care must be meticulous, as there is reduced sensation in the lower extremities.

Older adults are much more likely to suffer from chronic disease than are younger individuals. These chronic conditions can affect any body system and are rarely cured, only symptomatically controlled. Some of the more common chronic diseases of elderly persons are Parkinson's disease, dementias, congestive heart failure, chronic obstructive pulmonary disease, arthritis, and diabetes mellitus. See Chapter 27.

FIGURE 23-5   Guidelines for Helping Persons Who Are Blind

- Talk to the person in a normal tone of voice. The fact that sight is impaired is no indication that hearing is also impaired.
- When offering assistance, do so directly.
- In guiding the person, permit the person to take your arm. Never grab the person's arm.
- In walking with the person, proceed at a normal pace. Hesitate slightly before stepping up and down.
- Be explicit in giving directions to the person.
- There is no need to avoid use of the word see when talking with a person who is blind.
- When assisting the person to a chair, place his or her hand on the back or arm of the chair.
- When leaving the person after conversing together, advise that you are leaving so that the person does not continue the conversation when no one is listening.
- Never leave a person who is blind in an open area. Lead him or her to the side of a room, to a chair, or to some landmark from which he or she can obtain direction.
- A half-open door is one of the most dangerous obstacles that people who are blind encounter.
- When serving food to the person, identify each item as you place it on the table. Call attention to food placement by using the numbers of an imaginary clock. For example, "The green beans are at two o'clock."
- Be sure to make the person aware of other guests.

Adapted from *Health Promotion Strategies through the Life Span* (7th ed.), by R. B. Murray and J. P. Zentner, 2001, Upper Saddle River, NJ: Prentice-Hall.

FIGURE 23-6   Guidelines for Communicating with Persons Who Are Hearing Impaired

- When you meet a person who seems inattentive or slow to understand, you consider the possibility that hearing, rather than manners or intellect, may be at fault.
- Remember that persons who are hearing impaired may depend on reading your lips. You can help by always trying to speak in a good light and by facing the person and the light as you speak.
- When in a group that includes a person who is hearing impaired, try to carry on your conversation with others in such a way that your lips can be seen.
- Speak distinctly but naturally. Try not to speak too rapidly.
- Do not start to speak to the person abruptly. Attract the person's attention first by facing the person and looking straight into his or her eyes. If necessary, lightly touch one of the person's hands or shoulders.
- If the person to whom you are speaking has one "good" ear, always stand on that side when you speak. Do not be afraid to ask a person who has an obvious hearing loss whether his or her hearing is better in one ear than in the other.
- Facial expressions are important clues to meaning.
- In conversation with a person who is very deaf, jot down key words on paper.
- Many people who are hearing impaired are sensitive about their disability and will pretend to understand you even when they do not. Repeat your meaning in different words until it gets across.
- Teach family members that they do not have to exclude the persons who are hearing impaired from all forms of entertainment involving speech or music. Even persons who are profoundly deaf can feel rhythm, and many are good and eager dancers.
- Use common sense and tact in determining which of these suggestions apply to particular persons.

Adapted from *Health Promotion Strategies through the Life Span* (7th ed.), by R. B. Murray and J. P. Zentner, 2001, Upper Saddle River, NJ: Prentice-Hall.

Cancer

The CDC (1999) published data indicating that for those 65–74 cancer rates more than doubled from rates of the previous decade, for those 75–84 rates more than tripled, and for those over 85 years old cancer rates were 4.5 times higher than for people aged 55–64. Fifty percent of all cancers are diagnosed in people over 65 years of age. Gambassi (1998) collected data on 13,625 cancer patients aged 65 and older and found they were grossly undermedicated for pain and those over 85 as well as African Americans frequently received nothing for pain. Reasons for the increased risk of cancer in elders are currently being researched. One possible reason is the accumulated exposure to carcinogens over time. Another might be the long latent period some cancers require before appear-

ing; for example, skin cancer due to sun exposure may appear 40 years after exposure (Sarna, 1995). Yet another theory regarding increased cancer rates in elders is that aging changes the immune system, resulting in a decreased ability of the elderly body to detect and eliminate cancer cells.

The community health nurse's role remains as advocate, educator, support, and resource person. The nurse holds a unique place in this relationship with the client,

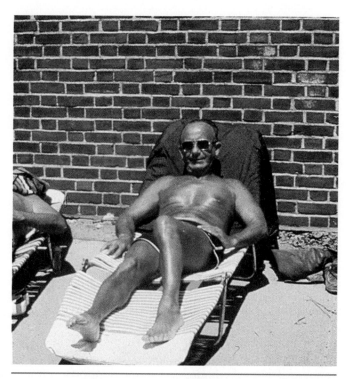

Cancer caused by sun exposure may take years to appear. Courtesy of Phoenix Society for Burn Survivors, Inc.

family, and those resources needed to maintain optimal health in the client.

Ageism

Ageism is a major social risk for the older adult. This term refers to discrimination based on age. Older adults are characterized as senile, useless, dependent, and sick (Bee, 1998). Although publicly denounced by gerontologists, ageism continues to affect society. There have been some advances in improving the image of older adults, but there is still a tendency, even among those who work with elders, to view elders as asexual, unemployable, unintelligent, and socially incompetent. This notion that all older individuals are essentially the same is a form of ageism and is more difficult to correct than blatant prejudice. Older people themselves are often as guilty of ageist attitudes as are younger adults (Murray & Zentner, 2001). The medical profession is also guilty of ageist assumptions when making decisions about treatable conditions. Too often incontinence, memory changes, sexual dysfunction, or preoccupation with death are considered a normal result of aging and are either not treated or are not treated vigorously. Ageism is prominent among health care professionals as well, affecting the quality of physical and psychological care received by elders (Ward, 2000; Wilkes, LeMiere, & Walker, 1998). In addition, research indicates that while elder abuse is a widespread practice in our society, it is often not diagnosed by family physicians (Swagerty, Takahashi, & Evans, 1999).

Closely connected with ageism is the issue of independence. Although only 5% of older people are in institutions and only 10% show even mild to moderate memory loss, the misconception continues that old people are incompetent, sick, senile, and dependent on others to function successfully (Murray & Zentner, 2001). Because of the societal orientation to youth and the fast pace of today's world, older adults often feel they are not respected or valued. Without clear guidelines regarding their role in society, many older adults opt out and become dependent, relying on others to make decisions for them. One of the nurse's roles in caring for the older adult is to promote the client's abilities and potential and to assist in promoting optimal functioning.

When an elderly person becomes unable to remain at home because of the need for extensive nursing care, however, the community health nurse can be of great assistance in helping the family or individual choose a nursing home or convalescent care center. This is one of the most dreaded decisions a family makes regarding an elderly family member. Often, the family has maintained the client for years in an informal caretaking situation with some assistance from friends, home health agencies, and other organizations. Research shows that the caregiver burden contributes to an increased risk of institutionalization in the United States (Ryan & Scullion, 2000). When the decision is made, the caregivers need as much support and guidance during the transition as does the client.

Bereavement

A primary social risk factor for the older adult is the risk of the death of a spouse or partner. This can occur in other life stages but is more common in older adulthood. Usually, bereavement does not permanently affect the health of an older adult, but it can produce physiological symptoms and a great deal of psychological distress (Bee, 1998). Although suddenly single status disrupts established couple-based relationships, the changes can sometimes produce positive results. Relatives and friends may become closer and more supportive; a move to a smaller residence may involve the individual in more neighborhood socializing; and being alone may stimulate the client into making new contacts and broadening life interests.

Spirituality

The nurse is in a unique position to address spirituality with the older adult. Older adults often express a desire to discuss spiritual matters. More than religious affiliation or rituals, spirituality reaches the deeper aspects of an individual's capacity for love, well-being, and meaning in life (Klaas, 1998). A large number of elderly individuals see religion as a means of coping with life's difficulties and turn to their clergy and church community in times of need. Recognition of this aspect of a person's life is important. Hicks (1999) reported that quality care to enhance elders' well-being and sense of inner peace include spiritually focused nursing interventions such as silent witnessing, serving as a liaison, and active listening.

Safety

Many aspects of aging threaten the safety of elders. For some it may be diminishing sight, hearing, sense of touch, and sensitivity to hot and cold. For others it may be a loss of physical strength, chronic illness, or dementia. Fuller (2000) reported that falls are the number one cause of accidental death in persons over 65. In persons over 75, falls account for 70% of accidental deaths. One-third of elderly persons in the community fall every year. Risk factors include housebound status, living alone, use of a cane or walker, acute or chronic illness, four or more medications, cognitive impairment, sensory deficits, foot problems, and difficulty rising from a chair.

Aging Successfully

Aging successfully is difficult to define. There is the **inner aspect of aging,** one's relationship and contentment with self, and the **outer** (or **social**) **aspect of aging,** one's relationship with society as one ages. No one theory of aging explains the process completely. Common theories are considered to represent only some of many possible patterns of aging. Some researchers prefer to look at successful aging with regard to the individual's personality makeup. Although there have been several definitions of personalities and how successfully or unsuccessfully they age, the emerging truism for personality and aging seems to be that older people become more of who they were (Bee, 1998). Persons continue to develop and grow, but personality characteristics are only emphasized, and drastic changes in basic personality are

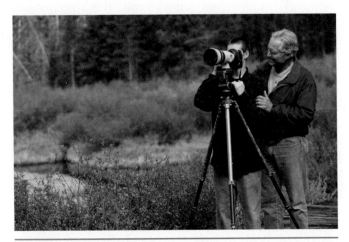

An older adult can serve as mentor to younger adults.
Courtesy of PhotoDisc.

not made. The talkative, flexible, social personality will become more so in older age as appropriate to physical status and life situation. If the older adult is rigid, conservative, and opinionated, it is probable that those same traits were present in younger life, but to a lesser degree. Perhaps the younger individual sublimated these traits to make them more acceptable or less obvious than they are in old age.

In the near future older adults will garner more and more attention from community health nurses as the baby-boom generation moves into the geriatric cohort. These nurses will research, create, administer, and provide services that include, in part, policymaking, promoting, and maintaining healthy active elders, creating community supports, and assisting in a healthy death transition. As finite resources are distributed among those in need, community health nurses will be instrumental in creating care and policies that promote the health of older adults, which in turn promotes health in the population at large.

Community health nurses can help reduce the risk of falls in the home by assisting the elder to eliminate environmental hazards, improving home supports, referrals for opportunities for socialization, balance training, medication modification, and educating the family about monitoring for risk factors. The nurse, again, is invaluable not only in identifying those individuals who are at risk for isolation, but also in serving as an advocate to obtain necessary services.

THE NURSING PROCESS AND THE ADULT YEARS

The community health nurse provides care to adult clients in all three developmental stages. It is helpful to use the nursing process in addressing health and well-being and determining those nursing functions that are most common to each of the developmental stages of adulthood.

Implications for Community Nursing Practice

Health promotion and protection is a primary function of community health nurses. Health protection occurs at three levels: primary, secondary, and tertiary. Primary prevention usually involves educating clients about health issues to maintain or enhance their level of wellness. Examples include developing a curriculum for educating young adults about sexually transmitted diseases, educational promotions for adequate exercise in middle-aged adults, and teaching the elderly about environmental hazards that may induce falls. Secondary prevention involves screening for or educating about diseases for early detection and intervention. Examples include screening for cervical cancer in young adults, for

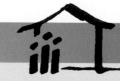

COMMUNITY NURSING VIEW

Pilar, a 55-year-old woman, comes to a blood pressure clinic operated by a community health nurse. She complains of vague headaches, feeling tired all the time, and having no energy. She has not had a menstrual period for two years and has occasional hot flashes and sweating. She recently began wearing bifocals and has had some trouble adjusting to them. She states she feels "blue" and uninterested in her usual activities, including sexual activity with her husband.

Pilar works for an insurance company in a sedentary job that is not particularly challenging. She does not exercise regularly: "Walks around the neighborhood now and then." She states that she loves to cook and misses having her two children home to cook for. The children are attending college some distance away. Because he is unable to safely live alone, her 87-year-old father recently moved in with her and her husband. Her father is on a restricted diet and cannot eat the type of food Pilar enjoys preparing, such as casseroles and meats and poultry with heavy sauces.

Nursing Considerations

Assessment

- In assessing this client, what data can be drawn from the interview to assist the nurse in the care plan?
- What additional questions might the nurse ask in order to formulate the nursing care plan?

- In what developmental stage is this client? Can you identify the developmental tasks she is trying to accomplish?
- In the review of the client's problems, which of her statements requires top priority? Why?

Diagnosis

- Do any of this client's problems cluster around and pertain to a single nursing diagnosis?
- Can you identify four nursing diagnoses from the information presented in the case study?

Outcome Identification

- What outcomes can the nurse expect if the plan is successful?

Planning/Interventions

- What should be the nurse's first step in forming a plan to assist this client?
- Identify interventions for each of the nursing diagnoses you have listed.

Evaluation

- Identify evaluation methods that would enable the nurse to determine whether Pilar is succeeding or failing with regard to the nursing plan.

---

colorectal cancer in middle-aged adults, and sensory deficits in elderly adults. Tertiary prevention occurs when a disease or disability is well established and involves rehabilitation or restoring the client to an optimal level of functioning (Lindeman & McAthie, 1999). Examples include treating prostate cancer in a young adult male, diabetic education in a middle-aged diabetic adult, and nursing home policies for care of frail elderly clients. The community health nurse is a vital component of health promotion and disease prevention for adults residing in the community and health within the community in general.

Community health nurses are actively involved at the micro- and macrolevels of health care, wielding a powerful influence on community health-related needs. This is done via formal and informal research as well as during the provision of care. At the macrolevel they create, administer and enforce public policy providing for the

health of adults in a variety of venues such as environmental contamination, public safety, adequate housing, disease and birth control, adequate sources of water, and innumerable health-related services. The role of the community health nurse in adult health care is limited only by imagination.

KEY CONCEPTS

- Several theories of growth and development must be considered because no one theory adequately explains the adult years.
- Adults in each stage of development—young, middle, and older—proceed through tasks and accomplish age-related skills before progressing to the next stage of adulthood.

Out
of the Box

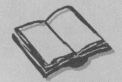

Foundations Enhancing Health in Young Adulthood

Community health nurses are actively and courageously paving the way for healthy young adulthood by providing diligent, effective and creative care to teens. While adolescent behaviors are often addressed in the media, when it comes to seeking health care, they are a silent and neglected cohort, despite vast physical/mental changes, concerns, and risks. An example of nurse-led care for adolescents began in 1990 in Flagstaff, Arizona. During a youth town hall meeting, several area teens expressed desires for free, confidential health care services, particularly related to the issues of sexuality, pregnancy, violence, and substance abuse. Initially the county Department of Health Services and a Behavioral Health Center collaborated to start the Teen Wellness Clinic in which pregnancy testing and counseling were provided. The services quickly expanded to provide primary health care services for youth ages 13–19 years. Care provided by a community health nurse, two family nurse practitioners, and a behavioral health specialist now includes physical, behavioral, mental health, and social needs. All services are free and confidential, except in the case of physical illness not related to sexual activity. In this situation, parents must be contacted for consent to treat.

Seventy-five percent of client visits involved pregnancy issues when the clinic first started. Now, 10 years later, data show just 50% of visits address reproduction and pregnancy, sexually transmitted diseases (STDs), and other physical problems while 50% of the visits address behavioral and mental health issues. Based on the success of the Teen Wellness Clinic, in 2000 funding was received to focus more on the needs of adolescent males. This clinic has been a primary factor in decreasing the teen pregnancy rate in the county and in fact has become the medical home for many at-risk, disenfranchised adolescents who would otherwise not be served or served minimally.

The clinic is open two afternoons a week from 2 P.M. until 6 P.M. on a first-come, first-served, walk-in basis. Despite the fact that clients are growing in numbers (nearly 150 are seen in a month), no teen is ever turned away. They may have to return for examinations but will always have at least the opportunity to talk with the community health nurse manager, the nurse practitioner, or the behavioral health specialist. The clinic focuses on assessment of physical and psychological issues as well as works in collaboration with other local health care agencies for appropriate referrals as necessary. The community health nurse manager is responsible for referral and follow-up for the teens seen in the clinic by the nurse practitioner and the behavioral health specialist. This community health nurse is also responsible for accountability to the various funding agencies. The Teen Wellness Clinic in Flagstaff, Arizona, is a model for an effective nurse-run community intervention that maximizes the potential for experiencing a healthy young adulthood by serving adolescents, particularly those at risk. ■

—Kathy Ingelse, FNP, MS
Teen Wellness Clinic

◆ Particular risk factors and conditions apply to each life stage, including emotional, mental, physical, spiritual, and social risks. Some risk factors are present through all stages of adulthood.

◆ Healthy relationships in the adult years are a vital part of successful aging.

◆ The stages of adult development give nurses valuable information for providing care to young, middle, and older adults.

RESOURCES

ACROSS ADULTHOOD

Harvard School of Public Health: www.hsph.harvard.edu
Health concerns across the life span: www.cmwf.org/programs
Directory of Health and Human Services Data Resources:
   http://www.hhs.gov/aspe/minority/mintoc
Section on Geriatrics, American Physical Therapy Association:
   www.geriatricspt.org

Wellness Web: www.wellnessweb.com
Your Health Daily: www.yourhealthdaily.com

ADDICTIONS

Addiction Search: www.addictionsearch.com
National Center on Addiction and Substance Abuse:
    www.casacolumbia.org

MENTAL HEALTH

Center for Addictions and Mental Health Resources:
    www.camh.net/resources
Mental Help Net: www.mentalhelp.net
National Strategy for Suicide Prevention:
    www.mentalhealth.org/suicideprevention
Older Adults: Depression and Suicide Facts:
    www.nimh.nih.gov/publicat/depoldermenu.cfm

NUTRITION

Food and Nutrition Information Center: www.nal.usda.gov/fnic

OLDER ADULTHOOD

Administration on Aging: www.aoa.dhhs.gov
American Association of Retired Persons: www.aarp.org
Seniors—Senior Site: www.seniorsite.com

YOUNG ADULTHOOD

Go Ask Alice: www.goaskalice.columbia.edu
Parent Soup: www.parentsoup.com

Chapter

24

FRAMEWORKS FOR ASSESSING FAMILIES

Janice E. Hitchcock, RN, DNSc

One of the most important aspects of nursing is the emphasis placed on the family unit. The family—along with the individual, group, and community—is nursing's client or recipient of care.

—*Friedman, 1998, p. 3*

COMPETENCIES

Upon completion of this chapter, the reader should be able to:

- Identify the difference between family as context and family as client.
- Recount definitions of family including a definition that encompasses the changing family structure.
- List a variety of family forms.
- Detail nursing theories that provide guidance for understanding families, including those of Neuman, King, Roy, and Rogers.
- Discuss social science theories that help to explain family dynamics, processes, and tasks, including developmental theory, systems theory, structural-functional framework, and interactional theory.
- Explain the contribution of family system theories to the understanding of the family.
- Describe theories that focus on the interaction between family and community.
- Discuss the difference between the nurse as caregiver and the family as caregiver to family members.
- Detail cultural aspects of the family and their impact on family life.
- Explain the importance of working in partnership with families.
- Delineate the dimensions of the nursing process—assessment, diagnosis, planning, intervention, and evaluation—as they apply to family nursing.

KEY TERMS

assimilated family style	ecosystem
biological mother	energy
blended (or binuclear) family	entropy
boundary	equifinality
caregiver	equilibrium
contextual family structure	equipotentiality
contextual stimuli	exosystem
contextualism	extended family
developmental tasks	external family structure
developmental theory	family
differentiation	family acculturative styles
ecological approach	family as client
ecomap	family as context

family function
family health tree
family interactional theories
family of origin (or orientation)
family of procreation
family strengths
family structure
family systems theories
feedback
flow and transformation
focal stimuli
focal system
general systems theory
genogram
hierarchy of systems
input
integrated bicultural family style
internal family structure
macrosystem
marginalized family style
mesosystem
microsystem

morphogenesis
morphostasis
negentropy
network therapy
nuclear family
openness/closedness
output
patterns
physical environment
psychological environment
residual stimuli
rules
separatist family style
social environment
structural-functional framework
subsystems
suprasystem
surrogate mother
system
traditional family
traditional-oriented nonresistive style
transactional field theory
wider family

Families are society's most basic small group. Each person's perception of life and the world is the product of both interactions within the cultural milieu of family and the individual's innate patterns and characteristics. Many nurses have worked primarily in inpatient settings and with individuals rather than with the total family constellation. Much of the emphasis in nursing education has been on the individual rather than on the family or community. With the changes that have occurred in health care, nursing will direct more of its energies toward work with families in home or community settings.

Gilliss (1999) describes two ways that nurses identify families. The first is family as context; the second is family as client. When families are treated as the context within which individuals are assessed, the emphasis is primarily on the individual, keeping in mind that he or she is a part of a larger system, the family (**family as context**). This is a generalist practice view that may be used

REFLECTIVE THINKING

Family Patterns

Perhaps the first time you became aware of your family's patterns occurred when, as a child, you visited a friend or relative and noticed the patterns and characteristics of this other family. Remember such an occasion now.

- Did the family eat foods that were different from those to which you were accustomed?
- How did parents and children interact?
- What were forbidden and permitted topics of conversation?
- What else about the family seemed different from life in your family?

in other nursing specialty areas as well (Gilliss, 1999). Conversely, when the nurse treats the family as a set of interacting parts and emphasizes assessment of the dynamics among these parts rather than the individual parts themselves (family members), the family as a whole, rather than the individual members, becomes the client (**family as client**). These nurses are specialists in family care although they may be generalists in other areas of practice (Gilliss, 1999). The nurse must grasp the interacting aspects of the family, whether to understand the context within which the individual lives and to which he or she reacts or to work with the family as client.

The purpose of this chapter is to give the nurse direction, via the understanding of family theories, for family assessment, planning, intervention, and evaluation. Caring, both for families and in families, is explored, as are **patterns** (family behaviors, beliefs, and values that together make up the uniqueness that is the family) and structure of the family in U.S. society; family system concepts; life cycle development; and variations on family forms and developmental patterns. The impact of culture on the family is also addressed. The reader also can expect to receive new insights into his or her own family system. Although much of this chapter is theoretical, it is important that nurses use theory in conjunction with an understanding of the subjective perspectives of families. The lived experience of the family must be the basis of care.

DEFINITION OF THE FAMILY

Families are defined in many ways. Definitions of **traditional families** usually cite the presence of children, legal marriage, blood kinship bonds that include inheritance

transfers ensuring intergenerational continuity, and a lifestyle that has its genesis in the family (Marciano & Sussman, 1991). The U.S. Bureau of the Census (1999) reflects this tradition, defining the **family** as "a group of two or more persons related by birth, marriage, or adoption and residing together in a household" (p. 6). However, this narrow definition does not address the many variations of family structures present in today's society. To address these changing family forms, Marciano (1991) has introduced the concept of **wider family,** a family that "emerges from lifestyle, is voluntary, and independent of necessary biological or kin connections" (p. 160). Wider families do not always share a common dwelling, although some do. Kin (those related by blood) families and wider families can coexist together. A wider family may be time limited and exist only to meet a particular need: for instance, a foster mother who cares for a child with AIDS. This concept of family accommodates such configurations as two divorced mothers and their children living together, gay or lesbian couples with or without children, group homes that may or may not provide individual living areas, some Big Sister/Big Brother relationships, and many self-help groups. In summary, a wider family is voluntary, unstructured, and family oriented; is not rule bound; and may be time limited. Whall (1999) offers a definition of family that encompasses this perspective:

The family is a self-identified group of two or more individuals whose association is characterized by special terms, who may or may not be related by bloodlines or law, but who function in such a way that they consider themselves to be a family. (p. 4)

This definition reflects the perspective of family to be presented in this text: It does not insist on or exclude blood kinship ties or the presence of children, and it acknowledges the subjective nature of family for many groups. Some other terms associated with definitions of

REFLECTIVE THINKING

Family Exploration

- How many of your extended family can you identify?
- Can you relate your family of origin and/or procreation to the text definition of family?
- What families do you know—either personally or in your clinical setting—that fit the definition of a wider family?
- Discuss these families with your colleagues. What implications do these different family constellations have for your practice?

the family and to which the literature frequently refers are as follows:

- **Nuclear family.** Composed of husband, wife, and their immediate children (natural, adopted, or both).

- **Family of origin (or orientation).** The family unit into which a person is born.

- **Family of procreation.** The family created for the purpose of raising children.

- **Extended family.** Traditionally, those members of the nuclear family and other blood-related persons, usually from family of origin (grandparents, aunts, uncles, cousins), called "kin." More recently, people who identify themselves as "family" but are not necessarily related by blood or through adoption. An example might be a group of lesbians and perhaps some male friends who have agreed to share in the responsibility of raising the child of one of their members.

- **Blended (or binuclear) family.** The combination of two divorced families through remarriage.

Varieties of Family Forms

Until recently, the nuclear (traditional) family was considered the most common and ideal, implying that they are the only valid family form (Carter & McGoldrick, 1999). Terminology commonly used in conjunction with divorce and remarriage has negative connotations (e.g., stepchild, broken home, failed marriage, stepparent, ex-spouse), and members of families that have been generated through remarriage, called blended families, are not routinely accorded the courtesies afforded to members of the original nuclear family (e.g., invitations to open school night, weddings, and other family and community events). Households with more than two adults living in intimate relationships or with homosexual couples are often denied legal rights that most citizens take for

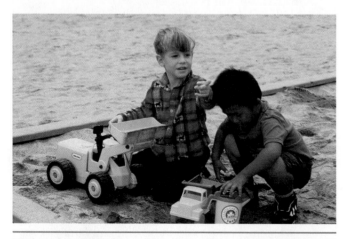

Through remarriage, these boys became members of a blended family.

granted (e.g., insurance coverage, recognition as next of kin in health care situations). The historical bias toward viewing the nuclear family as the only legitimate form of family has led many health care workers and researchers to form negative stereotypes of other family forms and to treat individuals in other kinds of families in both subtly and overtly demeaning ways. Instead of working with the needs and perceptions of the family, they consider their task one of facilitating family adjustment to the system. Although social systems are slowly catching up with family changes, the daily experience of millions of children and adults often continues to be one of alienation.

Harway and Wexler (1996) encourage health professionals to look for the strengths and resources of nontraditional families rather than for their pathology. They propose a taxonomy of normative families that is not dependent on a traditional family perspective. The dimensions of their taxonomy are biological relationship (both, one, or neither parent related), marital status (single, married, or cohabiting parents), sexual orientation (heterosexual, gay, or lesbian), and gender roles/employment status (traditional or nontraditional). When this perspective is used, all family forms become normative.

Studies point to the probability that families will continue to vary from the nuclear configuration. Aerts (1993) notes that, in addition to common differences such as single-parent and blended families, at the levels of social and legal considerations, at the very least, recent advances in reproductive technologies have created an artificial distinction between a **surrogate mother** (a woman who, for someone other than herself, carries a child conceived from an egg not always her own) and **biological mother** (a woman who gives birth to and raises her own children). The option to have a pregnancy via a surrogate mother leads to additional forms of family variation. A same- or opposite-sex couple may have a child that is conceived from their own or another person's or people's sperm and egg and nurtured in someone else's uterus. Such possibilities give rise to new considerations. For instance, problems can arise when the surrogate mother refuses to give up the child or when the growing child wants to know about his or her biological parents. In today's world, almost any imaginable combination of family form is possible and is practiced somewhere. Figure 24-1 lists some of the more common configurations.

Staples (1989) summarized the expected trends for families for the next 25 years as follows:

> Sexual relations will precede marriage: people will have a trial period of cohabitation before entering into marriage, and they will increasingly delay marriage until their late twenties or early thirties; the divorce rate will continue to increase, and remarriage will occur more slowly; couples will limit their families to one or two children; and the dual wage earner family will be the norm for almost all households. (p. 167)

Her predictions are proving to be accurate. Thus, while many family options will be available, most individuals will continue to marry and bear children. Lesbians, more often than gay men, come to their relationships with children or give birth to children in the context of the homosexual relationship. Hare and Richards (1993) found that when one or both partners bring children into a lesbian relationship, lesbian families resemble heterosexual stepfamilies. They also noted that children born in the context of a lesbian relationship resembled those born in the context of a nuclear family. If such a marriage/partnership dissolves, the children of the lesbian partners may go on to spend most of their lives in single-parent or blended families. Chan, Raboy, and Patterson (1998) note that "research has provided no evidence of significant disadvantages suffered by children of lesbian mothers as compared with those of heterosexual mothers" (p. 443).

Such family changes create many issues. For instance, divorce has several stages. Before the actual divorce is the decision to divorce. Then the breakup of the system begins, first with discussion and planning of the divorce and then with the separation. The final stage is the actual divorce and all the related legal and emotional considerations. Families who then remarry also undergo a process in order to achieve a positively blended family. Once they enter the new relationship, they must conceptualize and plan the new marriage and family. Then, in the remarriage, they must reconstruct the family. To successfully complete this process, they must recover from the loss of the first marriage and recommit to dealing with the complexity and ambiguity of a new family. They must realize that it takes time to adjust to new roles, boundaries, space, time, membership, and authority. Affective issues such as guilt, loyalty, conflicts, desire for mutuality, and unresolvable past hurts must be addressed.

FIGURE 24-1 Varieties of Family Forms

Legally married

Traditional nuclear

Binuclear or blended

- Co-parenting
- Joint custody
- One member of the original family remarried
- Both members of the original family remarried

Dual-career

Both in same household

Commuter

Adoptive

Foster

Voluntary childlessness

Unmarried

Never married

- Voluntary singlehood, with or without children
- Involuntary singlehood, with or without children

Cohabitation, with or without children

Same-sex relationship

Formally married

Widowed

Divorced

- Custodial parent
- Joint custody of children
- Noncustodial parent

Multi-adult household

Communes and intentional communities

Multilateral marriage, in which three or more people consider themselves to have a primary relationship with at least two other individuals in the group (Macklin, 1987)

Extramarital sex

- Swinging
- Sexually open marriage
- Coprimary relationships, in which one or both members maintain a primary relationship with at least two partners who may or may not know about the other (Macklin, 1987)
- Home-sharing individuals, with or without children

Extended family (e.g., grandparents, parents, and children; adult children moving home; siblings living together, with or without partners or children)

✳ DECISION MAKING

Domestic Partnerships

Some counties in the United States have domestic partnership registration bills that allow any couple living together in a committed relationship, including same-sex couples, to register as domestic partners. These partners have three specific rights: (1) the right to visit each other in the hospital, (2) the right to will property to one another, and (3) the right to conservatorship if one partner becomes incapacitated (Associated Press, 1994). Without these assurances, unmarried people, particularly gay men and lesbians, who cannot legally marry, may face difficulties related to their partners' not being considered next of kin. For instance, a gay man may lose all access to his partner during severe illness and may be ineligible to inherit when his partner dies.

- Should unmarried people in a committed relationship be allowed to legally register their partnership?

FIGURE 24-2 Major Issues in Remarriage

1. **Initial Family Issues**
   - Name for the new parent
   - Affection for the new parent and the absent parent (conflict between biological parent and stepparent)
   - Loss of the natural parent (grief for the previous family structure)
   - Unrealistic belief in instant love of new family members
   - Fantasy about the old family structure (reconciliation fantasy)

2. **Developing Family Issues**
   - Discipline by the stepparent
   - Confusion over family roles
   - Sibling conflict
   - Competition for time
   - Extended kinship network
   - Sexual conflicts as result of more sexually charged atmosphere of the new family
   - Changes over time (at least two years needed for basic remarriage reorganization)
   - Exit and entry of children (visits to noncustodial parents [exit] and returns to custodial home [entry])

3. **Feelings about Self and Others**
   - Society's concept of the remarriage family
   - Familial self-concept
   - Individual self-concept (whether person feels an accepted part of the family)

4. **Adult Issues**
   - Effects of parenting on the new marital relationship
   - Financial concerns
   - Continuing adult conflict
   - Competition of the noncustodial parent

From "Twenty Major Issues in Remarriage Families" by W. M. Walsh, 1992, *Journal of Counseling and Development, 70,* pp. 709–715.

ics and family processes. There are also several theories that provide insight into the interrelationship between the family and the larger community. These theories are important to understand because they give direction to the nursing care of families. Although no one theory completely addresses all dimensions of the family or fully explains family dynamics and behaviors, knowing the basic precepts of these theories helps the nurse to effectively assess families.

Nursing Theories

Some nursing theories and conceptual models address the family either directly or indirectly. Although most nursing theories began with a focus on the individual, with the family being viewed as only a part of the client's context, some have enlarged their conceptual bases to include the family as client.

Neuman's System Model

Neuman's system model has a family systems approach as its foundation. The ways that family members express themselves influence the whole and create the basic structure of the family. All transactions take place vis-à-vis this structure and are directed toward keeping the structure stable as it moves between stability (wellness) and instability (illness). The major goal of the nurse, therefore, is to help stabilize the family system within its environment (Neuman, 1983). Herrick and Goodykoontz (1999) have illustrated the application of Neuman's model. They note that it is a "valuable tool to assist the child psychiatric nurse in assessing a child or adolescent and the family because of its holistic and systemic perspectives" (p. 82).

King's Open Systems Model

As do most nursing theorists, King (1981) views the family as context (environment) but also recognizes it as client. She believes that nurses are partners with families. Her theory of goal attainment "assumes that family nursing consists of helping these individuals to reach goals

Finally, there must be acceptance of a different model of family with permeable boundaries (McGoldrick & Carter, 1999). Figure 24-2 identifies some of the issues that must be addressed in blended families.

THEORETICAL FOUNDATIONS IN FAMILY NURSING

All families share certain characteristics. Every family can be characterized as a social system with certain structures and functions that move through recognizable stages. A number of theories in nursing, social sciences, and family systems theory give insight into these family dynam-

REFLECTIVE THINKING

Family and Nursing Theory

- Choose a nursing theory. How would you explain your family in terms of that theory?
- Do some theories or models fit your family life better than others, or do they all seem to have relevance to your life experiences?

Perspectives... ✳

INSIGHTS OF A NURSING FACULTY MEMBER

The community health nursing (CHN) practicum is a challenging course to teach and, from a student perspective, a difficult course to take because of the generalist nature of this practice setting. Students often comment on the difficult nature of the course and the amorphous feeling of being held accountable for diverse content areas. I also remembered this feeling as a nursing student and as a practitioner in CHN. Therefore, as a clinical professor in CHN, I decided to examine this problem and try a new way to facilitate student learning.

I believed the CHN practicum would be enhanced by using a nursing theory, as it would provide more structure and parameters to the course. As an educator, I had participated in incorporating nursing theory into classes and curriculum design. However, I had never employed a non-eclectic approach of using one nursing theorist in a course or curriculum. I wanted to use just one theorist because I believed using an eclectic approach or expecting students to use a theorist of their choice would increase the difficulty of this course.

Five years ago I began using the theory of Imogene King in teaching the CHN practicum. My rationale for using King's theory of goal attainment was threefold: (1) Goal attainment and quality outcomes have become almost synonymous in the health care field; (2) King's theory provides a framework for looking at both the dynamics of interacting systems and mutual interactions or transactions between client, client's family, and the health care system; and (3) King assumes that the client has the right to self-determination. All of the above are consistent with principles and concepts in CHN practice, and all three provide parameters for the practitioner. By using King's theory, the student is provided with a perspective from which to practice. The theoretical base for nursing process demonstrates a way for students to interact purposefully with clients. The student learns that the theory involves a process focused on the goal or outcome that is an effective way of measuring nursing care.

The metaparadigm of Person has special significance for students in the CHN practicum. Frequently, values of client and student conflict, and priorities for prevention and promotion activities differ. For example, the student, wanting to educate about healthful living and to see change occur, may not understand why a mother will not keep medical appointments for her children, whereas the mother is more concerned about how she is going to feed and clothe her chil-

dren. Inherent in King's theory is a basic respect for the capacity of human beings to think, acquire and use knowledge, make choices, and select courses of action (King, 1986). By using King's model, the student incorporates these beliefs about the rights of clients. Students become partners in health care with their clients and respect clients' decisions.

Feedback from the students has been very positive. They find that they can more easily organize their thinking about client assessment, planning, and interventions. They also use King's framework to evaluate their work and as a reminder to focus on client needs and the implications of client interactions and transactions. As one student said, the theory acknowledges "clients as able to set goals and make decisions about their care, which are right for them, without creating value judgments over what is 'right or wrong' " (Baker, 1996, p. 20).

—Laurel Freed, RN, CPHN, MSN

INSIGHTS OF A NURSING STUDENT

I was introduced to King's theory of nursing as a senior student in the RN-BSN program at Sonoma State University and began to use the theory in my nursing practice during my community health nursing practicum. Applying this theory to my practice helped in organizing my care and clinical decision making. It also freed me to provide the education, instructional support, resourcing, and referrals that were truly going to make a difference in my clients' lives. It was not just a "Band-Aid" approach, but one wherein clients participated and were empowered to make decisions regarding their lives and health and the lives and health of their families.

As nurses, we must remember that our clients are biopsychosocial, spiritual individuals, rather than a series of tasks that must be completed in a given period of time. They are sentient beings, bringing with them pasts full of experiences and views of the future that are uniquely their own. These experiences and views will color the present choices they make. An experience I had illustrates this concept and how the application of King's theory of nursing helped in the establishment of a therapeutic relationship with a young developing family.

(continues)

Perspectives... ✳

INSIGHTS OF A NURSING FACULTY MEMBER (continued)

The referral came from an OB/GYN physician at the county hospital. He was concerned that Susan was not keeping her routine OB appointments. She had been drinking prior to her last appointment, and the physician had arranged for her to be driven home. She was at approximately 32 weeks' gestation with twins. She was 24 years old, para III, gravida I, unmarried, but living with her boyfriend. Her young son was almost 2 years old.

Upon attempting a home visit at the address noted on the referral, I found that the family had recently moved, leaving a large pile of debris behind. The next week another referral came from the county hospital as a result of the premature birth of female twins at 35 weeks' gestation. I was able to locate the mother at the new address noted on the hospital referral. They had no telephone. The first visit was extremely strained. Susan came to the door of the large house in front of the studio apartment where she, her boyfriend, and young son lived. She did not invite me in or volunteer any personal information, although she did briefly respond to questions. I introduced myself and offered community health assistance in preparing for bringing her twins home from the hospital. I told her I would visit with her again the next week and asked her to be thinking of questions she might have or areas where she would like my help. She immediately responded that she needed assistance with obtaining car seats in which to bring home the girls. I was elated! This was a good start. We had developed mutual goal number one!

As the weeks went on and the infants came home, she showed no evidence of drinking, and we continued to explore the problems of parenthood, birth con-

trol, cramped living space, lack of transportation, and available educational opportunities. We set several mutual goals. She liked the infants to be weighed and measured. It was encouraging to see their weekly growth. She needed respite care for her toddler son. We set goals around finding him a Head Start program and arranging transportation for him to get there and back home. Toward the end of my semester with her, we even began exploring ways for her to obtain her high-school graduate equivalency diploma.

During our visits, it was important for me to take cues from Susan and to be sure that I was not imposing my agenda on her. The goals we set had to be ones that she valued and that would empower her to take charge of her own decision making, for both herself and her children. As a nurse, I could guide her with information, but, ultimately, the choices she made were her own. Without this approach, I believe I would not have gotten a foot in the door, much less made any permanent difference in this young family's life.

This example illustrates on multiple levels the natural fit of King's theory of nursing in a community health setting. It shows use of her concepts of interaction, transaction, and mutual goal setting and demonstrates the interrelatedness of personal, interpersonal, and social systems. The use of King's theory in community health nursing helps to organize and guide nursing decisions along the continuum of care and facilitates recognition of the client's right and responsibility to actively participate in the decision-making process.

—Deborah Baker, RN, BSN

through improved interaction or communication" (Friedmann, 1999, p. 15). Mutual goal setting requires decision making, which King (1994) sees as a collaborative process "between nurse and nurse, nurse and physician, nurse and family, and allied health workers" (p. 31).

Roy's Adaptation Model

Roy (1983) believes that the family can be the unit of analysis and the adaptive system that is assessed. Studies have supported this assertion (Blue et al., 1994; Silva, 1999). Enhancement or modification of the **focal stimuli** (factors that precipitate an adaptive response), **contextual stimuli** (all other factors that contribute to the behavior),

and **residual stimuli** (factors that may affect behavior but for which effects are not validated) promotes adaptation of the family system. For example, the nurse's assessment of a family's coping skills and the environmental context within which the family faces the death of a member provides the data needed to facilitate a positive adaptation to the changes engendered by the crisis.

Rogers' Life Process Model

Rogers' (1992) concepts of integrality (the continuous, mutual human field and environmental field process), resonancy (continuous change from lower to higher frequency wave patterns in human and environmental fields),

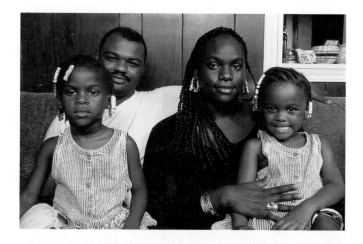

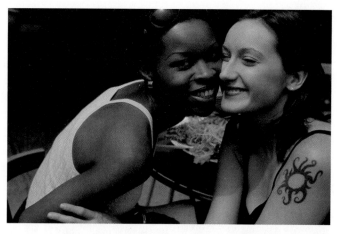

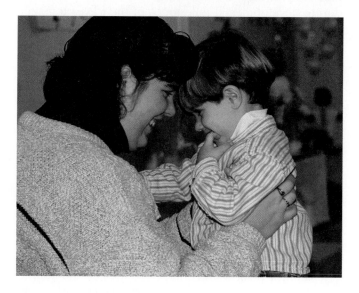

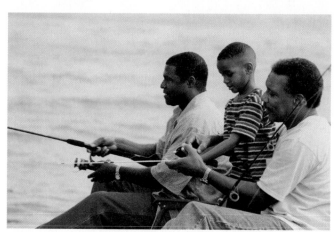

Different Family Configurations.

and helicy (the continuous, innovative, unpredictable, increasing diversity of human and environmental field patterns) can be used to describe the family as well as the individual. She states that the family can be the field of study and describes the family as an "irreducible, pandimensional, negentropic family energy field" (Whall, 1999, p. 10). Thus, the energy generated by family dynamics influences all family members. Family members learn from one another in ways that are unique to that family.

Social Science Theories

A number of theories that come out of social science research help explain families. For purposes of this text, four will be examined: developmental, general systems, structural-functional, and interactional. When using these theories as frameworks for nursing care, the nurse must take into account cultural and ethnic differences that may be present. For instance, the developmental tasks identified by the theorists do not take into account the impact

on four- to eight-year-old girls (including the lifelong effects on their familial relationships) of the ritual of female genital mutilation. This rite, practiced primarily in Africa, is practiced by some immigrants from African countries who live in the United States (Barstow, 1998).

Developmental Theory

Developmental theory, also known as the life cycle approach, purports that families evolve through typical developmental stages and experience growth and development much in the same way as do individuals: Each stage is characterized by specific issues and tasks. The ways that tasks at each stage are resolved help determine the family's capability for handling the challenges of the next stage.

The life cycle approach is useful because it assists the nurse in planning client care that is family oriented and appropriate to the family's stage of development. Perhaps the best-known formulation of the developmental

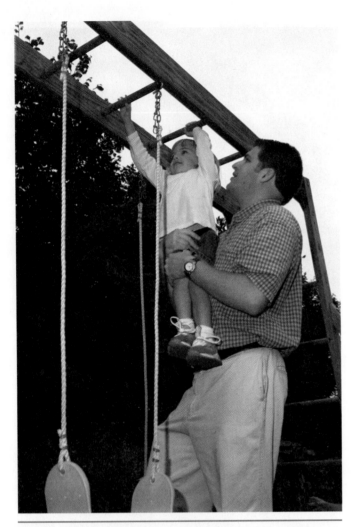

This father must balance the tug of war between home life, career, and finding time for himself.

stages comes from Duvall (1977; Duvall & Miller, 1985). Each stage has certain requisite tasks that must be completed before movement to the next stage is possible. Her model has limited value, however, because it presupposes a two-parent nuclear family and begins with marriage. Her perspective maintains that the nuclear family is the norm and that most young adults marry in their early twenties before or instead of developing a career of their own. Life cycle changes are linked primarily to child-rearing activities. Today, the majority of family forms do not fit this configuration.

In the past, women moved from their families of origin directly to marriage. If there was a break between the two, women worked only while waiting to marry. Now, women often begin their careers before marriage and continue them after the birth of children (Fulmer, 1999; Rubin & Riney, 1994). Childrearing today occupies less than half of the adult life span prior to old age (Carter & McGoldrick, 1999) such that childrearing is no longer the central focus of the life cycle. Today's women must think about career goals in ways that past generations of women never even

considered. This change in life situation has prompted women to insist on a new phase in the life cycle, that "phase in which the young adult leaves the parent's home, establishes personal goals, and starts a career" (Carter & McGoldrick, 1989, p. 11). Carter and McGoldrick (1999) describe six stages of the family life cycle that take into account the reality of today's young adult. Table 24-1 compares Duvall and Miller's (1985) and Carter and McGoldrick's (1999) stages of family development and lists the accompanying tasks of each stage.

Wallerstein (1995, 1996) and Wallerstein and Blakeslee (1995), from Wallerstein's research designed to "illuminate the interior domains of happy marriages" (Wallerstein, 1995, p. 640), suggest psychological tasks that couples must address early in marriage and again during developmental milestones of their lives together. These tasks are stated here in the form of questions that the nurse can use when assessing the psychological health of the family. Each one is then briefly discussed.

1. Has the couple separated psychologically from their families of origin and begun to "create a new and different kind of connectedness that will maintain the generational ties" (Wallerstein, 1995, p. 642)? Women tend to have a more difficult time separating from their families of origin. Particularly if the woman is a child of divorce, there is often overdependence of the mother on the daughter and resulting guilt, compassion, and love that cements the two together. Dysfunctional family dynamics also generate guilt about separation. While a connectedness should remain between parents and adult children, it must be redefined together by the couple. These issues reemerge with pregnancy and the arrival of children and at the time of the death of a parent.

2. Is the couple able to build a marital identity? The task is to develop a sense of "we-ness." The partners identify not only with each other but also with the marriage. They create an empathy with one another

---

REFLECTIVE THINKING

Family Development

- Did you have an opportunity to live and learn as a single young adult, or did you move directly into a committed relationship? How have life choices in this regard affected your life?
- How well do you think you and your family have completed your family tasks of development?

TABLE 24-1 Comparison of Duvall and Miller, Carter and McGoldrick Family Life Cycle Stages and Tasks

STAGES		TASKS
DUVALL AND MILLER (1985)	**CARTER AND MCGOLDRICK (1999)**	
No stage identified, although Duvall considers this the time of "being launched."	1. The unattached young adult	Successful separation of parent and young adult from one another
1. The beginning family or the stage of marriage	2. The new couple	Committing to a new family system
2. Childbearing families	3. Families with young children	Accepting new members into the system
3. Families with preschool children		
4. Families with school-age children		
5. Families with teenagers	4. Families with adolescents	Increasing flexibility of family boundaries to permit children's independence and grandparents' frailties
6. Families launching young adults	5. Launching children and moving on	Accepting many exits or entrances into the family system
7. Middle-age parents (empty nest up to retirement)		
8. Retirement to death of both spouses	6. Families in later life	Accepting shifting generational roles and death

From Family Nursing: Theory and Practice *(4th ed., p. 83), by M. M. Friedman, 1998, Stamford: CT: Appleton & Lange;* Families in Health and Illness: Perspectives on Coping and Intervention, *by C. B. Danielson, B. Hamel-Bissell, and P. Winstead-Fry, 1993, St. Louis, MO: Mosby-Yearbook;* Marriage and Family Development *(6th ed.), by E. M. Duvall and B. C. Miller, 1985, New York: Harper and Row, Copyright © 1985 by Harper & Row, Reprinted by permission of Addison-Wesley Educational Publishers, Inc.; and* The Expanded Family Life Cycle, *by B. Carter and M. McGoldrick, 1999, Boston: Allyn and Bacon, Copyright © 1999 by Allyn & Bacon. Adapted by permission.*

whereby they listen to and are concerned about each other's needs. At the same time, the partners must maintain autonomy and set boundaries to allow themselves private and protected space. Weness, then, does not mean merging with one another. There is a continued tension between togetherness and autonomy, and differentness is acknowledged and welcomed.

3. Have the partners established a sexual life as a couple? Partners need to develop their own patterns that gratify both people, restore the core relationship, renew love, and counter the stresses and disappointments of life. The couple's sex life is the most vulnerable part of the relationship because it is "uniquely sensitive to events and mood changes that originate in all the other domains of individual and family life" (Wallerstein & Blakeslee, 1995, p. 223), such as work, childbirth, responsibilities to children, illness, and fatigue.

4. Is the marriage a zone of safety and nurturance, where the partners can express all the dimensions of feelings and experience aging and being human?

Development of this safe place involves working out that which is unsafe as well as coming to understand and accept one another: "Learning to disagree and to stand one's ground without fear of dire consequences" (Wallerstein, 1996, p. 224) is important. Trusting one another is crucial.

5. Can the couple expand to psychologically accommodate children and at the same time safeguard their own private sphere? The couple must work to keep their own relationship alive. The parents' inner psychological and emotional lives are forever changed when the dyad becomes a triad with the birth of a baby. The couple must face their internal conflicts and make room for the child yet not allow the child to take over the marriage (Wallerstein & Blakeslee, 1995).

6. Has the couple built a relationship that is fun and interesting for them? Boredom can debilitate a relationship, as can constant serenity. A certain tension is necessary to prevent tedium, but not to the degree of generating anxiety.

7. Is the couple able to confront and master life crises and maintain the strength of the marital bond during

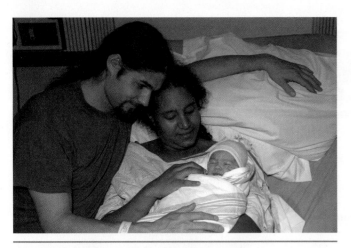

Often a baby brings the family together.

adversity? There are several dimensions of coping with crisis. First, the partners must realistically acknowledge and think about the consequences to self and other family members in order to make rational plans. They must also protect one another from blame and self-blame. Another important dimension is keeping perspective by letting in some pleasure and humor so that the crisis does not totally dominate. Equally important is making a strong effort to keep destructive impulses from getting out of control. It is important to recognize that the impulses are responses to the crisis. Finally, it is important that the partners intervene at an early stage, when the potential for a crisis is first seen (Wallerstein & Blakeslee, 1995).

8. Is the couple able to nurture and comfort each other? Partners need to be able to accurately assess the cause of each other's suffering and make genuine efforts to relieve or head off that suffering. It is important to provide for a partner's dependency needs and help bolster battered self-esteem (Wallerstein & Blakeslee, 1995).

9. Is the couple able to maintain a "vision of the other that combines early idealizations with a firm grasp of the present reality" (Wallerstein, 1995, p. 649)? An important way to mute the disappointments and rage inherent in all close relationships is to maintain the ability to associate the past with the present. This ability increases in importance over time.

Although there seems to be a beginning and an end to the family life cycle (i.e., beginning with leaving home and ending with death), it is important to remember the continuity that characterizes families. Among some families, behavior is influenced by belief in life after death. Others believe that people live on through the acts they commit in life. Young adults are part of a family with a long ancestral history; the couple's children constitute the couple's link with the future. The interaction and complementarity that exist between the different generations constitute another set of factors that contribute to the patterns, behaviors, and relationships in the contemporary family.

The complementary nature of the **developmental tasks** (the work that must be completed at each stage of development before movement to the next stage is possible) of the different generations makes it useful to conceptualize family as a three-generation system moving through time. Carter and McGoldrick (1999) note the overlapping of life changes among generations. Combrinck-Graham (1985) describes a family life spiral whereby the life cycle is not seen as linear (see Figure 24-3). She defines death as a life change event rather than a life cycle event, acknowledging that death can happen at any time during the life cycle. She notes that life cycle events in different generations frequently happen concurrently. For example, the middle years of childhood occur at the same time that parents are settling down in marriage and that grandparents are planning for retirement. Marriage courtship generally occurs during the middle adulthood of parents and late adulthood of grandparents. When a child begins life, the roles of parent and grandparent emerge. The first two phases tend to distance the generations because each member is working on his or her own changes. The third phase, which involves childbirth, tends to bring families closer together, however.

Resolution of Developmental Tasks

The degree to which developmental tasks are successfully resolved by the family in different generations affects the functional and dysfunctional aspects of family life. Anxiety is generated when developmental tasks are resolved poorly; this anxiety is cumulative over generations in a family and, like heavy baggage, is carried from one generation to the next. Anxiety within the family is a continuous drain on the energy available for meeting the challenges of family life. Dysfunctional perceptions and behavior perpetuate. For example, a family for which pregnancy and birth have been problematic may

---

REFLECTIVE THINKING

Life Cycle Events

- What has been your experience with life cycle events? Did they bring your family closer together or move it more apart?
- Did the birth of a child bring your family closer together?

FIGURE 24-3 Family Life Spiral

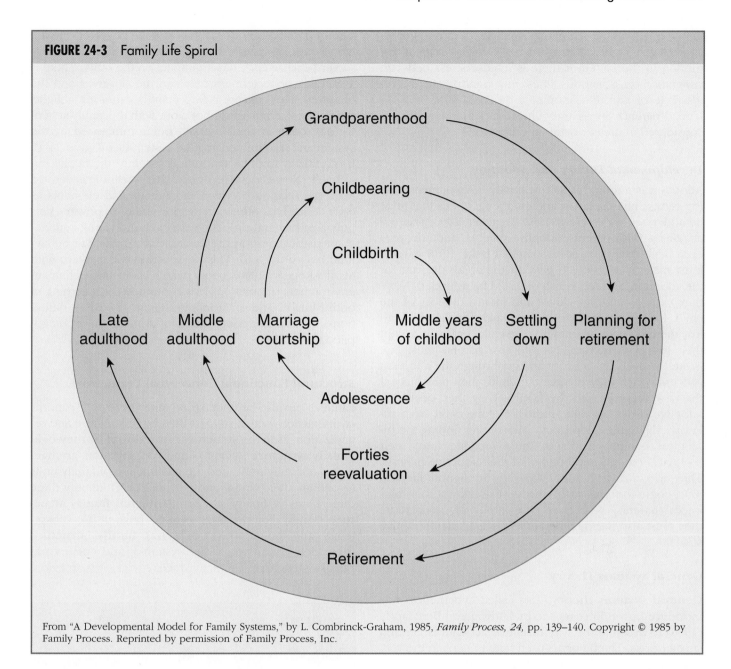

From "A Developmental Model for Family Systems," by L. Combrinck-Graham, 1985, *Family Process, 24*, pp. 139–140. Copyright © 1985 by Family Process. Reprinted by permission of Family Process, Inc.

discover during the process of examining its history that there is a family secret that the grandparents are reluctant to discuss. The secret may involve the great grandmother, who had a child before she was married and who was ostracized by her family and the community. Even though the family members of ensuing generations did not know the details of the traumatic incident, the anxiety generated by the event was passed down and was felt in different ways by the women during pregnancy and birth. Difficult labor, excessive bleeding, or sickness during pregnancy or crises in the family when a member is pregnant are some of the ways this phenomenon might manifest.

When a family is experiencing simultaneous crises in two generations, the anxiety generated may be more

than the family can deal with at one time. If the family is conceptualized as a large emotional web, it is easier to understand how reverberations in one part of the web affect all the other parts. For instance, the death of a grandparent at the same time as the birth of a child may disrupt the closeness of the three generations and manifest at a later time in the life cycle.

Predictable developmental transitions as well as unpredictable life events such as untimely death, divorce, severe illness, war, and the like, all create stress for the family. The stress level in a particular family involves stressful events that are occurring in a particular generation over time as well as those that are occurring in the different generations at the same time. An understanding of the interactions between these stressful events can help explain why a seemingly small stress in one generation (e.g., a child's starting school) can lead to great disruption in the system if there is intense stress between generations (e.g., serious illness in a grandparent and remarriage of and relocation to a different state by a divorced parent). Stress and vulnerability in family life are considered in greater detail in Chapter 25.

Developmental Theory and Adoption

Adoption is another aspect of family development having certain phases, tasks, and emotional issues that must be addressed (Rosenberg, 1992; Treacher, 2000; Triseliotis, 2000). Birth parents, adoptive parents, and adoptees each have their own developmental tasks. Birth parents must make a decision to give up the child, prepare for the adoption, and relinquish the child for adoption. Next, they must resume their lives and mourn the loss of the child. Later, they may decide to search for the child, allow themselves to be found by the child, or finally accept their loss with tranquillity. Adoptive parents must first make the decision to adopt and go through the adoption process. Once they receive the child, they must accept the new member into the family. They then deal with adoptive issues throughout the life of the child, from acknowledging the adoption to considering finding the biological parents. Adoptees must separate from their biological parents and bond with their adoptive parents. They, too, deal with adoptive issues throughout life and must come to terms with whether to seek out their biological parents. With their own family of procreation, they must also decide whether to disclose their adoptive status.

General Systems Theory

General systems theory, also called cybernetics, was introduced over 50 years ago by Ludwig von Bertalanffy (1950) to describe the way units interact with larger and smaller units. The theory is used here to explain the way the family interacts with its members and with society. This theory is useful in family assessment because it emphasizes the interdependence of the family's parts and asserts both that the whole of the family is greater than the sum of its parts and that whatever affects the family as a whole affects each of its parts. According to this theory, then, one cannot understand the family simply by knowing each of the members. The interrelationship of the members of the family with each other and with the larger society must be addressed. As originally conceived, systems theory is mechanistic in that it suggests that an individual can observe the system in interaction from outside the system. Becvar and Becvar (2000) present another dimension, which they call "cybernetics of cybernetics" (p. 7), that has relevance for nurses in interaction with clients. This perspective emphasizes that the

system (family) is not separate from the observer (nurse), who is also a system. In fact, there is no objective observer because each has an impact on the other. There is a mutual connectedness between the observer and the observed. This concept is important because it highlights the notion that nurses cannot work with the family system (or any other system) without being influenced by the system and also influencing the system (see Figure 24-4). It is a fallacy to think that one is "seeing" the family objectively. Nurses must recognize that "meaning is derived from the relation between individuals and elements as each defines the other. . . . Responsibility or power exists only as a bilateral process, with each individual and element participating in the creation of a particular behavioral reality" (p. 66). This perspective is consistent with Martha Rogers' (1990) theory, which characterizes human-environment transactions as a continuous repatterning of both humans and environment. Figure 24-5 lists definitions of the major components of systems theory as applied to families.

Structural-Functional Conceptual Framework

Families can also be understood in terms of their patterns of interaction, which suggest their basic structure and organization, as in the **structural-functional framework. Family structure** refers to family organization, arrangements of family units, and the relationship of family units to one another. Wright and Leahey (1994) identify three dimensions of family structure: **internal family structure** (family composition, gender, rank order, subsystems, and boundaries), **external family structure** (extended family and larger systems), and **contextual family structure** (ethnicity, race, social class, religion,

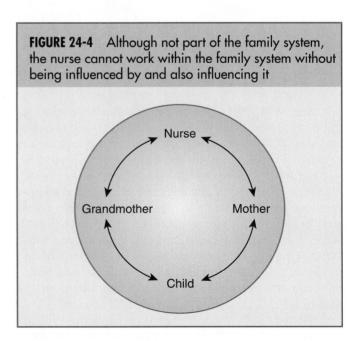

FIGURE 24-4 Although not part of the family system, the nurse cannot work within the family system without being influenced by and also influencing it

FIGURE 24-5 Definitions of the Major Components of Systems Theory as Applied to Families

Boundaries. Each system has an imaginary demarcation line that is made up of rules and separates the **focal system** from its environment. This boundary may be more or less open. Families with open boundaries can utilize information and energy from their environment to maintain greater equilibrium or to grow. If the boundary is too porous, however, there can be so much input that the family may lose its identity (e.g., be so involved with community agencies that they depend on the agency to direct their lives). If the family boundary is too closed, the family is isolated from their environment and cannot use the services of the community to support them in times of need.

Differentiation. Refers to a living system's capability and propensity to progressively and serially "advance to a higher order of complexity and organization" (Friedman, 1998, p. 159). A normal social system has a natural tendency to grow (called morphogenesis), but a balance between stability (morphostasis) and morphogenesis is needed for the system to differentiate.

Energy. Energy is needed to meet the demands for system integrity. The more open the system, the more input needed from the environment to maintain high energy levels.

Entropy. Tending toward maximum disorder and disintegration. Occurs when the system is either too open or too closed, causing family dysfunction.

Equifinality. The quality of there being a characteristic final state regardless of initial state. For instance, people tend to develop habitual ways of behaving and communicating so that whatever the topic, their way of dealing with it will be the same.

Equilibrium. Self-regulation, or adaptation that results from a dynamic balance or steady state. Because the balance is dynamic, it is always reestablishing itself.

Equipotentiality. The quality of different end states being possible from the same initial conditions.

Feedback. The process of providing a circular loop so that the system can receive and respond to its own output. A self-corrective process whereby the system adjusts both internally and externally: internally by making changes in the subsystems as necessary and externally by modifying boundaries.

Feedback can be negative or positive. Positive feedback refers to input that is returned to the system as information that moves the system toward change. Negative feedback promotes equilibrium and stability, not change. An analogy would be a laboratory test labeled "negative" that indicates no body changes or "positive" that indicates a change from the normal.

Flow and transformation. The process whereby input flows through the system either in its original state or, in some cases, transformed so that the system can use it.

Hierarchy of systems. The level of influence of one system with respect to another. The closer the supra- or subsystem to the focal system, the greater the influence. With the family as a focal system, each of the suprasystems and subsystems must be considered. For example, the individual member's system would be a close subsystem of the family, and the community would be a closer suprasystem than the system of the universe.

Input. Energy, matter, and information that the system must receive and process in order to survive.

Morphogenesis. Process of growth, creativity, innovation, and change. In a well-functioning system, cannot be separated from morphostasis.

Morphostasis. A system's tendency toward stability, a state of dynamic equilibrium. In a well-functioning system, cannot be separated from morphogenesis.

Negentropy. Tending toward maximum order; appropriate balance between openness and closedness is maintained.

Openness/closedness. Extent to which a system permits or screens out input, or new information, into the system.

Output. The result of the system's processing of input. It is released into the environment as matter, energy, or information.

Rules. Characteristic relationship patterns by which a system operates. They both express the values of the system and the roles appropriate to behavior within the system and distinguish the system from other systems and, therefore, form the system boundaries.

Subsystems. The smaller units or systems of which a system (the family) consists (i.e., individual members, sibling, spouse, parent-child, extended family relationships).

Suprasystem. The larger system, such as the community (churches, schools, hospitals, businesses, clubs) of which smaller systems (the family) are a part.

System. "A goal-directed unit made up of interdependent, interacting parts that endures over a period of time" (Friedman, 1998, p. 156). Systems are made up of a hierarchy of systems that consist of suprasystems and subsystems. The particular system under study at a specific time is called the focal system. In this chapter, the focal system is the family.

Adapted from *Behavioral Systems and Nursing,* by J. R. Auger, 1976, Englewood Cliffs, NJ: Prentice-Hall; *Family Therapy: A Systematic Integration* (4th ed.), by D. S. Becvar and R. J. Becvar, 2000, Boston: Allyn & Bacon; and *Family Nursing: Theory and Practice,* by M. M. Friedman, Stamford, CT: Appleton & Lange.

and environment). **Family functions** are interdependent with structure. They have to do with the ways individuals behave in relation to one another. Family functions are discussed in Chapter 25. Although the structural-functional approach does not address the importance of growth and change within a family over time, it more fully explains the relationship between family and environment than does developmental theory.

Family Interactional Theories

Family interactional theories focus primarily on the way that family members relate to the family and·on internal family dynamics. These dynamics, which are further discussed in Chapter 25, consist of role playing, status relations, communication patterns, decision making, coping patterns, and socialization. This approach, while useful in assessing and explaining these dimensions, is limited because it does not take into account the way the family interfaces with society.

Family Systems Theories

Family systems theories, which arise from sociology and psychology, are related to general systems theory, the structural-functional framework, and developmental theory. But family systems theories tend to focus on ways to change "dysfunctional" families (Whall, 1991). Whall identifies three therapeutic approaches. In the first, Haley proposes approaching the family as a unit. He emphasizes "the need for discovering the social situation which makes the problem possible" (p. 323). He considers the "family a living and somewhat open system that must accommodate growth needs" (p. 323).

Minuchin's approach is directed more toward open systems (Whall, 1991) and family structural concerns. He believes that the individual is influenced by and influences constantly recurring sequences of interaction; the individual is reflective of the family system of which he or she is a part; stress in one part of the system affects other parts of the system (see Figure 24-6); and changes in family structure contribute to changes in the behavior of individuals within a given system.

Finally, Framo, as discussed in Whall (1991), is interested in the way the past affects the present. His is a closed-system perspective, the focus being on the way that family history affects the family in all of its facets. Family environment is not extensively addressed.

Much research is still needed to identify ways that family systems theories can be utilized in nursing practice. At present, the theories that originated in the social sciences (developmental, systems, structural-functional, and interactional) continue to offer the best guidance for the community health nurse in the provision of health care.

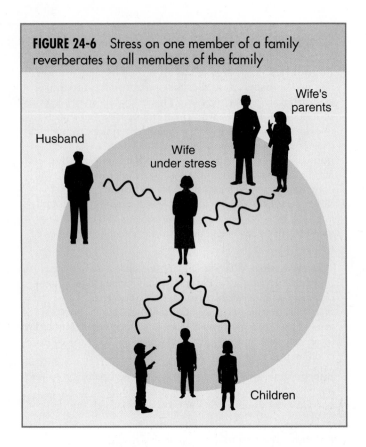

FIGURE 24-6   Stress on one member of a family reverberates to all members of the family

Husband
Wife's parents
Wife under stress
Children

INTERACTION BETWEEN THE FAMILY AND THE SOCIAL SYSTEM OUTSIDE THE FAMILY

Three approaches provide focus primarily on interactions between the family and the larger community. They are the ecological approach, network therapy, and the transactional field approach (Spiegel, 1982).

Ecological Approach

The **ecological approach** incorporates developmental, systems, and situational perspectives. This theoretical perspective emphasizes the interrelationship of these dimensions. Bronfenbrenner (1977) has delineated the ecology of human behavior. The **ecosystem** is composed of four systems. The first is the **microsystem,** which is the immediate setting within which the person fulfills his or her roles (family, school, business, and the like). The next system is the **mesosystem,** which is the interrelationships of the major settings of the person's life. The third system is the **exosystem,** which includes the major institutions of the society (neighborhoods, mass media, and all levels of government). The final system is the **macrosystem,** which "encompasses the overarching institutional patterns of the culture" (p. 24). The family is viewed as nesting within the larger systems and actively influencing and being influenced by them (see Figure 24-7). Szapoeznik and Kurtines (1993) have taken

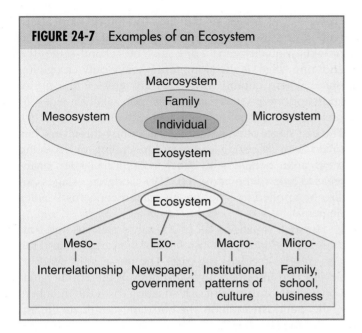

FIGURE 24-7 Examples of an Ecosystem

the concept one step further. They use the term **contextualism** to explain the idea of understanding the individual in the context of the family and the family in the context of the culture. This concept reflects a true ecological perspective. It is a particularly useful concept for community health nurses to keep in mind.

Network Therapy

Network therapy, or social networking, focuses on the natural relationship systems of individuals and families. The family network is a relatively invisible but real structure within which the family is embedded. Networks can be either functional or dysfunctional. "A well-functioning network mediates stress, facilitates communication, and interprets the environment in an effective manner. Dysfunctional networks tend to be rigid and constraining and are characterized by depersonalization and alienation" (Becvar & Becvar, 2000, p. 310). Family networks can be mapped. Members include people within the household, emotionally significant people outside the household, casual relationships, and distant relationships. A distinction is drawn between family and nonfamily members and those people whom one dislikes or with whom one feels uncomfortable and those about whom one feels more positive. In a therapeutic setting, the goals are to resolve the family crisis through resolution of problems with the network and to ensure that the network is a positive resource for the family.

Transactional Field Approach

Transaction "denotes system in process with system, where no entity can be located as first or final cause" (Spiegel, 1982, p. 35). In the **transactional field theory**

the individual is viewed in the context of his transactional field (made up of all aspects of the person's life, including physical, psychological, social, and cultural) and the family group in interaction with other social groups and in interaction with the universe. Spiegel believes that institutions are culturally anchored. In terms of his theory, he defines culture as a "set of beliefs and values about the nature of the world and human existence" (p. 36). An awareness of the system's culture, particularly the values of the dominant culture versus the value patterns of the family, is thus important.

CARING AND FAMILY NURSING

As described in Chapter 1, caring encompasses both affective and instrumental dimensions. There is a tendency in the caring literature to focus on the affective dimension when the subject is the caring nurse and on the instrumental (work) dimension when the subject is the family caregiver (Pepin, 1992). Family caregivers need emotional support as well as family behavioral management skill training. For instance, Arai, Sugiura, Washio, Miura, and Kudo (2001) found that depressed caregivers tend to discontinue care for disabled elderly at home. This information suggests that attention to the affective needs of caregivers is very important. These findings are supported by Brinson and Brink (2000) and Chang (1999).

The caring nurse relates to individuals within the context of the family. Therefore, the nurse, when caring for a family, will exhibit the same behaviors as when caring for an individual. Given the complexity of the family context, the implementation of these behaviors is crucial to accurate and adequate assessment of the family and to

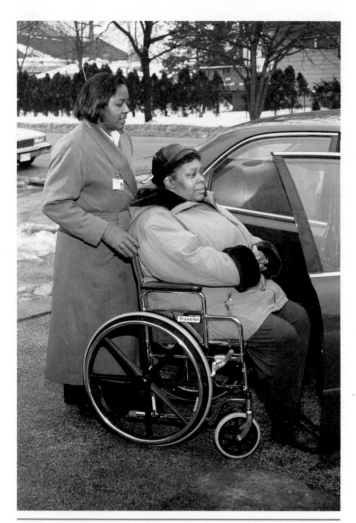

This caregiver takes care of her mother as well as works full time and takes care of her children. The community health nurse must watch for role strain in caregivers.

implementation of appropriate interventions. Many times, it is the caregiver and other family members, rather than the client, on whom nursing care will be focused.

Family caregiving usually involves a primary **caregiver,** often a woman, who cares for the chronically ill spouse, child, or parent. Care may be intermittent, such as shopping or financial management, or may include in-home assistance requiring a regular time commitment. Often, intimate personal and health care are necessary activities. The more time consuming the care, the less likely it is that the affective aspects of daily living will be addressed (Pepin, 1992).

Lindgren (1993) has defined a caregiving career that gives a perspective for the lived experience of a family caring for a member with dementia. She describes three stages: encounter, enduring, and exit. These stages provide important information for nursing assessment and the development of appropriate interventions for the caregiver. The first stage, the encounter stage, is characterized by "the need for rapid adjustment to major

changes and losses in the life, for information about pathologies and illness characteristics, and instruction on providing quality care" (p. 219). The second stage, the enduring stage, is the "long-term, heavy-duty caregiving phase where coping with everyday stress is the norm, and supportive interventions are more likely needed to prevent the caregivers' physical exhaustion" (p. 219). The exit stage, often not thought about by caregivers, has to do with "assisting caregivers in ending or reducing their career demands by either institutionalization or increased help in the home" (p. 219). Lindgren's stages can also be applied to other health-related concerns besides dementia.

In such situations, all of a family's patterns and routines are disrupted, not just those of the caregiver and the person who receives the care. The nurse must work to develop an informed understanding of the family situation and the meaning of that situation to all the members of the family. In addition, the nurse must evaluate the impact of the situation on the family dynamics. Family caregiving skills are also important to assess (see Research Focus). Brinson and Brink (2000) identified coping strategies of rural family caregivers caring for an elderly relative in a home hospice situation. These included (1) support from a variety of sources, including other family members and neighbors and hospice caregivers; (2) adaptive activities such as laughter, reasoning, respite, working through it, taking one day at a time, and establishing a routine; (3) support from religious faith; and (4) avoidance, such as not thinking about it, not asking about what to expect, keeping busy, and use of medications.

While similar strategies are used in other cultures, there are some important considerations regarding caregiving that must be addressed. For instance, in most countries, women have the major responsibility for elder care in their families. In Nigeria, where polygamy is common, grandparents reside with the son, and it is often the third wife who provides them with care, as well as her husband, who is usually much older than she (Johnson & Climo, 2000).

In Taiwan, a daughter moves to her husband's home and becomes the caregiver for the family (Chou, LaMontagne, & Hepworth, 1999; Johnson & Climo, 2000). In Ireland, there is pressure to retain one son at home to provide financial and physical assistance to the family. In all three cultures, as well as others, a lower status is given to those who provide physical care than to those who provide financial support. "The lower status according to physical help means that it is relegated more frequently to women than to men" (Johnson & Climo, 2000, p. 688). While caring is applicable to all of the nursing process, two specific aspects that are expressions of caring are attending to family cultural perspectives and working in partnership with the family to provide family care. Additional information about caregiving can be found in Chapter 27.

RESEARCH FOCUS

Family Caregiving Skill: Development of the Concept

Study Problem/Purpose

To develop the concept of family caregiving skill.

Methods

The initial theoretical phase of concept development consisted of literature review and analysis of existing definitions of skill in light of interview data and clinical observations. The result was to name a concept and gain a preliminary appreciation of what the properties and dimensions of the caregiving skill might be. This report is about the empirical phase, which consisted of an in-depth qualitative analysis of the data. The data base consisted of interviews of 10 client/caregiver dyads. In addition, the combined data set (130 interviews with 30 clients and 29 caregivers) from two previous studies were used because they provided previously unanalyzed data on family caregiving skills. The majority of participants were women. Caregivers had a mean age of 53 years and the clients a mean age of 60 years. Most were white. The clients were being treated with chemotherapy for the first time for solid tumors or lymphoma. Clients were recruited through medical oncology practices and clinics. A grounded-theory approach was used.

Findings

Sixty-three indicators of caregiving skill were identified and categorized into one of nine caregiving processes: monitoring (observing how the care receiver was doing or "keeping an eye on things" to ensure that changes in the ill person's condition were noticed), interpreting (the process of making sense of what was observed), making decisions (the process of choosing a course of action based on one's observa-tions and interpretations of the situation), taking action (the process of carrying out caregiving decisions and instructions), making adjustments (the process of progressively refining caregiving actions until a strategy that worked well was found), providing hands-on care (the process of carrying out nursing and medical procedures), accessing resources (the process of obtaining what was needed to provide care), working together with the ill person (the process of sharing illness-related care in a way that was sensitive to the personhood of both care receiver and caregiver), and negotiating the health care system (the process of ensuring that the care receiver's needs were met adequately). The indicators are observable characteristics of caregiving that signify the level of skillfulness with which each caregiving process is carried out.

Interpretation

Family caregiving skill was defined as the "ability to engage effectively and smoothly in nine core caregiving processes" (p. 199). Three properties of family caregiving were identified: (1) a blend of previously developed skills, (2) integrating knowledge about the ill person with knowledge about specifics of illness care, and (3) caregiving skill developed over time and with experience.

"Study results suggest that clinicians should assess multiple caregiving processes and target their interventions to processes with which a caregiver needs help" (p. 201). Coaching for skill development may be needed and it requires both time and continuity in the helping relationship.

Source: Schumacher, K. I., Stewart, B. J., Archbold, P. G., Dodd, M. J., & Dibble, S. L. (2000). Family caregiving skill: Development of the concept. Research in Nursing and Health, 23, 191–203.

CULTURAL CONSIDERATIONS

The cultural milieu within the family develops from the blending of patterns of the two families of origin in the context of the larger society. Although it is helpful to understand the beliefs and values of the traditional culture of the families of origin and those of the dominant society, caring nurses recognize the importance of allowing the uniqueness of the family to become evident and of presenting oneself as a learner in the process of understanding the family as a cultural system. Cuellar and Glazer (1996) have hypothesized five types of **family acculturative styles.** They are as follows:

> **Traditional-oriented nonresistive style.** First-generation parents and children "who are traditionally oriented with regard to that culture and have minimal exposure to the majority culture" (p. 20).

They are open to acculturation but have had little association with the host country.

Integrated bicultural family style. Fairly equal integration of elements of both cultures resulting in a balanced orientation and acceptance of two or more cultures.

Assimilated family style. Full assimilation within the host culture with little residual traditional orientation or character.

Separatist family style. Discomfort with assimilation and active resistance and opposition to acculturation forces and pressures.

Marginalized family style. "Some or all of the family members seem to have lost their identity with both the traditional and the majority culture" (p. 21).

Most traditional cultures see health as "a state of balance with the family, community, and the forces of the natural world" (Cuellar & Glazer, 1996, p. 99) and see illness as a state of imbalance (Spector, 2000). Ways of maintaining or restoring this balance vary from culture to culture. Within families where different cultures are represented, many variations on health beliefs and practices may exist. Spector notes that "ethnic beliefs and practices related to health and illness of the family are more in tune with the mother's family than with the father's" (p. 29), because the nurturer of the family tends to be the mother. Knowledge of factors such as family health practices (discussed in Chapter 25), socioeconomic status, political and historical background, and migration patterns can assist the nurse in balancing his or her general understanding of the family's culture with the unique patterns and experiences of the actual human network.

People who are secure and comfortable in their own cultural identities are more likely to be flexible and open to people of different cultural backgrounds. Respectful and sensitive behavior by the nurse can help shape the family's self-perceptions and minimize the possibility that the family will themselves participate in discriminatory behavior in the future. A basic requirement for the caring nurse is to develop the sensitivity and respect necessary for successful relationships with clients of different ethnic and socioeconomic backgrounds.

Nurses should be wary of believing they have expertise simply because they have cognitive understanding of a particular culture's traditional values. A certain amount of knowledge can be helpful, but without the openness to learn about the uniqueness of a particular family from the family itself, cognitive knowledge can become a barrier and a deterrent. The possibility of overidentification with the client family on the part of the provider must also be kept in mind, especially if family and provider are from similar ethnic or socioeconomic backgrounds.

Families are not immune to stereotyping the behavior of the human service provider. Families may also present caricatures and exaggerations of their ethnicity in their interactions with providers, a phenomenon that can be viewed as another manifestation of the family's themes and patterns.

Knowledge of socioeconomic factors is also helpful in understanding people of different cultures. For example, families from rural areas will be different from urban families within the same culture. And some families have more in common with families from other cultures than they do with families of their own culture.

The family's migration experience is another important dimension to be considered. Millions of individuals in different parts of the world migrate each year. For some, the move is the result of a lengthy planning process; for others, it represents a rapid uprooting necessitated by tur-

---

REFLECTIVE THINKING

Family Differentness

Some families move from one country to another or from one section of the country to another for employment or because they are in the military.

- Whom do you know who has moved here from another country?
- What were their reasons for moving?
- How have they adapted to their new environment?
- Do you see differences between those who chose to come here versus those who were forced to do so for political or economic reasons?
- How does cultural, ethnic, or religious background facilitate or impede a family's adjustment and adaptation to a new living situation?
- In what ways is their way of life similar or different from yours?
- How comfortable are they about their move?
- Are they different from you in ways they express themselves?
- What is your reaction to these similarities or differences?
- How do their health beliefs and practices differ from your own?
- From where did your health beliefs and practices come?
- Do your health beliefs and practices have a scientific basis?

moil and crisis in their native land. Migrants differ in other ways as well. Some may come from cultures in which mobility is common and may move within the boundaries of the same culture; others may leave a society that has been highly sedentary for generations. These factors and others affect the process and problems the family experiences in the new environment. There are often generational differences regarding the place of cultural beliefs in family life. Children and grandchildren of immigrants tend to take on many of the values and attitudes of the dominant culture, values that may conflict with the cultural beliefs of the parents. For instance, there may be a great deal of conflict if a child plans to marry an individual who is from another cultural or ethnic background.

Many immigrants have had little or no experience with Western medicine. They enter our health care system with their own health beliefs and customs for preventing and dealing with illness. In order to effectively treat and educate these clients, the nurse must understand their points of view. The ability to integrate Western interventions with traditional cultural therapies is an important skill for nurses to have.

PARTNERSHIPS IN FAMILY NURSING

Family-centered care emphasizes the central role of the family rather than that of any individual within the family. It is not enough to identify the family member who plays a central role; one must also identify the interaction among the members in relation to one another. To provide effective and acceptable care, the nurse must work in partnership with the family in an atmosphere of mutual respect and cooperation, recognizing the family's central role in guiding the person's selection and use of health care services (Wright & Leahey, 2000).

FAMILY ASSESSMENT

Wright and Leahey (2000) note that there are no family assessment models that explain all family phenomena. They have developed a framework that encompasses structural, developmental, and functional categories. This model includes assessment of both internal family functioning as well as its relationship to community resources and activities. It also includes assessment of the impact of the community on the family and of the family on the community. The nurse enters the family system with the intent of assisting the family in its quest to promote health and alleviate illness. Problem solving is accomplished through application of the nursing process, with the family, rather than the individual, being the unit of focus.

Wright and Leahey (2000) have developed a family assessment guide for use by nurses. As illustrated in Figure 24-8, the model consists of three major categories: structural, developmental, and functional. These categories reflect major components of family theories previously described. Each category is made up of several dimensions (external, internal, etc.), each of which has several subcategories. Although assessment of every element is not always necessary, following this guide ensures that data about the family are not presented as isolated facts. The nurse is able to develop an integrated picture of the many dimensions of the family.

Petze (1991) notes that most nursing care deals with family transitions, such as losses, occupational changes, parenthood, adulthood, retirement, or illness. Nursing care acts as a bridge to facilitate family reflection, problem solving, planning, and evaluation of outcomes, enabling the family members to regain their sense of competency and control of the situation or events for both the present and the future. Figure 24-9 lists ways that nurses assist the family toward competent behavior.

Family Environment

Major components of family assessment are the physical, psychological, and social dimensions of the environment within which the family lives. The community health nurse has a responsibility to assess each of these aspects because each has an impact on the family. A more extensive discussion of community assessment is presented in Chapter 15.

Physical Environment

The **physical environment** includes the dwelling and the conditions both inside and outside. Size, number of rooms, orderliness, cleanliness, condition of the yard, furnishings, plumbing, heat, health and safety hazards, and presence or absence of smoke detectors and fire extinguishers all provide important information regarding the status of the family. Some families may have spacious homes but be unable to buy food or to pay for telephone service or basic utilities such as heat and

---

※ **DECISION MAKING**

Family Competence

Consider each of the 10 ways that nurses assist the family toward competent behavior (as noted in Figure 24-9).

◆ What questions could you ask of family members to elicit related information?

FIGURE 24-8   Family Assessment Guide

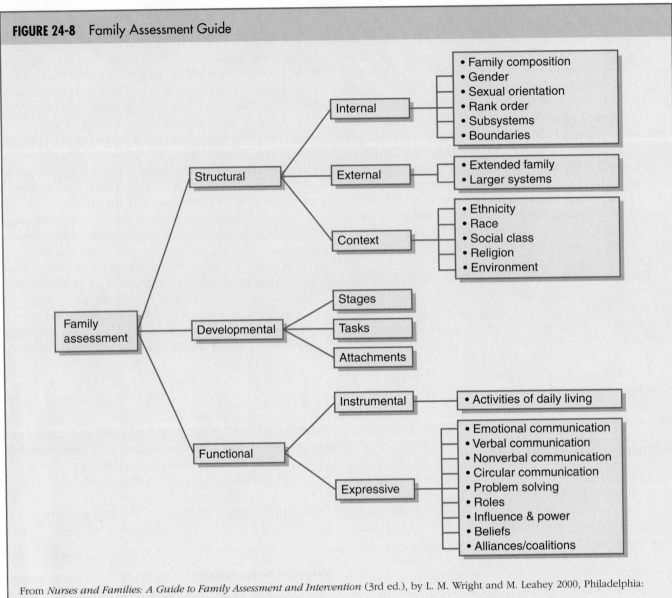

From *Nurses and Families: A Guide to Family Assessment and Intervention* (3rd ed.), by L. M. Wright and M. Leahey 2000, Philadelphia: F. A. Davis.

FIGURE 24-9   Ways in Which Nurses Assist the Family toward Competent Behavior

1. Help members to clarify goals and needs.

2. Introduce or reinforce effective communication patterns, coping skills, and behaviors.

3. Encourage a safe and nurturing environment for communication activities.

4. Guide toward congruence between individual and family goals, needs, and activities.

5. Discuss and enumerate the behaviors, statements, and actions that are evidence of both functional and dysfunctional coping.

6. Provide direct physical and emotional care when needed.

7. Foster educational and informational exchange.

8. Identify additional appropriate resources.

9. Offer compassionate but honest support.

10. Help family members identify contributions they are able to make to the family process and the ill family member and contributions they expect to receive from others.

From "Health Promotion for the Family," by C. F. Petze, 1991, in B. W. Spradley (Ed.), *Readings in Community Health Nursing* (4th ed., pp. 355–364), New York: J. B. Lippincott.

REFLECTIVE THINKING

Your Family's Competence

Think of your own family.

- How does your family deal with stress?
- How do your family activities influence your nutritional status?
- Who works in the family? How much?
- How do family work patterns affect the family's level of functioning?
- What is the use of alcohol, tobacco, caffeine, or other legal or illegal drugs in your family?
- Are rest and sleep patterns consistent and adequate, or are there frequent interruptions or barriers to adequate rest?
- Does your family exercise adequately and make appropriate use of leisure activities?
- How well do they follow appropriate safety practices?

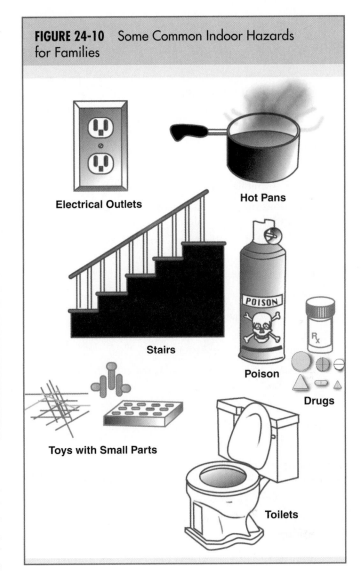

FIGURE 24-10 Some Common Indoor Hazards for Families

Electrical Outlets · Hot Pans · Stairs · Poison · Drugs · Toys with Small Parts · Toilets

lights. Other families may have homes that are small and crowded but where everyone feels secure and comfortable. An important component to assess is the presence of safety hazards and family plan for emergencies such as fire or earthquake. Figures 24-10 and 24-11 identify some of the more common hazards for which the nurse can look when assessing the family's home.

Other physical aspects of the environment to be assessed are the neighborhood and air and water quality. Information about the neighborhood can be obtained via observation when driving in the area and by asking questions of family members.

Are schools, churches, hospitals, stores, and the like easily accessible?

Is public transportation available?

What types of homes occupy the area?

How well do family members know their neighbors?

What is the crime rate in the neighborhood?

Air and water quality also can be assessed by asking questions.

What are the air, water, and noise pollution levels?

What is the quality of sanitation?

Each of these areas should be addressed according to the needs of the family. In addition, family members should be asked about their perceptions and knowl-

edge of these issues. It is the family's perspective about the environment that will most influence both the way the family functions within that environment and the degree to which family members will respond to nursing interventions.

Psychological Environment

Significant aspects of the **psychological environment** include developmental stages, family dynamics, and emotional strengths, already discussed in this chapter. Communication patterns, including verbal and nonverbal communication, both within and outside the family, family roles, and coping strategies also provide important clues to the health of the family. These factors are discussed in Chapter 25.

Social Environment

Social environment includes religion, race, culture, social class, economic status, and external resources such

---

FIGURE 24-11   Potential Physical Environmental Hazards for Families

- Lack of barriers to stairs or upper story porches when children are in the environment
- Swimming pools without barriers to prevent children or animals from falling in
- Presence of lead-based paint (usually in older homes)
- Loose throw rugs
- Broken furniture, stairs, stair railings, or floorboards
- Hazardous materials, such as cleaning materials or medications, within children's reach
- Plumbing that does not allow for sanitary disposal of human wastes
- Toys in walkways
- Overcrowding
- Absence of fire alarms in the home, lack of a fire plan
- Lack of a disaster plan for earthquake, tornado, hurricane, or other disaster
- Lack of a poison control plan (posted telephone numbers)
- Numerous house pets such as cats, chickens, or dogs
- Lack of fenced-in yard for small children
- Lack of childproof electrical outlets
- Proximity to a heavily traveled highway

REFLECTIVE THINKING

Assessing the Home Environment

Look at your own home environment.

- How would you assess its physical components? Psychological components? Social components?

---

as school, church, and health resources. It is important to learn about the family's perception of these areas.

- What is the kind and level of religious involvement of the family?
- How do the family's cultural values affect family members?
- What is the pattern of the family's social relations?
- What is the family's financial status?
- How involved is the family in organizations and institutions outside of the family?
- How does the family manage health and illness experiences?

Such questions help clarify the context of the family and provide information regarding family strengths and resources and well as family deficits.

Family Strengths

Often, the health provider—as well as the family itself—tends to look only at the problems and conflicts within a family. To know the full extent of the way a family functions, however, the nurse must also assess

family strengths. Otto (1963) identified family strengths as follows:

- The ability to provide for the physical, emotional, and spiritual needs of a family
- Sensitivity to the needs of family members
- The ability to communicate effectively
- The ability to provide support, security, and encouragement
- The ability to initiate and maintain growth-producing relationships and experiences within and outside of the family
- The capacity to create and maintain constructive and responsible community relationships in the neighborhood, the school, and town, local, and state governments
- The ability to grow with and through children
- The ability for self-help and the ability to accept help when appropriate
- The ability to perform family roles flexibly
- Respect for the individuality of each family member
- The ability to use a crisis or seemingly injurious experience as a means of growth
- A concern for family unity, loyalty, and interfamily cooperation

Although all these strengths are important to healthy family functioning, it is unlikely that any given family will have all of them. The degree to which they do manifest these behaviors, however, gives the nurse clues as to how well the family is managing its life. Some families may be dealing with many serious problems, but if they exhibit a number of the aforementioned strengths, they can cope with little or no outside intervention. Other families may need extensive help, even in the face of fewer or less serious problems, because they have fewer strengths.

Feeley and Gottlieb (2000) note that clinical practice has been dominated by the "deficit-, disorder-, or problem-oriented approach" (p. 9). This approach fails to appreciate the family's strengths and suggests that the family lacks the ability to solve its own problems without the help of a professional. Feeley and Gottlieb recommend a strength-based approach that they believe requires a "major conceptual shift in how the clinician views families, the nature of the clinician's relationship with the family and how the clinician then works with the families" (p. 10). This approach emphasizes a partnership between nurse and client. The nurse "recognizes and uses strengths and positive forces in the individual-family situation as a basis of action" (p. 11). They identify three strategies in using strengths. The first is identifying strengths and providing positive feedback to the clients. This approach helps develop the relationship and motivates clients to participate in meeting their health care needs. Second, client strengths are developed by "(a) helping a family transfer the use of a strength from one context to another, (b) turning a deficit into a strength, and (c) developing knowledge or competency" (p. 15). The third strategy is calling forth strengths, that is, emphasizing strengths in the family of which the family, itself, may or may not have been aware. These approaches support collaboration with the family in a positive way that allows family members to recognize and use their own abilities to solve health problems.

Assessment Tools

Two of the most useful and most commonly used family assessment tools are the genogram and the ecomap. A **genogram** is a tangible and graphic picture outlining a family's patterns over a period of time, usually three generations (McGoldrick, Gerson, & Shellenburger, 1999). It is a way to map the structure of the family, to record family information (e.g., significant life events, cultural and religious identification, occupations, place of residence), and to delineate relationships. By adding major dimensions of the family's health history, the genogram becomes a **family health tree** from which knowledge can be gained about genetic and familial diseases. Environmental and occupational diseases; psychosocial problems such as obesity, anorexia nervosa, and mental illness; and infectious diseases also can be noted. Family risk factors and strengths can be added to the genogram by soliciting information from the family regarding things such as the way the family manages stress and leisure and the frequency of physical exams, testicular exams, Pap smears, and exercise among family members. Resulting information can help the nurse identify areas of risk and ability, facilitate the family's awareness of the situation, and work with the family to plan appropriate interventions (Friedman, 1998; McGoldrick et al., 1999). Figure 24-12 identifies the common genogram symbols. Figure 24-13 is an example of a genogram/family health tree.

The **ecomap** is a visual depiction of the family members' contact with larger systems through a graphic

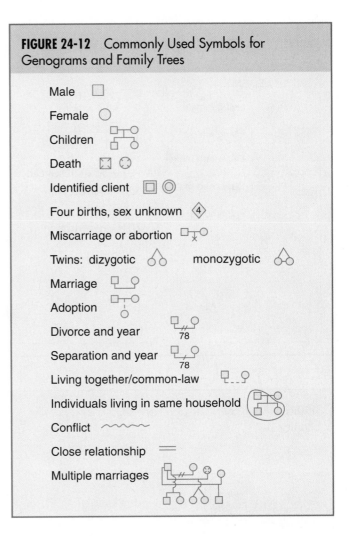

FIGURE 24-12 Commonly Used Symbols for Genograms and Family Trees

Male □
Female ○
Children
Death ⊠ ⊘
Identified client □ ◎
Four births, sex unknown ④
Miscarriage or abortion
Twins: dizygotic   monozygotic
Marriage
Adoption
Divorce and year   78
Separation and year   78
Living together/common-law
Individuals living in same household
Conflict ∿∿∿
Close relationship =
Multiple marriages

description of its relationship and interaction with its immediate external environment (Friedman, 1998; Wright & Leahey, 2000). After the nurse develops an ecomap with the family, she or he can use the information to identify interactive family strengths, conflicts in need of mediation, connections to be made, and resources to be sought and mobilized. Figure 24-14 shows symbols and forms used in a ecomap. A completed ecomap, based on the Community Nursing View, can be found in Figure 24-18.

Both the genogram and ecomap are useful tools during an early interview with a family. The whole family can become engaged in completing each tool so that family members' involvement in their own health care is facilitated from the beginning of the relationship. Wright and Leahey (2000) note that the visual gestalt conveyed through the use of these tools provides information more simply and usefully than can words. They "act as constant visual reminders for nurses to 'think family' " (p. 87).

Other tools that are vitally important to nursing assessment are observation of the family and their environment and the family interview. The previous discussion of family environment addressed the many aspects of the family

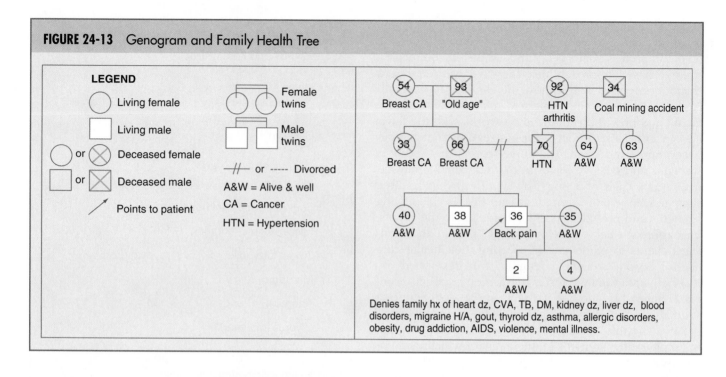

FIGURE 24-13 Genogram and Family Health Tree

FIGURE 24-14 Symbols and Forms Used in a Family Ecomap

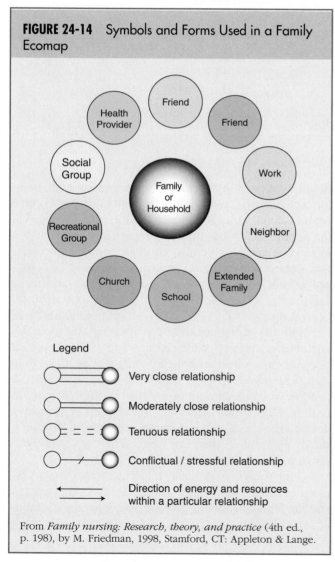

From *Family nursing: Research, theory, and practice* (4th ed., p. 198), by M. Friedman, 1998, Stamford, CT: Appleton & Lange.

that can be assessed through observation. The family interview within the context of the home visit is explored in Chapter 22. Analysis of the information gained from all the tools together provides the basis for the identification of nursing diagnoses.

FAMILY DIAGNOSIS

There are two major systems of nursing diagnosis. The North American Nursing Diagnosis Association (NANDA) has been developing nursing diagnostic labels and defining characteristics since the 1970s. The Omaha system, which also began development in the 1970s, focuses more directly on the needs of community health nurses.

The NANDA System

Family nursing diagnoses are not yet well developed. At present, they can be best used to identify problems of the individual within the family. Nurses should be prepared to devise their own diagnoses when the focus is on the family as client. Malone (1998) notes that few of the NANDA-approved diagnostic categories address family concerns, and "the need to communicate what nurses do and with whom remains" (p. 329). Only one, *family coping: potential for growth*, implies health-promoting concepts. Further, Geissler (1991) and Giger and Davidhizar (1999) note that the diagnostic categories do not facilitate culturally sensitive nursing care. For example, *impaired communication related to foreign language barrier* assumes that the recipient of health care is at fault; there is no acknowledgment that the nurse is equally unable to communicate with the client. Andrews (1995) suggests that it might be

---

FIGURE 24-15 NANDA Family Diagnostic Categories

- Interrupted family processes
- Impaired parenting
- Anticipatory grieving
- Compromised family coping
- Decisional conflict
- Dysfunctional grieving
- Family coping: readiness for enhanced
- Health-seeking behaviors
- Impaired home maintenance management
- Impaired social interaction
- Impaired verbal communication
- Disabled family coping
- Deficient knowledge
- Parental role conflict
- Sexual dysfunction

From *NANDA Nursing Diagnosis: Diagnoses and Classification* 2001–2002 by North American Nursing Diagnosis Association, 2000, Philadelphia, PA: Author.

✳ DECISION MAKING

Developing a Diagnosis

You are visiting the Klee family for the first time. You know from the referral that they have no health insurance and that Ida Klee is a single parent with a six-year-old daughter, Patty, who has asthma. Ida is two months pregnant and is undecided about whether to terminate her pregnancy. She says she is always tired and that her daughter gets on her nerves. She has slapped her daughter a few times. Patty is in the first grade and is having trouble reading and concentrating. Ida has little time to help her and spends a lot of time in bed when she is not working as a waitress.

◆ Using the NANDA nursing diagnosis system, identify one or two applicable nursing diagnoses.

◆ Using the Omaha nursing diagnosis system:

  Which domains would you address?

  What problems can you identify?

  Which modifiers would you use?

  If you have identified active problems, what are the signs and symptoms?

◆ With which of the two systems did it seem easier to work?

---

more appropriate to discuss the nurse's "knowledge deficits" of the client's culture. Figure 24-15 lists selected NANDA nursing diagnoses related to the family.

The Omaha System

The Omaha system is particularly appropriate for use in community health nursing. The system was developed by community health nurses to specifically meet their needs for accurately diagnosing problems and strengths and for consistently documenting findings. The Omaha system consists of three parts: the problem classification scheme, the intervention scheme, and the problem rating scale for outcomes (Martin & Scheet, 1992). The problem classification scheme is divided into four levels. The first level is called the *domain* and includes the four general areas of community health practice: environmental, psychosocial, physiological, and health-related behaviors. The second level, called the *problem,* consists of 40 nursing diagnoses that nurses are licensed to assign and treat and that are amenable to nursing intervention. They are stated from the client's perspective and are accompanied by one modifier from each of two sets. The third level identifies *modifiers,* or terms used in conjunction with the problems. The first set describes the degree of severity of such aspects as risk factors and signs and symptoms (i.e., Health Promotion, Potential Deficit/Impairment, and Deficit/Impairment/Actual). The second set identifies ownership of the problem: that is, whether it is an individual or a family problem.

Signs and symptoms are the fourth level. They are used only with actual deficits. Signs are the objective evidence of a client's problem, and symptoms are the subjective evidence of a client's problem reported by the client or another significant person. Each domain includes a number of problems and each includes one problem identified as "other" in order to accommodate a problem not in the classification. Figure 24-16 lists some of the 40 problems along with the modifiers and some problem-specific signs and symptoms.

The intervention scheme arranges nursing actions or activities in a systematic way at three different levels. All interventions include a "category," a "target," and, usually, "client-specific information." The categories are the first level and are divided into "four broad areas that provide a structure for describing community health nursing actions or activities (i.e., Health Teaching, Guidance, and Counseling; Treatments and Procedures; Case Management; and Surveillance)" (Martin & Scheet, 1992, p. 84). The targets are "the 62 objects of nursing actions or activities that serve to further describe interventions" (p. 84). These include such things as coping skills, family planning, and ostomy care. The third level, client-specific information, is generated by the community health nurse

FIGURE 24-16 Examples of Omaha System

Environmental Domain

Problem 04

Neighborhood/workplace safety. Freedom from injury or loss as it relates to the community/place of employment

Modifier

Health Promotion   Family

Potential Deficit   Individual

Deficit

Signs/Symptoms

01. high crime rate

02. high pollution level

03. uncontrolled animals

04. physical hazards

05. unsafe play areas

06. other

Psychosocial Domain

Problem 11

Grief. Keen mental suffering or distress over affliction or loss

Modifier

Health Promotion Family

Potential Impairment   Individual

Impairment

Signs/Symptoms

01. fails to recognize normal grief responses

02. difficulty coping with grief responses

03. difficulty expressing grief responses

04. conflicting stages of grief process among family/individual

05. other

Physiological Domain

Problem 28

Respiration. The exchange of oxygen and carbon dioxide in the body

Modifier

Health Promotion   Family

Potential Impairment   Individual

Impairment

Signs/Symptoms

01. abnormal breath patterns

02. unable to breathe independently

03. cough

04. unable to cough/expectorate independently

05. cyanosis

06. abnormal sputum

07. noisy respirations

08. rhinorrhea

09. abnormal breath sounds

10. other

Health-Related Behaviors Domain

Problem 38

Personal hygiene. Individual practice conducive to health and cleanliness

Modifier

Health Promotion   Family

Potential Impairment   Individual

Impairment

Signs/Symptoms

01. inadequate laundering of clothing

02. inadequate bathing

03. body odor

04. inadequate shampooing/combing of hair

05. inadequate brushing/flossing/mouth care

06. other

From *The Omaha System,* by K. S. Martin & N. J. Scheet, 1992, Philadelphia: W. B. Saunders. Used with permission.

or other health care practitioner and is the detailed portion of the care plan. For more detailed information, see Martin and Scheet (1992).

The problem rating scale for outcomes "provides a framework for evaluating the client's problem-specific knowledge, behavior, and status at regular or predictable time intervals" (Martin & Scheet, 1992, p. 93). These components can be assessed on a continuum that provides five degrees of response, from the most negative to the most positive state of a problem.

PLANNING AND INTERVENTION

Perhaps the most important aspect of the planning and intervention part of the nursing process is planning in partnership with the family. As previously stated, it is critical that the nurse work with the family members to identify their concerns and to plan intervention strategies. It has long been noted, and is important to recognize, that for the health provider "empowerment of clients and changing their victim status means giving up our position as benefactors" (Pinderhughes, 1983, p. 337). It is not always easy to let go of the wish to rescue the family, but it is in the family's best interest to do so. Malone (1998) notes that "an alliance with the family is a prerequisite for quality care" (p. 329). From this perspective, partnership with the family is necessary at every step, and assessment and intervention occur simultaneously in a dynamic process. Further, interventions are planned taking into account family priorities and filling information gaps in the family's knowledge base so that intervention decisions are made from a position of knowledge. Interventions address primary, secondary, or tertiary levels of prevention.

Primary Prevention

Primary prevention encompasses health promotion and disease prevention. It identifies actions taken to prevent the occurrence of health problems in families. One of the major nursing activities in this realm is that of anticipatory guidance. Activities might include, for example, providing information about normative changes that can be expected in a child's growth so that parents are prepared for the changes and are ready to deal with them when they occur. Another activity might be helping a family prepare for the changes that will occur when a member returns home after a period of time spent in a mental institution or prison. *Healthy People 2010* (U.S. Department of Health and Human Services, [USDHHS], 2000) addresses primary prevention for families in most of its objectives. While the emphasis of the plan is more on individuals, the impact for families is great. For instance, the implementation of programs to reduce teenage and unintended pregnancies or alcohol-related motor vehicle accident deaths has important implications for family life.

Of particular concern is the assessment of the family and home environment with an eye to prevent falls. In the elderly, particularly, falls contribute significantly to mortality and morbidity (Rawsky, 1998). Objective 15-27 of *Healthy People 2010* has set 3.0 deaths/100,000 by falls as their goal. In 1998, there were 4.7/100,000 (USDHHS, 2000). In one study of emergency room admissions, it was found that approximately one-half of the admissions had undocumented histories of falls (Edelberg, Lyman, & Wei, 1998). There are many conditions that set the stage for falls in the home. These include age (changes in neuromuscular and cardiac homeostatic mechanisms), neurological conditions (gait and balance disorders), foot disorders and poorly fitting footwear, syncope, medications (particularly sedatives, hypnotics, antidepressants, anxiolytics, cardiovascular agents, and alcohol), postural hypotension, and environmental risk factors. Given these conditions, a client evaluation should include a physical examination that targets possible causes of a fall or suggests there could be a fall and direct observation of mobility and performance. Laboratory tests may also help to explain the cause of a fall. In addition to hospital admission for serious falls, treatment should include a home safety evaluation, strength and range-of-motion exercises, and provision for assistive devises such as canes or walkers, grab bars, or handrails. Physical and occupational therapy may be helpful to "improve activities of daily living or teach new approaches to performing them safely" (p. 43). A complete medication review is indicated to determine if dosage adjustments or substitutions may be necessary (Edelberg, 2001; Enevold & Courts, 2000; Resnick, 1999).

One example of a primary preventive program that encompasses the community and has a major impact on the family can be seen in Out of the Box, Community Partnership to Promote Family Health.

✳ DECISION MAKING

Sibling Rivalry

When assessing a family composed of a single parent with two girls, ages one and three years, you recognize that the mother is devoting all her time to the one-year-old, who has spina bifida. The mother states that the three-year-old is driving her crazy with constant "unnecessary" demands for attention. You identify that the mother needs help in recognizing the impact of her younger child's illness on her older daughter.

- In discussion with the mother, what strategies would you propose that would enable her to attend to both children in a more equitable way so that more extensive acting out by the older child is averted?

- What level of prevention does this example illustrate?

✳ DECISION MAKING

Fall Prevention

Mr. Avery, an 80-year-old man with macular degeneration, diabetes, and hypertension, lives alone. He has complained that he sometimes feels dizzy when he gets up from a chair. On your first visit to his home, you notice that he has throw rugs on his hardwood floors, there are no hand rails in his tub, and the light by the stairs is very dim.

- How would you discuss these issues with the client?

- What plan would you like to make with the client?

COMMUNITY NURSING VIEW

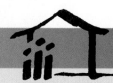

Maria Perez is a 22-year-old mother of three children: Manuel, age 5 years, Mae, age 3 1/2 years, and Rosarie, a 1-week-old newborn who is still in the hospital because of a chronic lung problem. When she goes home in a few days, Rosarie will need oxygen PRN. Maria has expressed concern that she will not be able to manage the oxygen equipment and will not know when Rosarie needs oxygen. Maria and her 25-year-old husband, Jamie, live in a three-room house. Maria and Jamie sleep in one bedroom, where Rosarie will also stay when she comes home. The other children, along with their grandmother, Maria's mother, sleep on a daybed in the living room. Alice, the grandmother, is 47 years old and has lived with the family since her husband's death three years ago from complications of diabetes. He was 51 years old. Maria's husband has been unable to work for the past month because of a back injury incurred in his work as a farm laborer. They do not know when he will recover enough to return to work. He is very depressed and worried about his condition and, although he does not hit Maria or the children, he frequently lashes out verbally in anger when the children become noisy or Maria reaches out to him with affection. His parents live a few blocks away and visit frequently. Maria wishes they would come less often. They spoil the children and often disapprove of the way Maria cares for the household. Manuel and Mae have a yard in which to play, but it is mostly dirt, and an old refrigerator is lying on the ground. The yard is not fenced in, and the family lives on a rather busy street. The children are friendly and playful. Manuel, who is in kindergarten, is very serious and watchful of his sister. Maria says he has become more protective since her husband became disabled. Maria has two sisters and three brothers. Jamie has one brother and three sisters. They live too far away to visit often, but both Maria and Jamie are close to all their siblings. Figures 24-17 and 24-18 illustrate a genogram and an ecomap, respectively, for the Perez family.

Nursing Considerations

Assessment

- What is the Perez family form?
- According to Duvall and Miller (1985) and Carter and McGoldrick (1999), in which stage is the Perez family? What are their developmental tasks?

- Where would you place the Perez family in terms of Combrinck-Graham's (1985) family life cycle?
- Describe the family in terms of systems definitions.
- How well do you think the Perez family is carrying out their family functions?
- What environmental hazards can you identify in the Perez family?
- What family strengths can you identify?
- What cultural considerations must you address in order to work effectively with the Perez family?
- Using Wright and Leahey's (2000) family assessment guide, identify the structural, functional, and developmental dimensions that are important to the understanding of the Perez family.

Diagnosis

- What family nursing diagnoses would you assign to this family? Provide your rationale.

Outcome Identification

- Given the diagnoses you have identified, what outcomes do you expect?

Planning/Interventions

- How would you begin to develop a partnership with the Perez family in order to identify the family's health goals?
- What aspects of their situation might put you at risk for wanting to "rescue" the Perez family?
- Identify primary, secondary, and tertiary interventions for the Perez family.

Evaluation

- Given the interventions identified previously, what might you look for that would enable you to assess the effectiveness of your interventions?
- In order to answer all the preceding questions more fully, what additional information do you need?

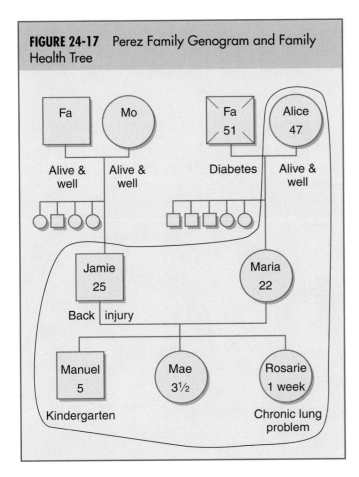

FIGURE 24-17 Perez Family Genogram and Family Health Tree

Secondary Prevention

Secondary prevention has to do with the early recognition and treatment of existing health problems. A family perspective requires examining the interactive problems that suggest family dysfunction as well as the concerns of individuals within the family. *Healthy People 2010* (USD-HHS, 2000) emphasizes screening examinations that can detect problems early and prevent long-term and costly care that drains families resources. Such screening examinations include mammography, Pap smears, and fecal occult blood testing.

Tertiary Prevention

Tertiary prevention has to do with the rehabilitative level of health care. In families, the focus is on preventing the return of the problem. An example might be helping a homeless family, through facilitating the family's connection to appropriate community services, find permanent housing as well as employment that will enable the family to maintain housing.

EVALUATION

Evaluation begins with an examination of the outcomes of the objectives of care defined in the planning and intervention phase and identification of additional data needed

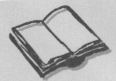

Out of the Box

Community Partnership to Promote Family Health

A partnership between a college of health and human sciences and an inner city middle school was developed to enhance the health and well-being of families in their community. The overall goals were to reduce health risks among youth.

To assure the success of the partnership and future program endeavors, all stakeholders were involved. These included teachers, staff, parents, middle school students, and faculty affiliated with the university. An initial community assessment was conducted to elicit community strengths and assets. Assets included "the ability to network with families, intentionally related to achieving a healthier community, a sense of pride and willingness to act for the better" (p. 75). Needs identified were "health services (and education) for students, staff, and parents, support groups for special concerns related to children with asthma, attention deficit disorder, and developmental delay" (p. 75).

The program delivered both quality health services and health education with emphasis on health promotion to a vulnerable population. Nursing, medicine, social work, physical therapy, and respiratory therapy were all involved in the partnership. The services were tailored to the multidimensional needs of school-aged youth and their families and were developmentally, culturally, and contextually appropriate. With the involvement of other disciplines has come the continuous evolution of consultation and referral networks. "These networks often expand mentoring opportunities for graduate students, faculty, and community leaders" (p. 78).

Evaluation is underway to assess the effectiveness of interventions used, and focus groups will be used to assess the desires and willingness of the community to make health a priority. Factors that have helped to make the project successful have been the mutual commitment and participation of the partners and frequent communication among the stakeholders.

Source: Pittman, K. P., Wold, J. L., Wilson, A. H., Huff, C., & Williams, S. (2000). Community connections: Promoting family health. Family and Community Health, 23, 72–78. ■

FIGURE 24-18 The Perez Family Ecomap

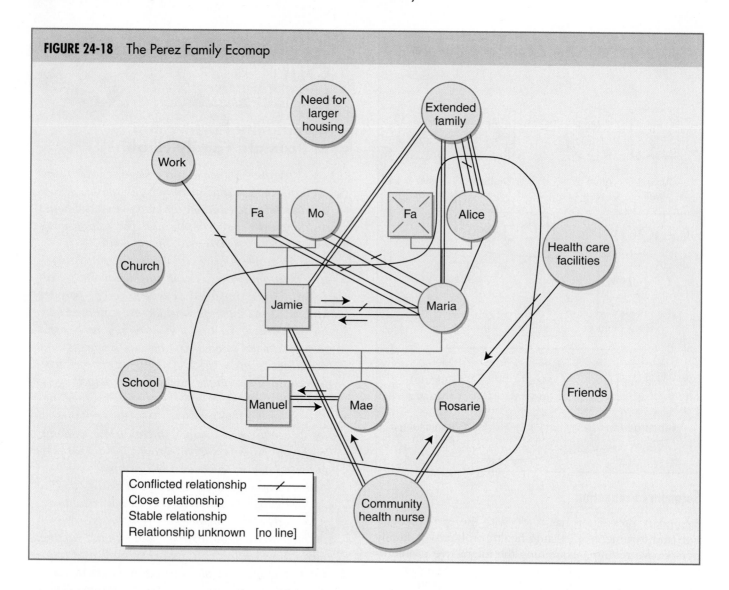

for further assessment. If measurable objectives have been developed, they provide the criteria for measuring the effectiveness of the outcome of the intervention. This process is ongoing in that every new piece of data adds a dimension to that which is already known and forces a new evaluation of the status of needed family care.

KEY CONCEPTS

♦ Families can be identified in two ways: family as context and family as client.

♦ The wider family concept addresses changing family forms and takes into account lifestyles that are independent of biological or kin connections.

♦ It is important to understand a variety of family theories because they give direction to nursing care of families, and no one theory addresses all dimensions of the family or fully explains family dynamics and behavior.

♦ Some nursing theories have enlarged their conceptual base to include the family as client.

♦ Four theories from the social sciences have major relevance to nursing. They are developmental, general systems, structural-functional, and interactional theories.

♦ The stages of family development and the accompanying tasks of each stage guide the nurse in assessing the family.

♦ Rather than a linear event, the family life cycle can be conceptualized as a life spiral wherein family members move closer together or farther apart depending on the life events that are occurring.

♦ Ecological approaches to the family focus on the way the family interacts with their environment.

♦ The cultural milieu within the family develops from the blending of patterns of the two families of origin within the context of the larger society.

♦ Family caregiving must be considered from the point of view of both the nurse as caregiver and the family as caregiver to family members.

◆ To provide effective and acceptable care, the provider must work in partnership with the family in an atmosphere of mutual respect and cooperation.

◆ Family assessment includes an assessment of internal family functioning and of the relationship of the family to community resources and activities.

◆ In order to understand the way a family works, the nurse must assess family strengths as well as problems and conflicts.

◆ Two of the most useful assessment tools for families are the genogram and the ecogram.

◆ The Omaha system of nursing diagnoses is more useful to community health nurses working with families than is the NANDA system of nursing diagnoses.

◆ It is critical that the nurse work with family members to identify their concerns and to plan intervention strategies, rather than focusing on concerns from the nurse's perspective.

◆ Evaluation is an ongoing process in that every new piece of data adds a dimension to that which is already known and forces a new evaluation of the status of needed family care.

Note: The author acknowledges Joan Heron, retired Professor of Nursing, California State University, Fresno, for her significant contributions to the development of this chapter.

RESOURCES

Administration for Children and Families, Department of Health and Human Services: http://www.acf.dhhs.gov
National Council on Family Relations: http://www.ncfr.com
Gay and lesbian parenting: http://www.apa.org/pi/parent.html

MAKING THE CONNECTION

We strongly believe that individual development takes place in the context of significant emotional relationships and that the most significant relationships are family relationships whether by blood, adoption, marriage, or commitment.

—Carter & McGoldrick, 1999b, p. 5

COMPETENCIES

Upon completion of this chapter, the reader should be able to:

- Identify the characteristics of a healthy family.
- Discuss five functions of the family.
- Identify components of family process, including roles, values, communication, and power.
- Understand the resiliency model of family stress, adjustment, and adaptation.
- Identify three types of family crisis.
- Explain the dynamics of vulnerable families.
- Define four specific behaviors that occur in vulnerable families: family myths, scapegoating, triangling, and pseudomutuality.
- Understand the circumplex model of marital and family systems.
- Understand the McMaster model of family functioning.

KEY TERMS

achieved role	informal roles
affective function	instrumental functions
bonadaptation	legitimate power
chaotic family	maladaptation
circumplex model of marital and family systems	McMaster model of family functioning (MMFF)
decision making	nonlegitimate power
disengaged family	power
economic function	power bases
enmeshed family	power outcomes
expressive functions	power processes
family cohesion	pseudomutuality
family communication	reproductive function
family flexibility	resiliency model of family stress, adjustment, and adaptation
family functions	
family myths	
family networks	role accountability
family process	role allocation
family roles	role complementarity
family values	role conflict
first-order change	role enactment
formal roles	role flexibility
health care function	

role strain
role stress
rules
scapegoating

second-order change
socialization
triangling
vulnerable families

In Chapter 24 family structure (composition, type, size, marital status, and social network) was discussed. This chapter considers the functions and processes of the family. Family roles, communication patterns, power structures, values, and family functions in both healthy and dysfunctional modes are considered, and family stress and crisis theory are also explored.

THE HEALTHY FAMILY

Understanding the characteristics of a healthy family is helpful in understanding the many dimensions of the family in its adaptive and maladaptive states. Pratt (1976) refers to families that exhibit healthy characteristics as the "energized family" (p. 3). Curran (1983) and, more recently, the U.S. Department of Health and Human Services (USDHHS, 1990) and Walsh (1998) have conceptualized traits of healthy family processes that support Pratt's description. Some of the major characteristics reflecting the multidimensional nature of a healthy family are:

- Flexible and egalitarian family relationships concerning power, divisions of tasks and activities, role patterns and organization of family tasks, affirmation, support and respect for one another, and trusting relationships among members.
- Sense of play and humor; joint participation in structured and unstructured events. There exists a balance of interaction among family members whereby work and other activities are not allowed to infringe routinely on family time.
- Respect for individual differences, autonomy, separate needs, and privacy. The development and well-being of members of each generation are fostered. Members' contacts are supportive and facilitative, not overwhelming and limiting.
- Connectedness and commitment of members as a caring, mutually supportive unit. Cliques within the family are discouraged. Rituals and traditions are important. There are parental leadership and authority, as well as nurturance, protection, and socialization of children and caretaking of other vulnerable family members. There are adequate resources for basic economic security.
- Communication patterns that foster conversation with family members and effective listening skills; characterized by clarity of rules and expectations,

pleasurable interactions, and a range of emotional expression and empathic responsiveness.

- Family coping skills developed by the family for creative problem solving. Effective conflict resolution processes master normative and nonnormative challenges and transitions across the life cycle. The family is able to admit the need for and seek help with problems.

- Shared belief system that includes a spiritual core and an ability to teach a sense of right and wrong and that fosters mutual trust, connectedness with past and future generations, ethical values, and concern for the larger community.

- Links with the broader community, such as membership and leadership participation in groups and activities that bear on family needs. The family receives enrichment from outside sources and initiates growth-producing relationships in the neighborhood, town, and the wider society. Adequate resources for psychosocial support are available from extended kin and friendship networks and from community and larger social systems, (Pratt, 1976; Curran, 1983; Walsh, 1998).

Although it is important to understand these healthy characteristics, it is equally important to remember that each family is unique and addresses these components in its own way. The nurse must not be quick to assume dysfunction in a family because the family's interaction seems different from that of the nurse's family. On the other hand, nurses should not normalize behavior because it seems familiar or represents that which they be-

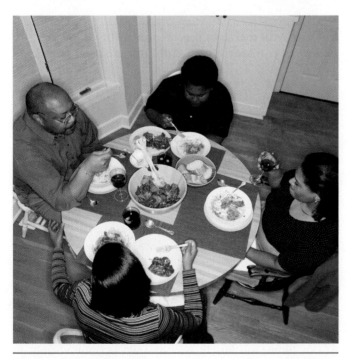

A sense of connectedness is important for a family.
Photo courtesy of PhotoDisc.

> ### REFLECTIVE THINKING
>
> #### Personal Family Dynamics
>
> Consider the dynamics within your own family of origin.
> - Identify behaviors that affirm and support your family.
> - Are there other behaviors that interfere with family growth?
> - Can you identify accepted family behaviors that, on the basis of the list of characteristics of a healthy family, you can now identify as dysfunctional behavior?

lieve to be "good" behavior. For example, an interpretation of conflict avoidance as family harmony prevents the nurse from exploring the family's concerns regarding conflict.

FAMILY FUNCTIONS

Family functions refer to "how families go about meeting the needs of individuals and meeting the purposes of the broader society" (Hanson, 2001, p. 175). They can be divided into two basic aspects of instrumental and expressive (Wright & Leahey, 2000). **Instrumental functions** are those that pertain to activities of daily living. **Expressive functions** have to do with the affective dimension of the family. Friedman (1998) identifies five major family functions important for nurses to understand in their work with families. These functions incorporate both instrumental and expressive components. The functions are:

- Affective
- Socialization and social placement
- Reproductive
- Economic
- Health care

Affective Function

The **affective function** has to do with affirmation, support, and respect for one another (Curran, 1983). It is one of the most vital and rewarding functions for the formation and continuation of the family unit. The family is able to express a full range of emotions (Janosik & Green, 1992). Although the affective function is important to all families, families who must focus on the more basic functions of physical maintenance may have little energy to give to it (Friedman, 1998).

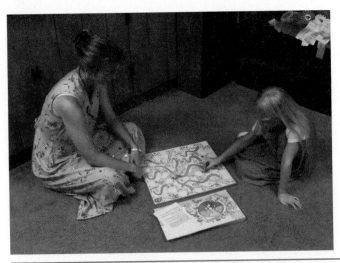

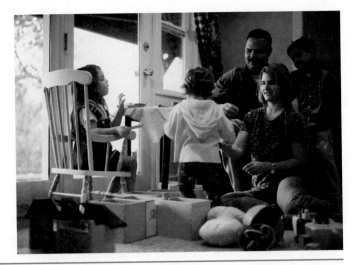

Working and playing together are important for a healthy family.
Photo courtesy of PhotoDisc.

Socialization and Social Placement

Socialization is a lifelong process of assuming the norms and values for the many family roles that are required of family members. These roles include those of child, teenager, parent, grandparent, employed person, bride or groom, and retired person. The family is the major setting and parents are the primary agents of socialization (Hanson, 2001). The family is responsible for transforming the infant into a social being who can assume adult social roles. In today's world, this function is shared with many institutions outside the family, such as school, day care centers, churches, and health and human service agencies. However, the family continues to play a crucial role in the transmission of the family cultural heritage and the indoctrination regarding controls and values related to what is right and wrong.

Studies have delineated some important implications of these socialization functions with regard to the health of families. Bisagni and Eckenrode (1995) found that a strong work identity helped divorced women adjust to their changed marital status.

Davis (2000) found that women from Vietnam living in the United States consider the family to be a stabilizing influence. They stress the importance of having family involved in health care and are concerned that their ethnic roots and culture will be forgotten as their children and grandchildren grow up in the United States. See the Research Focus.

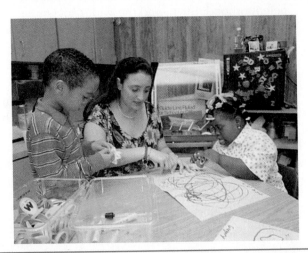

Day care often shares the responsibility with the parent of transforming a child into a social being.

Reproductive Function

The continuity of both the family and society continues to be ensured through the **reproductive function,** although this function is carried out very differently today than in previous generations. Whereas people of earlier generations considered it their responsibility to marry, have many children, and not raise children outside of marriage, today there are many single-parent families (Anderson, 1999) and couples without children. Many parents and children have come together through adoption, artificial insemination, or other technological means that may or may not include a second parent. Procreation will continue to be a family function; but it is increasingly being seen as irresponsible to bear more than two children, particularly in developing countries, and many couples are choosing to have no children.

Economic Function

Achievement of economic survival, known as the **economic function,** although important to any family, has changed in the way it is accomplished (Hanson, 2001). At one time, the family was its own economic unit, in which all members worked together to meet their basic needs. Children were an economic resource because

Convergence of Health and Family in Vietnamese Culture

Study Problem/Purpose

Examines family structure and intersections of health and family structure in the Vietnamese culture.

Methods

A phenomenological approach was used in which Vietnamese women discussed how family is perceived. Network sampling yielded 15 participants, women identifying themselves as living in the Vietnamese ethnic group and willing to converse in English. The study lasted 18 months and included visits to neighborhood resources used by the women. Often, visits took place in women's homes and lasted 2–3 hours. Emerging themes were followed up in one to three telephone conversations or interviews. These interviews "focused on health and illness experiences and were initiated through general questions about childhood events" (p. 139). The women were encouraged to describe life stories and memories.

Findings

Definition of family: Many family members were often present during interviews. Family was described as paramount and a stabilizing influence in an uncertain world. Family members are more apt to share and help each other than in other cultures. Family life is guided "by strong traditions that determine the hierarchy of structure and of responsibility" (p. 141).

Connectedness: "The Vietnamese view children and child rearing as great blessings, involving all family members" (p. 142). Privacy is rare. In Vietnam, houses are small and always open. Visiting with other families is frequent throughout the day. Family members' connectedness is important during illness or hospitalization.

All for the family good: There is an expectation of contributing to the family's well-being. Family members "are taught to place the requirements of other members ahead of their own" (p. 144). Regarding health, "one should take care of oneself to best attend to the rest of the family" (p. 145).

Wisdom of elders: The greater the age, the greater the care and respect that was given. If parents lived in the same geographic area, visiting was frequent. "The wisdom of elders, including parents, uncles, and grandparents, reportedly guides issues about life, marriage, and discipline" (p. 146). Marriage is the only consideration for moving away from home. "Otherwise, it is deemed selfish. In Vietnam, when a woman marries, she leaves the family village and goes to the home of her husband. She then becomes responsible not only for her husband and their future children but also for a new family" (p. 146). Parents sacrifice for their young children, and in return grown children are expected to see to the parents' needs. Remembrance of deceased elders is culminated in memory day, the day the family member died. It is considered more important than birthdays. Discipline of children is harsh and often physical. It is not considered abusive.

Continuity of values: Families have concern about the exposure of their children and grandchildren to what they see as a very unstructured American society. They fear that their ethnic roots and culture will be forgotten.

Implications

"The importance of family for the Vietnamese client should be given deference in any health care setting. . . . Separation of family members can create an enormous degree of stress and anxiety" (p. 153). Incorporate family members into the health care situation whenever possible. Decisions about health care may not be easily made without input from family members.

"Greater research into Vietnamese family life in the United States, particularly on how the family and health intersect, is needed . . . also more information regarding the effect of American culture on traditional Vietnamese family structure and functions is critical. . . . Research that examines the connection between ethnic identity and family structure over time would be invaluable to the further development of family therapy" (pp. 153–154).

Source: Davis, R. E. (2000). The convergence of health and family in the Vietnamese culture. Journal of Family Nursing, 6, 136–156.

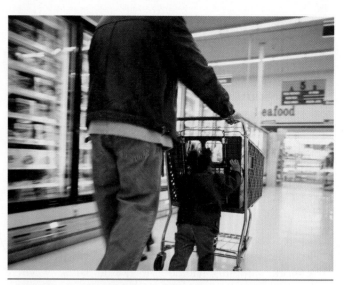

Family roles must be flexible when parents work outside the home. Photo courtesy of PhotoDisc.

they could work the land and care for aging family members. In contemporary times, families, at least in developed countries, do not need each other in the same ways. There are many community resources from which they can seek help to meet their financial obligations until they are able to fulfill that responsibility themselves (e.g., Medicaid, Medicare, and Aid to Families with Dependent Children). Women no longer must depend on marriage for economic security. Children do not contribute economically as they did in the past. Two-earner families are becoming more common. In the past, such couples might have considered the possibility of both working but usually agreed that they would have children and one parent would stay home with the children. Now, such couples are more likely to question whether to have children rather than whether to work (Strober, 1988). Studies (Moorehouse, 1993) suggest that this change is a positive one when family roles become more flexible and there is cooperation among family members

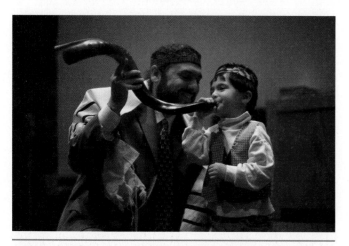

The family often is the vehicle by which cultural heritage is passed down to future generations. Photo courtesy of PhotoDisc.

to complete family tasks. In many families, however, the woman who works outside the home has most of the domestic work waiting for her when she comes home (Arrighi & Maume, 2000).

Health Care Function

The **health care function** involves both the provision of physical necessities to keep the family healthy, such as food, clothing, shelter, and protection against danger, and health care and health practices that influence the family health status. Conceptualization of health and illness varies widely among cultures, regions, and families (see Chapter 8). Healthy families manage their own health care in collaboration with health professionals. "Energized" families are assertive in seeking and verifying information, making appropriate decisions, and negotiating assertively with the health care system. The nurse can assist families in this respect by reinforcing their right and responsibility to be actively involved in their own health care. Other factors important in determining the family's health are nutrition communication, recreation, sleep and rest patterns, problem solving, sexuality, of time and space, coping with stress, hygiene and safety, spirituality, illness, care, health promotion and protection, and emotional health of family members and the family's health environment, which includes exposure to smoke, herbicides and pesticides, asbestos, noise pollution, and other potential hazards (Hanson, 2001).

Healthy families participate in preventive measures to protect their health and prevent illness. They observe good dental health practices; have periodic screening procedures such as mammograms, Pap smears, breast and testicular examinations, and vision and hearing examinations; and keep their immunizations up to date.

FAMILY PROCESS

Hanson (2001) describes **family process** as "the ongoing interaction between family members through which they accomplish their instrumental and expressive tasks" (p. 87). She points out that, although families may have the same structure and may function in similar ways, they interact very differently in terms of roles, communication, power, decision making, marital satisfaction, and coping strategies. For purposes of this chapter, discussion will focus on roles, values, communication, power, and coping strategies.

Family Roles

Family roles can be described as the "patterns engaged in by family members to perform family functions" (Becvar & Becvar, 2000, p. 328). Walsh (1993) notes that role allocation and role accountability are two important aspects of role functioning. **Role allocation** is "concerned with the family's pattern in assigning roles" (p. 148), and **role accountability** "looks at the procedures in the family for making sure that functions are fulfilled" (p. 148). In a healthy family, allocation is reasonable, and accountability is clear. For instance, a seven-year-old son is expected to clean his room every week to earn his allowance. An inappropriate allocation would be if this child were expected to care for a three-year-old sibling.

Other important concepts are role enactment, role stress, role strain, and role conflict. **Role enactment** concerns that which a person actually does in a particular role position. **Formal roles** consist of activities commonly assigned to a specific role (e.g., mother as nurturer). An **achieved role** includes activities not ordi-

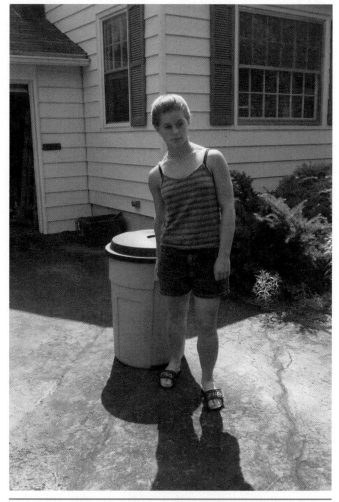

Role allocation must be clearly delineated and reasonable, with accountability clear.

narily assigned (e.g., daughter taking on the role of a deceased mother) (Janosik & Green, 1992). **Role stress** occurs when the family creates difficult, conflicting, or impossible demands for a family member. **Role strain** is generated from the stress and reflected in feelings of frustration and tension. **Role conflict** occurs when one is confronted with incompatible expectations (Friedman, 1998). As an illustration of these concepts, consider the following. Julie works fulltime, has a four-year-old child, and is taking classes to become a teacher (role enactment as mother and student). Her husband, Jim, is a fireman who is at work for several days at a time. When Jim is away, Julie has difficulty taking her daughter to preschool and getting to work on time (role stress). Because she is sometimes late to work, she is unable to leave to get to class (role conflict). She is feeling discouraged about passing her course (role strain).

In a healthy family, there must be mutual agreement about a role or modification of a role (**role complementarity**). The family must be open to shifts in role behavior to keep the family equilibrium (**role flexibility**).

REFLECTIVE THINKING

Personal Health Beliefs

Consider your own health beliefs.

- From where did they come? What influence did your family have on their development?
- With several classmates, preferably representing different cultural backgrounds, share your health beliefs and practices. How does your understanding of healthy behavior compare with theirs?
- Which of your health beliefs differ from those of a family with whom you have worked or are working? Discuss this experience with your classmates.

If one member of the family is ill or away, other members must be willing to carry out the functions usually performed by that member. For instance, when the mother is sick, the father or a friend must take the children to school, and older children must be enlisted to do some of the household chores usually carried out by the mother.

Family Position

In families, individuals have a formal place (e.g., mother or father) that is associated with related roles. Examples of attached roles include, traditionally, father as breadwinner and mother as homemaker or, more currently, both parents as breadwinners and homemakers. Each family develops its own roles that meet the family's needs. Single-parent families require that the parent play the parts of both mother and father. Gay and lesbian families often work out individualistic positions within the family that do not fit traditional categories. Blended families have one blood parent and one stepparent. Some of the conflict that occurs in these families results from lack of clarity about family positions. "You're not my mother [or father]!" is a frequent comment in blended and gay and lesbian families.

Formal and Informal Roles

There are standard formal roles in every family. These are roles explicitly given to family members as needed to keep the family functioning. They include breadwinner, child-rearer, homemaker, cook, and financial manager. **Informal roles** are covert and are used to meet the emotional needs of the individual and to maintain the family equilibrium (Friedman, 1998). Informal roles can be adaptive or detrimental to the well-being of the family, depending on the unconscious purpose of their use. Examples of these roles are *harmonizer* (mediates the

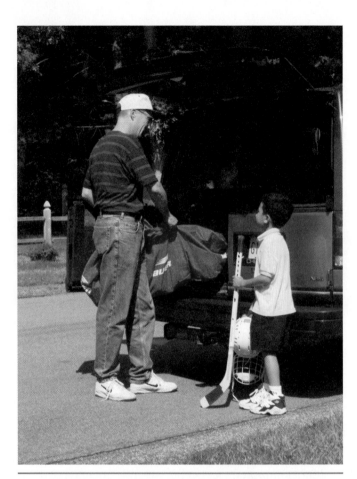

Coordination of children's extracurricular activities may be considered a formal role in some families.

differences that exist between other members by jesting or smoothing over disagreements), *blocker* (tends toward the negative regarding all ideas), *dominator* (tries to assert authority or superiority by manipulating the family or certain members), *martyr* (wants nothing for self but sacrifices everything for the sake of other family members), *caretaker* (member who is called on to nurture and care for other members in need), *coordinator* (organizes and plans family activities), and *go-between* (family "switchboard" [often the mother], who transmits and monitors communication throughout the family) (Friedman, 1998).

Role expectations can be quite different depending on the culture of the family. Garbarino (1993) notes the wide variability of the role of fatherhood in different cultures. Whereas some cultures bind fathers to children, others hardly acknowledge the necessity of fathers with regard to childrearing, leaving that role to mother.

Values

Family values are "a family's system of ideas, attitudes, and beliefs about the worth or priority of entities, or ideas that bind together the members of a family in a common culture" (Hanson, 2001, p. 420). Values, along with atti-

---

✳ DECISION MAKING

Family Roles

Mrs. Strong has told you that her husband is very strict with their children. He is angry that their five-year-old son likes to play with his sister's dolls and has told him not to do so any more. She would like to discuss the situation with her husband, but because he makes all the family decisions, she does not think she should bring it up.

◆ How would you describe the family roles? Role flexibility? Role strain?

◆ How would you explore the situation with Mrs. Strong?

◆ Should an attempt be made to help Mrs. Strong become more assertive in her marital relationship?

REFLECTIVE THINKING

Family Values

- Identify some values that a family might have that would conflict with your own values about families.
- As a nurse, how would you work with a family whose members held such values?

---

tudes and beliefs, are fundamental to all that people do. Values influence family members' understanding of the world, their place in the world, and the ways to reach their goals and aspirations (Friedman, 1998). As families grow and change over time, so, too, do their values. Family values are an amalgam of society's values and the family's own subculture and are passed on by the family of origin down through the generations. Problems arise when there is a conflict between either society and subculture values or subculture values and the realities of the family's life. For instance, in a family in which the homemaker role is valued but, because of economic necessity, the wife must work outside the home, the husband may feel less of a man because he cannot, by himself, provide for the family. His wife may in turn resent the disruption to her preferred way of life.

Communication

Family communication "describes the exchange of information in the instrumental and affective dimensions of family life" (Becvar & Becvar, 2000, p. 328). Every family provides a context for learning to communicate. Our communication skills include both the general cultural language (e.g., English in the United States) and continuously created shared meanings (e.g., nicknames for family members, funny words for familiar things, particular ways to express feelings or conflict). Each family has learned these things differently. For example, whereas one family may consider it natural to hug people upon initial meeting, another may find such behavior to be personally invasive and may instead prefer to shake hands.

Communication is symbolic, and family members must have a shared understanding of which behaviors represent love, anger, fun, and the like. If communication is vague or distorted or left unresolved, disagreement and confusion will result (Walsh, 1998). See Chapter 10 for more information regarding the communication process.

Family Communication Rules

All families have rules that help the family organize itself. **Rules** are the specific implicit or explicit regulations re-

garding what is acceptable or unacceptable and to which the family is expected to adhere. Some rules are about communication. For instance, a common rule has to do with management of anger. The rule in one family might be that anger is to be avoided at all costs and that it is considered a breach of family loyalty to express anger to a family member. In another family, anger might be an acceptable and respected emotion to be expressed as openly as possible in order to deal with the issue that precipitated the anger. These are opposing rules by which to live, and problems could develop if members from these two families tried to resolve a conflict. To achieve conflict resolution in such a circumstance, the individuals must understand the rules that they have brought with them from their families of origin.

Communication rules sometimes carry anxiety and shame (Carson & Arnold, 1996). Most families have taboo topics that either cannot be discussed at all or can be discussed only under special circumstances. Sexual or financial topics often fall in one of these categories. Severely problematic behaviors such as incest or alcoholism are also frequently taboo topics. Some topics can be discussed only at certain times, in certain places, or in certain ways. "Don't bother your father while he's reading the paper" is a statement that illustrates this rule.

Sometimes, certain members of the family are not allowed to know family information. Statements illustrative of this rule include "You can talk to me about the fact that you're gay, but don't tell your father" and "We don't want Jenny to know that she's adopted until she's older."

Family Communication Networks

Family networks are the patterns of communication that families develop in order to deal with the needs of family living, particularly needs of regulating time and space, sharing resources, and organizing activities. They are a vital part of the decision-making process and are related to the power dynamics of the family (Galvin & Brommel, 1986). Networks take many configurations,

---

REFLECTIVE THINKING

Your Communication Networks

- What type of communication network do you see in your own family?
- Compare your family network of communication with the networks of several of your classmates. How are they similar or different?
- What implications do your discoveries have for nursing care of families?

but, in reality, most communication takes place in subsystems (e.g., parent, child, siblings, and spouses) (Friedman, 1998). It is therefore important to recognize family coalitions. Nurses must identify the family communication network in order to pinpoint the key communicators in the family. If these members are ignored, interventions are unlikely to be effective.

Power in Families

Family power is a dynamic and multidimensional process (Hanson, 2001). **Power** is the reflection of unwritten family rules and values and is crucial in establishing and maintaining family communication channels and networks. Power structures vary greatly from family to family and may be functional or dysfunctional; however, they all involve a relationship whereby one member exerts greater control in the relationship than do other members (Friedman, 1998). In a well-functioning family,

there is a clear hierarchy of power, whereby the parents take leadership in an egalitarian coalition. Children's contributions influence decisions and become more nearly equal as the children grow toward adulthood (Beavers & Hampson, 1993).

Decision making and authority are important components of power. **Decision making** is the process of "gaining the assent and commitment of family members to carry out a course of action or to maintain the status quo" (Friedman, 1998, p. 267). Authority, or **legitimate power,** refers to the shared agreement among family members to designate a person to be the leader and to make the decisions. Legitimate power is held only when other family members willingly confer authority on a member. **Nonlegitimate power** may be characterized as "domination" or exploitation, which suggests power against another's will.

Friedman (1998) identifies three areas of assessment regarding power. These are **power bases** (sources from which family members' power is derived), **power outcomes** (who makes the final decisions or ultimately possesses the control), and **power,** or decision-making, **processes** (processes used in arriving at family decisions). Figure 25-1 summarizes power bases, and Figure 25-2 summarizes decision-making processes.

Some situational changes affect the power structure of a family. For instance, when the family breadwinner becomes ill and can no longer work, another family member or community agencies must take on that responsibility. The power associated with providing financial security is taken away from the sick family member.

Feminist theorists look at power issues in heterosexual families in terms of male domination, seeing this behavior as a reflection of male domination in the larger society. They believe domination to be neither natural nor inevitable but recognize its prevalence in society (Walsh, 1998).

Power configurations change over time as a result of family developmental changes. As children grow, they

---

FIGURE 25-1   Family Power Bases

Legitimate power or authority. Shared belief and perception of family members that one person has the right to control another member's behavior.

Helpless or powerless power. Power of the powerless; based on the generally accepted right of those in need or of the helpless to expect assistance from those in a position to render it.

Referent power. Power persons have over others because family members positively identify with them.

Resource and expert power. Power related to having the greater number of valued resources in a relationship.

Reward power. Expectation that the influencing, dominant person will do something positive in response to another person's compliance.

Coercive or dominance power. Based on belief that the person with power will punish (through threats, coercion, or violence) other individuals if they do not comply.

Informational power. An individual is convinced of the "rightness" of the sender's message because of a careful and successful explanation of the necessity for change; similar but more limited than referent power.

Affective power. Power derived through the manipulation of a family member by bestowing or withdrawing affection and warmth.

Tension management power. Control that one person achieves by managing the present tensions and conflicts in the family.

From *Family Nursing* (4th ed., p. 269) by M. M. Friedman, 1998, Norwalk, CT: Appleton & Lange. Reprinted with permission of Pearsen Education, Inc.

FIGURE 25-2   Power, or Decision-Making, Processes

Decision making by consensus. Course of action mutually agreed on by all involved. Equal commitment to the decision and satisfaction among all family members.

Decision making by accommodation. One or more of the family members make concessions, either willingly or unwillingly. Some members assent in order to allow a decision to be reached.

De facto decision making. Things are allowed "to just happen" without planning.

From *Family Nursing* (4th ed., pp. 272–273), by M. M. Friedman, 1998, Norwalk, CT: Appleton & Lange. Reprinted with permission of Pearsen Education, Inc.

can manage and demand more power. Adolescents, who by definition are attempting to develop individual identity, tend to challenge the family power status quo by rebelling against the family system. Such changes in children affect parents, who must adjust their patterns of power interactions with their children. Families have varying abilities to make such adjustments (Petro, 1999). Power struggles develop when an issue becomes important to one or more family members. If exploration of alternatives does not work, various power maneuvers result, and family intimacy is affected. Variables affecting family power structures include all components of family structure, function, and process (e.g., power hierarchy, communication network, family coalitions, developmental stages, cultural and religious backgrounds).

FAMILY STRESS AND COPING

Although all families face stressful situations, families vary in how well they cope with stressors. All families "fight to remain stable and resistant to systematic changes in the family's instituted patterns of behavior" (McCubbin & McCubbin, 1989, p. 38). Family adjustment is usually minor, but some events necessitate drastic changes.

One of the most studied life events requiring substantial family change is the birth of a child. Shapiro, Gottman, and Carrere (2000) found a 67% decline in marital satisfaction following their transition to parenthood. The couple did not report the decline until one to two years after the birth. The decline was steeper if the "husband expressed negativity toward the wife, the husband expressed disappointment in the marriage, or both the husband and the wife felt their lives were chaotic" (p. 65).

Family Resiliency Model

McCubbin and McCubbin (1989, 1993) and McCubbin (1993) have explicated the **resiliency model of family stress, adjustment, and adaptation.** This model emphasizes family adaptation and enumerates family types and levels of vulnerability. The model is depicted in Figure 25-3.

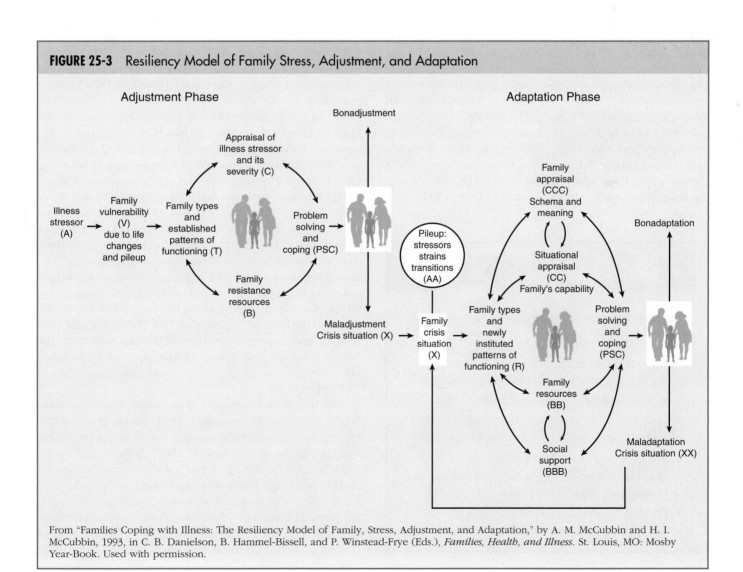

FIGURE 25-3 Resiliency Model of Family Stress, Adjustment, and Adaptation

From "Families Coping with Illness: The Resiliency Model of Family, Stress, Adjustment, and Adaptation," by A. M. McCubbin and H. I. McCubbin, 1993, in C. B. Danielson, B. Hammel-Bissell, and P. Winstead-Frye (Eds.), *Families, Health, and Illness*. St. Louis, MO: Mosby Year-Book. Used with permission.

In this model, there are two phases of family response to life events and changes. In the first phase, the adjustment phase, the stressor (A) (in Figure 25-3 it is illness, but it could be any stressor) interacts with the family's vulnerability (V). The stressor can be at any level of severity, and the level of family vulnerability will depend on the pileup of family stresses and changes that are occurring at the time the new stress emerges. The family vulnerability interacts with the family's typology (T), which is manifested by the family's established patterns of functioning. These components interact, in turn, with (B) the family resistance resources: that is, their capabilities and strengths; (C), the family's appraisal of the stressor; and (PSC), the problem-solving and coping strategies used by the family. For instance, a family in which the mother becomes ill and unable to work or to care for the children (stressor) will be more vulnerable (V) if she is the sole adult in the family than if there are other family members who can carry out those family functions. The family will manage better in either case if their established pattern of functioning (T) is to seek support outside the family when necessary. Their ability to communicate with one another openly about family needs (B) will affect how well they can deal with the changes in the family activities. All of the above affects their appraisal of the family stressor (C). Is it a catastrophic change with which the family cannot cope, or is it a manageable situation that requires some feasible shifts in family responsibilities? If the shifts needed to accommodate the mother's illness are relatively simple, the family will adjust and move on. Most often, more complex changes must occur. For instance, a severe or chronic illness creates a crisis or a maladjustment situation (X) that initiates the adaptation phase (McCubbin & McCubbin, 1993).

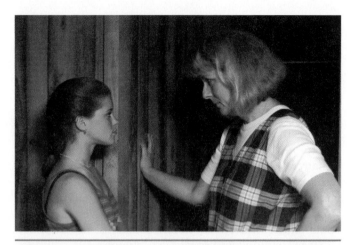

Making small adjustments in family power configurations is necessary to provide opportunities for children to develop their own identities.

In the adaptation phase, the stressors (AA) from the illness and other family difficulties interact with (R), the family's level of resiliency. That is, their established patterns of functioning combined with the new patterns they may have established in response to the new stressor (the mother's illness). (R) interacts with (BB), the family resources, which are supported by the degree of support from outside the family (BBB) and the family's appraisals. A situational appraisal (CC) is determined by how the family perceives the relationship between the family's resources and the demands of the situation. For instance, if the mother's illness lasts long and she has no health or disability insurance, the family may believe that their financial resources are not adequate to support the family because they are not willing to turn to others for help, or they may see that this situation is not overwhelming because they realize that they can seek agency assistance or help from family members to get them through this difficult time. This situational appraisal (CC) interacts with the family's schema appraisal (CCC), which consists of their values, goals, priorities, and rules. These interactions create the meaning the family gives to the illness and the changes it has produced. The family problem-solving and coping repertoire (PSC) interacts with the family resource and appraisal components to facilitate family response to the crisis situation (McCubbin & McCubbin, 1993).

In health care settings, the model serves to assist health providers in assessing what "family types, capabilities, and strengths are needed, called on, or created to manage illness in the family" (McCubbin & McCubbin, 1993, p. 22) The model allows for a systematic diagnosis and evaluation of the family functioning under stress and for the development of intervention strategies. Interacting personalities, individuals, and family unit characteristics influence each other to shape the family's course of changing itself. The result may be successful adaptation

REFLECTIVE THINKING

Family Power Dynamics

- How would you assess the power dynamics in your own family?
- Do you use the same or different strategies in your nonfamily relationships?
- Compare your perceptions of family power with those of some of your classmates. How are they similar or different?
- Do you believe that your family is male dominated? Why or why not?
- Do you believe the families of your friends are male dominated?

FIGURE 25-4 Keys to Family Resilience

Family belief systems

- Making meaning of adversity
- Positive outlook
- Transcendence and spirituality

Organizational patterns

- Flexibility
- Connectedness
- Social and economic resources

Communication processes

- Clarity
- Open emotional expression
- Collaborative problem solving

From *Strengthening Family Resilience*, p. 24, by F. Walsh, 1998, New York: Guilford.

(**bonadaptation**), whereby the family is able to stabilize itself in a growth-producing way, or unsuccessful adaptation (**maladaptation**), whereby the result is a more chaotic state, family growth and development are sacrificed, and the "family's overall sense of well-being, trust, and sense of order and coherence becomes very low" (McCubbin & McCubbin, 1993, p. 25). Walsh (1998) has identified keys to family resilience. These are listed in Figure 25-4.

Although the nurse's first intervention response is likely to be a focus on problem solving to deal with the immediate crisis, all the interactive factors in the family must be considered if the family is to make the needed changes in its system and if the nurse is to facilitate family adaptation to its changed circumstances. Specific ways to intervene in crisis are discussed in Chapter 29.

VULNERABLE FAMILIES

Vulnerable families are those whose physical and emotional resources are so insufficient that critical tasks and family functions are threatened. All families lose their equilibrium from time to time, often because of illness or disability. Sometimes, crisis can be overwhelming for even the healthiest family. Healthy families, however, take appropriate actions to solve their problems. Vulnerable families have few resources to help them maintain balance in the family so that even appropriate actions are usually not enough. Vulnerable families' attempts to offset their difficulties tend to be inappropriate or distorted and do not serve to solve their problems (Janosik, 1994). For instance, a healthy family having a parent diagnosed

with Alzheimer's disease would reach out to community resources and friends. The family would be assertive in seeking out needed support. A marginal family would marshal all family members to take care of the diagnosed member. Although the family members do a good job of caretaking, they hesitate to use community resources or, in many cases, are unaware of those resources available to them and tend to burn out before trying other things. Disorganized families may tend to blame others for their problems, and some members may drink heavily to avoid dealing with their difficulties. These are the families in which addiction, violence, low stress tolerance, and impulsivity further strain meager resources (Janosik, 1994). As a result, they live from crisis to crisis, never really learning from their experiences. They use community services only when their crises reach such magnitude that they have to seek outside help.

Friedman (1998) has delineated adaptive strategies of vulnerable families. She notes that such families (1) deny problems and exploit one or more family members in physical and or nonphysical ways, using scapegoating, threats, child abuse and neglect, abuse of parents, or spousal violence; (2) deny family problems and use adaptive mechanisms such as family myths, threats, emotional distancing, triangling, and pseudomutuality that impair the family's ability to meet their adaptive function; (3) separate or lose family members (via abandonment, institutionalization, divorce, physical absence of family members, substance abuse); and (4) exhibit submission to marked domination.

Family myths are longstanding family beliefs that shape family members' interactions with one another and with the outside world (Carson & Arnold, 1996). The beliefs are unchallenged by family members, who distort their perceptions, if necessary, to keep the myth secure. Myths are established early in the life cycle to defend against the unpleasant realities of life. The more myths the family has, the less effectively family members can perform family tasks and functions because they judge family situations in terms of the myth rather than reality. Statements reflecting common myths include "We're a happy family," "We like to do things together," and "Gina needs to be protected because she is the weak child in the family." The function of family myths is to cement the cohesiveness of the family. However, myths cause the family to respond to life events in a stereotypical manner. In times of crisis, alternative approaches to problem solving are not used, and family growth is stifled.

Triangling is bringing a third person into a difficult dyadic relationship to absorb and reduce the tension (Carter & McGoldrick, 1999a). Although triangling occurs in all families to some extent, it is not helpful if of long duration. Conflicts are not addressed, and long-term emotional needs of family members are harmed. An example of this dynamic would be two parents focusing on a child's misbehavior rather than addressing their own conflicts. In this situation, the effects of triangling would likely surface when the child leaves home and the parents are forced to deal with one another. Divorce may occur if the parents continue to be unable to resolve their problems with each other. Of particular concern to the community health nurse is the potential for being drawn into the family as the third member of a triangle. One member of the family may seek out the nurse to tell her or him of the problems in the family or of a particular conflict with a family member. The nurse may be asked to keep the information a secret or to be the problem solver. Although the nurse may be tempted to do as asked in order to maintain a positive relationship with the client, such an approach is not effective and undermines the family's ability to manage its own problems. The nurse must make it clear to clients that they must deal with family members directly. In some instances, it may be necessary for the nurse to act as mediator, but never as a member of the triangle (see Figure 25-5).

Scapegoating occurs when hostility and frustration exist in a family, usually the marital dyad, and a third person, usually a child, becomes the target of blame for the problem (Townsend, 2000; Varcarolis, 1998). One member of the family is "chosen" to be negatively labeled and stigmatized while the rest of the family achieves unity and cohesiveness. "The identified patient" is an example of a scapegoat; all the pathology is placed on one member, and that member is identified as the cause of all the family's problems. Scapegoating hides actual family problems such as marital conflict. Children are the most common choices to be scapegoats because they are less significant to family survival than are parents. The scapegoat internalizes the role and behaves as expected. As a reward, he or she gets much attention, albeit negative attention, and is exempt from all responsibility except playing the role. If the scapegoat leaves the family or refuses to play the role, the family will choose another scapegoat to maintain family balance.

Pseudomutuality is a long-term dysfunctional adaptive strategy that maintains family homeostasis at the expense of meeting the family's affective function. Families totally focus on the whole. Although the family presents a face of solidarity and cohesiveness, individual identity is viewed by the family as a threat to the family. These families lack humor and spontaneity, and their roles are rigidly assigned and maintained. Problems are denied, and the family believes in the desirability and appropriateness of this role structure (Becvar & Becvar, 2000). A member who does not wish to participate is seen as a threat to the family solidarity and is coerced into staying involved.

Heiney (1999) has outlined characteristics useful in assessing vulnerable families with regard to their functional and dysfunctional dimensions (see Table 25-1). Families who are homeless are one sample of vulnerable families. A program that has been developed to decrease their vulnerability is the Aftercare Project in San Francisco. See "Out of the Box" for details of their program.

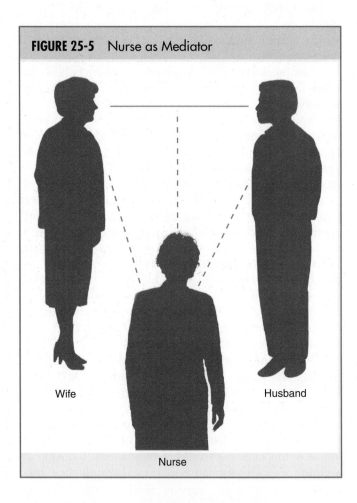

FIGURE 25-5 Nurse as Mediator

Wife

Husband

Nurse

✴ DECISION MAKING

Family Dynamic

You are meeting with Ms. Bates and Ms. White. They are a lesbian couple who coparent their son, Trent. Ms. White is the biological mother. When Ms. White steps out to the restroom, Ms. Bates takes the moment to plead with you to urge Ms. White to be less controlling and let Ms. Bates spend more time with Trent.

◆ What is the dynamic at work in this situation?

◆ How do you respond to Ms. Bates?

◆ How do you respond to the request when Ms. White returns?

TABLE 25-1 Assessment Summary for Functional versus Dysfunctional Family Characteristics

FUNCTIONAL	DYSFUNCTIONAL
Emotional system	**Emotional system**
Independence encouraged	Dependence encouraged
Positive self-esteem prompted	One person "identified" as problem
Positive conflict resolution	Negative conflict resolution
Adapts to change	Repetitive, rigid use of ineffective coping
Differentiation	**Lack of differentiation**
Relationships foster emotional maturity	Emotional immaturity encouraged
Thoughts separated from feelings	Thoughts and feelings enmeshed
Sense of separateness among family members	Sense of fusion
Differences of opinion allowed and encouraged	Differences of opinion unacceptable
Problem solving used to generate solutions to concerns	Family members do not think through alternatives to problems
Absence of triangling	**Triangling**
Patterns of interaction among family members are flexible and adaptive to the situation	Patterns of interaction among family members are fixed and rigid

From "Assessing and Intervening with Dysfunctional Families," by S. P. Heiney, 1999, In G. D. Wagner and R. J. Alexander (Eds.), Readings in Family Nursing (p. 397), Philadelphia: J. B. Lippincott. Copyright 1999 by J. B. Lippincott. Used with permission.

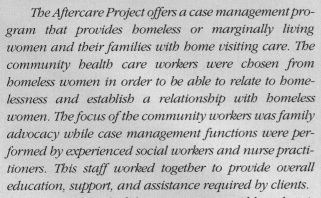

Out
of the Box

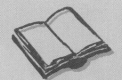

The Aftercare Project offers a case management program that provides homeless or marginally living women and their families with home visiting care. The community health care workers were chosen from homeless women in order to be able to relate to homelessness and establish a relationship with homeless women. The focus of the community workers was family advocacy while case management functions were performed by experienced social workers and nurse practitioners. This staff worked together to provide overall education, support, and assistance required by clients.

"A major goal of the project was to address barriers to care and to expand outreach for childbearing families that were or had been homeless" (p. 23). The program's purpose was also to ensure healthy babies and family cohesion. To these ends, in addition to home visits, a weekly support group was offered in which the clients could discuss their problems and receive emergency services as necessary. Referrals were offered to clients. Most were for housing and shelter, food, furniture, clothing, prenatal care, mental health of substance abuse, domestic violence counseling, state benefits, parenting classes, pediatric health care, and legal assistance for immigration issues.

Although a weekly schedule of home visits was planned, this plan was altered because of the difficulty in contacting the women and the part-time status of the community workers. In the new plan, the client families were "contacted biweekly through a combination of home visits, office visits, and phone conversations" (p. 24).

Eighty-eight percent of families enrolled in the Aftercare Project received prenatal care in their first trimester and 92% of newborns weighed over 3000 g and were free of substances. A majority of the participants obtained permanent housing. The use of the community health care workers was very successful.

When project funding ended, the Perinatal Services Project was developed. This program was developed to achieve healthy birth outcomes through work with the entire family, as in the original project. However, it is extended to encourage the development of children from birth to age five.

Source: Murrell, N. L., Scherzer, T., Ryan, M., Frappier, N., Abrams, A., & Roberts, C. (2000). The Aftercare Project: An intervention for homeless childbearing families. Community Health, 23(3), 17–27. ■

MODELS OF FAMILY FUNCTIONING

Through years of research, models have been developed that depict the range of family functioning. Two are discussed here because of their pertinence to community health nursing. They are the circumplex model of marital and family systems and the McMaster model of family functioning (MMFF).

Circumplex Model of Marital and Family Systems

The **circumplex model of marital and family systems** identifies three critical variables that influence family adaptation (McCubbin, 1989; Olson, 1993). It is useful for the nurse to understand this model because it pro-

vides a conceptual frame of reference for assessing the family. Unfortunately, like most studies, it has focused on two-parent, middle-class, Caucasian families (Moriarty, 1990; Crosbie-Burnett & Helmbrecht, 1993). However, the dynamics presented have relevance for all family structures.

The circumplex model (see Figure 25-6) provides a map of 16 types of marriages and family system attributes that, throughout the life cycle, characterize patterns of family life that mediate or buffer stressors and demands (McCubbin, 1989). It illustrates four types of balanced relationships and four types of unbalanced relationships.

The three critical variables that influence family adaptation are the dimensions of cohesion, flexibility, and communication. **Family cohesion** is the emotional

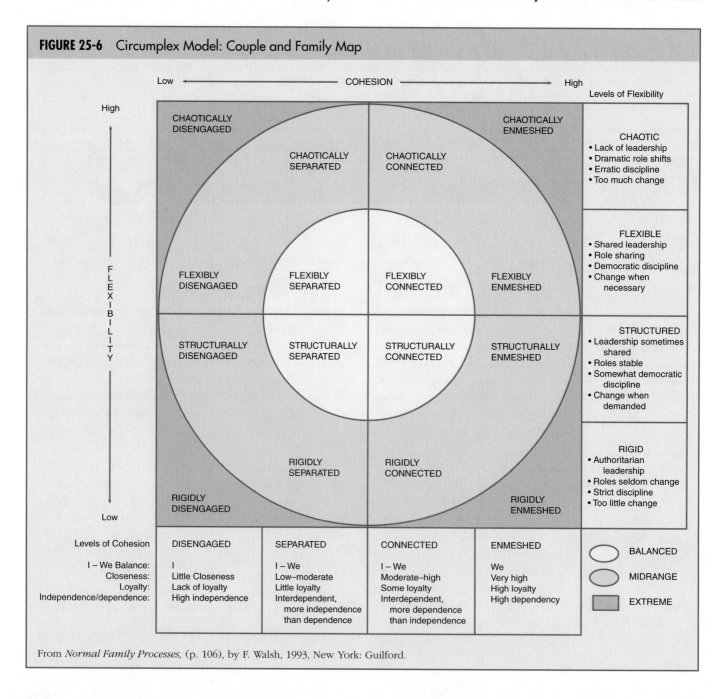

FIGURE 25-6 Circumplex Model: Couple and Family Map

From *Normal Family Processes*, (p. 106), by F. Walsh, 1993, New York: Guilford.

bonding among family members (Olson, 1993). Cohesion can be measured in terms of emotional bonding, boundaries, coalitions, time, space, friends, decision making, interests, and recreation. There are four levels of cohesion, ranging from disengaged to enmeshed. Optimal family function is in the middle. Optimally functioning families are able to experience and balance a degree of separateness and connectedness. That is, members need and want time apart, but times together are also important.

The second dimension of the circumplex model, **family flexibility,** refers to the amount of change in the family's leadership, role relationships, and relationship rules (Olson, 1993). Functional families have the ability to change when necessary, whereas unbalanced (dysfunctional) families tend to be either rigid or chaotic.

Family communication is considered a facilitating dimension. As one would expect, balanced systems tend to have good communication, whereas extreme systems do not.

Olson (1993) identifies two ways that families change. **First-order change** is change in the degree of family functioning but not in the family system. An example would be allowing an adolescent to stay out later at night and to use the family car, thus increasing his or her autonomy and independence but not significantly changing the family system.

Second-order change occurs in times of stress or crisis and is change in established family patterns. Change is greater in the balanced system, which is more flexible and able to make appropriate changes. For instance, when a breadwinner dies, another family member must take on this role. If no one is willing or able to do so, the very survival of the family is threatened.

Zacks, Green, and Marrow (1988) note that lesbian couples report higher satisfaction on the variables of cohesion, flexibility, and communication than do heterosexual couples. They suggest that this outcome may be the case because, as women, lesbians have superior relational skills and more egalitarian relationships. In addition, because there are no legal sanctions against ending dysfunctional relationships, these couples are more likely to separate and it may be more likely that it is the well-functioning relationships that endure.

Riper (2000) notes that the family variables described by McCubbin (1989) and Olsen (1993) may play a "critical role in determining how siblings or children with Down syndrome respond" (p. 279). Three components of the model were significantly associated with sibling self-being. These were family demands (family vulnerability due to life changes and milieu), family resources, and family problem-solving and coping.

Nursing interventions based on using the circumplex model would focus on moving rigid or chaotic families closer to the center of the model. That is, in rigid families, the nurse would promote interaction flexibility through improved communication and negotiated decision making. The nurse must be careful not to push for change too fast, because doing so could increase the

✳ DECISION MAKING

Example of the Circumplex Model

The Martin family leads a very busy life. Both parents work, and all three children go to school and are active in a variety of school activities. On some days, the Martins see one another only in the morning, when they are preparing for the day's activities. Meals are often eaten on the run. Mrs. Martin, who is attending school part time, tells you she is feeling overwhelmed and wishes that the family would help her more with the household tasks.

◆ Where would you place this family in the circumplex model?

◆ How would you advise Mrs. Martin regarding her concerns about managing the household?

family's resistance to a nursing action perceived as threatening. Members of a **chaotic family** will need help in developing structure, order, and predictability in their interactions. These families tend to be crisis prone: Members rebound from one crisis to another. Emphasis would be on helping the adults to accept their leadership roles in the family and to become consistent and democratic with regard to demands and discipline.

A **disengaged family** is distanced or totally cut off from family relationships. Intervention would be directed toward the separated level of the cohesion dimension of family functioning, facilitating much separateness but some connectedness and some joint decision making among family members.

Enmeshed families sacrifice individual needs for the group. Little personal separateness or privacy is allowed. Boundaries are blurred, sometimes to the extent of fusion, so that the individual has little sense of self. Attention is focused inside the family, and there are few outside friendships or interests. Intervention would be directed toward the connected level of the cohesion dimension of family functioning, facilitating a balance between emotional closeness and respect for separateness and encouraging outside friendships. The enmeshed family may try to involve the nurse in family activities and may have difficulty understanding why the nurse cannot meet with the family as often as the family would like.

McMaster Model of Family Functioning

The **McMaster model of family functioning (MMFF),** named for the university where work on the model took place, is based on a systems approach. It describes a set of positive characteristics of a healthy family, focusing on "the dimensions of functioning that are seen as having the most impact on the emotional and physical health or problems of family members" (Epstein, Bishop, Ryan, Miller, & Keitner, 1993, p. 139). Each characteristic can range in quality from "most ineffective" to "most effective." The model acknowledges that judgments of health and normality are relative to the culture of the family and that family values must be taken into account in the assessment of each dimension. Focus is on the following six dimensions:

- *Problem solving:* A family's ability to resolve problems to a level that maintains effective family functioning (Epstein et al., 1993). Problems are either instrumental (mechanical in nature, such as provision of money, food, housing, and the like) or affective (emotional in nature, such as anger or depression). Families with instrumental problems rarely deal effectively with affective problems. Those with affective problems, however, may deal adequately with instrumental problems. A sequence of seven steps describes effective problem solving: (1) identifying the problem and communicating with appropriate people about the problem, (2) creative brainstorming, (3) developing a set of possible alternative solutions, (4) deciding on one of the alternatives, (5) initiating and carrying out the action required by the alternative, (6) monitoring to ensure that the action is carried out, and (7) evaluating the effectiveness of the problem-solving process (see Figure 25-7). These steps become less systematic and fewer are accomplished as functioning becomes less effective (Walsh, 1998).

- *Communication:* Exchange of information within a family (Epstein et al., 1993). As does problem solving, communication has instrumental and affective areas. Two other aspects that are assessed are the clarity of communication (whether messages are clearly stated or camouflaged, muddied, or vague) and the directness or indirectness of communication (whether messages go to the appropriate targets or tend to be deflected to others).

- *Role function:* Repetitive patterns of behavior by which family members fulfill family functions (Epstein et al., 1993). Five family functions similar to those described earlier are identified as the basis for necessary family roles: (1) provision of resources, (2) nurturance and support, (3) adult sexual gratification, (4) personal development, and (5) maintenance and management of the family system. The fifth function includes decision making, boundaries and family membership, behavioral control, household finance functions, and health-related functions. Two additional

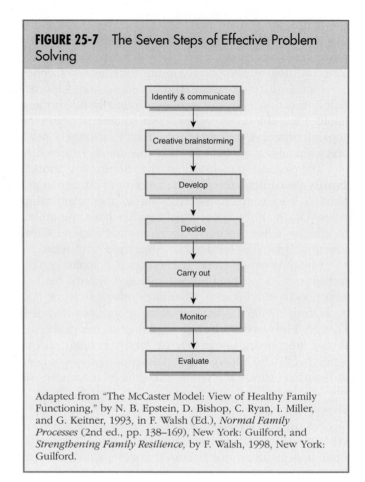

FIGURE 25-7 The Seven Steps of Effective Problem Solving

Identify & communicate

Creative brainstorming

Develop

Decide

Carry out

Monitor

Evaluate

Adapted from "The McCaster Model: View of Healthy Family Functioning," by N. B. Epstein, D. Bishop, C. Ryan, I. Miller, and G. Keitner, 1993, in F. Walsh (Ed.), *Normal Family Processes* (2nd ed., pp. 138–169), New York: Guilford, and *Strengthening Family Resilience,* by F. Walsh, 1998, New York: Guilford.

aspects of role functioning, role allocation and role accountability, were previously described.

- *Affective responsiveness:* "The ability to respond to a given stimulus with the appropriate quality and quantity of feelings" (Epstein et al., 1993, p. 149). There are two dimensions to responsiveness: responding with a full spectrum of feelings and experiencing feelings consistent with the stimulus or situational context. Also to be considered is the degree of affective response along a continuum from absence of response through reasonable or expected response to overresponse. Although overall patterns of family response are considered, this dimension focuses on the behaviors of individual members more than the other dimensions do. Two categories of affect are identified: welfare emotions (affection, warmth, tenderness, support, love, consolation, happiness, and joy) and emergency emotions (anger, fear, sadness, disappointment, and depression). A healthy family can express the full range of emotions and experiences those emotions appropriately, with responses being of reasonable intensity and duration.

- *Affective involvement:* "The extent to which the family shows interest in and values the particular

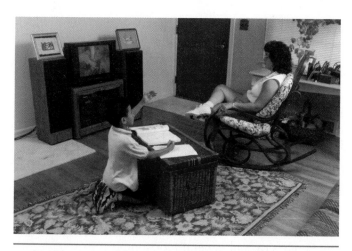

Lack of interested involvement may result in less effective family functioning.

activities and interests of individual family members" (Epstein et al., 1993, p. 150). The focus is on the amount of interest as well as the manner whereby interest is shown and the quality of investment in one another. Styles can range from a total lack of involvement to extreme involvement. Six types of involvement are identified, with empathic involvement being considered optimal for health. Moving away from empathic involvement in either direction results in less effective family functioning in this area. The six types of involvement are:

1. Lack of involvement: no interest or investment in one another.

2. Involvement devoid of feelings: some interest and/or investment in one another, although interest is primarily intellectual in nature.

3. Narcissistic involvement: interest in others only to the degree that their behavior reflects on the self.

4. Empathic involvement: interest and/or investment in one another for the sake of the others.

5. Overinvolvement: excessive interest and/or investment in one another.

6. Symbiotic involvement: extreme and pathological interest and/or investment in others; seen only in very disturbed relationships characterized by marked difficulty in differentiating one person from another.

- *Behavior control:* "The pattern a family adopts for handling behavior in three areas: physically dangerous situations, situations that involve the meeting and expressing of psychobiological needs and drives, and situations involving interpersonal socializing behavior both between family members and with people outside the family" (Epstein et al., 1993, p. 152). The focus is on standards or rules

the family sets and the freedom allowed around the standard. Four styles of behavior control are identified: (1) rigid—narrow and specific standards and minimal negotiation or variation; (2) flexible—reasonable standards with opportunity for

---

✳ DECISION MAKING

Example of the McMaster Model of Family Functioning

The Ming family is an Asian American family consisting of Peter and Martha, parents of Jennifer (13 years old) and Ben (9 years old). Peter's widowed mother, Amelia, lives with the family. Peter works long hours during the week but is home on the weekends. There is some conflict between Martha and Amelia because Amelia tends to favor Ben and ignore Jennifer. Martha has discussed her concerns with Peter, and he understands but is not willing to talk with his mother about the issue. Other than that, the family identifies no ongoing family problems. The usual conflicts of daily living come and go, but the family works them out. Because Peter is essentially unavailable during the week, family members have an agreement that they will spend every Saturday together in some family activity. They realize that this pattern will change as Ben and Jennifer grow older and want to spend more time with their friends. Although family members express love for one another, their expressions tend to be reserved. There is little hugging or kissing in front of others, although Martha does express affection to her children. The children know that they are loved.

- How would you assess the problem-solving abilities of the family?

- How would you describe the level of instrumental and affective communication in the family?

- How do the Mings manage their family functions and family roles?

- How would you describe the affective responsiveness and involvement in the Ming family?

- How would you describe the standards and rules of the family?

- What is your overall assessment of the general functioning of the Ming family?

- What additional information do you need to more fully assess this family in the six dimensions of family functioning?

negotiation and change (considered the most effective style); (3) laissez-faire—no standards held and total latitude allowed regardless of context; and (4) chaotic—unpredictable and random shifting between other styles such that family members do not know which standards to apply or how much negotiation is possible (considered the least effective style).

Stevenson-Hinde and Akister (1996) note a seventh dimension, *general functioning,* which is an independent encapsulation of the other six dimensions. In a formalized way, these dimensions can be assessed through the use of two psychometric tools, the Family Assessment Device (FAD), which is a self-report measure that can be completed by families and scored on each of the MMFF dimensions, and the Clinical Rating Scale (CRS), which can be rated by observers during a semistructured family interview. Although these measurements are more suited for research purposes, the dimensions themselves provide useful guidelines for nurses when doing family assessments. Figure 25-8 lists suggested questions to raise with family members in order to assess the family on the basic six dimensions of family functions. These questions only propose general themes to explore. Each nurse must find wording that feels comfortable. Questions would be raised as appropriate and in no specific order. Each family is different. Specific questions will depend on the focus and needs of the assessment. Family responses can provide data that enable the nurse to assess the family's overall general functioning.

FIGURE 25-8 McMaster Model Family Assessment Questions

Problem Solving

- What do you think are your most important family problems?

- Do you discuss these problems with anyone? If you do, with whom do you discuss them?

- How do you resolve problems?

- Can you give me an example of one family problem and how you resolved it?

Communication

- How would you describe the ways you communicate with one another? Could you give me an example?

Nursing note: Observation of family interaction is important. Observe how members communicate. Do they communicate clearly or masked, directly or indirectly? Do they communicate the same way or differently with different family members?

Role Function

- How would you describe your ability to provide for your family in terms of food, clothing, money, and shelter? (Although you may observe the family situation with regard to these factors, it is important to also learn the family's perspective.)

- How do you experience and provide nurturance and support within the family?

To adults in the family:

- Do you have any sexual concerns? How satisfied are you with your sex life? What are your plans for educating your children about sexuality?

- What concerns do you have about raising your children? (Consider their responses in terms of physical, emotional, educational, and social development.)

- How are you managing regarding your job, career, recreational activities, and social activities?

- What concerns do you have regarding the discipline of your children? How do you discipline your children?

- Who makes the decisions in the family? Who takes care of the family finances? Who makes health-related decisions?

- Describe your relationships with people outside of the family. How are these relationships decided on among family members?

Nursing note: Through the answers of family members and your own observations, you can identify the family's pattern of assigning roles, their procedures for ensuring that functions are fulfilled, and whether they are in fact fulfilling the necessary family functions.

Affective Responsiveness

- How would you describe your family regarding its ability to express and receive feelings such as affection, warmth, anger, and sadness?

Nursing note: Observe the degree to which their verbal statements reflect their actual behaviors.

Affective Involvement

- How do family members show interest in and value activities and interests of other family members?

Nursing note: Observe the degree to which their verbal statements reflect their actual behaviors.

Behavior Control

- What kinds of standards and rules does your family have about socializing with others, managing potentially dangerous situations (such as children's speaking to strangers), and expressing feelings and needs.

Nursing note: Observe the degree to which their verbal statements reflect their actual behaviors.

Perspectives...

There is so much to learn and much joy to be found in sharing the knowledge acquired in nursing school. Although I recall several experiences that provided me the opportunity to share this knowledge, one in particular stands out. During my community health rotation, I was assigned to a teenager in her eighth month of pregnancy with her first child. With my heart's desire focusing on this particular population, I was delighted to take on this case. My eagerness to learn everything possible about teenage pregnancy encouraged me to search for and study all materials and information on pregnancy and adolescence that I could locate.

When it came time to make my first home visit, I felt extremely nervous because I had no idea what to expect. My mind became preoccupied with various questions such as did I know enough material about teenage pregnancy to teach about it, was I prepared to answer pertinent questions, and would my teaching style be compatible with her learning style? Despite these questions and self-doubt, my enthusiasm and determination continued. I approached this first visit with the goal of establishing a caring, trusting, and helping relationship. I realized that obtaining a complete and thorough family assessment would be essential to providing quality care and would also enable me to view the world through the eyes of my client.

As we exchanged relevant information, we identified many of her questions, concerns, and desires encompassing family and maternal health issues as well as issues surrounding the growth and development of her baby. Her primary concern focused on nutrition and the growth of her baby. I agreed that nutrition is an important aspect of prenatal education geared toward maintaining the health of the adolescent and her baby. The girl's diet must be sufficient to provide the nutritional needs of her own changing body as well as the additional nutritional needs of her growing baby. Nutrition education is a significant factor in contributing to the prevention of complications associated with teen pregnancy, such as iron deficiency anemia and low birthweight infants. Nurses working with this population play an instrumental role in providing such prenatal education.

Another significant concern she disclosed included all of the emotions she was experiencing during her pregnancy. Although some of her feelings were normal and associated with physical and hormonal changes during pregnancy, most of them were brought on by external factors such as family difficulties. Upon listening to her express her profound emotions, the effects these feelings were having in her relationships with her mate, parents, relatives, and friends became apparent. During this visit, we discussed sources of stress, feelings associated with stress *and* with pregnancy, and several techniques she could implement to reduce stress. After our discussion, it was apparent that my client and I had developed trusting, open lines of communication, with her sharing her complicated family dynamics and fluctuating feelings toward her pregnancy. I felt honored that my client would confide in me regarding this part of her life and that I could have a positive influence on her pregnancy and the health of her baby. What a reward!

As the visit progressed, I presented her a list of topics related to health maintenance and pregnancy—topics that I had planned to cover during our home visits. However, I soon realized that not all of these topics were compatible with her unique needs. To meet these needs and motivate learning, I thus had her choose from the list those topics about which *she* desired more education. Once I gained a better understanding of her learning desires, I constructed an outline of the topics she had chosen. I prioritized the contents of this teaching plan in order of importance and to correspond with her stage of pregnancy. During our first visit, we discussed fetal development during the eighth month, feelings associated with pregnancy, stress reduction techniques, and maternal-fetal nutrition. In the weeks that followed, I provided her an abundance of information, from exercises for childbirth preparation to ninth-month fetal development. During our last visit, which was approximately a week and a half before her due date, we discussed the labor-and-delivery process, newborn information (feeding and safety issues), and normal growth and development after birth. From this experience, I quickly learned the importance of flexibility, understanding the client's needs, and client involvement in planning of care.

This first experience provided me with increased confidence in my communication skills and personal abilities. I conquered my anxieties by allowing my self-determination and devotion to this particular population to empower me. With this motivation, I was able to fulfill my goal to build a trusting relationship with my client and to provide her the best quality of care by first assessing her learning needs and then effectively meeting those needs. I believe that maintaining confidence in oneself is an essential component of goal attainment. To all students who explore community health nursing, you *do* possess the knowledge and capabilities to overcome any new and unfamiliar challenges and to attain your goals. Best of luck!

—Alisa A. Muir, Sonoma State University,
BSN Nursing Student

COMMUNITY NURSING VIEW

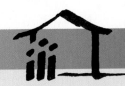

When making a second visit to the Perez family (Chapter 24), you notice some bruises on Manuel's (the son's) back. The mother, Maria, is not sure how the bruises got there but says that Manuel was complaining of a stomachache the night before and that Alice (the maternal grandmother) thought he might have some food stuck in his stomach. Maria further states that Alice may have pinched Manuel's back to loosen the food. Maria seems distracted and unconcerned about the bruises.

Maria's main concerns today are the family's finances and Jamie's (her husband's) depression. She says that Jamie's disability payments do not provide enough money to make it through the week. Neither she nor Jamie wants to borrow money from their parents, although Alice does contribute to the household expenses. Maria realizes that she needs to return to work as soon as Rosarie, her newborn, is settled at home and Alice is comfortable caring for her. Maria looks forward to working, but the idea seems to contribute to Jamie's depression, although he will not talk about it. Maria asks you to tell Jamie that it would be a good idea for her to go back to work because they need the money.

When you talk with Jamie, he has little to say except that he wants to get back to work. He knows that Maria is thinking about going back to work, but he wants her to stay home and care for the children. He does not believe that Alice can do the job as well as Maria. He also wants to be more involved with Manuel. He believes that the boy needs more male influence, particularly living in a family that is primarily female.

Nursing Considerations

Assessment

◆ What elements of a healthy family can you identify?

◆ How well is the Perez family carrying out the five major functions of the family?

◆ What impact does the Perez family's level of functioning have on the family's ability to effectively manage the lives of the family's members?

◆ What information do you have about the internal, external, and contextual family structure of the Perez family? What additional information

do you need? How will you elicit this information from the family? Which family members do you need to talk with?

◆ What are some of the role issues in the Perez family? What are some power issues? How do they affect the family?

◆ What family values can you identify? How do they affect the family's health and health care practices?

◆ What are some of the communication patterns in the Perez family? Which are functional? Dysfunctional?

◆ What additional information do you need to evaluate the meaning of the bruises on Manuel's back?

◆ How would you assess the family in terms of the family resiliency model? The circumplex model? The McMaster model?

◆ Do you think your assessment of the priorities for the Perez family are the same as those of the family? Why or why not?

Diagnosis

◆ Identify at least three nursing diagnoses that you consider to be a priority for this family.

Outcome Identification

◆ What outcomes can you expect for this family?

Planning/Interventions

◆ What might you do to resolve differences?

◆ Over time, what other issues would you want to work on with the Perez family?

◆ What aspects of family dynamics would be important to consider when implementing a plan of care so as to avoid undermining the care provided?

◆ What specific interventions would you want to implement for each of the nursing diagnoses?

Evaluation

◆ How will you know if your interventions have been successful?

These models provide information about important dimensions of family dynamics. The community health nurse can use this information to evaluate family needs and determine both problems and strengths in families. With the data obtained, nursing diagnoses can be made and appropriate plans and interventions developed with the family.

KEY CONCEPTS

◆ The healthy family has certain identifiable characteristics that reflect its multidimensional nature. It is important to keep in mind that each family is unique and addresses these dimensions in its own way.

◆ Five major family functions are important in the nurse's work with families: the affective, socialization, economic, reproductive, and health care functions.

◆ Family process comprises several interacting dimensions that facilitate the development of family life. The major structural components are role, communication, values, power, decision making, and coping. Each of these is multifaceted.

◆ The resiliency model of family stress, adjustment, and adaptation emphasizes family adaptation and enumerates family types and levels of vulnerability. This model helps nurses deal with families in crisis.

◆ Vulnerable families are those who have lost their equilibrium. They are vulnerable to life stresses to a greater or lesser extent depending on whether they usually function at a healthy, marginal, or dysfunctional level.

◆ A typology of dysfunctional family strategies can be delineated. Four behaviors of particular interest are family myths, scapegoating, triangling, and pseudomutuality.

◆ The circumplex model of marital and family systems characterizes patterns of family life that mediate or buffer stressors and demands. The three critical dimensions of this model are cohesion, flexibility, and communication.

◆ The McMaster model of family functioning provides a view of healthy family functioning. It centers around six dimensions of family functioning: (1) problem solving, (2) communication, (3) roles, (4) affective responsiveness, (5) affective involvement, and (6) behavior control.

RESOURCES

American Association of Marriage and Family Therapy:
   http://www.aamft.org
Families and children:
   http://www.nih.gov
   http://www.acf.dhhs.gov

Unit

VI

CARING FOR VULNERABLE POPULATIONS

U*nit VI provides insight into a variety of vulnerable populations with whom the community health nurse works including those populations suffering from communicable disease, chronic disease, developmental disabilities, mental illness, family violence, and substance abuse.*

IN THIS UNIT

Chapter
26

COMMUNICABLE DISEASES

Rebekah Jo Damazo, RN, MSN

MAKING THE CONNECTION

Chapter 14 Epidemiology

Figure 22-6 Recommended Childhood Immunization Schedule

The History of Medicine:
- *2000 B.C.—Here, eat this root.*
- *1000 A.D.—That root is heathen, Here, say this prayer.*
- *1850 A.D.—That prayer is superstition. Here, drink this potion.*
- *1920 A.D.—That potion is snake oil. Here, swallow this pill.*
- *1945 A.D.—That pill is ineffective. Here, take this penicillin.*
- *1955 A.D.—Oops . . . bugs mutated. Here, take this tetracycline.*
- *1960–1990—39 more "oops" . . . Here, take this more powerful antibiotic.*
- *2000 A.D.—The bugs have won! Here, eat this root.*

—Anonymous

COMPETENCIES

Upon completion of this chapter, the reader should be able to:

- Recount the history of communicable diseases and identify efforts throughout history to control these diseases.
- Recognize the importance of a global perspective on communicable disease control.
- Identify modes of transmission for communicable diseases.
- Explain the difference between acquired, natural, and active immunity.
- Describe vaccine-preventable diseases and the role immunization plays in keeping diseases under control.
- Recognize the causative agents and signs and symptoms of common sexually transmitted diseases.
- Describe appropriate nursing interventions for controlling human immunodeficiency virus (HIV) infection.
- Delineate the three levels of prevention as they pertain to sexually transmitted diseases.
- Understand the reasons for the emergence of new viruses and drug-resistant bacteria that are reversing human victories over infectious disease.
- Summarize barriers to the control of communicable diseases.
- Explain the community health nurse's role relevant to communicable disease control.

KEY TERMS

acquired immunity	epidemic
active immunity	eradication
agents	fecal/oral transmission
airborne transmission	horizontal transmission
carrier	host
Centers for Disease Control and Prevention (CDC)	immunity
	indirect transmission
communicable disease	mode of transmission
contacts	mutation
direct transmission	natural immunity
emerging diseases	nosocomial infection
endemic	pathogenicity
environment	reservoir

surveillance	virulence
vector	zoonosis
vertical transmission	

The discussion of **communicable disease,** illness in a susceptible host and caused by a potentially harmful organism or its toxic products, has moved from the public health journal to the evening news and from the microscope to the big screen as new killer strains of both viruses and bacteria appear to be winning the war aimed at disease eradication. **Eradication** is the extermination of an infectious agent and, thus, the irreversible termination of that agent's ability to transmit infection (Chin, 2000). Only a few years ago, after eradicating smallpox from the planet, epidemiologists promised to move forward on eradicating other fatal communicable diseases. This battle rages on as scientists attempt to gain the high ground in the fight with microorganisms.

This chapter presents the background for nurses' involvement in the control and surveillance of communicable disease. One of the earliest functions of the community health nurse was caring for individuals with communicable diseases. The focus later changed to the prevention of diseases through early treatment, reporting, and immunization. This chapter also presents an overview of emerging infections as well as infectious **agents** (organisms that transfer disease from the environment to the host) that have been known to people for centuries. Also included is a review of the natural history of communicable disease and a discussion of prevention measures effective in controlling disease transmission. Finally, the chapter summarizes disease transmission, immunity, disease reporting, and the characteristics of select communicable diseases. The beginning community health nurse will be able to utilize the specific principles presented as they pertain to communicable diseases in general and to those diseases reviewed in particular.

HISTORICAL PERSPECTIVES ON COMMUNICABLE DISEASE AND COMMUNITY HEALTH NURSING

Community health nursing and communicable diseases share a long history. As discussed in Chapter 2, tracking case contacts, monitoring infectious disease, and recording disease statistics have been a part of the nurse's responsibilities from the earliest years of professional nursing. Case **contacts** are persons who have been exposed to an infectious agent or environment and who thus have the potential for developing an infectious disease. For years, nurses have been dedicated to improving the health of individuals, families, and communities. The control of the spread of disease plays a large role in this task.

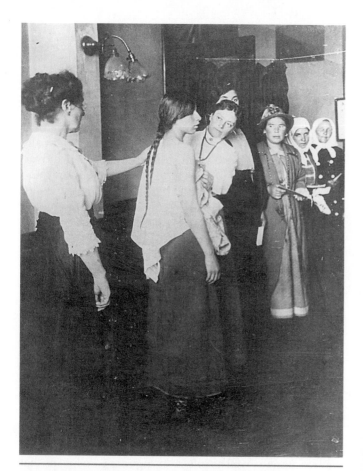

Immigrants were required to pass a physical examination while at Ellis Island to interrupt the spread of infection between countries. Photo courtesy of the Ellis Island Immigration Museum, U.S. Department of the Interior.

With the growth of urban areas in the early part of the 19th century, epidemics swept through communities. An **epidemic** exists when the number of cases of an infectious agent or disease is clearly in excess of that which is normally expected. Hospitals were unsanitary hotbeds of infection and often were considered places where people went to die. The terrible conditions in the nation's hospitals, the growing fear of epidemics, and the improved understanding of disease origins brought about health care reform efforts in the late 1800s. Just as the cities in the United States began to gain a grasp on infection, a new wave of immigrants poured into the country from Europe.

Because of the number of immigrants settling in East Coast cities, overcrowding and sanitation became an issue. Despite public health efforts to control the emergence of new diseases and epidemics, communicable diseases were once again on the rise. Community health nurses were fearless in their pursuit of disease. They carried the black satchel containing necessary equipment wherever there was reported illness. Responsible for keeping everything from measles to diphtheria in check, community health nurses exposed themselves to virulent

infections in an effort to assist the sick and prevent further spread of disease.

In 1900, epidemics of communicable disease ravaged U.S. communities and were the leading cause of death in the United States and throughout the world. Although today infectious diseases have taken a backseat to heart disease, cancer, and stroke in the United States, they remain the leading cause of death worldwide. An army of new and reemerging diseases is today threatening the health of the world's citizens (WHO, 1997b).

Community health nurses are taking action to become knowledgeable about the types of diseases that threaten the health of communities in order to play a role in the diagnosis, treatment, control, and prevention of infectious disease.

CHANGING WORLD OF INFECTIOUS DISEASE

Within the past decade, human beings have been forced to focus on their vulnerability on the planet. As people, we must recognize that we are not unlike all other living things when it comes to basic survival instincts and de-

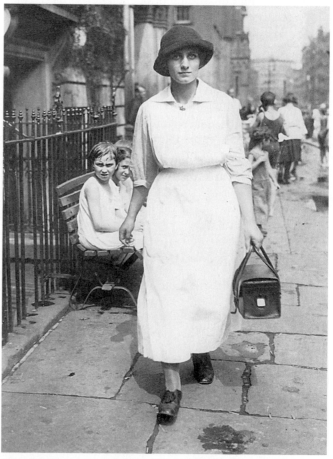

The visiting nurse service served as a first line of defense in the fight against communicable disease of the era. Photo courtesy of the Visiting Nurse Service of New York.

sires, including fundamental needs such as shelter, food, and safety as well as the desire to perpetuate our species. Microorganisms that cause disease in humans neither seek special revenge against nor hold any malice toward humans; they are merely engaged in a struggle for survival and species perpetuation. Many of these organisms have simply found the human body to be a convenient halfway house well suited for their biological life cycles (Hanlon & Pickett, 1979). In the past 20 years, at least 30 new disease-causing organisms have been identified, including the human immunodeficiency (HIV), hepatitis C, and ebola viruses and the bacterium that causes Lyme disease. Microbial predators are everywhere, and there exists a constant struggle for individual survival.

Today's hospitals are considered a breeding ground for infection. **Nosocomial infections,** infections that develop in a health care setting and that were not present in the client at the time of admission, are feared among clients and health care professionals alike. Super strains of extremely virulent bacteria and viruses make a hospital stay potentially lethal. Hospitalized individuals are more than normally susceptible to infection, are exposed to more infectious agents from both hospital staff and other clients, are given more broad-spectrum antibiotics and immunosuppressive drugs, and are subjected to more invasive procedures and surgeries that make them vulnerable to disease. Nosocomial infections cause substantial morbidity and mortality, prolong the hospital stay of affected patients, and increase direct patient care costs (Girou et al., 2000). Since 1970, the National Nosocomial Infections Surveillance System (NNIS) has collected and analyzed data on the frequency of nosocomial infections in U.S. hospitals.

Striking episodes of deadly infectious disease emergence have become commonplace. One need only pick up the latest news magazine or turn on the television to hear reports of "flesh-eating" bacteria, multidrug-resistant tuberculosis, hantavirus, and food or waterborne illnesses such as the infamous "fast-food bacteria," *Escherichia coli* O157:H7. These microorganisms will take every opportunity possible to develop a biological association with the human host and are spreading with astounding vigor. Communicable disease organisms require a continuous commitment to their control. It has become evident that **mutation,** organism adaptation that results in a modification in the makeup of subsequent generations of the organism, and change are "facts of nature" and that the human species will continue to be challenged by mutant microbes with unpredictable manifestations. The **Centers for Disease Control and Prevention (CDC)**—the governmental agency with the mission of promoting health and quality of life by preventing and controlling disease, injury, and disability— has stated that emerging infections lead the list of urgent threats to the world's population (CDC, 1998a). Figure 26-1 shows the global microbial threats in the 1990s.

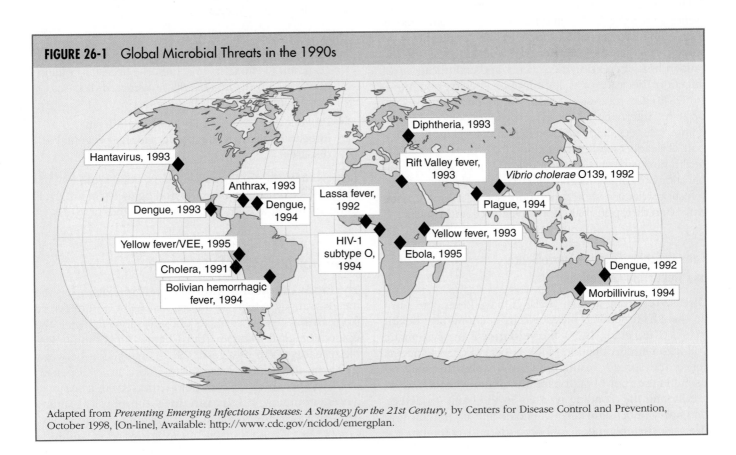

FIGURE 26-1 Global Microbial Threats in the 1990s

Adapted from *Preventing Emerging Infectious Diseases: A Strategy for the 21st Century,* by Centers for Disease Control and Prevention, October 1998, [On-line], Available: http://www.cdc.gov/ncidod/emergplan.

United States citizens take a measure of assurance in existing public health programs that have led to high immunization rates, early detection methods, and readily available pharmacological agents useful in the control of infectious disease. It should be recognized, however, that because of relatively inexpensive, rapid travel opportunities, disease can disseminate quickly around the globe. New patterns of human movement, growing populations and urbanization, climate changes, and changing sexual mores have set in motion a perfect situation for the development of emerging infectious disease. The Institute of Medicine has defined **emerging diseases** as "diseases of infectious origin whose incidence in humans has increased within the past two decades or threatens to increase in the near future" (CDC, 1998a, p. 1). It is imperative that public health agencies maintain the infrastructure necessary for early detection and treatment of emerging infectious disease.

GLOBAL PERSPECTIVES FOR COMMUNICABLE DISEASE CONTROL

Communicable diseases are a growing threat to communities worldwide. Microbes do not stop at border crossings or immigration checkpoints. Old infections such as tuberculosis (TB), diphtheria, and cholera have resurfaced with increased virulence and drug resistance. Deadly new infections such as acquired immunodeficiency syndrome (AIDS) and hantavirus have emerged as frightening counterparts to more primitive infections. In some cases, diseases such as AIDS and TB coexist in the human host, increasing the severity and complications of infection. Because of today's mobile society, communicable diseases cannot be sealed within one country, city, or state. International travel of businesspersons, immigrants, refugees, and vacationers has assisted in the transport of deadly diseases throughout the world. Community health nurses must take a worldview as they study the implications of communicable diseases in local communities. Infectious disease should be addressed as a global issue with shared responsibility for surveillance and control.

Communicable Disease Surveillance and Reporting Guidelines

Disease reporting and surveillance have been core public health functions practiced by community health nurses (Kuss et al., 1997). **Surveillance** is the systematic collection and evaluation of all aspects of disease occurrence and spread, resulting in information that may be useful in the control of disease. Community health nurses are among the frontline workers in the battle to detect, diagnose, and, ultimately, eliminate the communicable diseases that plague neighborhoods and communities. Community health nurses play an important role in disease surveillance by investigating sources of disease outbreaks, collecting data, reporting cases, and providing information to the public about disease morbidity and mortality within the local community.

In 1878, Congress authorized the U.S. Marine Service (forerunner of the Public Health Service) to collect morbidity reports regarding cholera, smallpox, plague, and yellow fever from U.S. consuls overseas. This information was to be used to institute quarantine measures developed to prevent the spread of disease from other countries to the United States. The law was later expanded to prevent the spread of disease among the states. Thus began the evolution of communicable disease reporting in the United States. Requirements for disease reporting in the United States are mandated by state laws and regulations. State health departments report nationally notifiable diseases to the CDC in Atlanta, Georgia. Seventy-four infectious diseases are designated as notifiable at the national level (CDC, 2002) (see Figure 26-2). Community health nurses are involved in the surveillance system at many different levels including disease outbreak investigation and reporting, immunization, contact tracing, and collection of vital statistics.

Healthy People 2010: Objectives for Communicable Diseases:

Healthy People 2010 summary goals in the area of communicable diseases include:

- Reduce foodborne illness.
- Promote responsible sexual behaviors, strengthen community capacity, and increase access to quality services to prevent sexually transmitted diseases (STDs) and their complications.
- Prevent disease, disability, and death from infectious diseases, including vaccine-preventable diseases.

Achievement of these objectives is dependent on the ability of health care providers and agencies at all levels to be aware of, access, and report objective progress.

MODES OF DISEASE TRANSMISSION

The **mode of transmission** of a particular disease is the mechanism by which an infectious agent is transferred from an infected host to an uninfected host. Recall the epidemiological triangle from Chapter 14. Communicable diseases occur as a result of the interaction between an agent, the causative organism, and a **host** (a person or living species capable of being infected) in a supportive environment. **Environment** is the physical setting that provides the context for agent-host interaction. Community health nurses must be aware of different modes of transmission to be able to understand the most

FIGURE 26-2 Nationally Notifiable Infectious Diseases: United States, 2002

Acquired Immunodeficiency Syndrome (AIDS)

Anthrax

Botulism

- Botulism, foodborne
- Botulism, infant
- Botulism, other (wound and unspecified)

Brucellosis

Chancroid

Chlamydia trachomatis, genital infections

Cholera

Coccidioidomycosis

Cryptosporidiosis

Cyclosporiasis

Diphtheria

Ehrlichiosis

- Ehrlichiosis, human granulocytic
- Ehrlichiosis, human monocytic
- Ehrlichiosis, human, other or unspecified agent

Encephalitis, Arboviral

- Encephalitis, California serogroup viral
- Encephalitis, Eastern equine
- Encephalitis, Powassan
- Encephalitis, St. Louis
- Encephalitis, Western equine
- Encephalitis, West Nile

Enterohemorrhagic *Escherichia coli*

- Enterohemorrhagic *Escherichia coli,* O157:H7
- Enterohemorrhagic *Escherichia coli,* shiga toxin positive, serogroup non-O157

Giardiasis

Gonorrhea

Haemophilus influenzae, invasive disease

Hansen disease (leprosy)

Hantavirus pulmonary syndrome

Hemolytic uremic syndrome, postdiarrheal

Hepatitis, viral, acute

- Hepatitis A, acute
- Hepatitis B, acute
- Hepatitis B virus, perinatal infection
- Hepatitis, C; non A, non B, acute

HIV infection

- HIV infection, adult (≥13 years)
- HIV infection, pediatric (<13 years)

Legionellosis

Listeriosis

Lyme disease

Malaria

Measles

Meningococcal disease

Mumps

Pertussis

Plague

Poliomyelitis, paralytic

Psittacosis

Q fever

Rabies

- Rabies, animal
- Rabies, human

Rocky Mountain spotted fever

Rubella

Rubella, congenital syndrome

Salmonellosis

Shigellosis

Streptococcal disease, invasive, Group A

Streptococcal toxic-shock syndrome

Streptococcus pneumoniae, drug resistant, invasive disease

Streptococcus pneumoniae, invasive in children <5 years

Syphilis

- Syphilis, primary
- Syphilis, secondary
- Syphilis, latent
- Syphilis, early latent
- Syphilis, late latent
- Syphilis, latent unknown duration
- Neurosyphilis
- Syphilis, late, non-neurological

Syphilis, congenital

- Syphilitic stillbirth

Tetanus

Toxic shock syndrome

Trichinosis

Tuberculosis

Tularemia

Typhoid fever

Varicella (deaths only)

Yellow fever

NOTE: Although not a nationally notifiable disease, CSTE recommends reporting of cases of Varicella (chickenpox) via the National Notifiable Diseases Surveillance System (NNDSS).

From Centers for Disease Control and Prevention, January 15, 2002 [On-line]. Available: http://www.cdc.gov/epo/dphsi/phs/infdis.htm.

efficient and effective methods to interrupt disease occurrence and to prevent transmission between hosts.

Disease transmission can take place either horizontally or vertically (Gordis, 1996). In **vertical transmission,** disease is transmitted between parent and child. In some cases when a parent has an infectious disease, the disease may be spread to offspring via sperm, placenta, breast milk, or contact with the vaginal canal at birth. Examples of organisms and diseases transmitted vertically include: HIV, herpes, and syphilis. **Horizontal transmission** is the transport of infectious agents from person to person. The transport of infectious agents between hosts can be accomplished in a number of ways: direct transmission, indirect transmission, airborne transmission, and fecal/oral transmission. Figure 26-3 illustrates the concepts of vertical and horizontal transmission.

Direct Transmission and Indirect Transmission

Direct transmission is the immediate transfer of disease from the infected host to the susceptible host. Transmission of sexually transmitted disease is a prime example of direct transmission. Direct projection of droplet infection into the conjunctiva or mucous membranes of the nose, mouth, or eye during sneezing or coughing is also considered direct transmission. Direct transmission can be implicated in the spread of numerous communicable diseases such as impetigo, scabies, and anthrax. Direct inoculation is the direct transfer of infection from a host via a vehicle that penetrates the susceptible host's natural barriers to disease, such as the skin. An example of direct inoculation would be a needle stick received by a health care worker caring for an infected person.

Indirect transmission occurs when the human host has contact with vehicles or vectors that support and transport the infectious agent. Lyme disease is a classic example of indirect transmission, where the organism is transported to the host via the deer tick. Fleas were the

vectors that transmitted bubonic plague from infected rats to the human host, another example of the indirect transmission of disease.

Airborne Transmission

Airborne transmission occurs when microorganisms are suspended in the air and spread to a suitable port of entry. This type of transmission occurs primarily through droplet nuclei or aerosols. Particle size influences how long the organism can remain airborne. The longer the particle is suspended, the greater the chance it will find an available port of entry to the human host. An example of an organism that relies on airborne transmission is measles. Contaminated droplets containing the measles virus are contained in the spray from sneezing. The droplet can find a portal of entry through the mucous membranes or conjunctiva. Droplets that do not remain airborne or settle out are excluded from this category (Chin, 2000).

Fecal/Oral Transmission

Fecal/oral transmission of an infectious agent occurs directly when the hands or other objects are contaminated with organisms from human or animal feces and then placed in the mouth. Fecal/oral transmission can also occur indirectly via the ingestion of water or food that has been contaminated with fecal particles, as when a restaurant worker fails to properly clean hands and under nails after defecation and before returning to work. Oral-genital sexual activity can also result in fecal/oral transmission of disease. Good handwashing and thorough washing and cooking of food help to decrease the potential spread of disease. Examples of diseases spread through this method of transmission are hemolytic uremic syndrome (caused by the bacterium *E. coli* O157:H7) and hepatitis A.

IMMUNITY

Immunity refers to the resistance of the host to disease. One of the ways communicable diseases are controlled is through efforts directed at strengthening the host. There are three ways that the host may develop immunity, or protection from infectious diseases:

- **Acquired immunity.** The transfer of antibodies from mother to child via the placenta or breastfeeding. If a mother has developed antibodies to particular agents, she can pass on short-term immunity to the newborn child. This ability to provide immunity to neonates, who typically are vulnerable to infectious disease, is an important reason for the community health nurse

---

FIGURE 26-3 Modes of Transmission

Vertical Transmission

Infection from parent to child via sperm, placenta, breast milk, or contact in the vaginal canal at birth

Horizontal Transmission

Person-to-person spread of infection through one or more of the following routes:

- Direct
- Indirect
- Airborne
- Fecal/oral

TABLE 26-1 Recommendations for Routine Immunization of HIV-Infected Children

VACCINE	HIV INFECTION	
	KNOWN ASYMPTOMATIC	SYMPTOMATIC
DTP	Yes	Yes
OPV	Contraindicated	Contraindicated
IPV	Yes	Yes
MMR	Yes	Yes*
Hib	Yes	Yes
Pneumococcal	Yes	Yes
Influenza	Yes	Yes
Hepatitis B	Yes	Yes

Should be considered.

From The Manual for the Surveillance of Vaccine-Preventable Diseases, *by Centers for Disease Control and Prevention, 1999, Atlanta, GA: Author.*

to educate women about the benefits of breastfeeding.

- **Natural immunity.** The development of antibodies that protect against subsequent infections as a result of the host's having acquired an infection. Diseases such as diphtheria, measles, and pertussis are good examples of diseases that produce lifelong immunity. Not all organisms, however, produce natural immunity in the host. Most sexually transmitted diseases do not provide natural immunity. Thus, without appropriate treatment, reinfection is common.

- **Active immunity.** Vaccination of the host. Properly administered immunizations provide the host with lifelong protection from disease. United States policy requires documentation of active immunity in children prior to school entrance. Recommendations for immunization of HIV-infected children are listed in Table 26-1. The recommended pediatric immunization schedule and the adolescent and adult immunization recommendations can be found in Figure 22-6.

VACCINE-PREVENTABLE DISEASES

History is full of colorful examples of individuals who were victims of infectious diseases that were rampant around the world until the mid-1950s. Franklin D. Roosevelt was infected with paralytic polio at the height of his political career, and it is reported that Wild Bill Hickock's only son was a victim of diphtheria. Few households escaped the wrath of the "hard" measles (rubeola), German measles (rubella), and mumps. Hospitals had entire wards dedicated to the care of whooping cough (pertussis) victims. It is easy to forget the devastation these diseases caused before the widespread development of vaccines that now prevent their occurrence. National immunization programs have been so successful that parents today no longer fear these diseases.

Authorities in virtually every nation of the world recommend routine immunization of children as the best way to prevent illness and death caused by certain infections. Some individuals have not taken advantage of the availability of vaccinations at relatively low cost throughout the United States. Missed opportunities for vaccination have also impeded progress in the national campaign to have every child immunized by age 2. Missed opportunities for immunization occur when a child in need of immunization seeks health care but does not receive needed immunizations.

Contraindications to Immunization

Community health nurses must be aware of the relatively few contraindications to immunization and must take advantage of every possible opportunity to provide immunizations to individuals seeking care. There are only two permanent contraindications to vaccination:

- Severe allergy to a vaccine component or following a prior dose of a vaccine
- Encephalopathy without a known cause and occurring within seven days of a dose of pertussis vaccine

Four vaccine contraindications that are generally temporary are:

- Pregnancy
- Immunosuppression
- Severe illness
- Recent receipt of blood products

Live vaccines should not be given until these conditions are resolved (CDC, 2000e). Mild common illnesses such as otitis media, upper respiratory infections, colds, and diarrhea are *not* contraindications to immunization. In communities with poor immunization rates, barriers to successful immunization should be assessed and, where possible, removed. Vaccination status should be assessed at all health visits in an effort to complete necessary immunizations. Health departments and clinics should be flexible in scheduling appointments and should not penalize individuals who do not have transportation or adequate financial resources. Community health nurses play a vital role in ensuring that all infants and children

Adults and Immunization

Many adults forget their vulnerability to disease and may fail to take necessary precautions to protect themselves from infection and, possibly, death and to interrupt the spread of disease.

- When was the last time you had a tetanus immunization?
- Have you been protected against hepatitis A and B?
- Should you have a flu shot?

are given the opportunity to be protected from unnecessary illness.

Development of a National Immunization Program

The first support for a national immunization program developed after the licensure of inactivated poliomyelitis vaccine (IPV) in 1955. In the two-week period following the successful field trial of this important vaccine, approximately 4 million doses of vaccine were administered, primarily to elementary school children. On April 25, 1955, however, an infant with paralytic poliomyelitis was admitted to a Chicago hospital. The disease case was important because it occurred exactly nine days after the child was immunized with the IPV vaccine. Five additional cases of poliomyelitis were reported the following day. All of the children received vaccine that was produced by one manufacturer. In each case, the paralysis developed first in the limb where the vaccine was administered. On April 27, 1955, the surgeon general asked the manufacturer to recall all remaining lots of vaccine (CDC, 1999b).

As a result of these vaccine-related events, state health officers were asked to designate a polio reporting officer responsible for reporting cases of poliomyelitis among vaccinated persons. Case reports were sent to the poliomyelitis surveillance unit, where the data were analyzed and disseminated via poliomyelitis surveillance reports. The first report was published only three days after surveillance activity began. Case data confirmed suspicion that the problems were confined to one vaccine manufacturer.

Without the rapid instigation of a surveillance program, the manufacture of poliomyelitis vaccine might have been halted entirely. Important aspects of modern public health surveillance include data collection, data analysis, and rapid dissemination of information (CDC, 1999b).

The National Immunization Program (NIP) at the CDC performs national surveillance for measles, mumps, rubella, congenital rubella syndrome, diphtheria, tetanus, pertussis, poliomyelitis, and varicella. The National Center for Infectious Diseases at the CDC is responsible for surveillance of other vaccine-preventable diseases such as hepatitis A and B, *Haemophilus influenzae* type b (Hib) invasive disease, influenza, and pneumococcal disease. Cases are reported to state health departments and then to the National Notifiable Diseases Surveillance System. The collected data are analyzed and then published in the *Morbidity and Mortality Weekly Report (MMWR)*. Reported cases of selected vaccine-preventable diseases from 1990 to 1998 are shown in Table 26-2 (CDC, 1999).

Development of New Vaccines

Campaigns to promote the widespread vaccination of children, as well as school entrance requirements, have resulted in tremendous decreases in the morbidity and mortality related to vaccine-preventable diseases in the

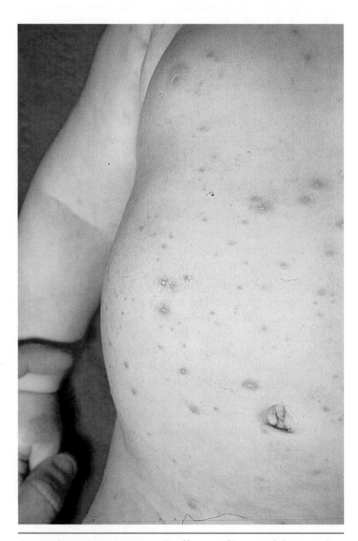

A vaccine to prevent varicella was licensed for use in the United States in 1995. Photo courtesy of Robert A. Silverman, MD, Clinical Associate Professor, Department of Pediatrics, Georgetown University.

TABLE 26-2 Reported Cases of Selected Vaccine-Preventable Diseases, 1990–1998*

DISEASE	1990	1991	1992	1993	1994	1995	1996	1997	1998
Measles	27,786	9,643	2,237	312	963	309	508	138	89
Rubella	1,125	1,401	160	192	227	128	238	181	345
Congenital rubella syndrome	11	47	11	5	7	6	4	5	6
Poliomyelitis, paralytic[†]	6	10	6	4	8	6	5	3	1
Diphtheria	4	5	4	—	2	—	2	4	1
Tetanus	64	57	45	48	51	41	36	50	34
H. influenzae invasive disease (aged < 5 yr)[φ]	nn	1,540[φ]	592[φ]	435[φ]	284[‡]	193[‡]	143[‡]	139[‡]	150[‡]
Pertussis	4,570	2,719	4,083	6,586	4,617	5,137	7,796	6,564	6,279
Mumps	5,292	4,264	2,572	1,692	1,537	906	7751	683	606
Hepatitis B	21,102	18,003	16,126	13,361	12,517	10,805	10,637	10,416	8,651

*1998 data are provisional. Confirmed and unknown case status only. nn = not nationally notifiable.

[†]No cases were wild virus associated. Data from previous years subject to change due to delayed reporting.

[φ]Invasive disease including type b, other types, untyped, and untypable strains; only cases due to type b are preventable by vaccine.

[‡]Includes type b and unknown serotype.

From CDC Manual for the Surveillance of Vaccine Preventable Diseases, *by Centers for Disease Control and Prevention, 1999, Atlanta, GA: Author.*

United States. Diseases that in recent history were recognized as leading causes of death and disability among children, such as diphtheria and congenital rubella syndrome, are now almost nonexistent.

Until the development of the Hib vaccine in the 1980s, *H. influenzae* type b was the most frequent cause of bacterial meningitis among children and resulted in approximately 900 deaths each year (CDC, 1999b). Until 1995, most individuals expected to develop varicella (chickenpox) at some time in their life. There were an estimated 4 million cases of varicella in the United States in the early 1990s (CDC, 1999b). Although varicella has traditionally been considered a mild illness with predictable outbreaks among school children each spring, 100 deaths with varicella as the underlying cause were reported annually. In March 1995, the live attenuated varicella vaccine was licensed for use in the United States. Immunity has been shown to persist in 20-year follow-up studies in Japan and 10-year follow-up studies in the United States. Studies have also shown fewer and milder cases of shingles, a reblossoming of infection from the dormant virus (Plotkin, 1996).

Another vaccine licensed for use in persons two years of age and older is the hepatitis A vaccine. This vaccine provides long-term protection against the hepatitis A virus. Children and adults need a two-shot series of hepatitis A vaccine in a six-month interval for sustained protection. Two inactivated hepatitis A vaccines are currently commercially available: Havrix (SmithKline Beecham) and Vaqta (Merck and Company). Surveillance will be important to monitor the impact of these vaccines.

In addition to the availability of new vaccines, recommendations for administration of standard vaccines have changed. Recommendations for the use of IPV for all four doses of polio vaccination come as a direct result of the eradication of "wild polio" virus from the Western Hemisphere and as a result of potential vaccine complications from previous vaccines (CDC, 2000a). A new acellular pertussis vaccine is now available in combination with diphtheria and tetanus (DTaP). This vaccine produces fewer reactions (Peters, 1997a). The recommended immunization schedule is shown in Figure 22-6.

Centers for Disease Control and Prevention Disease Reduction Goals

The CDC's 2000 and 2010 disease reduction goals (see Table 26-3) represent remarkable progress toward the eradication of vaccine-preventable diseases. To consolidate national efforts and promote further reductions in disease incidence, the Childhood Immunization Initiative (CII) established goals for the elimination of indigenous acquisition of six vaccine-preventable diseases by 1996. The goals established by the CII were interim milestones toward the *Healthy People 2010* health objectives for the United States. The *Healthy People 2010* objectives

TABLE 26-3 Disease Reduction and Elimination Goals: 2000 and 2010

DISEASE	2000 GOALS	2010 GOALS
Congenital Rubella syndrome	No goal established	0*
Diphtheria	0[†]	0[‡]
H. influenzae type b invasive disease	No goal established[§]	0
Hepatitis B	40 per 100,000 population	0[‖]
Measles	0	0
Mumps	500	0
Pertussis	1000	2,000[#]
Polio (wild-type virus)	0	0**
Rubella	0	0
Tetanus	0[†]	0[‡]
Varicella	No goal established	400,000

*From: National Congenital Rubella Syndrome Registry.

[†]*Among persons = 25 years of age.*

[‡]*Among persons < 35 years of age.*

[§]*Although no goal was established specifically for Hib, Healthy People sets a goal for reduction in the incidence of bacterial meningitis from 6.3 per 100,000 population (1986) to no more than 4.7 per 100,000 by the year 2000.*

[‖]*Among persons < 25 years of age.*

[#]*Among children < 7 years of age.*

**Polio expected to be eradicated by the year 2000.

From Manual for the Surveillance of Vaccine Preventable Diseases *by Centers for Disease Control and Prevention, 1999, Atlanta, GA: Author.*

include disease elimination objectives for diphtheria and tetanus (among persons 25 years of age and younger), polio, measles, rubella, and congenital rubella syndrome. Also included are disease reduction goals for mumps, pertussis, and hepatitis B. Although no specific disease reduction or elimination goal for *H. influenzae* type b infection was established by the *Healthy People 2010* objectives, there is a goal for the reduction of bacterial meningitis, to no more than 4.7 cases per 100,000 people, from a baseline of 6.3 per 100,000 in 1986.

Great challenges remain in meeting the disease reduction and elimination goals established by *Healthy People 2010* objectives. Achievement of disease reduction goals depends on several factors, including maintenance of high vaccination coverage among children, development of improved strategies to encourage appropriate vaccination of adults, accurate and timely diagnosis and reporting of suspected cases, and thorough

case investigations (CDC, 1999b). Community health nurses can take an active role in ensuring the success of immunization programs by working to eliminate barriers to immunization.

Immunization is the most effective disease control measure in limiting the spread of these diseases. Educational measures are important to inform the public of the hazards of vaccine-preventable diseases and the necessity for immunization. Preventing and controlling the transmission of vaccine-preventable diseases in this century will require the continuous efforts of public health personnel.

SEXUALLY TRANSMITTED DISEASE

In the United States, more than 65 million people are currently living with an incurable sexually transmitted disease (STD) (CDC, 2000f). Fifteen million individuals become infected with one or more STDs each year. Nearly half of these individuals will suffer from lifelong infections (Cates, 1999). Despite the widespread prevalence of STDs, they are one of the most underrecognized problems in our country. STDs add billions of dollars to the nation's health care costs each year. In spite of this, most people in the United States are unaware of both the risks and consequences surrounding all but the most prominent STD: HIV (CDC, 2000f). Figure 26-4 illustrates the number of new STD cases annually.

Many people with these infections are difficult to track because they are asymptomatic and may go undiagnosed and untreated. The close physical contact and sharing of fluids associated with sexual activity provide perfect conditions for the direct transmission of infectious organisms. STDs hold the distinction of occupying 5 of the nation's 10 most frequently reported diseases.

The roots of today's STD epidemic developed in the 1960s when postwar baby boomers explored newfound freedoms. Birth control pills came into widespread use and barrier contraceptives, and the disease protection they offered, were cast aside for the freedom and assurance that came with the oral contraceptive. "Venereal disease" appeared to be well controlled with the use of antibiotics. No one could have predicted the vengeance with which STDs would again explode onto the infectious disease scene. AIDS would draw the attention of the nation as thousands became infected with the deadly disease. While AIDS got all of the media attention, other STDs—such as hepatitis B, herpes virus, and human papillomavirus—spread silently until the 1990s, when they began to be reported in epidemic proportions.

The spectrum of consequences to this national epidemic ranges from mild symptoms to serious and long-term consequences such as cervical, liver, and other cancers; reproductive health problems; and possibly death. Societal problems, behavioral and social stereotypes, and unbalanced mass media messages present bar-

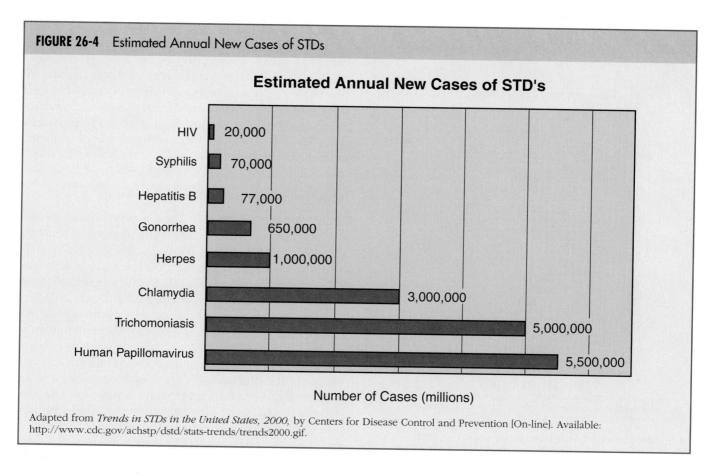

FIGURE 26-4 Estimated Annual New Cases of STDs

Adapted from *Trends in STDs in the United States, 2000,* by Centers for Disease Control and Prevention [On-line]. Available: http://www.cdc.gov/achstp/dstd/stats-trends/trends2000.gif.

riers to the prevention and control of STDs at all levels. These barriers contribute to the "hidden" nature of these diseases and impede important dialog within the community which would facilitate primary prevention efforts for risk reduction (Donovan, 1997; Eng and Butler, 1996).

The rates of curable STDs in the United States are the highest in the developed world and are higher than in some developing regions. Community health nurses can support STD control through primary prevention programs where individuals are educated about high-risk behaviors. Secondary prevention should include case contact notification and effective case management of individuals affected by disease.

Populations at Increased Risk

Adolescents, young adults, women, minorities, substance abusers, and persons of low socioeconomic status are listed among those at the greatest risk for the development of STDs and AIDS. Sexually transmitted diseases are most prevalent among teenagers and young adults under age 25. Teenage girls are particularly vulnerable to infection because of immature reproductive systems (Donovan, 1993). Women are more likely than men to acquire an STD after exposure to infection because of anatomical differences that augment transmission and support "silent" infection. In addition, women tend to suffer more devastating consequences of untreated infection, such as

infertility and cervical cancer (Donovan, 1993). Intravenous drug use and heterosexual contact are responsible for the greatest proportion of AIDS among women (see Figure 26-5). Increased rates of infection among African American and Hispanic women are remarkable. Although African American and Hispanic women made up only 21% of all U.S. women, they constituted the majority of reported AIDS cases among women in 1999 (CDC, 2000c).

The use of illicit drugs and the STD epidemic have expanded together in the United States. Blood-borne diseases such as hepatitis B and AIDS can be transmitted when needles are shared. Poverty tends to create an environment that supports the spread of disease: Crowded neighborhoods with high rates of drug use, infection, and delayed health-seeking behaviors contribute to the spread of STDs in this population.

Prevention of Sexually Transmitted Disease

Sexually transmitted diseases significantly impact health care costs in the United States. In 1994, experts estimated that the health care costs associated with a select group of STDs other than HIV/AIDS carried a $10 billion price tag, with HIV/AIDS adding an additional $6.7 billion (Eng & Butler, 1996). Costs could be decreased significantly via effective primary prevention, including education about ways to prevent the spread of infection and the

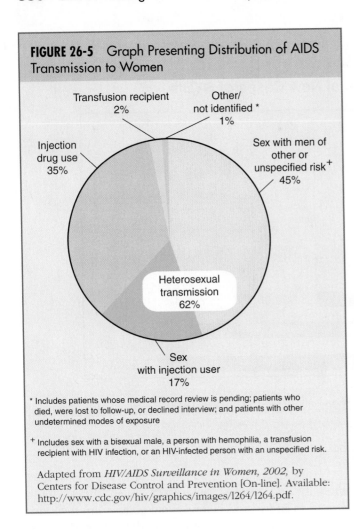

FIGURE 26-5 Graph Presenting Distribution of AIDS Transmission to Women

Transfusion recipient 2%

Other/ not identified * 1%

Injection drug use 35%

Sex with men of other or unspecified risk+ 45%

Heterosexual transmission 62%

Sex with injection user 17%

* Includes patients whose medical record review is pending; patients who died, were lost to follow-up, or declined interview; and patients with other undetermined modes of exposure

+ Includes sex with a bisexual male, a person with hemophilia, a transfusion recipient with HIV infection, or an HIV-infected person with an unspecified risk.

Adapted from *HIV/AIDS Surveillance in Women, 2002,* by Centers for Disease Control and Prevention [On-line]. Available: http://www.cdc.gov/hiv/graphics/images/1264/1264.pdf.

availability of immunization for some diseases, and via secondary prevention efforts that support detection, treatment, and effective case management of STDs in their early stages. Tertiary prevention to support appropriate long-term treatment and management of chronic infection will provide the most optimal health outcomes. This approach is especially important with viral STDs, which may present lifelong symptoms. Prevention of STDs will be discussed in more detail in the section "The Role of the Community Health Nurse in the Prevention of STDs."

Sexually transmitted diseases are classified into two main categories: viral and nonviral. Whereas nonviral STDs can usually be treated without long-term consequences, viral illnesses have no cure.

Viral Sexually Transmitted Diseases

When viral STDs are diagnosed, individuals face a lifetime of outbreaks and the need for both infection and symptom management. Public health efforts focus on primary prevention, with the goal of preventing disease occurrence. The emergence of AIDS in the 1980s forced a

reluctant public to face the deadly consequences of viral STD infection. Research shows that STDs appear to increase in areas where AIDS is common (Henderson, 1997). Although AIDS has received the most attention in this category because of its mortality statistics, other viral infections such as hepatitis B, herpes simplex 2, and human papillomavirus are epidemic within world populations and account for larger numbers of infected individuals.

Acquired Immunodeficiency Syndrome

Human immunodeficiency virus is responsible for the development of AIDS, a devastating illness that was first recognized in 1981 (Chin, 2000). A retrovirus, HIV infects a cell and uses an enzyme called reverse transcriptase. This enzyme then transcribes the viral genome onto the cell's DNA, resulting in viral replication by the infected cell. Although the virus is able to attack numerous types of cells, the CD4, or helper T-cell, is where the greatest damage from infection occurs. These cells are the body's defense against infection and cancer. In HIV-positive individuals, the numbers of CD4 cells decrease with time, thus rendering the infected person vulnerable to disease. Without the CD4 cells, the body becomes a host for opportunistic infections. Several opportunistic infections and cancers were considered specific indicators of AIDS and were included in the initial case definition published by the CDC in 1982. This definition was revised in 1987 and again in 1993 (CDC, 2000a) as more information about the disease became available. Effective January 1, 2000, the surveillance case definition for HIV infection was revised to reflect advances in laboratory HIV virologic tests. The definition incorporates the reporting criteria for HIV infection and AIDS into a single case definition for adults and children (CDC, 1999a). The disease causes a gradual destruction of the immune system and progresses at a different pace in each infected person. Opportunistic infections often occur only in the advanced stages of AIDS, causing a delay in diagnostic classification of the disease. With the revision of surveillance case definitions in 1993, a CD4 cell count of fewer than 200 cells/mm^3, regardless of an individual's clinical status, is now considered an AIDS case (Chin, 2000). Most individuals who die from AIDS do so as a result of

---

REFLECTIVE THINKING

Caring for Clients with AIDS

- What are your feelings about providing nursing care to an HIV/AIDS-infected person?
- What are your risks for developing HIV infection as a health care worker?

opportunistic infections or cancer rather than the virus itself. Because of their associated low resistance to disease, persons with AIDS have become "incubators" for diseases once thought to be controlled, such as TB.

Human immunodeficiency virus can be subdivided into two types of infection: HIV-1 and HIV-2. Although the two types of infection have similar characteristics, the pathogenicity of HIV-2 appears to be less than that of HIV-1. **Pathogenicity** is the ability or power of an infectious agent to produce disease. Individuals infected with HIV-2 take longer to develop AIDS, and the disease progresses at a slower pace. United States blood centers have been testing for HIV-1 infection since 1985 and for HIV-2 since 1992. Those individuals listed in Figure 26-6 should request an HIV-2 enzyme immunoassay, or EIA.

Transmission

Early in the epidemic, AIDS was thought to be a disease of homosexual men. First documented with rare manifestations of *Pneumocystis carinii* pneumonia and Kaposi's sarcoma in previously healthy, young homosexual

---

FIGURE 26-6 Indications for HIV-2 Testing

Persons for Whom HIV-2 Testing Is Indicated

- Those who have sex with or share needles with West Africans
- Persons who have received blood transfusions in West Africa
- Children born to HIV-2-infected mothers
- Those with conditions suggestive of HIV infection (such as an AIDS-associated opportunistic disease) for whom HIV-1 testing is not positive
- Persons whose blood specimens are reactive on HIV-1 EIA testing and exhibit certain unusual indeterminate patterns on HIV-1 Western blot

---

men in San Francisco and New York, AIDS is now recognized as a disease and has been recorded in almost all countries. It affects men, women, and children of all races and sexual orientation and from all social classes

---

RESEARCH FOCUS

Individual and Community Risks of Measles and Pertussis Associated with Personal Exemptions to Immunization

Study Problem/Purpose

This study evaluated whether children aged 3–18 whose parents chose not to allow them to be vaccinated for religious or philosophical reasons (exemptors) were at greater risk for the development of measles or pertussis. In addition, the study evaluated whether the community was at greater risk for disease development when exposed to exemptors.

Methods

To assess individual risk, children aged 3–18 represented the cohort from which researchers retrospectively calculated the incidence rates for measles and pertussis from 1987 to 1998. Measles and pertussis are notifiable at both the state and national level. Cases were confirmed by evaluating case reports filled out by public health nurses from local health departments. For both diseases, case report forms documented demographic data and included immunization status.

To assess community risk, the researchers analyzed whether the frequency of exemptors in a county was predictive of the average annual incidence rate for measles and pertussis among vaccinated children in 1987–1998.

Findings

Exemptors were 22.2 times more likely to acquire measles and 5.9 times more likely to acquire pertussis than vaccinated children. Communities and schools with high numbers of exemptors were at greater risk for an outbreak. In addition, this study provides specific evidence suggesting that personal exemptors put vaccinated children at risk of acquiring measles and pertussis. At least 11% of vaccinated children in measles outbreaks acquired infection through contact with an exemptor.

Implications

The decision to forgo vaccination must balance individual rights with social responsibility. The health of an individual in the community is dependent on the health of the rest of the community. Until vaccines become available that are 100% effective or a disease is eradicated, an increase in exemptors has the potential to precipitate communitywide outbreaks of vaccine-preventable diseases. Public health personnel should recognize the potential effect of exemptors in outbreaks and parents should be educated about the risks involved in not vaccinating their children.

Source: From Feikin, D. R., Lezotte, D. C., Hamman, R. F., Salmon, D. A., Chen, R. T., & Hoffman, R. E. (2000). Individual and community risks of measles and pertussis associated with personal exemptions to immunization. Journal of the American Medical Association, *284, 3145–3150.*

with equally devastating consequences (Chin, 2000). No cure has been found, and no vaccine is available to prevent this fatal disease.

Human immunodeficiency virus is found in the blood, semen, and vaginal secretions of an infected person and is not transmitted via casual contact such as hugging, touching, or shaking hands. Transmission from blood transfusions has been rare since HIV screening of all blood and blood products was instituted in March 1985. All blood collected in the United States is now screened for six infectious agents: HIV-1, HIV-2, HTLV-1 (human T-cell lymphotropic virus), hepatitis B virus, hepatitis C virus, and the syphilis spirochete. All potential donors are interviewed before they are tested and are informed that if they have a risk factor for HIV, they should not donate. Every unit of blood with a positive result from HIV-antibody testing is discarded, and future donations are not accepted from those persons. It is estimated that the risk of acquiring infection from a blood transfusion is now 1 in 225,000 units (CDC, 2000b).

Transmission of HIV can occur via:

- Sexual contact involving exchange of body fluids with an infected individual
- Blood transfusion prior to 1985
- Exposure to blood products or tissues of an infected person
- Perinatal transmission from an infected mother to the fetus during pregnancy, delivery, or breastfeeding
- Sharing needles or syringes with an infected person

While the risk of sexually transmitted infection via sexual intercourse is lower than with other STDs, the presence of a concurrent STD, particularly if it is one that produces an ulcer, such as herpes or chancroid, can significantly assist the transmission of disease (Chin, 2000).

It is important that the community health nurse be aware that the HIV virus is principally spread via unprotected sex and needle sharing with an HIV-infected person.

All pregnant women should be informed about the risk of HIV transmission to their babies and of treatment options that have been shown to be effective in preventing the vertical transmission of the AIDS virus. Although blood transfusions served as a mode of transmission when the virus was first discovered, persons who received blood transfusions after 1985 have a very limited risk of acquiring the infection.

It is equally important that community health nurses be able to dispel the myths surrounding this disease by informing the populations they serve that HIV is not transmitted via casual contact or insect bites or stings. Table 26-4 shows the HIV exposure groups that account for most cases of AIDS in the United States. Studies conducted by the CDC show no evidence of HIV transmission via insect vectors. Reasons transmission via insects is unlikely include the following: The amount of virus circulating in the blood of HIV-infected individuals is very low compared with levels observed for other viruses known to be transmitted by insects; mosquitoes do not regurgitate blood into the next victim they bite; and the saliva of mosquitoes does not contain the virus (CDC, 2000a). Furthermore, the virus cannot reproduce in insects.

Symptoms

Within the first two to four weeks, persons infected with HIV experience a flulike illness. Reported symptoms include fever, sore throat, swollen lymph nodes, headache, muscle and joint pains, and nausea and vomiting. Some individuals report open ulcers in the mouth and a viral rash. As antibodies are produced to combat the initial infection, infected persons enter a symptom-free phase. The time from HIV infection to the development of AIDS varies from less than 1 year to more than 10 years. Dur-

TABLE 26-4 AIDS Cases by Exposure Category*

EXPOSURE CATEGORY	MALE	FEMALE	TOTALS[†]
Men who have sex with men	348,657	—	348,657
Injecting drug use	137,650	51,592	189,242
Men who have sex with men and inject drugs	47,820	—	47,820
Hemophilia/coagulation disorder	4,847	274	5,121
Heterosexual contact	27,952	50,257	78,210
Recipient of blood transfusion, blood components, or tissue	4,920	3,746	8,666
Risk not reported or identified	48,343	19,042	67,387

*Numbers are based on AIDS cases reported to the CDC through June 2000 among persons aged 13 years, by sex and exposure category (www.cdc.gov/hiv/stats/exposure.htm).
[†]Includes three persons whose sex is unknown.

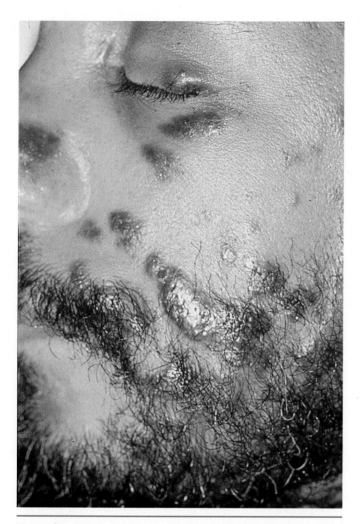

Kaposi's sarcoma. Photo courtesy of Robert A. Silverman, MD, Clinical Associate Professor, Department of Pediatrics, Georgetown University.

ing the symptom-free phase, individuals often feel completely healthy. Those individuals who are carrying the virus but are not symptomatic are the most dangerous for the spread of infection. Transmission of the virus is possible even in the symptom-free period. Recognition of early symptoms is critical to control the spread of infection. The virus lies dormant until the disease weakens and destroys the immune system and the body is unable to combat opportunistic disease.

Onset of AIDS is usually insidious, with vague symptoms such as anorexia and lymphadenopathy. Individuals typically experience one symptom and then, as the disease progresses, tend to develop clusters of symptoms that indicate the presence of AIDS. The percentage of individuals infected with HIV who go on to develop AIDS is not known. Approximately 20% of infected persons have developed AIDS within 5 years of the initial infection. Seventy percent will develop AIDS by the 15th year following exposure. The long dormant phase characteristic of the infection has changed the focus from acute illness care to chronic disease management of the infection.

Diagnosis

The ELISA (enzyme-linked immunosorbent assay) and Western blot antibody tests are the most common tests used to diagnose HIV infection. Testing can be done in most doctors' offices or health clinics and should be accompanied by counseling. If they have particular concerns about confidentiality, individuals can be tested anonymously at many sites. Antibodies to HIV generally do not reach detectable levels until one to three months following infection and may take as long as six months to be generated in quantities large enough to show up in standard blood tests. Persons exposed to HIV should be tested as soon as they are likely to have developed HIV antibodies to the virus. Secondary prevention is dependent on early diagnosis and appropriate treatment in the early stages of infection. High-risk behaviors may be averted in individuals who test positive for HIV.

Since 1998, clients in public health programs can be tested using one of many rapid HIV tests. The availability of rapid tests allows clients to receive the results of HIV testing on the day of the test. Persons whose rapid HIV test results are negative can be given a definite negative result and no follow-up is necessary. Persons whose rapid HIV test is positive should have the diagnosis confirmed using a standard test such as the Western blot.

All babies born to HIV-infected mothers carry their mothers' antibodies to HIV for several months. If these babies lack symptoms, a definitive diagnosis of HIV infection via the use of standard antibody tests cannot be made until after 15 months of age. By then, babies are unlikely to still carry their mothers' antibodies and, if they are infected, will have produced their own.

Treatment

Medical treatments for AIDS have improved dramatically since the disease was first identified. In the mid-1990s, protease inhibitors were first marketed. Researchers subsequently discovered that a combination of protease inhibitors and reverse transcriptase inhibitors could eliminate traces of HIV from the blood (Leccese, 1997). This combination therapy has resulted in remarkable improvement in individuals infected with HIV. Members of the International AIDS Society published an article that described how to implement treatment with a combination of three anti-AIDS drugs (Carpenter et al., 1997). A drawback to the combination therapy regime is cost. Combination therapy is estimated to cost approximately $15,000 per client per year (Leccese, 1997). The high cost of therapy may hinder availability of the drugs to individuals with limited financial resources. As a result of new treatment modalities, the AIDS death rate was down 19% in 1996 as compared with 1995 figures. Unfortunately, despite new treatment options for AIDS, individuals continue to become infected. As of June 2000 (CDC, 2000a) 753,907 AIDS cases had been reported to the CDC.

Because of the increase in cases of HIV/AIDS among women of childbearing age, there has also been an increase in cases among infants and children. Most of these children were infected via vertical transmission during pregnancy, delivery, or breastfeeding. In June 1994, a U.S. Public Health Service Task Force recommended AZT (zidovudine) for pregnant women infected with the AIDS virus. Research has shown that treatment with AZT can substantially reduce the risk of mother-child transmission of HIV. Treatment during pregnancy can help an HIV-infected woman protect her baby from becoming infected. Without treatment, more than one-third of all babies born to HIV-infected women will have the virus and eventually will get sick (Bloom et al., 1995). Community health nurses must educate pregnant clients about the substantial decrease in the risk of mother-child transmission associated with AZT therapy during pregnancy. Women who fall into risk categories for HIV infection should be tested during pregnancy to decrease the possibility of vertically transmitting the disease.

For a number of years, postexposure prophylaxis (PEP) has been available to health care workers who are stuck with needles contaminated with HIV-positive blood. The results have been promising, with the CDC reporting that as many as 79% of health care workers who utilized PEP did not develop HIV infection. The general populace is questioning why PEP is not being made routinely available to individuals at high risk for developing HIV infection. In some areas, PEP is offered to rape victims. The CDC published guidelines for the use of PEP in 1998. Postexposure treatment consists of a combination of AZT and lamivudine for four weeks. In some cases, a protease inhibitor such as indinavir is added to the treatment regime. Controversy surrounds the potential widespread use of PEP because it is feared that individuals will abandon safe-sex practices (Leccese, 1997).

Prevention

The only way to absolutely prevent HIV infection is to abstain from sexual intercourse or to maintain a mutually monogamous sexual relationship with an uninfected person (see Figure 26-7). Primary prevention measures include education about the need to use barrier methods such as condoms (male and female) to curb the potential spread of infection between sexual partners. Secondary prevention measures include increased availability of low-cost AIDS testing. Because of the high number of drug-addicted individuals at risk due to needle sharing, drug treatment facilities should be increased. Needle exchange programs have been effective in certain areas; such programs are not widely accepted, however, despite evidence that their presence dramatically decreases the rates of HIV infection.

All pregnant women should be informed about the risk of HIV transmission during the perinatal period and offered HIV testing and treatment when indicated.

FIGURE 26-7   Preventing the Spread of HIV

The following prevention measures apply to personal sex practices and intravenous drug use:

- To prevent sexual transmission of HIV, abstain from sex with an infected person.

- Ask about the sexual history of current and future sex partners.

- Reduce the number of sex partners to minimize the risk.

- Always use a condom from start to finish during any type of sex (vaginal, anal, or oral). Use latex condoms rather than natural-membrane condoms. If used properly, latex condoms offer protection against sexually transmitted disease agents including HIV.

- Use only water-based lubricants. Do not use saliva or oil-based lubricants such as petroleum jelly or vegetable shortening. If you decide to use a spermicide along with a condom, it is preferable to use spermicide in the vagina according to manufacturer's instructions.

- Avoid anal or rough vaginal intercourse. Do not do anything that could tear the skin or the moist lining of the genitals, anus, or mouth and cause bleeding.

- Condoms should be used even for oral sex.

- Avoid deep, wet, or "French" kissing with an infected person. Possible trauma to the mouth may occur, which could result in the exchange of blood. It is safe, however, to hug, cuddle, rub, or dry kiss your partner.

- Avoid alcohol and illicit drugs. Alcohol and drugs can impair your immune system and your judgment. If you use drugs, do not share "injecting drug works." Do not share needles, syringes, or cookers.

- Do not share personal items such as toothbrushes, razors, and devices used during sex, which may be contaminated with blood, semen, or vaginal fluids.

- If you are infected with HIV or have engaged in sex or needle-sharing behaviors that lead to infection with HIV, do not donate blood, plasma, sperm, body organs, or tissues.

Adapted from *HIV/AIDS Prevention Statistics,* by Centers for Disease Control and Prevention, 1997, Atlanta, GA: author.

It is well known that women with HIV can reduce the risk of vertical transmission of the virus to their unborn child by 66% if placed on a treatment regime using AZT during the perinatal period. A 1999 study in Uganda found that a single dose of nevirapine given to HIV-infected mothers during labor followed by a single dose given to the newborn within three days of birth gave better results than the AZT regime. Only 13.1% of these infants became infected with HIV (Chin, 2000). This is particularly good news because the cost of nevirapine is only $4 per dose. From a global perspective this new, lower cost treatment has given new hope to those third world countries struggling with high infection rates and few resources.

Health care workers should protect themselves from occupationally acquired HIV infection by using Universal Precautions (see Figure 26-8). All individuals who test positive for HIV should be checked for other STDs. Researchers have demonstrated that when STDs are present, HIV transmission is two to five times greater than in populations where other STDs are not present. Further, evidence is increasing that when STDs are treated, there is a reduced risk of HIV transmission (Henderson, 1997). Tertiary prevention includes connecting clients with appropriate support agencies and informing clients of new treatments and programs that improve long-term health outcomes of infected individuals.

Surveillance and prevention measures associated with infectious diseases include partner or contact notification. Experts have opposing opinions about how HIV should be managed in the United States. Some experts believe that the federal government has indirectly contributed to the growth of the AIDS epidemic by forgoing recognized public health practices, including partner notification. Instead, individuals' privacy rights have superseded accepted public health procedures. AIDS activists have asserted that AIDS testing and reporting are civil rights issues rather than a public health issue. The stigma associated with HIV and the fear of discrimination have led gay rights organizations to keep routine testing and mandated reporting politically charged issues. However, because of voluntary testing and notification, thousands of individuals who are unaware of their HIV status are being denied early treatment, which has been proven to extend life, and may unknowingly be infecting others. Coburn and Pelosi (1997) comment that "never before in medical history have we given the responsibility of controlling an epidemic to the individuals infected with the disease" (p. 24).

As of June 30, 2000, 35 areas had laws or regulations requiring confidential reporting by name of all persons with confirmed HIV infection, in addition to reporting of persons with AIDS. Connecticut required reporting by name of HIV infection only for children less than 13 years of age; and Oregon required reporting for children less than 6 years of age.

Human Papillomavirus

Genital warts are caused by the human papillomavirus (HPV), the name for a group of viruses that includes more than 60 different types, approximately 20 of which infect the anal and genital areas. Experts estimate that as many as 20 million Americans are infected with HPV, and the incidence of the diseases it causes appears to be increasing (Cates, 1999).

Transmission

Genital warts are highly infectious, with two-thirds of individuals who have sexual contact with infected individuals developing the disease. As many as 5.5 million people become infected in the United States each year (Cates, 1999).

Symptoms

Most HPV infections have no visible signs or symptoms. The fact that many people infected with HPV are asymptomatic contributes to the rampant spread of this infection, particularly among young people. Only approximately one-third of women experience symptoms with the HPV infection. Warts start to appear approximately two months

FIGURE 26-8 Universal Blood and Body Fluid Precautions

- Special training and education programs
- Use of protective equipment such as gloves, gowns, eye protection, and face masks
- Handwashing after each patient contact
- Proper handling and disposal of sharps
- Engineering control, such as special sharps containers and safety cabinets for biologicals
- Programs of immunization, such as hepatitis B vaccine for employees
- Proper contaminated waste disposal
- Use of disinfectants
- Proper labeling and signs

Adapted from "Universal Precautions for Prevention of Transmission of HIV, Hepatitis B Virus and Other Bloodborne Pathogens in Health Care Settings" by Centers for Disease Control and Prevention, 1988, *Morbidity and Mortality Weekly Report, 37*, pp. 377–382.

REFLECTIVE THINKING

AIDS Mandatory Partner Notification

- Do you think there should be mandatory partner notification and reporting of AIDS cases?
- Do the rights of HIV-positive individuals to determine whether they will be tested outweigh the rights of those at risk for acquiring infection, such as unborn children?
- Will the latest therapies, which rely on early diagnosis, change reporting laws?

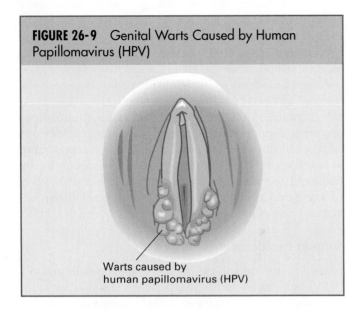

FIGURE 26-9 Genital Warts Caused by Human Papillomavirus (HPV)

Warts caused by human papillomavirus (HPV)

after initial exposure to an infected person. The warts are typically small and may occur in clusters around the genital area and anus. In women, warts may develop in the vagina, where they are hard to detect, and they may also appear on the vaginal lips (see Figure 26-9). In men, warts typically are detected on the penis but may be found on the scrotum or around the anus. Rarely, genital warts also can develop in the mouth or throat of a person who has had oral sexual contact with an infected person. Genital warts often occur in groups and can be very tiny or can accumulate into large masses on genital tissues. Warts may spontaneously resolve, but recurrence is common. In some cases, warts may eventually develop fleshy, small, raised growths with a cauliflower-like appearance. As the warts shed their outer layer, they spread infection. People who develop genital warts have a high risk for developing certain cancers such as cancer of the cervix, anus, penis, and vulva. In both developed and developing countries, more than 90% of the new cases of cervical cancer are due to sexually transmitted human papillomavirus infection of the cervix (WHO, 1997a).

Diagnosis

Health care providers conducting routine examinations of clients should check for abnormal tissue or the presence of genital warts. Clinical observation can be enhanced via the use of acetic acid stain and colposcopy or androscopy for the detection of subtle lesions. Individuals with documented HPV infection should be encouraged to have frequent screening examinations so that if cancer does develop, it will be diagnosed in the early stages. The Pap smear is designed to detect precancerous changes in the cervix of women and may show changes caused by HPV infection. Biopsy should be reserved for use with clients where the diagnosis is uncertain. In spite of the connection between certain subtypes of the dis-

ease and cervical cancer, there is no indication for viral subtyping of HPV during routine diagnosis and treatment (Miller & Brodell, 1996).

Treatment

Genital warts can be removed or destroyed via chemical applications, cryotherapy, laser, or electrosurgery. Removal of genital warts does *not* constitute a cure, and new outbreaks may occur months and years after the initial treatment. Removal of warts does, however, reduce the risk of transmitting the disease to uninfected sexual partners.

The main goal of therapy is to treat symptomatic, visable lesions. The CDC now recommends patient-applied medications to treat HPV (CDC, 1998b). Two patient-applied medications—podofilox (Condylox) and imiquimod (Aldara)—are available for patients to use in the management of HPV.

Herpes Simplex Virus 2 (HSV-2)

Herpes is recognized as a chronic, lifelong infection. Genital herpes is a contagious viral infection that affects an estimated 23% of adult Americans. Genital herpes is the most common cause of genital ulcers in the United States. An estimated 40 million individuals are affected by this disease, and there are approximately 500,000 new cases of infection each year (Eng & Butler, 1996). The infection is caused by the herpes simplex virus (HSV). There are two types of HSV, and both can cause the symptoms of genital herpes. Type 1 HSV most commonly causes sores on the lips (known as fever blisters or cold sores) but can cause genital infections as well. Type 2 HSV most often causes genital sores but can also infect the mouth. Both types of HSV can produce sores in and around the vaginal area (see Figure 26-10), on the penis, around the anal opening, and on the buttocks or thighs. Occasionally, sores also appear on other parts of the body where broken skin has come into contact with HSV. The virus remains in certain nerve cells of the body for life, causing periodic symptoms in some people.

Transmission

It is possible to become infected with HSV through oral, anal, or vaginal sex. Genital herpes infection usually is acquired via sexual contact with someone who has an active outbreak of herpes lesions in the genital area. Changing sexual practices have supported the spread of HSV-1 below the waist and HSV-2 above the waist, via oral-genital sex or self-inoculation. Because HSV lesions are ulcerative, individuals with HSV are at increased risk for contracting HIV. If lesions are present, HSV may be diagnosed via clinical examination. It is important to remember that the virus may be transmitted to uninfected individuals even when no visible lesions are present (Chin, 2000).

Newborns may be infected with HSV-2 via direct contact with lesions during the birthing process. Direct

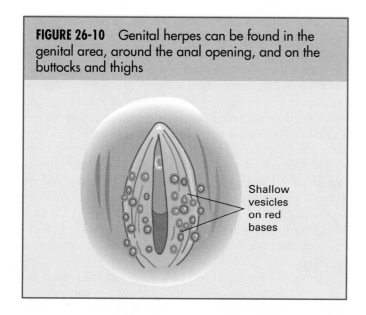

FIGURE 26-10 Genital herpes can be found in the genital area, around the anal opening, and on the buttocks and thighs

Shallow vesicles on red bases

newborn contact can result in severe consequences for the neonate, including neurological damage or death. If herpes lesions are present on the mother, exposure can be eliminated by delivering the baby via cesarean section.

Symptoms

Herpes is similar to other STDs in that many people have no symptoms of infection. Furthermore, symptoms vary in those individuals who do show signs of infection. Early symptoms include a burning sensation in the genitals, low-back pain, and dysuria. Flulike symptoms may accompany the initial outbreak. Symptoms are typically reported within 2–20 days after having sex with an infected individual. After the initial symptoms, small, red bumps appear in the infected area and develop into painful vesicles or blisters, which then crust over, scab, and heal. After the lesions resolve, the virus remains in the body, and recurrent episodes of active disease may occur at any time. Outbreaks are frequently associated with stress and overexertion.

Diagnosis

Confirmation of HSV infection is possible via laboratory examination of fluid from the vesicles. The most accurate method of diagnosis is viral culture. A new lesion is swabbed or scraped, and the sample is added to a laboratory culture containing healthy cells. When examined under a microscope after one or two days, the cells show changes that indicate growth of the herpes virus. Blood tests can confirm the presence of HSV antibodies but do not detect active disease.

Treatment

Herpes is a lifelong infection with no known cure. It is possible to treat the painful symptoms of herpes, however. During an outbreak, clients can speed healing by keeping the area clean and avoiding touching the lesion,

remembering to wash hands after contact with lesions to prevent the spread of infection. Acyclovir (Zovirax), when taken regularly, interferes with the virus's ability to reproduce itself. It also shortens the duration of the outbreak, reduces the number of outbreaks, and reduces symptoms. Acyclovir can be taken orally or is available in a cream.

Two new antiviral drugs, famciclovir (Famvir) and valacyclovir (Valtrex), have been added to the treatment options for individuals with genital herpes. Suppressive therapy reduces the frequency of recurrence by up to 75% in persons who have six or more outbreaks per year. Treatment also reduces viral shedding between outbreaks. Intravenous antiviral drugs are also available but should only be used in patients with severe or complicated infections (Miller & Brodell, 1996).

Bacterial Sexually Transmitted Diseases

Bacterial STDs, including syphilis and gonorrhea, have been documented for hundreds of years. They differ from viral STDs in their susceptibility to treatment. Bacterial STD infections can be treated with antibiotics and, in most cases, can be cured.

Chlamydia

Genital chlamydial infection is caused by the bacterium *Chlamydia trachomatis*. More than 3 million new cases of chlamydia are reported each year. The volume of cases makes chlamydia the most frequently reported STD in the United States. The annual cost of chlamydial infections and their sequelae is estimated to exceed $2 billion. The side effects of this bacterial infection can lead to pelvic inflammatory disease (PID), a leading cause of infertility (Chin, 2000; Cates, 1999).

Transmission

Chlamydia is transmitted during vaginal or anal sexual contact with an infected partner. A pregnant woman may pass the infection to her newborn during delivery, with subsequent neonatal eye infection or pneumonia.

Symptoms

Three-quarters of the women and 50% of the men who have chlamydia are symptom free. The majority of cases go undiagnosed. If symptoms are experienced, they commonly include discharge and a burning sensation when urinating. Women with chlamydia report low-back pain and pain during intercourse. Men experience itching and burning around the penis and, on occasion, swelling of the testicles. Chlamydial infections are often acquired concurrently with *Neisseria gonorrhoeae* and may persist after the gonorrhea is treated. It is estimated that 45% of those women diagnosed with chlamydia also are infected with gonorrhea (Chin, 2000).

Diagnosis

Chlamydia is diagnosed via cervical smear and culture.

Treatment

A single dose of azithromycin is effective treatment for chlamydia. A full seven days of treatment with doxycycline twice a day can also kill the bacteria causing the disease. For newborns and pregnant women, erythromycin is the drug of choice. All sex partners of a person with chlamydial infection should be evaluated and treated to prevent reinfection and further spread of the disease.

Chlamydia and gonorrhea are often found together, and because their symptoms and clinical manifestation are difficult to distinguish, treatment for both conditions is recommended when one is suspected (Chin, 2000). Because of the increasing drug resistance of many of the organisms that cause STDs, it is important that all medication be taken according to directions.

Syphilis

Syphilis is caused by a spirochete called *Treponema pallidum*. Syphilis is a serious disease that, when left untreated, can have debilitating and deadly consequences. Some historians believe that syphilis emerged as a new disease as early as the 15th century. According to one theory, early explorers like Christopher Columbus were responsible for bringing the disease from the New World and transmitting it throughout Europe. For many years, *syphilis* was a catchall term for sexually transmitted disease. Physicians assumed that gonorrhea and syphilis were the same thing until 1837, when a researcher reported differences in the two diseases. In 1906, Wasserman developed a blood test for syphilis, leading to advances in treatment including Salvarsan, an arsenic compound. With the introduction of penicillin in 1943, a once deadly infection became curable. Although syphilis appeared to be controlled for many years, there was a dramatic rise in cases of primary and secondary syphilis in the 1970s and 1980s. Like those at high risk for other STDs, people at increased risk for syphilis are those who have had multiple sex partners, have sexual relations with an infected partner, have a history of STD, and do not use condoms. Despite effective treatment, syphilis continues to be a common STD.

After the introduction of penicillin in the 1940s, the near elimination of syphilis in 1957 has been followed by cyclic national epidemics every 7–10 years (CDC, 1998a). The most recent epidemic occurred in 1990. Since then, syphilis rates have declined 88% (CDC, 2000f).

Transmission

The bacterium spreads from the sores of an infected person to the mucous membranes of the genital area, the mouth, or the anus of a sexual partner. It also can pass through broken skin on other parts of the body. The syphilis bacterium is very fragile, and the infection is rarely, if ever, spread by contact with objects such as toilet seats or towels. A pregnant woman with syphilis can pass the bacterium to her unborn child, who may be born with serious mental and physical problems as a result of this infection. The most common way to get syphilis is to have sex with someone who has an active infection. The rise in horizontal transmission of this disease resulted in an equally dramatic increase in the number of infants born with congenital syphilis acquired via vertical transmission. The first decline in the number of reported cases of syphilis occurred in 1994 ("AIDS Fear Brings Syphilis Decline," 1994), with a corresponding decline in the number of reported cases of congenital syphilis.

In 1999, 556 cases of congenital syphilis were reported. Peaks in congenital syphilis usually occur one year after peaks in primary and secondary syphilis (CDC, 2000f).

Symptoms

Syphilis is characterized by three distinct stages. The first stage, considered the primary stage, is distinguished by a painless lesion or chancre appearing at the site where the bacterium first entered the body. The sore usually appears between 10 and 90 days after contact with an infected person. The lesion may go unnoticed and is particularly difficult to discern in women because it can present inside the vagina, where it is not easily seen without a pelvic examination. The lesion can also be found on the penis or inside the mouth or anus. When syphilis goes unnoticed in the primary stage, it progresses to the second stage of infection, known as secondary syphilis (see Figure 26-11). Secondary syphilis presents as numerous, highly infectious lesions and may include flulike symptoms and even hair loss. Another recognizable feature of this stage is the characteristic rash on the palms of the hands and the soles of the feet.

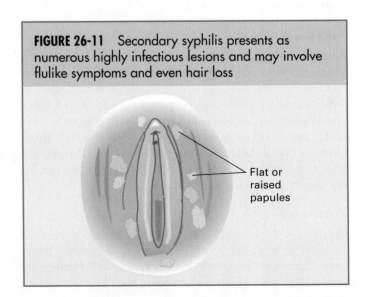

FIGURE 26-11 Secondary syphilis presents as numerous highly infectious lesions and may involve flulike symptoms and even hair loss

Flat or raised papules

A generalized rash occurs in some individuals. Tertiary infection is extremely rare and appears 3–10 years after the initial stages of disease. Irreversible complications of this stage include mental deterioration and loss of vision, balance, and sensation.

Diagnosis

Diagnosis of syphilis can by made at any stage of the disease via the VDRL (Venereal Disease Research Laboratory) or the RPR (Rapid Plasma Reagin) test. Both of these tests are relatively inexpensive and easy to access. Recent studies support the critical need for early diagnosis of syphilis because it seems to be a marker for the prevalence of HIV infection. Individuals who are HIV positive may present with syphilis that has already progressed to the secondary stage, with the course of the disease advancing at an accelerated pace (Hutchinson, Hook, Shepherd, Verley, & Rompalo, 1994). Because of the serious complications to the fetus of the woman with syphilis, it is recommended that all women be screened for the disease in the first trimester of pregnancy (Chin, 2000). Annual screening is recommended for sexually active and high-risk individuals.

Treatment

Penicillin G, administered by injection, is the drug of choice in the treatment of syphilis at all stages. Other antibiotics can be used for patients allergic to penicillin. A person usually can no longer transmit syphilis 24 hours after beginning therapy. It is important to retest clients to eliminate the potential for treatment failure. Although proper treatment in all stages of syphilis will cure the disease, the damage done to organs, primarily in late syphilis, cannot be reversed.

Gonorrhea

Neisseria gonorrhoeae is a common sexually transmitted disease that affects approximately 1 million Americans each year. Because of a lack of symptoms, the disease may go unnoticed. Gonorrhea is caused by the gonococcus bacterium, which grows and multiplies quickly in moist, warm areas of the body, such as the cervix, urethra, mouth, or rectum. In women, the cervix is the most common site of infection. However, the disease can spread to the uterus and fallopian tubes, resulting in PID, which, in turn, can cause infertility and ectopic pregnancy.

Transmission

Most commonly transmitted during genital sexual activity, gonorrhea can also be passed from the genitals of one partner to the throat of the other during oral sex (pharyngeal gonorrhea). Gonorrhea of the rectum can occur in people who practice anal intercourse and may also occur in women as a result of the spread of infection from the vaginal area. Gonorrhea can be passed from an infected woman to her newborn infant during delivery. When the infection occurs in children, it is most commonly due to sexual abuse. It is important to recognize the existence of a chronic **carrier** state, which can develop in both men and women with gonorrhea. A **carrier** can harbor an infectious agent without showing noticeable signs of disease or infection. The carrier state can be temporary or chronic.

Symptoms

It is estimated that 25%–80% of infected women have no symptoms of infection. Symptoms in women present initially as a mild cervicitis or urethritis. Men typically present with a purulent discharge or dysuria. Complications of the disease occur if the disease goes untreated. Pelvic inflammatory disease, endometriosis, and infertility are recognized complications of untreated disease. Newborns born to infected mothers and exposed to the infection in the birth canal are at high risk for the development of conjunctivitis. If not promptly treated, this infection can cause blindness in the newborn.

Diagnosis

Gonorrhea is diagnosed via a microscopic examination of exudate and via bacterial cultures. Because of the growing number of antibiotic-resistant gonorrhea strains, it is important to test organisms for sensitivity to specific antibiotics to prevent ineffective treatment and relapse of disease.

Treatment

Gonorrhea is treated with antibiotics that have been shown to be effective against the strain of gonorrhea cultured in the laboratory. Current antibiotics in widespread use for the treatment of gonorrhea include many of the cephalosporins and, most recently, azithromycin (Chin, 2000). Because of the high probability that individuals infected with gonorrhea are also infected with chlamydia, treatment regimes which include agents that are effective against both organisms should be routine. The development of antibiotic-resistant strains of *N. gonorrhoeae* have complicated the treatment picture.

Trichomoniasis

Trichomonas vaginalis ("trich") causes a common STD that attacks as many as 2–3 million Americans each year. Trichomoniasis is found worldwide and is a frequent disease of adults. Approximately 20% of females will become infected with *T. vaginalis* during their reproductive years (Chin, 2000).

Transmission

Transmission of the bacterium occurs via sex with an infected individual.

TABLE 26-5 Summary of Sexually Transmitted Disease

DISEASE	INCUBATION PERIOD*	SYMPTOMS	DIAGNOSIS	TREATMENT	NURSING ROLE
Bacterial					
Chlamydia	7–14 days	*Women:* vaginal discharge, itching, burning of the vagina, pelvic inflammatory disease (PID). Women are often asymptomatic. *Men:* penile discharge dysuria, burning or itching at the urethral opening, epididymitis. Men are often asymptomatic.	Vaginal culture; Gram stain of endocervical or urethral discharge	Tetracycline, doxycycline, or azithromycin	Partner notification; educate client regarding barrier methods to prevent reinfection and avoid sex until therapy is complete and both partners are asymptomatic; educate client about the importance of following medication instructions and completing therapy; recommend HIV testing.
Gonorrhea	2–21 days	*Women:* May be asymptomatic; abdominal pain, dysuria; vaginal discharge *Men:* urethritis, discharge, dysuria and frequency, epididymitis; may be asymptomatic	Culture and sensitivity	Doxycycline, spectinomycin, or ceftriaxone	Partner notification and screening; educate client regarding barrier methods to prevent reinfection and avoid sex until therapy is complete and both partners are asymptomatic; educate client about the importance of following medication instructions and completing therapy; recommend HIV testing; reevaluate if symptoms persist.
Syphilis, primary	10–90 days	Primary syphilis: painless chancre	VDRL (reactive 14 days after appearance of chancre)	Benzathine penicillin G	Partner notification and screening; recommend HIV testing; reevaluate at 3- and 6-month intervals.
Syphilis, secondary	6 weeks–6 months	Fever, malaise, headache, sore throat, rash	Clinical signs and symptoms	Benzathine penicillin G	Partner notification and screening; recommend HIV testing.
Syphilis, tertiary	Within 1 year of infection	Early latency period; individuals are often asymptomatic; however, lesions may reoccur.	VDRL	Benzathine penicillin G	Partner notification and screening; recommend HIV testing.

	After 1 year from date of original infection	Late latency period, asymptomatic; noninfectious except to fetus of pregnant women	Examine cerebral spinal fluid cell count and VDRL		Partner notification; educate client regarding barrier methods to prevent reinfection and avoid sex until therapy is complete and both partners are asymptomatic; educate client about the importance of following medication instructions and completing therapy; recommend HIV testing.
	Late active, 2–40 years	Gummas of skin, bone and mucous membranes, heart, liver; paresis, optic atrophy; aortic aneurysm, aortic valve insufficiency			
Chancroid	3–7 days	Irregular papule that progresses to deep very painful ulcer that drains blood or pus; inguinal tenderness and dysuria	Examine lesion	Azithromycin, erythromycin, or ceftriaxone	
Viral					
Hepatitis B virus (HBV)	4 weeks	Variation of symptoms between subclinical infection to cirrhosis, liver cancer	Serum IgM alpha HBc	No cure; treatment is palliative	Partner notification; educate client regarding barrier methods; educate client about the importance of immunization; recommend HIV testing.
Genital warts (human papillomavirus)	Varies from 4 weeks to 9 months	Varies between subclinical infection, cauliflower lesions in varying numbers near vaginal opening, anus, penis, vagina, cervix. Certain types increase risk of cervical cancer.	Pap smear; visual inspection of lesions	No cure; lesions may disappear without treatment; removal of lesions or topical medication	Partner notification; educate client regarding barrier methods to prevent reinfection; recommend HIV testing and importance of annual Pap smear.
Genital herpes: herpes simplex	2–20 days	Vesicles which progress to painful ulcerations of vagina, labia, perineum, penis, or anus. Lesions last for weeks and reinfection is common. Virus may be present at times individual is asymptomatic.	Presence of vesicles; viral culture if lesion is present	No cure; acyclovir, famcyclovir, and valacyclovir may minimize symptoms and duration of lesions	Partner notification; educate client regarding barrier methods; recommend HIV testing and annual Pap smear.

*Numbers are approximate.

Symptoms

Many individuals experience no symptoms. Trichomoniasis often presents as an unusual vaginitis in women. The thin, foamy, vaginal discharge has a characteristic greenish yellow color and a very foul odor. Women with symptoms may experience vaginal or vulval redness accompanied by small petechial or punctate red spots. Other common symptoms are itching, burning, and painful urination. Men experience mild symptoms and may complain of a "tingling" inside the penis. Trichomoniasis may coexist with gonorrhea and may facilitate HIV infection. When trichomoniasis is diagnosed, a complete STD check is recommended. When symptoms occur, they usually appear within 4–20 days of exposure, although symptoms can appear years after infection.

Diagnosis

Either microscopic examination or a culture of the discharge can confirm the diagnosis. The infection is often diagnosed by being observed on a routine Pap smear.

Treatment

A single dose of metronidazole (Flagyl) is effective in treating most cases of trichomoniasis. Although symptoms of trichomoniasis in men may disappear within a few weeks without treatment, men can transmit the disease to their sex partners even when symptoms are not present. It is therefore preferable to treat both partners to eliminate the organism.

Role of the Community Health Nurse in the Prevention of Sexually Transmitted Diseases

Prevention of all STDs involves educating the public about the frequency and the often deadly consequences of these diseases, both to individuals and to newborns exposed to the various infections during pregnancy or vaginal delivery.

Primary-prevention efforts currently focus on educating health care providers and the public about the signs of STDs, instructing individuals on ways to avoid exposure, and emphasizing the need for regular checkups. Community health nurses can help prevent the spread of sexually transmitted infection by promoting safe-sex behavior and the need for correct and consistent condom use. Prevention efforts should also include education about immunization, when appropriate. Individuals should be educated about the potential spread of these infections via oral or anal sex and, in some cases, IV drug use or sharing of body fluids. Young people should be taught about the risks of having multiple sex partners and participating in casual sexual activity and of the health value of delaying the initiation of sexual activity. Clients should be warned about new evidence that suggests increased risk of HIV infection in

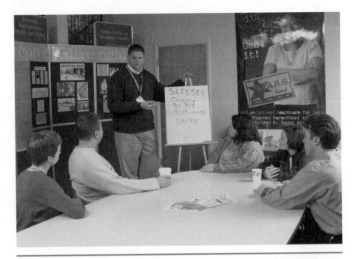

The community health nurse must take advantage of every opportunity to counsel on safe-sex practices.

individuals who have a history of STD. In their rush to help young clients prevent unwanted pregnancy, nurses must not forget to inform the public that oral contraceptives provide no protection against STDs and must be used with a form of barrier protection to defend against STD transmission.

Secondary-prevention efforts focus on early detection and treatment of infection as well as on partner notification to prevent further spread. Encouraging pregnant women to be screened for HIV infection to prevent the vertical transmission of infection is part of secondary prevention.

Tertiary-prevention efforts focus on minimizing and managing the effects of chronic STDs such as herpes, HIV infection, and untreated syphilis. Information provided to the public should take into consideration cultural differences: Educational materials and the manner whereby information is discussed should always be culturally appropriate. Table 26-5 summarizes selected STDs.

EMERGING INFECTIONS

In the United States, documented emerging infections include a variety of bacterial, parasitic, and viral diseases. In addition to infections classified in these documented categories, other types of agents, such as prions detected in the investigation of "mad cow disease," provide a constant challenge to disease investigators. The recent occurrence of Ebola-Reston virus in a quarantined population of primates located in a Texas holding station indicates the importance of understanding **zoonosis,** the transmission of infection from animals to humans, and the related potential threat to human survival (Strausbaugh, 1997). Other cases support the disregard agents have exhibited for geographic boundaries and barriers. "Raccoon rabies," once thought to be confined to the eastern United States, has spread westward (Deasy, 1996), and Lyme disease, once recognized only in Connecticut, has spread via the deer tick to dozens of states and countries, constituting a dramatic example of how an organism can become global within a decade. Food-borne illnesses such as hepatitis A and cyclospora infection transmitted via food processed in countries outside the United States illustrate the fact that contamination that takes place in one part of the globe can quickly be transmitted to human hosts in other parts of the world and be responsible for widespread illness (Getty, 1997).

Examples of pathogens that are resurgent (emerging with increased virulence) are listed in Table 26-6. **Virulence** is the degree of pathogenicity of the agent. Outbreaks of ebola and plague continue to surface throughout the world, and drug-resistant strains of agents have become increasingly common in the United States.

Factors Contributing to the Emergence of Infectious Disease

Human behavior plays a critical role in creating an optimal environment for the development and spread of new organisms. International travel, changing sexual mores, and high-risk behaviors create a vulnerable human host susceptible to disease organisms. Increased population and urbanization throughout the world provide for a changing ecology and an environment that supports the zoonotic transmission of disease. As humans expand their habitats into forests, jungles, and deserts, they come into contact with disease-causing organisms and the **vectors** (agents that actively carry a pathogen to a susceptible host) that transmit them. In many areas of the world, urban development has caused overcrowding, poor sanitation, and unclean drinking water. These conditions play a direct role in the transmission of disease (Lederberg & Shope, 1992; CDC, 1998a). The factors in disease emergence are as follows:

- Societal events: impoverishment, war or civil conflict, population growth, migration, urban decay
- Health care: new medical devices, organ or tissue transplantation, immunosuppressive drugs, widespread use of antibiotics
- Food production: globalization of food supplies, changes in food processing and packing methods
- Human behavior: sexual behavior, drug use, travel, diet, outdoor recreation, use of child care facilities
- Environmental changes: deforestation/reforestation, changes in water ecosystems, flood/drought, famine, global warming
- Public health infrastructure: curtailment or reduction in prevention programs, inadequate communicable disease surveillance, lack of trained personnel
- Microbial adaptation and change: changes in virulence and toxin production, development of drug resistance, microbes as cofactors in chronic diseases

The CDC (1998a) has developed a plan designed to prepare the United States for potential epidemics resulting

---

TABLE 26-6 Examples of Resurgent/Reemerging Infections and Factors Contributing to Their Reemergence

AGENT	FACTORS IN REEMERGENCE
Rabies	Breakdown in public health measures; changes in land use; travel
Dengue and dengue hemorrhagic fever	Transportation; travel and migration; urbanization
Acanthamebiasis	Introduction of soft contact lenses
Malaria	Favorable conditions for mosquito vector
Giardiasis	Increased use of child care facilities
Plague	Economic development; land use
Diphtheria	Interruption of immunization program due to political changes
Tuberculosis	Human demographics and behavior; industry and technology; international commerce and travel; breakdown of public health measures; microbial adaptation
Pertussis	Refusal to vaccinate because of the belief that vaccines are not safe
E. coli O157:H7	Food processing and shipment
Cholera	Travel; a new strain introduced to South America from Asia by ship

From ProMED: Pathogenic microbes and infectious diseases, *[On-line]. Available: www.fas.org/promed.*

from emerging infectious diseases: *Preventing Emerging Infectious Diseases: A Strategy for the 21st Century.* Four goals are outlined in this plan in an attempt to revitalize our nation's ability to identify and contain infectious agents that pose a potential threat to our populace. The goals are related to surveillance and response, applied research, prevention and control, and infrastructure. Each of these areas holds equal importance in the challenging fight against emerging infections (CDC, 1998a).

Emerging infections were brought into the spotlight within the medical community after the 1992 Institute of Medicine (IOM) report entitled *Emerging Infections: Microbial Threats to Health in the United States* (Lederberg & Shope, 1992). Along with the ability to recognize emerging infections, community health nurses have the additional obligation of participating in effective surveillance, treatment, and case management of these diseases.

Examples of Emerging Infections

Ebola

Ebola burst on the communicable disease frontier in April 1995, with remarkable outbreaks of severe hemorrhagic fever in Kikwit, Democratic Republic of the Congo (formerly Zaire) (Rodier, 1997). The disease has a rapid incubation period, and, in Zaire, the virus had a case fatality of more than 90%. Much of what is known about the Ebola virus was developed by the CDC Infectious Disease Surveillance Team that rushed to Kikwit in an effort to track the evolution of this fatal disease.

Transmission

The virus is spread from person to person by direct contact with infected blood, secretions, organs, or semen. Epidemics have resulted from person-to-person transmission, nosocomial transmission, and laboratory infections. After infection, the virus spreads through the blood and is replicated in many organs (Chin, 2000).

Symptoms

Infected individuals manifest bleeding in the mucosa, abdomen, pericardium, and vagina. Bleeding, shock, and acute respiratory disorder are the causes of fatality among those infected with the Ebola virus. When the illness is severe, infected persons sustain high fevers and become delirious and difficult to control (Chin, 2000).

Diagnosis

Ebola is diagnosed via the ELISA test for the specific immunoglobulin G (IgG) antibody.

Treatment

There is no known cure for Ebola.

Prevention

The basic method of prevention and control is the interruption of person-to-person spread of the virus.

Multidrug-Resistant Tuberculosis

"In hospitals alone, an estimated one million bacterial infections are occurring worldwide every day, and most of these are drug resistant" (WHO, 1997b). The incidence of TB in the United States increased 20% between 1985 and 1992 (CDC, 1998a) but declined from 1992 to 1997 (CDC, 1998c). The increase can be attributed to a number of factors, including the HIV epidemic, the deterioration in local public health infrastructure, immigration from countries where TB is **endemic** (i.e., prevalent), and increasing poverty and homelessness. The later decline was a result of prompt identification and reporting of cases and close follow-up to ensure completion of treatment. The alarming rise in new cases of TB was particularly troubling because a growing percentage of cases are resistant to traditional drug therapy. When an individual has TB and does not complete the recommended course of medication therapy (six months), resistant strains of the organisms develop. Tubercle bacillus mutations are responsible for reported drug resistance in TB. Using only one drug to treat TB disease can create a population of tubercle bacilli that are resistant to that particular drug. Drug resistance is costly to the individual and society. Figure 26-12 demonstrates the dramatic increase in treatment cost for multidrug-resistant TB.

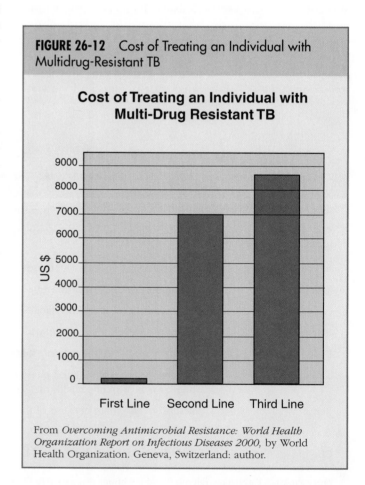

FIGURE 26-12 Cost of Treating an Individual with Multidrug-Resistant TB

From *Overcoming Antimicrobial Resistance: World Health Organization Report on Infectious Diseases 2000,* by World Health Organization. Geneva, Switzerland: author.

Symptoms

Common symptoms of TB include fever, cough, hemoptysis, fatigue, weight loss, and chest pain.

Diagnosis

Drug resistance is confirmed by laboratory culture and sensitivity.

Treatment

Currently, a four-drug regime (isoniazid, rifampin, pyrazinamide, and ethambutol or streptomycin) is considered essential in preventing multidrug-resistant cases (NJMC National Tuberculosis Center, 2001). Direct observed therapy (DOT) has shown promising results in ensuring that individuals comply with the full course of drug therapy and, thus, in decreasing the threat of resistant organisms.

Prevention

Primary-prevention measures involve educating the public about the necessity to complete drug therapy. Secondary prevention includes minimizing the disease's ability to spread within the community. The nosocomial spread of drug-resistant organisms has created the need for special isolation protocols including negative-pressure rooms with sophisticated air exchange systems that prevent the nosocomial spread of disease within the hospital population. In addition, DOT has proved useful in preventing treatment failures in individuals with poor compliance records.

Hantavirus Pulmonary Syndrome

In 1993 a cluster of deaths in New Mexico set in motion a local, state, and federal investigation that lead to the identification of the lethal hantavirus. Hantavirus pulmonary syndrome (HPS) is a serious, potentially lethal respiratory disease. The number of cases and the geographic locations where the disease is found have increased dramatically since hantavirus was first identified in 1993. A total of 350–400 cases of HPS have been confirmed (WHO, 1997b). Of these cases, approximately 45% were fatal. The high mortality associated with this syndrome is generally thought to be due to the sudden onset of respiratory distress and pulmonary edema in previously healthy young people. The average age of victims of this disease is 37 years.

Transmission

The disease is caused by a hantavirus that is carried by rodents, primarily the deer mouse, and subsequently passed on to humans through infected rodent feces, urine, and saliva. Breathing the virus is the most common way that the virus is spread from rodents to people. The virus enters the air in an aerosol often caused by sweeping the rodent's fecal droppings or urine in an attempt to clean an outdoor area. Transmission is believed to be primarily from rodent to person. After the investigation of outbreaks in Argentina and Chile in 1995, however, strong evidence now suggests the possibility of person-to-person transmission (CDC, 1999a). Transmission is also possible through direct contact with contaminated materials or a rodent's bite (Chin, 2000).

Symptoms

Hantavirus infection is characterized by a febrile illness (temperature greater than 101.0°F) and bilateral diffuse interstitial edema accompanied by shortness of breath that requires supplemental oxygen within 72 hours of hospitalization, all occurring in a previously healthy person. Respiratory symptoms are often accompanied by headache; abdominal, joint, and low-back pain; and, occasionally, nausea and vomiting.

Diagnosis

ELISA and/or Western blot can establish the diagnosis of hantavirus infection by demonstrating specific IgM antibodies.

Treatment

Treatment for hantavirus infection is currently limited to supportive care. This includes controlling for fever, providing respiratory support, observing and treating for hypertension and hemorrhage, and administering medication to control pulmonary edema and other complications. Critical care unit services are essential for acutely ill clients.

Prevention

Strict barrier nursing techniques are now recommended for management of confirmed or suspected cases of hantavirus infection. Control measures focus on educating the public about the importance of rodent control in endemic areas. It is important to reduce those areas in and around buildings that may prove an attractive habitat for rodents. It is recommended that disinfectants such as chlorine bleach solution be used to decontaminate areas with potentially infectious droppings *prior* to cleaning. Surgical masks or other protective clothing may also be appropriate for cleaning high-risk areas. Figure 26-13 lists recommendations to minimize the risk of hantavirus infection. Public health workers investigating outbreaks must use caution to protect themselves during disease investigation.

E. coli:O157:H7

Escherichi coli is an emerging cause of foodborne illness. In early 1993, hamburgers contaminated with this bacterial strain caused a multistate outbreak of severe bloody diarrhea and serious kidney disease. More than 700 children and adults were affected, and four children died during this outbreak. After this episode, which was

> **FIGURE 26-13** Recommendations to Minimize Risk of Hantavirus Infection
>
> - Air out abandoned or unused cabins before occupying. Inspect premises for rodents and do not occupy if there is evidence of rodent infestation.
> - If sleeping outdoors, check potential campsites for rodent droppings or habitat.
> - Avoid sleeping near woodpiles, garbage sites, or other areas that may be attractive to rodents.
> - Avoid sleeping on the bare ground. If possible, sleep on elevated cots or mats.
> - Store food in rodent-proof containers and dispose of garbage promptly.
> - Do not seek out or disturb rodents, burrows, or dens.
>
> Adapted from "Hantavirus Pulmonary Syndrome—Chile, 1997" by Centers for Disease Control and Prevention, 1997, *Morbidity and Mortality Weekly Report, 46,* p. 949.

> **FIGURE 26-14** Ways to Prevent *E. coli* O157: H7 Infection
>
> - Cook ground beef or hamburger until the meat is gray or brown and the juices run clear. The inside of the meat should be hot.
> - Send undercooked hamburger received in a restaurant back for further cooking.
> - Consume only pasteurized milk and milk products. Avoid raw milk.
> - Infected persons should wash hands carefully to prevent spread of infection.
> - Drink municipal water that has been treated with adequate levels of chlorine.

linked to undercooked hamburgers served at a fast-food chain in Seattle, Washington, the syndrome began to be referred to as "fast-food syndrome." *Escherichia coli* O157:H7 is one of hundreds of strains of *E. coli* bacteria. Most of the strains are harmless, but this strain is especially virulent and produces a toxin that can lead to severe illness and death.

Transmission

Transmission occurs via ingestion of contaminated foods.

Symptoms

Though sometimes asymptomatic, infection with the *E. coli* O157:H7 virus often causes bloody diarrhea and abdominal cramps. In 2%–7% of cases, particularly in children under 5 years of age, the infection can lead to hemolytic uremic syndrome, which can cause kidney failure. The illness resolves in 5–10 days. The increasing numbers of commonly consumed food items contaminated with infectious agents place large numbers of persons at risk (CDC, 1996b).

Diagnosis

Stool cultures are helpful to confirm the presence of the virus. The clinical picture assists in diagnosis.

Treatment

Treatment varies depending on the severity of the illness. Fluid and electrolyte replacement is indicated when watery diarrhea is present or if there are signs of dehydration.

Prevention

Radiation of beef has been suggested as a public health prevention measure to kill the bacteria in the nation's food supply. Adequate handwashing and proper cooking prevent the disease. Figure 26-14 lists the steps that individuals can take to prevent *E. coli* infection.

Lyme Disease

Lyme disease was first recognized in 1975 after a puzzling outbreak of arthritis in children near Lyme, Connecticut. By 1993, Lyme disease had been reported in 44 states and has become the most commonly reported vector-borne infectious disease in the United States (CDC, 1997b).

Transmission

The disease agent is carried by ticks and is transmitted when an individual is bitten by the deer tick.

Symptoms

Lyme disease is a multisystem disorder caused by *Borrelia burgdorferi,* a spirochete. This spirochete is transmitted from mammal to mammal by a small, hard tick. Erythema migrans, or the "bull's-eye" rash that has become a characteristic finding in the disease, appears at the site of the tick bite after approximately one week in some infected individuals (Walker et al., 1996). This infection presents as flulike symptoms indistinguishable from those of many other illnesses. Recurrent arthritis, neurological symptoms, heart problems, and severe fatigue are commonly reported by infected individuals.

Diagnosis

Lyme disease is difficult to diagnose because many of the symptoms mimic those of other diseases. The only distinctive hallmark that seems to be unique to Lyme disease is the erythema migrans rash. However, the rash is absent in at least 25% of cases. Isolation of the agent from a skin biopsy or blood or serological evidence from serum samples confirms the diagnosis. In cases in which the diagnosis of late Lyme disease is considered, isolation of the organism from the client is rare, and laboratory support for the diagnosis depends on serological assay. The ELISA test followed by Western blot for positive or borderline reactions is the recommended diagnostic procedure (Walker et al., 1996).

Treatment

Effective treatment is essential in preventing long-term consequences of the infection. Antibiotics such as doxycyline or amoxicillin taken over a two-week period usually prevent the development of arthritis or other serious health problems. Early diagnosis is critical because the sooner the antibiotic therapy is started, the more complete the recovery. In many cases, Lyme disease is only considered after every other option has been explored, causing a delay in effective treatment.

Prevention

Prevention efforts focus on avoiding tick-endemic areas, wearing long sleeves and long pants in endemic areas, inspecting for the tiny (pinhead-sized) deer tick, and applying tick repellent when going outside. Infection usually takes place in the summer, when people venture into forested areas for recreation. People should be educated about the possibility of Lyme disease and the need to check for ticks after outdoor activity in a wooded area. Researchers believe that a tick must be attached for many hours to be able to transmit Lyme disease and that prompt tick removal can thus prevent infection (CDC, 1998a). Ticks should be removed with tweezers using steady gentle pulling. Because the infection can be transmitted from the tick's body fluids, the tick's body should not be squeezed during the removal process (Mandell, Bennett, & Dolin, 1995).

The CDC's Advisory Committee on Immunization Practices (ACIP) provides recommendations for use of a newly developed recombinant outer-surface protein A (rOspA) Lyme disease vaccine (LYMErix, SmithKline Beecham Pharmaceuticals) for persons aged 15–70 years in the United States. The purpose of these recommendations is to provide health care providers, public health authorities, and the public with guidance regarding the risk for acquiring Lyme disease and the role of vaccination as an adjunct to preventing Lyme disease. Decisions regarding vaccine use should be based on a thorough assessment of individual risk, which should include evaluation of the geographic area and the person's activities and behaviors relating to tick exposure (CDC, 1999b).

OTHER COMMUNICABLE DISEASES

Tuberculosis

Evidence suggests that *Mycobacterium tuberculosis* (TB) has been around for centuries. Traces of lesions from tuberculosis have been isolated from the lungs of Egyptian mummies. With the flurry of research and funding for the AIDS epidemic, tuberculosis has been called the "forgotten plague."

The incidence of TB increased at an alarming rate between 1985 and 1992. During this period, the number of TB cases increased by 20% among the general population and by 35% among children. Since 1992, there has been a 31% decrease in the number of reported cases of TB. This reduction can be attributed to effective TB control programs that include early identification, appropriate therapy, and assurance that therapy has been completed. Following the resurgence of TB and the emergence of multidrug-resistant TB as a public health threat, federal resources were delegated to rebuild the public health infrastructure. The subsequent 31% decrease in TB cases from 1992 to 1998 is a notable public health achievement (CDC, 2001b).

Though the United States has experienced success in TB control, this must be balanced with the increase in disease rate among foreign-born persons. Persons born in Asia, Africa, or Latin America, where TB rates are 5–30 times higher than U.S. rates, are at increased risk for the development of TB. The TB case rate for foreign-born persons is at least 4–5 times higher than for U.S.-born persons (CDC, 1999b).

Worldwide, 8 million cases and 2 million deaths per year have been attributed to TB. Global TB control efforts have been hampered by the lack of effective TB control programs. The World Health Organization (WHO) has developed several strategies to combat this pandemic (CDC, 2001b). The prevalence of TB among persons infected with HIV has been particularly notable. Approximately 10% of HIV-positive individuals are also infected with TB.

Transmission

When an infected individual coughs or sneezes, droplet nuclei containing tubercle bacilli may be expelled in the air. For the TB organism to be transmitted, another person must inhale the droplet nuclei.

Symptoms

Symptoms of TB include fatigue, weight loss, night sweats and chills, and persistent coughing accompanied by blood-streaked sputum. Most people who become infected with the TB organism do not progress to the active-disease stage. They remain asymptomatic and noninfectious. These individuals, who have positive skin tests but negative chest x-rays, retain a lifelong risk of developing TB. Preventive therapy is recommended to minimize the risk of developing active TB. Without treatment, active TB is usually fatal. It should be remembered that TB is not exclusively a pulmonary disease; it is a systemic disease that can affect any body organ or system. Extrapulmonary TB is most often seen in persons with HIV infection. Clients with extrapulmonary TB should be tested for the HIV virus if HIV status is unknown.

Diagnosis

According to the National Tuberculosis Center, there are four steps in diagnosing TB disease: medical history, tuberculin skin test, chest x-ray, and bacteriologic examination. Persons who report exposure to a TB-infected person or symptoms of TB or who have risk factors for developing TB should be given a tuberculin skin test. The Mantoux skin test is the preferred type of screening test because it is more accurate than other available skin tests. If a person tests positive on the skin test, a chest x-ray is used to evaluate whether the person has pulmonary TB disease. The bacteriologic examination of sputum is necessary to confirm active TB disease. Persons with positive smears are considered infectious. The specimen should be sent for culture and sensitivity analysis to determine whether it contains *M. tuberculosis* and, if it does, drug resistance (NJMC National Tuberculosis Center, 2001). High-risk groups that should be screened for tuberculosis are listed in Figure 26-15.

Treatment

Treatment for TB is lengthy when compared with that for other infectious diseases. Preventive therapy can be effective in preventing active disease. Skin testing can identify appropriate candidates for prevention therapy. To prevent the development of TB disease, the typical regime requires 6 months of chemotherapy treatment, usually with isoniazid, in persons with documented TB infection. Children should receive 9 months of preventive therapy, and individuals with HIV should receive 12 months of preventive therapy.

If infection progresses to active TB disease, health care providers must prescribe an adequate treatment regime. If treatment is not continued long enough, some of the TB organisms will survive, and the potential for relapse increases. In most areas of the country, TB disease treatment should include four drugs: isoniazid, rifampin,

pyrazinamide, and either ethambutol or streptomycin for a minimum of six months. This regime may be changed on the basis of reliable culture and sensitivity results. Clients who do not take the treatment as prescribed may relapse and develop drug resistance. Direct observed therapy (DOT) is one way to ensure that clients adhere to drug treatment requirements and has proved to be cost effective in the treatment of TB disease (NJMC National Tuberculosis Center, 2001).

Prevention

Primary prevention efforts include health promotion and education. Immunization is not widely used in the United States except in well-defined circumstances, because the incidence of TB is relatively low. Skin testing is commonly used as a control measure aimed at early detection. Chemoprophylaxis is widely used for prevention of active TB. Isoniazid (INH), an anti-tuberculin drug, is the most common form of prophylaxis. Adequate chemotherapy and instructing the person who has symptoms suggestive of TB to cover the nose and mouth when coughing, laughing, or sneezing can reduce transmission of TB. Ultraviolet light and sunlight, as well as adequate ventilation, can further reduce transmission. Secondary-prevention efforts focus on screening members of high-risk populations (see Figure 26-15) and on early diagnosis and treatment. Tertiary prevention involves monitoring long-term health status and direct observed therapy.

Role of the Health Department in Prevention of Tuberculosis

Early reporting of suspected or confirmed TB cases is important for the control of TB. The public health department provides clients and clinicians with access to resources for assistance in case management and contact identification. The health department conducts contact investigations to determine who has been exposed to TB so that tuberculin skin testing can be performed and, when indicated, preventive therapy can be initiated.

Role of Community Health Nurse in Prevention of Tuberculosis

Community health nurses are often the individuals responsible for skin testing, reading, and referral. The nurse should be aware of persons who are at risk for infection and instigate screening clinics to facilitate early diagnosis in high-risk populations. Community health nurses have maintained growing case loads of persons with TB disease in varying stages. The nurse must understand the distinction between TB infection and disease as well as mode of TB transmission. Identification of contacts of individuals with TB disease enables the nurse to recommend preventive therapy and interrupt the spread of infection.

FIGURE 26-15 High-Risk Groups to Screen for Tuberculosis

- People with HIV infection
- Close contacts of infectious tuberculosis cases
- People with medical conditions that increase the risk of tuberculosis
- Immigrants from countries where TB is endemic
- Low-income populations
- Alcoholics and IV-drug users
- Residents of long-term care facilities
- Individuals living in congregate settings (e.g., shelters, prisons, and hospitals)
- Health care workers and others who provide service to high-risk groups

The community health nurse is frequently the health professional responsible for DOT in noncompliant individuals. The importance of ensuring that the community is safe by documenting that infected individuals have completed adequate treatment cannot be overstated. Community health nurses are also responsible for educating clients regarding medications, including appropriate dosages and potential side effects. A symptoms checklist, administered periodically by community health nurses, is an effective way of documenting effectiveness of treatment and adverse side effects of medication. The American Nurses Association (ANA) has developed a position statement on tuberculosis and public health nursing. Relevant points are summarized in Figure 26-16. Community health nurses should participate with other health care workers in having annual purified protein derivative (PPD) skin tests. A checklist for tuberculin skin testing is provided in Figure 26-17.

Use of Bacillus Calmette-Guerin Vaccine

In many parts of the world, Bacillus Calmette-Guerin (BCG) vaccine is routinely used to prevent serious complications of TB. Immigrants should be asked whether they have received BCG vaccine before they are given a Mantoux skin test. The BCG vaccine is not recommended as a preventive strategy in the control of TB in the United States because of its interference with tuberculin skin testing. Although evidence is conflicting, research indicates that neither TB infection nor pulmonary TB is completely prevented by the BCG vaccine. Some studies suggest that BCG vaccination does lessen the likelihood of disseminated TB and TB meningitis in infants. Therefore, BCG may be indicated for infants and children living in households where they have close contact with an individual who has persistently untreated or ineffectively treated, sputum-positive tuberculosis, especially multidrug-resistant TB infection (Chin, 2000).

Hepatitis

Hepatitis, an inflammatory condition of the liver, can be caused by several bacterial or viral infections, fungal or parasitic infection, alcohol, drugs, or chemical toxins. The inflammation destroys patches of liver tissue and can ultimately cause death. Despite the many origins of this disease condition, the symptoms, diagnosis, and treatment methods are similar and are discussed here in general terms.

Symptoms

Symptoms associated with hepatitis depend on the type and severity of infection. The infection may be mild and, in some cases, can go undetected or it may be severe and life threatening. Hepatitis symptoms include jaundice, hepatomegaly, anorexia, muscle aches, nausea, vomiting, changes in taste and smell, clay-colored stools, and tea-colored urine. Physical examination may be perfectly normal, although enlarged lymph nodes, liver, and spleen are common findings.

FIGURE 26-16 ANA Position Statement on Tuberculosis and Public Health Nursing

- The use of a nursing care management model
- Supervision of unlicensed assistive personnel
- Enhancement of role in surveillance, assessment, treatment, and evaluation activities
- Collaboration with other agencies to "encourage research on the development and implementation of different treatment models of care" (p. 1).
- Innovative demonstration projects
- Nursing research initiatives on the effectiveness of different treatment modalities and documentation of the "most effective control measures which will prevent the transmission of TB to nurses providing treatment" (p. 1).

Adapted from *Position Statement on Tuberculosis and Public Health Nursing,* by American Nurses Association, 1997 [On-line]. Available: http://www.ana.org/readroom/position/blood/bltbhl.htm.

FIGURE 26-17 TB Skin Testing Recommendations

Mantoux tuberculin testing is the standard used to identify persons infected with TB.

1. Inject 0.1 ml of purified protein derivative (PPD) containing 5 tuberculin units (TU) intradermally into the forearm.
2. Document the site location in the client's record.
3. Read the test 48 to 72 hours later.
4. Measure and record the induration (not the erythema) in millimeters:

- Reactions of ≥5 mm are classified as positive in the following groups:

Persons who are close contacts of a person with infectious TB

Persons with known or suspected HIV

Persons with chest x-rays suggestive of previous TB

Intravenous drug users

- A reaction of ≥10 mm is positive for all other persons who do not meet previous criteria but have other risk factors for TB.
- A reaction of ≥15 mm is positive for all persons who are not in a high-risk category.
- Persons with positive PPD skin tests should undergo a chest x-ray to rule out the possibility of active TB.

Perspectives... *

Anna said she was 65, but she looked much older. Her wrinkled face, stooped posture, and tired eyes told of a hard life. Her eyes refused to brighten, even with the good news.

"Anna, I've got great news! The sputum cultures were all negative. Your tuberculosis is no longer infectious. Aren't you excited?" As I explained the results of the lab report, Anna seemed annoyed, restless. She lit a cigarette.

"I saw Hitler, heard him speak. You ever meet anyone before who actually heard Hitler speak? He was a crazy man. Even though I was only thirteen, I could tell he was crazy . . . and all those blonde German goons goose steppin' around like they were better than the rest of us! It was somethin' to see, I'll give him that." Anna's voice trailed off.

"Anna, have you been taking your medicine?" I was now becoming upset. "There are too many pills in your bottles. You should only have six left and I count at least 10. How're we gonna get rid of the TB if you don't take your meds?"

"Whatever you say," Anna replied, puffing on her cigarette. "It's a cockroach, this disease. Keeps people nosing around into a person's business, sticking their heads into my things. It's a roach I tell you!"

"Anna," I questioned as I caught a whiff of her breath, "have you been drinking?"

"Just a little brandy . . . to help the pills go down," she chuckled.

"Hey, I'm a nurse too. Fancy that . . . I was a darn good nurse, too. Worked nights for 20 years, when my Jack was small. A nurse and a mother! Now you've got somethin' to tell your friends about old Anna!"

"Anna, time to take your pills, and now I have to come back tomorrow," I scolded. "It's because you've been drinking and not taking the pills. Anna you've got to take the pills so we can keep the negative cultures. You've got to help me or we'll never get 'the cockroach' off your back! I only have two weeks of clinical left, and I'd like to end on a happy note."

"A happy note," she repeated. "Okay, I'll take my pills . . . sing a few bars too," Anna laughed. "I'll sing for the roach and you!"

It was two days before graduation when the public health nurse called. "I thought you might want to know," she said slowly. "Anna died this morning. She liked you. Well, I just thought you might want to know."

I wish I'd asked her where . . . where she'd heard Hitler speak.

—Anonymous

Diagnosis

Laboratory studies reveal high liver function tests. Symptoms, physical examination, and laboratory findings cannot distinguish between the different types of viral hepatitis. Hepatitis serology laboratory tests are needed to make the specific diagnosis.

Treatment

Because hepatitis is a viral illness, there is no treatment. In mild cases, the liver is usually able to regenerate its tissue, but severe cases can lead to cirrhosis and chronic liver disease. Vaccines are now available for hepatitis A and B.

Most hepatitis infections are caused by viruses, which researchers named alphabetically as they were identified. The first hepatitis virus described was, of course, hepatitis A; hepatitis B was the next discovered. The identification of another hepatitis virus that tested negative for hepatitis type A and B was subsequently called hepatitis non-A, non-B. As researchers studied these viruses, hepatitis C was isolated and replaced the non-A, non-B classification. In recent years, hepatitis viruses D through G have been described, and the list continues to grow. Al-

though the viruses have similar clinical presentations, each differs in etiology, prevention, and control (Chin, 2000). Hepatitis viruses A through E are discussed next.

Hepatitis A

Transmission

Hepatitis A is caused by oral ingestion of the hepatitis A virus (HAV), which is found in the stool of persons with hepatitis A. It is usually spread from person to person by putting something in the mouth that has been contaminated with the stool of a person with hepatitis A. Because the virus is transmitted via the fecal/oral route, it is easily spread in areas where there are poor sanitary conditions or where good personal hygiene is not observed. Persons with HAV can spread the virus to others who live in the same household or with whom they have sexual contact. Casual contact, as in the office, factory, or school setting, does not spread the virus. Individuals working in day care centers or children attending day care centers, however, are at high risk for developing the disease.

The source of infection is either contact with an infected person or direct contact with infected fecal material that has entered food or water supplies. Outbreaks have been related to sewage-contaminated water, infected food handlers (who do not wash their hands after using the bathroom), and shellfish caught in waters contaminated by sewage (Chin, 2000). Hepatitis A is easily spread between family members if good handwashing is not a common practice before handling food and after using the bathroom.

Prevention

Hepatitis A infection typically resolves and does not result in chronic hepatitis. Deaths from HAV can occur, but they are rare. Individuals at high risk for acquiring the infection should take advantage of the hepatitis A vaccine. If persons are aware of exposure to hepatitis, immunoglobulin (Ig) can be administered to prevent the disease or to minimize symptoms. The benefit of Ig administration is protection against HAV for three to five months, depending on the dosage. It can be given before exposure to HAV or within two weeks after exposure. Travelers to areas with high rates of HAV should receive Ig if they did not receive the hepatitis A vaccine. Of the more than 10 million estimated people worldwide who acquire HAV each year, most recover within three to six months (Shovein, Damazo, & Hyams, 2000). Groups at high risk for contracting HAV are listed in Figure 26-18.

Hepatitis B

Transmission

Hepatitis B is sometimes referred to as "serum hepatitis" because it is spread via direct contact with infected blood. Blood transfusions, once a common source of hepatitis B

FIGURE 26-18 High-Risk Groups for Hepatitis A

- Day care workers
- Persons who work with HAV-infected animals or with HAV in a research setting. (Hepatitis A vaccine is not generally recommended for health care workers.)
- Persons with clotting factor disorders such as hemophilia
- Persons traveling or working in countries with high rates of HAV, such as Central or South America, the Caribbean, Mexico, Asia (except Japan), Africa, and southern or eastern Europe. (The first dose should be given at least four weeks before travel.)
- Persons who live in communities with high rates of HAV
- Men who have sex with men
- Persons who use illicit drugs
- Persons with chronic liver disease

High-risk individuals over 2 years of age should get the hepatitis A vaccine.

---

infection, are now considered safe owing to current screening tests. Hepatitis B virus (HBV) is carried in the blood and body fluids of an infected person. Considered the most prevalent of the hepatitis viruses, HBV is transmitted sexually, through shared needles, and from mother to child. The virus can pass between people through breaks in the skin, mouth, vagina, or penis. Hepatitis B is unlike hepatitis A in that a person can harbor HBV without being actively infected and can spread it to others (LaPook, 1995).

Hepatitis B is considered extremely contagious and is very hardy. Dried blood outside the body and containing HBV has been shown to be infectious up to a week or longer. Although most individuals infected with HBV recover fully, 6%–10% of infected individuals do not completely recover and become carriers (Stein, 1993). Carriers can transmit the infection to others throughout their lifetimes. This fact is important to remember because vertical transmission remains a primary cause of new infections. Hepatitis B is potentially lethal, and it is estimated that each year in the United States approximately 150,000 persons are infected, 11,000 persons are hospitalized, and 300–400 persons die from acute fulminant hepatitis.

A variable portion of persons with acute HBV infection develop chronic infection. Chronic HBV infection is defined as the presence of hepatitis B surface antigen (HBsAg) in serum for at least six months. The risk of developing chronic infection is age dependent and greatest for infants, who have a 90% chance of developing chronic infection if infected at birth. Overall, 30%–50% of children and 5%–10% of adults with acute infection will develop chronic infection (Edmunds, Medley, Nokes, Hall, E. Whittle, 1993). Persons with chronic HBV infection are at increased risk of developing chronic liver disease or primary hepatocellular carcinoma. Approximately 1–1.25 million people in the United States have chronic HBV infection, and 5000–6000 people die each year from HBV-induced chronic liver disease.

Chronic HBV infections are often detected via screening programs such as blood bank serological testing and refugee health screening. Cases of chronic HBV infection are not reportable to the National Notifiable Disease Surveillance System (NNDSS) (CDC, 2001a). Individuals with chronic disease are at increased risk of developing cirrhosis and liver cancer.

Persons with chronic HBV infection are a primary reservoir for transmission of HBV infections. A **reservoir** is any host or environment in which an infectious agent normally lives and multiplies. Any person testing positive for HBsAg is potentially infectious to both household and sexual contacts. These contacts should receive appropriate prophylaxis. Although chronic HBV infections are not reportable to NNDSS, all states are encouraged to make HBsAg positivity among pregnant women reportable. Pregnant women who are HBsAg positive may pass on the infection to their newborn infants, and prevention of perinatal HBV transmission requires intensive case management.

Prevention

Over the past 10 years, the most frequently reported risk factor for acute HBV was heterosexual activity (41%), followed by intravenous drug use (15%), homosexual activity (9%), household contact with a person with HBV (2%), and health care employment (1%). Many persons with HBV do not identify risk factors (31%), and their sources of infection may be other infected persons who are asymptomatic (CDC, 1997c). Efforts at disease control focus on prevention. Primary prevention is central to the prevention of this disease. A vaccine against HBV has been available since 1982. This vaccine requires three injections at specified intervals and is now part of routine immunization schedules for children. Immunization is encouraged in adolescents prior to the onset of sexual activity. Health care workers should also take advantage of immunization to prevent HBV. Screening of high-risk populations can assist in the early detection of disease and is an important component of secondary prevention. Tertiary prevention involves minimizing the effects of the disease, primarily liver damage caused by the infection.

Hepatitis C

Transmission

Hepatitis C virus (HCV) was not identified until 1988, when researchers realized it was responsible for most of what had been known as non-A, non-B hepatitis. Specifically, HCV was responsible for most cases of posttrans-

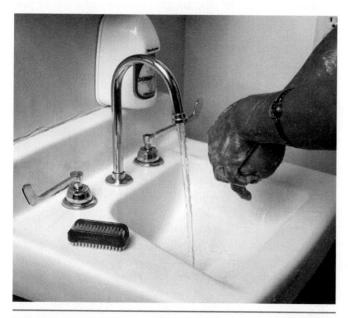

It is very important to stress handwashing to control the spread of communicable disease.

fusion hepatitis. The identification of the virus led to the development of a blood test in 1990, which has been useful in reducing, though not eliminating, the number of HCV infections among transfusion recipients. Currently in the United States, HCV is responsible for approximately 20% of acute viral hepatitis cases, of which fewer than 5% can be related to blood transfusions. Prevalence of HCV disease is highest among intravenous drug users and hemophiliacs (Chin, 2000). As with other forms of hepatitis, the disease may be spread through sexual contact. It is important to note that individuals with HCV have high rates of chronic disease in more than 60% of cases (Chin, 2000). Individuals who develop chronic disease are at increased risk for cirrhosis and liver cancer.

Prevention

Education and screening are important to prevent new cases and to minimize the effects of disease via early detection. Tertiary prevention is necessary to assist clients with chronic disease to be aware of risks, resources, and support systems. Many new support groups have formed to assist clients in living with HCV.

Hepatitis D

Transmission

Hepatitis D virus (HDV), or delta hepatitis, occurs only in clients with HBV and can cause a more serious form of hepatitis than is found with HBV alone (LaPook, 1995). Hepatitis D magnifies HBV's severity and can "coinfect" during the initial HBV episode or "superinfect" by infecting individuals with chronic HBV. Hepatitis D is considered the most severe form of hepatitis, killing 20%–25% of those it infects (Stein, 1993).

Prevention

Prevention of HBV via vaccination will also prevent coinfection with HDV. However, neither the HBV vaccination nor hepatitis B immunoglobulin (HBIg) will protect the HBV carrier from super infection with HDV (Chin, 2000).

Hepatitis E

Transmission

The clinical course of hepatitis E virus (HEV) is similar to that of hepatitis A. Outbreaks of disease occur most frequently in developing countries with inadequate sanitation. The disease is transmitted primarily through the fecal contamination of food or water. Hepatitis E is an acute infection that does not progress to the carrier state but can be fatal in up to 20% of pregnant women (Chin, 2000).

Prevention

Prevention should focus on improving sanitation and providing education about the importance of clean wa-

TABLE 26-7 Hepatitis Facts*

TYPES OF HEPATITIS	INCUBATION PERIOD	MODE OF TRANSMISSION	PREVENTION	POSSIBLE COMPLICATIONS
A	15–50 days	• Fecal-oral through contaminated food or water • Poor hygiene	• Immunize • Education on proper food handling	
B	45–180 days	• Unsafe sex • Poor hygiene • Body secretions • Blood transfusions • Contaminated needles	• Immunize • Educate to prevent exposures to blood and body fluids • Needle exchange programs • Identify carriers	• May become chronic • Cirrhosis • Liver cancer
C	2 weeks–6 months	• IV drug use • Blood transfusions	• Educate to prevent exposures to blood and body fluids • Needle exchange programs • Identify carriers	• May become chronic • Cirrhosis • Liver cancer
D	2–8 weeks	• Blood • Contaminated needles • Limited to those who have had HBV	• Immunize against HBV • Educate to prevent exposures to blood and body fluids • Needle exchange programs • Identify HBV carriers	• May become chronic • Cirrhosis
E	15–64 days	• Fecal-oral through contaminated water	• Vaccine is being developed • Practice sanitation • Travelers should be made aware of the risk of infection	• May be fatal in pregnant women

*Hepatitis symptoms: *Some individuals are asymptomatic—however, most viral hepatitis infections present with fever, chills, nausea, vomiting, diarrhea and fatigue. Individuals also report dark urine, jaundice, abdominal pain, anorexia, muscle aches, and light (clay-colored) stool.*

ter supplies and proper food handling and storage. Table 26-7 compares the different types of hepatitis.

Food- and Water-Borne Infections

The reporting of food- and water-borne diseases in the United States began more than 50 years ago when state and territorial health officers, concerned about the high morbidity and mortality associated with typhoid fever and infantile diarrhea, recommended that cases of "enteric fever" be investigated and reported. The purpose of investigating and reporting these cases was to obtain information regarding the role of food, milk, and water in outbreaks of intestinal illness as the basis for public health action. Beginning in 1923, the Public Health Service published summaries of outbreaks of gastrointesti-

nal illness attributed to milk. In 1938, it added summaries of outbreaks caused by all foods. These early surveillance efforts led to the enactment of important public health measures (e.g., the Model Milk Ordinance) that had a profound influence in decreasing the incidence of enteric diseases, particularly those transmitted by milk and water (CDC, 1996b).

Transmission

Water-borne pathogens typically enter water supplies via human or animal fecal contamination. Americans are so accustomed to safe, clean, and plentiful water supplies that the possibility of contamination is not considered until a problem arises. However, a clear appearance to water does not always indicate safety as drinking water, and outbreaks of gastrointestinal illness due to contaminated municipal water still occur in the United States.

Many of these outbreaks are associated with viral and parasitic infectious agents, such as cryptosporidium. The largest recorded water-borne disease outbreak in U.S. history occurred in Milwaukee, Wisconsin, in April 1993. The disease was cryptosporidiosis, a parasitic infection of the small intestine that can produce severe watery diarrhea. This outbreak of cryptosporidiosis affected over 400,000 people, and more than 4400 people were hospitalized.

Symptoms

Each year in the United States, water- and food-borne infections cause mild to severe illness in millions of people and are responsible for thousands of deaths. Symptoms range from mild to violent and severe gastrointestinal symptoms.

Diagnosis

Many food- and water-borne illnesses go undiagnosed and are in many cases unreported. Diagnosis can be confirmed via laboratory culture of suspected sources of infection.

Treatment

Treatment for food- and water-borne infections varies depending on the organism and the severity of illness. Fluid and electrolyte replacement is indicated in cases of severe diarrhea or vomiting.

Prevention

Preventing food-borne illness is a complex process. Despite public health efforts to maintain healthy food and water sources, many old disease scenarios have resurfaced as new challenges to health officials. Consumers obtain food after it has passed through a long chain of industrial production, with each link in the chain providing the opportunity for contamination. Investigation of disease outbreaks should focus not only on identifying the infectious organism and likely food source but also on examining the industrial process that allowed the organism to survive the food production process and, ultimately, infect the human host (Tauxe, 1997).

Although substantial progress has been made in preventing food- and water-borne illnesses in the United States, new infections are emerging that threaten the health of consumers. Approximately 400–500 food-borne disease outbreaks are reported each year (CDC, 1996b). *Escherichia coli* O157:H7, discussed earlier in this chapter, is one of the new food-borne pathogens that have emerged. The 1997 recall of 1.2 million pounds of hamburger that was distributed by a single processing plant in Nebraska and linked to an outbreak of *E. coli* O157:H7 infection emphasizes the potential health and economic

impact of food-processing and distribution practices (Satchell & Hedges, 1997). Cyclospora was responsible for a 1996 outbreak of illness, the food source of which was traced to imported Guatemalan raspberries (Ackers & Herwaldt, 1997). Hepatitis A was transmitted to more than 150 Michigan school children and teachers after they ingested frozen strawberries imported from Mexico (CDC, 1997b).

Consumer education is key in food safety and the prevention of food-borne illnesses. Foods contaminated with emerging pathogens usually look, smell, and taste normal, and the pathogen often survives traditional preparation techniques. Thorough cooking will kill almost all food-borne bacteria, viruses, and parasites and is an important step in the prevention of disease. Figure 26-19 lists 10 "golden rules" of safe food preparation.

There are several reasons for the emerging risks of food- and water-borne diseases. First, the food supply in the United States is changing. The way animals are raised has changed the picture of food-borne illness. Healthy animals have now been implicated in the spread of disease.

An example of the changing food-borne illness picture is the emergence of a new variant of a human disease called Cruetzfeldt-Jakob disease. Since 1996, evidence has been increasing for a causal relationship between ongoing outbreaks in Europe of a disease in cattle called bovine spongiform encephalopathy (BSE, or "mad cow disease") and new variant Cruetzfeldt-Jakob disease (nvCJD). Both disorders are invariably fatal brain diseases with unusually long incubation periods measured in years and are caused by an unconventional transmissible agent, the prion.

Although there is strong evidence that the agent responsible for these human cases was the same agent re-

---

FIGURE 26-19 Ten Golden Rules of Food Preparation

1. Choose food processed for safety.
2. Cook food thoroughly.
3. Eat cooked foods immediately.
4. Store cooked foods carefully.
5. Reheat cooked foods thoroughly.
6. Avoid contact between raw food and cooked food.
7. Wash hands repeatedly.
8. Keep all kitchen surfaces meticulously clean.
9. Protect food from insects, rodents, and other animals.
10. Use safe water.

From *The WHO Golden Rules for Safe Food Preparation*, by the World Health Organization, 2000 [On-line]. Available: http://www.who.int/fsf/gldnrls.htm. Used with permission.

sponsible for the BSE outbreaks in cattle, the specific foods that might be associated with the transmission of the agent from cattle to humans are unknown.

Should you be concerned about the recent headlines concerning mad cow disease? To reduce the possible current risk of acquiring CJD from food, travelers to Europe should be advised to consider either (1) avoiding beef and beef products altogether or (2) selecting beef or beef products, such as solid pieces of muscle meat (versus beef products such as burgers and sausages), that might have a reduced opportunity for contamination with tissues that might harbor the BSE agent. Milk and milk products from cows are not believed to pose any risk for transmitting the BSE agent.

The CDC monitors the trends and current incidence of CJD in the United States by analyzing death certificate information from U.S. multiple cause-of-death data, compiled by the National Center for Health Statistics, CDC. A summary of these data was published in the *Journal of the American Medical Association* on November 8, 2000 (Vol. 284, No. 18, pp. 2322–2323; available at http://jama.ama-assn.org/issues/v284n18/ffull/jlt1108-6.html.

Second, citizens' expectation of having fresh produce all seasons of the year has led to the import of more than 30 billion tons of food each year, including fruits, vegetables, seafood, and canned goods. These food items are often raised in developing countries where sanitation is inadequate. Some of this imported food is irrigated or rinsed with contaminated water or shipped in ice made from contaminated water that has been implicated in the spread of disease (Tauxe, 1997). Third, consumers eat out more frequently and consume processed foods in higher quantities. Finally, new pathogens that can cause disease have been identified. Policies regarding the safe handling of food should include evaluation of food production and shipping in all countries that serve as suppliers to the U.S. food stock.

Pediculosis

Few contagious situations evoke the kind of response that comes with a diagnosis of pediculosis. Simply the idea of having bugs crawling on the skin or in one's hair brings about the sensation of itching. Public health nurses and school nurses are particularly familiar with the contagious nature of pediculosis and the ability of these parasites to spread rapidly.

Pediculosis refers to an infestation of lice, which are easily spread via person-to-person contact. There are three types of lice: Head lice (*Pediculus humanus capitus*) are primarily found in children who share combs or hats; pubic lice (*Phthirus pubis*), also known as pubic crabs, are frequently found in adults and are transmitted primarily by sexual contact with an infected person (Chin, 2000); and body lice (*Pediculus humanus corpo-*

sis) are transmitted through infected clothing and linen. Poor hygiene is implicated only in the spread of body lice and is most frequently found in individuals who do not wash their clothes regularly.

Transmission

Although pediculosis infestations are considered very contagious, it is important to remember that lice do not typically jump from person to person. All three parasites are transmitted via close body contact with an infested person. They may also be transmitted by contact with shared items such as bed sheets, clothing, combs, or brushes. Younger children, who play and work closely together and are likely to share clothing and combs, are more susceptible to disease than older children or adolescents, so outbreaks tend to be rare after grade 6. Pubic crabs are found in adult populations and are transmitted by sexual contact.

Symptoms

Symptoms of infection are an itching or prickling sensation. In *P. humanus corposis* infestation, the nits are laid in the seams of clothing and cause itching when in contact with the skin. *Phthirus pubis* infestation causes anogenital itching.

Diagnosis

Pediculus humanus capitis is accompanied by the appearance of nits, or white spheres, on the hair at the back of the head and neck and behind the ears.

Treatment

Pesticidal shampoos are recommended in the treatment of head lice. Products vary slightly and should be used as directed. Treatment must be accompanied by removal of the nits (egg cases) that attach to the hair shaft. Clients should be instructed in the proper treatment of this condition:

- Prior to the use of pesticidal shampoos, notify health provider if the affected individual has asthma, allergies, or neurological conditions.
- Read and follow the manufacturer's label before applying the product.
- Nit removal can be accomplished by methodical "picking" of the eggs from the hair shaft. Eggs that are not removed are likely to hatch and cause reinfestation.
- Clothing, linens, and toys should be washed in hot water and dried at a high heat; if washing is not practical, these items should be vacuumed. Upholstery (both home and car) should also be vacuumed and the vacuum bag discarded. Brushes and combs should be washed in very hot water.

✳ DECISION MAKING

Controlling a Head Lice Outbreak

You are the school nurse at Hometown Elementary. Mrs. Jones, a third grade teacher, reports that white spots are visible in the hair of four of her students, one of whom complains of severe itching of the scalp. After examining the heads of the four children, you confirm that all four of the children have head lice. You contact the children's parents, and all four children are sent home with treatment recommendations and instructions. Each child in Mrs. Jones's class is then checked for head lice. After screening the entire class, you find three more children with visible nits in their hair. These children are also sent home with treatment recommendations and instructions.

◆ What primary prevention measures might have prevented this outbreak? What secondary and tertiary interventions are indicated?

◆ What actions will you take to protect the school community?

◆ What agent, host, and environmental factors may contribute to the transmission of disease in this setting?

◆ What social and cultural considerations may influence the effectiveness of treatment?

◆ Does the school nurse's responsibility stop after excluding the affected children from school?

Prevention

Lice can infect people of all socioeconomic groups and can infect people who take particular care to practice good hygiene as well as those who do not. In fact, some clinicians report that lice prefer clean hair. Children should be taught to keep combs, brushes, and caps to themselves. Screening of children with symptoms and isolating those infected from school populations until successful treatment is possible are recommended.

Scabies

Scabies is a parasitic disease in which tiny mites burrow under the skin. Although scabies mites are difficult to spot, infestation can be recognized by the characteristic burrows that contain the mites and their eggs. These burrows look like tracks, or small lines that resemble scratches, across the surface of the skin. Lesions are typically visible in the webs of the fingers, on the anterior surface of the wrists, on the buttocks, on the axillae, and along the beltline.

Transmission

Scabies mites can live for only a brief time away from the host, and the infection is transmitted between persons only via close skin-to-skin contact (Chin, 2000).

Symptoms

Scabies is characterized by intense itching, especially at night.

Diagnosis

Scabies should be suspected when clients complain of intense itching. The rash is typically found between fingers and toes and on wrists, armpits, genitals, and the lower buttocks. Dark ink applied to skin areas of suspected infestation helps locate the burrow sites of scabies mites. The presence of scabies is confirmed by applying a drop of sterile mineral oil to the affected area. A scraping from this area is then examined under a microscope. Scabies is often accompanied by bacterial infections and is easily confused with other skin diseases.

Treatment

Treatment is indicated for all persons who may have come into close contact with an infested individual. Over-the-counter insecticide lotion treatments are available for killing the mites. Treatment of infants, young children, nursing mothers, pregnant women, elderly individuals, and people with skin diseases requires the consultation of a physician before starting treatment. The rash may take two to six weeks to develop (Chin, 2000). Treatment should include a thorough housecleaning, including washing all bed linens, bath towels, and clothing in hot water. Vacuuming of furniture and mattresses and immediately discarding the vacuum bag can prevent the spread of scabies from furniture and other items.

Prevention

If an infested person is in a school or institutional setting, the individual should be excluded until 24 hours after treatment has been completed. Persons who have had direct contact with the infected person should be notified and may need treatment.

Influenza

Influenza, or "the flu," is an acute viral illness, prevalent during the winter and early spring. Because of the short incubation period (one to three days), epidemics can develop rapidly, and severe complications and death have been known to accompany infection. Severe illness and death occur primarily in elderly persons and are due to viral or bacterial respiratory complications. Each flu season is unique and brings a new strain of illness (Peters, 1997b).

Three types of influenza virus are recognized: A, B, and C. Of the three types, A is the most common and is the type usually associated with epidemics, complications, and death (Hemming, Palmer, Sinnot, & Glaser, 1997).

Transmission

Influenza is commonly spread through airborne droplets, nasopharyngeal secretions, and contact with contaminated materials. Transmission is facilitated by closed spaces such as those found in schools, school buses, hospitals, and nursing homes (Chin, 2000).

Symptoms

Influenza is an acute viral illness characterized by muscle aches, fever, fatigue, headache, sore throat, and cough. Symptoms usually last from two to four days but may linger for up to two weeks. Influenza pneumonia may develop when the influenza virus attacks the lower airways and lungs (Hemming et al., 1997).

Diagnosis

The diagnosis of influenza is clinical, based on client history and symptoms.

Treatment

Treatment of influenza is symptomatic unless complications develop. Persons at high risk for complications should seek treatment early. See Figure 26-20.

FIGURE 26-20 Persons Who Should Get the Influenza Vaccine

- Persons 65 years of age and older
- Residents of nursing homes and other chronic care facilities that house persons of any age with chronic medical conditions
- Adults and children with chronic pulmonary or cardiovascular disorders, including children with asthma
- Adults and children who required regular medical follow-up or hospitalization during the preceding year because of chronic metabolic diseases (including diabetes mellitus), renal dysfunction, hemoglobinopathies, or immunosuppression (including immunosuppression caused by medications)
- Children and adolescents (6 months to 18 years of age) who are receiving long-term aspirin therapy and might therefore be at risk for developing Reye syndrome after influenza
- Women who will be in the second or third trimester of pregnancy during the influenza season

---

Prevention

Anyone over age 6 months who is at increased risk of developing the complications of influenza (see Figure 26-20) should have a flu shot. Changes in antigenic properties that occur from year to year, called antigenic drift, require the preparation of a new vaccine each year. Vaccines typically contain two type A and one type B virus strains. Because of antigenic changes in the virus, antibodies produced as a result of influenza infection or vaccination containing earlier strains may not protect against viruses circulating in subsequent years. Thus vaccination each year is necessary to prevent infection. When the match between the vaccine strain and circulating viruses is good, influenza vaccine is approximately 70% effective in preventing illness (Peters, 1997b). Secondary prevention involves early diagnosis and treatment of symptoms to prevent complications of the disease.

Rabies

Over the past 30 years, reported cases of animal rabies in the United States have increased from fewer than 5000 per year in the early 1960s to almost 10,000 per year in the mid-1990s, with 1994 recording the highest annual mortality since 1979. Most of the increase is attributable to the spread of raccoon rabies from Florida to the northeastern states (Rupprecht & Smith, 1994) and the growing incidence of coyote rabies in southern Texas (Deasy, 1996). Human rabies is a preventable disease when it is recognized and appropriate therapy is initiated. If symptoms develop, rabies will invariably result in death.

Rabies is primarily an animal disease that may be transmitted to humans. Although rabies is often thought of as a disease passed from domesticated animals to humans, there has been a shift in disease prevalence to wildlife. In the United States, the most frequently reported rabid wild animals are raccoons, skunks, foxes, and bats. Because of increased urban expansion into the habitats of wild animals, humans are at increased risk of coming in contact with rabid animals. In New York and Massachusetts, where raccoon rabies is prevalent, oral immunization of these animal vectors is being tested. Areas that have instigated oral immunization programs have had decreased episodes of rabies (Uhaa et al., 1992). Bats have been implicated in several recent rabies deaths, and the CDC recommends that when a bat is physically present and the possibility of a bite exists, postexposure prophylaxis should be given (CDC, 1996a). In North America, the spread of infection follows a cycle in which the infection is passed from animal to animal via bites or scratches. In the United States, cats pose a greater risk for rabies than do dogs. In many developing countries, however, the dog is still the main vector in the spread of disease (Deasy, 1996).

Transmission

Rabies is transmitted to humans via an animal scratch or bite. A bite by a rabid animal carries a much greater risk of infection than does a scratch. The rabies virus enters the body where there is direct saliva contact with broken skin or mucous membranes.

Diagnosis

Diagnosis is based on history of exposure to infection, the occurrence of characteristic signs and symptoms, and laboratory tests.

Symptoms

The incubation period in humans ranges from 5 days to more than 1 year, with 2 months being the average. Initially, clients report vague symptoms that last from 2 to 10 days. The client may complain of fever, headache, malaise, and decreased appetite, and pain, itching, or numbness is often present at the site of the wound. As the disease progresses, clients develop difficulty swallowing and are unable to swallow their saliva. A characteristic of the infection is that the sight of water terrifies the individual. Paralysis, agitation, and disorientation are followed by coma and death from complications.

Treatment

There is no known, effective treatment for rabies once the symptoms of the illness have developed. Because of the frightening mortality associated with this disease—essentially 100%—all individuals who have come in contact with an infected animal or person should receive postexposure prophylaxis. The decision on whether to initiate postexposure prophylaxis treatment should be based on the guidelines of the Advisory Committee on Immunization Practices of the Public Health Service and should be coordinated with local health officials and animal control authorities. Management of animal bites is important and is outlined in Figure 26-21.

Prevention

Nurses can educate clients about the need to vaccinate pets to ensure a healthy neighborhood. Prevention of human rabies requires both animal control and public awareness. Consumers should be educated about the importance of rabies prevention. The public should avoid unnecessary contact with wild animals (particularly bats, raccoons, coyotes, and skunks) and should be aware of the signs displayed by rabid animals, such as daytime appearance by normally nocturnal animals. Domestic animals should be routinely vaccinated to prevent rabies.

Preexposure vaccination should be considered for individuals whose occupations, avocations, or activities place them at frequent risk of exposure to rabies virus or

---

FIGURE 26-21 Checklist for Treatment of Animal Bites

- Immediately clean and flush the wound (first aid).
- Under medical supervision, thoroughly clean the wound.
- Administer rabies immune globulin and/or vaccine as indicated.
- Administer tetanus prophylaxis and antibacterial treatment when required.
- Unless unavoidable, do not suture or close the wound.

Control of Communicable Diseases Manual (17th ed.), by J. Chin (Ed.), 2000, Washington, DC: American Public Health Association.

---

to potentially rabid animals. Occupations considered at risk are hunters, forest rangers, taxidermists, laboratory workers, stock breeders, slaughterhouse workers, and veterinarians.

COMMUNITY HEALTH NURSE RESPONSIBILITIES AND OPPORTUNITIES RELEVANT TO COMMUNICABLE DISEASE

Community health nurses must arm themselves with information about new and emerging infectious diseases. It is often the nurse who has the initial contact with clients, and an informed nurse can be instrumental in preventing the unnecessary spread of disease throughout a community. Practicing community health nurses may encounter new disease entities that have not yet been identified or adequately described. Recognizing infectious disease conditions is a challenge and responsibility of nurses working to protect the health of communities.

Community health nurses should be aware of epidemiological principles so that they can use this knowledge to interrupt the chain of infection relative to communicable disease. Strengthening the host through immunization and education, controlling the environment through protection of food and water supplies, and controlling transmission of agents between infected hosts by promoting both barrier methods to prevent STDs and needle-exchange programs to protect intravenous drug users are part of the nurse's responsibility in the control of communicable disease.

Awareness of core public health functions such as disease surveillance and reporting is key in the control of communicable diseases. Core public health functions include the surveillance of disease. In order to interrupt the spread of infection, community health nurses must rely on their knowledge of the nursing process to assess agent, host, and environmental factors that may be contributing to the development of specific disease condi-

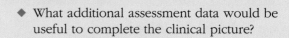

COMMUNITY NURSING VIEW

A public health nurse is working at a local health department's sexually transmitted disease clinic. A 14-year-old girl, Amy, arrives early for her appointment at the clinic. She seems nervous and upset. While taking a health history, the nurse learns that this young woman has been sexually active for approximately 6 months. Amy reports only one sexual partner, her 21-year-old boyfriend, Jimmy. She has been using oral contraceptives to prevent pregnancy and reports reliable compliance. Two weeks ago, however, she noticed a lesion on her "privates." She says the lesion is extremely painful and causes irritation and burning when she urinates. She has also developed a "smelly" vaginal discharge, which Jimmy does not like. He says she stinks, which is what brought her to the clinic today. When questioned about the number of sexual partners Jimmy has had, she replies, blushing, "I'm his first."

On physical examination, the nurse finds the following:

- A small, ulcerated lesion, now crusted over on the labia minora
- A red and inflamed perineal region
- A greenish, foamy, vaginal discharge accompanied by a fishy odor

Cultures and a Pap test were obtained, and all other physical findings were normal.

Nursing Considerations

Assessment

- What is your initial assessment of Amy's situation?

- What additional assessment data would be useful to complete the clinical picture?

Diagnosis

- What is the likely diagnosis?
- What levels of prevention are appropriate to prevent the spread of infection?

Outcome Identification

- What might be your short- and long-term goals in this situation?

Planning/Interventions

- How might you involve the client in decision making?
- What are the treatment options? What nursing actions will ensure treatment compliance?
- What responsibilities do you have in this situation with regard to reporting, contact notification, and client education?

Evaluation

- How might you evaluate your success in this situation?
- What follow-up care and referrals are indicated?

---

tions. At the same time, the nurse plans and implements control procedures that serve to protect the health of the community. Evaluation of the effectiveness of disease surveillance and control is often apparent when local, state, and national morbidity and mortality statistics are reviewed.

Educating consumers about basic sanitation principles related to food preparation as well as the importance of handwashing will help reduce the spread of infection. Information regarding Universal Precautions (see Figure 26-8) should be available to health care worker and consumer alike to assist in the fight against AIDS and other bloodborne infections. Whereas nurses in acute-care settings often rely on medications and treatments to fight disease, nurses working in the community are aware of the need to return to basic principles to keep the public healthy. Water supplies protected from

contamination, appropriate waste control, knowledgeable food growers and handlers, and a public informed of barriers that can interrupt the spread of infection, such as safe-sex practices and proper handwashing and food storage and handling in the home, can go a long way toward curbing communicable disease.

Primary Prevention

Community health nurses can be active participants in the education of individuals, families, and communities. Informing individuals of disease risk and ways to prevent disease occurrence is a valuable link for the prevention of disease. Immunizations are by far the most cost-effective way to prevent the occurrence of infectious diseases. Strengthening the host to resist infection interrupts the spread of infections and supports primary prevention

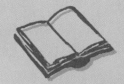

Out
of the Box

Spring S.T.I.N.G. Weekend

Communities can put research into practice by empowering citizens to take control of their health through communitywide prevention efforts. West Nile virus is a threatening new mosquito-borne disease that was seen for the first time in the Eastern United States in 1999. West Nile virus has been commonly found in humans and birds and other vertebrates in Africa, Eastern Europe, West Asia, and the Middle East but until 1999 had not previously been documented in the Western Hemisphere.

It is not known from where the U.S. virus originated, but it is most closely related genetically to strains found in the Middle East. Several people in New York State acquired this new virus and died as a result of encephalitis caused by infection with the West Nile virus. It is possible to minimize the chance that people will contract West Nile virus.

Westchester County, New York, is encouraging citizens to join a S.T.I.N.G. effort to address the West Nile encephalitis outbreak. Citizens of Westchester County are encouraged to control mosquitoes at an early stage to prevent illness due to West Nile virus. The county has a 24-hour West Nile information line that provides information on the virus and how to protect against mosquito

bites. Residents are encouraged to report dead birds, especially crows, which are also affected by this virus.

The Department of Health for Westchester County is holding a spring S.T.I.N.G. weekend to get citizens involved. It encourages people to:

1. *Survey the property around their home to eliminate potential mosquito breeding grounds.*
2. *Organize neighborhood clean-up squads to work together to clean up breeding grounds in the neighborhood.*
3. *Partner with other community organizations to tackle bigger areas in the community.*

Citizens are informed about how to control mosquitoes, which serve as the vector for this deadly disease:

1. *Get rid of water-holding containers.*
2. *Cover trash containers to keep out the rain.*
3. *Drill holes in the bottoms of recycling containers.*
4. *Clean roof gutters and remove standing water.*
5. *Drain the water in birdbaths and plant pots twice a week.*
6. *Sweep the driveway after it rains to eliminate puddles.*

Read about the spring S.T.I.N.G. weekend at www.westchestergov.com/health/Westnile.htm. ∎

---

efforts. Community health nurses must be creative and innovative in an effort to make immunizations available to all populations and attempt to break down the barriers to timely immunizations. An example of one community's effort at prevention of a threatening new mosquito disease is described in "Out of the Box."

Secondary Prevention

Disease treatment or secondary prevention should focus on minimizing the effects of agents on both host and environment. Particularly in the age of emerging infections, nurses should be leaders in early recognition and treatment of infection to minimize the potential long-term effects of these diseases. AIDS is an example of how early intervention and treatment can change the natural history of disease and increase individual health potential.

Tertiary Prevention

Effective case management can help to eliminate the debilitating effects of disease. CHNs should be aware of

agencies and other resources that can assist clients in the management of disease. Many of the communicable diseases that affect communities are chronic and the focus is on management. For example, community health nurses should be aware of the latest treatments to minimize symptoms and outbreaks of genital herpes. Individuals with AIDS may need assistance in managing medications and assistance with finances. Community health nurses can greatly assist these individuals in maintaining their current lifestyle.

Nurses can be instrumental in the development of public health policy at every level, from local to international. Awareness of community needs and issues ensures accurate information for policy development that will help maintain the public health infrastructure. Nurses can also be involved in the research and investigation of disease, leading to increased understanding and information to support disease treatment and control. Finally, it is imperative that nurses document the cost effectiveness of routine case management efforts made on behalf of the community to ensure adequate financial resources and personnel in the future.

KEY CONCEPTS

◆ Emerging infections pose a threat to populations throughout the world. A global perspective is necessary in addressing infectious disease concerns. Global transmission of communicable disease is a reality and must be recognized.

◆ Immunization is the most effective prevention against communicable disease.

◆ Educating clients and health care providers about the use and misuse of antibiotics in the treatment of disease is necessary to control the emergence of drug-resistant microbes.

◆ Sexually transmitted diseases constitute one of the most serious communicable disease problems in the United States. Community health nurses can have a direct role in stopping the spread of infection by educating clients about STD prevention.

◆ Early detection and case management of HIV-infected persons can help prolong the symptom-free period in AIDS. Pregnant women should be told about the possibility of AIDS transmission to the fetus during pregnancy, delivery, and breastfeeding. Testing for AIDS should be available to all pregnant women, who should also be educated about treatment to stop the transmission of infection.

◆ Direct observed therapy has been effective in slowing the spread of multidrug-resistant TB.

◆ Nurses must remain alert to new clusters of symptoms and must practice appropriate Universal Precautions.

◆ Nurses should be involved in policy setting related to surveillance, disease reporting, and treatment options because they are the frontline workers in disease investigation and case management.

RESOURCES

Centers for Disease Control and Prevention: http://www.cdc.gov
Connection between HIV/STD and AIDS: http://www.cdcnpin.org
Epidemic: The world of infectious disease: http://www.amnh.org/exhibitions/epidemic
Infectious disease report: http://www.who.int/infectious-disease-report
Morbidity and Mortality Weekly Report: http://www.cdc.gov/mmwr
Women's health initiative: http://www.nhlbi.nih.gov/whi
World Health Organization: http://www.who.org

EMERGING INFECTIONS

Hantavirus: http://www.cdc.gov/ncidod/diseases/hanta/hps
http://www.hantavirus.net
Lyme disease: http://www.cdc.gov/ncidod/dvbid/lyme
Mad cow disease: http://www.pbs.org/wgbh/nova/madcow
STDs: http://www.ashastd.org, http://www.herpes-coldsores.com/std,
http://www.intelihealth.com/IH/ihtIH/8799/9339/10672.html
West Nile virus: http://www.westchestergov.com

Chapter

27

CHRONIC ILLNESS

Doris Callaghan RN, BScN MSc

MAKING THE CONNECTION

Having a serious chronic illness often crystallizes vital lessons about living that otherwise may remain opaque.

—Charmaz, 1991, p. vii

COMPETENCIES

Upon completion of this chapter, the reader should be able to:

- Define chronic illness.
- Discuss the epidemiology of chronic illness.
- Identify the most common conditions that result in chronic illness.
- Discuss the concept of empowerment in the context of chronic illness.
- Understand the implications of chronic illness for ill individuals and their families.
- Describe the strategies employed by clients and families in living with a chronic illness.
- Understand the value of the perspective of the person with a chronic illness on the experience.
- Understand the health promotive role of community health nurses in relation to chronic illness.
- Identify primary, secondary, and tertiary preventive approaches for chronic illness.
- Describe the national *Healthy People 2010* objectives that are related to chronic illness.

KEY TERMS

approach strategy	disability
biographical disruption	handicap
	impairment
biographical work	insider's perspective
chronic disease	normalizing
chronic illness	power resources
circular questioning	powerlessness
coping	uncertainty

Chronic illness, a social phenomenon that accompanies a disease that cannot be cured and extends over a period of time, has challenged the lives of people for centuries. Major advances in health care technology and in the acute care of clients have occurred in the past few decades. During this proliferation of cure interventions, the care of people with chronic illnesses has received little attention from health care professionals and researchers. More recently, many Western nations have recognized chronic illness as an important issue in the health of their people [U.S. Department of Health and Human Services (USDHHS), 1992; USDHHS, 2000a; Epp, 1986]. This increasing interest in chronic illness can be attributed to several factors, including the increased occurrence of chronic illnesses, soaring costs of

health care, and the World Health Organization's (WHO, 1978, 1985) promotion of health for all.

Chronic illnesses do not respond well to prevalent curative medical interventions. Chronic illness care requires a rethinking of the traditional acute health care approaches with which health care providers are most familiar. The purpose of this chapter is to provide the nurse with an opportunity to explore the challenges faced by people who experience a chronic physical illness. The associated role of community health nurses will be discussed, as will the epidemiology of **chronic disease,** a long-term physiological disorder.

DEFINITION OF CHRONIC ILLNESS

Conrad (1987) distinguishes between a disease and an illness. A disease is "an undesirable physiological process;" an illness is "profoundly social, more to do with perception, behavior and experience than with physiological process" (p. 2). An illness may become chronic when it cannot be cured and continues over an extended period. Miller (2000a) defines chronic illness as "an altered health state that will not be cured by a simple surgical procedure or short course of medical therapy" (p. 4). Chronic illness represents long-term or permanent disability that hinders peoples' physical, psychological, or social functioning (Hymovich & Hagopian, 1992). The WHO (1980) presents a system of classification of related concepts including impairment, disability, and handicap. **Impairment** is defined as an abnormality of body structure and appearance or disturbance of organs or systems resulting from any cause. A **disability** results from impairment and is a restriction or lack of ability to perform an activity in a manner or within a range considered normal. The disadvantages resulting from impairments and disabilities are classified as **handicaps** (WHO, 1980).

These academic definitions attempt to clarify the concept of chronic illness, but it is the individual experiencing the illness who can best define the meaning. Conrad (1987, 1990) labels this view as the **"insider's perspective,"** which he defines as focusing on people's lived experiences in relation to the illness. Conrad (1987) writes:

REFLECTIVE THINKING

Chronically Ill Friends and Family

Think about friends or family members whom you would consider to be chronically ill.

- How do you think the chronic illness affects their lives?
- How does the chronic illness affect your perception of them?

An insider's perspective focuses directly and explicitly on the subjective experience of living with and in spite of illness. It focuses specifically on the perspectives of people with illness and attempts to examine the illness experience in a more inductive manner. (p. 2)

It is important to acknowledge that many people who have a chronic illness see themselves as healthy. Being diagnosed with a chronic illness does not exclude the experience of feeling well (Charmaz, 1991; Lindsey, 1996). The highly individual nature of responses to chronic illness emphasizes the need for nurses to assess and understand the subjective experience of the client.

EPIDEMIOLOGY

The USDHHS (1992) classifies heart disease, cancer, stroke, lung, and liver disease and also chronic and disabling conditions such as diabetes mellitus, arthritis, deformities or orthopedic impairments, hearing and speech impairments, and mental retardation as chronic illnesses (p. 73). As is evident in this classification, the concept of chronic illness encompasses many different disease processes. Each has its own natural history. Pathogenic processes of diseases such as coronary heart disease and some cancers begin early in life and have progressed extensively prior to clinical manifestations. Causality of chronic diseases is associated with several factors rather than a single causative agent. Causality is frequently related to factors in lifestyle, genetics, or environment and is completely unknown in some conditions. This variability of causality makes the epidemiological study of chronic illness complex and specific to the disease being considered. The incidence and prevalence of chronic illnesses are difficult to estimate, because these conditions are not reported to official agencies as part of a disease surveillance program.

A vital part of epidemiology is risk factor identification, which can lead to risk reduction through specific in-

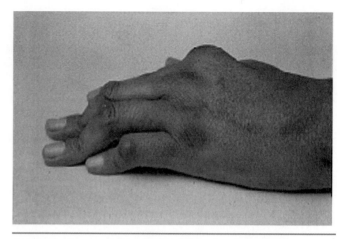

Arthritis is considered a chronic health problem. Courtesy of Arthritis Foundation.

terventions. Such interventions aim to reduce morbidity and mortality related to chronic illness. Risk factors can be classified as modifiable or nonmodifiable. For example, modifiable risk factors for stroke include high cholesterol, hypertension, cigarette smoking, and obesity. The nonmodifiable risks factors are heredity, race, age, and gender (Brillhart, 2000). Although each chronic disease must be considered individually, the risk factors of dietary practices and smoking are significant in several common chronic diseases including heart disease and stroke, cancer, lung disease, and diabetes mellitus.

MORBIDITY

"Chronic illnesses are currently the prevalent form of illness in developed countries" (Harkness, 1995, p. 141). Table 27-1 identifies the 10 major causes of chronic health problems in the United States in 1996. The four leading causes of chronic health problems are arthritis, chronic sinusitis, deformities and orthopedic impairments, and high blood pressure. Although many of the 10 leading causes of chronic health problems are not life threatening, they have a significant impact on peoples' lives and on health care costs. Life-threatening chronic conditions are also prevalent in the United States, with about 12 million people affected by heart conditions. Approximately 10.5 million people have diabetes mellitus (USDHHS, 2000a). Over the past two decades, the incidence of cancer has increased, with approximately 16 million new cancer cases diagnosed since 1990 (American Cancer Society, 2002). Figure 27-1 reveals a similar picture in Canada, where arthritis/rheumatism, nonarthritic back problems, high blood pressure, and migraine headaches are the four most prevalent chronic conditions in people 12 years and older (Statistics Canada, 2001). In developing countries, the incidence of chronic illness is lower as infectious diseases remain the major health challenge (Conrad & Gallagher, 1993).

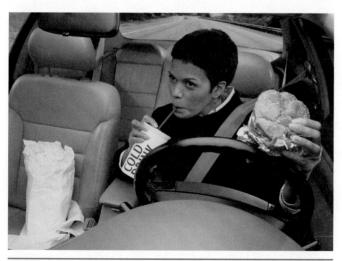

Dietary intake high in saturated fats is a modifiable risk factor. Courtesy of Photodisc.

TABLE 27-1 Chronic Illnesses with Highest Prevalence Rates per 1000 Persons by Age: United States, 1996

		NUMBER OF CHRONIC CONDITIONS PER 1000 PERSONS					
RANK	CHRONIC CONDITION	ALL AGES	UNDER 18 YEARS	18–44 YEARS	45–64 YEARS	65–74	75 YEARS AND OVER
1	Arthritis	127.3	1.9	50.1	240.1	453.1	523.6
2	Chronic sinusitis	125.5	63.9	144.7	174.1	127.0	103.5
3	Deformity and orthopedic Impairment	111.6	25.9	122.4	177.8	175.1	133.5
4	High blood pressure	107.1	0.5	49.6	214.1	356.0	373.8
5	Hay fever or allergic rhinitis without asthma	89.8	58.7	109.4	104.8	61.9	75.7
6	Hearing impairment	83.4	12.6	41.9	131.5	255.2	369.8
7	Heart disease	78.2	23.6	39.3	116.4	238.2	310.7
8	Asthma	55.2	62.0	56.9	48.6	43.7	48.0
9	Chronic bronchitis	53.5	57.3	45.4	59.1	60.7	67.3
10	Migraine headache	43.7	15.2	60.0	57.9	28.6	28.4

Adapted from Current Estimates from the National Health Interview Survey, *1996 (pp. 81, 82), by National Center for Health Statistics, 1999. Hyattsville, MD. Public Health Service.*

FIGURE 27-1 Prevalence of Chronic Conditions, Population Aged 12 or Older, Canada, 1998–1999

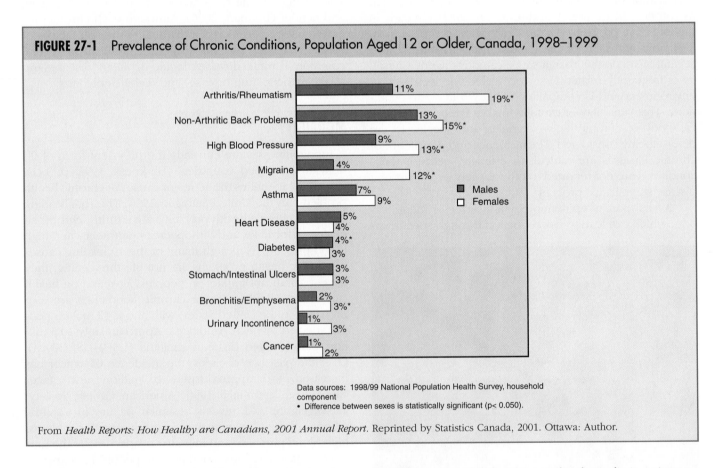

Data sources: 1998/99 National Population Health Survey, household component
• Difference between sexes is statistically significant (p< 0.050).

From *Health Reports: How Healthy are Canadians, 2001 Annual Report.* Reprinted by Statistics Canada, 2001. Ottawa: Author.

The incidence of chronic health problems is related to gender. In the United States, of the four most prevalent chronic health conditions, there is a higher incidence of arthritis, chronic sinusitis, and high blood pressure in females than in males in those aged 65 years and older, al-though the rate of deformities and orthopedic impairments is only slightly higher in females. See Figure 27-2. Interestingly, a similar pattern exists for those under 65 where 8 of the 10 most prevalent chronic conditions are more common in females than in males. Only hearing impair-

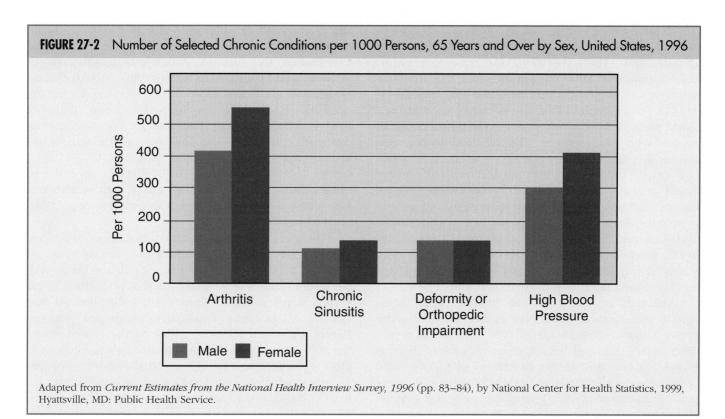

FIGURE 27-2 Number of Selected Chronic Conditions per 1000 Persons, 65 Years and Over by Sex, United States, 1996

Adapted from *Current Estimates from the National Health Interview Survey, 1996* (pp. 83–84), by National Center for Health Statistics, 1999, Hyattsville, MD: Public Health Service.

TABLE 27-2 Limitation of Activity Caused by Chronic Conditions, According to Selected Characteristics, 1996

AGE*	PERCENT OF POPULATION WITH LIMITATION IN MAJOR ACTIVITY[†]			
	MALE	**FEMALE**	**WHITE**	**BLACK**
Total	9.7	10.2	9.7	12.5
under 18 years	5.5	3.2	4.1	6.2
18–44 years	7.1	7.0	6.8	10.0
45–64 years	16.7	16.4	15.7	23.7
65–69 years	25.9	26.9	25.2	37.2
70 years and over	15.1	22.2	18.6	27.1

Age adjusted to the 1970 civilian noninstitutionalized population.

†Limitation in major activity includes those people unable to carry on usual activities for their age: working, keeping house, going to school, or living independently.

Adapted from *Current Estimates from the National Health Interview Survey, 1996 (p. 105), by National Center for Health Statistics, 1999. Hyattsville, MD: Public Health Service.*

ment and heart disease are more prevalent in males than females. The higher rate for chronic conditions in older females is important as their life expectancy is longer as compared to males. In 1998, life expectancy for females was 79.5 years compared with 73.8 years for males (National Center for Health Statistics, 2000). This same gender relationship is evident in Canada, where in 1998/99 the most commonly identified chronic conditions were overall more prevalent in females than in males aged 12 or older, except for heart disease and diabetes, where the prevalence in males was slightly higher (Statistics Canada, 2001).

The significance of chronic illness is reflected in the effect it has on the person's ability to carry out daily functions of life. Limitation of activity accompanies many chronic illnesses and presents another perspective on the prevalence of chronic illness. Table 27-2 illustrates limitation of activity according to sex and age and race and age. Although the total numbers of females and males with limitation of activity are similar, the trend is higher for females over the age of 70 years. Limitations of activity are higher for African Americans of all ages than for Caucasians (National Center for Health Statistics, 1999a).

Chronic health problems are more prevalent in people with the lowest income (USDHHS, 2000a; Statistics Canada, 2001). The USDHHS (2000a) states that "population groups that suffer the worst health status are those that have the highest poverty rates and least education" (p. 12). For example, heart disease, diabetes, and high blood pressure have a higher than average incidence in people with low incomes. The relationship between chronic illness and poverty is not completely understood. Low income may contribute to the occurrence of chronic illness or it may be the product of poor health. "Higher incomes permit increased access to medical care, enable people to afford better housing and live in safer neighborhoods and increase the opportunity to engage in health promoting behaviors" (USDHHS, 2000a, p. 12). Whatever the relationship, poverty is an important factor for the community health nurse to consider.

Although occurring among people of all ages, chronic conditions have a higher incidence among older persons. In the United States in 1996, the chronic conditions of arthritis, high blood pressure, hearing impairments, and heart disease occurred more frequently in the population over 65 years of age. Deformities and orthopedic impairments were higher in the age group 45 years and older. See Table 27-1. "In 1995, among noninstitutionalized persons 70 years of age and over, 79% reported at least one of seven chronic conditions common among the elderly. The majority of persons 70 years of age and over reported arthritis, and approximately one third reported hypertension. Diabetes was reported by 11 percent" (USDHHS, 1999a, p. 3). This relationship is especially significant in light of the "graying" of the population in the industrialized world. The U.S. population is experiencing an aging trend. In 2000, approximately 12 out of every 100 Americans were 65 years of age or older (U.S. Bureau of the Census, 2000). Predictions indicate that, by the year 2030, "20 out of 100 persons will be 65 years of age or over, and 2 out of 100 will be 85 years of age and over" (USDHHS, 1999a, p. 17). Similar demographic patterns exist in other western nations (Statistics Canada, 2000b). Such demographic changes are likely to be accompanied by an increased incidence of chronic illnesses. There will be a corresponding increased need for nurses to work in health promotion, prevention, and acute care with people who are chronically ill and a need for health care dollars to be allocated to chronic illness.

MORTALITY

Many conditions listed among the leading causes of death in both the United States and Canada are chronic diseases (National Center for Health Statistics, 2000; Statistics Canada, 2000a). "Every year, chronic disease claim the lives of more than 1.7 million Americans. These diseases are responsible for 7 out of every 10 deaths in the United States" (USDHHS, 1999c, p. vii). Diseases of the heart, malignant neoplasms, cerebrovascular diseases, chronic obstructive pulmonary diseases, diabetes mellitus, nephritis, nephrotic syndrome and nephrosis, chronic liver disease and cirrhosis, Alzheimer's disease, atherosclerosis, and hypertension with or without renal disease are chronic conditions listed among the top 15 leading causes of death in the United States in 1998. See Table 27-3. In 1998, mortality rates for each of the leading causes of death for the total population except for Alzheimer's disease were higher for males than females (National Center for Health Statistics, 2000). The leading cause of cancer deaths in 1998 for both males and females was lung and bronchus cancer (American Cancer Society, 2002). See Figures 27-3 and 27-4.

There are differences in mortality rates among races. The mortality rate was higher for the African American population than for the Caucasian population for most of the leading causes of death for the total population in the United States in 1998. Chronic pulmonary disease, suicide, and Alzheimer's disease were exceptions (National Center for Health Statistics, 2000). In the United States, the 1996 age-adjusted death rate among American Indians for unintentional injuries and diabetes were approximately double the rate for Caucasians and the rate for liver cirrhosis was nearly triple the rate for Caucasians. The overall death rate for all causes for Hispanic Americans was lower than for non-Hispanic white Americans. However, the death rate due to homicide was eight times higher for Hispanic males aged 15–24 years and four times higher for those aged 25–44 than for non-Hispanic white American males of similar ages. The death rate for human immunodeficiency virus (HIV) infection for Hispanic males aged 25–44 years was double the rate for Hispanic white American males of similar age. The age-adjusted death rates for cancer and heart disease for Asian Americans were 39% and 45% lower than the rates for Caucasians (USDHHS, 1998).

Years of potential life lost (YPLL) is a measure of premature mortality that is calculated over the age range from birth to 75 years of age. Because YPLL reflects the effect of chronic conditions on the population below the age of 75, it is an important aspect of mortality rates. Table 27-4 illustrates the YPLL for deaths resulting from selected illnesses in the United States in 1995. Malignant neoplasms and diseases of the heart were the chronic conditions that accounted for the greatest number of YPLL as a result of premature death. However, HIV infection, cerebrovascular diseases, chronic pulmonary diseases, diabetes mellitus, and chronic liver disease and cirrhosis also had a significant impact (USDHHS, 1998).

Mortality figures are changing, and between 1997 and 1998 the mortality rate in eight of the leading causes of death in the United States declined. Death rates for all of the chronic conditions declined during this time except chronic obstructive lung disease and hypertension, which rose by 4.8% and 4.3%, respectively. The death rate for diabetes rose only slightly. See Table 27-1. Rates for HIV infection have changed significantly, falling from

TABLE 27-3 Percent of Total Deaths, Death Rates, Age-Adjusted Death Rates for 1998, Percent Change in Age-Adjusted Death Rates from 1997 to 1998 and 1979 to 1998, and Ratio of Age-Adjusted Death Rates by Race and Sex for 15 Leading Causes of Death for Population in 1998: United States*

| | | | | AGE-ADJUSTED DEATH RATE | | | | |
| | | | | | PERCENT CHANGE | | RATIO | |
RANK	CAUSE OF DEATH†	PERCENT OF TOTAL DEATHS	DEATH RATE	1998	1997–1998	1979–1998	MALE TO FEMALE	BLACK TO WHITE
	All causes	100.0	864.7	471.7	−1.5	−18.2	1.6	1.5
1	Diseases of heart	31.0	268.2	126.6	−3.0	−36.5	1.8	1.5
2	Malignant neoplasms, including neoplasms of lymphatic and hematopoietic tissues	23.2	200.3	123.6	−1.6	−5.5	1.4	1.3
3	Cerebrovascular diseases	6.8	58.6	25.1	−3.1	−39.7	1.1	1.8
4	Chronic obstructive pulmonary diseases and allied conditions	4.8	41.7	21.3	0.9	45.9	1.4	0.8
5	Accidents and adverse effects	4.2	36.2	30.1	0	−29.8	2.4	1.2
	Motor vehicle accidents	1.9	16.1	15.6	−1.9	−32.8	2.2	1.1
	All other accidents and adverse effects	2.3	20.1	14.4	1.4	−26.5	2.7	1.4
6	Pneumonia and influenza	3.9	34.0	13.2	2.3	17.9	1.5	1.4
7	Diabetes mellitus	2.8	24.0	13.6	0.7	38.8	1.2	2.4
8	Suicide	1.3	11.3	10.4	−1.9	−11.1	4.3	0.5
9	Nephritis, nephritic syndrome, and nephrosis	1.1	9.7	4.4	0	2.3	1.5	2.5
10	Chronic liver disease and cirrhosis	1.1	9.3	7.2	−2.7	−40.0	2.3	1.1
11	Septicemia	1.0	8.8	4.4	4.8	91.3	1.2	2.7
12	Alzheimer's disease	1.0	8.4	2.6	−3.7	1,200.0	0.9	0.7
13	Homicide and legal intervention	0.8	6.8	7.3	−8.8	−28.4	3.5	5.7
14	Atherosclerosis	0.7	5.7	1.9	−9.5	−66.7	1.3	1.0
15	Hypertension with or without renal disease	0.6	5.3	2.4	4.3	26.3	1.1	3.8
	All other causes	15.8	136.6	NA	NA	NA	NA	NA

*Death rates on an annual basis per 100,000 population; age-adjusted rates per 100,000 U.S. standard population; see Technical notes.
NA = category not applicable.
Rank based on number of deaths.
†Based on International Classification of Diseases, 9th rev., 1975.

Reprinted from Deaths: Final Data for 1998, 2000, National Vital Statistics Reports, 48(11), p. 5.

FIGURE 27-3 Age Adjusted Cancer Rates, Males by Site, U.S., 1930–1997

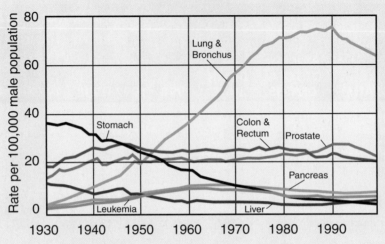

Age-Adjusted Cancer Death Rates,* for Males by Site, U.S., 1930–1997

*Per 100,000, age-adjusted to the 1970 US standard population.
Note: Due to changes in ICD coding, numerator information has changed over time. Rates for cancers of the liver, lung & bronchus, and colon & rectum are affected by these coding changes.

From *Cancer Facts and Figures 2000,* by American Cancer Society, 2000, Atlanta, GA: Author. Reprinted with permission of American Cancer Society, Inc.

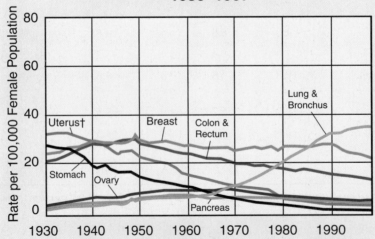

Age-Adjusted Cancer Death Rates,* for Females by Site, U.S., 1930–1997

*Per 100,000, age-adjusted to the 1970 US standard population.
†Uterus cancer death rates are for uterine cervix corpus combined. **Note:** Due to changes in ICD coding, numerator information has changed over time. Rates for cancers of the uterus, ovary, lung & bronchus, and colon & rectum are affected by these coding changes.

From *Cancer Facts and Figures 2000,* by American Cancer Society, 2000, Atlanta, GA: Author. Reprinted with permission of American Cancer Society, Inc.

TABLE 27-4 Years of Potential Life Lost Before Age 75 for Selected Causes of Death: United States, 1995

CONDITION	YEARS LOST PER 100,000 POPULATION UNDER 75 YEARS OF AGE (ALL RACES)
Malignant neoplasms	1587.7
Diseases of heart	1259.2
Unintentional injuries	1155.5
Human immunodeficiency virus	570.3
Homicide	436.4
Suicide	405.6
Cerebrovascular diseases	211.5
Chronic obstructive pulmonary diseases	161.4
Diabetes mellitus	149.9
Chronic liver disease and cirrhosis	149.7
Pneumonia and influenza	115.3

Adapted from Health, United States, 1998 *(p. 115), by National Center for Health Statistics, 1998, Hyattsville, MD: Public Health Service.*

the ranks of the 15 leading causes of death for the first time since 1987. The death rate for HIV infection fell 20.7% between 1997 to 1998. However, HIV infection remained the leading cause of death for African Americans aged 25–44 years. The downward trend in mortality rates for diseases of the heart, cerebrovascular disease, and atherosclerosis has been observed consistently since 1950 (National Center for Health Statistics, 2000). This trend has largely been attributed to public education regarding disease risk factors, lifestyle changes, and medical advances in treatment. Although progress has been made in decreasing the death rate from these diseases, heart and cerebrovascular diseases remain among the top three killers of Americans.

A CARING, EMPOWERING PERSPECTIVE

Chronic illness increases the vulnerability of individuals and groups (Charmaz, 1991; Hymovich & Hagopian, 1992). Situations such as poverty, lack of available resources, and inadequate health care coverage add to this vulnerability. The WHO (1974) identified the care of vulnerable groups as fundamental to community health nursing.

The need for community health nurses is increasing as health care reform shifts the care of people with chronic illness from institutions to their own homes. Provision of nursing services in the community includes health education, screening, referrals, direct home care,

discharge planning, and case management. To provide appropriate care, the nurse should be knowledgeable about the possible impact of chronic illness on the individual, the family, and the community. The nurse must consider the insider's perspective regarding chronic illness, whether this is the perspective of the individual, the family, an aggregate, or the community.

Important concepts underlying effective assessment, planning, and intervention by community health nurses include caring and empowerment. Valuing the client's lived experience is fundamental to caring and empowerment and moves nursing care away from a focus on technology and cure (Watson, 1988; Benner & Wrubel, 1989; Baker, 1996). Technology and cure interventions simply do not serve many people with chronic illness well. The incurability of chronic illnesses shifts the focus to the caring aspect of health care, and nurses are key providers of this care. Chapter 1 explores the foundations of a caring nursing practice.

The concept of empowerment is central to humanizing nursing care. Assumptions of empowerment that are fundamental to working with individuals and their families include the assumptions that (Labonte, 1990; Fahlberg, Poulin, Girdano, & Dusek, 1991):

- People themselves are the most capable of identifying both their own problems and their own solutions to those problems.

- There are multiple ways of viewing reality, and people know their own realities best.

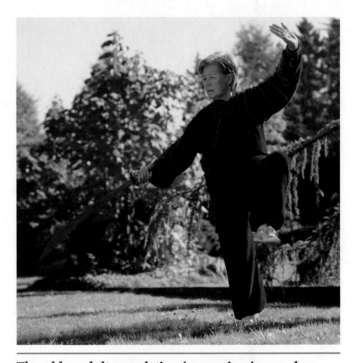

The older adult population is growing in number and the incidence of chronic health problems is likely to increase. The community health nurse should offer primary prevention techniques, including keeping active. Courtesy of Photodisc.

Developing a personal philosophy based on the assumptions of empowerment requires restructuring the traditional hierarchical structure of the nurse-client relationship to one of partnership between the individual, the family, and the nurse. In a partnership, the nurse shares power with the individual and the family. Power is integral to the empowerment of the client, and important aspects include "providing for and caring for self, directing others regarding self-care, and being the ultimate decision maker regarding care. With power comes the ability to effect change or prevent it" (Miller, 2000a, p. 4).

In their study of attitudes toward client expertise in chronic illness, Thorne, Nyhlin, and Paterson (2000) found that "the general pattern of health care interactions described by all participants was characterized by a pervasive attitude of disbelief in their [participants'] competence to make decisions on their own behalf" (p. 305).

As individuals with chronic illness and their families experience an extended period of time living with an illness, they become experts in their own care. They want

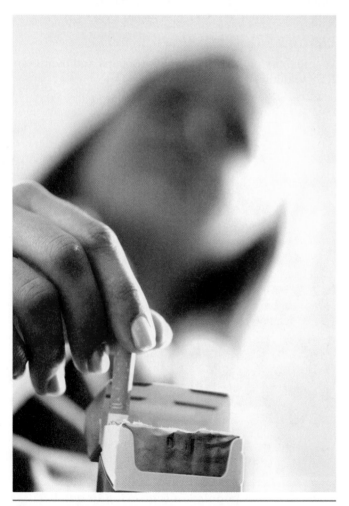

Tobacco-related deaths from heart disease and cancer are likely to increase unless preventative measures are effective in decreasing the incidence of tobacco use. Courtesy of Photodisc.

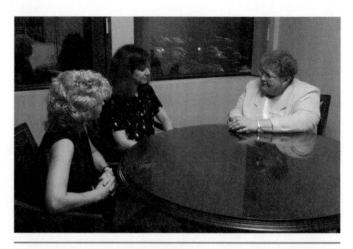

Demonstrating respect for the family's lived experience is an important role for the community health nurse.

their knowledge and ability acknowledged and respected by health care professionals (Callaghan, 1992; Corbin & Strauss, 1988; Thorne, 1993; Thorne et al., 2000). Shifting focus to the lived experience of individuals and their families enables a nurse to recognize their expertise and their ability to make the choices that best meet their needs. This approach requires the nurse to trust that people themselves are experts about their health needs. Partnership allows individuals and their families to (Lindsey, 1993; Thorne, 1993):

- Develop confidence in their abilities related to their own health.

- Be involved in setting their health goals, thus increasing the probability that they will attend to the goals.

- Identify the best approach for attending to their health.

Thorne et al. (2000) advise that health care relationships in the context of the chronic illness experience are very important. Respect, trust, and a partnership between the nurse and client are integral to a positive relationship.

Nurses who base their practice on the concepts of caring and empowerment support the healing of clients and their families (see Figure 27-5). Participants in Lindsey's (1995, p. 303) study offer these suggestions for promoting healing in people with chronic illnesses:

"Ask me what I need, give me a sense of partnership. Don't be afraid to lose control. I would like to tell them [health professionals] to have the courage to be real with us. I wish they wouldn't hide their feelings of powerless [sic] behind their arrogance."

"The most important thing they [health professionals] can do for me is just listen, listen and try to get some sense of my story."

"The most help he [the physician] ever gave me was one day when he said 'Look, I know you will

FIGURE 27-5 Tips for Nurses Working in Partnership with Their Clients

- Listen to what clients have to say.
- Respect and value what they say.
- Support them in making choices based on their own experience and their own expertise.

be the one to know what is right for you.' That level of respect."

"Being able to pose questions rather than give answers, to promote self-exploration and self-examination. I am talking about challenging questions that can only be done in an atmosphere of trust and respect which has to be built up over time."

"Be willing [health professionals] to take risks with people, to move into the unknown, and to be trusting."

These suggestions are reflected in the Parents As Teachers program at the Center for Children with Chronic Illness and Disability at the University of Minnesota. See Out of the Box.

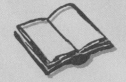

Out
of the Box

Parents As Teachers

The Center for Children with Chronic Illness and Disability (C3ID) at the University of Minnesota, Minneapolis, Minnesota, focuses on "maximizing the developmental potential of all children and adolescents with chronic illnesses and disabilities and their families (p. 1)." In addition to rehabilitation and research, the center educates physicians, nurses, and other health care professionals. The concept of client as expert is embraced in the Parents As Teachers program. In this program, the parents of children with disabilities teach health care workers about issues the child and their family encounter in daily life. The family's experiences with the health care system highlights what works well and areas for improvement.

Source: Division of General Pediatric and Adolescent Health and the Regents of the University of Minnesota. (2001). Center for Children with Chronic Illness and Disability. [On-line]. Available: http://www.peds.umn.Edu/peds-adol/cc.html. ■

Despite major technological advances in medical interventions during the last few decades, the incidence of chronic illness continues to have a major impact on the lives of people. When working with clients who are living with a chronic illness, nurses need to understand and acknowledge the impact the illness has on all dimensions of the lives of the individual and the family.

IMPACT OF CHRONIC ILLNESS

The experience of chronic illness permeates all aspects of a person's life, including physical, psychosocial, spiritual, and economic. King (cited in Michael, 1996), the editor in chief of the *Diabetes Interview,* tells his story of having diabetes:

> Many people think diabetes is just a disease, but it's not. It is much more than that. A disease is something that happens to your body. Diabetes affects every aspect of your whole life. It's more than a medical problem, it takes over your mind too. It's more than a simple adjustment of medicine and nutrition; it requires a complete retraining of your lifestyle. Nothing is spared; no part of your life is left unscathed. (p. 2)

Quality of life is a concept that appears frequently in health-related literature. Many research studies have attempted to quantify and measure quality of life. Meeberg (1993) suggests that there are as many definitions of quality of life as there are people who use the term. She cautions that quality of life assessments are vulnerable to the individual researcher's beliefs and biases. In considering the quality of a client's life, the community health nurse must be aware of its subjective and individual nature. This concept becomes congruent with client-centered nursing if considered within a definition offered by Meeberg. She defines quality of life as "a feeling of overall life satisfaction, as determined by the mentally alert individual whose life is being evaluated. Other people, preferably those from outside that person's living situation, must also agree that the individual's living conditions are non-life-threatening and are adequate in meeting that individual's basic needs" (p. 37).

Trajectory is a term that can be used to describe the progression of a chronic illness in a person's life. "An illness can be seen as a trajectory if one thinks of it as a process that begins with some physiological change and alteration in health status and continues through life with a positive or negative resolution" (White & Lubkin, 1997, p. 53). The illness trajectory, including management of the illness and eventual outcomes, can be influenced by the client, family, health care professionals, and any other person involved with the client (Corbin & Strauss, 1988, 1992). Corbin and Strauss (1988, 1992) developed a Chronic Illness Trajectory Framework which has been expanded and applied to working with older clients in the community (Corbin & Cherry, 1997). See Table 27-5.

TABLE 27-5 Trajectory Phases

PHASE	DEFINITION	GOAL OF MANAGEMENT
Pretrajectory	Genetic factors or lifestyle behaviors that place an individual or community at risk for the development of a chronic condition.	Prevent onset of chronic illness.
Trajectory onset	Appearance of noticeable symptoms, includes period of diagnostic workup and announcement by biographical limbo as person begins to discover and cope with implications of diagnosis.	Form appropriate trajectory projection and scheme.
Stable	Illness course and symptoms are under control. Biography and everyday life activities are being managed within limitations of illness. Illness management centered in the home.	Maintain stability of illness, biography, and everyday life activities.
Unstable	Period of inability to keep symptoms under control or reactivation of illness. Biographical disruption and difficulty in carrying out everyday life activities. Adjustments being made in regimen with care usually taking place at home.	Return to stable.
Acute	Severe and unrelieved symptoms or the development of illness complications necessitating hospitalization or bed rest to bring illness course under control. Biography and everyday life activities temporarily placed on hold or drastically cut back.	Bring illness under control and resume normal biography and everyday life activities.
Crisis	Critical or life-threatening situation requiring emergency treatment or care. Biography and everyday life activities suspended until crisis passes.	Remove life threat.
Comeback	A gradual return to an acceptable way of life within limits imposed by disability or illness. Involves physical healing, limitations stretching through rehabilitative procedures, psychosocial coming to terms, and biographical reengagement with adjustments in everyday life activities.	Set in motion and keep going the trajectory projection and scheme.
Downward	Illness course characterized by rapid or gradual physical decline accompanied by increasing disability or difficulty in controlling symptoms. Requires biographical adjustment and alterations in everyday life activity with each major downward step.	To adapt to increasing disability with each major downward turn.
Dying	Final days or weeks before death. Characterized by gradual or rapid shutting down of body processes, biographical disengagement and closure, and relinquishment of everyday life interests and activities.	To bring closure, let go, and die peacefully.

From "Caring for the Aged in the Community," by J. Corbin and J. Cherry, 1997, in E. Swanson and T. Tripp-Reimer (Eds.), Advances in Gerontological Nursing: Chronic Illness and the Older Adult *(pp. 62–81), New York: Springer Publishing Company. Reprinted by permission of Springer Publishing Company.*

Corbin (1998) suggests that "shaping a trajectory takes place within a context which consists of: projected outcomes, biographical factors (lives over time), and larger societal issues, like economic and political trends. It is expected that illness and illness management shape lives, and in turn, what persons want and expect out of their lives affects illness management and ultimately its course" (p. 37). An understanding of the illness trajectory can assist the nursing in working with the clients and their family. Depending on the phase of illness that the client is experiencing, the nurse may be involved with direct care, referrals, education, and assisting the client and family to acquire resources (Corbin & Cherry, 1997).

Perhaps the most important understanding of the impact that chronic illness has on people comes from accounts of people's experiences (Callaghan & Williams,

REFLECTIVE THINKING

Clients with Chronic Illness

Think of clients with whom you have worked who have a chronic illness.

- How did the illness affect their lives?
- In the context of chronic illness, what does empowerment mean to you?
- Give some examples of clients who have been experts in their health care and how you have worked in partnership with them.

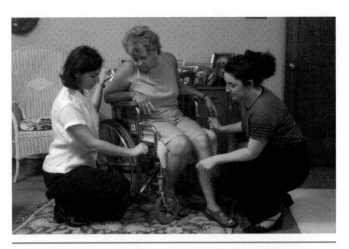

The community health nurse can help caregivers learn to care for a family member who has just returned home from a rehabilitation center.

1994). The person's view of the effect illness has on his or her life may be very different from the view of health professionals, friends, and family. People living with chronic illness develop a personal knowledge of their illness. Michael (1996) found the people in her study "knew their illness better than the health care professionals did. This presented a problem, because many health care professionals were unwilling to acknowledge participants' insights and disregarded what they said" (p. 262). People's perspective on their illness will also determine how they live with it. Charmaz (1991) suggests that "how people think about and categorize their illness reflects how they treat it" (p. 67). In considering the lived experience of chronic illness, the nurse needs to recognize that each individual has a unique story of the effect of illness on his or her life.

Physical Aspects

The variety of diseases that can result in chronic illness is reflected in the complexity of physical challenges that can accompany chronic illness. Most often the onset of physical symptoms is the first sign that something is wrong. The characteristics of the physical symptoms depend on the specific disease process, and, even within a specific illness, the symptoms may range from a sudden onset with accelerated progression to an insidious onset with slow progression. The specific physical challenges experienced during any of the trajectory phases can be diverse, including physical immobility, pain, fatigue, disfigurement, and deformities. The physical aspects of chronic illness can limit the client's independence, and this limitation can affect self-esteem and overall life satisfaction. In addition, physical challenges may affect sexuality and may limit the individual's ability to participate in a sexual relationship.

Historically, nurses have been educated about the care of people with the physical challenges related to diseases. Besides assisting clients in living with their physi-

cal challenges, the nurse must recognize the interrelationship between physical and psychosocial aspects of an illness. One difficult facet of chronic illness is its ongoing nature. Chronic illnesses cannot be cured and do not always respond to therapeutic interventions. Physical deterioration can occur despite efforts to treat the illness. This deterioration can be challenging and discouraging for the person with the illness, the family, and the nurse.

Psychosocial Aspects

The psychosocial challenges of chronic illness have been the focus of many studies. Several concepts related to the psychosocial aspects of chronic illness have been identified. Three frequently addressed concepts include uncertainty, powerlessness, and biographical disruption (Strauss, 1975; Charmaz, 1983, 1991; Conrad, 1987; Corbin & Strauss, 1987, 1988; Thorne, 1993).

Uncertainty

"**Uncertainty** is the inability to determine the meaning of events. . . . The decision maker is unable to accurately predict events" (Mishel & Braden, 1988, p. 98). Mishel (1999) states that "uncertainty is a constant experience in chronic illness due to the unpredictable and inconsistent symptom onset, continual questions about recurrence or exacerbation, and unknown future due to living with debilitating conditions" (p. 269)

Diagnosis is a critical occurrence in the lives of people with chronic illness and has a major impact on them. Conrad (1987) proposed that there is prediagnosis uncertainty, when the person does not know what is wrong; medical uncertainty, when physicians try to diagnose the problem; and uncertainty that accompanies the diagnosis itself. Diagnosis is often a time when the client and family must adjust to the treatment regimen and begin to integrate illness into their lives.

Commonalities in the diagnosis experience exist despite the many different diagnoses classified as chronic illness. Although for some diseases, such as diabetes mellitus or stroke, the diagnosis is usually early in the illness, others, such as multiple sclerosis, result in delays and prolonged prediagnosis testing procedures and even incorrect diagnoses. Thorne (1993), in her study of participants with a variety of chronic illnesses, found that often "the diagnostic testing process was an intensely difficult and confusing time, characterized by serious doubts about the benevolence or competence of health professionals as well as questions about their own [the clients'] sanity" (p. 21). Thorne suggests that the diagnostic event can mean an end to a long and frustrating diagnosis process, and many clients and families consider this a critical turning point in their lives. She writes:

> Although the diagnosis represented the possibility of finally taking some action from the patient and family point of view, many found that the health care professional lost interest in their case once the diagnosis deemed the condition to be chronic. (pp. 27–28).

As a way of dealing with uncertainty at the time of diagnosis, people may rely primarily on knowledge provided by professionals. However, as they live with the illness they learn about it. In her study, Michael (1996) found that for the participants' "going to the doctor, attending support group meetings and reading about the illness [were] helpful, but much of what they learned came from trial and error" (p. 262). Nurses must support clients and their families through their diagnosis experience and explore the impact it has on their lives. Listening to the client and family can help them make meaning of the experience.

Day-to-day living with a chronic illness can bring new uncertainties. The continuous ups and downs of the illness present a sense of uncertainty, which can cause people to isolate themselves (Miller, 2000a). Charmaz (1983) concluded that since many chronic illnesses have an unpredictable course, the accompanying uncertainty and fear cause some people to restrict their lives more than they need. Restrictions in the lives of people with a chronic illness are sometimes set in motion by professionals when clients are not given sufficient information and treatment.

An understanding of uncertainty as it relates to chronic illness will help the nurse to view the client's care from a holistic perspective. Nurses need to assess the client's and the family's experience and help them in developing strategies for living with the uncertainty. Client strategies may include becoming more informed about the illness, searching for additional treatments, undertaking stress-reduction techniques, and seeking support from others including family, friends, people with the same illness, and health care professionals.

Powerlessness

The unpredictable challenges that accompany chronic illness can promote a sense of powerlessness. Miller (2000a) describes **powerlessness** as "the perception that one lacks the capacity or authority to act to affect an outcome" and suggests that in chronic illness it can be related to "remissions and exacerbations or, in some instances, to progressive physical deterioration" (p. 4). Hymovich and Hagopian (1992) suggest that powerlessness encompasses helplessness, hopelessness, and loss of control and can manifest as passivity, nonparticipation in care and decision making, dependence on others, and verbal expression of loss of control (p. 158). See Figure 27-6 for suggested nursing strategies aimed at decreasing feelings of powerlessness in persons affected by Acquired Immunodeficiency Syndrome (AIDS).

FIGURE 27-6 Nursing Strategies for Empowering Persons Affected by Acquired Immunodeficiency Syndrome (AIDS)

The nurse can coach clients and their families to:

- recognize potentialities and tap sources of power
- to acknowledge the options that are available
- to sort through the multiple illness demands to set goals and plan for future potentialities.

Nurses can help clients become competent in self-care and symptom management.

Adapted from: "Empowering Persons Affected by Acquired Immunodeficiency Syndrome," by J. Bennett, 2000, in J. Miller (Ed.), *Coping with Chronic Illness* (3rd ed.), Philadelphia, PA: F. A. Davis, p. 388.

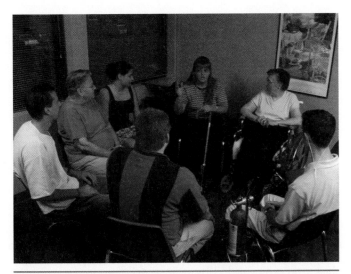

This support group of people with chronic illnesses is listening to a speaker discuss ways to relax.

Biographical Disruption

Biographical disruption is a concept that has emerged from the foundational research on chronic illness (Charmaz, 1983, 1991; Corbin & Strauss, 1988). Corbin and Strauss (1988) call biography a life course: "life stretching over a number of years and life evolving around a continual stream of experiences that result in a unique identity" (p. 50). They suggest that chronic illness is often accompanied by changes or disruption in biography (biographical disruption). The changes may include alterations in clients' perception of themselves as a person; in the concept of their body, which may not function as it once did; and in their sense of biographical time. Time takes on new meaning for people, as their past abilities and performances may be very different from those of the present. Lengthy treatment regimens such as kidney dialysis impinge on a person's life routine and can disrupt biographical time (pp. 52–65). Corbin and Strauss allege that health care professionals fall short of being aware of the biographical disruptions being experienced by people with chronic illness because of the focus on the medical model and acute care. Taking a holistic approach to the care of people requires that the nurse have an awareness of the client's biographical processes.

In her study, Charmaz (1983) found that, as the participants became more dependent and immobilized as a result of chronic illness, they suffered from a loss of self in which they lost not only self-esteem but also self-identity. Their diminished sense of self resulted in the participants' leading restricted lives, experiencing social isolation, being discredited, and burdening others. These experiences occurred even when the impairments were not visible. Loss of self-esteem related to the chronic illness experience crosses ethnocultural boundaries (Anderson, 1991).

Spiritual Aspects

"Spirituality is a belief in or relationship with some higher power, creative force, divine being, or an infinite source of energy" (Kozier, Erb, Berman & Burke, 2000, p. 220). Spiritual belief can influence a client's feelings about his or her illness and help the client cope with the challenges of chronic illness. It can provide a sense of hope and a purpose for one's life.

Miller (2000a) describes the client's belief system that includes spirituality as a resource. She writes:

> The chronically ill person needs relief from the isolation of suffering, and having a relationship with God may alleviate the feelings of aloneness. Some individuals may find meaning in the misfortune of chronic illness through religion and faith. (p. 14)

In turn, the invasiveness of chronic illness in the lives of people impinges on their spirituality. There can be a

---

✴ DECISION MAKING

Persons with Disabilities and Society

The United States and Canada have attempted to remove barriers in the environment for individuals with disabilities (e.g., by installing ramps to buildings, leveling curbs, establishing designated parking spaces).

◆ What measures can society take to address the issue of psychosocial suffering of people with chronic illness?

REFLECTIVE THINKING

Sense of Self

Anderson (1991) poses two thought-provoking questions for consideration by all health care professionals. Think about these two questions (p. 715):

- Why do health care providers, whose mandate it is to care for patients, interact with them in ways that sometimes reinforce the devalued sense of self?
- Why are health care services not structured to enable people to manage their chronic illness in ways that foster their feelings of self-worth?

✳ DECISION MAKING

Spirituality and the Client with Chronic Illness

Mary is a 35-year-old woman with two children: a 3-year-old and a newborn. During her recent pregnancy, she was diagnosed with breast cancer. When you make a postnatal visit to her home, you find that she is very upset. Mary tells you that she has always been a devout Christian and has in the past been able to draw strength from prayer. Now, with what has happened to her, she doubts if God exists.

◆ What would you do in this situation?

◆ What words of comfort could you offer Mary?

strengthening of spirituality or a turning away. Hymovich and Hagopian (1992) suggest that people who are chronically ill can experience spiritual distress,

> which can be characterized in ways such as questioning the meaning of suffering, the meaning of one's existence, or the moral and ethical implications of the therapeutic regimen. . . . Spiritual distress can cause nightmares and sleep disturbances or alterations in behavior and mood as evidenced by crying, anger, withdrawal, anxiety, hostility, or apathy. (p. 127)

Sterling-Fisher (1998) states that "it is very important for nurses to be familiar and comfortable with spirituality" (p. 244).

However, spirituality is a concept that nurses do not always feel comfortable discussing with clients, although it is a significant factor in how people come to live with their chronic illness. An awareness of the client's spirituality provides a basis for holistic nursing care. Walton (1996) suggests that nurses who practice holistically "can connect intimately with patients and facilitate their spiritual relationships with self, higher power, and others" (p. 247). Lindsey (1996), in her study of the experience of health within chronic illness, found that participants "attributed their experiences of feeling healthy to an awareness of their spirituality, with a sense of connectedness, wholeness, harmony and peacefulness." Nurses need to understand what experiences give meaning to life for clients and their families and promote such experiences. In studying the meaning of spirituality to the elderly, Bauer and Barron (1995) found that participants in their study saw caring and communication skills as important aspects of spiritual care nursing interventions. The participants wanted nurses to be "attentive, respectful, caring and hopeful" (p. 277).

Economic Aspects

Chronic illness has economic implications for individuals, their families, and society. Although health care insurance covers costs such as hospitalization, doctors' visits, and home nursing care, there are many costs that the ill person must assume. Hymovich and Hagopian (1992) refer to such costs as indirect costs, which include special diets, special equipment, vocational rehabilitation, time lost from work, travel expenses, telephone calls, and insurance.

The total amount of uninsured costs are difficult to measure, although the National Center for Health Statistics found that, in 1998, 20% of all personal health expenditures were paid "out of pocket" (USDHHS, 2000b, p. 13) The challenges faced by individuals and their families are compounded by uninsured expenses.

Chronic illness can have a direct effect on the occupation and employment of the ill individual. Equal opportunity in employment is required by law in some developed nations (*Canadian Charter of Rights and Freedom,* 1982; *Americans with Disabilities Act,* 1990). Although such laws exist to protect the individual from discrimination on the basis of disability, they do not preclude all challenges in the work environment. Symptoms associated with the illness can affect the individual's job performance and influence the attitude of co-workers. Complex treatment regimens do not always fit into work routines and may require a change of occupation. A progression of the illness can lead to unemployment. Charmaz (1991) suggests that financial pressures of the illness often force ill people to struggle to work and remain independent as long as possible, sometimes to the detriment of their health.

The Centers for Disease Control and Prevention (CDC) reports that "medical care costs for people with

✳ DECISION MAKING

Employment and the Person with Chronic Illness

You have worked with Sam, a 28-year-old single man, for several years. Sam has developed rheumatoid arthritis and will require more frequent rest periods while at work. In addition, he will need to stay home and rest when the disease flares up.

◆ What special considerations (such as work schedules and working conditions) do you think could be made for Sam?

◆ Would you be prepared to make changes in your own work situation to accommodate his needs?

chronic diseases total more than $400 billion annually, more than 60% of total medical care expenditures" (US-DHHS, 1999b, p. vii). In 1998, health insurance paid 33% of personal health care expenditures, and the federal and local government paid 10% (USDHHS, 2000b). Chronic illness and disability continue to be important factors in the nation's economy. The estimated annual costs of selected conditions in the United States include cardiovascular disease, $287 billion; cancer, $107 billion; and diabetes mellitus, $100 billion (USDHHS, 1999b).

Governments in the United States and other developed nations are trying to contain and reduce health care costs through health care reform. One strategy is to keep people who are chronically ill at home rather than in institutions. Although such initiatives are less costly to the government and may be more desirable to the client, there is a risk of shifting the burden of care to family caregivers.

LIVING WITH A CHRONIC ILLNESS

Chronic illness is a significant event that can affect all aspects of life, including physical, psychological, spiritual, social, and occupational (Strauss, 1975; Gerhardt, 1990). In his classic work, Strauss (1975) proposes seven key challenges faced by people who are chronically ill:

- Prevention and management of medical crises
- Control of symptoms
- Carrying out and managing prescribed regimens
- Preventing or living with social isolation
- Shaping the course of the illness
- **Normalizing** style of life and interactions with others (a coping strategy used by people to control the impact of chronic illness on their lives)
- Ensuring adequate funding

In response to these challenges, people with chronic illnesses, their families, and friends must develop basic strategies for day-to-day living. Among the basic strategies are approaches for self-care and symptom management. Exercise, healthy eating, and smoking cessation are examples of self-care strategies that not only promote health and prevent disease but in some instances can also help alleviate disease symptoms. Clients who develop a chronic illness are often highly motivated to explore numerous options with regard to living with their illness. The options are varied and include the traditional medical approaches such as medications as well as an increasing number of nontraditional approaches like healing touch. Clients may require the assistance of others, including health care professionals, to determine which approaches best suit their needs. See Chapter 11 for health promotion and disease prevention strategies.

Corbin and Strauss (1988) have made a substantial contribution to the understanding of chronic illness. They introduced the concept of "work" to portray what it is that the client and family do in attending the challenges of chronic illness. They describe this chronic illness work as maintenance of both physical health status and emotional stability. The intensity of this work varies with the course of the illness and with the impact it has on personal relationships and personal identities. Life with a chronic illness can be complex, and clients and their families must be considered on an individual basis. The nurse must be aware of the specific **biographical work** being done by people and must support them and assist them in finding other resources to help meet the psychological challenges of their illness.

Consideration of the insider's view of illness supports beliefs related to the client's culture. Citing the work of Grace and Zola, Peters (1998) identifies three cross-cultural issues that may affect the way a person views his or her illness (pp. 36–37):

- *Culturally perceived causes of disability.* Some cultures may view the chronic illness as a form of punishment for wrongdoing. Others consider it an honor, as may be the case with Mexican Americans who have children with a chronic illness.
- *Expectation for survival.* Cultures with limited resources may redirect resources from the person with an illness to stronger members.
- *Appropriate social roles.* In some cultures, family resources are not allocated to the education or achievement of girls or women. Chronic illness may reinforce this belief.

Cultural aspects of health remain important in developing countries despite an emergence of Western curative health approaches (Airhihenbuwa & Harrison, 1993; Conrad & Gallagher, 1993). A system has developed in which Western medicine is incorporated alongside the traditional approach to medicine that is rooted in the country's culture. For example, Subedi and Subedi (1993) found that the people of Nepal use Western and traditional medicine at different points of their illness. Early in an illness, the Nepalese use traditional cultural approaches. Modern health care services are, for the most part, sought only as a last resort. Nursing care that is based on the assumptions of empowerment respects the beliefs of others regardless of whether these beliefs are related to culture or religion (see Chapter 8).

Coping

Coping is a term commonly used to describe a strategy for living with a chronic illness (Hymovich & Hagopian, 1992; Miller, 2000a). Miller (2000b) defines coping as "dealing with situations that present a threat to the individual to resolve uncomfortable feelings such as anxiety, fear, grief, and guilt" (p. 22). Miller suggests that coping strategies used by people who are chronically ill are

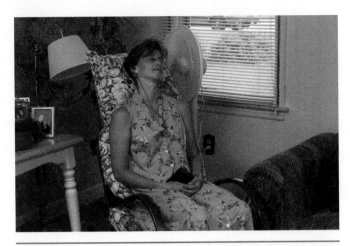

Listening to relaxation tapes is a way of coping with chronic illness.

more likely to be effective when they are **approach strategies.** Approach coping strategies signify an effort to confront the challenges of the illness and include (pp. 38–39):

- Seeking information and help
- Gaining strength from spirituality
- Using methods of diversion
- Expressing feelings, emotions, and concerns
- Maintaining control
- Using relaxation and positive-thinking techniques
- Maintaining realistic independence but remaining positive about depending on others if necessary
- Maintaining social activities
- Seeking help
- Setting goals and using problem solving
- Using humor
- Conserving energy
- Engaging in activity covering up disability, discomfort
- Finding comfort in the realization that other people have the same illness

Lazarus and Folkman (1984) criticize the traditional view of coping because it focuses on successful adaptation to a stressor such as illness. Moving away from the view of coping as either an effective or an ineffective outcome, they present coping as a process. Lazarus and Folkman define coping as "constantly changing cognitive and behavioral efforts to manage specific external and/or internal demands that are appraised as taxing or exceeding the resources of the person" (p. 141). This view of coping considers what "the person actually thinks or does in a specific context" and allows for "change in coping thoughts and acts as a stressful encounter unfolds" (p. 142). The way a person copes may vary from situa-

tion to situation. They suggest that the way a person copes is determined in part by:

- Personal resources such as health, energy, existential beliefs
- Personal commitments
- Problem-solving skills
- Social skills
- Social support
- Material resources

Supporting clients and families in their efforts to cope with a chronic illness is important. The nurse must explore with them the need for referral to specific services such as counseling and stress management.

Normalizing

"The chief business of a chronically ill person is not just to stay alive or keep symptoms under control, but to live as normally as possible despite his symptoms and disease" (Strauss, 1975, p. 58). This process of normalizing is an effort to minimize the social effects of the illness (Thorne, 1993). People with chronic illness use various strategies to normalize their lives, including (Strauss, 1975; Charmaz, 1991; Hymovich & Hagopian, 1992):

- Making efforts to keep symptoms invisible
- Engaging in their preillness activities
- Maintaining social relationships

The effects of a chronic illness can be visible, such as disfigurement, changes in physical characteristics, and limitation in body functions, or invisible, such as pain or fatigue. Although having a visible illness makes it more difficult for the person to pass as being well, it does justify the need for assistance and elicit sympathetic responses. Being visibly ill, however, can result in penalties, including stigmatization and discrimination, being labeled as disabled, and being considered less competent (Saylor & Yoder, 1998). In a literature review related to the stigma of visible and invisible chronic conditions, Joachim and Acorn (2000) revealed a lack of research and understanding about the "stigmatized state" (p. 247). Charmaz (1991) proposes that having an invisible illness allows the person the option of either disclosure or nondisclosure of the illness. Nondisclosure allows the person to pass for normal but can result in stress for the individual with a risk of being found out and discredited. Disclosure of the illness can be accompanied by stigmatization, especially with certain chronic illnesses, such as epilepsy or AIDS. In addition, the invisible nature of the illness means the person may have difficulty legitimizing the illness. Others may not take the effects of the illness seriously (Strauss, 1975; Thorne, 1993). Thorne (1993) suggests that health care professionals exhibit these same prejudices toward the chronically ill. Nurses must consider if these prejudices exist in their own practice. It is important that the nurse be aware of the possible negative reactions of others to people with chronic illnesses. In assisting clients, the nurse must explore with them the possible impact of a visible illness on relationships with others and also the potential outcomes of disclosure or nondisclosure of an invisible illness.

Managing the Treatment

Treatment regimens can be complex and can require significant amounts of time, energy, and money. Examples include home blood glucose monitoring for diabetes and hemodialysis for renal failure. Maintaining client compliance with or adherence to treatment recommendations has long been a goal of health care professionals. Individuals who do not adhere to their treatment regimen risk increasing the negative effects of their illness. Nevertheless, the incidence of failure to adhere to the treatment regimen is high (Hymovich & Hagopian, 1992; Blevins, Berg, & Dunbar-Jacob, 1998).

The client's decision to alter the treatment regimen takes on a different meaning when considered from his or her perspective (Roberson, 1992; Thorne, 1993; Blevins et al. 1998). In her study, Callaghan (1992) found that participants wanted their expertise to be an integral part of their treatment plan. When health care professionals disregarded their ideas, participants who felt capable of making decisions about their care customized their treatment regimen to suit their needs, without the professionals' consent. If a client does not adhere to treatment regimens, the client may have different expectations than health care professionals and may be making an effort to exert some control over the impact of the illness on his or her life (Roberson, 1992; Blevins et al., 1998).

Wuest (1993) expresses concern about the use of the term *noncompliance* to label clients who do not follow their prescribed treatment regimen. She states that this term comes from the medical model and is grounded in a patriarchal worldview. Feminist thought may offer an alternative perspective on ways to work in partnership with the client regarding the issues that arise from prescribed treatment. Wuest writes:

This [feminist thought] requires an entrance into a dialogue with those for whom we care, a dialogue that ultimately leads to understanding personal, social, and political factors that determine what this person [the client] views as possible and desirable at this point in time. (p. 23)

Considering clients' perspectives on their ability to live with their treatment regimen is a vital aspect of nursing care that seeks to involve clients in the decision making. Coates and Boore (1995) advise nurses to support the efforts of people in their self-management of chronic illness. They write:

If patients are to be given the opportunity to be active participants in care, they must also be given the right to decline to follow therapy or to modify it without recrimination. If patients and health professionals are to be partners in care, both partners must have equal power. This necessitates a change in attitude of nurses and other health care professionals which is reflected in interaction between the partners in care. (p. 636).

Role of the Family

The role of the family changes and takes on new significance in the face of chronic illness. Strauss (1975) proposes that other people associated with the ill person, including the family, act as various agents:

People act as rescuing agents (saving a diabetic individual from dying when he is in a coma), or as protective agents (accompanying an epileptic person so that if he begins to fall he can be eased to the ground), or as assisting agents (helping with a regimen), or as control agents (making the person stay with his regimen), and so on. (p. 8)

Strauss submits that health professionals play a secondary role in the day-to-day lives of people with chronic illness. He advises professionals to "see with some directness and clarity the social and psychological problems faced by the chronically ill and their immediate families in their daily lives" (p. 7).

Families can enable the individual with a chronic illness to relinquish obligations such as maintaining a job, getting an education, and providing child care. (Charmaz, 1991). Charmaz states that the family can provide a major buffer against social isolation from friends, associates, and neighbors. Families can help fill the time and break the routine of the day-to-day challenges of the illness.

Family Caregivers

Family members often become caregivers for the ill person. Caring for a loved one can be a rewarding experience. Enjoyment can result from keeping the care receiver at home and from fulfilling a sense of duty and love (Cohen, Pushkar Gold, Shulman, & Zucchero, 1994). Home can be perceived as a place of healing. A challenging aspect of family caregiving, however, is the demanding nature of the commitment. Spousal relationships are tested, as an intrusive illness often affects the ability of the ill person to share in the partnership of the marital relationship. Mobilizing, bathing, dressing, and feeding the ill person can be physically demanding. The caregiver role is sometimes carried out in addition to employment, child rearing, and other household tasks. *Caregiver burden* is a term commonly used to describe the challenges that accompany the caregiving. In their study, Boland and Sims (1996) found that the 24-hour commitment of the caregiver

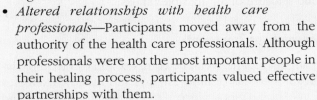

RESEARCH FOCUS

Experiences of Chronically Ill: A Covert Caring for the Self

Study Problem/Purpose

To examine, explore, and understand the meaning of experience for people living with a chronic illness.

Methods

This qualitative study was an interpretive phenomenological inquiry. Each of the eight participants had a different chronic illness. The researcher and each participant engaged in a conversational relationship. Data interpretation followed the guidelines for phenomenological analysis.

Findings

Four themes of covert caring for the self emerged from the data:

- *Taking control*—Participants acquired the strength to take control of their care and to assert their own authority.
- *Seeking knowledge*—Participants began to read about their illnesses as well as about healing, personal growth, metaphysics, and spiritual awareness and became committed to help others with chronic illnesses.
- *Accessing alternate healing modalities*—Participants explored and engaged in nonmedical forms of healing. All participants attained their greatest relief and healing from these other modalities. The cost of alternate care was paid by the participants, adding to their financial burden. Fearing ridicule, they did not

inform their professional caregivers of their use of other healers and healing methods.

- *Altered relationships with health care professionals*—Participants moved away from the authority of the health care professionals. Although professionals were not the most important people in their healing process, participants valued effective partnerships with them.

Implications

Health care professionals potentially can be support and facilitate different health and healing practices for people with chronic illnesses.

Consideration should be given to covering the cost of alternate healing practices as are the more traditional medical services.

Nurses need to move from a dominant expert model of care to client-directed care guided by these principles:

- Acknowledge and respect client wisdom and expertise.
- Respect client authority.
- Participate in a client-directed model of care.
- Value multiple forms of healing.
- Recognize and adopt a holistic approach to health and healing.
- Acknowledge the different philosophies and religions of the world, particularly as they relate to healing the mind, body, and spirit.

Source: Lindsey, E. (1997). Experiences of the chronically ill: A covert caring for the self. Journal of Holistic Health, 15(3), 227–242.

---

experience strained the physical and mental health of the participants. Caregivers become vulnerable to injuries, exhaustion, social isolation, and despair (Lubkin & Payne, 1998). Financial hardship is another risk as the family caregivers spend their time in this unpaid labor. This aspect of caregiving receives little political attention, because the family caregiver role is predominantly a female one and society may view this as a natural role for women.

Rutman's (1995) study of women caregivers revealed that they experienced powerlessness when (p. 22):

- Their competence and expertise as a caregiver were not recognized or respected
- There was a lack of control (either over the care receiver's disease process or over the care choices) or a need to relinquish control

- They were unable to prevent harm from befalling the care receiver
- The system was bureaucratic and lacked resources; the needs of caregiver and care receiver apparently did not come first

The caregivers in Rutman's (1995) study provided the following suggestions for improving the caregiving experience:

- Enhanced resources to ensure quality care facilities and environments
- Enhanced public recognition for caregiving work
- Respect for caregivers
- Access to education and information

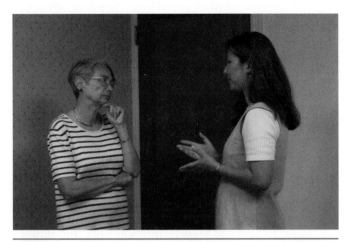

Offering support to the caregiver of a chronically ill client is important.

- Enhanced communication and working in partnership—families, parents, and professionals
- Support for caregivers—developing and strengthening peer support and networking within communities

Understanding the family's perspective is fundamental to an effective partnership between health care professionals and family caregivers. Some families rise to meet the challenge that illness presents. The stresses and difficulties overwhelm others and consequently can lead to neglect, abuse, or disintegration of the family unit. With an increasing number of caregivers in the community, nurses must recognize their needs in addition to those of the recipient of care. The principles of empowerment discussed earlier in this chapter are a sound basis for working in partnership with the caregiver, the care receiver, and other family members. The knowledge and expertise of caregivers in caring for their family member must be acknowledged and valued. Given and Given (1998) advise attention to health promotion as a means

REFLECTIVE THINKING

The Caregiver of a Chronically Ill Client

- Think of someone you know who is caring for a chronically ill family member. How do you think the experience has influenced his or her life?
- Imagine that a member of your family has become ill and you are required to provide the care. How would this situation affect your life?

of contributing to the health and well-being of family caregivers. Caregivers can be assisted through the provision of information, support, and resources. Community resources such as support groups and respite care can help the caregiver with the challenges of the role. Additional information about caregiving can be found in Chapter 24.

HEALTH PROMOTION AND DISEASE PREVENTION: THE NURSE'S ROLE

Community health nursing can be guided by the global commitment to achieve health for all by the year 2000 (WHO, 1978). The United States and Canada have been among the leaders in this movement, as evidenced by the *Healthy People 2010* document (USDHHS, 2000a), the Epp Report (Epp, 1986), and the Ottawa Charter (WHO, 1986). The Ottawa Charter identifies the prerequisites to achieving health for all as peace, shelter, education, food, income, a stable ecosystem, sustainable resources, social justice, and equity (WHO, 1986).

The 1993 *World Development Report* highlights the importance of the "good" health of citizens for the economic well-being of a country. Although many of the world's developing countries have made a commitment to health for all, the challenges are enormous. The report states:

> Rapid progress in reducing child mortality and fertility rates will create new demands on health care systems as the aging of populations brings forth costly noncommunicable diseases of adults and the elderly. (World Bank, 1993, p. 3)

However, in developing nations the toll from childhood and infectious diseases remains high and adds to the health care demands that accompany a significant increase in life expectancy. The problems of controlling health care costs and ensuring the accessibility of health care to the overall population are common to both developing and developed nations.

The *Healthy People 2010* report recommends health promotion and preventive services at primary, secondary, and tertiary levels of prevention (USDHHS, 2000a). The recommended services include education, counseling, screening, immunization, and chemoprophylactic interventions. Priority care should focus on the most prevalent chronic conditions: heart disease and stroke, cancer, diabetes, and chronic disabling conditions. The *Healthy People 2010* document identifies that significant progress has been made in improving the nation's health since the implementation of the *Healthy People 2000* goals and objectives. Death from coronary heart disease and stroke has declined. Significant advances have been attained in cancer diagnosis and treatment. However, diabetes and other chronic conditions "continue to present a serious obstacle to public health" (USDHHS, 2000a,

Perspectives... ✳

INSIGHTS OF A CAREGIVER

My wife, [Louise], has Huntington's disease. It is an inherited disorder affecting the nervous system. It causes progressive deterioration of physical and mental capabilities, leading ultimately to severe incapacitation and eventual death, usually 15 to 20 years after the onset. Louise also has irritable bowel syndrome. This means most of her day at home is spent in the bathroom, a behavior she has great difficulty controlling on her own. Louise is 60 years old.

Onset for my wife occurred about 10 years ago. She can no longer perform the role of homemaker. Maintaining our home requires a reasonably reliable income. I am self-employed and work as a home-based businessman. It is essential I continue to be the breadwinner. This is becoming most challenging and stressful. Having my work in the same place as where I carry out most of my caregiving definitely has its shortcomings. Work often takes a back seat.

Without full daytime care for my wife, I am unable to generate full-time earnings. I am working to about 50% capacity. Every hour not worked is an hour of lost income plus the deterioration of my reputation of getting the job done on time.

I cannot complain about the caliber of home care and assistance we are presently receiving. But what is not available is full-time care to enable me to work away from home and to expand my business. Admis-sion to a care facility is at least a year away. As my wife's disease progresses, my opportunity for full employment decreases. She cannot be left alone without an element of risk. If she were to require more assistance because of an accident, I would definitely be unable to care for her. To hire full-time help would cost me most of any additional income from full-time work. Unemployment is not a choice. Caregiving and working are full-time jobs. There is only one of me.

Abandonment is a choice. Then I know she will be looked after. But the outcomes, for me, are not what I want. The percentage of male caregivers of those with Huntington's disease who make this choice is very high. I don't want to be part of that statistic. In all honesty, though, the thought has occurred to me.

Huntington's disease has affected our whole family. It has put a great emotional and physical strain on my wife and me. Our children are at risk as well. One has been tested positive as carrying the Huntington's gene, one tested negative, and two are undecided about being tested. We have 10 grandchildren. Seven are at risk. Is caregiving ever going to be over for me? I do know I have to continue earning a living for a long while yet.

—Henry Ficke (1995)

---

p. 3). In addition, HIV/AIDS remains a serious health issue for the nation. Reduction of risk factors for chronic illness require further attention related to a 50% increase in obesity over the past 20 years, a sedentary lifestyle in 40% of adults, and an increase in smoking among adolescents (USDHHS, 2000a).

Health promotion is central to the work of community health nurses in caring for people with chronic illness [American Public Health Association (APHA), 1981; American Nurses Association, 1986; Canadian Public Health Association, 1990]. The APHA suggests that health promotion can be accomplished by nurses who work with individuals, families, aggregates, and multidisciplinary teams. The APHA includes identifying groups at risk for illness, disability, and premature death as a key element of the nurse's role. The nurse is responsible for directing resources toward these groups (APHA, 1981, p. 4). The Canadian Public Health Associ-ation (1990) considers the nurses' health-promotive roles from a health determinant basis. They see the nurse's role as (p. 7):

1. Assisting communities, families, and individuals in taking responsibility for maintaining and improving their knowledge of, their control over, and their influence on health determinants.

2. Facilitating and mediating to enhance community, group, or individual strategies that help society anticipate, cope with, and manage maturational changes and the environment.

3. Encouraging communities', families', and individuals' ability to balance choices with social responsibility to create a healthier future.

4. Initiating and participating in health-promotion activities in partnership with others, including the community, colleagues, and other sectors.

Community health nurses act as resource managers, planners, and coordinators as they help individuals and their families explore health-promotive and disease-preventive community resources. Resources vary from community to community; however, there are national resources related to the most prevalent chronic illnesses. In the United States, these include, for example, the American Diabetes Association, the American Heart Association, the American Cancer Society, the Multiple Sclerosis Society, the Kidney Foundation, and the Cystic Fibrosis Foundation. Equivalent resources exist internationally in Canada, Britain, and other developed nations. Many of these national organizations have local chapters in communities, making their services more accessible. These organizations address a variety of goals such as health promotion, public education at all levels of prevention, fund raising, support of research, and some direct client and family services.

Within the context of health care reform, community health nurses have a role in policy development and planning and in the delivery of preventive programs and services. In addition, they have a role in research that considers the effectiveness of health promotion and prevention and facilitation of the transfer of research into practice. Chronic illness issues are complex and varied: for example, accessibility of community resources, economic challenges for individuals and families, and availability of long-term care support services. Funding for research, screening, public education, and societal concerns such as poverty are examples of other issues that require community health nurse involvement. The Washington State Core Government Public Health Functions Task Force states that "efforts to promote personal health, protect community health, and prevent disease are known to be effective. Yet, only 3% of current health system care dollars are spent on these services" (Washington Department of Health, 1993, p. 5). Nurses working in the community must raise the awareness of key policymakers in all levels of government of the need for a more equitable distribution of resources between the acute-care and health-promotive and health-preventive aspects of chronic illness. Community planning and evaluation are integral to policy development. See Chapter 16.

The key to successful health promotion and disease prevention is partnership between community health nurses and members of the community. The nurse should encourage people to actively participate in identifying and taking ownership of community health issues. Issues related to chronic illness prevention may include the lack of parks and playgrounds, availability of cigarettes to underage smokers, tobacco advertising, high cost of fruits and vegetables, and need for access to land for gardens. The nurse serves as a resource by educating community members about the political process as it relates to health issues, about successful communication with the health care and political systems, and about

strategies for participating in decisions concerning health issues (Canadian Public Health Association, 1990, p. 9).

Primary Prevention

Primary prevention focuses on taking measures to alter risk factors before the disease has begun. The increasing incidence of chronic illness, the lack of curative interventions, and the requirement for long-term care have resulted in great expense to the health care systems of many nations. Consequently, primary prevention is a vital approach to chronic illness.

Primary prevention strategies focus on environmental or behavioral risk factors that are modifiable. These measures need to be implemented before the disease has developed. For example, preventive measures for heart disease and stroke should be aimed at children and adolescents because physiological changes related to these conditions may begin in these age groups. Community health nurses have long been involved in a variety of strategies aimed at disease prevention. These include immunization, health education, and counseling. Immunization against infectious disease such as polio or measles prevents the associated sequelae that can lead to chronic disability. Community health nurses educate and counsel clients and their families about the reduction of modifiable risk factors related to chronic illness and disability. The nurse encourages changes in lifestyle activities not conducive to good health and supports those that are (Canadian Public Health Association, 1990). Adequate nutrition, exercise, sleep, stress reduction, and self-care are important aspects of this education and counseling.

It is important to apply the principles of empowerment to health education. Traditional models of teaching and learning have had limited success with the need for lifestyle and behavioral changes often associated with

---

✳ DECISION MAKING

The Community Health Nurse and Political Involvement

Nurses are increasingly becoming involved in political action related to health care. Your city needs more green space to provide an area where people can be physically active.

◆ As a community health nurse what could you do to influence the local city government in addressing this issue?

◆ How might you gather support from other nurses in your community?

chronic illness prevention and with living with an illness (Fahlerg et al., 1991; Funnel et al., 1991). Education at the level of primary prevention addresses the general lifestyle issues that are considered risk factors for chronic illness. Preventive measures are very specific to the chronic illness being considered. However, dietary practices and smoking are risk factors for several chronic illnesses, including heart disease and stroke, cancer, and lung disease. Education related to the risks associated with smoking, obesity, and dietary fat intake is important in the prevention of chronic illness.

Secondary Prevention

Secondary prevention focuses on early disease detection through screening programs as well as early treatment of the disease. For example, screening for high cholesterol and high blood pressure, in addition to implementing primary-prevention strategies, has resulted in a steady

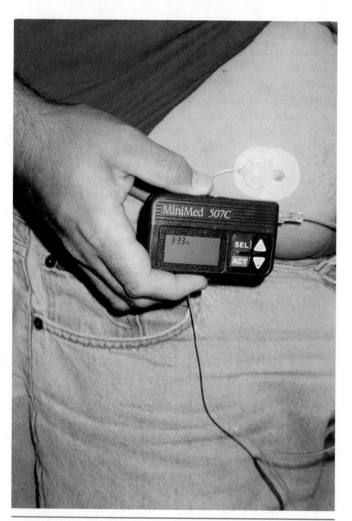

This person manages his diabetes using an insulin pump.

decline in the number of deaths from heart disease and stroke over the past two decades (USDHHS, 2000a). Education about the importance of taking advantage of available screening techniques such as mammograms, Pap smears, examinations for prostatic cancer, and regular physical examinations is an approach aimed at secondary prevention. Through early diagnosis, treatment can be implemented to slow the progression of an existing disease and to minimize damage caused by the disease. Early diagnosis is especially significant for chronic illnesses that may have an insidious onset, with a significant progression of the disease prior to the appearance of clinical signs and symptoms. Risk factor modification strategies aimed at asymptomatic adults become secondary prevention for chronic illnesses in which physiological changes leading to the disease begin in early childhood or adolescence, for example heart disease, stroke, and some cancers.

Tertiary Prevention

Tertiary prevention focuses on rehabilitation and restoration after an illness has occurred to minimize morbidity and benefit the client's life. Rehabilitation following a heart attack or stroke, prevention of complications related to immobility in individuals with disabilities, and regular eye examinations for people with diabetes mellitus are examples. Important aspects of tertiary prevention address the physical and psychosocial challenges associated with chronic illness. Self-help or support groups can offer clients and their families considerable psychosocial support. Such groups are an important resource, and they exist in many communities. Some examples are the Stroke Club, the Hospice Association, and the Arthritis Society.

Client education is an important preventive strategy in chronic illness as clients learn to live with the illness and to manage challenging symptoms and complex treatment regimens. Funnel (2000) reinforces the need for patient-centered education. She writes, "the best thing you can do for your patients with chronic disease is to let them run with the ball" (p. 47). Empowering client education respects the knowledge and ability of the client. The nurse must work with the client to set goals and to explore strategies for meeting these goals. In this partnership, the client and nurse are valued as resources and both share the responsibility for treatment and outcomes (Funnel et al., 1991). Chapters 11 and 12 provide further discussion of client education.

The community health nurse assists individuals and their families in determining what resources may be of value to them and how they can use these services. Nurses become involved in the referral process, if necessary. Dialogue with clients and their families focuses on the exploration of their expectations related to these resources. Involvement with these resources takes time, energy, and sometimes money, a fact that clients and their families must consider.

Tertiary prevention requires community health nurses to work directly with people with chronic illnesses. This work involves assessment, planning, and intervention with individuals and their families. In all aspects of nursing care, the lived experience of individuals and their families must guide nurses as they work in partnership. In this way, the beliefs and assumptions that underlie caring and empowerment are applied.

Assessment and interventions can be focused on the individual with the chronic illness. However, this approach must be considered in the context of the family. Although individuals themselves can best elucidate the challenges they experience and the effect of the chronic illness on all aspects of their lives, it is important for the nurse to be aware of certain assessment factors that pertain to people with chronic illness. Chapters 21, 24, and 25 offer assessment tools for use with individuals and families. Assessment should reflect the whole client and seek to understand the totality of his or her illness experience, including the physical, psychological, social, spiritual, and environmental dimensions. An assessment should reveal the client's challenges as well as personal resources.

Miller (2000a) refers to personal resources as **power resources.** She advocates that nurses assess the person's power resources, which can be compromised by illness. Power resources include physical strength, psychological stamina, social support, positive self-concept, energy, knowledge and insight, motivation, and a belief system. People who are chronically ill have a vast capacity for coping, but Miller advises that nurses who do not recognize helpful coping behaviors may not adequately help clients face the challenges that accompany illness. She believes that people look to nurses to help them face the challenges of long-term health problems (pp. 9–15).

Nursing interventions need to be considered from a holistic perspective in partnership with the client. Many people with a chronic illness use healing modalities not prescribed by their physicians to assist them with the physical and psychological challenges of their illness (Lindsey, 1993; Thorne, 1993; Thorne et al., 2000). A variety of healing modalities are used such as special diets, chiropractic care, naturopathy, stress management, biofeedback, Therapeutic Touch, and visualization. Healing modalities that are of ethnic origin are intrinsic to many cultures (see Chapter 12); for example, acupuncture is part of Asian cultures, and healing circles are part of some Native American cultures. Although research evidence is only now being accumulated on the effectiveness of these various healing modalities, people are turning to them with increasing frequency. Neuberger and Woods (1998) suggest that these therapies attract people with chronic illness for several reasons, including cultural or ethnic beliefs, frustration with the health care

they are receiving, or the ineffectiveness of medically ordered treatment.

Thorne (1993) found that most of the participants in her study had pursued a course of therapy not prescribed by their physician. These therapies were often successful in helping them with symptom relief. When participants encountered negative attitudes to this therapy from health care professionals, the participants questioned the assumed superiority of traditional health care. Similarly, Lindsey (1993) found that, as participants in her study explored nonprescribed healing modalities, their relationships with health care professionals often became unsatisfactory. She suggests that these different healing modalities provide people an opportunity to "look far beyond their physical limitations, and to begin to acknowledge and embrace other important aspects of their lives" (p. 113). The community nurse needs to be aware of the wide range of healing modalities and take care not to judge or ridicule the client's use of them. Nurses must acknowledge the cultural aspects of healing that clients bring to their experience and use this knowledge in the care provided.

The fact that clients and their families seek the assistance of other therapists in no way devalues the nurse's role. The move to other therapies may signify that individuals are taking responsibility and control for their own healing (Lindsey, 1993). In this light, the nurse can be helpful in exploring other methods of healing with clients and their families when they express an interest. The nurse has a responsibility to advocate for clients and families with regard to all therapies. Health goals, alternatives, and methods of evaluating the treatment should be determined by clients, their families, and the nurse. This strategy should apply to both prescribed medical therapies and other healing modalities.

People with chronic illnesses most often continue to live in their homes with their families and are sometimes cared for by family members. Even when the family does not become involved with the direct treatment regimen or care of the ill person, each family member and the family as a unit experience the illness. A framework offered by Hartrick et al. (1994) focuses on the family's health and illness experiences and attends to the interdependent nature of assessment and intervention. Such a framework, based on health promotion and partnership, is useful for community health nurses working with families challenged by a chronic illness. Central to this framework is **circular questioning.** Wright and Leahey (2000) note that the effect of circular questions is to introduce new cognitive connections that pave the way for new or different family behaviors. Tomm (1988) describes circular questions as questions that are neutral, accepting, and exploratory. Such questions are based on the assumption that "everything is connected to everything else" and reveal patterns that connect "persons, objects, actions, perceptions, ideas, feelings, events, beliefs, context, and so on, in recurrent circuits" (p. 7). Examples of circular

TABLE 27-6 Health-Promoting Family Nursing Assessment: The Framework

COMPONENT	STRATEGIC ELEMENTS	HEALTH-PROMOTION PRINCIPLES
Listening to the family	• Eliciting different family member perceptions • Gaining an understanding of the family story • The family as experts in their own health experience	• People without power have as much capacity as the powerful to assess their own health needs. • Every person and family lives within a social historical context that helps shape their identity and social relationships. • Diversity is positively valued.
Participatory dialogue	• Posing circular questions to elucidate the taken-for-granted family patterns and interactions • Family members critically reflecting on the circular questions and posing questions of their own	• Relationships between people and groups need to be arranged to provide an equal balance of power. • Empowerment describes our intentional efforts to create more equitable relationships with greater equity in resources, status, and authority.
Pattern recognition	• In collaboration, identifying the family's behaviors • In collaboration, recognizing the family's patterns and themes based on their beliefs and values • Cocreating the family's story	• The power of defining health problems belongs to those experiencing the problem. • Professional expertise and skills are used in new ways.
Envisioning action and positive change	• Making informed choices • Taking action • Reflecting on the action • Taking renewed action	• All people have strengths and are capable of determining their own needs, finding their own answers, and solving their own problems. • The people involved are the chief actors.

From "Family Nursing Assessment: Meeting the Challenge of Health Promotion," by G. Hartrick, A. E. Lindsey, and M. Hills, 1994, Journal of Advanced Nursing, 20, pp. 85–91. *Reprinted with permission of Blackwell Science Limited.*

questions include: Who in the family is most fearful about the stroke? Who is best at helping other family members deal with the fear? How does he or she do this? What do you do when you are afraid?

The Hartrick et al. (1994) framework consists of four interdependent components, all occurring together throughout both the assessment and the intervention process (see Table 27-6). The four components are:

1. *Listening to the family.* The nurse listens to the family's story to gain an understanding of the family's experience with the chronic illness. Listening enables family members, including the ill individual, to become aware of important aspects of the illness. By focusing on both the individual and the family experiences, the nurse offers an opportunity for people to be experts in their own health. As the nurse and family listen to the family members' stories about their perceptions, needs, and healing experiences, they all gain a better understanding of the family's experience.

2. *Participatory dialogue.* Hartrick et al. (1994) advocate the use of circular questions to elicit the fam-

ily's beliefs, values, and experiences of illness. Circular questions serve both as assessment questions and interventions. The questions assess each member's perceptions of relationships, experience, or beliefs. This dialogue enables the family to gain insight into how their patterns and interactions are affecting their experience with chronic illness. This awareness enables the family to "maintain or change existing family patterns and behaviors" (p. 15).

3. *Pattern recognition.* The nurse and the family explore, examine, and create the picture of the family's experience. "Through critical reflection, the nurse assists family members to express, elaborate, and externalize their feeling and understandings about the family and about their health situation" (p. 16). In this way, the nurse can assist the family in understanding their own health story.

4. *Envisioning action and positive change.* With the understanding gained about their experience with chronic illness, the family is able to make more informed health choices and to make the changes they want in their situation.

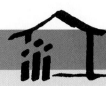

COMMUNITY NURSING VIEW

Onya is a 34-year-old married mother of three children aged 10, 6, and 1. Although she has had symptoms for several years, she has been diagnosed with multiple sclerosis only recently. She is currently in remission but has some residual effects including fatigue, altered gait, and diplopia. Onya stays at home to care for the children and manage the home. The two older children attend school. Until the birth of her last child, Onya had taken responsibility for transporting the children to school and to their extracurricular activities. She finds that she can no longer drive because of her diplopia. Charles, her husband, expresses concern about Onya's condition and displays caring behaviors toward her. Charles is a company executive, and his job frequently requires out-of-town meetings. He expresses how much he values Onya's ability to manage the household when he is not at home.

Nursing Considerations

Assessment

◆ What psychosocial challenges do you think Onya may be facing?

◆ What challenges could be present for this family?

◆ Using the Hartrick, Lindsey, and Hills (1994) assessment framework (Table 27-6), what information do you need to gather?

◆ What other information would you want to assess about this family?

Diagnosis

◆ What NANDA and Omaha nursing diagnoses can you identify?

Outcome Identification

◆ Given the diagnoses you have identified, what outcomes do you expect?

Planning/Interventions

◆ Using the Hartrick et al. (1994) assessment framework (Table 27-6), how might you work with this family?

◆ What preventive measures would be appropriate for Onya and her family? What would be the level of prevention?

Evaluation

◆ What outcome measures will tell you if you have achieved your goals?

KEY CONCEPTS

◆ A chronic illness can affect all aspects of a person's life.

◆ The chronic illnesses of heart disease and stroke, cancer, and diabetes are among the leading causes of death in North America.

◆ The incurability of chronic illness minimizes the importance of curative approaches. The focus shifts to the caring aspect of nursing.

◆ Empowerment of clients and families is central to effective nursing approaches.

◆ The most important aspect of understanding the impact of chronic illness on people is that of the person's lived experience.

◆ Diagnosis is a critical time in the lives of people with chronic illness.

◆ Psychosocial aspects of chronic illness include uncertainty, powerlessness, and biographical work.

◆ Spirituality can be a resource for people with chronic illness.

◆ Chronic illness challenges the economic status of people through the added expense of uninsured expenditures and the effects on employment.

◆ Chronic illness is costly to society as a whole.

◆ Chronic illness has an impact on relationships and roles within the family.

◆ Normalization is a strategy used by individuals and families to live with the challenges presented by the chronic illness.

◆ Nonadherence to prescribed treatment may reflect a person's efforts to control the illness and to adjust treatment regimens to suit personal needs.

◆ The role of the community health nurse in relation to chronic illness includes health promotion and prevention.

◆ The primary, secondary, and tertiary prevention of chronic illness is a significant aspect of the community health nurse's role.

◆ The incurability and increasing incidence of chronic illness and the high cost of related care reinforce the need for primary prevention.

◆ The *Healthy People 2010* report (USDHHS, 2000a) provides guidelines for the implementation of health promotion and preventive strategies for the most prevalent chronic conditions: heart disease and stroke, cancer, and diabetes and other disabling diseases.

RESOURCES

Cancer Net—National Cancer Institute, National Institute for Health
http://cancer.gov/cancer_information

Center for Disease Control and Prevention:
National Center for Health Statistics
http://www.cdc.gov/nchs
National Center for Chronic Disease Prevention and Health Promotion
http://www.cdc.gov/nccdphp/index.htm
National Center for Infectious Diseases
http://cdc.gov/ncidod/diseases/cfs/index.htm
Colorado Health Site
http://www.coloradohealthnet.org
Tobacco Information and Prevention Source
http://www.cdc.gov/tobacco/ibdex.htm

28

DEVELOPMENTAL DISORDERS

Deborah Klaas, RN, PhD

MAKING THE CONNECTION

It was as if a curtain had lifted before her eyes. The life she had thought forever closed to her daughter spread out its great pastoral vista. After all, she thought, why not?

—Spencer, 1960

COMPETENCIES

Upon completion of this chapter, the reader should be able to:

- Define the term developmental disorders.
- Define the term *developmental disabilities* as a legal term.
- Compare the two definitions and classifications of mental retardation. Consider the influence on the practitioner of the choice of definition and classification.
- Compare the major conditions subsumed under developmental disability and define the commonalities of care or service needs.
- Identify the attitudinal, social, and legal changes leading to improved conditions for persons with mental retardation and other developmental disabilities.
- Delineate the influence of the normalization principle on the systems of services for people with developmental disabilities.
- Explain the rationale for the developmental approach to nursing care of the developmentally disabled child, particularly the child with mental retardation. Consider the need for nursing assessment of adaptive skills through the life cycle of the person with a developmental disability.
- Describe the prevention programs and note the nursing role in primary-, secondary-, and tertiary-prevention activities.
- Delineate the impact of developmental disability on the family. Consider the role of the community health nurse in assisting the family.
- Describe nursing goals for family care specific to the presence of a member with a developmental disability.
- Cite the preparation needed by the person with a disability to maintain health and safety in community living.
- Cite the special supports that may be needed by parents with mental retardation.
- Outline some of the weaknesses of community health and service systems for people with developmental disabilities who are lower functioning, mentally ill, or elderly.
- Discuss the future for people with developmental disabilities and the importance of nurse advocacy to maintain their participation in the community.

KEY TERMS

activity center
Asperger's disorder
attention-deficit/hyperactivity disorder (ADHD)
Autistic disorder
autistic spectrum disorder
behavior modification
case management
cerebral palsy
childhood disintegrative disorder
continuum of care
deinstitutionalization
developmental approach to care
developmental assessment
developmental disorder
developmental model of service
early intervention
epilepsy
inclusion
interdisciplinary services
mainstreaming
medical assistive device
mental retardation
newborn screening
normalization
pervasive developmental disorders
pervasive developmental disorder not otherwise specified
prenatal diagnosis
prevention
Rhett's disorder
self-care
sheltered employment
small-group residence
statis epilepticus
supported employment
technology assisted
transition

People with developmental disabilities have benefited from changing social attitudes over the past 40 years of advocacy and reform. New federal and state laws were passed and funding was allocated to provide increased diagnostic services, research, health and habilitation programs, education, community residential services, and work training programs. The civil rights of all persons with disability were guaranteed. Children with significant problems entered public schools. Children and adults with disabilities left institutions for community residence. People with developmental disabilities gained opportunities formerly denied them for personal relationships, marriage, and family life.

Community health nurses offer clients with developmental disabilities and their families support, education, direct care, and linkage to resources as people with disabilities enter schools, workforces, and community residences as well as throughout the life span. An overarching goal is to assist the client to acquire, maintain, and improve health and functioning. This chapter offers community health nurses information, principles, and perspectives for working with people with developmental disabilities. Advocacy by nurses for these populations is especially vital as dwindling health care dollars create an atmosphere of competition for finite resources. Opportunities for community health nurses to make vital and powerful contributions to those with developmental disorders are rich and abundant.

DEVELOPMENTAL DISORDERS

The term **developmental disorder** refers to "a severe, chronic disability of an individual 5 years of age or older that (*Developmental Disabilities Assistance and Bill of Rights Act,* 1996, Section 102):

(a) Is attributable to a mental and/or physical impairment or combination of mental and physical impairments.

(b) Is manifested before the individual attains age 22.

(c) Is likely to continue indefinitely.

(d) Results in substantial functional limitations in three or more of the following areas of major life activity: self-care, receptive and expressive language, learning, mobility, self-direction, capacity for independent living, economic self-sufficiency.

(e) Reflects the individual's need for a combination and sequence of special, interdisciplinary or generic services, supports, or other assistance that is of life-long or extended duration and is individually planned and coordinated." This includes persons from birth to five years of age who have substantial developmental delays, congenital or acquired conditions with a high probability of developmental disabilities if services are not provided.

Developmental disorders, then, encompass single impairments or groupings of physical, emotional, intellectual, or sensory impairments that may begin from prenatal development to young adulthood. These disorders are likely to continue indefinitely. The *International Classification of Impairments, Disabilities and Handicaps* (ICIDH, 2001), a classification of functioning and disability is currently being revised and is scheduled to be implemented in May 2001.

Developmental disability is a legal definition first introduced in 1970 for the purpose of identifying groups of people requiring similar services. When determining eligibility for services, states or other jurisdictions may include different combinations of conditions in their definition of developmental disability.

The most common conditions included in the legal definition of developmental disability are mental retardation, epilepsy, cerebral palsy, and pervasive developmental disorders, including autism. The legal definition of developmental disability may also include other neurological conditions of sufficient severity to require services similar to those required by persons with mental retardation. Some of these can be learning disability, attention-deficit/hyperactivity disorder, and deaf-blindness. Infants and children with conditions placing them at risk for developmental disability may be included.

Nearly four million citizens of the United States have developmental disorders. The Centers for Disease Control and Prevention (CDC, 2001) estimates approximately 17% of children under 18 are affected and of those 2% are severely affected. Thirty-six billion dollars in state and federal funds are spent each year on special education for those between the ages of 3 and 21 (CDC, 2000). In 1998 Congress passed the Birth Defects Prevention Act authorizing the CDC to collect, analyze, and publicize data on birth defects through regional centers and to educate the public about prevention (CDC, 1998).

Primary objectives of *Healthy People 2010* (2000) include:

1. Reducing numbers of children and adolescents with developmental disabilities reported to be unhappy or depressed

2. Increasing the proportion of adults with disabilities who participate in social activities

3. Increasing numbers of adults with disabilities reporting emotional support and satisfaction with life

4. Reducing numbers of developmentally disabled persons in congregate care facilities

5. Increasing numbers of children and youth who spend at least 80% of their time in regular education programs

6. Reducing numbers of disabled persons who report not having assistive devices and technology needed

7. Reducing environmental barriers to participation in home, school, work, or community activities

8. Increasing numbers of public health surveillance and health promotion programs for people with disabilities and their caregivers

The term *developmental disability* has acquired a clinical meaning. In developmental pediatrics the term refers to a disability or disorder arising from central neurological damage, pathology, or defect that is permanent and chronic.

Developmental disorders and ensuing disabilities vary greatly in effect and severity. Although developmental disorders are permanent, some individual's ability to cope and adapt diminishes or precludes the likelihood of the disorder becoming a disability. Discussion of all developmental disorders and their cause, prevalence, characteristics, and treatment is beyond the scope of a single chapter. Therefore, three forms—mental retardation, epilepsy, and cerebral palsy—will be briefly reviewed to illustrate the broad spectrum of developmental disorders.

It is also important to know that **pervasive developmental disorders** include autistic disorder, Rhett's disorders, childhood disintegrative disorder, Asperger's disorder, and pervasive developmental disorder not otherwise specified [American Psychiatric Association (APA), 2000]. **Autism spectrum disorders (ASDs)** are a group of related disorders including pervasive developmental disorders not otherwise specified, Asperger's disorder, and autistic disorder. Autistic spectrum disorders are lifelong developmental disabilities caused by brain abnormalities. Lifelong care and services are generally required because there is no cure and little is known about the etiology. In some cases medications can reduce symptoms and early, intensive special education can greatly enhance chances for near-normal function and life skills achievement. The financial costs of special education are high, but it is even higher for residential education, which can cost from $80,000 to $100,000 per year (CDC, 2001).

Autistic disorder is a group of behaviors that have in common serious developmental abnormalities in social interaction and communication. Behaviors reveal marked restrictions in interests and activities which are remarkably pronounced, repetitive, and stereotyped; the individual is often intensely focused on and preoccupied with these. Three-quarters of children with autistic disorder have mental retardation, generally at the moderate level, and nearly one-quarter develop seizures. Median rates of autistic disorder in epidemiological studies are 5 persons per 10,000 with a range from 2 to 20 per 10,000 (APA, 2000).

Rhett's disorder involves the development of multiple functional deficits after five months but before four years of normal development in infancy. Although born with a normal head circumference, between the ages of 5 and 48 months, the head circumferences of these children decelerates. The disorder has been reported only in females and is rare. Stereotyped hand movements (e.g., wringing, handwashing) develop along with impairments in social interaction, communication, and psychomotor skills. Mental retardation is usually severe to profound.

Similarly, after at least two years of normal development but before 10 years of age **childhood disintegrative disorder** manifests itself as a marked regression in function, is associated with severe mental retardation, and resembles autistic disorder. The disorder is rare and is more common in males. **Asperger's disorder** involves impairment in social interaction plus restricted, repetitive, and stereotyped patterns of behavior, interests, and activities but without deficits in language or cognitive skills. **Pervasive developmental disorder not otherwise specified** involves severe and pervasive problems in social and communication skills as well as stereotyped behavior, interests, and activities; however, the specific diagnostic criteria for the other four pervasive developmental disorders are not met (APA, 2000).

Mental Retardation

The APA describes **mental retardation** as significantly below average intellectual abilities occurring before 18 years of age and associated with significant limitations in adaptive functioning in at least two of the following skills: communication, self-care, home living, social/interpersonal, use of community resources, self-direction, functional academic, work, leisure, health, and safety. Below-average intellectual abilities are defined by intelligence quotients (IQ) of not more than 70. Mental retardation is then further categorized as mild, moderate, severe, or profound based on IQ (see Table 28-1) (APA, 2000). The APA system provides objective measures used for diagnosing, etiology study, epidemiology, and determining level of function and interventions. The community health nurse uses these objective measures for diagnoses, research, identifying appropriate interventions, and evaluation.

The American Association on Mental Retardation (AAMR) emphasizes problems in adaptive skills as opposed to a specific intelligence quotient favored by the APA. The AAMR denies that mental retardation is a mental or medical disorder, rather that is simply a state of functioning that is limited by intelligence and adaptive skills. Mental retardation "reflects the fit between the capabilities of individuals and the structure and expectations of their environment" (AAMR, 2000, p. 1). Further, the AAMR emphasizes that adaptive limitations are often accompanied by strengths in other aspects of the individual. An essential consideration for health care professionals is that with appropriate supports it is likely that the person with mental retardation will improve their skills over time. This is crucial information for caregivers, lawmakers, and educators.

An individual's capabilities should be evaluated to customize a program of support. Levels of support that may be needed in the areas of communication, self-care, home living, social/interpersonal behavior, use of community resources, self-direction, work, leisure, health, and safety vary despite similar IQ scores. For example, a person with mild mental retardation may need extensive support in social, work, leisure, and academic functions as opposed to an individual with profound mental retardation. The AAMR emphasizes the use of culturally appropriate assessments and consideration of personal strengths, with an expectation of improvement in function with sustained efforts and support (AAMR, 2000). Community health nurses use this system to evaluate adaptive skills, identify needed support and interventions, evaluate outcomes, and generate culturally appropriate nursing interventions with the client and family.

In 1998 the AAMR generated a broad range of policy statements relevant to those who have mental retardation and those who care for and coexist with them. Guidelines to professional conduct provide principles for making decisions involving ethical dilemmas affecting the well-being of those with mental retardation, institutions of business, and the social good (Figure 28-1). Note these guidelines mirror those of any encounter between a health care professional and a client.

TABLE 28-1	Severity of Mental Retardation
Mild	IQ 50–55 to 70
Moderate	IQ 35–40 to 50–55
Severe	IQ 20–25 to 35–40
Profound	IQ less than 20

Source: American Psychiatric Association. (2000). DSM-IV TR diagnostic and statistical manual of mental disorders (4th ed.). Washington DC: American Psychiatric Association.

FIGURE 28-1 AAMR Guidelines for Professional Conduct

1. The practitioner objectively solicits, honors, and respects the unique needs, values, and choices of the persons being served.

2. The practitioner communicates fully and honestly in the performance of his or her responsibilities and provides sufficient information to enable individuals being supported and others to make their own informed decisions to the best of their ability.

3. The practitioner protects the dignity, privacy, and confidentiality of individuals being supported and makes full disclosure about any limitations on his or her ability to guarantee full confidentiality.

4. The practitioner is alert to situations that may cause a conflict of interest or have the appearance of a conflict. When a real or potential conflict of interest arises, the practitioner not only acts in the best interest of individuals being supported but also provides full disclosure.

5. The practitioner seeks to present and promptly respond to signs of abuse and/or exploitation and does not engage in sexual, physical, or mental abuse.

6. The practitioner assumes responsibility and accountability for person competence in practice based on the professional standards of his or her respective field, continually striving to increase professional knowledge and skills and to apply them in practice.

7. The practitioner exercises professional judgment within the limits of his or her qualifications and collaborates with others, seeks counsel, or makes referrals as appropriate.

8. The practitioner fulfills commitments in good faith and in a timely manner.

9. The practitioner conducts his or her practice with honesty, integrity, and fairness.

10. The practitioner provides services in a manner that is sensitive to cultural differences and does not discriminate against individuals on the basis of race, ethnicity, creed, religion, sex, age, sexual orientation, national origin, or mental or physical disability.

Adapted from *AAMR Fact Sheet,* 2000, on-line, available: www.aamr.org.

plinary communication. Community health nurses will benefit from both systems when providing care for the person with mental retardation. In addition, nurses can benefit from an historical perspective of the treatment of those who are mentally retarded (see Table 28-2).

Role of IQ Tests

Most systems of definition and classification of mental retardation rely on standard IQ tests, which do not directly measure intelligence but measure knowledge and skills considered related to intelligence by a particular culture. The tester must account adequately for gender, culture, age, or race variation. The relevant characteristics of the individual being assessed should be represented in the population on which the tests are based to avoid bias. The examiner should be from the same cultural group as the person examined or at least should be familiar with that cultural group.

Controversy still exists over the use of standard IQ tests. Some researchers contend that such tests best predict achievement in Caucasian children. Other researchers

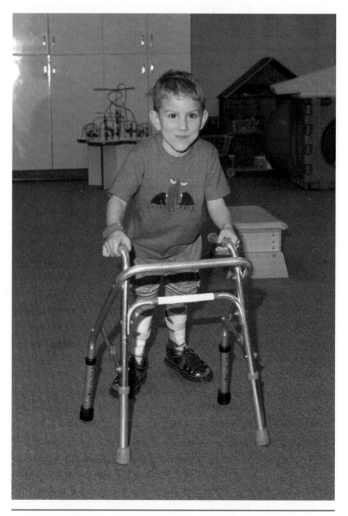

In conclusion, the APA and AAMR differently influence nurses' perceptions of clients with mental retardation. Focusing on a diagnosis and IQ level ignores the potential for improved function and quality of life. Alternatively, underlying all developmental disorders is a neurological condition that requires ongoing medical care and assessment. Medical interventions may be required versus a change in support. Further, IQ levels and diagnostic criteria are important for research and interdisci-

Do you know anyone who has a developmental disorder? What has been done to help that person?

TABLE 28-2 Partial History of Treatment for Those Who are Mentally Retarded

1547	Bedlam is declared a hospital exclusively for the "insane"
1768	The Public Hospital for Persons of Insane and Disordered Minds opens in Williamsburg, Virginia
1824–1870	Several "Lunatic and Feeble Minded Asylums" open in eastern states
1842	P. T. Barnum opens the American Museum in New York and exhibits "freaks"
1852	Harvey Wilbur identifies four types of "idiocy" (stimulative, higher grade, lower grade, incurables)
1876	The Association of Medical Officers of American Institutions for Idiotic and Feeble-Minded Persons established (later know as the American Association on Mental Retardation)
1882	U.S. Congress passes the Undesirables Act (eugenics—methods of controlling population characteristics through selective breeding)
1894	Kansas State Asylum for Idiotic and Imbecile Youth begins castrations
1900–1930	Marriage, childbirth, and living in society prohibited for "mentally defective, feeble minded" persons—tens of thousands institutionalized—seen as burden, menace to society and civilization, and responsible for societal problems
1930–1950	The "science" of eugenics discredited; however, children and adults with disabilities still seen as sick, subhuman, and a menace and institutionalized
1950–1970	Consumer advocacy movement began, resulting in development of service programs and legislation to improve institutions; people began returning to communities
1970–2001	Multiple laws passed protecting constitutional rights of persons with developmental disabilities and providing improved services, funding, education, wholistic care and community living; increase in self-advocacy groups

Source: Life Stream (www.lifestreaminc.com/history.htm) and An American history of mental retardation (http://members.aol.com/MRandDD).

assert that some tests are equally good predictors for African American, Caucasian, or Mexican American children (Kramer, Allen, & Gergen, 1995). Nurses administering standard tests or assessing adaptive skills consider cultural factors as part of the assessment process. The Association of Retarded Citizens (ARC) notes that the term "mental age" used in intelligence testing compares an individual's score to the average score attained by persons of a certain age in a sample population:

Saying that an older person with mental retardation is like a person of a younger age or has the "mind" or "understanding" of a younger person is incorrect usage of the term. The mental age only refers to the intelligence test score. It does not describe the level and nature of the person's experience and functioning in aspects of community life (ARC, 2001, Introduction to Mental Retardation, publication no. 101-2, p. 2).

Characteristics

Children or adults with mental retardation learn more slowly than children whose IQ falls within the normal range. The individual rate of learning depends on the degree of impairment but all require more repetition and instruction to learn. People with mental retardation do not generalize well and may need to learn what to do in each new situation. They do not recall information easily and have difficulty thinking abstractly or critically.

People with mental retardation are slow to develop speech and language, depending on the degree of impairment. Motor development is slow, and the child is late in sitting, walking, running, and acquiring self-help skills. Movements may be uncoordinated, and these kinds of physical problems may inhibit clear enunciation. Determining an etiology of mental retardation may occur through associated problems and disorders such as dysmorphic features, and a greater likelihood of neuromuscular, visual, auditory, cardiovascular, speech, and language problems, epilepsy, and behavioral and mental disorders (APA, 2000).

Children and adults are frequently aware of their difficulties and suffer from societal stigma. Often this awareness begins during the school years when children are either segregated into special education classes or mainstreamed into the regular classroom. Children and adults as well may struggle with painful feelings of rejection or low self-esteem. School and community health nurses play a significant role in tempering this stigma and the painful sequelae by providing education and support for clients with mental retardation, their families, educators, classmates, and the general public. Meaningful contributions to society by individuals with mental retardation are

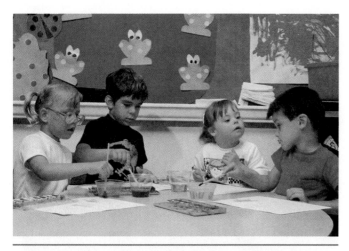

Children and adults with developmental disabilities should be encouraged to take pride in their accomplishments to promote a positive self-image.

common when they are provided with adequate resources. A positive self-image, healthy self-esteem, productivity, and pride in accomplishments are outcomes of efforts by and on behalf of those with mental retardation. Often obstacles to a healthy self-esteem lie with a society that stigmatizes differences through a lack of knowledge and understanding.

Prevalence

Based on the 1990 census, Batshaw (1997) reported an estimated 6.2–7.5 million people have mental retardation, approximately 2.5%–3% of the U.S. population. Research completed by the Metropolitan Atlanta Developmental Disabilities Surveillance Program reported rates of mental retardation of 9.7 per 1000 children aged 3–10 years of age

(www.cdc.org). Mental retardation does not discriminate in terms of race, ethnicity, educational, social, or economic backgrounds. One out of 10 families in the United States will be affected by mental retardation (ARC, 2001).

Etiology

Over 500 genetic diseases are associated with mental retardation as well as hundreds of factors related to pregnancy, birth, childhood diseases, environmental factors, accidents, poverty, and cultural deprivation. Yet the cause remains unknown in nearly one-third of people affected (ARC, 2001). Table 28-3 represents some of the factors believed to cause mental retardation. Down syndrome, fetal alcohol syndrome, and fragile X are the three most common known etiologies for mental retardation (ARC, 2001).

Prevention

Many conditions leading to mental retardation are preventable and this is becoming increasingly true as research generates more evidence of cause and effect. Examples include measles encephalitis prevented by immunization, fetal alcohol syndrome prevented by abstention from alcohol during pregnancy, head injury prevented by many child safety measures, including abuse prevention, lead poisoning prevented by environmental sanitation measures, and genetic disorders prevented by preconception genetic counseling. Literally thousands of cases of mental retardation are prevented yearly through these and related preventative measures. Community health nurses provide services in many programs of primary prevention that reduce the incidence of conditions leading to mental retardation. See Chapters 11 & 22.

TABLE 28-3 Known Causes of Mental Retardation

Unexplained		The largest category and a catchall for undiagnosed incidences of mental retardation
Trauma	Examples:	intracranial hemorrhage before or after birth
Infectious	Examples:	congenital rubella, meningitis, congenital cytomegalovirus, encephalitis, congenital toxoplasmosis, listeriosis, human immunodeficiency syndrome
Chromosomal *a*	Examples:	Down syndrome, fragile X syndrome, chromosomal translocations, Klinefelter's syndrome, Prader-Willi syndrome, cri du chat syndrome
Genetic	Examples:	Tay-Sachs, phenylketonuria, galactosemia, Rhett's disorder, Hunter's disease, Hurler's syndrome, Sanfilippo's disease, Lesch-Nyhan disease, tuberous sclerosis
Metabolic	Examples:	Reye's syndrome, hypernatremic dehydration, hypoglycemia, hypothyroid
Toxic	Examples:	intrauterine exposure to alcohol, cocaine, amphetamines, and other drugs; methylmercury poisoning; lead poisoning
Nutritional	Examples:	kwashiorkor, marasmus, malnutrition
Environmental	Examples:	poverty, low socioeconomic status

Source: Adapted from C. E. Koop, www.drkoop.com/conditions/ency/article/001523.htm.

Treatment and Management

Because of the complexity of and multisystem involvement in mental retardation, management and treatment require an interdisciplinary approach. Some conditions associated with mental retardation are treatable, such as phenylketonuria and galactosemia, in which mental retardation can be prevented by dietary treatment, or some forms of hydrocephalus, in which shunting can prevent mental retardation. If no treatable etiology is identified, management is directed to maintaining or improving health, correcting any treatable associated conditions, and providing programs of early developmental stimulation and special education. Community health nurses working with children and adults with mental retardation, in addition to providing health care, define adaptive skill levels and help the family and client obtain education, services, and support needed to maximize individual potentials.

Epilepsy

Epilepsy is the oldest known brain disorder, having been first documented 3000 years ago. As early as 400 B.C. Hippocrates noted it was a disorder of the brain, but epilepsy was not scientifically studied until the mid-1800s [Epilepsy Foundation of America (EFA), 2001]. Throughout history epilepsy was believed to have either a positive or a negative divine cause. Much of the stigma associated with epilepsy is rooted in these beliefs. Epilepsy is a condition characterized by recurrent abnormal electrical discharges from neurons in the cortex of the brain that cause seizures. Thus, the seizures are symptoms of an underlying neurological disorder. Epilepsy is actually a group of symptoms reflecting multiple disorders of the brain (Smelzer & Bare, 2000). The International Classification of Seizures and the International League Against Epilepsy classify two general categories of seizures: partial and generalized. The difference between the two categories is simply the area of the brain affected. Partial seizures affect one limited area of the brain while generalized seizures affect the entire brain (ILAE, 2002; ICS, 2002).

Characteristics

People with epilepsy manifest a variety of seizure types. Persons experiencing partial seizures may maintain consciousness (simple partial) or have impaired consciousness. Simple partial seizures involve a range of unusual events such as distortions in visual, tactile, aural, gustatory, and olfactory senses; sudden jerky movement of a part of the body; or uncomfortable affective sensations such as fear. These experiences may be called "auras" if followed by another seizure. Complex partial seizures involve impaired consciousness and a purposeless, complex motor act. The person may appear bewildered or stunned and does not recall the episode afterward. Partial seizures are the most common form (62%) of epilepsy (EFA, 2001). Generalized seizures include absence seizures, which are brief losses of consciousness exhibited by star-

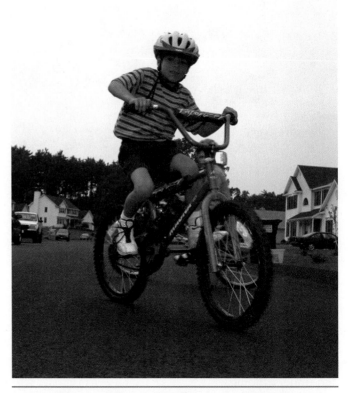

Encouraging parents to ensure their child wears a safety helmet while bike riding is a primary prevention technique that may reduce the risk for severe head injury and developmental disorders.

ing into space with possible rolling of eyes upward. A tonic-clonic seizure involves loss of consciousness in which the body falls and becomes rigid followed by a jerking or twitching of extremities. Subdivided within the two categories are over 30 different types of seizures. **Statis epilepticus** describes recurrent seizures with no recovery in between. This condition is a medical emergency because it can cause permanent brain damage or death.

Parents should fully inform the child's teacher of symptoms and frequency of seizures and any first aid that might be required. Adults may or may not inform employers depending on the type of seizures they have, their job, and their relationship with the employer. Dissolution of stigma surrounding epilepsy is occurring as the result of openness, honesty, and scientific advances. However, some stigma remains, negatively impacting socialization, career opportunities, and personal freedom. Further negative influences may occur as family members and friends impose unnecessary activity restrictions in an effort to protect the individual with epilepsy.

Prevalence

The National Institute of Neurological Disorders and Strokes (NINDS) and the EFA estimate 2 million citizens of the United States (more than 1%) have epilepsy, and the World Health Organization (WHO) estimates 40 million people worldwide (1% of worldwide disease) have epilepsy (1997). Approximately 50% of newly diagnosed cases are children [National Information Center for Children and Youth with Disabilities (NICHCY), 2001]. Epilepsy can occur at any age, but more than 50% of cases are diagnosed before 10 years of age. Frequently, as the individual ages, epilepsy disappears. This occurs most often when seizures start in childhood and can be well controlled with medication. Epilepsy occurs more frequently in some countries due to genetic predispositions (EFA, 2001), but overall, epilepsy is the most common serious brain disorder in every country in the world (*WHO/ILAE/IBE/global campaign against epilepsy,* 1997). Due to the prevalence of this neurological disorder, "epileptology" is emerging as a distinct discipline (Engel, 1999).

Etiology

Anything that disturbs the normal neuronal activity in the brain can lead to seizures. Imbalances in neurotransmitters and abnormal neurological wiring can lead to the development of epilepsy. Gamma-aminobutyric acid (GABA) seems to be an important neurotransmitter in tracking seizure etiology, and its study has led to a variety of antiepileptic drugs. Sometimes injury and abnormal nerve regeneration follows brain injury leading to epilepsy. Causes of brain injury are innumerable and include factors such as stroke, malnutrition, hypoxia, hemorrhage, infection, and accidents. The NINDS reports that genetic abnormalities may be some of the most important factors contributing to epilepsy. Researchers indicate that genetic predispositions to seizures often need an environmental trigger to become evident. Further, genetic influences may significantly affect the effectiveness of antiepileptic drugs. Epilepsy may develop due to brain damage from a wide variety of diseases, such as alcoholism, Alzheimer's disease, AIDs, celiac disease, parasites, and brain tumors. Finally, no link to cause has been established for nearly half of all persons experiencing seizures (NINDS, 2001).

Glascoe (1999) found that parents may not share their worries unless specifically questioned by a health care provider. See Research Focus.

RESEARCH FOCUS

Using Parents' Concerns to Detect and Address Developmental and Behavioral Problems

Study Problem/Purpose

Only half of all children with disabilities are identified before school entrance. This study describes the effectiveness of using parents' concerns to identify children with disabilities before school entrance.

Methods

More than 900 families, roughly representative of the national demography, were recruited from private pediatric practices throughout the United States. Twenty-three percent were low income, 22% were African American, 14% were Hispanic or of another ethnic group, and 64% were white. Parents' concerns were sought with a standardized surveillance tool, the Parents' Evaluations of Developmental Status (PEDS). This tool categorizes and interprets parents' concerns about their child. Formal testing was also done for each child by licensed psychologists blinded either to parents' concerns or to their significance. Psychologists formally measured child development using a battery of standardized tests.

Findings

Parents' concerns, regardless of education or experience in parenting, met standards for developmental screening accuracy. Sensitivity ranged from 74% to 79%, and specificity ranged from 70% to 80%. Reasons parents gave for not sharing their concerns with health care providers previously included lack of confidence in their own perceptions and trust that if the problems were real, they would be detected by professionals independently.

Implications

Parents may not share their worries unless specifically questioned by a health care provider. Systematically eliciting this information from parents can be a cost-effective, efficient, and accurate way of identifying children for further screening, referral, or simply close monitoring. In some cases it may result in offering parents reassurance that development of their child is proceeding normally.

Source: Glascoe, S. F. (1999). Using parents' concerns to detect and address developmental and behavioral problems. Journal of the Society of Pediatric Nursing, 4, *24–36.*

Perception of Mental Retardation

The parents and siblings of a child being provided dietary treatment for a metabolic disorder underwent psychological testing as part of the evaluation of treatment outcomes. The mother's IQ scores placed her in the moderate to mild range of mental retardation.

The young woman was beautiful, wore stylish and expensive clothes, and was well groomed. Her manner was sweetly dignified. She asked questions that encouraged the other person to talk at length while she listened attentively.

Her husband, a prominent professional man, explained that his wife's family had accepted her condition and had provided every advantage. She went to private school with no suggestion of "special" classes. She took art classes at the local community college so she could be perceived as having gone to college. Her family carefully trained her in social skills and household care.

She was unable to plan and shop for an elaborate meal or manage her child's special diet, but she had a housekeeper to assist her. She could not chair a committee meeting, but she presided well at their dinner parties.

Her husband esteemed her for what she was: a loving wife, mother, and graceful companion. Their common interests were their children, extended families, social life, and travel. Her husband helped her to avoid situations she could not handle.

- Should this woman be considered mentally retarded? Consider her ability to meet social and cultural expectations. Consider her support system.
- How might your perception of her be influenced by applying to her the system of definition and classification of the American Psychiatric Association? Of the American Association on Mental Retardation?

Treatment

Seizures can be eliminated or reduced with medication and/or surgery in 70%–80% of person's with epilepsy. However, nearly three-quarters of the 40 million people with epilepsy worldwide do not receive any treatment; most reside in developing countries (*WHO/ILAE/IBE global campaign against epilepsy,* 1997). There is no cure for epilepsy, but treatment is accomplished mainly with medications, although surgery has also been successful. Drugs are prescribed alone or in combination and may require more than one trial to find the drug most effective for an individual. Side effects of antiepileptic drugs are numerous and range from mild to severe (Kee & Hayes, 2000). As a result, some people requiring large doses of medication to prevent seizures opt for a lesser dose with only partial seizure control.

Surgery is a last resort for clients unresponsive to medications who have clearly delineated and confined injured brain tissue. A further requirement is that the surgery can be performed without damaging personality or life functions. *Epilepsy and Brain Mapping Program* (2000) reports 83% of clients undergoing temporal resections are seizure free and 97% are significantly improved. Seizures occurring in the frontal lobe are significantly reduced in 85% of clients undergoing surgical resection. Little research is available on nontraditional methods of seizure reduction such as biofeedback, acupuncture, meditation, and ketogenic diets. Generally they are used in conjunction with antiepileptic drugs.

Nurses in multiple settings assist and support clients with epilepsy and their families in preventing and controlling seizures and successfully managing the multiple sequelae of epilepsy. Nursing interventions include reducing the fear associated with seizures, improving coping mechanisms, fostering a positive mental outlook, and improvements and maintenance in self-care through education of clients and families. Community health nurses also need to consider financial consequences of epilepsy, the possibility of a need for vocational rehabilitation, ongoing evaluation, and genetic counseling for clients (Smelzer & Bare, 2000). As in care for all developmental disorders, a primary responsibility of the community health nurse is facilitating empowerment of those with epilepsy and their families.

Cerebral Palsy

Cerebral palsy refers to a group of chronic, nonprogressive conditions affecting body movement and muscle coordination (United Cerebral Palsy, 2001), usually occurring before, during, or immediately after birth or during the first few years of life. Approximately 80% of people acquired cerebral palsy before or within the first month of birth (CDC, 2001) and for many the cause is unknown. The resulting abnormal control of movement is not caused by problems in the muscles or nerves; rather it is the result of damage to specific motor areas of the brain. It may or may not be associated with intellectual deficiencies.

The disorder was first documented in the 1860s by a physician named William Little and for years after was called Little's disease. Fifty percent of people with cerebral palsy use special assistance devices for mobility and nearly 70% have other disabilities, primarily impaired intellect. Although there is no cure for cerebral palsy, life-skills training and therapy can improve function and life quality significantly. Studies show that cerebral palsy has the highest lifetime costs per case and half of these costs are borne by families (CDC, 2001).

Characteristics

There are four major types of cerebral palsy [American Cerebral Palsy Information Center (ACPIC), 2001; CDC, 2001]:

1. *Spastic:* Also called hypertonic, this type of cerebral palsy is characterized by stiff and difficult movements or an overabundance of muscle tone and possible uncontrollable tremors. There are five subtypes based on the affected limbs: diplegia, hemiplegia, quadriplegia, monoplegia, and triplegia. Spastic cerebral palsy accounts for 70%–80% of all cerebral palsy.

2. *Athetoid:* Also called dyskinetic, hypotonic, dystonic cerebral palsy, this is characterized by uncontrolled, slow, writhing movements usually of the feet, arms, or legs and in some cases facial muscles affecting speech (dysarthria). Types of movement or postures include athetosis, tremor, dystonia, choreiform, and rigidity. Athetoid cerebral palsy is the second most common type of cerebral palsy accounting for 10%–20% of persons affected by cerebral palsy.

3. *Ataxic:* Characterized by a lack of coordination, depth perception, and balance. "Intention tremors" may occur as an individual initiates a voluntary movement. Ataxic cerebral palsy accounts for 5%–10% of all persons with cerebral palsy.

4. *Mixed form:* Two or more types of cerebral palsy occur in the same person. This type of cerebral palsy is becoming more common as diagnostic techniques improve. The most common type of mixed-form cerebral palsy combines spastic and athetoid movements.

Symptoms and severity of cerebral palsy vary greatly in affected individuals. Although not a progressive disorder, symptoms may change with time. Cerebral palsy does not always cause a profound handicap nor is it contagious or genetic.

Anee Stanford, a person with cerebral palsy and the creator of Cerebral Palsy Information Central (www.geocities.com/HotSprings/Sauna/4441), developed a list of terms commonly used when describing people with cerebral palsy. She reminds us that it is important to remember the individual with cerebral palsy often experiences the disorder not as a physical deficit but as a physical variation.

Prevalence

Cerebral palsy is second only to mental retardation in frequency of developmental disorders. Five thousand infants in the United States are diagnosed each year, and an additional 1200–1500 preschool children are also recognized as having cerebral palsy (United Cerebral Palsy, 2001). A review of the literature indicated rates of cerebral palsy ranging from 1.5 to 2.8 persons per thousand (Rapp & Torres, 2000). Estimates indicate approximately 500,000 children and adults in the United States have cerebral palsy. Researchers reported a gradual increase in the incidence of cerebral palsy from the mid-1960s to the mid-1980s, after which levels were reported down 0.5 persons per thousand births (Rapp & Torres, 2000). Much of the earlier increase in cases has been attributed to increased survival rates of low-birthweight neonates. The increased incidence of multiple births in the last third of the 20th century contributed significantly to the numbers of low-birthweight infants (Keith, Ozeszczuk, & Keith, 2000). An increase in the number of adults with cerebral palsy follows improved survival rates of affected infants.

Etiology

Ten percent to 20% of children acquire cerebral palsy after birth from such things as infections, trauma, vascular problems, anoxia, and neoplasms (ACPIC, 2001). Prenatal causes include anoxia; maternal infections such as rubella, toxoplasmosis, and herpes simplex; metabolic disorders such as asthma, diabetes, and heart conditions; Rh factor; and abdominal injury during pregnancy. Perinatal causes include anoxia, analgesics, trauma, jaundice, and low birthweight due to prematurity, multiple births, and other complications. Causes of acquired cerebral palsy occurring before three years of age include brain trauma, infections of the central nervous system (CNS), vascular problems, anoxia, and neoplasms. From this list it becomes obvious that optimal well-being before conception, adequate prenatal care, and protecting infants from accidents and injury are primary ways to prevent cerebral palsy. Often the cause cannot be determined.

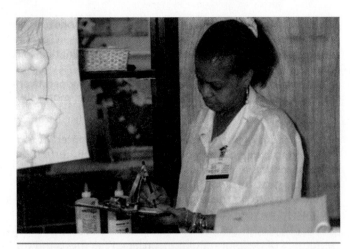

By observing and recording the behavior and actions of children, the school nurse and teacher are in a prime position to identify developmental problems.

Treatment

The United Cerebral Palsy Association notes that *management* is a better word than *treatment* for those with cerebral palsy (United Cerebral Palsy, 2001). The goal of management is assisting the individual to achieve maximum potential and independence, beginning with early identification. Management is conducted by an interdisciplinary team of physicians; nurses; physical, occupational, recreation, and speech therapists; educators; social workers; and other professionals. Community health nurses are vital members of this team and serve to prevent, identify, intervene, and provide long-term follow-up. Prevention may involve such things as facilitating prenatal care, teaching child care and safety, or providing adequate immunizations. The nurse may also identify affected children through assessment, act as a case manager, provide personal care and resource information, support and educate clients and families in the home or organizational settings as well as in school systems, or provide care and consultation in an adult care setting (Dzienkowski, Smith, Dillow, & Yucha, 1996).

Diazepam, baclofen, and dantrolene are the drugs most commonly prescribed for short-term reduction of spasticity, although the side effects can be significant and long-term effectiveness has not been clearly demonstrated. Anticholinergics have been used to reduce abnormal movements associated with athetoid cerebral palsy. Alcohol injections ("washes") have been used to weaken a spastic muscle in an effort to correct developing contractures. Surgery is also performed to correct contractures, reduce leg spasticity, and stimulate or resect certain parts of the brain. Results are mixed and some approaches remain controversial. Various forms of therapy, including physical, occupational, and speech, are of prime importance to the individual with cerebral palsy and may continue intermittently throughout life. Most therapy is performed in the home (ACPIC, 2001).

Attention-Deficit/Hyperactivity Disorder

Attention-deficit/hyperactivity disorder (ADHD) is one of the most common childhood behavioral disorders and may affect more than 2 million children and adolescents in the United States (CDC, 2001). The National Institutes of Health (NIH) notes children with ADHD have pronounced impairments and can experience long-term adverse effects on academic performance, vocational success, and social-emotional development. ADHD has a profound impact on individuals, families, schools, and society (NIH, 1998). Although the disorder is controversial, it is one of the most widely researched in the field of mental health, with more compelling data than for most other mental disorders (Goldman, 1998). For more information the reader is referred to Chapter 22.

Commonalities of the Developmental Disorders

Characteristics that developmental disorders generally have in common are as follows:

- A significant number of conditions leading to developmental disability are preventable.
- Developmental disorders originate in the nervous system, are permanent and nonstatic, and have effects ranging from mild challenges to profoundly disabling. Associated problems often occur throughout the life of the affected individual but may be prevented or successfully treated with appropriate interventions.
- The changing nature of developmental disorders requires ongoing assessment and understanding of cognitive, physical, behavioral, emotional, social, and spiritual health.
- Interdisciplinary services are usually needed to assist individuals with developmental disorders to lead productive lives.
- Community health nurses approach and treat these individuals and families holistically with an emphasis on empowerment for maximizing health, quality of life, and productivity.
- The degree of disability for a person with a developmental disorder is determined by the environment. A disorder that is disabling in one situation may be enabling in another.

REFLECTIVE THINKING

Managing Attention-Deficit/Hyperactivity Disorder

The school nurse organized a meeting with Mike's teacher and mother and arranged for Mike's doctor to participate over a speaker telephone. Mike's distractibility had recently increased. He was not doing his work, and he was joining other boys in rowdy behavior at the end of the school day. Mike's mother was surprised. She thought he was improving, as his hyperactivity had decreased since he turned 12. At Mike's request his dosage of stimulant medication was being slowly decreased.

The nurse acknowledged the reduction of hyperactivity but clarified that Mike still needed help to attend and focus adequately. The nurse and his teacher knew that Mike was embarrassed about his school work and thought that he might be clowning to cover his feelings.

Mike's doctor was reluctant to increase his medication and was of the opinion that Mike was capable of better regulation of his attention and behavior. Mike's teacher and mother agreed. Mike's mother indicated that she would initiate interventions needed to get Mike back on track. She proposed to increase his time in productive activity and to decrease his time in unsupervised activity.

His mother obtained a paper route for Mike, and he began to deliver papers as he walked home from school. She took two afternoons off from work to accompany him as he learned his route. As a reinforcement, she paid a college student to meet Mike at home afterward to coach him and his friends in soccer or baseball. She sat with him for half an hour after supper to help him organize his homework and stay on task.

Mike began to complete his work. His disruptive behavior at school diminished as he participated more in school sports. Mike was proud of his ability to handle school work and his paper route. He agreed to stay on his medication until the end of the school year.

- What is the role of the nurse in assisting the child with attention disorder? The role of the family?
- How might persons not familiar with the disorder interpret Mike's behavior?
- Consider the amount and types of environmental structuring provided to help Mike. Do you think medication alone would be effective? Why or why not?

PRINCIPLES AND PERSPECTIVES

Changing social attitudes after World War II led to the development and dissemination of important principles of service to persons with disabilities and their families. These principles developed from the advocacy of families, particularly those with members with mental retardation, and their supporters. Their advocacy arose from their moral conviction that persons with developmental disorders must have the same human rights and range of services as their nonhandicapped fellow citizens. Indeed, this spirit continues today, illustrated in the following quote from *Healthy People 2010* (2000): "the underlying premise of Healthy People 2010 is that the health of the individual is almost inseparable from the health of the larger community and that the health of every community in every State and territory determines the overall health status of the Nation" (p. 2).

Civil Rights

Internationally, the 1970s ushered in a human rights perspective for persons with disabilities. Two declarations were adopted by the United Nations General Assembly: (1) the Declarations on the Rights of Mentally Retarded Persons in 1971 and (2) the Declaration of the Rights of Disabled Persons in 1975. These involved recognition of and advocacy for those with disabilities having the same political and civil rights as others, such as rights to education, medical services, economic and social security, employment, self-sufficiency, legal representation, living and participating fully in communities, and protection from exploitation, abuse, and degrading behavior (Persons with Disabilities, 2001). In 1975, federal law granted all students between the ages of 6 and 18 the right to appropriate public education in the least restrictive environment possible regardless of physical or mental

Individuals with Developmental Disabilities

Think about a person you know who has a developmental disability.

- How does he or she express what it is like to have the condition?
- What is the person's adaptation in the home and community?
- What system of supports is available to the person? Can you suggest other supports that would help the person become more fully integrated into the community?

disabilities. Amendments has since been made expanding eligible ages and services (Knoblauch, 1998). The civil rights of all persons with disabilities were made explicit in the Americans with Disabilities Act of 1990. The intent was that all persons with developmental disabilities be as fully integrated into the community as possible fostered through adequate opportunities for employment, public services, public accommodations, telecommunications, and miscellaneous (largely protective measures) (Job Accommodation Network, 2001). Most states now have protection and advocacy agencies responsible for pursuing legal, administrative, and other remedies to protect the rights of persons with disabilities.

The civil rights of people with developmental disorders are often unthinkingly and casually violated by family, friends, or officials. The community health nurse is aware and prepared to intervene in situations such as the following:

- Removal of a child from a home due to mental retardation of a parent
- Residential rules that violate adult residents' rights to associate with friends, have consensual sexual relationships, or travel in the community
- Refusal of health care providers to accept treatment consent of an adult with a disability although the person has no cognitive limitations
- Clients and families who are unaware of their civil rights

Normalization

The principle of **normalization** originated in the Scandinavian countries in the 1960s and was promoted in the United States by Wolfensberger: "Normalization is

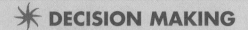

The Experience of Living with Golden Har's Syndrome

I was diagnosed at birth with Golden Har's syndrome, a disorder for which the etiology is unknown. This disorder occurs in approximately 1 in 5600 births. The severity of the disorder varies tremendously, but I was born lacking any vestibular or mandibular structure on the right side of my face, called hemifacial microsomia. Living with this anomaly is a constant challenge. It is incredibly disruptive to my self-image and fosters anxiety, isolation, and an intense need for acceptance. I have undergone eight major surgeries to rebuild my face and achieve bilateral symmetry. The excellent nursing care I received during this gradual reconstruction has deeply inspired me to reciprocate this excellence.

When I began nursing school, it was very difficult for me to reveal my disability to my classmates. However, I decided that if I was going to spend three years with them, I'd better make myself comfortable early. Although my grades were excellent, I felt somewhat inferior to the others because I have only half of my hearing: I do not have a right ear. It was incredibly frustrating struggling with hearing through stethoscopes, essential tools in nursing, that were so easily manipulated by everyone else. I considered purchasing a hearing-enhanced stethoscope; however, I was not prepared to spend $400 on this piece of equipment. I was determined, though, and perseverance and encouragement from my family led to mastery of the stethoscope and continuation in the nursing program in good standing.

—Claudia Florke, 2001, nursing student, Sonoma State University

- How does Claudia express what it is like to have a disability?
- What kind of adaptations has Claudia made as the result of her disability?
- What system of supports is available to Claudia and can you think of other supports that would facilitate her progression in the nursing program?

utilization of means which are as culturally normative as possible, in order to establish and/or maintain personal behavior and characteristics which are as culturally normative as possible" (Wolfensberger, 1972, p. 28). This statement has had a significant influence on attitudes toward persons with mental retardation as well as toward people with other disabilities. The statement and its corollaries underlie significant positive changes in developmental disability service systems in the United States.

The principle of normalization requires that people with any type of disability be permitted to live a life that offers every possible advantage and opportunity enjoyed by people without disabilities. Normalization means persons with disabilities are provided with appropriate developmental experiences with the supports necessary to maximize benefit, exercise self-advocacy, and advocate for civil rights. Efforts to move people from institutions to communities have succeeded such that generally people are housed in institutions only if they require a level of care that cannot be acquired in the community. An ongoing problem is a lack of community services or a complexity and confusion of services that impede normalization. In 2000 President Clinton signed the Developmental Disabilities Assistance and Bill of Rights Act. It expanded services and included a performance-based accountability requirement for those providing services (*Statement by the president,* 2000).

The theme of the International Day of Disabled Persons in 1999 was "accessibility" and served as a reminder that normalization is still often an ideal rather than a fact. Lack of access creates experiences of discrimination and lost opportunity. Community health nurses significantly contribute to rectifying some of these problems through client and family interventions, advocacy, and public education about normalization. Understanding the principles of normalization empowers clients and families to be effective civil rights advocates and to formulate long-term goals for life in the community.

Developmental Perspectives

Development as used in this chapter incorporates two concepts: a **developmental model of service** used to design service systems and the **developmental approach to care** of the individual. These concepts form the basis for most programs and care for people with developmental disabilities.

The Developmental Model of Services

In 1977 the Health Services Extension Act mandated standards for community preventive health services. An outgrowth of this act was the multiagency development of Model Standards for Community Preventive Health Services published in 1979 (Clark, 1999). In 2000 the *Health Communities 2000: Model Standards* was developed and serves as a structure for *Healthy People 2010.* It is based on the premise that community partnerships are some of the most effective tools for improving health in communities.

The Developmental Approach to Care

The developmental approach to care is based on theories of normal development. Changes occurring throughout the life span are considered from a biological, psychological, and ecologic-social perspective. To gain a holistic understanding of individuals and groups, multiple theories are employed to explain total development (Murray & Zenter, 2001). The developmental approach to care of those with developmental disorders then emphasizes the likenesses between the disabled person and the nondisabled person, particularly in the early years of life. Developmental stages are the same for all, differing only in rates of or a halt in progression. Interventions for those with cognitive impairments are based on developmental level instead of chronological age. Goals are formulated based on an expected rate of development and any associated problems. Ideally, the individual's physical and social environments are structured to facilitate development in the most beneficial ways.

Interdisciplinary Services, Continuum of Care, and Case Management

The complex, varied, and changing problems of many people with developmental disorders require the services of an array of specialists over a long period of time.

Interdisciplinary services involve specialists from varying disciplines collaborating as a team to address problems and potential problems of the individual with developmental disabilities. Examples of interdisciplinary team activities include medical care, school placement, respite care, behavior problems, vocational planning, out-of-home placement, rights advocacy, home care, and social and spiritual support. Team composition and leadership depend on client and family needs. The need for interdisciplinary services on a broader level is illustrated by the Administration on Developmental Disabilities' (ADD, 1999) goal to partner with state governments, local communities, and the private sector to promote each individual's opportunities to reach maximum potential through all elements of the life cycle.

Continuum of care refers to the succession of services needed by the individual and family as needs fluctuate with ongoing growth and development. For example, many children require special school services. As they move into adolescence and young adulthood, they may require training in social and vocational skills. Community living skills may become a priority in late adolescence and young adulthood. The complexity of maintaining appropriate ongoing interdisciplinary services and continuity of care requires expert coordination, generally achieved through **case management.**

Community health nurses have been performing the functions of case management for more than a hundred years (Clark, 1999). They identify, create, coordinate, and implement appropriate health and support services to address client needs, advocate for clients and families, create and maintain comprehensive care plans, and serve as team members—all functions of care managers. Further they are active in mobilizing public support for these services.

Prevention of Developmental Disorders

The term **prevention** in discussion of developmental disorders refers to interventions prior to or in the course of the disorder. Primary prevention involves implementing measures that prevent disabilities from occurring. Secondary prevention refers to measures to detect and treat disabilities early in their course to maximize an individual's ability to reach full potential. Tertiary preventative measures prevent or limit related disabilities or conditions once a disability has occurred (tertiary prevention).

Government mandates for preventive initiatives began increasing in the 1960s beginning with the Maternal and Child Health and Mental Retardation Planning Amendments in 1963. These amendments to the Social Security Act of 1935 assisted states and communities in preventing mental retardation through improved maternal/child health care programs (Clemen-Stone, McGuire, & Eigsti, 1998). Currently a major goal of the U.S. Department of Health and Human Services (USDHHS, 2000), Administration of Developmental Disabilities, is a partnership with state governments, local communities, and the private sector to provide services and increase knowledge for primary, secondary, and tertiary prevention of developmental disabilities. Steps to accomplish these goals include $122,275,000 for funding four major grant programs nationwide. These include (1) state developmental disabilities councils, (2) a protection and advocacy council, (3) university-affiliated programs for education, and (4) research, services, and monies for de-

velopment of improved policies for national and state organizations (ADD, 2000).

The CDC provides prevention research and services. For example, the CDC has determined that the leading cause of infant mortality in the United States is birth defects and the cause of 70% of birth defects is unknown. Subsequently, Congress passed the Birth Defects Prevention Act of 1998 authorizing the CDC to collect data, operate regional centers for epidemiological research, and educate the public about the prevention of birth defects. The Developmental Disabilities branch of the CDC conducts surveillance and epidemiological research to identify trends, causes and risk factors, prevention, and effective treatment of developmental disorders.

Healthy People 2010 is a collaboration of 350 national organizations and 250 state agencies representing public health, mental health, substance abuse, and environmental agencies. Two goals for those with disabilities are (1) to increase quality and years of healthy life and (2) to eliminate health disparities directly related to varying levels of prevention. Disabilities are increasing for those under 45 years of age, and many of these people do not have access to health services (*Healthy People 2010,* 2000).

The focus and philosophy of community health nurses is on prevention and maximizing the potential of individuals and groups who have acquired disabilities by whatever means. Much of this occurs through individual, family, and public education, assessments, interventions, and referral to appropriate resources. For example, educating teens about smoking, safe sex, and substance abuse may reduce rates of pregnancy and improve the health of the teen who becomes pregnant as well as the fetus. Low-birthweight infants are born more frequently to mothers who have low prepregnancy weights and/or use tobacco, alcohol, or illegal substances. Low birthweight is associated with long-term disabilities such as cerebral palsy, autism, mental retardation, and other developmental disabilities (*Healthy People 2010,* 2000). Early and adequate prenatal care reduces the risk of infant mortality and morbidity. Since the time of Lillian Wald in the early 1900s, periodic nurse contacts with pregnant and newly delivered women in populations of greatest risk reduced the risk of infant mortality and morbidity.

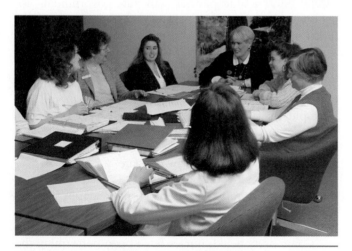

The members of the interdisciplinary team will vary depending on the needs of the client.

THE NURSING ROLE IN DEVELOPMENTAL DISABILITIES

Community health nurses provide services to clients with developmental disorders and their families in many different practice settings. Further they have been instrumental in creating and influencing laws and community services. Community health nurse roles include direct caregiving, rehabilitation, counseling, teacher, advocate, case manager, resource expert, and communication facilitator. The primary goal is to maximize the potential of clients and their families to live a healthy, active, and productive life.

Prenatal Diagnosis

Prenatal diagnosis involves examination of the fetus to detect abnormalities by numerous means, such as fetoscopy, amniocentesis, maternal blood test, chorionic villus biopsy, ultrasound, magnetic resonance imaging (MRI) or x-ray, fetal blood sampling, fetal muscle or skin biopsy, and fetal echocardiography. Abnormalities that can be detected are inborn errors of metabolism, chromosomal abnormalities, cancers, heart disease, tumors, twin transfusion and perfusion problems, neural tube defects, omphalocele, gastroschisis, and hydrocephalus (Center for Fetal Diagnosis and Treatment, 2001). Fetal surgery now includes cellular transplantations for hemoglobinopathies, inborn errors of metabolism, and immune deficiencies plus thoracoamniotic and vesicoamniotic shunting. Open fetal surgery is performed only rarely for life-threatening conditions. Women are referred for prenatal diagnostic procedures because of advanced maternal age, personal or family history of a genetic disorder, or problems suspected from the history or physical findings.

Community health nurses do not impose personal beliefs about pregnancy termination onto the family. Cultural and religious beliefs as well as related emotional and social factors have an influence on a family's decision to continue or terminate a pregnancy. After exploring alternatives with the family, their decision must be respected and supported. Opinions about abortion vary widely within cultural groups and families as well.

Early Identification of Developmental Problems

Early identification of children with variations of development or developmental delays is important in order to intervene as quickly as possible to prevent or remediate problems—a form of secondary prevention. Community health nurses, working with persons from other disciplines, provide early identification through developmental assessment, history, and examination.

Newborn Screening

Newborn screening for certain treatable disorders began in the 1960s. Although these programs have been highly successful, some infants still do not have access to these services. A goal of *Healthy People 2010* is that all newborns are screened at birth for conditions mandated by their state, follow-up diagnostic testing for positive screens is performed within the appropriate time frame,

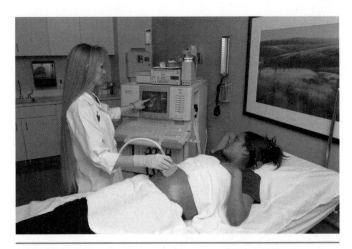

The nurse should encourage prenatal testing as some disorders can be detected before the baby is born. Research may offer hope of therapies to treat an affected fetus.

and infants diagnosed with disorders are enrolled with appropriate services in a timely manner. All states require newborns to be screened for certain genetic conditions such as phenylketonuria (PKU) and hypothyroidism. Many states also require screening for sickle cell disease and most screen for galactosemia. Postdelivery interventions treat these diseases to prevent related developmental disorders. Among other diseases screened by certain states are congenital adrenal hyperplasia, homocystinuria, maple syrup urine disease, biotinidase deficiency, tyrosinemia, cystic fibrosis, congenital infections, and other metabolic disorders (*Healthy People 2010,* 2000). Unfortunately the occurrence of appropriate follow-up testing and preventive treatment is uneven (Council of Regional Networks for Genetic Services, 1998).

Nurses must be sensitive to the special issues raised for these families as well as for those families who received a prenatal diagnosis. Because most of these conditions have a genetic basis, the families may face difficult reproductive decisions relating to the risk of occurrence in subsequent children or in other relatives. For families with an affected infant, there may be no guarantee of assistance with special treatment costs. Also, although new laws may help, the diagnosis, once recorded in the health record, may expose the family to risk of loss of or increased costs of health insurance.

Developmental Surveillance

The developmental outcome for the child rests in the interplay between the child and the physical, sociopolitical, spiritual, cultural, and emotional environment. A nurturing environment often leads to fulfillment of the child's potential while a dysfunctional environment can lead to insufficient development.

REFLECTIVE THINKING

Termination of Pregnancy

Think about a couple's decision to abort a defective fetus.

• How will you react when they discuss their options and decision with you?

• How will you counsel the couple if your personal beliefs differ from theirs?

Example child risk factors include prematurity; maternal smoking or drug or alcohol abuse during pregnancy; infections; chronic illness; injury; inadequate nutrition; genetic or metabolic disorders; war; lack of financial and social support; temperamental differences between parent and child; abuse and neglect; and inadequate interdisciplinary health care communication, educational opportunities, community resources, and law enforcement for equal opportunities.

Community health nurses can explore parental views and concerns about development with each family contact and coordinate care through case management. *Healthy People 2010* suggests children with special needs should have:

1. Care provided in their community accommodating insurance policies and Medicaid

2. Family-centered care, meaning the family is the center of strength and support

3. Continuous care with the same primary pediatric health care professionals from infancy through transitions to adulthood

4. Comprehensive health care 24 hours a day addressing primary, secondary, and tertiary needs

5. Care coordination linking families to support, community-based services and centralized information

6. Compassionate caregivers

7. Culturally appropriate, respectful, and linguistically competent care

Developmental Assessment

Nurses use a number of **developmental assessment** tools. The well child receives periodic screening with global screening instruments such as the Denver Developmental Screening Test II, designed to identify the child needing further investigation. Children with specific risk conditions, including concerns identified at the periodic screening, receive additional screening by health professionals for development, nutrition, behavior, parenting, mental health, medical status, or vision and hearing. Par-

ent education and resource coordination are offered, often by nurses. Children who have health and development problems are monitored by some of the more comprehensive instruments suitable for children with risk conditions, such as the Bayley Scales of Infant Development II (Black & Matula, 2002).

Nurses providing developmental assessment recognize the value of parental involvement in the test situation. Parents are entitled to a careful explanation of the tests, their purpose, and how well their child performed. They may need time and repeated evaluation before recognizing a delay and accepting the need for further evaluation. When the child is known to be delayed, the reassessment can be a time of disappointment, discouragement, and grieving. It is important for the nurse to acknowledge parental feelings, provide support, assist parents to identify their contributions to positive development in the child, and provide needed education.

Interdisciplinary Evaluation

Because the etiologies of developmental disabilities are multiple and diverse, a standard medical evaluation is not possible. General diagnostic elements include the medical and family history, neurodevelopmental assessment, physical examination, and appropriate laboratory tests.

When delays are noted, additional assessment by multiple disciplines are completed based on the delays involved. Psychologists, audiologists, optometrists, speech, physical and occupational therapists, geneticists, and educators are among those enlisted to perform assessments. The nurse contributes culturally competent health appraisal, developmental assessment, and assessment of the client's special care needs and of the family's ability to provide needed care. In addition, the nurse is essential in assisting the family to identify and use all available resources. Figure 28-2 identifies some developmental assessment instruments.

Cultural Factors

To be effective, the nurse needs to understand the particular cultural system of the family. The United States is a country of great diversity, requiring nurses to have knowledge of the assumptions, values, and beliefs of their own culture in addition to learning the same about cultures with whom they work. Each cultural group has its own longstanding, distinctive cultural beliefs, values, assumptions, practices, and group relationships that determine the way members define and address the needs of persons with developmental disorders. However, it should be kept in mind that within each cultural group there is great diversity to avoid harmful stereotyping. For example, the dominant Northern European culture in the United States varies greatly by region, religion, habits, and many other respects, not unlike cultures around the

FIGURE 28-2 Examples of Screening and Assessment Instruments

There are many instruments now available to screen and assess children or to structure and monitor developmental programs. Listed are a few examples of instruments commonly used by community health nurses or by advanced practice nurses.

Examples of Instruments Used to Screen the Well Child

1. Denver Developmental Screening Test II (DDST). Examiner tests well child, 2 weeks to 6 years.

   Denver Pre-screen Questionnaire. Rating by parents of child, 3 months to 6 years.

   > W. K. Frankenberg, J. B. Dodds, A. Fandal, E. Kazuk, and M. Cohrs
   > ADOCA Publishing Foundation
   > 5100 Lincoln St.
   > Denver, CO 80212

2. Ages and Stages Questionnaires (ASQ). Parents respond to questionnaires (for children 4 months to 48 months).

   > D. Bricker, J. Squires, and L. Mounts
   > Paul H. Brookes Publishing Co.
   > PO Box 10624
   > Baltimore, MD 21285-0624

3. Developmental Profile II. Rating from birth to 9 years. Parents report development in physical, self-help, social, academic, and communication skills.

   > G. Alpern, T. Boll, and M. Shearer
   > Psychological Development Publications
   > PO Box 3198
   > Aspen, CO 81612

4. Home Observation for Measurement of the Environment (HOME). Birth to 3; 3 to 6 years.

   Examiner assesses home environment and parent and child interactions.

   > B. Caldwell and R. Bradley
   > University of Arkansas at Little Rock
   > 23rd and University Ave.
   > Little Rock, AR 72204

Examples of Instruments Employed with Children at Risk or with Developmental Problems

1. Bayley Scales of Infant Development II. Examiner tests child, 1 month to 42 months.

   > N. Bayley and 1993 revision team
   > The Psychological Corporation
   > 7500 Old Oak Blvd.
   > Cleveland, OH 44130

2. Mullen. An examiner offers stimulus materials to child and records child's responses.

   > E. Mullen
   > American Guidance Service
   > 4021 Woodland Rd.
   > Circle Pines, MN 55014-1796

3. Nursing Child Assessment Satellite Training (NCAST).

   Feeding scale. Examiner assesses child and parent interaction in feeding situation.

   Teaching scale. Examiner assesses child and parent interaction in teaching situation.

   > K. Barnard
   > NCAST
   > University of Washington
   > WJ-10
   > Seattle, WA 98195

4. Eyeberg Child Behavior Inventory. Parent or other adult rates child's conduct (2 to 16 years).

   > S. Eyeburg
   > Department of Medical Psychology
   > School of Medicine, The Oregon Health Sciences
   >   University
   > 3181 SW Sam Jackson Park Road
   > Portland, OR 97201

5. Achenbach Child Behavior Check List

   Rating of child's behavior (4 to 18 years).

   > T. Achenbach
   > Department of Psychiatry
   > University of Vermont
   > Burlington, VT 05401

Examples of Instruments Useful for Assessing Adaptive Skills

1. Nursing history and assessment forms.

   Numerous forms are found in nursing texts or clinical procedures manuals that guide assessment of client self-care skills, social skills, level of understanding, and mental status.

2. American Association on Mental Deficiency (AAMD) Adaptive Behavior Scales for Children and Adults. One standard scale and two school-use scales. Observation or self-report may be used. Scales designed to assess persons with mental retardation or emotional maladjustment.

   > Publishers Test Services
   > 2500 Garden Road
   > Monterey, CA 93940

3. Vineland Adaptive Behavior Scales, 1984 edition.

   Observation or semi-structured interview of persons birth to 19 years. Survey form or expanded form for program planning available.

   > S. Sparrow, D. Balla, and D. Cicchetti
   > American Guidance Services Publisher's Building
   > Circle Pines, MN 55014-1796

Courtesy of Forrest Bennett, MD, Professor of Pediatrics, Clinical Training Unit, University of Washington. Used with permission.

REFLECTIVE THINKING

Cultural Response to Disability

A Native American couple had a baby born with congenital absence of the eyes. They refused to take the baby home from the hospital. Threats of prosecution for abandonment did not deter them, and the baby was placed in foster care. The local public health nurse told the hospital personnel that the baby's great-grandmother was responsible for the parents' decision. She had reminded all the relatives that the customary and only appropriate response to the birth of such a baby was to place it out in the desert to die, "face down in the sand." Whatever their personal feelings, the parents had accepted the decision that the baby had no place in the family or community.

- Does this family's culturally sanctioned action differ from "decision not to treat" or "do not resuscitate"?

FIGURE 28-3 Adapted from Explanatory Model for Culturally Competent Care

- What do you feel caused this condition?
- When and how did this condition begin?
- Why do you think it started when it did?
- How has this condition affected you or this child physically? How has it affected you or your child mentally?
- Do you feel upset about this condition?
- Has the condition interfered with you or your child's play or forced you to make changes in your or your child's lifestyle?
- What course has this condition taken?
- Do you notice this condition all the time?
- Do you or does your child sometimes do better than others?
- How do you think this condition should be treated?
- What do you think we can do to treat this condition?
- What are your expectations?
- Do you think this condition is curable?
- What are your expectations of the outcome of this condition?

Luckmann, J. (1999). *Transcultural Communication in Nursing*. Clifton Park, NY: Delmar Learning.

---

world. Luckmann (1999) reported the explanatory model as a means to elicit views of illness. See Figure 28-3.

Respectful exploration of these questions with the family or knowledgeable members of the culture can help the nurse assess the cultural influences on individual family decisions related to care of the client. Understanding the cultural values and beliefs enables the nurse to work more productively with the client and the family.

Planning with the Family

The goal of community health nursing is to assist the person with a disability attain the highest possible level of health and social functioning. Nursing specific to developmental disability includes:

1. Helping parents develop an individualized, flexible care plan to guide care for their child
2. Assisting and supporting parents to teach their child self-care and appropriate social behavior
3. Providing information on community resources for parents and their children or adult clients and assisting in linking clients with resources
4. Teaching the adult client healthy self-care.

Self-care is an important focus for client and family. **Self-care** is the individual's ability to achieve and sustain maximum health, well-being, and safety. Thus, self-care is a key element for living as independently as possible in the least restrictive environment.

The Nursing Health Care Plan

The child with a disability has the same basic health needs as any other. Routine health maintenance procedures can be forgotten in the context of completing therapies, treating acute illnesses, or controlling seizures. The nursing health care plan provides a means to avoid oversights by articulating the multiple elements necessary to maintain wellness in a person with a disability.

The nursing care plan not only contains the actions initiated by medicine and nursing but also provides written coordination of the entire health care team for any particular client—an essential component for holistic care:

The written plan of care communicates the patient's past and present health status and current needs to all members of the healthcare team. It identifies problems solved and those yet to be solved, approaches that have been successful, and patterns of patient responses. The plan of care documents patient care in areas of liability, accountability and quality improvement. It also provides a mechanism to help ensure continuity of care. (Doenges, Moorhouse, & Geissler, 2000, pp. 7–8)

Objectives specific to the client's diagnosis should be included. For example, children with ADHD are at increased risk for sleep difficulties, depression, anxiety, obsessions, and eventual substance abuse (Kewley & Latham, 2000). Care plans will specify close surveillance for those risks. A client with seizures may be at risk for perceptual/cognitive impairment, emotional difficulties, various forms of injury, and tracheobronchial obstruction. The nursing care plan provides anticipatory guidance to prevent these things from occurring or treating them should they occur.

The nursing plan will also specify removal of any barriers that might prevent the child from acquiring the education needed to achieve maximum potential. Parents may be told that glasses are not necessary for a child who cannot learn to read. This perspective is short-sighted and ignores the fact that good vision facilitates optimal learning and reduced vision is a barrier. Likewise, hearing aids and sign language training should be provided as early as possible to the child with hearing impairment or delayed language. Environmental stimuli are critical to language development for the young child. Without it they will not learn to speak (Wong, 1999). Adaptive equipment should be provided to the child with motor delays so that he or she is upright and mobile at the same developmental level as other children of the same age. Resistive, hyperactive, or withdrawn behaviors that interfere with learning should be addressed in the plan. Isolation from new experiences or new roles, particularly in adolescence, may delay social role learning. Isolation may occur as a perceived protective measure, outright exclusion, or a lack of facilities to accommodate special needs. Whatever the reason, nurses provide the needed information to prevent or ameliorate this problem. Nurses and families should strive to identify and include in the plan all procedures, supports, and experiences that promote health and social development.

Teaching Health Self-Care

Slow development or multiple problems involving the child may disrupt normal parenting roles and should be empathetically and directly addressed by the nurse. Realistic parental expectations strengthen family coping and facilitate effective parental teaching. Following assessment, the nurse can help parents gain a clear and realistic understanding of ways they can enhance their child's development, projected rates of development, and risks for associated problems. Parents can be taught

specific techniques to address problem behaviors that may interfere with the child achieving full capabilities (see Figure 28-4). **Behavior modification** is based on

---

FIGURE 28-4 Designing a Behavioral Program

Jean is a 4-year-old girl with mild mental retardation and a seizure disorder. Her indulgent parents report to the community health nurse that she ignores most requests and is not mastering the self-help skills that she should. They want assistance in improving her cooperation.

1. Review client and family situation.

The nurse reviewed Jean's health history and performed a developmental assessment. Jean functions near age 3 in most skills and has no physical limitations. Her seizures are controlled. She is capable of understanding and obeying simple requests. Her parents are very motivated to help her.

2. Identify target behaviors.

After much discussion, Jean's parents decide that they want Jean to comply with requests to come to them, to go to her room, and to sit at the table. They select coming when called as the first behavior to increase.

3. Obtain a baseline.

Jean's parents record the events surrounding her behavior: the parents' request to come; her response of compliance or noncompliance; and the consequences (i.e., what the parents do). They record for five days and learn that Jean complies with a request to come once in 10 times. They also learn that when she complies, they tend to take her behavior for granted. When she does not, they tend to scold or go to her.

4. Set the behavioral goal and select the reinforcement.

The parents and nurse state the goal as "Jean will come within 20 seconds of being called 95% of the time." Reinforcement for coming is a smile and a pat every time and a small food treat given intermittently. Noncompliance is ignored.

5. Schedule the plan and record results each time.

The parents specify that they will make eight trials (i.e., requests to come) per day at times when Jean is not engrossed in a favorite activity. After one week, the recording indicates that Jean is coming when called 75% of the time. The parents are pleased and are motivated to continue.

6. Review plan, evaluate, and make appropriate changes.

After two weeks, compliance is at 90%. The parents are confident that they understand how to set appropriate behavior goals and reinforce consistently. They plan to continue the program until Jean complies with their requests 95% of the time.

the principle that behaviors can be molded through rewards and setting limits. These simple procedures can be readily taught, although most parents use this technique at some time during childrearing. Desired developmentally appropriate behavior is rewarded systematically and either undesirable behavior is ignored or limits with natural consequences are set (Varcarolis, 1998).

The nurse also needs to consider the attitudes, knowledge, resources, and willingness to commit of the parents. Expectations for parents of a developmentally disabled child can be overwhelming, and every effort should be made to support them, avoid requiring what may not be possible, and provide resources as they are needed. While labels for disorders serve to facilitate diagnosis, treatment, prognosis, communication, and research, they also bring with them stereotypes, misunderstanding, and a good deal of discrimination. Parents and children should be taught healthy ways to deal with the misunderstanding and fear associated with stigma.

Serious and intractable behaviors require expert intervention involving the interdisciplinary team and particularly a behavioral specialist. Examples of potentially dangerous behaviors include extreme hyperactivity, purposeful self-injury, rumination, and assaultive and deeply withdrawn behavior. For example, the child with autism may be at risk for serious injury from self-injurious behavior, inability to trust and communicate, and inadequate processing of sensory stimulation (Townsend, 2000). Often these behaviors require specialized help from psychologists, behavioral specialists, and occupational therapists. Family members and school personnel can be trained in individualized and specialized behavior management techniques.

Family Support

Most parents and other family members experience shock, denial, anger, helplessness, sorrow, and other strong emotions following the realization that something is wrong with their child. Circumstances surrounding the disability may give rise to feelings of guilt, shame, and isolation. The response of each family is uniquely influenced by many factors, including the child's diagnosis and gender, family belief system, attitudes of relatives and community members, community resources, and economic circumstances. The nurse offers emotional support by encouraging open discussion among family members, reflecting and helping them grieve and clarify feelings and regain a sense of control over their lives. Specialized counseling can be accomplished by certified and advanced-practice nurses and other appropriate resources. See Figure 28-5.

Siblings of a child with a developmental disability may need special attention. They may be confused about the cause of the disability and feel somehow to blame.

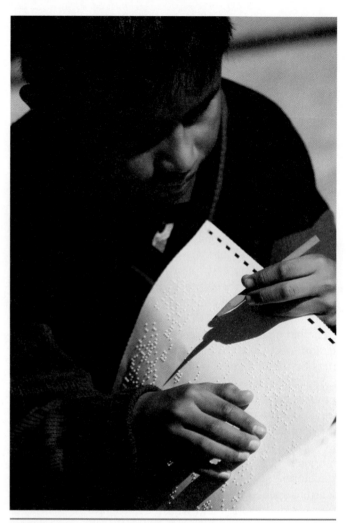

Blindness should not hinder educational achievement. This boy is taking a test in braille.

They may wish to avoid any identification with their sibling or feel resentful of the time and attention the parents must devote to him or her. They may mirror any feeling of shame or stigma evident in the parents. Parents may need guidance in determining how much to do for their special needs child without neglecting other children. They may feel guilty about decisions to use respite care and attending to the needs of other children (Wittert, 2001). Nurses can provide reassurance that these decisions maintain family balance.

Often nurses come into contact with these families at a time of crisis, such as during diagnosis, illness, or trauma. Assessment of the child's and family's ability to cope with daily needs and challenges is important. Empathetically listening to and acknowledging the demands of raising a special needs child may comfort parents. Nurses educate families about the disabilities, educational rights, respite and home care resources, special services, financial assistance resources, community support groups, and pub-

FIGURE 28-5 On Chronic Sorrow

Chronic Sorrow is a term coined by sociologist Simon Olshansky to describe the long-term reaction of parents who have a child with a disability. This pervasive reaction is often not recognized or understood by those around the parents—professionals, family, and friends. These feelings of chronic sorrow are normal and to be expected and accepted given the life-long implications for the family and child. Many factors can affect the intensity and exhibition of chronic sorrow: the parents' personalities, the severity of the disability, the nature of the disability, and the adequacy of support and services provided. Chronic sorrow does not mean that the parents do not love or feel pride in their child. These and many other feelings exist alongside the sadness. It is as if many threads are woven side by side, bright and dark, in the fabric of the parents' lives. They coexist; they do not blend into one color or feeling.

Because ours is such a "can do" society, there is pressure on parents to quickly put their feelings of sadness away or deny them. Parents are told to "think positively" and "to get on with your lives." They are told that God has "selected" them to receive this special child because they are such strong people. These kinds of comments, while well meant, deny the validity or parental long-term grieving. The discomfort of observing pain in those we care about can be part of the reason for such comments from others.

Grieving, however, is a process that takes time, often years. It is a prickly bush that one must go through, not jump over. However, there are ways to support the process of grieving. Most parents found support in a community of people who understand because they too have lived the experience. It is lonely to be the only family on the block with a child with a disability. Being part of a support group or organization helps to combat feelings of isolation.

Engaging in personal activities that do not center on the family member with a disability can help increase feelings of competency and self-worth. Counseling, especially at times of significant stressful milestones, can be useful.

Chronic sorrow becomes a permanent part of the personality structure of most parents who have a child with a disability. It is a normal response. Its thread narrows and widens depending on life situations; most often, it is accepted with courage. And, although permanent, it is not the dominant force in interactions with our children.

The dominant forces are love and feelings of connectedness to them.

Adapted from L. Sarasquetta, Spring 1998, *Hydrocephalus Association Newsletter*. [On-line]. Available: www.hydroassoc.org/newsletter/.

---

lished resources (Wittert, 2001). Certain developmental milestones create increased stressor for the child and family (e.g., entering school, adolescent sexual interests, exiting school as a young adult, aging parents). The community health nurse can prepare the family so they are able to anticipate and better manage these added challenges.

Organized groups of parents and siblings exist in every state. Family or individual counseling may be available through local developmental disorder service programs, religious affiliations, local mental health agencies, or other social services. Most states have public and private financial resources to assist with expenses associated with many disabilities. Persons under 18 receive benefits based on the income and resources of the family. Local health and human services agencies are usually the initial contact for obtaining information and services. See Figure 28-6.

THE EARLY YEARS

The period of maximum brain growth is from birth to 3 years. The experiences of the child during this period influence emotional, physical, cognitive, and social

FIGURE 28-6 National Information Center for Children and Youth with Disabilities

The National Information Center for Children and Youth with Disabilities (NICHCY) provides information to assist parents, educators, caregivers, advocates, and others in helping children and youth with disabilities become participating members of the school and community. Information Specialists are available to answer questions. The center provides information on specific disabilities, organizations supporting persons with disabilities, public agencies, legislation, materials for parents, resources for adults with disabilities, news digests, and other data bases. The center offers material in Spanish also. It is operated by the Academy for Educational Development through a cooperative agreement with the U.S. Department of Education.

P.O. Box 1492, Washington, DC 20013-1492
1-800-695-0285 (Toll Free, Voice/TT)
or search their web page
http://www.NICHCY.org
E-Mail: NICHCY@aed.org

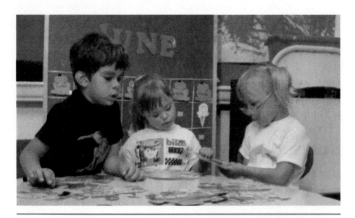

One of the objectives of *Healthy People 2010* is to provide access to preschool programs for children with developmental disorders that will prepare them for school.

development. Special supports for the child at risk or the child with a disability should be provided as soon as possible.

Early Intervention

Early intervention in the context of this chapter means to provide to the infant or child and family an individual development program with associated social support services for the purpose of preventing or ameliorating disability, maximizing potential, and enhancing parental skills and family adjustment.

Several federal laws and amendments mandate all state education agencies to serve children with disabilities from age 3 to young adulthood. Part 303 of the Individuals with Disabilities Education Act of 1997 addressed early intervention programs for infants and toddlers with disabilities. The purpose was to implement, enhance, and improve statewide, comprehensive, coordinated, multidisciplinary, interagency systems of early intervention services; to facilitate payments from federal, state, local, and private sources; and enhance identification and evaluation and meet the needs of underrepresented populations with disabilities (e.g., minority, low income, inner city, and rural). Developmental delays associated with disabilities include cognitive, physical, communication, social or emotional, and adaptive or a condition with a high probability of subsequent delays. Intervention services are identified on an individualized family service plan that delineates goals and identifies child and family strengths and resources (IDEA, 1990).

Health Care

An objective from *Healthy People 2010* is to increase access to a "medical home" for children with special health care needs. "Medical home" refers to medical care for in-

fants and children that is accessible, continuous, comprehensive, family centered, coordinated, and compassionate (*Healthy People 2010,* 2000). To this end, advanced-practice nurses working in programs treating infants and toddlers with developmental delays provide physical and developmental assessment of the family's ability to provide medical, nursing, or other health care procedures themselves. Children who have fragile health or are **technology assisted** (i.e., dependent upon a device that substitutes for a body function) are also served. Nurses assist the family and program team to develop the individual family service plan, including the nursing care plan. Nurses teach the family any needed health care procedures and may be the primary caregiver in the family or act as consultant to the family or other health team members. Because many early intervention procedures or therapies are provided as part of daily child care, cultural differences in practices of feeding, toilet training, discipline, sick-child care, or social training are taken into account when planning with the family.

THE SCHOOL YEARS AND TRANSITION TO ADULTHOOD

During the school years, the child with a developmental disability comes into contact with peers and the wider community. In this setting, he or she strives to develop the skills for optimal ability to successfully cope with the challenges of adulthood.

Legal Supports

Since the passage of the Education for All Handicapped Children Act (1975) and successor acts, all states accepting federal funds must provide a free and appropriate education to all children with disabilities. Related services such as transportation or physical or speech therapy must also be provided. A standard classroom teacher, special education teacher, and representative of the school district must assess the student's educational needs and with the parents develop an individual education plan (IEP). The IEP should contain annual goals and short-term objectives and be based on the child's needs determined by a formal assessment conducted at least every three years. The school is required to seek parental consent (PACER, 1995) for this plan. The IEP must include the transition services needed for postschool objectives such as employment, additional schooling, community participation, or independent living. See Figure 28-7.

Education must be offered in the least restrictive environment. **Mainstreaming, or inclusion,** meaning the most contact possible with children who do not have disabilities, is required. Children with physical disabilities or mild mental retardation may be served in regular classrooms with any needed physical or educational assis-

FIGURE 28-7 An Example of an Individual Education Plan

Child's Name: Justin W.   Age: 4 years, 2 months

Center City Public School District

September 17, 2001

Present Level of Functioning

Social development: Justin does not play with other children. He never approaches another child and runs away every time a child approaches him.

Annual Goals

Justin will learn to play cooperatively with other children.

Short-Term Objectives

Justin will play next to other children during highly preferred activities (for example, sandbox, sensory table, finger painting) for two 10-minute periods each day.

Special Services

School district will provide transportation to and from community preschool placement, and school district will pay Justin's tuition for a half-day program at the Learning Center Community Preschool.

Speech therapist will visit the preschool once a week to work with Justin and to meet with the teacher.

Behavior management program will be coordinated by classroom teacher and itinerant special education teacher.

Beginning and Duration of Services

Justin will begin attending the Learning Center on October 5. Other services will be in place by October 12. Placement and services will be reevaluated by April 5, 20xx.

Evaluation

Justin will be reassessed on the Preschool Profile in March. A graph will be kept showing the amount of time Justin spent playing next to children each day.

From *The Exceptional Child: Inclusion in Early Childhood Education,* by K. E. Allen and I. S. Schwartz, 1996, Clifton Park, NY: Delmar Learning.

Parents are in a strong position to obtain these services for their child because the law outlines the rights of the child and an appeals process that must be followed if the parents are dissatisfied with their child's education. States and local districts vary in what is offered within a particular school system, and this is further influenced by funds available to run school programs. Nurses encourage parents to examine their local programs in order to decide what is best for their child and to pursue legal recourse if federally mandated programs are not forthcoming.

Health Care

An objective of *Healthy People 2010* is increasing the service systems for children with special health care needs. These health services include education; promotion; preventive and primary care; screenings for vision, hearing, speech, and language; assessment of physical and psychosocial milestones; diagnostic and therapeutic services; and habilitation and rehabilitation services. Early intervention is stressed.

School nurses often participate in the IEP, contributing essential information about accessibility and safety of the school environment, health services, and health education. Children with **medical assistive devices** such as gastrostomies and oxygen machines may attend school. School nurses consult with the family, physician, home health nurse, and equipment personnel to establish an appropriate care plan integrating direct-care procedures within the school setting.

School nurses are participating in a wide variety of health care related to developmentally disabled students. Hansma (1997) reported that school nurses conducted staff in-services about adapting disaster plans to the needs

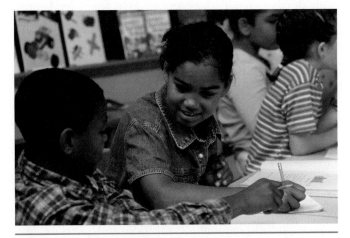

Children with developmental disorders may be served by and encouraged to participate in traditional classrooms depending on the severity of their disability.

tance. Children with significant behavior difficulties or with moderate or severe mental retardation may be served in contained classrooms with scheduled classes or activities with nonhandicapped peers. Children with the need for pervasive supports have been and may still be served in "development centers" where their special physical needs are addressed, but the trend is to place these children in classrooms attached to regular schools. *Healthy People 2010* set an objective to increase the proportion of children and youth with disabilities who spend at least 80% of their time in regular education programs.

of severely handicapped students, stocked classrooms with emergency kits specific to handicapped students' needs, trained school staff in first aid, and conducted classroom inspections for repairs and supplies specific to children with special needs. Increasingly, nurses are becoming familiar with instructive devices and computer-driven environmental controls designed to enhance the learning and function of children with disabilities. School nurses are members of the interdisciplinary team and help ensure that the adaptive technology is comfortably and safely incorporated into the school and home environment of the child (Hansma, 1997).

Self-Care Education

Children and adolescents in the general population require significant health education. For the developmentally disabled child or adolescent, health education issues are greatly compounded relative to the degree the person is affected. For example, children with cerebral palsy or spina bifida must learn to manage orthopedic devices, skin care, or bowel and bladder routines. The child with epilepsy must learn to manage medications and maintain good oral health. School nurses advocate for or develop general and individualized curricula that teach proper terminology, identification of common and special health problems, and appropriate self-care. Some people with developmental disabilities are at risk for obesity due to reduced motor activity or opportunities for motor activity, while others are at risk for nutritional deficits due to high metabolic demands, poor oral health, and/or problems with ingestion.

Sex education is often neglected because of erroneous beliefs that people with disabilities are not interested in, able, or likely to reproduce. A policy statement by the American Academy of Pediatrics (1996) strongly advocated sex education for children and adolescents with developmental disorders to help them lead more fulfilling lives and protect them from exploitation, unplanned pregnancies, and sexually transmitted diseases. Sex education will increase chances that they perceive themselves as attractive members of their gender with expectations of satisfying adult relationships and assert themselves in protecting their bodies and reporting violations (Wolbring, 2000). Some parents tend to view their disabled children as children for life and so are uncomfortable or do not know how to teach them about sex [American Academy of Pediatrics (AAP), 1996]. Information should be tailored to the understanding level of the child and offered concretely, unambiguously, and repeatedly. The AAP suggests parents teach children about appropriate expressions of affection and pleasure, expectations for privacy, modestly and public behavior, their right to refuse touching, and reporting violations.

Sex education curricula have been developed for use by parents, nurses, and teachers. Updated resources may be located through the NICHCY (2001).

Ninety percent of people with developmental disorders will experience sexual abuse at some point in their lives. (See Table 28-4.) Forty-nine percent will experience 10 or more abusive incidents. People with mental retardation are more vulnerable, and it has been estimated that only 3% of these cases are ever disclosed (Valenti-Hein & Schwartz, 1995). Because of these statistics, it is imperative that community health nurses recognize the signs and symptoms of sexual abuse in populations who are mentally retarded. In an effort to curb sexual abuse and exploitation and improve reporting, the ARC recommends educating individuals and service providers, improving investigation and prosecution procedures, providing a safe environment for disclosure, and improving background checking policies for employment. Finally, employers are urged to turn over suspected abusers and employees with criminal backgrounds to the police instead of simply firing the employee (ARC, 1997).

Like all children and adolescents, those with developmental disabilities need education on drug, alcohol, and tobacco abuse, conflict resolution, and violence prevention. School nurses teach and counsel the individual student on those matters and promote curricula for the classroom.

The school years can be a time when peers increasingly exclude the child with developmental disorders from group activities. The ARC notes that associating with people without disabilities provides opportunities for interaction and helps the person with a disability develop appropriate social skills, self-esteem, self-worth, and friendships. Inclusion in recreational programs also assists with physical fitness and energy (ARC, 1998). To compensate schools for this exclusion, the nurse can help the parents seek social and recreational opportunities for the client through sports such as Special Olympics, arts and crafts, parent- or church-sponsored activities, private lessons such as horseback riding and martial arts, and public recreation programs such as the YMCA or YWCA and city or community programs. Teenagers may attend conferences sponsored by organizations for the challenged such as the Spina Bifida Association of America, Down Syndrome Congress, or United Cerebral Palsy. Many organizations offering opportunities for self-advocacy exist for youth and young adults. These can be accessed through NICHCY. Although much progress has been made in establishing equal rights for persons with disabilities, discrimination of a more subtle kind continues to exist. Bogdan and Taylor (1999) argue that being *in* the community is different from being *part* of the community. They note that being part of the com-

TABLE 28-4 Sexual Exploitation and Abuse of Persons with Developmental Disorders

POTENTIAL VULNERABLE SITUATIONS

Traits of Some Persons That May Increase Vulnerability

Normal sexual development and drives but limited social opportunities	Ability to find a suitable partner may be limited by factors beyond the individual's control, such as physical attributes, societal rejection and devaluation, or restricted lifestyle. The person may tolerate someone who is exploitive or abusive in order to maintain the relationship.
Desire to be considered normal	Having a boyfriend or girlfriend or having a baby is evidence of normality. The individual may accept someone unsuitable or exploitive in order to be considered normal.
Trust and affection for the abuser	The person is easily persuaded to keep the abuse secret.
Limited ability to perceive an inappropriate social situation, limited understanding of the acts and their consequences, or socialized to be compliant and obedient	The individual is readily tricked and exploited by persons offering favors, professing affection, or exerting authority over the person.
Limited or no communication	The individual is unable to report abuse.
Physically unable to escape unwanted attention or assault	The person may have inadequate community living skills and may be unable to travel safely in the community. The living or work situation may be unsafe.

Environmental Risk Factors

Isolated living site	Individual loses oversight protection of friends, family, or neighbors.
Multiple caregivers	Lack of attachment between individual and care providers increases risk of detachment and indifferent care and supervision.
Situation discourages independence	Individual does not learn how to resist abuse or seek help.
Individual devalued by significant people in his or her environment	Persons defined as "other," "less than," or "unworthy" are likely to become targets for abuse.

munity means having meaningful relationships with community members, contributing, recognizing that people are more than victims, and eventually doing away with concepts like normalization, integration, quality of life, and inclusion.

Transition Services

The Individuals with Disabilities and Education Act (IDEA) defines **transition** as

a coordinated set of activities for a student, designed within an outcome-oriented process, that promotes movement from school to post-school activities, including postsecondary education, vocational training, integrated employment (in-

cluding supported employment), continuing and adult education, adult services, independent living, or community participation (*Federal Register,* 1999).

Transition services were developed to assist students with disabilities to move successfully into life after public schools. The goal is to facilitate opportunities to achieve potential for self-care, independence, and community integration. Planning for the school-to-community transition is part of the IEP process. Additionally, an individual rehabilitation plan (IHP) that offers training and needed support services can be developed.

Graduates of special education programs are prepared for various levels of employment. Many enter competitive employment. Others obtain **supported employment** at which a job coach or other support ensures success at a competitive job. Still others train for

Out
of the Box

Teaching Real-World Safety to Young Adults with Developmental Disabilities

Community health nurses can collaborate with special education teachers to develop primary preventative programs such as the following.

The Community Transition Program housed on the Sacramento City College campus in California is an innovative and effective program for young adults with developmental disabilities who are moving from the relatively sheltered public school system into the community. This is a time of great growth and development, but unfortunately the new roles and independence also place them at serious risk for victimization by predators. In response to these risks, teachers in the transition program developed a plan to assess, improve, and maintain the personal safety and reporting skills of these youths as they move into the community setting.

Following thorough classroom safety training, transition students are given opportunities for making safe choices in potentially dangerous real-life situations in the community. In collaboration with community transition teachers and the campus police, drama students at Sacramento City College are oriented and instructed about a staged victimization attempt. Drama students' roles are to act as an individual preying on the unsuspecting transition student. The campus police are given dates and times of these activities and an instructor, unbeknownst to transition student, directly observes the process. Consequences are set for various responses the transition student has to the staged victimization attempt. An example follows: A drama student approaches a transition student at a bus stop and says he remembers seeing the transition student around. The drama student offers a ride in his car, which is parked down the street.

Possible Outcomes

Student accepts ride and leaves with the drama student to go to car. In response a familiar staff would casually walk by and say "Hello, where are you going?" to the transition student. The drama student then suddenly runs away, leaving the transition student a little stunned or scared. The staff asks the transition student about what happened, giving the student plenty of time to think about what happened and why. The staff person guides the student to report accurate information to the appropriate person. When the student realizes he or she made a dangerous mistake, the staff person reassures him or her that they will continue to practice saying no to people who are trying to trick, take advantage of, or hurt others.

Student refuses to accept ride. Staff assesses if the transition student appropriately reports the occurrence and reinforces refusing the ride as a good choice. If the transition student fails to report, they will be prompted. For example, staff may announce to the class that someone has been trying to lure students into their car by offering the student a ride, then robbing them. When a report is drawn from a student in this way, the importance of instant reporting is stressed, followed by an opportunity to practice this again in the community. Staff may also give a great deal of attention to the situation when it is appropriately reported and take a description of the drama student, warning other classmates to beware of the person described.

It is often difficult for students with developmental disabilities to generalize classroom learning by applying it in relevant real-life situations. This program creatively and realistically integrates classroom learning with life in the community. Thus, students' skills for living safely in the community are significantly enhanced. ■

—Susan Whaley, MA, Special Education
Stacey Hoffman, MA, Special Education
Community Transition Program Teachers

sheltered employment at a work center where supports are available and individual productivity may be set at noncompetitive levels. Persons needing extensive or pervasive supports may enter an **activity center** and continue to be taught self-care, social skills, homemaking, and leisure activities skills. *Healthy People 2010* aims to eliminate disparities in employment rates for adults with developmental disorders.

Perspectives...

INSIGHTS OF A RESIDENT IN A SMALL GROUP HOME

I didn't like being cooped up at the Developmental Center (large state residential facility). I felt I was locked away in a home away from home, in a strange place. Now Pat is a nice house mother to me. I'm glad she took me in. Our house is nice and clean and I am living with my old friend Lloyd that I knew back at Bentley. He lets me help feed his dog at night. We share our dog. North Bay Regional Center helped buy our new house.

Work is wonderful. It's making me blossom into a nice woman. The workshop has plenty of windows I can see out of. I'm happy to be back in freedomland now with no locked doors or high windows and I am surrounded by lovely dogs. I went to my first Special Olympics. I have good relaxation in my own private bedroom with my own TV and tapes. I'm glad I can go out in my electric wheelchair in my neighborhood safely.

It took me five years to get out of Sonoma. It was real hard. I won't ever have to go back again. My social worker, Blenda, helped me. Other people should get the chance to be on their own.

—Beth Ratto

Reprinted by permission from the North Bay Regional Center Newsletter, Napa, California, September, 1997, p. 2

ADULTHOOD

Most adults with developmental disorders will live independently and will no longer be perceived as needing services. Persons with more severe mental retardation and/or multiple disabilities need strong support to move from home into independent living, semi-independent living, or community residential programs. Many will continue to live with their families.

A proportion of adults with developmental disabilities who are unable to earn enough to become totally self-supporting may rely on some government or community benefits, in whole or in part. The standard benefits available to eligible persons may include Supplemental Security Income (SSI), Social Security Disability Income (SSDI), Medicare, Medicaid (in California, MediCAL), or community assistance. Obtaining and maintaining benefits can be difficult and confusing. Community health nurses help adults identify programs for which they are eligible and services available to assist with application for and maintenance of the benefits.

Residential Services

Since the 1970s programs of **deinstitutionalization** have increasingly and in huge numbers moved persons from large institutions into smaller community settings. Many state-operated institutions have closed, and nine states have institution-free service delivery systems. Government funds are increasingly being diverted to residential alternatives in community and family settings. Since 1980 there has been a 10-fold increase in group homes and supervised apartments. The percentage of institutionalized persons with mental illness and mental retardation has decreased 75% in the last 30 years [National Institute of Disability and Rehabilitation Research (NIDRR), 2001]. There remain reports, however, that children ready for discharge remain institutionalized (Priaulx, 2000).

Each state defines and licenses residential programs; terminology and regulations differ from state to state. Some areas have programs offering training in independent living with placement in supervised apartments or shared housing. Most areas offer licensed family care or foster care for persons of all ages. **Small-group residences,** housing with paid staff serving no more than 15 residents, are common. In some communities no more than six clients may be served in one small-group residence. See Table 28-5.

Health Care

Interdisciplinary teams may be needed in adulthood as well. Depending on the disorder, multiple considerations must be weighed in terms of health care. Examples include specialized dental care, isolation, psychiatric disorders, challenged motoric function, transportation, and continued or new problems with seeing and hearing. Coordination of these services is often not as easily accomplished as in a one-system school setting. Further services may not be as readily available or monetarily compensated as they were at a younger age. It is imperative that individuals continue to receive services to maintain as independent a lifestyle as possible. There is currently a waiting list of 52,000–87,000 for residential housing out of the family home (Heller & Factor, 2001). Bogdan and Taylor (1999) noted that solving problems for those with developmental disorders addresses problems of the community at large.

Community health nurses may be frustrated when finding that easily accessible, comprehensive health care services for adults with complex problems associated with their diagnoses continue to be difficult to obtain. The Americans with Disabilities Act (1990) mandated legislation to make society more accessible for those with disabilities; however, it did not address rights to coordinated, comprehensive, and easily accessible holistic

TABLE 28-5 Residential Options for Persons with Developmental Disorders

Residential services, terminology, and regulations differ from state to state. Services can be for profit, nonprofit, or tax supported.

SMALL RESIDENTIAL FACILITIES: 16 OR FEWER PERSONS	
Supported living	The individual lives in the same type of housing as others in the community and receives as much support as desired or needed.
Supervised living	The individual lives in regular housing, and staff from a support program monitor and continue to train the client for community living.
Child or adult foster home	The individual lives as a member of the family. Usually, the home serves no more than six residents. Some homes are licensed to care for fragile children or adults, and the service provider performs care and necessary treatments such as gastrostomy feedings. In some areas, the provider must be a licensed nurse. In others, lay providers are trained and nurses visit to consult or monitor care.
Group home	Staff provide care, supervision, and training. Some homes provide specialized care for persons with physical limitations, dietary needs, or behavior problems.
Personal care home	Staff provide personal assistance but no training.
Boarding home	Room and board are provided, but no personal care or training is offered.
Intermediate care facility (ICF/MR or DD)	Staff provide 24-hour care and training with registered nurse to supervise health care services.
LARGE RESIDENTIAL FACILITIES: 16 OR MORE PERSONS	
State-supported or private developmental centers (formerly called institutions)	Staff provide 24-hour care and training with available intermediate care and often skilled nursing care.
Group homes	Offer similar services as small-group homes.
Intermediate-care facilities (ICFs)	Regular ICFs may admit a person with a developmental disability.

health care. In 2000 the Developmental Disabilities Assistance and Bill of Rights Act took steps to address this problem by focusing, in part, on accountability criteria for those performing services for persons with developmental disorders. Under any system, the community health nurse is a key person to assess the special needs of adult clients, provide or obtain health care, and secure specialty services. The nurse may be the primary health care provider, the case manager, or the consultant to residential or work programs or to agencies serving people with disabilities. Whatever the setting, nurse advocacy for client health care may be the crucial element in obtaining comprehensive care.

Nursing Process

Although the nursing process for clients with disabilities is the same as for any client, special attention is needed for the following:

- *Communication.* Extra time may be needed to talk effectively with clients with limited understanding.

Use more direct than open-ended questions. Sentences should be short, with concrete, simple terminology. Request feedback frequently. Talking at a higher volume does nothing to increase understanding.

- *Data collection.* Make extra effort to obtain *all* prior medical records. Clients may not be able to give an adequate history. Medical records are rarely transferred when clients change residence. It is not unusual to find surgical scars and be unable to determine what procedures were done or when. Sources for more complete oral or recorded information may be relatives, residential service providers, friends, former or current care providers, case managers, or program directors.

- *Review latest literature on the client's particular disability.* New findings may dictate a changed approach to care.

- *Record the current level of self-care and other adaptive skills at each contact.* Physical, emotional, or degenerative conditions that the client is unable to identify may be expressed as loss of adaptive skills.

- *Nursing diagnoses.* In addition to health, diagnoses are usually needed to address self-care, motor problems, social and behavioral issues, communication, emotional status, and family coping issues. If working with an interdisciplinary team, medical diagnoses may be the most beneficial to team communication.

- *Nursing plans/interventions.* Confer with the client and care providers. Ensure that health-related interventions serve to promote social integration, age-appropriate behavior, health, and self-advocacy. Copies of the plan should be provided to the client, associated members of a health care team and any significant persons the client indicates. If pertinent, facilitate obtaining identification.

- *Evaluation.* Evaluate the plan and its effectiveness frequently. Restructure the plan as needed and update adaptive skills level as well as health status.

- *Client assistance.* Encourage the client with cognitive limitations to identify a trusted and willing person to assist with access to health care and implementation of health care recommendations.

Behavior Disorders and Mental Illness

Clients with developmental disorders may also exhibit behavior problems or signs of mental illness. These difficulties present additional challenges to the client, family, and community health nurse.

Behavior Disorders

Adults with developmental disabilities who come to the attention of the community health nurse because of behavior problems are likely to be persons with mental retardation, severe pervasive developmental disability, or multiple disabilities. They may be persons with a behavior disorder related to the diagnosis, as in fragile X syndrome. Problem behaviors can include inability to cooperate, temper outbursts, regression in skills, withdrawal, aggression toward others or self, impulsiveness, repetitive behaviors, and hyperactivity.

Nurses who work with clients exhibiting behavioral problems need to gain an in-depth understanding of the behavior content and context. This may be accomplished through observation, gaining an understanding of the client's perspective, talking with involved others in different settings, assessing for precipitating factors, reviewing the client's health history and current status, and assessing adaptive behaviors. Disruptive and aggressive behaviors may be substitutes for communication in those who lack communication skills (APA, 2000). Often physical problems that the client cannot identify or report, such as a headache, dysmenorrhea, toothache, or constipation, can be the source of the behavior. Environmental changes frequently evoke behavior problems such as a change in roommate, daily routines, diet, or recreation. A loss such as quarrel with a friend, change of instructor, or death in the family can also trigger behavior problems, as can abuse. Correcting the underlying problem, rapidly establishing new, stable routines or instituting a short-term behavioral program often resolves the situation.

Because behavior problems can be a symptom of illness, emotional problems, or both, services of an interdisciplinary medical-behavioral team should be sought. The community health nurse may identify, obtain, and coordinate the services of the appropriate specialist.

Mental Illness

Individuals with mental retardation are three or four times more likely to have mental disorders (APA, 2000), and mental disorders occur more frequently for all persons with all developmental disorders. For instance, frustrations related to communication, motor, cognitive, and emotional problems as well as pervasive societal stigma and discrimination often preempt mental illness: Susceptibility to certain mental illnesses accompany certain diagnoses. Identification may be complicated by modification of symptoms due to the disability and the possibility of an inadequate history. Axis I and II diagnoses (APA, 2000) in those with developmental disorders do not differ from the population at large.

Treatment for mental disorders in persons with developmental disorders parallels treatment for the same disorders in the general population but is complicated when there are problems of communication and multiple pharmacological interventions are already in use. Often mental health needs can be met in the community setting, but hospitalization for acute illness may be necessary. Community health nurses may be the first to identify a need for psychiatric intervention.

Nursing Care

Finding ways to resolve mental illness in those with developmental disorders takes special considerations (Coerver, 1999). Nursing care can occur in day treatment programs, residential settings, outpatient clinics, client homes, and rehabilitation programs. It has been suggested that mental illness be *perceived* as a disability with a wide range of services needed, often for long periods of time and best accomplished in the community. Further, skill enhancement and support are essential (Stewart & Laraia, 1998). Community health nurses consider the individual, family, and community when assessing and promoting mental health for their clients. As in psychiatric nursing, community health nurses frame their advocacy and interventions with a focus on strengths, empowerment, and self-esteem. For more information about mental illness, see Chapter 29.

Family Life

Like the general population, persons with developmental disorders mature, form relationships, marry, and have children. Rarely does this fact attract public attention unless the disability is mental retardation. Sex, marriage, and procreation are major concerns for parents of mentally retarded children. Schwier (1995) interviewed people with disabilities and clearly documented their wishes to live full lives, including having loving human relationships. Public, professional, and family concerns center on parents with mental retardation. Two issues are of greatest concern: (1) prevention of genetic transmission of mental retardation (a form of eugenics) and (2) the ability of parents with mental retardation to provide adequate care for their children (Brown, 2001). Sterilization of citizens with mental retardation and informed consent for this procedure continue to be a perplexing social issue.

When a parent's disorder is due to genetic factors, offspring may be at risk. Parents with mental retardation due to genetic factors have a 42% chance of having an affected child. When only one parent has genetic mental retardation, the chances are approximately 20%. Historically, parent rights have been removed without regard for actual parenting abilities (Ingram, 1993). The ability of these parents to care for their child is difficult to predict, yet many are capable of raising and loving their own children.

Community health nurses working with these families are in a key position to assess parenting skills, educate and empower clients to make sound, appropriate health care and childrearing decisions; and monitor the welfare and development of the children. They promote socialization by demonstrating interactions with the child, and teaching recognition of illness and environmental hazards, preventive care, and use of health care. Community health nurses advocate for addressing socioeconomic issues that hinder a parent's ability to provide adequate child care, encourage work centers or educational departments to offer specialized training to parents with cognitive limitations, and facilitate parental use of resources such as food programs. They promote social support such as arranging for help from a relative or friend to guide parents in day-to-day child care. Parenting needs differ little in content from those of any parents but may require more individualized, intensive support services. Throughout the United States there are programs offering in-home or classroom tutoring to parents with mental retardation. Help may be obtained through social service agencies, hospital educational programs, community mental health centers, state-run programs, child protective services, or Head Start. Many parents with mental retardation are closely scrutinized and live in fear of having their children taken away. Young people considering marriage and childbirth are encouraged to participate in educational resources about family life and parenting. Sheerin (1998) reviewed literature throughout the 1900s regarding parents with mental retardation and found that although they may be predisposed to problems, they can be good parents given support and training.

OLD AGE

With improvements in care and technology, persons with developmental disorders are living longer, as is the population of the United States in general. The U.S. Bureau of the Census estimates that by 2011 there will be over 30 million elderly. Estimates place the numbers of adults with developmental disorders over 60 at approximately 526,000, with expectations that numbers will reach 1,065,000 by 2030 (Heller & Factor, 2001). Persons with developmental disorders face all the age-related health conditions of their nondisabled cohort, and certain disabilities are associated with increased risks for specific age-related diseases. Life expectancies are similar for

---

✳ DECISION MAKING

Mario

Mario, a middle-aged man with severe mental retardation and related cardiac problems, had always lived at home. The family had never sought services, and Mario was not known to any agency. After his mother died, his father assumed his care. A neighbor, aware of the father's failing health and Mario's progressively poorer care, including missed medications and inappropriate diet, notified the community health nurse in the agency serving people with developmental disabilities. When the nurse called on the father to provide information about services, he became indignant. He said, "We Italians take care of our own." It was obvious, however, that extensive support was needed to maintain Mario in the family home.

♦ How would you proceed?

♦ How can the father's culture-based plan of care be acknowledged?

♦ Who might you enlist to talk with the father about Mario's future care?

♦ What resources for care can you define?

COMMUNITY NURSING VIEW

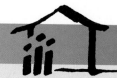

Mrs. Palma has come with her daughter, Mary, to talk to the community health nurse at the local agency serving persons with developmental disability. Mrs. Palma is considering having Mary sterilized and wants the nurse to advise how to go about it. Mary, now 20, has cerebral palsy and is mildly mentally retarded. She ambulates with a cane. She has dysarthria but can be readily understood.

Mrs. Palma, 50, is a widow with two sons married and living out of the home. Her large extended family is Filipino and Catholic; they are well-educated, with ample incomes.

Mary completed high school in special classes. Her general level of understanding is similar to that of a 12-year-old. She attends a work center that offers training in workplace behavior and specific job skills. Her mother permitted her to enter the work center against family advice because Mary was lonely and bored and wanted something to do. The family objected because of unsupervised contacts with male co-workers and because they do not expect a family member with physical difficulties to work.

Mrs. Palma is very distressed because Mary has paired off with a young man at the work center. This situation is bad enough, but pregnancy would be a disgrace.

Mrs. Palma is very angry with the work center staff. They tell her that Mary is an adult and is free to choose to have a boyfriend and to be sexually active. They say it is not normalizing to expect Mary to stay home with her mother. They expect to train her in community living skills needed for apartment living and for a job. Mrs. Palma has tried to tell them this plan is inappropriate. A Filipina of good family lives at home until marriage, and, of course, Mary will never marry.

Mrs. Palma reports that Mary's judgment is poor. She has never gone out alone. She is very careless about bathing, menstrual hygiene, and dental care. She doesn't even hang up her clothes. Her mother is sure that Mary cannot manage more complicated responsibilities, and she plans to consult her attorney and obtain conservatorship. Despite her religious beliefs, she thinks sterilization is the way to protect Mary.

Mary is quietly defiant. She is proud of having a boyfriend as other girls do. She thinks she would like a big wedding like her cousins have had. She is willing to learn to improve her grooming in order to look pretty. She thinks it might be fun to have a little baby after she is married.

Nursing Considerations

Use family development theory, the principle of normalization, and the concept of self-care to develop the nursing process suitable for this case.

Assessment

- What further data from the family, Mary, and the work center would be useful?
- What is the family life cycle stage?
- Has Mary's disability significantly altered the usual pattern?
- How can nursing intervention encourage the most normal pattern?
- What is normalization from the point of view of Mrs. Palma, Mary, and the work center staff?
- What is Mary capable of learning?
- What are her legal rights?

Diagnosis

- What diagnoses can be formulated concerning family function?
- Does Mary have self-care deficits that can be defined and addressed by nursing interventions?
- What self-care requisites may Mary face in the future?
- What should the nursing plan include?

Outcome Identification

- What are the desired outcomes?

Planning/Interventions

- What objectives can be formulated that meet the criteria for success as defined by Mary? By Mrs. Palma?
- What nursing interventions can be applied?
- How are interventions made compatible with the principle of normalization?
- What resources may be used?

Evaluation

- How and on what time table can the plan be reviewed by the Palma family?
- Have the criteria for success been met? If they have, what new goals may be considered?

adults with mental retardation and the general population unless there is severe cognitive impairment, Down syndrome, cerebral palsy, or multiple disabilities (Heller & Factor, 2001). Persons with Down syndrome may experience age-related changes earlier, and they are at greater risk of developing Alzheimer's disease after the age of 40. Risk of Alzheimer's disease is also higher for individuals with head injuries, especially severe and multiple (ARC, 2000). Major health concerns for aging persons with developmental disorders are nutrition and exercise (Heller & Factor, 2001). Women with mental retardation have higher obesity rates than other women. As persons with mental retardation experience the death of their parents, there is evidence that siblings are taking responsibility for their well-being, playing advocate, supervisory, and mediator roles (Bigby, 1998).

Lacy (2000) noted that aging and cerebral palsy lead to unanticipated problems, and recently research seems to support this. Spasticity and other muscular problems may lead to contractures and a decline in ability to ambulate and maintain balance over time. Additionally, medical professionals may wrongly link speech impairments to cognitive impairment. It often takes longer to assess an elder with cerebral palsy, and adhering to time constraints of managed care may make adequate assessment a challenge. Nearly 300,000 senior citizens in the United States have epilepsy. Statistics show that epilepsy is as likely to begin after age 60 as in the first 10 years of life (EFA, 2001). The majority of senior citizens who develop epilepsy and are otherwise in good physical and mental health continue to live independently.

Community health nurses pay special attention to the specific developmental disorder and its impact as the client ages. For instance, a senior citizen with epilepsy may maintain independence with education and interventions addressing environmental safety, emergency communication protocols, and assessment of medication sensitivity, toxicity, and interactions (EFA, 2001). Services and supports that may enable adults with developmental disabilities to age in place include assistance with personal care as needed, assistive devices to promote mobility, maintaining and improving function, environmental accommodations and communication, home health care, and in-home support (Heller & Factor, 2001). Community health nurses are instrumental in providing appropriate linkages to aging services, recreational programs, and later-life planning resources. Often aging parents have concerns about care for their developmentally disabled older child once they have died. Community health nurses can assist parents to access resources to help with future residential, legal, and financial plans for their child. In addition to NICHCY, an information resource for families and professionals is the National Institute for Life Planning for Persons with Disabilities, 513 Carriage Lane, Twin Fall, Idaho 83301.

THE FUTURE

Persons with developmental disabilities are increasingly reaping the benefits of improved legislation proclaiming and legally enforcing their civil rights. As a result, they are moving into communities, schools, and work places in ever-greater and more productive numbers.

Forty years is a relatively brief time to establish the attitudes and social changes that have been so beneficial to persons with developmental disorders. Despite adverse economic and political conditions and subtle and not so subtle stigma and discrimination, persons with disabilities and their families have increasingly become self-advocates. Women and men with disabilities speak for themselves through organizations such as People First International or TASH: The Association for Persons with Severe Handicaps. Community health nurses and other health professionals serve as advocates from a personal and professional platform. People thus united can retain and expand the systems of individual and family supports that accept and maintain people with developmental disorders in the community for a more harmonious, productive, and inclusive world.

KEY CONCEPTS

◆ Developmental disorders encompass single or groupings of impairments that may begin prenatally to young adulthood and are likely to continue indefinitely.

◆ *Developmental disability* as a legal term groups people with similar service needs but with different medical diagnoses. *Developmental disability* employed as a clinical term refers to persons with permanent central nervous system conditions that vary in severity, in degree of resulting handicap, and in expression over time. The most common conditions regarded as developmental disabilities are mental retardation, epilepsy, autism, cerebral palsy, and learning disability.

◆ Changing social attitudes and general acceptance of the principle of normalization led to increased services, support for community living, and affirmation of the legal rights of all persons with developmental disabilities.

◆ A significant number of conditions leading to and problems associated with developmental disorders are preventable or remediable. Community health nurses provide preventive interventions in most interactions with individuals and families.

◆ The goal of community health nursing is to promote the highest level of health and social functioning of persons with developmental disabilities. Nurses define and address the developmental, health, cognitive, social, behavioral, and emotional issues related to a particular disability at a particular point in the client's life. The nurse participates in or organizes the interdisciplinary services that may be needed to solve complex health problems. Individual nursing care plans are needed over the life span in response to changing health care needs.

◆ Early and sustained support to at-risk or delayed infants and their families promotes optimal child health and development and family functioning.

◆ Individual education plans for school children with developmental disability must include instruction on health, self-care, family life and sex, and self-protection.

◆ Persons with developmental disability are at risk of behavior problems and mental illness. Nurses promote client mental health by supporting self-determination, optimal living conditions, and satisfactory social relations.

◆ Parents with mental retardation and other developmental disabilities can be good parents. Some may require extensive family supports to be successful. Nurses are key persons to identify the need and organize supports.

◆ Older persons with developmental disabilities are at risk of specific health problems related to their diagnoses as well as health problems related to aging. Specialized health and community support services will be needed in their communities.

◆ Current benign attitudes toward persons with mental retardation and other developmental disorders can return to more negative ones in response to political or economic pressures. Supports may be curtailed or withdrawn. Nurses and other citizens advocate for the rights of all people with developmental disorders.

RESOURCES

ATTENTION-DEFICIT HYPERACTIVITY DISORDER

CHADD (Children and Adults with Attention Deficit Disorder): www.chadd.org
National Attention Deficit Disorder Association: www.add.org

BIRTH DEFECTS

March of Dimes Birth Defects Foundation: www.modimes.org
National Easter Seal Society: www.seals.org

Cerebral Palsy
United Cerebral Palsy Association: www.ucpa.org
American Cerebral Palsy Information Center: www.cerebralpalsy.org
Cerebral Palsy Information Center: www.geocities.com/HotSprings/Sauna/4441/CPIC

DEVELOPMENTAL DISORDERS

Administration of Developmental Disabilities: www.act.dhhs.gov/programs/add/pmsoz
Center for Disease Control, Birth Defects and Pediatric Genetics: www.cdc.gov/ncbddd/bd
CDC, Developmental Disabilities Branch: www.cdc.gov/ncbddd/dd
Institute on Disability and Human Development: www.uic.edu/depts/idhd/toc
Individuals with Disabilities Act: www.ideapractices.org
International Classification of Impairments, Disabilities and Handicaps: www.who.int/icidh
National Information Center for Children and Youth with Disabilities: www.nichcy.org
National Institute of Disability and Rehabilitation Research: www.ed.gov/offices/OSERS/NIDRR
National Institute for Neurological Disorders and Strokes: www.ninds.nih.gov
Internet Resources Concerning People with Developmental Disabilities: http://soeweb.syr.edu/thechp/internet.html
Council for Exceptional Children: www.cec.sped.org
National Parent Information Network: www.npin.org

DOWN SYNDROME

National Down Syndrome Society: www.ndss.org

EPILEPSY

Epilepsy Foundation of America: www.efa.org
Epilepsy and Brain Mapping Program: www.epipro.com

HEAD/SPINAL CORD INJURY

National Spinal Cord Injury Association: www.spinalcord.org
Spina Bifida Association of America: www.sbaa.org

HEALTHY PEOPLE 2010

http://health.gov/healthypeople

LEARNING DISABILITIES/DYSLEXIA

Learning Disabilities Association: www.ldanatl.org
National Center for Learning Disabilities: www.ncld.org
Orton Dyslexia Society: www.selu.edu/Academics/ Education/TEC/orton
Recording for the Blind/Dyslexic: www.rfbd.org
International Dyslexia Association: www.interdys.org

MENTAL RETARDATION

Association of Retarded Citizens: www.thearc.org
American Association on Mental Retardation: www.aamr.org

PERVASIVE DEVELOPMENTAL DELAY/AUTISM/HYPERLEXIA

Autism Society of America: www.autism-society.org
Autism Research Institute: www.autism.org
American Hyperlexia Association: www.hyperlexia.org

TOURETTE'S SYNDROME

Tourette's Syndrome Association: http://tsa-usa.org

VISUAL IMPAIRMENT

American Council for the Blind: www.acb.org

Chapter

29

MENTAL HEALTH AND ILLNESS

David Becker, MS, RN, CS

MAKING THE CONNECTION

We cannot live only for ourselves. A thousand fibers connect us with our fellow men. And among those fibers, as sympathetic threads, our actions run as causes, and they come back to us as effects.

—*Herman Melville (1819–1891)*

COMPETENCIES

Upon completion of this chapter, the reader should be able to:

- Identify selected historical, political, and economic foundations of the concept of community mental health.
- Discuss the relationships among the various nursing, behavioral, and biological concepts and theories that guide the nurse in community mental health work.
- Identify the range of settings in which the community health nurse works with mental health clients.
- Discuss the nursing health promotion/illness prevention activities that address the continuum of mental illness in the community.
- Describe the importance of interdisciplinary teamwork in mental health nursing in the community.
- Discuss the adaptations required by clients with major mental illness in order to function in the community.

KEY TERMS

deinstitutionalization	operant conditioning
ego	psychoanalysis
id	psychotherapy
mental hygiene movement	stigma
neurotransmitter	superego

It is not supposed to work this way: The most severely ill among us not only have multiple illnesses but also are less likely to receive any treatment. The National Comorbidity Survey (Kessler et al., 1994) discovered a much greater prevalence of mental illness in the general population than had been thought. Nearly 50% of those surveyed had or once had a diagnosable mental health disorder. Fourteen percent of the population had a history of three or more disorders over a lifetime. The majority of people with severe mental health disorders had more than one diagnosis. Most significantly, less than 40% of those who had ever had a diagnosable disorder had received any treatment. Community health nurses are uniquely positioned to reach out to those who are suffering from mental illness, uncovering and removing the barriers to mental health. Skilled and accessible, nurses are often more acceptable to clients who fear or

---

REFLECTIVE THINKING

Judging vs. Assessing

- What are my beliefs and values relating to mental health and mental illness?
- How do I know when I am being judgmental, and how do I avoid judging my clients' choices and behavior?
- How can I periodically evaluate my assumptions about a client's situation against his or her own experience of the world?
- How do I work with people who are different?
- How can I make professional assessments, as opposed to personal judgments?

---

have given up on professionals specializing in mental health.

This chapter will discuss the foundations for caring, including nursing theories, for clients who are mentally ill. The community nurse's role is discussed, including basic screening and assessment, support interventions, and advanced psychiatric mental health nursing.

The poem in the accompanying perspectives box was written by one of the clients of a large state mental hospital as he contemplated what it might be like to enter what was to him an unfamiliar and unwelcoming place that we call "the community." Listening to our clients' voices is essential in developing, implementing, and evaluating community practice and programs. Keep listening for them, in the following pages, in other media, and in your practice.

FOUNDATIONS OF CARING

The practice of the community health nurse working with clients who are mentally ill must be guided by an understanding of history, politics, economics, and biology. Nursing theories as well as principles developed by the allied health disciplines of psychiatry, psychology, and social work also apply to mental health work.

While some progress was noted in levels at which people sought help for severe and persistent mental disorders, there was a decline in the proportion of pediatric and family nurse practitioners who typically inquire about parent-child relationships or in the proportion of nurse practitioners who asked adult clients about cognitive, emotional, or behavioral functioning. This was offset by an increase in treatment and referrals. The best outcome was in terms of suicide prevention. The suicide rate declined for targeted populations, and by 1997 the age-adjusted suicide rate in the total population had met its target for the decade. These and other goals have now been adjusted toward further improvements.

In a landmark report to the nation, the Surgeon General of the United States gathered the conclusions of recent research into the causes of, impact of, and best response to mental health issues. The key points of the report are listed in Figure 29-1. Community health nurses should keep these ideas in mind as they approach mental health needs and should be prepared to help clients, family members, and the general public to learn them as well.

Community health nurses can make great contributions toward achieving the mental health objectives in a variety of ways, including, for example, reducing the incidence of depression in women (statistics show that women suffer from depression at twice the rate of men) and reducing the adolescent suicide attempt rates, which by 1995 had increased 200% from 1990 (U.S. Department of Health and Human Services [USDHHS], 1996). Nurses work in a variety of community settings, putting them in a position to identify problems and intervene, often before others in the family or the health care system are likely to recognize that there is a problem.

Historical Foundations

Attitudes toward the care and treatment of mentally ill persons have nearly always differed from those with recognized physical disease. For many people, a "sick mind" has different connotations than a sick body, and the difference has existed for centuries. Behavioral symptoms of what we now understand to be psychoneurobiological conditions were seen as evidence of demonic possession or at least grave sin. The struggles that early psychiatrists had with laypeople and the clergy for the right to treat the mentally ill led to further isolation of both the treater and the treated (Porter, 1989).

Community health nurses serving psychiatric and mental health clients are part of a historical alteration in the way humanity deals with mental health and mental illness. The current shift of mental health care to community agencies has been called the "third psychiatry revolution" (Kaplan, Sadock, & Grebb, 1998).

Moral Treatment and Psychoanalysis: The First and Second Revolutions

The first revolution occurred in the mid to late 18th century, as Western culture shifted its thinking about those who behaved in a difficult, dangerous, or worrisome way. After persecuting some and either hiding or ignoring others, society finally established asylums where rational, moral treatment was employed to restore reason.

FIGURE 29-1 What Everyone Needs to Know

In 1999 the Surgeon General of the United States issued the first Surgeon General's Report on Mental Health. It contained the following key messages for the nation:

- Mental health is fundamental to health.
- Mental disorders are real health conditions.
- The efficacy of mental health treatments is well documented.
- A range of treatments exists for most mental disorders; thus the explicit recommendation of the report to the nations is to seek help if you have a mental health problem or think you have symptoms of a mental disorder.

The following overarching themes run throughout the Surgeon General's report:

- A public health perspective, attending to the health of a population in its entirety, must identify risk factors, mount preventive interventions, and actively promote good mental health.
- Mental disorders are disabling.
- Mental health and mental illness are points on a continuum.
- Mind and body are inseparable.

From *Mental Health: A Report of the Surgeon General,* by D. Satcher, 1999, Washington, DC: Public Health Service, U.S. Department of Health and Human Services.

Perspectives...

INSIGHTS OF AN AGNEWS STATE RESIDENT

They're closing Agnews State
Where we hid empty wine bottles
In laundry baskets.
They're closing Agnews State
Where old men passed out flowers
In the canteen.
They're closing Agnews State
Where volunteers from the Red Cross
Cared enough to dance with you.
They're closing Agnews State
Where the gophers pop their heads out of lawns
And say "hi" to you.
They're closing Agnews State
Where Billy Hamilton broke a window
After every shock treatment.
They're closing Agnews State
And opening up lonely hearts' clubs.

—Yoga Bare (1974)
"Requiem for Agnews State"

As historian Porter (1989) put it: "The madhouse should thus become a reform school" (p. 19). Late-19th century advances in science brought the second revolution, when the increasing power and prestige of medicine were applied to the issue. In the first half of this century, Freud and others shifted mainstream thinking about the cause of madness away from moral laxness to illnesses caused by unresolved infantile conflicts due to faulty parenting. Through all this, society tended to blame those suffering for causing the condition.

Sigmund Freud (1938) developed the concepts that explained mental illness as being caused by faulty mental mechanisms. **Psychoanalysis** offered hope in the form of a "talking cure." As a treatment technique, psychoanalysis uses free association and the interpretation of dreams to trace emotions and behaviors to repressed drives and instincts. By making the client aware of the existence, origins, and inappropriate expression of these unconscious processes, psychoanalysis helps the client eliminate or diminish undesirable affects.

By the end of World War II, the asylums begun in the 18th century had evolved to very large state hospitals. In these institutions, psychoanalysis met with limited success in the vast majority of patients with serious mental illness. Thus, the third revolution, which had begun with a prewar **mental hygiene movement,** a movement emphasizing education and public awareness techniques to promote prevention and effective treatment, gained momentum in conjunction with the great advances in the use of psychotropic drugs.

Community Mental Health Movement: The Third Revolution

This third revolution, the community mental health movement, is concerned with the prevention and treatment of mental illness and with the rehabilitation of former psychiatric clients through the use of organized community programs, including community health nursing. Some of these programs are specialized community psychiatric/mental health services, staffed by advanced practice mental health nurses. Other programs are more general, such as senior centers or home nursing agencies. The focus of this chapter is on community health nurses working with psychiatric/mental health clients in the latter type of agency. Community health nurses serve in what could be described as the area of overlap between community health nursing and community mental health. See Figure 29-2.

The historical shifts in attitudes and approaches to mental health and mental illness illustrate that physical punishment, isolation, work farms, and long-term corrective relationships with a therapist have each, in turn, been accepted as correct responses to the phenomenon of mental illness. Considering the historical perspective helps nurses understand why many clients and families of mental health clients feel shame, mistrust, or anger dealing with members of the health professions, especially those in mental health. The disgrace or reproach experienced by mentally ill persons and their families is referred to as **stigma.** Community health nurses may encounter this in the form of hostility in dealing with clients, their families, and members of the community.

REFLECTIVE THINKING

Personal Experience with Mental Illness

While in nursing school you become good friends with another student. One day she tells you she was institutionalized for "being crazy." She tells you it was a terrible experience. She was locked up and put on medications. She says she has never shared this experience with anyone.

- How do you feel, and what do you think about hearing words like *crazy*?
- How does knowing her history affect your feelings toward her and toward her becoming a nurse?
- Do you worry about her decompensating again?
- Do you ever worry about becoming mentally ill yourself?
- Is anyone in your family mentally ill?
- What hunches do you have about the reasons she may have for telling you?
- What do you say to her?

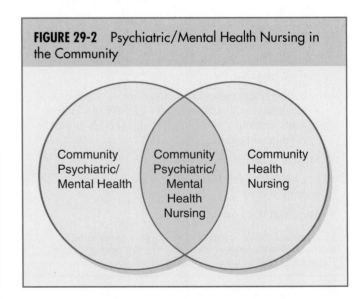

FIGURE 29-2 Psychiatric/Mental Health Nursing in the Community

For this reason it is useful to emphasize the community health nurse's identification with health promotion activities such as prenatal and well-child clinics, which are less threatening to clients and do not carry the stigma of the mental health system.

Even though science has provided a better understanding of the psychoneurobiological processes that are now thought to cause mental illness, historical attitudes based on faulty understanding continue to influence health professionals as well as the general population. The nurse, through a self-examination of prejudices and attitudes, can begin to prepare to correct the misunderstandings of clients, their families, the community, and other health care workers. From a historical perspective, a community in which families are not blamed, treatment is not feared, and clients and those who serve them are not stigmatized is long overdue.

Theories and Concepts from Allied Disciplines

Nursing practice in community mental health involves much greater interdisciplinary teamwork than in typical nursing settings. A fundamental understanding of psychiatry, psychology, social work, and rehabilitation therapies is necessary to achieve an effective interdisciplinary practice. Conversely, the nurse must be prepared to present a theoretically based nursing view to colleagues from other disciplines. Creating or maintaining such a team is a continuing challenge in today's rapidly changing health care environment. The following overview of the theories that contribute to community health nursing is offered as a brief reminder. For a more comprehensive review of these theories, the student should consult a psychiatric nursing text or the theorist's original works.

Psychodynamic Theories

Sigmund Freud (1938) postulated the existence of a set of mental structures: the **superego,** or conscience; the unconscious **id;** and the **ego,** which mediates between the id and the superego. Examining these can lead to uncovering unconscious conflict among them. Such conflicts, Freud claimed, are the source of mental illness. Through psychoanalysis, the client can gain insight, that is, can bring these unconscious conflicts into conscious awareness and thus be cured. Although the theories of traditional psychoanalytic treatment offer little for nurses, the vocabulary developed to explain Freud's theories is still widely used to describe clients' defense mechanisms, personality development, and relationships with others.

Social-Interpersonal Theories

Evolving from psychoanalytic theory, social-interpersonal theories emphasize the developmental influences of family and society. Mental health problems are seen to be, at their core, interpersonal problems. Improvement in interpersonal functioning is the means toward meeting psychosocial needs and decreasing mental health problems. Self-actualization is the ultimate fulfillment of a hierarchy of needs (Maslow, 1962). These ideas guide many nursing concepts and interventions. Sullivan (1953) is best known for his creative psychotherapy working with severely disturbed patients. Unlike Freud, Sullivan thought that even the most psychotic patients suffering from schizophrenia could be reached through the human relationship of **psychotherapy,** the process of addressing symptom relief, resolution of problems or personal growth through interacting in a prescribed way with a therapist. Peplau used Sullivan's concepts to develop a theory conceptualizing nursing as an interpersonal relationship (Meleis, 1997). Social theory provides nurses with a framework for personal interventions with clients and families and for community and political action.

Behavioral Theories

Many of the theories previously mentioned were of little interest to B. F. Skinner (1953) and the behaviorists who followed. In their view, observable behavior is the only certain foundation for assessing a client's state. Behavioral change is the only appropriate goal. **Operant conditioning** is the concept of seeking to discover what elicits a particular behavior in the first place and what subsequently reinforces it. These reinforcements can be manipulated to shape behavior and thereby to improve the client's functioning. Nurses use behavior theory to understand and manage behavioral symptoms and to teach appropriate life skills.

Neurobiological Concepts

Over time, practitioners using a medical model have used all of the foregoing theories, sometimes in combination, often with a preference for one or the other. As it is evolving, however, the medical model increasingly addresses emotional and behavioral problems as illnesses like any other. Assessment of clients is based on their symptoms. The problem addressed is an illness caused by a pathological process: lesion, toxin, or abnormality of neuroanatomy or **neurotransmitter.** The neurotransmitters are nervous system chemicals that facilitate the transmission of impulses across the synapses between neurons and are the subject of a great deal of current research. In this model, symptoms of disease are to be measured, then managed, while a cure is sought.

Nurses use these neurobiological concepts to care for clients taking powerful psychotropic drugs (and occasionally other somatic treatments) now widely used to treat mental illness. New classes of drugs such as selective serotonin reuptake inhibitors (SSRIs) and atypical antipsychotic drugs have increased the effectiveness of possible treatments available. New applications for old drugs such as using anticonvulsants as mood stabilizers have broadened the range of treatments. The very rapid changes in psychopharmacology practice means that nurses must ensure that they have access to the latest findings in the biological factors of mental disorders.

Nursing Theories

Nursing theories and conceptual models are often given limited attention in community mental health nursing. Nursing theorists who emphasize caring and principles of communication and relationship in their models have particular relevance to mental health nursing. These theorists (Watson, Leininger, Neuman, Peplau, Orlando, & Benner) stress that care provided through the nurse-client relationship is a core component and the basis of excellence in nursing practice. Both objective and subjective (feelings and intuitions) observations by the nurse are of value (Meleis, 1997). The nurse is both an observer and a participant in the therapeutic relationship. The nurse relates to the client as a complete human being while directing nursing interventions on the symptomatic level.

There are useful principles in most nursing theories. For the community health nurse working with mentally ill clients, the theories of Peplau and Orem may be most practical. The nurse-patient relationship is central

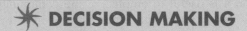

✳ DECISION MAKING

Family Disruption

You have been working with a family in which the mother has not left the house in six months and the 26-year-old single daughter is three months pregnant. The daughter wants the mother to be with her when she has her baby. The mother would like to accompany her daughter but is afraid to leave the house, let alone go to the hospital with her daughter.

◆ Given your knowledge of treatment of phobic disorders, what steps would you take to set mutual goals in this family?

◆ Do you think it is possible to meet the daughter's request? Why? Why not?

to Peplau's (1952) nursing theory. She shifted the focus of interest from what the nurse does *for* the client to what the nurse can do *with* the client, such as mutually set goals and other interactions. She identified the stages of the nurse-client relationship as orientation, introduction, working, and termination. Orem, Taylor, and Renpenning's (2001) concepts of self-care can be easily adopted by the community health nurse, especially in addressing the needs of the chronically mentally ill.

CURRENT INFLUENCES ON COMMUNITY MENTAL HEALTH

Political, economic, and cultural events have greatly influenced the way society attempts to assist its members with mental illness. The following factors have had great impact on increasing the mental health aspects of the community health nurse's work.

Prevalence

Social, economic, and medical advances such as improvements in nutrition and the control of infectious disease have changed the profile of disability in developed nations. In a landmark study of the global burden of disease, Murray (1996) measured years of life lost to premature death and years lived with a disability of specified severity and duration. They calculated this using a unit of measure called the disability-adjusted life year (DALY). They found that in established market economies such as the United States the burden of mental illness (including

FIGURE 29-3 Change in the Rank Order of Disease Burden for 15 Leading Causes, 1990–2020

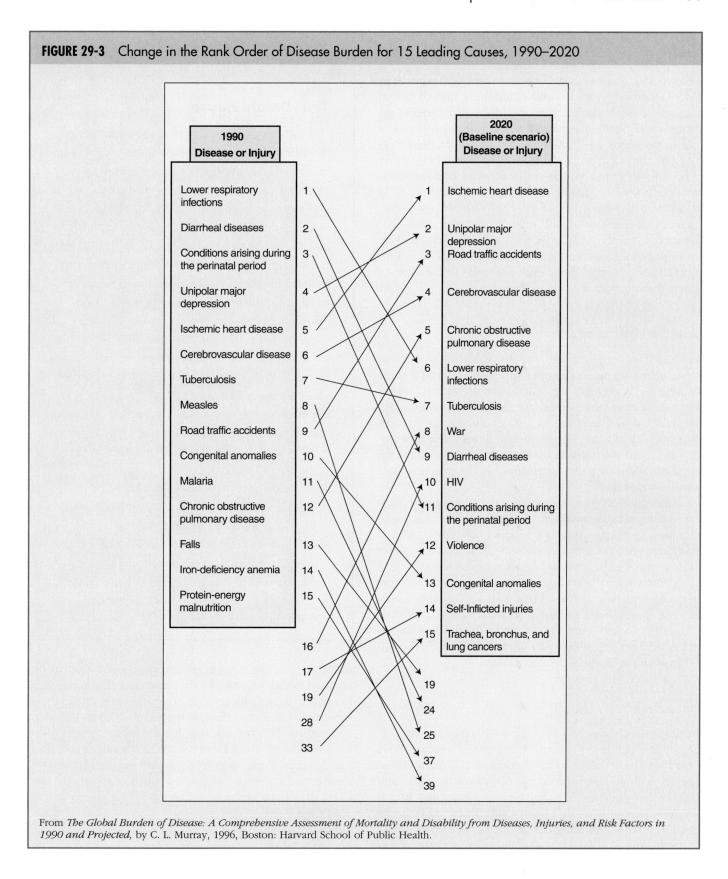

From *The Global Burden of Disease: A Comprehensive Assessment of Mortality and Disability from Diseases, Injuries, and Risk Factors in 1990 and Projected,* by C. L. Murray, 1996, Boston: Harvard School of Public Health.

suicide) accounted for 15.4% of total DALYs. That is more than cancer or any other category except cardiovascular conditions. Alcohol and other drug abuse together accounted for 6.2%, making it the fourth in rank among causes of disease burden. They predict that, by 2020, unipolar major depression will be the second leading cause of disability burden, measured in DALYs, in both developed and developing regions (see Figure 29-3).

Community Mental Health Reform

In response to the problems of what were seen to be expensive and dehumanizing large state mental hospitals, in 1963 Congress began to fund community mental health centers. These agencies were established to provide inpatient and outpatient services to specific geographic areas and populations of 75,000–200,000 as an alternative to long-term inpatient hospitalization. Twenty-four-hour emergency services and partial hospitalization options (day, evening, aftercare, halfway houses) were offered. This legislation helped to transform the way society treats mentally ill persons. Unfortunately, political and economic constraints, such as the expense of public funding for free-standing mental health centers, have always limited full realization of the intended benefits of community mental health reform.

Deinstitutionalization

In the 1960s, legal reforms making it harder to commit someone to hospitalization involuntarily, political actions limiting the budgets of the state hospitals, and the promise (which many say went unfulfilled) of the community mental health centers led to a great shift in the lives of patients with chronic, severe mental illness. The new initiative, called **deinstitutionalization,** was to discharge large numbers of patients from public mental hospitals into communities.

Deinstitutionalization requires that a range of supportive services be available and utilized. In most communities, adequate services to meet the needs of the clients are not present. As a result, these former clients often regress, exhibiting increased symptoms and related problems such as homelessness and petty crime. Unfortunately, jails have replaced hospitals for many mentally ill. The Department of Justice (Ditton, 1999) estimates that in 1998 there were 283,800 mentally ill offenders incarcerated in the nation's prisons and jails, while the latest psychiatric hospital census showed 61,772.

Economic Factors

Insurance and other third-party payors provide less coverage for treatment of mental illness and substance abuse than they do for other medical conditions. Private insurers often limit coverage to 30–60 inpatient days, and Medicare requires a 50% copayment for mental health services. Recognizing that mentally ill people are stigmatized and have limited access to the services they need, many have called for equitable coverage and the elimination of special restrictions and controls on psychiatric care. Barreira and Cohen (2000) note that while spending on general medical care has stayed relatively constant during the last decade, spending on psychiatric care was

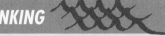

REFLECTIVE THINKING

Your Dream House

You just bought your dream house. It has all the features you want, including a quiet neighborhood, good schools, and friendly neighbors. You've settled in to raise your family and just now learn that the city is holding hearings on a plan to establish a transitional residence (halfway house) one block from your home. The facility will be in a large single-family house and will serve six psychiatric patients who need preparation for fully independent living. You understand how important and effective these programs are and that the same things that attracted you to the neighborhood make it a great choice for the program. You are concerned about its impact on your family. Your neighbors expect you to go to the hearings and demonstrate against the plan.

- How do you feel about having a halfway house in the next block?
- What do you think about the idea of speaking out, pro or con, about the halfway house at a public hearing?
- What do you think about the idea of participating at a demonstration, either supporting or opposing, the halfway house?
- How does the pressure from neighbors influence your decision?

reduced 30%. By subcontracting psychiatric care to behavioral health managed-care organizations, commercial insurance organizations and government agencies have moved financial and clinical responsibilities to for-profit companies. The bottom line for decisions moved away from the client, away from the client's family, away from the clinician, even away from client's insurers or government payer, to a separate profit-making company that the client may have never heard of.

Consumer Activism

The foremost example of effective consumer involvement in mental health is the National Alliance for the Mentally Ill (NAMI). NAMI was formed in 1979 by people who wanted to learn how to help themselves and their mentally ill relatives. For decades, parents had been blamed for their children's mental disorders. Through the supportive networks formed by NAMI, families find the courage and hope to advocate for needed changes in public policy and attitudes. By working together, this group and those like it support one another, provide information to other consumers regarding services available, advise professionals and politicians regarding needed services, and advocate for effective humane services (NAMI, 2000).

Cultural Factors

Culture is an observable manifestation of inner life as displayed by manners, customs, skills, language, parent-child interactions, beliefs, and social life. Because mental health and illness are often demonstrated in terms of behavior, an understanding of cultural factors is often necessary to make sense of a client's behavior and to plan interventions that are appropriate for a particular client.

Too often, nurses with a background in the dominant culture are unaware of their own cultural heritage and especially of its unexamined customs, beliefs, manners, and so on. Keeping mindful of their own cultural heritage allows nurses to better assist clients from another culture.

Research in anthropology, ethnopsychiatry, and transcultural nursing informs nursing practice in several ways. Nurses can find data on culture-specific concepts of space, time orientation, language, and health beliefs and practices to guide their work with specific groups. (See Chapter 8.)

Symptoms of the major mental disorders exist among all cultures (Kaplan et al., 1998). Although the presenting symptoms generally conform to the diagnostic categories of the *Diagnostic and Statistical Manual of Mental Disorders,* commonly called the DSM (American Psychiatric Association [APA], 2000), clients and their families may use indigenous labels to describe their experience of a mental illness. Many of these labels have been cataloged in a Glossary of Culture-Bound Syndromes in the fourth edition of the DSM.

International Trends

Although culture, politics, economics, geography, and health systems all influence variations in the manifestation of mental illness, certain symptoms exist in all societies. These include:

- Anxiety—a response to perceived threats to self-esteem, identity, or physical well being
- Mania—a disturbance of affect manifest by abnormal and persistent elevation of mild, expansiveness, and/or irritability

- Depression—a common mood or affective disorder that can affect all aspects of perception and functioning
- Suicidal ideation—thoughts of killing oneself
- Somatization—expression of psychological stress through physical symptoms
- Persecutory delusions—a false belief that one is being singled out for harm by others
- Thought disorders

Although labels and prescriptions vary, recognizing a problem and making an attempt at treatment are universal. Societies that do not stigmatize persons with mental illness have much better treatment outcomes than societies that do, because such persons are quickly reintegrated into society (Kaplan et al., 1998).

Many of the more developed nations of the world have been moving mental health activities from institution-based to community-based care for reasons similar to those of the United States. In a large, multinational European study, Dowrick, et al (2000) considered the effectiveness and acceptability of two simple interventions for care of community residents with depression but without psychosis or substance abuse. He found that simple, problem-oriented care, provided primarily through home visits, was as effective as group psychotherapy and was more acceptable to clients. Clients were more likely to complete treatment at home than in groups and had slightly better outcomes 12 months after treatment. Both groups did better than clients who received no treatment.

Some developing countries have been focusing on fostering mental health activities as an integral part of community-based care out of necessity as well as tradition. Not only is community-based care attractive economically, but also it is more acceptable to many who have not become accustomed to the institutional approach to care more common in industrialized countries. Immigration is an increasingly important cultural influence in the United States. The U.S. Bureau of the Census (Brittingham, 2000) reported that, in 1999, 26.4 million foreign-born people resided in the United States. This represents 9.7% of the total U.S. population. Immigrants and refugees have often experienced extreme stress. The circumstances surrounding immigration, the resources available to immigrants, and their reception in the new country influence health and well-being. Guarnaccia and Lopez (1998) studied the mental health and adjustment of immigrant and refugee children. In spite of the stresses associated with immigration, they did not find evidence for increased levels of mental illness among this group. However, they did find that discrimination, especially for immigrants in racial minority groups, was associated with poor mental health. Walker and Jaranson (1999) note the increased frequency of post-traumatic stress disorder (PTSD) and depression among those who migrate because of war and ethnic strife.

STIGMA

Stigma is a powerful, pervasive force that prevents people from acknowledging their own mental health problems or accepting care and treatment. To reduce the burden of mental illness and to provide the resources needed to more fully understand the causes, prevention, and treatment of these disorders, stigma must no longer be tolerated. Community health nurses are potentially influential agents of change in this regard. Nurses should model appropriately respectful, hopeful, and compassionate regard for members of society burdened with mental illnesses. They should also confront discrimination and disrespect. People are not diseases. Just as no one should be referred to as a "paraplegic," no one should be called a "maniac" or a "schizophrenic."

SETTINGS FOR COMMUNITY MENTAL HEALTH NURSING PRACTICE

Full participation in community mental health interdisciplinary teams can mean weaving a fabric of relationships within a nursing system, an interdisciplinary team, and, perhaps most important, a community. To that end, nurses attempt to locate themselves so as to facilitate the client's access to services and to maximize the benefit of nursing resources. Community health nurses are key because access is often enhanced when nurses operate within the client's daily social environment: home, school, or job site.

Prevention efforts located nearest to the client can best support and preserve critical family and social resource networks. Thus, nursing can be practiced in battered women's shelters, food programs for the homeless, senior centers and residences, jails, health maintenance organizations and primary care clinics, occupational health and employee assistance programs, immigrant and cultural centers, and on home visits. Some clinical nurse specialists in psychiatric or mental health nursing work in community settings. Most often, however, it is community health nurses who are found in these sites, providing comprehensive nursing care that includes elements of psychiatric and mental health nursing.

One effective model of practice has been for many nurses to work together, often with other health disciplines, at agencies organized for treatment and support of the clients. These service agencies most often work with individuals who have severe and chronic mental health disorders. Outpatient clinics in mental health centers, rehabilitation centers, and therapeutic foster care all employ nurses as part of interdisciplinary teams.

Out
of the Box

Out of Darkness

The shortcomings of large institutions in providing care to people with severe and persistent mental illnesses have been recognized for a long time. But establishing community alternatives has not been as easy. Societal, governmental, and professional resistance has largely kept the ideal from coming to fruition. Susie Kim, RN, DNSc, FAAN, has created a notable exception in her model for nurse-managed community psychosocial rehabilitation programs.

Dr. Kim established an effective mental health nursing program that has grown to 15 sites in the Republic of Korea. Operating from nursing centers or a church, the model utilizes volunteer professionals, cultural traditions, and a form of psychosocial rehabilitation. The World Health Organization is studying the feasibility of replicating this low-cost arrangement in other countries.

The goals of the program are to rehabilitate long-term psychiatric clients to decrease hospitalizations and to maximize the individual's psychosocial function. Teaching the client to rehabilitate himself and to restructure a client's environment is central to their efforts. Three types of interventions are employed. First, home visits deliver care and treatment but also teach families to support clients who are developing coping and stress reduction skills. Second, day care in the nursing centers offers a milieu for practicing social skills. Third, during weekend seminars, clients' families learn specific rehabilitation skills.

While the program's dependence on family support and care reflects Korean culture practice, the model may be generally applicable to both developed and developing nations. In the face of social stigma and severe economic constraints, these nurses demonstrate the profession's role in caring and advocating for persons with severe, persistent mental illnesses. ∎

Source: Kim, S. (1998). Out of darkness. Reflections, 24, 8–12.

In many communities, a network of supervised living accommodations provides a range of services geared toward assisting persons in the transition from inpatient hospitalization toward full independence. Nurses play key roles in partial hospitalization programs and can be an important adjunct to such a network. Some communities provide day hospitals, sometimes called adult day treatment programs, where patients attend during business hours and return to family homes, group homes, or independent living arrangements for some meals and to sleep. Night care serves clients who can function in supervised work settings during the day but require more structure than can be provided by other living arrangements. When psychiatric/mental health nurses are not employed within these settings, community health nurses are called on to provide care and consultation regarding clients' nursing and health care needs. See Chapters 19 and 20 for further discussion of the roles and specialties for community health nursing practice. Although more mental health issues are associated with at-risk populations in community setting than ever before, mental health and illness are major aspects of nursing in all settings and roles.

HEALTH PROMOTION/ILLNESS PREVENTION IN COMMUNITY HEALTH NURSING PRACTICE

The goal of prevention is to decrease the onset (incidence), duration (prevalence), and residual disability of mental disorders in the community. Community health nurses can actively work toward prevention of mental disorders through primary, secondary, and tertiary prevention activities.

The range of mental health and illness phenomena of concern to nurses is illustrated in Figure 29-4. Two diagnostic classification systems, the Omaha system (Martin & Scheet, 1992) and the North American Nursing Diagnosis Association (NANDA, 2001) system, are commonly used by community health nurses to name actual or potential client mental health problems. Advanced-practice nurses certified in psychiatric nursing use the *Diagnostic and Statistical Manual of Mental Disorders,* fourth edition text revision (DSM-IV) (APA, 2000) to diagnose mental health problems.

Primary Prevention

The goal of primary prevention is to prevent the onset of mental health disorders. Nursing primary-prevention activities target groups at risk through mental health education programs. Examples include:

- Teaching parenting skills and child development to teen parents
- Teaching the psychobiological effects of alcohol and drugs to young people in schools

- Developing social support systems to reduce the effects of psychosocial stress on persons at high risk: e.g., safer sex groups for HIV-negative gay men
- Anticipatory guidance programs to assist people in preparing for expected stressful situations: e.g., training young people to run peer counseling programs at high schools to address issues such as family abuse, street violence, date rape, peer pressure, and conflict mediation
- Crisis intervention after stressful life events, such as group disasters or the death of a child due to gang violence

Primary-prevention programs also aim to eradicate stressful agents and to reduce stress. Examples of specific strategies nurses employ to help decrease the risk of mental

---

FIGURE 29-4 Mental Health and Illness: Phenomena of Concern to Nurses

Actual or potential mental health problems of clients pertaining to:

- The maintenance of optimal health and well-being and the prevention of psychobiological illness
- Self-care limitations or impaired functioning related to mental and emotional distress
- Deficits in the functioning of significant biological, emotional, and cognitive systems
- Emotional stress or crisis components of illness, pain, and disability
- Self-concept changes, developmental issues, and life process changes
- Problems related to emotions such as anxiety, anger, sadness, loneliness, and grief
- Physical symptoms that occur along with altered psychological functioning
- Alterations in thinking, perceiving, symbolizing, communicating, and decision making
- Difficulties in relating to others
- Behaviors and mental states that indicate the client is a danger to self or others or has a severe disability
- Interpersonal, systemic, sociocultural, spiritual, or environmental circumstances or events that affect the mental and emotional well-being of the individual, family, or community
- Symptom management, side effects/toxicities associated with psychopharmacologic interventions and other aspects of the treatment regimen

From *Scope and Standards of Psychiatric-Mental Health Nursing Practice.* Reprinted with permission from American Nurses Association, American Psychiatric Nurses Association, and International Society of Psychiatric-Mental Health Nurses. Copyright 2000 by American Nurses Publishing, American Nurses Foundation/American Nurses Association.

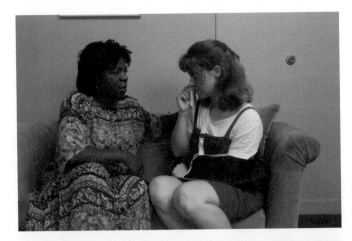

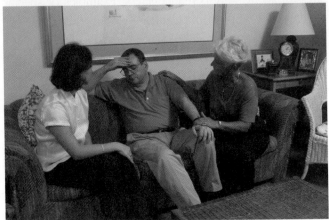

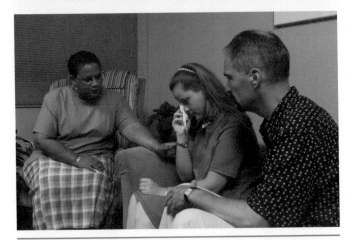

Community health nurses can be found in different settings assisting those who are in need of psychiatric help.

retardation and other cognitive disorders in children include assisting families to reduce lead exposure in their housing and counseling prenatal clients to abstain from drug and alcohol use and to improve their nutrition via education.

Disaster

Mental illness is sometimes conceived of as a severe disruption that exceeds the coping ability of an *individual*. The World Health Organization (WHO, 1992) definition of disaster is "a severe disruption, ecological and psychosocial, which greatly exceeds the coping ability of the affected *community*" (italics added). When we think of disasters, we commonly think of hurricanes, floods, the widely publicized terrorist bombing, and the World Trade Center disaster. On a slightly smaller scale, events such as the kidnapping of a child or the suicide of a popular teen can also have a serious emotional impact on a community. The disaster plan for any community should include preparing for responses to the emotional reactions to disaster. An effective response cannot only prevent many long-term effects such as PTSD or major depression; it can also contribute to short-term general recovery by maintaining the abilities of a community's members to attend to themselves, their families, and their neighbors. Care for the caregivers is a priority.

A community health nurse who needs to make a referral to or consult with mental health professionals in a disaster can reach them through the Red Cross or other lead relief organization. According to the Suggested Mental Health Response Plan (APA, 1993), participating mental health professionals can be expected to make themselves available to speak with groups of community workers, to visit community centers to provide direct services and backup services, and to take referrals.

Planning for and responding to disasters is not the only way in which the impact of disasters can be mitigated. Prevention of disasters can also be addressed by support for public health and safety programs such as industrial safety, fire safety, and violence prevention.

Secondary Prevention

Secondary prevention is the early identification and prompt treatment of an illness or a disorder. The goals are to reduce the number of cases in the population at risk and to shorten the illness's duration. Secondary-prevention nursing targets individuals and groups in whom a high risk for illness or illness symptoms has been assessed. Nursing activities include the provision of or referral for treatment and other services, including:

- Ongoing assessment of infants prenatally exposed to drugs and alcohol: e.g., during visits to clients' homes, residential drug treatment programs, family shelters, and foster care programs
- Provision of care to individuals through individual or group counseling, medication administration, crisis intervention: e.g., staffing suicide prevention hotlines or shelters for abused women
- Case management of emotionally ill children living with their families

Tertiary Prevention

The goal of tertiary prevention is to reduce the prevalence of residential defects and disabilities caused by severe or chronic mental illness. Nursing tertiary-prevention interventions focus on client rehabilitation and the prevention of complications. Nursing activities address the medical, psychiatric, and social needs of persistently mentally ill persons. Examples include:

- Teaching clients daily living skills to support their highest level of functional capacity and independence
- Case management of the persistently mentally ill: e.g., referral to and monitoring effectiveness of various community mental health programs, making referrals to support services such as assistance with household chores and other activities of daily living, encouraging social activities

SUICIDE

Suicide is a tragic and potentially preventable public health problem. According to the National Institute of Mental Health (1999), suicide was the ninth leading cause of death in the United States in 1996. Suicide accounts for approximately 31,000, or 1.3%, of all deaths, which is about the same number as deaths from AIDS/HIV (see Figure 29-5). In addition, suicide impacts families, schools, and communities in a devastating manner.

While it is difficult to determine definitively the rates of suicidal behavior for lesbian and gay individuals, studies have shown that there is a disproportionate number

who do attempt suicide (Saulnier, 1998). Most attempts occur before the age of 21. Stressful life events are precipitant causes in both heterosexual and homosexual suicides, but adolescents who are concerned about their sexual orientation have some unique stresses. They are often rejected in school and frequently believe that they have no one to which they can turn. Some turn to alcohol to fog their concerns about themselves. They tend to feel separated and emotionally isolated from others. In many parts of the United States, there are no social groups available to help them feel more accepted.

Suicide and related actions, sometimes called parasuicide behavior, is complex. Suicide itself, the intentional taking of one's own life, is sometimes preceded by other associated activities. Suicide attempts are sometimes interpreted as "just a call for help" but always demand careful evaluation and intervention. Other high-risk behaviors, such as unprotected sex with multiple partners or driving at high speed, often reflect unconscious and/or passive wishes to die. However, nurses should not presume that all self-destructive behavior is suicidal. Some clients injure themselves on purpose but without intention of killing themselves. They may be responding to delusions about body functions or to find relief from psychic pain. Intervention is needed in either case, but listening closely to the client is essential if the nurse is to understand the behavior and to respond appropriately. Risk factors for suicide, listed in Figure 29-6, are also complex. They vary with age, gender, and ethnic group, occur in combination, and probably change over time.

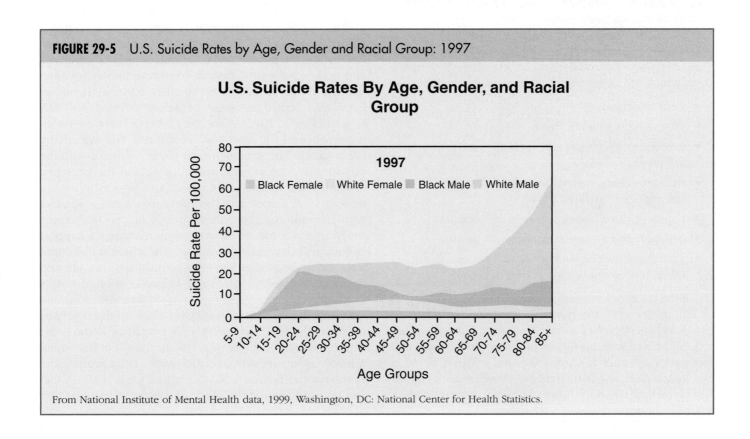

FIGURE 29-5 U.S. Suicide Rates by Age, Gender and Racial Group: 1997

From National Institute of Mental Health data, 1999, Washington, DC: National Center for Health Statistics.

FIGURE 29-6 Risk Factors for Suicide

- Depression
- Other diagnosable mental illness
- Substance abuse
- Alterations in neurotransmitters, especially decreased serotonin
- Prior suicide attempt
- Family history of mental or substance abuse
- Family violence, including physical or sexual abuse
- Firearms in the home
- Incarceration
- Exposure to suicidal behavior of others: family members, peers, news media, or fictional literature
- Adverse life events when present in combination with other risk factors

From *Suicide Facts,* by National Institute of Mental Health, 1999 [On-line]. Available: http://www.nimh.nih.gov/publicat/ suicidefacts.cfm.

Nursing Assessment and Intervention

It is difficult to separate assessment and intervention of the suicidal client. The nurse who assesses suicidal ideation begins intervention immediately to prevent any escalation of behavior. Assessment and intervention will be considered simultaneously.

When the nurse identifies that a client is depressed and manifesting other risk factors for suicide, an evaluation of suicide potential must be completed. Warning signs which are deserving of close attention include:

- Prior attempts
- Escalating substance abuse
- Comments about suicide, such as "I am going to kill myself"
- Behavior changes—particularly giving away belongings or making a will
- Expressions of hopelessness or helplessness
- Isolation and a preoccupation with death
- Situational events, such as death of a significant other, retirement (Frisch & Frisch, 2002)

If the client acknowledges suicidal ideation (thoughts of killing oneself), the nurse must determine if a plan exists and the degree of lethality involved. If the client has a detailed plan with no means of rescue, involving lethal methods, the means to carry it out, and a plan to do so in one to two days, she or he must be considered a high risk. Lethal methods include guns, hanging, knives, carbon

monoxide poisoning, drowning, and jumping from extreme heights.

Based on the known statistics of suicide, questions to ask when assessing for lethality include the following:

- Does the client have a detailed plan?
- Does the plan include a means of preventing discovery or rescue?
- Does the method of suicide involve a gun, a knife, hanging, carbon monoxide poisoning, drowning, or jumping from extreme height?
- Does the client have the means to carry out the plan (access to a gun or other weapon)?
- Does the client intend to carry out the plan within 24–48 hours?

Psychiatric referral should be sought for any high-risk client and the client needs to be carefully supervised until provisions can be made for ensuring safety. The nurse will save time if she or he is aware of the mental health laws pertaining to legal holds and hospitalization for clients who present as a danger to self.

If the client presents with low lethality, the nurse may utilize a suicide contract, make referrals as indicated, develop plans for increased support, and assess the need for medications. Lethality is assessed as low when the client thinks of suicide sporadically, has a vague plan with no time frame, considers methods such as wrist cutting, and has an available support system. Suicide contracts are most effective when the client has a relationship with the health care provider. A contract should be seen as an adjunct to a thorough assessment and a tool to provide an alternative to impulsive action. It is a written promise that the client will not harm himself before calling the provider. The contract should be reviewed and updated at established time intervals and at any time that the nurse observes, or the client feels, a change in emotional status or sense of safety (Firestone, 1997; Frisch & Frisch, 2002). A suicide prevention contract is an imperfect tool for assessing suicide risk and enhancing client safety. The strength of the client's alliance with the provider, the client's impulse control, and the presence of hallucinations and other risk factors affect the usefulness of such a contract. The client may need assistance with referrals for appropriate groups or psychotherapy. Referrals are a means of expanding the client's support system and decreasing isolation. The client will benefit from examining other ways to expand his or her life and develop alternatives to suicide. Depression often results in tunnel vision and feelings of worthlessness. Assisting the client in identifying friends, relatives, spiritual guides, or others the client has previously trusted or found to be supportive can be a first step toward the client becoming reinvolved in supportive relationships. The client should also have the numbers of suicide and crisis hotlines that can be used around the clock. If the nurse assesses that there is a need for psychoactive medications, consultation with the client and a psychiatrist is indicated. Psychoactive drugs, particularly antidepressants, have varying time frames before becoming effective, they are often sedatives for the first few weeks, they may have uncomfortable side effects, and some have frightening adverse reactions. Thorough client education is essential to the client's sense of well-being and his or her willingness to remain on the medication long enough to experience its benefits. If a client is experiencing suicidal ideation and is taking antidepressants, the nurse should coordinate the dispensing of the drug with the psychiatrist to reduce the potential of a lethal overdose.

When the client returns home after a suicide attempt, the environment should be made as safe as possible. Firearms should be removed and medications assessed so that there is no possibility of stockpiling them for a future attempt. The nurse should assess the social support system to determine how best to help reduce social isolation and to collaborate with those individuals, whether family or friends, about how they can act in the client's best interest (Frisch & Frisch, 2002).

NURSING ROLE AND IMPLICATIONS

This section discusses how some community health nurses employ the nursing process to address mental health needs of their clients and communities.

The scope of clinical practice is differentiated by the community setting and the nurse's educational preparation. Most community health nurses have a baccalaureate degree but may not have advanced or specialized training in the area of mental health. When working with clients with mental health disorders, the nurse functions at a *basic practice level*. Nurses work in concert with psychiatric and mental health staff, some of whom are psychiatric or mental health clinical nurse specialists. The ANA (1994) recognizes the following basic-level functions of psychiatric/mental health nurses as screening and assessment intake and evaluation.

Screening and Assessment Intake and Evaluation

Mental health evaluations are a routine component of individual and family assessment. The community health nurse may be the one to discover the compromised client and make referrals for care. Nurses practicing in the home often have access to first-hand data useful in identifying mental health disorders. Data collected by community health nurses during routine assessments of an individual's physical, functional, and nutritional status, medication and substance use, health beliefs, and domestic and family life may indicate the need to conduct more specific mental health status examinations. Al-

---

✳ DECISION MAKING

School Crisis Event

You are working in an inner city school where a third grader was shot but not killed on the playground by his stepfather in front of the other children.

◆ As the nurse, what can you do at a primary prevention level in response to this event? At a secondary level?

◆ When you learn that the child's mother has been long diagnosed as a schizophrenic and is dependent on the stepfather for her care, is there anything you can do to facilitate the situation at any level of prevention?

---

though nurses at the basic level are not specifically trained to do mental status examinations, information and observations gained during client and family interactions are used to make tentative nursing diagnoses. For example, assessment of the neuromental status of all clients admitted to the nurse's caseload may identify risk factors such as long-term use of psychotropic drugs, sleep disturbance and lack of appetite in the bereaved, or symptoms of combat stress in refugees and immigrants. In these cases, follow-up using more specialized tools or referral for a more comprehensive evaluation is indicated. See Figure 29-7 for a list of general assessment areas used in a mental health evaluation. See Appendix E for an example of a minimental health status exam.

Screening and assessment of clients with identified mental health problems must not be limited to psychosocial aspects. There are emerging data suggesting that mentally ill persons are at greater risk for cardiopulmonary disease and cancer. Statistics from the Massachusetts Department of Mental Health (Tye, 2001) reveal that their clients have substantially higher morbidity rates when compared to a nondisabled cohort. It is not clear why this is so. There are suggestions that differences may be due to psychotropic drugs, behavior and lifestyle factors such as smoking and eating habits, or problems with access to health care.

Many nurses use genograms or family health trees and ecomaps to assess an individual or family's general health, functioning, and resources. Genograms help nurses identify family members with histories of mental health disorders and psychiatric-related hospitalizations and those who have been on psychotropic drugs or in psychotherapy or counseling.

The ecomap is a diagram of a family's contacts with others outside the family. It provides a visual picture of significant relationships between the person or family

FIGURE 29-7 General Assessment Areas Used in Mental Health Evaluations

Assess the client's:

- Appearance—posture, poise, clothing, grooming

- Behavior and psychomotor activity—gestures, twitches, agitation, combativeness, gait, agility, restlessness, activity level

- Attitude toward the nurse—cooperative, hostile, guarded, evasive

- Mood—depressed, irritable, angry, sad, expansive, euphoric, frightened, anxious

- Affect—emotional responsiveness, range of facial expressions, depth of emotion, affect (for congruence with mood), dull/flat, appropriateness to the situation

- Speech—talkative, slow or rapid, monotonous, loud, whispered, mumbled, impaired

- Perceptual disturbances—visual, auditory, or sensory hallucinations

- Thought process—flight of ideas, slow or hesitant thinking, vague responses, unrelated, disconnected

- Content of thoughts—preoccupations, obsessions, compulsions, fantasies, recurrent ideas about suicide, homicide, hurting self, hypochondriacal symptoms, antisocial urges

- Alertness and level of consciousness—alert, lethargic, somnolent

- Orientation—to person, place, time

- Memory—changes in remote, recent past, and recent memories; immediate retention problems

- Environment—house cluttered, unkempt, clean

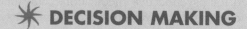

DECISION MAKING

Home Care with a Schizophrenic Client

You have made a home visit to Marie and her husband, Grant, who has recently returned home from a two-week stay in a psychiatric facility following his attempt to destroy all the electrical appliances in their home because they were "receiving messages from the government." He had stopped taking his medicine before the incident, and Marie hadn't realized how important it was for him to continue. Now that he is home, he's still not sure about the appliances and doesn't like the side effects of his medication.

◆ Following the suggestions for caring for the client with schizophrenia (Figure 29-11), which would be the best ways for you to work with the couple?

and others outside the immediate family and of the adequacy or lack of social support. Genograms and ecomaps are described in more detail in Chapter 24. Other mental health screening tools and techniques are available for use by community health nurses. These tools require basic orientation, but minimal training, to use.

The Posttraumatic Stress Disorder (PTSD) Screen for Newcomer Children was developed for nurses working with immigrant and refugee children who may have developed mental health symptoms after exposure to extreme stress in their country of origin (Golden, 1994) (See Figure 29-8). For more information about PTSD, see Chapter 30. Nurses may also administer standard rating scales to measure the severity of a psychiatric disorder and the effectiveness of treatment. The Hamilton Depressive Rating Scale and the Brief Psychotic Rating Scale are simple, statistically reliable tools that can be used by nurses to assess a client's symptoms and to communicate findings to others.

Whooley and Simon's (2000) Two-Question Case Finding Instrument should be part of most routine client

visits. It is designed to screen for depression in medical outpatients with two simple questions (see Figure 29-9).

The Abnormal Involuntary Movement Scale (AIMS) measures involuntary movements (see Figure 29-10) for clients at risk for tardive dyskinesia (TD). Often irreversible, TD is a side effect of many older antipsychotic medications. Although newer, atypical drugs have greatly decreased the incidence of TD, the new drugs are expensive and unfamiliar to some clinicians. Thus, they may not be used initially. All clients taking standard antipsychotic medications should have a baseline AIMS with periodic rescreening. Positive findings should be reported to the prescribing clinician immediately.

The complex nature of a more comprehensive assessment often justifies the nurse's consultation with specialized resources. The national goals set forth in *Healthy People 2010* (USDHHS, 2000) make it a high priority to increase the proportion of clinicians who routinely review the patient's cognitive, emotional, and behavioral functioning.

Nursing Support Interventions

Basic good listening and communication skills used to establish the therapeutic nurse-client relationship provide the foundation for counseling clients with mental illnesses. Many nurses may not recognize these support activities as significant interventions because they are so common to good nursing practice. Simple psychotherapeutic management techniques do not require advanced psychotherapy training. These and other skills important to the nurse-client relationship, which are discussed in Chapter 10, can be used by nurses who are supported by ongoing clinical supervision, the process by which

---

FIGURE 29-8 Posttraumatic Stress Disorder Screen for Newcomer Children

Does the child/or has the child ever:

( ) seemed unhappy

( ) cried excessively (unexplained)

( ) tried to or actually hurt self

( ) had peculiar or strange behavior

( ) seemed excessively restless

( ) displayed reckless or dangerous behavior

( ) wet or soiled pants at night or during day

( ) had sleeping problem (too much or too little, frequent nightmares)

( ) had eating problem (too much or too little, hoarding food)

Does the child have any of these problems at home or school?

( ) separation problem/school phobia

( ) poor grades

( ) difficulty concentrating—gets off task easily

( ) has to be coaxed to play or work with peers

( ) difficulty making friends

( ) disruptive in class

( ) arguing or fighting with classmates, teacher, siblings

( ) frequent suspensions from school

( ) refusing to obey parents

( ) excessive clinging to parent or teacher, (e.g., following parent to shower, bathroom)

( ) lying or stealing

( ) running away from home

( ) problems with police

( ) engaging in inappropriate sexual behavior

Has anyone in your family ever been treated or hospitalized for emotional problems such as depression, anxiety, mood swings, suicide attempts, or alcohol or drug abuse? If YES, explain.

FIGURE 29-9 Two-Question Depression Screening Tool

1. During the past month, have you often been bothered by feeling down, depressed, or hopeless?

   ☐ Yes   ☐ No

2. During the past month, have you often been bothered by having little interest or pleasure in doing things?

   ☐ Yes   ☐ No

If "no" to both, patient is unlikely to have major depression.

If "yes" to either, proceed with the follow-up clinical interview.

Follow-up Clinical Interview

The diagnosis of major depression requires five or more of the following nine symptoms, including depressed mood or anhedonia, during the same two-week period, causing clinically significant distress or impairment in social, occupational, or other important areas of functioning.

Symptom	DSM-IV Diagnostic Criteria for Major Depressive Episode
Depressed mood	Depressed mood most of the day, nearly every day
Anhedonia	Markedly diminished interest or pleasure in almost all activities
Weight change	Substantial unintentional weight loss or gain
Sleep disturbance	Insomnia or hypersomnia nearly every day
Psychomotor problems	Psychomotor agitation or retardation nearly every day
Lack of energy	Fatigue or loss of energy nearly every day
Excessive guilt	Feelings of worthlessness or excessive guilt nearly every day
Poor concentration	Diminished ability to think or concentrate nearly every day
Suicidal ideation	Recurrent thoughts of death or suicide

From "Primary Care: Managing Depression in Medical Outpatients," by M. A. Whooley and G. E. Simon, 2000, *New England Journal of Medicine, 343,* pp. 1942–1950. Copyright 2000 by Massachusetts Medical Society. All rights reserved.

FIGURE 29-10 Abnormal Involuntary Movement Scale (AIMS)

DEPARTMENT OF HUMAN SERVICES PUBLIC HEALTH SERVICE Alcohol, Drug Abuse, and Mental Health Administration NIMH Treatment Strategies in Schizophrenia Study **ABNORMAL INVOLUNTARY MOVEMENT SCALE (AIMS)**	PATIENT NUMBER – – – –	DATA GROUP aims	EVALUATION DATE — — — — — — $\overline{M}\ \overline{M}\ \overline{D}\ \overline{D}\ \overline{Y}\ \overline{Y}$
	PATIENT NAME		
	RATER NAME		

RATER NUMBER – – –	EVALUATION TYPE (Circle)			
	1 Baseline	4 Start double-blind	7 Start open meds	10 Early termination
	2 2-week minor	5 Major evaluation	8 During open meds	11 Study completion
	3	6 Other	9 Stop open meds	

INSTRUCTIONS:	Complete Examination Procedure (reverse side) before making ratings. MOVEMENT RATINGS: Rate highest severity observed.	Code:	1 = None 2 = Minimal, may be extreme normal	3 = Mild 4 = Moderate 5 = Severe

	1. Muscles of facial expression e.g., movements of forehead, eyebrows, periorbital area, cheeks; include frowning, blinking, smiling, grimacing	(Circle One) 1 2 3 4 5
FACIAL AND ORAL MOVEMENTS:	**2. Lips and perioral area** e.g., puckering, pouting, smacking	1 2 3 4 5
	3. Jaw e.g., biting, clenching, chewing, mouth opening, lateral movement	1 2 3 4 5
	4. Tongue Rate only increase in movement both in and out of mouth, NOT inability to sustain movement	1 2 3 4 5
EXTREMITY MOVEMENTS:	**5. Upper** (*arms, wrists, hands, fingers*) Include choreic movements (i.e., rapid, objectively purposeless, irregular, spontaneous), athetoid movements (i.e., slow, irregular, complex, serpentine) Do NOT include tremor (i.e., repetitive, regular, rhythmic)	1 2 3 4 5
	6. Lower (*legs, knees, ankles, toes*) e.g., lateral knee movement, foot tapping, heel dropping, foot squirming, inversion and eversion of foot	1 2 3 4 5
TRUNK MOVEMENTS:	**7. Neck, shoulders, hips** e.g., rocking, twisting, squirming, pelvic gyrations	1 2 3 4 5
GLOBAL JUDGMENTS:	**8. Severity of abnormal movements**	None, minimal — 1 Minimal — 2 Mild — 3 Moderate — 4 Severe — 5
	9. Incapacitation due to abnormal movements	None, minimal — 1 Minimal — 2 Mild — 3 Moderate — 4 Severe — 5
	10. Patient's awareness of abnormal movements Rate only patient's report	No awareness — 1 Aware, no distress — 2 Aware, mild distress — 3 Aware, moderate distress — 4 Aware, severe distress — 5
DENTAL STATUS:	**11. Current problem with teeth and/or dentures?**	No — 1 Yes — 2
	12. Does patient usually wear dentures?	No — 1 Yes — 2

(continues)

FIGURE 29-10 Abnormal Involuntary Movement Scale (AIMS) (continued)

EXAMINATION PROCEDURE

Either before or after completing the Examination Procedure observe the patient unobtrusively, at rest (e.g., in waiting room).

The chair to be used in this examination should be a hard, firm one without arms.

1. Ask patient to remove shoes and socks.

2. Ask patient whether there is anything in his/her mouth (i.e., gum, candy, etc.) and if there is, to remove it.

3. Ask patient about the *current* condition of his/her teeth. Ask patient if he/she wears dentures. Do teeth or dentures bother the patient *now?*

4. Ask patient whether he/she notices any movements in mouth, face, hands, or feet. If yes, ask to describe and to what extent they *currently* bother patient or interfere with his/her activities.

5. Have patient sit in chair with hands on knees, legs slightly apart, and feet flat on floor. (Look at entire body movements while in this position.)

6. Ask patient to sit with hands hanging unsupported: if male, between legs; if female and wearing a dress, hanging over knees. (Observe hands and other body areas.)

7. Ask patient to open mouth. (Observe tongue at rest within mouth.) Do this twice.

8. Ask patient to protrude tongue. (Observe abnormalities of tongue movement.) Do this twice.

9. Ask patient to tap thumb, with each finger, as rapidly as possible for 10 to 15 seconds: separately with right hand, then with left hand. (Observe each facial and leg movement.)

10. Flex and extend patient's left and right arms (one at a time). (Note any rigidity.)

11. Ask patient to stand up. (Observe in profile. Observe all body areas again, hips included.)

12. Ask patient to extend both arms outstretched in front with palms down. (Observe trunk, legs, and mouth.)

13. Have patient walk a few paces, turn, and walk back to chair. (Observe hands and gait.) Do this twice.

From *Abnormal Involuntary Movement Scale,* by W. Guy, 1976, Rockville, MD: National Institute of Mental Health.

---

one nurse confers with another (usually more advanced) regarding the nursing care of a client or clients. In the case of severe mental illness such as schizophrenia, severe depression, or bipolar disorder, such counseling is an adjunct to the primary, psychopharmacological treatment.

Psychoanalytic concepts that the nurse may have learned should not be used to make interpretive statements about the supposed unconscious motivations of a psychotic client. Any self-disclosure and admiring or social conversation should be worded so as to avoid overtones that the client may find seductive. See Figure 29-11 for techniques on handling experiences of a client with schizophrenia.

Psychobiological Interventions

Although psychopharmacological agents can greatly decrease or eliminate the most profound symptoms of major mental illnesses, many clients do not adhere to the optimal treatment regimen. Most often, problems with adherence can be traced to the client's experience with side effects of medication. Teaching clients about their medications and helping them to work with providers to manage the side effect symptoms are common and very important roles for the nurse.

Many home care clients referred for medical care present with mental health conditions. For example, HIV/AIDS and elderly clients may be taking as many as 10–15 different medications, including a number of psy-

chotropic drugs. A major component of home care is assessing these clients for overmedication, reviewing medications for compatibility and adverse side effects, and working with providers to address these concerns. Other psychobiological measures used by the community health nurse include relaxation techniques, diet and nutrition regulation, and rest-activity cycle monitoring.

Health Teaching

Client education is recognized as an integral part of nursing practice. It is one of the most important interventions nurses use to move clients toward self-care. Unfortunately,

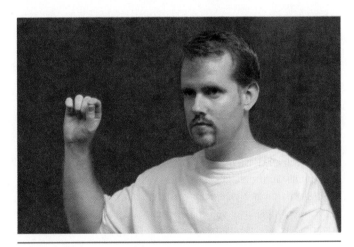

Client participating in AIMS test.

FIGURE 29-11 Caring for the Client with Schizophrenia

Patient's Experience	Nurse's Technique
Paranoia	• Maintain nonthreatening body position—side by side not face to face
	• Indirect speech content—verbal equivalent to above
	• Reciprocal emotional tone—help client to feel understood by mirroring his affect
	• Sharing mistrust—do not try to argue delusions away
	• Postpone psychoeducation until strong alliance is established
Denial of illness	• Avoid overzealous attack on denial—denial may be the best defense the client can mount
	• Provide alternative explanations—use indirect approach
Stigma	• Normalize behavior and attitudes—everyone has difficulties and struggles
	• Use your authority as a professional
	• Help client save face by tactful use of language to soften psychiatric terms
Demoralization	• Maintain a positive attitude
	• Make admiring and approving statements
	• Determine the origins of demoralization
Terror	• Reassurance
	• Companionship—offer a confident presence
	• Leave the client alone—avoid intrusive emotional reaching

From "Psychotherapeutic Management Techniques in the Treatment of Outpatients with Schizophrenia," by P. Weiden and L. Havens, 1994, *Hospital and Community Psychiatry, 45*(6), pp. 549–555. Adapted with permission of the American Psychiatric Association.

RESEARCH FOCUS

From Stigma to Strategy

Study Problem/Purpose

What is the impact of locally prepared public service advertising and curricula as a strategy to address stigma associated with mental illness?

Methods

Two community psychiatric nurses in a semirural area of Scotland used a community development model to address problems in the community regarding public attitudes associated with mental illness in the context of closing a psychiatric hospital and establishing community-based housing for the former patients. They tested two approaches. First, they prepared an advertisement for a local newspaper depicting the impact of stigma on families with mentally ill members. The second approach was an eight-session training package designed to raise awareness of mental illness among lay people who were students in a variety of community educational programs.

Findings

The newspaper advertisement ran once, in a distribution run of 13,000 copies. A sample of 246 residents was surveyed. Of 46 respondents who saw the ad, 3 of 4 reported a change in their attitude toward mental illness. The training package was evaluated by more rigorous measures. All students were surveyed before and after the training. An increase in awareness of the elements that reinforce stigma was demonstrated by 77.5% of students. Other measures showed significant change in attitude and opinion.

Implications

The study measured public awareness, not change in behavior, but does demonstrate the impact enthusiastic community health nurses can make working with a community health perspective and a small budget.

Source: Kaminski, P., & Harty, C. (1999). From stigma to strategy. Nursing Standard, 1(38), 36–40.

COMMUNITY NURSING VIEW

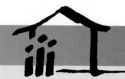

Esther Stuart is a 32-year-old African American who has been living with her 19-year-old married, unemployed partner, Daryl, for the past year. She was diagnosed with insulin-dependent diabetes mellitus six months ago and is poorly controlled. Her primary care provider notes that she has a history of schizophrenia. She was referred to the public health nurse because she is considering pregnancy. Esther is preoccupied with becoming pregnant, although she is using oral contraception. Esther tells the nurse she wants a child because so many of her neighbors have young children and having a child would allow her to develop friendships in her community and feel wanted. Esther's concerns include problems sleeping at night, chronic headaches, and a recent weight gain. She is 5 feet 4 inches tall and weighs 193 pounds. Esther and Daryl live in a neat one-bedroom apartment. Her mother lives in the same building "to keep an eye on me and make sure I'm doing OK." During the visits the nurse observes that Esther is not euphoric, depressed, or sad. Her behavior appears normal, her affect is constricted, and she is anxious. She enjoys seeing the nurse and tells her openly that she is schizophrenic. When the nurse reviews Esther's medications, she learns that Esther is taking Lithium, 300 mg TID, and 25 units of NPH insulin, BID; that she is followed at an outpatient mental health clinic; is not compliant taking her Lithium; and misses two out of every three scheduled appointments with her psychiatrist. Esther has been hospitalized two times within the past five months for ketoacidosis, using the emergency room for her care. When the nurse asks her about her diabetes, she is very knowledgeable. She tells the nurse that she was doing home glucose monitoring until the batteries in her machine died earlier this month and that she adjusts her insulin dose depending on how she feels, "my blood sugar being too high or too low." She follows no special diet and describes poor eating habits, frequently eating frozen or fast foods. In subsequent visits the nurse learns that Esther has two school-age children living with an aunt nearby.

Nursing Considerations

Assessment

- What areas should the nurse include in the mental health assessment? Are there any specific screening tools the nurse should use?
- What areas of risk should the nurse focus on in the assessment?
- What medication issues need to be considered with this client?
- What individual and family strengths can be identified?
- What cultural considerations need to be addressed in order to work effectively with this client and her family?

Diagnosis

- What nursing diagnoses can be assigned to this client and family?

Outcome Identification

- What measurable objectives would be used to evaluate the individual and family achievement of the best possible health outcomes?

Planning/Interventions

- How will the nursing plan address mental health, as well as other health concerns?
- What community resources would be appropriate to involve with this family?
- What nursing interventions should be included in the plan to address the nursing diagnoses?

Evaluation

- How will you know if your objectives have been met?
- In order to answer the above questions more fully, what additional information is needed?

---

client education is often neglected because of the pressures, time constraints, and multiple demands put on the nurse. Effective client education for the mentally ill has been lacking. See Chapters 10 and 11 for further discussions of teaching and health promotion, respectively.

Mental illness can disrupt almost every aspect of the life of the client and the client's family. Clients and families need to be educated about mental illness. As clients are defined

more as consumers of health care, the expectation is that they will have more questions and will be better informed than in the past. Content areas should include:

- The nature of mental illness, information about different diagnoses, major symptoms experienced, variability of experiences, probable causes, treatments options, prognosis

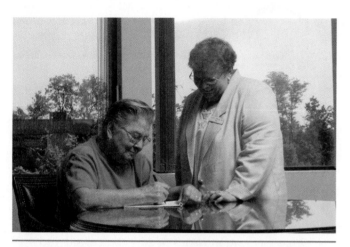

Providing encouragement to a client is an effective nursing intervention.

- Medications, actions, side effects, adherence to medication regimens
- Managing stress and using coping strategies
- Communication and relationship skills
- Community resources
- Impact of illness on family members
- Support networks

Case Management

Case management is key to successful rehabilitation for many clients with severe and chronic mental illness. Case managers provide continuity of care by following clients through all phases of care while helping them negotiate complex and fragmented systems. Case management includes assessing each client's needs, developing an individualized service plan with objectives related to needs, identifying strategies for achieving the stated objectives, and periodically evaluating the effectiveness of the services. Availability, accessibility, cost, and quality of care are central issues confronting the provision of case management services. Case managers ensure that the changing needs of their clients are addressed on an ongoing basis and appropriate choices are provided among the widest array of options for meeting those needs.

Murray and Baier (1993) describe the successful application of the concept to clients in a transitional residential program for chronically mentally ill homeless persons. Serving as coordinator, integrator, and advocate for health care needs of the chronically mentally ill is complex, given the pervasive nature of the disability. Whether serving as case manager or working with a case manager from another discipline, community health nurses employ the nursing process to periodically assess changes in clients' functional levels, medications, resources, skills, and self-esteem. As these elements change, so do the interventions required to meet the goals of psychiatric rehabilitation.

Self-Care Activities

Self-care activities are often disrupted in mental illness. Alterations in thinking processes can prevent clients from learning or performing activities of daily living. Whether the client is seen in day treatment, a halfway house, an outpatient clinic, a family home, or his or her own apartment, nurses can assess and teach personal hygiene, diet, recreation, shopping, and the use of public transportation. By modeling, directing, coaching, and supporting, nurses can use the person's real-world experience to help make the transition from dependent to increasingly independent arrangements.

Home Visits

The goal of psychiatric home visiting is to assist the client to remain in the community. The effectiveness of home visits and other nurse-based interventions is increasingly well recognized. In a prospective randomized trial, Rabins et al. (2000) studied the effect of the Psychogeriatric Assessment and Treatment in City Housing (PATCH) program. Depression and other mental illnesses are often unrecognized and undertreated, especially among the poor and elderly. To address this, residents at six large, urban apartment buildings were screened for symptoms of mental illness. At three sites, personnel were trained to recognize and refer residents who needed mental health care. Residents who were referred received weekly home visits. At 26-month follow-up, residents who received home visits had significantly fewer symptoms than did controls with psychiatric symptoms.

Taylor, Carson, and Bales (1999) discuss two elements particular to mental health visits. Psychiatric nursing visits require more time. They cite Ohlund's (1997) unpublished study benchmarking psychiatric home care, which found that mental health visits took longer than

---

REFLECTIVE THINKING

Disaster Nursing

Think about experiences you have had or have heard about in the news that describe a disaster situation.

- If you were called in as a community health nurse to participate in caring for the victims and their families, what would be your personal responses to the event?
- What concerns would you have about providing effective interventions?

other visits and impacted the productivity and pay of home care nurses. They also note the importance of recognizing the dynamics of the nurse-patient relationship and the implications for managers making assignments. See Chapter 21 for further discussion of the home visit.

Community Action

Concern for sociocultural factors that adversely affect the mental health of population groups and taking corrective action can mean getting involved with community planning boards, advisory groups, paraprofessionals, and other key people. Because community health nurses are identified with broad health concerns, their interest in and support for mental health issues help members of the public to see these issues as worthy of support.

ADVANCED PSYCHIATRIC/MENTAL HEALTH NURSING

Psychiatric/mental health advanced-practice nurses are prepared at the master's or higher level and are certified by a national credentialling body. They may also be referred to as clinical nurse specialists or certified specialists. Community health nurses will most often encounter the certified specialist as consultant-liaison. In this role, the specialist may provide direct care, from mental health promotion to illness rehabilitation, to clients who enter the health care system with physical illness, or indirect care by consulting and educating nurses and other caregivers. Other advanced-level functions include individual, family, and group psychotherapy. Many states have granted psychiatric/mental health advanced-practice nurses authority to write drug prescriptions.

◼ KEY CONCEPTS

- ◆ Treatment of psychiatric mental health clients has gone through three historical transformations. The most recent reform is the Community Mental Health Movement.

- ◆ Historical, political, and economic factors continue to greatly influence the concept and practice of community mental health nursing.

- ◆ Various nursing, behavioral, and biological theories give direction to the nursing care of the client with mental illness, and no one theory addresses all dimensions of community mental health nursing care.

- ◆ Community health nurses practice in a broad continuum of roles in the community, from generalist to specialist.

- ◆ Basic practice level includes screening and assessment, support interventions, psychobiological interventions, case management, and teaching self-care activities.

- ◆ Nurses provide services in a variety of community settings, including the client's home, shelters, outpatient clinics, aftercare agencies, jails, and senior centers.

- ◆ Nursing health promotion/illness prevention activities target and are directed toward the highest risk individuals and groups within the community.

- ◆ Advanced practice is differentiated by the nurse's educational preparation. The role of the clinical specialist is broad and includes consultant-liaison, direct care provider, and mental health educator.

Note: The author acknowledges the contribution of Baruch Golden, RN, CS, for his contribution to the first edition and for his continuing advice and support.

◼ RESOURCES

Alliance for Psychosocial Nursing: http://www.psychnurse.org
American Psychiatric Association: http://www.psych.org
American Psychiatric Nurses Association: http://www.apna.org
Association of Child and Adolescent Psychiatric Nurses: http://www.ispn-psych.org
California Chapter of American Psychiatric Nurses Association: http://www.calapna.org
Center for Mental Health Services, Substance Abuse and Mental Health Services Administration, U.S. Department of Health and Human Services: http://www.mentalhealth.org/cmhs
Clinical Resources in Psychiatry, Virtual Nursing College: http://www.langara.bc.ca/vnc/psych.htm
Correctional Medical Services: http://www.cmsstl.com
Internet Mental Health: http://www.mentalhealth.com
National Alliance for the Mentally Ill: http://www.nami.org
National Center for PTSD: http://www.ncptsd.org
National Commission on Correctional Health Care: http://www.ncchc.org
National Institute of Mental Health: http://www.nimh.nih.gov/practitioners/index.cfm
Online Dictionary of Mental Health: Psychiatric Nursing: http://www.human-nature.com/odmh/pnursing
Psychiatric Mental Health Nursing, 2nd edition, by Frisch & Frisch: http://www.delmarnursing.com/frisch
Psychiatric Nursing E-mail List: http://www.city.ac.uk/barts/psychiatric-nursing
Substance Abuse and Mental Health Services Administration, U.S. Department of Health and Human Services: http://www.samhsa.gov
WWW Sites for Violence Prevention (Occupational), National Institute for Occupational Safety and Health, Centers for Disease Control and Prevention: http://www.cdc.gov/niosh/violence.html

Chapter

30

FAMILY AND COMMUNITY VIOLENCE

Michelle Porter, RN, MSN, FNP

MAKING THE CONNECTION

"The community faces ethical dilemmas in deciding when and how to intervene in what is perceived as people's 'personal business.' The price of not intervening may be preventable death, serious injury, or persistent mental and physical health problems."

—Romans, Poore, & Martin (2000, p. 173)

COMPETENCIES

Upon completion of this chapter, the reader should be able to:

- Discuss selected international perspectives of family violence.
- Identify four theoretical frameworks that attempt to explain violence.
- Explain the impact of community violence on children.
- Discuss two issues related to guns and violence.
- Discuss reasons why individuals become gang members as they relate to the reasons why gangs commit crimes.
- Identify the various types of hate crimes.
- Discuss types of violence against women and their consequences.
- Explain the impact of sexual assault on survivors, perpetrators, and partners.
- Discuss the various types of abuse under the umbrella term *domestic violence.*
- Explain the cycle of domestic violence.
- Explain the concept of learned helplessness.
- Examine common myths surrounding sexual assault.
- Explain the primary forms of child abuse.
- Identify behavioral clues of child abuse.
- Consider how social environment, poverty, family stress, and violence might be linked.
- Discuss the nurse's role in working with elders and potentially abusive caregivers.
- Describe the extent of homicide in the community.
- Discuss the long-term effects of violence on individuals and communities.
- Identify reporting laws as they pertain to violent acts against children and adults.
- Describe primary, secondary, and tertiary community nursing interventions in the treatment of family violence.
- Discuss the importance of taking care of oneself when working with violent clients in order to maintain good nursing care.

KEY TERMS

acquaintance rape	child abuse
battered women	child neglect
batterer	date rape
domestic violence	rape
elder abuse	spiritual abuse
emotional abuse	spiritual terrorism
incest	spousal abuse
learned helplessness	terrorism
partner abuse	terrorist
patriarchy	trigger locks
posttraumatic stress disorder (PTSD)	wife abuse

The purposes of this chapter are to provide an overview of violence as it affects the individual, the family, and the community and to address the nursing process as it applies to those at risk for violence and to survivors. The chapter explores theories of violence; myths and realities surrounding violence; patterns of physical, sexual, and emotional abuse; and risk factors associated with homicidal behavior.

Violence is the intentional use of physical force against another person or against oneself, which either results in or has a high likelihood of resulting in injury, death, psychological harm, maldevelopment, or deprivation [U.S. Department of Health and Human Services (USDHHS), 1998]. Numerous sources indicate that some aspects of violence are on the decline. Firearm-related death rates for children and adolescents increased 31.8% in the six-year span between 1986 and 1992 but decreased each year from 1993 to 1997 [Bull et al., 2000; Fingerhut, Ingram, and Feldman, 1998; Centers for Disease Control and Prevention (CDC), 1999]. Although these death rates are encouraging, they must be contrasted with the reality that they are 71% higher than they were in the early 1980s (Fingerhut et al., 1998). Other intentional acts of violence—child abuse, domestic violence, sexual assault, and elder abuse—continue to rise (U.S. Department of Justice, 1998).

Given that the criminal justice system generally deals with violence after the fact, it is essential that other relevant sectors of society, including nursing, develop and deliver prevention strategies. Violent and abusive behavior is one of the 15 priority areas relating to specific problems, conditions, and diseases named in the *Healthy People 2010* report (USDHHS, 1998). The 1995 midcourse review shows that while suicide among adults, weapon carrying by adolescents, and rape have decreased, homicide, weapons-related violent deaths, assault injuries, and suicide attempts among adolescents have greatly increased (USDHHS, 1998).

What is the role of nursing in response to intentional violence? The definition of community health nursing given in Chapter 1 is certainly applicable to the provision of nursing care to survivors of violence as well as to interventions aimed at reducing potentially violent acts.

However, Perrin, Boyett, and McDermott (2000) discovered that many nurses are deficient in their knowledge, particularly of elder abuse and spousal abuse. It is recommended that nurses receive more education in these areas as well as being provided with opportunities to practice in real-life settings such as an abused women's shelter. In addition to providing care and prevention, there is a need for research to increase the knowledge base relevant to the community health nursing perspective in all areas of violence.

PERSPECTIVES ON VIOLENCE

Violence is making headlines across the United States. Public opinion polls evidence a growing concern regarding violence and public safety, although violence is hardly a new phenomenon. It has been and continues to be a popular theme in television, movies, music, and advertising.

Violence is embedded in our society and is not separate from us as individuals, as a community, or as a culture. Societal change begins with individual change. Community health nurses are in a position to teach nonviolent child-rearing practices, to educate families about the risk inherent in children's exposure to violent television and movie images, to counsel families at risk for violence, and to help link victims of violence to appropriate resources. Although this nursing intervention is only one aspect of addressing a complex cultural value system, it is a vital one.

International Perspective

Though it is known that domestic violence exists in most countries throughout the world, reliable statistics regarding the incidence and prevalence are lacking. The United Nations reports that somewhere "between 17% and 38% of the world's women have been physically assaulted by an intimate partner and it may be as high as 60% in many areas of the world" (Walker, 1999, p. 53). Lenore Walker (1999) makes the startling statement that "the single most powerful risk factor for becoming a victim of violence is to be a woman" (p. 23).

The Russian Federation's national report indicates that, in 1993, 14,500 women were killed by their male partner; in 1994 that figure rose to 15,000, and in 1995 the death rate rose to over 16,000. Nonfatal instances of domestic violence, also prevalent in Russia, are beginning to be publicly discussed. Reminiscent of the American domestic violence movement of the late sixties early seventies, hard-fought battles have won the right for a Russian woman to file a complaint when she is battered. Unfortunately, the police still have the right to refuse it. Factors thought to contribute to Russian male violence

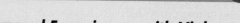

REFLECTIVE THINKING

Violence

The word *violence* means different things to different people depending on their own life experiences, personal encounters, stereotypes, and conditioning. What does violence mean to you?

- When you think of violence, what images come to mind?
- Consider the following variables: sex, age, race, class, educational background, neighborhood, city, state, country, and religious group. What are your particular stereotypes with regard to violence and each variable?
- How were these stereotypes formed?
- What behaviors do you consider to be violent?

REFLECTIVE THINKING

Personal Experiences with Violence

- How were you disciplined as a child?
- How did your family manage anger when you were a child? Is what you do when you are angry similar to or different from what adults in your family did when they were angry?
- As a child were you taught problem-solving skills?
- How many violent images were you exposed to in the past 24 hours? Consider television, movies, newspapers, magazines, radio, advertisements, public transportation, daily life, and neighbors.
- Have you ever had a violent impulse? Did you act on it? If not, what kept you from doing so?
- Under what circumstances, if any, would you justify the use of personal violence? To what degree? What might the consequences be for you and the person upon whom you inflict violence?

are not unlike those studied in the United States: poverty, alcohol abuse, housing shortages, and cultural/historical influences (Horne, 1999).

Women and children frequently suffer sexual violence and other forms of abuse as a part of war and brutal dictatorships. During the 15 years of Chile's Pinochet dictatorship women suffered sexual torture and the horror of being forced to watch as their children were tortured. The state used these methods to destroy families considered subversive (McWhirter, 1999). Under the Taliban, the radical Islamic movement that until recently controlled two-thirds of Afghanistan, women were not allowed to be in public unless accompanied by a male relative. When out, they had to be completely covered head to toe and wear shoes that made no noise. The women were not allowed to work or attend school. Only 20% of hospital beds were afforded to women while 70% were reserved for men. If a woman violated any of these laws, she was publicly beaten (Raselch, Bauer, Manos, and Iocopino, 1998). Japan has traditionally viewed domestic violence as violence inflicted on a parent, usually the mother, by a child—almost always a teenage son. Conflict between wives and their mother-in-laws often results in the physical abuse of the elder, 50% of whom are over 80 years of age. This dynamic is most likely linked to the cultural tradition of a wife being absorbed into the husband's family and being expected to care for his aging parents. The families are patriarchal, and male authority is not questioned. Because men maintain the family lineage, men are more valued than women. Incest is not considered a criminal act in Japan; there are no laws that punish a parent who sexually abuses his own child. Statistics regarding domestic violence and rape are lacking because of the silence around abuse. A Japanese saying provides an adequate summary of family abuse: A nail that sticks out will be struck down (Kozu, 1999).

A particular type of violence perpetrated on many children is female genital mutilation. While it is primarily a practice in many countries of Africa, it is also carried out in parts of the Middle East and Asia. With the many immigrants coming to the United States, Canada, Europe, New Zealand, and Australia from these countries, the practice is often continued in their adopted country. The World Health Organization (WHO) has a resolution calling on member states to establish national policies and practices to abolish female genital mutilation and other harmful traditional practices, and the International Council of Nurses (ICN) along with other international organizations has supported the abolishment of this practice. The degree to which the practice is integrated into many cultural beliefs makes it very difficult to stop. Some groups are trying by developing alternative initiation ceremonies in which dance, song, drumming, feasting, and other festivities substitute for genital mutilation. Information and education programs have been tried as well as targeting specific groups for training, such as providers, birth attendants, excisors, healers, religious and community leaders, law enforcers, media professionals, and legislators (Affara, 2000). For more information about female genital mutilation, see Chapter 8.

There is some financial help available for addressing these problems. The United Nations Development Fund for Women gives grants for programs to end violence against women in 21 countries. In 2001, they gave $1 million. Some of the work undertaken by the fund has been to "revise Thailand's penal code with relation to marital rate, forms of sexual violence that are not considered sexual intercourse, and child pornography; producing a 'soap opera' in Namibia to raise awareness about the impact on families of violence against women, stemming the trafficking of women and girls in Colombia, and establishing a network of community councils to address domestic violence" (United Nations, August 11, 2001, p. 6).

THEORIES OF VIOLENCE

A variety of theories attempt to explain violence, including biological, psychoanalytic, social learning, and feminist theories. No existing nursing theory explicitly addresses violence. This area remains in need of nursing research and theory development. No one theory explains the complex reasons one person behaves violently while another person does not. It may be that a combination of theories is most helpful.

Biological Theories

The biological perspective links violence to biological dysfunction. These theories are concerned with extreme acts of violence and tend to assume that aggression is innate and lesser forms of violence are normal.

Studies indicate a strong correlation between substance abuse and acts of violence (Lamberg, 1998a; Zoellner, Goodwin, and Foa, 2000; Abracen, Looman, & Anderson, 2000). Littrell and Littrell (1998) discuss alcohol as a potent antecedent of aggressive behavior. Its effect is compounded by social pressure and the aggressive disposition of the alcohol consumer. Lamberg (1998a) indicates that 25%–33% of persons who abused alcohol or other substances also reported violent acts.

Weapons, particularly firearms, account for a high percentage of all injury deaths in young people 1–19 years of age (Bull et al., 2000). The frequency of weapon carrying among adolescents is strongly correlated with substance abuse (DuRant, Krowchuk, Kreiter, Sinal, & Woods, 1999).

Psychoanalytic Theories

The psychoanalytic theories of violence have been advanced by such theorists as Freud, Storr, Kaplan, and Fromme, and for the most part they explain aggression as an instinctive drive in humans. Siann (1985) and Storr (1968) expanded on Freud's theory of aggression as in-

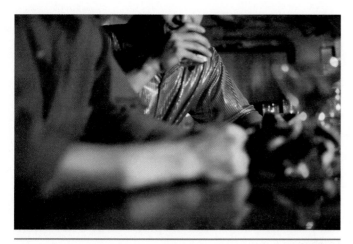

Alcohol is a potent antecedent of aggressive behavior.

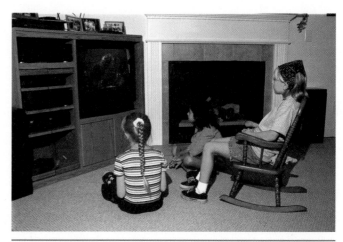

Do you think that television has contributed to a rise in violence?

stinctive by theorizing that aggression exists on a continuum of behavior from a normal to a pathological response. Siann hypothesized that the aggressive response is determined by each individual's early development. Kaplan (1975) and Fromme (1977) shared the theory that aggression results from thwarting a basic human need rather than from an instinctive drive.

These theories examined mothering styles and placed less emphasis on the parenting style of fathers or the effect of an absent father. Also these theories failed to explain the prevalence of violence perpetrated by men as compared with women.

Social Learning Theories

Social learning theory is a psychological theory incorporating sociological frameworks. Bandura (1973), Baron (1977), and other social scientists focus on violence as a learned response. If a child throws a tantrum whenever he or she wants something and the parents repeatedly give in, the child learns that aggressive behavior is effective. This learning can determine how the child will behave as an adult.

Modeling is another concept of socially learned behavior. When violent behavior is modeled and reinforced for children within their families, the children view it as a normal strategy to reduce stress, resolve conflicts, and get needs met. Violence can also be modeled and reinforced by aspects of the culture (school, church, neighborhood, and media). Mitka (2001) cites studies which link exposure to violent media with increased levels of aggression in children.

Feminist Theory

Feminist theory views violence within the family as a gender and power issue (Bogard, 1992; Dobash & Dobash, 1992). It focuses primarily on an analysis of violence against women and identifies **patriarchy,** a male-

dominated system in which males hold most of the power, as the root cause of this violence. Feminist theory rejects the notion that aspects of these roles are inherent, instead considering them socially constructed to maintain male power—not only in the family but in society at large. In this model, violence is seen as a social problem as well as a personal style of maintaining control over another person. The limitation of this model is its lack of application to other aspects of family violence such as elder abuse, sibling abuse, and child abuse.

COMMUNITY VIOLENCE

Family and street violence are interrelated. Studies have shown that men who are violent at home are likely to be violent outside the home (Walker, 1999).

Many factors have been identified that contribute to violence. These include influence of peers, unemployment, poverty, ethnic diversity, gun ownership, media violence, intrapersonal characteristics, and biological factors.

Guns and Violence

The United States is a violent country, with the highest rates of firearm-related deaths in the industrialized world (Bull et al., 2000). While guns and community violence are connected, there is considerable controversy regarding their management in society.

One of the arguments most often cited has to do with the second amendment's applicability to federal firearms control. Gun control advocates argue that "people who can bear arms" applies only to bearing arms in an organized militia, while gun rights advocates interpretation of "people" refers to all people, not just the militia (Henderson, 2000).

Beginning in the 1980s the medical community began to talk about an "epidemic" of gun violence (Henderson, 2000). They argue that a gun is an impulse weapon that can quickly commit a potentially irrevocable act. They also note that the use of a gun for suicide is more likely to be fatal than other means. (Henderson, 2000; Siebel, 2000). Other countries, such as Britain and Japan, have strict firearm controls and far lower homicide rates than the United States. The medical community have noted the tremendous costs to the community as a result of gun injuries. Webster (2002) reports on a Detroit news analysis of billing records in South East Michigan. They found that while only 7% of cases involved a firearm, these cases made up 25% or $53 million of the charges. The bill was about 4 times higher than for non-firearm injuries. Many of these bills do not get paid or are paid through medicaid, thus passing the cost on to taxpayers.

The nature of the injuries imply other costs. These include police investigations, emergency rescue services, coroner services, jails, security at schools and other public buildings, disability benefits and youth intervention programs. Neighborhoods where gun violence is common lose real estate value, and therefore reduce the community tax base.

One of the most recent concerns has been the use of **trigger locks** on guns. This is a "lock that fits into a gun trigger so that the gun cannot be fired until the lock is unlocked" (Henderson, 2000, p. 114). There are proposals in Congress calling for a requirement that trigger locks either be mandatory or be made available with each new gun sold. In 1997, most major handgun manufacturers agreed to voluntarily offer child safety locks for sale with new handguns, for the most part in order to prevent more restrictive legislation from becoming law. However, most have not been shipping them with their guns (Helpnetwork, 2002).

The original intent of gun ownership was for protection in the home. Gun advocates argue that owning a gun deters crime because most perpetrators do not want to deal with guns. They believe that being armed is having power to defend oneself and that such power should reside with the citizens (Powell, 1999). Those in favor of gun control note that too many children are victims of gun accidents resulting from careless gun storage and lack of parental guidance. Guns lend themselves to easy access to be stolen or used for suicide. Having a gun in the home is more perilous than protective (Brody, 1999).

Interventions that serve to reduce violence involve a multidisciplinary, multisectorial approach. D'Antonio (1999) suggests ways in which gun violence can be reduced. Community policing programs are important. These include having more police on foot throughout the community, holding open forums to work with citizens to find ways to prevent violence, establishing citizen advisory councils, and rehabilitating criminals rather than just punishing them. The neighborhood can help by making sure there is safe passage for children and becoming trained in conflict resolution to help avert violent confrontations. Conflict resolution can be taught in schools. This approach works best when it is followed up by the community becoming involved in children's lives.

Advertising similar to that which has worked with tobacco can be used to make violence socially unacceptable. Citizens action groups that pressure politicians to stop violence through the development of community programs are very important.

Other approaches not previously discussed include spiritual involvement that counters the disconnectedness of individuals that commit violent acts. Helping to develop their sense of self-respect and self-image is important, as is building positive attachments with families and helping to teach individuals self-respect (Rosado, 1999).

Nurses can be very instrumental in the above interventions. They see the result of violence first hand and can participate in many of the programs as well as work to change laws.

Gangs

A form of community violence that has escalated in recent years is that perpetrated by gangs. Gang members live in a "culture of guns and violence" (Christensen, 1999, p. 23) and can be found in every segment of society and every ethnic group is represented. They commit crimes to finance their activities, of which one of the main activities is selling drugs. Paramount to gang culture is respect, reputation, and revenge. When someone in a gang is disrespected, revenge, or retribution, is exacted in order to reestablish the reputation. Often, this retribution takes the form of shooting, not only the person or gang involved, but everyone in the immediate area. Most gang members are aged 16 or less. If they stay in the gang beyond their early twenties, they usually become career criminals. Perhaps after 16, they begin to see more options for themselves since they can then drive and work and have more freedom of choice.

There are many reasons why individuals become gang members. Parental abuse and neglect are major factors. In addition, many families who do care for their children are hampered because of poverty, unemployment, lack of education, or lack of support systems or they do not speak English or understand American customs. Therefore, they are unable to resolve problems before they become crises. Children feel out of place and want to belong somewhere. Gang membership gives them that feeling of belonging. Some children from well-functioning homes seek the excitement of gang life. When gang members are looked at from a mental health perspective, one sees many indicators of risk such as depression, bipolar disorder, posttraumatic stress disorder (PTSD), family involvement in the justice system, as well as child abuse (Christensen, 1999).

Women also join gangs. As reported in Hunt and Joe-Laidler (2001), female gang members are increasing and are 10%–30% of all gang members. Their reasons for becoming gang members are to have and create a sense of family and, sometimes, they bear children with the intent of bringing them up to become gang members.

Programs aimed at preventing children from becoming gang members need to start with young children and provide incentives that are more attractive than gang culture that help them to develop self-esteem. They need love, attention, and education. For those already in gangs, the process is more difficult. Anger management is important. Some just need to mature and graduate from the gangs on their own.

Hernandez (1998) suggests ways to end gang violence. First is to involve the whole community in a commitment to reown all of its children and plan for them. Next, is the need for a child advocate that will lobby for the special needs of gang-involved children, such as literacy programs and help for addiction. The third step is to develop alternative schools that provide such things as small student-teacher ratios, weekly support groups, ties to the business community to teach the students how to participate in a job interview and how to work, parent support group, and ties to cultural and athletic opportunities. Parents must be involved as partners in raising their children in hard environments. Children who come to school from the juvenile justice system need special help. That would include establishing a mentoring system for students on parole, establishing school liaisons who visit inmates at juvenile hall, and creating an on-going support group during school hours. Another important step is identifying learning disabilities among the children. These may have been the cause of their early difficulties with school and their lack of interest in education. Finally, there must be programs in place to aid in recovery from addiction.

There is no one solution that will work to prevent gang activity. The problem is too large and complex. The nurse, particularly the school health nurse, can play a large part in the development and facilitation of the necessary programs, but solutions can only be found by planning at a multidisciplinary level.

Terrorism

An important aspect of community violence is terrorism. **Terrorism** is defined by the Department of Defense as "the calculated use of violence or the threat of violence to inculcate fear, intended to coerce or to intimidate governments or societies in the pursuit of goals that are generally political, religious, or ideological" (Terrorism Research Center, 1997a, p. 1). Hoffman (1998) adds that terrorism is conducted by an organization which has an identifiable chain of command. A **terrorist** is defined as "a violent intellectual, prepared to use and indeed committed to using force in the attainment of his goals" (Hoffman, 1998, p. 43).

Terrorism is carried out through the use of nuclear, biological, chemical, incendiary, or conventional explosive agents. Any of these approaches is a threat to health, safety, food supply, property, or the environment. Until recently, the United States has viewed these terrorism attacks from a distance. Except for the bombing of the World Trade Center in New York City in 1993 and the Oklahoma Federal building in 1995, the United States and Canada have not had to experience terrorism first hand. Since September 11, 2001, when the World Trade Center was destroyed and the Pentagon attacked by terrorists who hijacked commercial airplanes filled with passengers and crashed them into these buildings, the world of U.S. citizens has changed forever. No longer is it possible to think of these acts of violence as being carried out in distant lands.

Bioterrorism is the major focus of public health. There is much controversy as to what degree public health could prepare for an attack. For instance, Henretig (2001) believes that bioterrorism does "pose a serious public health and security threat to our nation" (p. 718) and that a much larger budget is needed to prepare the public health infrastructure for an attack. He thinks that, in this process, the public health agency would be better prepared to serve all citizens at all times, not just be ready for a chemical or biological attack. However, Fee and Brown (2001) point out that preparations that were undertaken during the Cold War in the 1950s "narrowed the scope of public health activities, and failed to achieve sustained benefits for public health programs across the country" (p. 721). For more information about bioterrorism, see Chapter 9.

While nuclear attacks are possible, given that many countries have the ability to make the weapons, the more likely weapons are explosive devices that kill and injure masses of people. These attacks would strain all health facilities and create public health problems because of the effects on the environment and water supply.

While the results of a bioterrorist attack may sicken large numbers of people, other types of attacks lead to massive injuries and often the recovery of body parts during the rescue efforts. The rescue workers as well as the surviving victims and friends and relatives of every one affected are psychologically impacted. An important part of the recovery phase is to provide psychological services. See Chapter 29 for more information regarding psychological issues and interventions.

Many organizations are involved in both planning prevention strategies as well as coping with the results of an attack. The Federal Emergency Management Agency (FEMA) has developed new terrorism preparedness planning guidelines for state and local governments. The document can be seen at the FEMA website at www.fema.gov/pte/gaheop.htm. This document is the result of coordinated effort involving not only FEMA but also the National Emergency Management Association, the International Association of Emergency Managers, and the Federal Departments of Justice, Defense, Agriculture, Health and Human Services, and Veterans Affairs, the Environmental Protection Agency, and the Nuclear Regulatory Commission.

The Red Cross is one of the major agencies that provide aid following an attack. It works together with government, business, labor union, religious, and community organizations as well as other voluntary agencies to ensure a coordinated and efficient response to any disaster that strikes. As well as providing relief to victims of disaster, both locally and globally, the Red Cross is responsible for half of the nation's blood supply and blood products.

The impact of a terrorist attack on individuals and families is extensive. In a blink of an eye, parents lose children, children lose parents, one spouse loses the other. Emergency services are needed to place orphans temporarily and, later, permanently. Sometimes grandparents must take over raising a young child or children just as they were prepared to enjoy retirement. Mothers or fathers may suddenly become single parents. See Chapters 24 and 25 for more information about the consequences of disrupted family constellations and the importance of crisis intervention. School nurses and other community nurses must be on the alert for problem reactions of individuals and families following the attack and for years after.

Emergency and disaster response workers also need to take care of themselves. Following the attack of September 11, 2001, the USDHHS (2001) distributed on their website self-care tips for emergency and disaster response workers. They include information regarding normal reactions to a disaster event, signs that stress management assistance is needed, and ways to help manage stress. For more information, refer to www.mental-health.org/ cmhs/EmergencyServices/response.htm.

The future of terrorism, particularly in the United States, is unknown. The Terrorism Research Center (1997b) believes that terrorism will continue. Since the shock effect decreases with familiarity, the terrorist is likely to seek more unusual events to capture and hold public attention. The Center notes that "an effective antiterrorism program will reduce the likelihood of successful terrorist attacks but only if it is so deeply instilled that it is habitual" (p. 2).

Community violence can spill over into the workplace, including the hospital and places of worship.

In a 1998 study of 364 public health field workers, 139 reported 611 violent episodes, including weapon threats, physical attacks, and rape. A large percentage of mental health professionals, including nurses and physicians, have been assaulted in psychiatric inpatient and outpatient facilities (Lewis & Dehn, 1999; Nolan, Dallender, Soares, Thomsen, & Arnetz, 1999; Schulte, Nolt, Williams, Spinks & Hellsten, 1998). A survey of 127 emergency rooms found that almost one-half reported a physical assault on one or more staff members each month (Schulte et al., 1998). According to one study, while nurses working in the community area are assaulted less than those working in hospital settings, they are not immune (Nolan et al., 1999).

One study of all registered and licensed practical nurses in the state of Minnesota showed that the greater proportions of nurses worked in state, county, or city institutions, hospitals or long-term care institutions, and psychiatric and intensive care areas and on evening or night shifts. Most assailants were clients, although 3% were co-workers and 2% were visitors. The majority of assailants were white, male, middle-aged or elderly, and mentally impaired. The study showed that the presence of video monitors and security personnel might help to prevent the assaults, as might written procedures for assault prevention and policies of dealing with clients with repeated violent behavior. Working alone is also suggested as a risk factor (Lee, Gerberich, Waller, Anderson, & McGovern, 1999). Training workers in violence prevention and intervention and training managers in conflict resolution can help to reduce violence (Runyan, 2001).

Children's Exposure to Community Violence

Many children living in urban areas are exposed to violence daily. Many have lost friends, relatives, teachers, or neighbors to homicide. Song, Singer, and Anglin (1981) discuss one study of 3700 high school students which found a great deal of victimization at home, in school and in the community. Over 45% of urban children had witnessed a shooting, forty-seven percent of first and second graders had witnessed a shooting, and

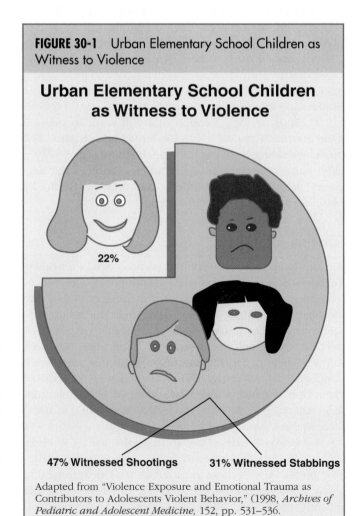

FIGURE 30-1 Urban Elementary School Children as Witness to Violence

Urban Elementary School Children as Witness to Violence

22%

47% Witnessed Shootings   31% Witnessed Stabbings

Adapted from "Violence Exposure and Emotional Trauma as Contributors to Adolescents Violent Behavior," (1998, *Archives of Pediatric and Adolescent Medicine,* 152, pp. 531–536.

FIGURE 30-2 Assessing a Child's Emotional Response to Witnessing Violence

Community health nurses will come in contact with children who have witnessed violence. Consider these aspects of assessment:

Is the child worried about being safe?

Is there a place where the child feels safe?

Is the child worrying about something bad happening to self or family?

Is the child sleeping through the night?

Is the child having nightmares?

Does the child have ideas about how to stay safe?

Is the child fearful of leaving home, of attending school?

Is the child preoccupied, having difficulty concentrating?

Has the child become incontinent?

Is the child eating, any significant weight gain/loss?

31% had witnessed a stabbing. See Figure 30-1. These children are at greater risk for the development of violent behaviors, psychological trauma, and impaired social functioning.

Urban children may live with the possibility of being shot in a drive-by as they walk home from school or even as they sit eating dinner in their homes. These realities rob them of any sense of safety or security. Witnessing violence places children at risk for the development of psychological trauma and the development of violent behaviors (Song et al., 1998). Figure 30-2 lists questions nurses can consider in their assessment of a child's level of stress secondary to exposure to a violent act. The needs of urban children and the epidemic of violence affecting their lives should be a top priority for nursing education, research, and practice.

HATE CRIMES

The Hate Crimes Statistics Act of 1990 was the first official recognition of the fact that there were crimes motivated by bias or hatred of minority groups occurring in the United States. As a result of this act, the FBI collects and reports on incidents of hate crimes. Bias-related, or hate, crimes reported to 10,730 law enforcement agencies in 1998 totaled 7755. The majority (4321) were racially motivated, and in 38% of the cases the crime was directed at an African American. In the 1260 assaults on homosexuals, 67% involved attacks on gay men and 18% of attacks were against lesbians. There are no clear statistics specific to hate crimes on bisexual, transvestite, or transsexual people. The majority of the 1390 assaults involving religious bias were against Jews and Catholics (*FBI Hate Crimes Statistics,* 1998).

In addition to overt acts of violence, widespread institutional prejudice also adversely affects racial, ethnic, religious, and sexual minorities. The implications for health care providers are poorly studied, and information on appropriate interventions and care is not available. This is an area in which nursing research is needed. Other issues appropriate to nursing research include motivation of perpetrators; the effect of hate on the victim's physical, mental, and spiritual health; support system needs; and prevention strategies.

VIOLENCE AGAINST WOMEN

The term *violence against women* is broad, encompassing physical violence, rape, homicide, genital mutilation, denial of rights based on gender, and female infanticide. Violence against women is often incorrectly viewed as a women's issue, but it is a community issue as well. Violence against women has emotional consequences affecting the victim and those who care about and depend on her. The financial consequence to society is high. Schroeder and Weber (1998) indicate that battery is an important cause of female employee absenteeism and accounts for over 28,000 emergency room visits annually with an estimated cost of 44 million health care dollars.

Nurses are encouraged to grapple with the bigger picture as a means of unlearning biased ways of viewing female victims, to redefine the notion of prevention, to develop strategies that empower women, and to participate in solutions that will bring about long-term societal change.

SEXUAL VIOLENCE

Sexual assault exists on a continuum of violence, including behaviors ranging from staring and voyeurism to rape of children (see Table 30-1). Most women experience more than one of these behaviors over the course of their lives, and the most recent assault may trigger memories of previous unresolved or never-acknowledged events. Sexually assaultive behaviors are intrusive and nonconsensual. They disregard a person's right to freedom from harassment and are potentially intimidating. They demonstrate a profound disrespect for the victims.

Emotional response may vary widely depending on whether the assault occurs when the victim is isolated, whether it is ongoing or progressive, how much contact there is with the perpetrator, whether the victim has self-defense skills, and how threatening the incident seems. See Figure 30-3 for an example.

TABLE 30-1   Continuum of Sexual Assault

TYPE	ACTIVITIES
Nonverbal	Voyeurism; exposure; stalking; suggestive looks or facial expressions such as licking lips, thrusting tongue out, smacking lips
Verbal	Suggestive noises such as grunting or sucking; sexist jokes; obscene phone calls
Unwanted contact	Slapping on buttocks; putting arm around a woman or a young girl and brushing her breasts in the process; touching genitals or the clothing over genitals
Harassment	Employer's negotiating job advancement on the basis of employee's willingness to cooperate in any of the activities on this continuum
Rape of adults	Sexual penetration of vagina, mouth, or rectum, without consent, using force or threat of force
Rape of children	Same as of adults, except victim is especially vulnerable because of size, age, dependency on adults, lack of power, and lack of comprehension

FIGURE 30-3   Example of Sexual Assault Awareness among Female Teenagers

The author taught sexual assault awareness to senior teens. During discussions of the continuum of violence, several similar examples arose repeatedly from young women in different schools. One example was that of walking past a construction site alone and having several men yell, whistle, comment about their bodies, and shout out sexually suggestive invitations. These young women reported a variety of feelings including anger, intimidation, and fear. When asked how they handled the situation, several women mentioned that they evaluated their environment to see if other people were around, then picked up their pace and checked behind them several times to be sure they weren't being followed. Some women wanted to yell at these men but believed it was unwise because they were alone.

SEXUAL ASSAULT

Healthy People 2010 (CDCP, 2001) define **rape** as "forced sexual intercourse including both psychological coercion and physical force. Forced sexual intercourse means vaginal, anal or oral penetration by the offender(s) and includes incidents of penetration by a foreign object." The National Incident–Based Reporting System (NIBRS), a statistical arm of the Uniform Crime Reporting Program, collects statistical information on sexual assault from law enforcement agencies. The categories it uses to define forcible sex offenses include forcible sex offenses, forcible rape (except statutory rape), forcible sodomy, sexual assault with an object, and forcible fondling (reported only if the sole sex offense committed since it is an element of all other categories). Figure 30-4 summarizes the NIBRS statistics from the July 2000 report (Snyder, 2000).

FIGURE 30-4   Sexual Assault Statistics

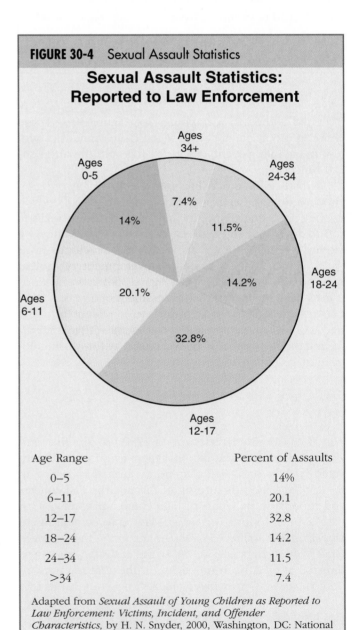

Sexual Assault Statistics: Reported to Law Enforcement

Age Range	Percent of Assaults
0–5	14%
6–11	20.1
12–17	32.8
18–24	14.2
24–34	11.5
>34	7.4

Adapted from *Sexual Assault of Young Children as Reported to Law Enforcement: Victims, Incident, and Offender Characteristics,* by H. N. Snyder, 2000, Washington, DC: National Center for Juvenile Justice.

Most rapes involve a man as the perpetrator and a woman as the victim. However, adult men are also raped by other men and are even more reluctant than women to report the assault. And women may be raped by women. **Incest,** the crime of sexual relations between persons related by blood, is another underreported form of rape.

The majority of rapes are not reported to law enforcement or health care providers (Feldhaus & Kaminsky, 1999). Three factors affect the likelihood of the assault being reported: the relationship of the perpetrator to the victim, the age of the victim, and the victim experiencing a series of rapes (Smith, Letourneau, Saunders, Kilpatrick, Resnick, & Best, 2000). A single assault committed by a stranger against a woman over the age of 18 is more likely to be reported than an **acquaintance** or **date rape.** In the latter, the perpetrator may be an individual in a position of confidence (priest, therapist, etc.), an acquaintance, family member, or intimate partner. The victim is often loathe to reveal that a rape has occurred.

REFLECTIVE THINKING

Sexual Assault

Popular novels, television, movies, and magazines continue to portray rape in a stereotypical manner. Answer the following questions based on stereotypes. Put aside what facts you might know. Try doing this with a partner—jot down your answers without conferring and then compare your responses.

Consider the victim.

- How old is the victim?
- Describe the victim's appearance: clothes, type and color of shoes and stockings, makeup, hairstyle and color, and race.
- What is the victim doing? Where?

Consider the rapist.

- Identify the rapist's age, race, and appearance, level of education, and employment.
- Where is the rapist? What is the rapist doing? Is there a weapon? What is it?
- Does the victim know the rapist?

Consider the circumstances.

- List the three most likely places this stereotypical rape would take place.
- What time of day is it?

Attitudes toward Rape Victims

It is not uncommon for people to consider the victim as being responsible for the rapist's behavior or to claim that the allegations are untrue. This attitude continues to influence the criminal justice system, the health care system, and the culture at large. Furthermore, these attitudes affect the psychological reactions of the victim after a rape or sexually assaultive incident. When a person is raped, a self-blaming, shamed response is in part a reaction to this legacy.

Myths and Realities

The myths surrounding sexual assault serve to keep the focus and blame on the victim. Some myths also serve as defense mechanisms against the fear of sexual assault. We think that if we can identify the things the victim did wrong, we can avoid those behaviors and successfully avoid sexual assault. Although the myths listed in Table 30-2 refer to rape, they are applicable to any type of sexual assault. As educators, nurses are in a position to provide accurate information about these topics and to eliminate misconceptions.

Victim Response to Sexual Assault

Rape and other forms of sexual assault abruptly alter the victim's life to varying degrees depending upon the nature and extent of the actual or threatened violence. Life events involving overwhelming threats to a person's physical or psychological integrity, including sexual assault, often result in posttraumatic stress disorder (Seedat & Stein, 2000). This disorder is discussed further with regard to long-term effects of violence.

Intervention for Survivors

Intervention during the period of crisis following the rape is vital and can help to reduce the severity of long-term consequences. The needs of the survivor are greatest during the first hours and days after the incident, but the victim might return to a state of crisis months or years later. Crisis intervention focuses on the assault and gives that trauma precedence over other issues in the client's life. The goal is to help the client cope. Rape temporarily alters a victim's sense of personal power and control and inhibits decision-making skills.

As the crisis phase subsides, the nurse can discuss activities that facilitate empowerment. Many victims find it helpful to take a self-defense or martial arts class. Other helpful activities include instruction in the proper use of pepper spray or mace, assertion training classes, or even weight lifting in order to feel physically stronger.

Nurses can contact a local rape crisis center for information regarding available services. See Appendix A for a national number that connects with area rape crisis centers.

TABLE 30-2 Rape Myths and Facts

MYTH	FACT
Sex is the motivation for rape.	Rape is an expression of power, anger, violence, and aggression—sex is the weapon.
Rape is an isolated event, a temporary loss of control or lapse in judgment on the part of the rapist.	A rapist is likely to have raped before and to repeat the act in the future. The average number of victims per rapist is seven (Thobaben, 1998).
Most rapes involve men of color raping white women.	Rape is primarily an intraracial crime. The myth of black men raping white women has been perpetuated by racist and sexist sentiments. It also masks the history of white men's sexual violence against women of color.
Rapists are mentally ill or developmentally disabled and are therefore not responsible for their acts.	Rapists cover the full range of age, race, culture, class, and intelligence, and only a minority are psychotic (Thobaben, 1998).
Women's behavior (e.g., manner of dress, makeup, use of language, walk, whereabouts, use of alcohol, etc.) evokes rape.	Persons of all ages are raped: infants, toddlers, children, adolescents, young women, middle-aged women, and elders. They are dressed in a wide variety of garb; 50% are raped in their homes; and the circumstances surrounding the rapes are as varied as the victims themselves.
The majority of rapes are committed by strangers.	The majority of rapes are committed by men known to the victim. Children are at greatest risk from sexual assaults by family members and caretakers. Adolescents and young adult women are most at risk for acquaintance and date rape. Adult women are most likely to be attacked by partners or ex-partners.

 DECISION MAKING

Helping a Rape Victim

You are a nurse in a well-child clinic. A mother asks you, "What would you do if you had been raped?" She is very nervous. She has red eyes and there are tears in them.

♦ How would you answer her?

♦ What would you do?

Partner Response to Rape

Rape usually has a devastating effect on the survivor's partner. While trying to deal with the survivor's emotional response, the partner must also deal with personal reactions ranging from shock to self-blame. Intimacy and sexual relations may be problematic for both partners. The survivor may have flashbacks that interfere with ability to respond to the partner or may have difficulty with sexual advances. Partners often feel that they are somehow being blamed for something they did not do, particularly if the survivor is displacing anger about the rape. The time it takes victims to recover can be surprising to

partners, who want their loved ones to be able to return to their former state of being in a short time. Frequently, there is no discussion around these issues, and the two are unable to support one another. The nurse can anticipate these problems and encourage discussion between the partners. Referral to a counselor who has expertise in this area may be indicated.

Sexual Offenders

Snyder (2000) found that 67% of sexual assaults handled by law enforcement primarily involved juveniles under the age of 12. The majority of these assaults were perpetrated by adult males who were acquaintances or family members. Strangers were the perpetrators in 3% of assaults involving children under the age of 6 and in 5% of the assaults on children aged 6–11. Stranger rape was found to be more prevalent among adult victims (27%). Juveniles under the age of 17 accounted for 23% of sexual assault; 16% of these offenders were under the age of 12. Psychosocial literature offers several theories to explain the preponderance of male sexual offenders. These include but are not limited to male promiscuity, the tendency to separate emotional contact and sexual contact, the desire to be in control, and a preference for partners who are younger, weaker, and immature (Hetherton,

1999). Women are also the perpetrators of sexual assault, although Hetherton's (1999) review of the literature on female perpetrators found themes of denial and minimization on the part of researchers, feminist organizations, and therapists. However, NIBRS statistics found that women committed 12% of the sexual assaults of children under the age of 6 and abused 6% of children aged 6–12.

Intervention for Sex Offenders

The role of the community health nurse with regard to sex offenders includes reporting suspected child sexual abuse, working with families in which a member is an offender and has been incarcerated, having contact with offenders in institutions, or working with a family with whom an offender has been reunited. It is important to be aware of treatment options and to be familiar with the concepts of intervention.

Current research on treatment outcomes among sex offenders (particularly child molesters) indicates that, to be effective, the treatment must be cognitive-behaviorally based and must include a relapse prevention component (Worling & Curwen, 2000). Specific treatment goals are reduction of deviant sexual arousal, enhancement of nondeviant sexual interest, improvement of social skills, and modification of distorted reasoning and beliefs (Worling & Curwen, 2000).

VIOLENCE IN INTIMATE RELATIONSHIPS

Violence occurring within the context of an intimate or familial relationship can be defined in many ways:

- **Domestic violence**—a broad term encompassing a spectrum of violence within a family.
- **Spousal abuse**—the physical, emotional, or sexual abuse perpetrated by either a husband or a wife against the marriage partner. This can also be referred to as marital rape.
- **Wife abuse**—the physical, emotional, or sexual abuse perpetrated by a husband against his wife.
- **Partner abuse**—the physical, emotional, or sexual abuse perpetrated by one partner in an intimate relationship against the other.
- **Battered women**—women who are in relationships in which battering is ongoing.
- **Child abuse**—physical or mental injury, sexual abuse or exploitation, negligent treatment, or maltreatment of a child by a person who is responsible for the child's health or welfare. (Child abuse will be discussed further later in the chapter.)
- **Elder abuse**—physical abuse, neglect, intimidation, cruel punishment, financial abuse, abandonment, isolation, or other treatment of an elder, resulting in physical harm or mental suffering. (Elder abuse will be discussed further later in the chapter.)

Domestic violence can take different forms but frequently involves a combination of assaultive acts, which may include sexual, physical, or emotional abuse or damage or destruction of property (see Table 30-3).

Dynamics of Intimate-Partner Violence

Partner abuse is frequently discussed in terms of males as perpetrators and females as victims, because these relationships constitute the greatest proportion of abusive relationships (Eyler & Cohen, 1999). This viewpoint does not negate or minimize violence that occurs in lesbian and gay

TABLE 30-3	Examples of Partner Violence
TYPE	**ACTIVITIES**
Sexual	Any sexual act or behavior without consent, from degrading name calling with sexual implications (such as whore, tramp, or slut) to rape.
Physical	Any forceful physical behavior such as slapping; shoving; pinching; poking; punching; kicking; spitting; throwing the person bodily; wrestling; pulling hair; throwing things at the person; denying the person sleep, food, or fluids or use of bathroom or confining the person in any manner. Harming self, partner, children, pets, or property.
Emotional	Verbal or behavioral actions that diminish another's self-worth and self-esteem. Examples include belittling name calling (e.g., "You're stupid," "You're ugly") or threatening actions such as taking the children and disappearing; leaving the relationship to be with someone else; or revealing personal or intimate information to others. Other emotional violence includes forcing someone to stay awake; forcing degrading behavior such as eating out of a pet dish; constant blame or ridicule; controlling behavior such as telling a person what to or not to wear, stopping partner from seeing friends or using the phone, timing absences from home, monitoring the mileage on the car.
Property	Breaking partner's special or treasured possessions; punching holes in walls; destroying furniture, doors, windows, or partner's vehicle; throwing things.

relationships or dismiss heterosexual relationships in which men are assaulted by women (Butler, 1995). Valente (2000) notes that, although women commit spousal abuse, they do not inflict the substantial injuries on men that men inflict on women. Figure 30-5 lists current facts concerning domestic violence against women. Table 30-4 lists numerous myths concerning partner abuse with regard to heterosexual couples in which the male is the perpetrator.

Lesbian Battering

The incidence of this violence in relationships is variously reported as from 17% to 26% (Loulan, 1987; Herek & Berril, 1992; Lie, Schlitt, Bush, Montagne, & Reyes, 1991). Less than a dozen academic studies examine the prevalence of battering among lesbian, gay, bisexual, and transgendered couples. There has been very little research on violence in lesbian relationships (Crowell & Burgess, 1996; Tjaden & Thoennes, 2000). Increasing numbers of lesbians are calling battered women's shelters seeking assistance. Lesbians may be less likely to identify themselves as victims secondary to protecting the image of lesbians in the community at large. The risk

FIGURE 30-5   Domestic Violence Fact Sheet
1. Domestic violence is more frequently committed than any other crime.
2. Domestic Violence is the second leading cause of injuries to women in the U.S.
3. Between 21% and 34% of women will be battered in their lifetime.
4. Women are 7–14 times more likely than men to be victims of severe physical assault from an intimate partner.
5. Murder of women by male partners accounts for one-third of all homicides against women.
6. In almost half of the cases of attempted suicide there is a diagnosis of domestic abuse.
From "Providing Medical Care and Advocacy for Survivors of Domestic Abuse," by S. A. Eisenstat and B. Zimmer, 1998, *Journal of Clinical Outcomes Management, 5,* pp. 54–64, "How to Assess and Intervene in Domestic Violence Situations," by K. Cassidy, 1999, *Home Health Care Nurse, 17,* pp. 665–671, "Screening Men for Partner Violence in a Primary Care Setting," by K. A. Oriel and M. F. Fleming, 1998. *Journal of Family Practice, 46,* pp. 493–498.

TABLE 30-4   Myths and Facts about Partner Abuse

MYTH	FACT
Battering happens primarily in low-income families.	Battering and other forms of abuse occur in all income groups. Poorer people rely more often on social service agencies, police, emergency rooms, and courts for assistance; hence statistics are higher for that population. Middle-class and upper-class individuals are more able to afford attorneys, private therapists, and personal physicians, consequently avoiding reports that contribute to statistical findings.
Battered women are masochistic. Why doesn't she leave?	Such questions maintain focus on the victim's behavior and ignore the fact that the batterer has no right to abuse. Many people stay in relationships, trying one thing after another, thinking their changes will stop the abuse. Some who are economically or emotionally dependent on the batterer feel trapped.
Women of color are battered more often than white women.	The myth is often linked with the socioeconomic myth that battering occurs only in low-income families. There are few comparative research studies that specifically explore domestic violence among various ethnic or cultural groups. Some studies have found that when controlling for social class, there is no difference between African American and European American couples with regard to incidence of abuse (Eyler & Cohen, 1999).
Men who beat women are mentally ill.	Studies have failed to identify any consistent psychiatric diagnosis among batterers, but common personality traits include a need for power and control and denial of the extent of violence and low self-esteem (Oriel & Fleming, 1998).
Battering occurs because the man is drunk and out of control.	The relationship between alcohol and battering is unclear, and current research shows a widely varying range of prevalence. Many abusive men do not drink.

of exposing oneself to a heterosexual agency may be perceived as greater than the risk of remaining silent. Battered lesbians need the same services as any other abused woman but are also dealing with the abuse of a homophobic society and the possibility of homophobia within the agency involved. Lesbians batter for the same reasons that men batter, and threat of violence is just as traumatizing to the victims as in other situations.

Gay Male Violence

Like abuse in the lesbian community, battering between gay male partners is poorly studied. Abused men are often afraid or embarrassed to tell anyone about the violence in their relationship. One partner is usually more violent than the other; the fact that the victim, like any battering victim, may engage in self-defense does not mean that the partners are equally violent. The estimates of annual rates of relationship violence for gay men is from 11% to 20% (Community United Against Violence, 1998; Tjaden & Thoennes, 2000).

Learned Helplessness

Learned helplessness, as applied to domestic violence by Walker (1979), describes the behavior resulting from learning that responses cannot control certain outcomes (Valente, 2000). Chronic feelings of powerlessness and decreasing motivation to respond ensue. These responses in turn lead to passivity, submissiveness, and helplessness.

Abuse occurs randomly and is not necessarily connected to any particular action or behavior. Abuse victims learn that, regardless of how they change or try to do things differently, the abuse continues. The victim cannot predict which responses will work in a given situation and avoids any unknown situations. To a person in a state of learned helplessness, the known—even the known violence—holds less fear than the unknown. Depression is well documented as a component of learned helplessness, although abused women frequently remain functional in terms of work, caring for their children, and performing activities of daily living (ADL). The combination of helplessness and depression places women and their children at high risk for self-harm.

Cycle of Violence

Walker (1979) proposed the cycle theory of violence. The cycle consists of three phrases: the tension-building phase, the battering incident or explosion, and the aftermath or honeymoon phase. The cycle is represented in Figure 30-6 and describes the usual process through which the individual passes.

FIGURE 30-6 Cycle of Violence

Phase One: Tension Building

Batterer Behavior	Victim Behavior
Irritable.	Avoids confrontation.
Tense.	Attempts to control environment to keep batterer calm.
Minor outbursts.	Makes excuses for his behavior.
Attempts to control rage or meter violence in small doses.	May provoke explosion to get explosion over with.

Phase Two: Explosion/Battering Incident

Batterer Behavior	Victim Behavior
Rage overrides control. Battering occurs. May be progressive and last for a number of hours.	May express rage, may fight back, though usually too fearful of more serious injury. If has the opportunity to leave, may hide until she feels batterer is back in control

Phase Three: Honeymoon Phase/Hearts and Flowers Phase

Batterer Behavior	Victim Behavior
Apologetic.	Wants to believe this is the last time.
Remorseful. Makes promises to get help, stop drinking, enter therapy, etc. Swears this will never happen again.	Accepts gifts, discusses plans for getting help.
Give gifts, helps around the house, mood lightens.	Moves into denial.

Return to Phase One—Cycles Shorten

Adapted from "The Cycle of Domestic Violence and the Barriers to Treatment," by L. A. Jensen, 2000, *Nurse Practitioner, 25*(5), pp. 26–29; *The Battered Woman,* by L. Walker, 1979, New York: Harper & Row.

Intervention with Intimate-Partner Violence Victims

Early identification of partner abuse is the first goal of intervention. Given the prevalence of intimate-partner violence, routine screening of all women should be part of the health history. The nurse's approach to exploring violence among family members must be nonjudgmental and empathetic in order to facilitate trust. Eisenstat and Zimmer (1998) document clues and physical signs that should raise the index of suspicion for abuse. These are listed in Figure 30-7.

Once alerted to the possibility of abuse, the nurse needs to address concerns to the victim directly and in a caring manner. This discussion should take place in a safe and private setting away from the suspected assailant. Questions can be intertwined with information about abuse in order to communicate an understanding of the issue and to indicate what kinds of assistance are available in the community, such as emergency shelters, counselors trained in intimate-partner violence, male anti-violence programs, and legal services to assist with restraining orders. Urge the client to have an intimate-partner violence plan. Preparation should consist of having the following items packed in a box or suitcase and kept in a safe and trusted place such as the home of a reliable neighbor, friend, or relative:

1. Identification: a duplicate driver's license, passport, and birth certificate
2. Cash: at least enough for a couple of nights shelter, food, perhaps a bus ticket
3. Emergency phone numbers: women's shelter, legal services
4. An extra set of car keys
5. Clothing for self and children

Risk Factors for Violence

There are certain characteristics that research has found to be strongly correlated with violent men. Oriel and Fleming (1998) analyzed 237 surveys designed to detect marital violence. They found three statistically significant predictors of violent behavior: depression, alcohol use, and personal history of abuse. Eyler and Cohen (1999) point to some common characteristics shared by abusive men, including rigid sex role stereotypes, low self-esteem, a need for power and control, and a tendency to minimize and deny their problem. See Figure 30-8 for a summary of these risk factors.

FIGURE 30-7 Indicators of Domestic Abuse

1. Complaints of insomnia and nightmares.
2. Passivity and lack of energy.
3. Somatic symptoms such as headaches, gastrointestinal complaints, asthma, chronic nonspecific pain.
4. Frequent emergency room visits with escalating injuries; explanations that fail to match injuries.
5. Depression, suicide attempts.
6. Substance abuse.
7. Anorexia, bulimia.
8. Sexual assault.
9. Suggestive injuries such as cigarette burns; black eyes; facial bruising or facial lacerations; injuries to the chest, back, breast, abdomen and/or genitalia; injury patterns that indicate use of belts, bites, hands, fists.
10. Anxiety, fear demonstrated when being interviewed.
11. Turning to partner before answering questions; visible fear when partner is in the room.
12. Partner consistently speaks for the person suspected of being abused.
13. The partner is overly solicitous and condescending to the partner who may be the victim of abuse.
14. One partner adheres rigidly to traditional roles and expects the other partner to meet needs and follow directions.

Adapted from "Providing Medical Care and Advocacy for Survivors of Domestic Violence," by S. A. Eisenstat and B. Zimmer, 1998, *Journal of Clinical Outcomes Management, 5,* pp. 54–64.

FIGURE 30-8 Characteristics of Batterers

Alcohol/Drug Abuse

History of Childhood Abuse

Witnessing Domestic Violence As a Child

Social Isolation

Rigid Sex Role Definition

Rigid Family Rules

History of Other Abusive Relationships

Low Self Esteem

Possessiveness

Jealousy

Adapted from "Male-Male Dimensions of Male-Female Battering: A New Look at Domestic Violence," by J. L. Jennings and C. M. Murphy, 2000, *Psychology of Men and Masculinity, 1*(1), pp. 21–29; "Case Studies in Partner Violence," by A. E. Eyler and M. Cohen, 1999, *American Family Physician, 60*(9), pp. 2569–2576. "Screening Men for Partner Violence in a Primary Care Setting," by K. A. Oriel and M. F. Fleming, 1998, *Journal of Family Practice, 46*(6), pp. 493–498.

Intervention for Batterers

Health professionals have traditionally not specifically focused on the **batterer,** one who beats, strikes, or pounds another person, as the problem in cases of family violence (Nicolette & Nuovo, 1999). Instead the violence has been viewed as a family problem and is frequently addressed by referral for family or couple therapy. Some believe that this approach sends a message of shared responsibility, deemphasizes the batterer's behavior, and ignores the very real danger to the victim. If the couple stays together, conjoint therapy may eventually play a role in treatment, but it is generally introduced after the batterer has addressed the violence in a treatment format. Eyler and Cohen (1999) also note the fact that the perpetrator may stop physical violence only to replace it with more subtle forms of violence such as psychological abuse and intimidation.

Safety for the victims of domestic violence is the first priority in the treatment of batterers. Currently the victim and children generally leave their home and find safety in a shelter. A consideration for future treatment programs for assailants might be a shelter in which the *batterers* are confined until it is determined that they are in control of their behavior. Programs designed to treat batterers are relatively new, and research regarding effective intervention is still in its infancy. Grass-roots antiviolence self-help collectives were the first wave of treatment for batterers. These programs grew out of the feminist movement and usually combined a social analysis of domestic violence with a counseling element emphasizing nonviolent masculinity.

In the early 1990s professional organizations took their first steps toward focusing on family violence as a health issue, and opportunities for professional training have increased Schroeder & Weber (1998). Likewise, the criminal justice system has developed training programs specific to domestic violence, and some progress is being made with regard to how battering is handled by the police and the courts. One such change is the institution of mandatory arrest laws for perpetrators of spousal abuse in some areas. Programs tend to exclude batterers who are mentally ill or developmentally disabled or who cannot admit their violence. Commonalities among treatment programs are listed in Figure 30-9.

Outcome studies are lacking, and it is difficult to say which approach works in the short or long term. It is also doubtful that any one approach will work for all offenders. We need to be able to identify what constitutes progress and when programs need to be altered to meet the needs of a particular participant. Eyler and Cohen (1999) also note the importance of being able to measure more subtle forms of violence that may replace physical abuse in the treated offender. Currently there are more questions than answers about what constitutes effective intervention and prevents recidivism. The issue of

FIGURE 30-9 Common Components of Treatment Programs for Batterers

Lethality assessment involves an assessment of the batterer's history with regard to the severity and frequency of the violence, substance abuse, psychiatric impairment, abuse toward children, current stressors, and access to victims. Higher levels of lethality may call for other forms of intervention. Lethality assessment should be ongoing throughout the course of treatment and the interventions adjusted to prevent further violence.

Group treatment is utilized because of its cost effectiveness and its potential for the batterers to gain insight into and to understand their behavior through interpersonal interaction and feedback.

Client accountability is an approach that holds the batterer accountable for past, present, and future actions. Minimization, projection of blame, and lack of motivation are addressed and challenged. If a batterer reoffends while in treatment, there must be a predictable and consistent response from the treating staff including making a report about the new offense. It is important that the legal system and the health care system coordinate their efforts.

The psychoeducational approach relies on the belief that violence is learned and can be unlearned. The goal is to teach new behaviors and attitudes that will prevent any future episodes of violence. Issues might include such things as: learning about the disinhibiting effects of drugs and alcohol; examining gender role socialization and the links to violence; defining what constitutes violence; examining the effects of violence on children; identifying how the media glamorize violence, including violence against women; learning techniques of stress management and anger management; and recognizing the covert ways in which society sanctions male violence and discourages male sensitivity.

Adapted from "Reframing Our Approach to Domestic Violence: The Cyclic Batterer Syndrome," by J. Nicollete and J. Nuovo, 1999, *American Family Physician, 60,* pp. 2498–2501.

domestic violence is coming more clearly into focus and is beginning to receive the attention it deserves.

Relationship Violence and Its Effects on the Family

The family is a complex system made up of individuals with multiple needs, different strengths, and varying coping mechanisms. Violence between partners was discussed earlier, but the impact on the family is deserving of further exploration.

Violence between parents or parental figures affects the children in a family. Although witnessing family violence is not always harmful, studies indicate that many children are negatively affected. Song et al. (1998) refer

RESEARCH FOCUS

Study Problem/Purpose

To examine the effectiveness of home visitation programs in preventing child abuse when domestic violence is a family dynamic. The study hypothesis was that home visitation is less effective in the presence of domestic violence.

Methods

This was a 15-year follow-up to the original research, which involved 324 mothers and their children who participated in a home visitation program between 1978 and 1980. The families were divided into four treatment groups; two of the groups received home visitation from nurses and two did not. At the 15-year follow-up the mothers were asked to recall the number of months they received Aid to Families with Dependent Children (AFDC) benefits, major life events, and domestic violence exposure. Mothers gave the researchers consent to review any Child Protective Services records.

Findings

Results demonstrated significantly fewer incidents of child abuse involving the mother as perpetrator in families who were receiving home visitation compared to families who did not. Almost half of the women reported some form of domestic violence following the birth of the study child. The home visitations had no impact on the domestic violence but there was less maltreatment of the children during the 15-year interval. The implication is that domestic violence limits the effectiveness of interventions designed to reduce child abuse.

Conclusion

Home visitation does have an impact on reducing child maltreatment but has no impact on the incidence of domestic violence. It is important to question how the nurse could have been more conscious of the domestic violence. How can the home visitation program, designed to educate mothers about appropriate child care, incorporate screening and intervention for domestic violence?

Source: EcKenrode, J., Ganzel, B., Henderson, C. R., Smith, E., Olds, D. L., Powers, J., Cole, R., Kitzman, H., & Sidora, K. (2000). Preventing child abuse and neglect with a program of nurse visitation. Journal of the American Medical Association, 284 (11), 1385–1391.

to a number of studies indicating that children who are exposed to spousal abuse have a variety of adjustment problems. Boys tend to demonstrate bullying behavior, temper tantrums, and cruel acts. Girls tend to exhibit anxiety, depression, perfectionism, and excessive neediness. When these children are adults, they will have a greater incidence of alcohol and drug dependency and will be more likely to abuse their children. Abused children are more likely than their nonabused peers to use aggression as a response to conflict or frustration, and the combination of witnessing violence and being the victim of abuse doubles the acceptability of violence as a solution to problems (Song et al., 1998).

Bethea (1999) cites studies showing that child abuse is 15 times more likely to occur in families where wife abuse is present. The community health nurse who identifies spousal battery must suspect abuse of children in the family. When children demonstrate behavioral problems, the nurse should obtain a careful history about family dynamics, including past or present violence.

CHILD ABUSE

Child abuse is another area in which nurses must examine their own biases and belief systems to avoid being blinded to possibilities. Any family of any race, class, income bracket, religious background, neighborhood, or sexual orientation can be violent or neglect their children. Keep family violence or neglect as an assessment possibility regardless of the external appearance of the family and their material possessions.

Characteristics of Child Abuse

Although the standards for what constitutes child abuse varies from state to state, there are four agreed-upon types of child abuse: physical abuse, emotional abuse, sexual abuse, and neglect. Table 30-5 identifies the physical and emotional indicators of child abuse. Each year approximately 160,000 children are severely abused, over 3 million are abused and or neglected, and 1000–2000 die as a result

TABLE 30-5 Indicators of Different Types of Child Abuse

TYPE	INDICATORS
Physical	History given fails to match injury Bruises on soft tissues and on multiple planes of the body: e.g., on the buttocks, lower back, cheeks, genitals Bruises in various stages of healing Finger marks on the neck indicative of choking Hand imprints on the face or body Human bites Cigarette, immersion, or scalding burns Unexplained fractures and pattern of healed fractures Bilateral black eyes Retinal detachment, dislocated lens, traumatic cataracts (shaken-baby syndrome) Subdural hematoma (shaken-baby syndrome) Abdominal injuries
Sexual	Child reports sexual abuse Frequent urinary tract infections Frequent yeast infections Sexually transmitted diseases Perianal bruising or tears Decreased anal tone Encopresis/enuresis at inappropriate developmental stage Genital pain or itching Genital trauma and/or bleeding Excessive masturbation Sexual acting out with younger children Age-inappropriate sexualized behavior or language Pregnancy Promiscuity, prostitution
Emotional	Failure to thrive Speech disorders Developmental delays Regression Poor social skills, antisocial behavior
Neglect	Lack of adult supervision, inappropriate supervision (e.g., children supervising children) Poor hygiene Hunger, distended abdomen, signs of malnutrition, anemia, stealing food Teeth in poor repair Clothing inappropriate to weather conditions
All types: emotional signs	Withdrawal, depression, suicidality, anxiety, or fear Self-destructive behaviors Substance abuse Sudden changes in behavior Sudden school difficulties Dramatic mood extremes Sleep disorders Nightmares Repeated runaway Aggression

of assault by their caretaker, generally a parent (Bethea, 1999). Children under the age of 5 are the most vulnerable to dying secondary to child abuse; 82% of fatalities involve children under five years of age and 41% involve children under one year of age (Nester, 1998). Although these numbers are staggering, they are thought by many to be a conservative estimate (Herman-Giddens, Brown, & Verbiest, 1999). In the United States, child neglect accounts for 56% of abuse, followed by physical, sexual, and emotional abuse (Mulryan, Catters, & Fagin, 2000).

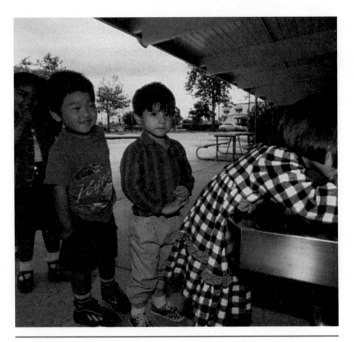

Child abuse can occur in any family regardless of race, class, income bracket, religious background, neighborhood, or sexual orientation.

Nursing Assessment

The community health nurse who works with families and individuals is in a position to recognize abuse and to advocate for the child. Advocacy is difficult, however, if the nurse cannot maintain the objectivity necessary for obtaining a history. Because a thorough history taking is an important aspect of advocacy, the nurse who finds it difficult to address the issue adequately should ask for assistance and consultation from another professional. Differentiating between abuse and discipline may also pose a problem. Any suspicious finding warrants a thorough history and a complete physical assessment to provide for the ultimate safety of the child.

There are specific characteristics that can be identified through assessment that increase the risk for child abuse. See Figure 30-10 for a list of these factors.

Discipline may be classified as abusive when a child is struck with objects such as cords, hairbrushes, or sticks; when the adult uses a fist, knee, or foot to hit the child; or when sensitive body parts such as the head, face, or abdomen are involved. In assessing any type of child injury, the nurse must remain alert to the possibility of abuse whenever the signs and symptoms fail to

Children are frequently referred to as innocent. They are also vulnerable by virtue of their size, age, basic dependency on adults, and lack of power. They are at greatest risk of being injured in their own home by a family member or other care provider. Research shows that child victims are three times more likely to be abused by their fathers than by their mothers (Bethea, 1999). Severe child abuse resulting in death is most commonly perpetrated by male caretakers and parents (Herman-Giddens et al., 1999).

There continues to be ambivalence about what constitutes child abuse from a community perspective. Children have been viewed as the property of their parents for centuries, and the community has been reluctant to interfere in matters concerning childrearing. Community endorsement contributes to the notion that parents have the right to use abusive forms of discipline with their own children. Definitions and perceptions of the seriousness of child abuse vary by culture, socioeconomic groups, and neighborhoods. Korbin, Coulton, Lindstrom-Ufuti, and Spilsbury (2000) review 10 studies that examine the definitions of child maltreatment among diverse populations. The variation in cultural, ethnic, and socioeconomic norms is striking and speaks to the importance of understanding the population being served if prevention and intervention efforts are to be successful.

FIGURE 30-10 Child Abuse Risk Factors

Unplanned, Unwanted Pregancy

Teenage Parent(s)

Single Parent

Closely Spaced Children

History of Child Abuse

Substance Abuse

Social Isolation

Poor Support System

Limited Knowledge of Child Development

Previous Report to Child Protective Services

Previous History of Child Abuse

Partner Violence

Young Children, Age Three and Under

Child is the Result of an Unwanted Pregancy

Sibling Younger than 18 Months Already in the Home

Children with Developmental Delays or Chronic Disease

Adapted from "Primary Prevention of Child Abuse," by L. Bethea, 1999, *American Family Physician, 59*(6), pp. 1577–1585; *The Nurse Practioner,* by C. B. Nester, 1998, PA: Springhouse Corporation; *Child Maltreatment,* by U.S. Department of Health and Human Services, 1998, *Reports from the States to the National Child Abuse and Neglect Data System,* Washington, DC: U.S. Government Printing Office.

match the history given by the child's caretaker or the description of the method of injury fails to match the child's developmental or motor skills.

Child Neglect

Child neglect and psychological maltreatment are diagnosed when the family fails to provide for a child's basic needs of food, clothing, shelter, supervision, education, emotional affection and stimulation, and health care. Child neglect is the most frequently reported form of child maltreatment.

The nursing assessment of child neglect may be problematic if the family is struggling with limited resources or physical disabilities. A careful history is important to determine if there are resources that are not being utilized to meet the child's needs. If the family does not have the resources to provide for the child's basic needs, the nurse can offer referrals to social service agencies that can assist. Depending on the particular manifestation of neglect, the nurse should assess what type of education and support the family might need to improve the care of the child. If, for instance, the neglect involves inadequate or inappropriate clothing, the nurse might explore how the parents see this problem, taking into consideration the issues raised in Figure 30-11.

The parents' childhoods should also be explored. If they were neglected, they may be parenting in the only way they know how. These are issues that have the potential to respond to education, counseling, and support. An important nursing intervention is teaching parents specific skills for increasing positive parent-child interactions, improving problem-solving abilities, and enhancing personal hygiene and nutritional skills. Family therapy may be another helpful adjunct if the family is amenable. Cultural and religious beliefs should be assessed because some behaviors that appear neglectful may stem from a family's belief system. If those beliefs are placing the child at risk, the nurse should consult with a child abuse specialist to determine how to proceed.

Neglect can be a precursor to other types of abuse: It might exist in tandem with other abuses or as a singular form of abuse. Though neglect is less externally dramatic than other forms of child abuse, the long-term sequelae and potential for adult dysfunction are serious (Bethea, 1999).

Physical Abuse

As shown in Table 30-5, certain types of injuries are characteristic of physical abuse. These include certain types and patterns of bruises, burns, fractures, and other injuries, as shown in Table 30-6. Bruises that are common in childhood are generally found over a bony prominence, such as an elbow, whereas bruising of soft tissue is suggestive of abuse. Scalding is the most common burn injury in children (Scales, Fleischer, & Sinal, 1999). An accidental burn that occurs from a splashdown of a hot

---

FIGURE 30-11 Points for the Nurse to Consider When Exploring Reasons for a Child's Inappropriate Clothing

- Is clothing too large, too small, or inappropriate for the child's developmental stage?

- Is the child dressing himself or herself without adult supervision or input?

- Is clothing being handed down and forced to fit?

- Do the parents have unrealistic expectations of the child's ability to cope with environmental realities such as cold weather?

- Is either parent abusing substances and thus depleting the family income and contributing to poor decision making?

TABLE 30-6 Patterns of Certain Abusive Injuries to Children

TYPE	PATTERN
Bruises	On soft tissue, especially lower back and buttocks; multiple sites; or in various stages of healing. Any bruising on an infant, though bleeding disorders should be ruled out.
Burns	On the back or buttocks, cigarette burns, branding types of burns such as those from a hot iron, comb, or curling iron; or glove-stocking pattern burns from immersion of the arms or legs in hot water.
Fractures	Spiral or transverse fractures of the humerus or femur and fractures of the scapula or sternum. Rib fractures in infants or children under 3 are almost always diagnostic of abuse, as are skull fractures or subdural hematomas in the first year of life, with irritability, vomiting, apnea, seizures, lethargy, poor feeding, or unexplained unconsciousness. There may be bruising on the shoulders, armpits, or abdomen where the baby was grabbed.
Abdominal	There may be no sign of external injury, or signs may be limited to mild bruising.

From "Differential Diagnosis of Abuse Injuries in Infants and Young Children," by B. W. Mayer and P. Burns, 2000, Nurse Practitioner, *25(10), pp. 15–35.*

✳ DECISION MAKING

"Problem Child"

You are making a first home visit to a family for postpartum follow-up. Their doctor was concerned about the family situation because the mother, Mary, had expressed concern that her husband, Jim, would not like it if the new baby cried much. He was very busy at work and needed his sleep and quiet time in the evening. They returned from the hospital two days ago with a newborn boy, Robert. There is also a three-year-old girl, Annette, in the family. Mary tells you that Robert is crying a lot and Annette is constantly bothering her and her husband for attention. She had no idea it would be so difficult. She has had little sleep since she got home. Her husband, who is Annette's stepfather, has been no help during the day. He is a stockbroker and is kept very busy. He is angry at Annette because she has been so clingy, but Mary tells you that she is relieved because Annette stayed away from him last evening. You note a large bruise on Annette's arm that looks like finger marks.

◆ Are there signs in this family that might suggest child abuse or potential abuse? What type of abuse?

◆ As the nurse, how would you proceed with the visit?

◆ What community resources might help?

◆ How would you follow up on the family after this visit?

---

liquid generally will be more severe on the upper body than on the lower body because the liquid cools as it moves downward. Intentional burns tend to be on the feet or the hands. Scales et al. (1999) may be referred to for ways the nurse can differentiate healing cigarette burns from impetigo or other skin lesions. Some cultures use folk remedies such as hot oils, herbs, or cupping that may imitate burn marks on a child's back. It is important to explore this possibility.

Abusive head trauma in infancy is the most common type of child abuse resulting in death (Duhaime, Christian, Rorke, & Zimmerman, 1999). Abusive head injury is also referred to as the shaken-baby syndrome, although Duhaime et al. (1999) make the point that this is a misnomer because the mechanism of injury may be either shaking or impact trauma. In either event, the trauma results in central nervous system damage.

Abdominal injuries are the second leading cause of death among abused children. Any abdominal injury of undetermined etiology should be assessed for abuse. These injuries may be secondary to the child's being kicked or punched in the abdomen (Mayer & Burns, 2000).

Sexual Abuse

Sexual abuse of children is any sexual act with a child. It may or may not involve violence; it may or may not involve force or coercion depending on the age of the child.

Male and female children of all ages, from infancy to adolescence, may be victims of sexual assault. Snyder's (2000) extensive statistical documentation indicates that 27% of victims under the age of 12 were male, whereas females are six times as likely as males to be the victims of sexual assaults. A male child is most likely to be a victim of sexual assault at age 4 and a female's year of greatest risk is age 14. Sexual abuse of both boys and girls is perpetrated by a male in 96% of the cases. A fraction of these (3%) are perpetrated by a stranger.

Emotional Abuse

Emotional abuse is a component of all forms of abuse in which verbal or behavioral actions diminish another's self-worth and self-esteem. In itself, it is the least reported form of abuse (Mulryan et al., 2000). When it exists alone, it can be difficult to identify and even more difficult to validate for the purposes of reporting. Observing family dynamics, particularly how children are talked to, disciplined, and attended to, offers clues to the emotional climate. Emotional abuse includes name calling, put-downs, and isolating, stigmatizing, humiliating, or ignoring the child.

Differentiating between a child who is emotionally abused and a child who is emotionally disturbed may be challenging because presentations are so similar. To further complicate matters, characteristics such as speech disorders, learning disabilities, and failure to thrive are identified in children who *may or may not* suffer from abuse or an emotional disorder. McAllister (2000) suggests that a detailed psychosocial assessment of the family may help differentiate between emotional abuse and an emotional disturbance. He generalizes that parents of emotionally disturbed children tend to recognize that there is a problem and seek help, whereas parents of emotionally abused children may deny that there is a problem and refuse help.

Parents who are emotionally abusive may benefit from nonjudgmental education and positive role modeling. They may need information about how to discourage behaviors without making the child feel like a bad person. Time-outs, loss of privileges, rewards for positive behaviors, and elimination of name calling and put-downs may be new concepts to the family. Parental education

RESEARCH FOCUS

Corporal Punishment and Primary Prevention of Physical Abuse

Study Problem/Purpose

To alert health providers that there is the potential for primary prevention of physical abuse by educating parents to end or reduce corporal punishment.

Methods

A 1999 special issue of *Child Abuse and Neglect, "A National Call to Action: Working Toward the Elimination of Child Maltreatment,"* was reviewed to assess the coverage of corporal punishment as a child abuse issue.

Findings

Corporal punishment was not addressed in any of the articles published in the special edition.

Implications

Parent education programs have ignored corporal punishment, thereby contributing to the American cultural belief that hitting children is sometimes necessary. Corporal punishment needs to be addressed as an aspect of violent socialization of children. Child maltreatment needs to be eliminated if we want to protect children from the risk of social and psychological problems associated with hurting children.

Source: Straus, M. A. (2000). Corporal punishment and primary prevention of physical abuse. Child Abuse and Neglect, 24(9), 1109–1114.

should include the impact that this type of treatment has on their child's self-esteem and emotional adjustment in later years. Parents may benefit from classes on parenting techniques in addition to family therapy.

Violence and Adolescents

Adolescents are often overlooked when family violence is assessed, yet statistics indicate that they experience disproportionately high levels of abuse (Christoffel, Spivack, & Witwer, 2000). Some warning signs of possible past or present abuse include behaviors such as chronically running away, sexual promiscuity (particularly prostitution), gang involvement, truancy, substance abuse, eating disorders, and self-abusive behaviors. Adolescents demonstrating these behaviors should always be carefully and privately assessed for an abuse history.

Adolescents between the ages of 12 and 19 years are more likely to be victims of violence than adults over the age of 19. According to Song et al. (1998), young people in this age group experience three times as many rapes and higher rates of severe violence than their adult counterparts.

Violence is a major cause of injury and death among adolescents, with homicide ranking as the second leading cause of death for all 15- to 19-year-olds in the United States. African American adolescent males between the ages of 15 and 19 are at greatest risk for fight-related assaults and death from homicide. Johnson, Fein, Campbell, and Ginsburg (1999) comment that the racial difference is related to poverty and when poverty is factored out the increase in African American statistics is nullified.

Urban youths have the highest rates of firearm-related homicides. Although nonurban areas have lower numbers of homicides, nonurban rates among teens are substantially higher in the United States than in many other industrialized nations (Johnson et al., 1999). Teen homicide victims are most likely to be killed by an acquaintance of the same race. In 35% of the cases the victim is also carrying a gun. Suicide ranks as the third leading cause of death among all adolescents and young adults aged 15–24 (Johnson et al., 1999). Bull et al. (2000) found an association between the legal purchase of a handgun and an increased risk of violent death through both homicide and suicide. Given these statistics, it is hard to believe that from 1993 to 1997 the firearm homicide rate for 15- to 24-year-olds fell by 29%. No source was found that explained this decline (Christoffel, Spivack, & Witwer, 2000).

Nursing Interventions

Nursing interventions for all types of child abuse have many commonalties. It is important to first develop a trusting relationship with the parents and the child. Be direct but supportive. Once a holistic history has been obtained, explore with the parents how the events that led to the abuse can be altered in the future and alternative strategies for managing the children. Health teaching is important, including parenting skill and information regarding basic growth and development. Many times, parents are not aware of what to expect from their child at different ages, and if they are expecting too much, the child cannot comply and the parents perceive this behavior as wrong and in need of punishment. For more information about parenting, see Chapter 22. Discussion of strategies for anger control is necessary. If possible, refer them to a group that teaches anger control. They can see that they are not the only ones with the problem and be helped by hearing other peoples' stories (Smith-DiJulio, 1998; Townsend, 2000; Urbancic, 2000).

It is important to discuss the laws on child abuse and help the family to be comfortable cooperating with Child Protective Services. If they can see this agency as providing help rather than punishment, they will be less likely to resist these services. Role model providing care to the child when possible. If the child needs hospitalization, encourage the involvement of the parents and use opportunities to teach them how to care for the child effectively. Assist parents to verbalize their understanding of the impact of abuse on their child and how they can prevent it in the future. Discuss the short- and long-term psychological effects on the child (Smith-DiJulio, 1998; Townsend, 2000; Urbancic, 2000).

Coordination of services to the family is a significant role of the community health nurse. Finding and monitoring attendance of the parents at parenting and anger management classes will be necessary. Often, the nurse acts as liaison with Child Protective Services. Other agencies that will be involved are the school and, sometimes, the church (Urbancic, 2000). It is vital that the nurse make sure that emotional and psychological support is adequately given to the child. Greenwalt, Sklare, and Portes (1998) point out that when the focus is on making the child safe and keeping the family together, this aspect of care is often overlooked.

Sexual Abuse

In addition to the above interventions, children who have been victims of child sexual abuse require some additional interventions. The child needs to be reassured that he or she is safe and that no one will hurt him or her again. Encourage the child to talk about his or her fears and concerns. It is particularly important to reassure him or her that he or she is not to blame and that his or her abuser did a bad thing to hurt him or her. Assess and strengthen the mother's coping ability by educating her about potential resources and the signs and symptoms of abuse that the child may exhibit and how to support the child. Be sure to assess the mother for her ability to cope with possible feelings of grief and betrayal. Counseling is likely to be necessary for both the parents and the child. Be sure that the child, if a girl, is examined for human papillomavirus (HPV). It may be a clue that sexual abuse has

taken place and puts the child at risk for cervical cancer (Toomey & Bernstein, 2001). The nurse can help the family to understand and accept therapeutic services which they may be reluctant to do in the beginning of treatment. The nurse can also provide information about referrals, such as a psychotherapist, mental health clinic, or community advocacy groups (Smith-DiJulio, 1998; Townsend, 2000; Urbancic, 2000).

ELDER ABUSE

The earliest research concerning elder abuse was completed in the 1970s. Current statistics suggest that 10% of the elder population is subject to caregiver abuse (Gray-Vickery, 2000). Elders are at greatest risk of being abused by a family member who is also the caregiver and lives with the victim (Gray-Vickery, 2000). Eighty percent of care in the home is provided by a woman, often a daughter. Sons are more likely to perpetrate active physical abuse; daughters are more likely to be responsible for emotional abuse or neglect. Husbands caring for their ailing wives are at high risk for caregiver overload and subsequent abuse secondary to limited nurturing experience, inadequate training, and limited support (Gray-Vickery, 2000). In general, caregivers are at greater risk to abuse if they do not know the normal physical and cognitive changes that accompany aging. Prevention of caregiver overload is one of the primary interventions the nurse can make to avoid elder abuse.

Nursing Assessment

Caregiver stress placing the elder at risk for abuse may be generated by events that are unrelated to the role of caretaking (Gray-Vickery, 2000). Typical caregiver stressors include marriage, divorce, pregnancy, substance abuse problems, job loss, and financial problems. Role-related stressors tend to be associated with the caregiver's perceptions of the role as a burden, increased dependency of the elder on the caregiver for activities of daily living, fecal or urinary incontinence, insomnia, and intellectual impairment. Another factor is the age of abusers. Many are elderly themselves and suffer from a variety of difficulties such as mental and physical impairment, low levels of social support, and substance abuse (Swagerty, Takahashi, & Evans, 1999).

Social isolation also places elders at greater risk for abuse. The socially isolated elder is not observed by others who might identify changes in behavior or appearance, and he or she has no one to talk to about possible mistreatment. The home health care or public health nurse is in a position to develop a relationship with the primary caregiver, to monitor for stressors, to assess the elder, and to promote self-care in the caretaker as well as in the elder when that is possible.

Elder abuse may be categorized as physical, financial, or psychological. Physical abuse includes physical or sexual assault, neglect, and medical mismanagement. Neglect, including self-neglect, accounts for the largest percentage of elder abuse reports, followed by physical, financial, and psychological abuse (Gray-Vickery, 2000). Table 30-7 gives examples of types of abuse in each category. Figure 30-12 lists signs of physical mistreatment in the elderly.

In cases of suspected abuse, assessment includes the elder's dependency needs, social situation, and relevant aspects of the history and physical examination. Culture, belief systems, and income must be evaluated as part of the assessment. Some folk treatments might be mistaken for abuse, and poverty may manifest in signs similar to neglect (e.g., unfilled prescriptions or inadequate diet). Certain religious beliefs involve the refusal of blood products or other medical interventions. The nurse will be challenged to respect the family's beliefs and maintain their dignity while assuring that the elder is not suffering or at risk secondary to these realities.

Assessing the potential for abuse is an important aspect of prevention. The nurse's assessment should include both the elder and the caretaker. When the caretaker is a family member, family dynamics should be explored. Allan, (1998) discusses the increase in caregiver roles by younger family members as older members live longer. This phenomenon increases the family's stress by taxing financial, emotional, and physical resources and makes the experience of caretaking a burden. This feeling of being burdened sets the stage for abusive behaviors. Families with long-term dysfunctional patterns are suspect for abuse potential as are caregivers with a history of having been abused themselves. Psychological problems and substance abuse in either the caretaker or the elder have also been found to be linked to abuse.

Evaluating the caregivers' concerns, their feelings about providing care for the family member, their ability to provide that care, and their need for support, counseling, or health care provides the nurse with the information needed to formulate prevention planning. Depending on what the family is comfortable with and is able to afford, the use of home health aides, sitters, temporary placement in an extended-care facility, or intermittent respite care by alternating family members and friends might be coordinated by the nurse. Figure 30-13 lists examples of assessment questions.

Longstanding dysfunctional family problems that create a potential for abuse should be identified and discussed. These may not be resolvable, but discussing them allows for supportive interventions such as counseling or shared responsibility for caregiving. The family can benefit from information about normal changes associated with aging as well as specific information about any existing illness or disability. Teaching specific skills needed to care for the elder and supervising return

---

✳ DECISION MAKING

An Ethical Issue

If an elder is determined to remain in a situation with abusive elements rather than be removed from the home and placed in an institution, should the right to autonomy and self-determination be honored?

◆ What is the nurse's legal obligation?

◆ What is the nurse's caring obligation?

◆ What factors other than safety are at issue?

TABLE 30-7 Examples of Three Types of Elder Abuse

TYPE	EXAMPLES
Physical	Slapping, punching, hitting with belts or other objects, etc.
	Physically restraining
	Isolating
	Withholding personal care—adequate food, clothing, medical attention, hygiene needs
	Sexual assault
Psychological	Verbal assault, humiliation, name calling, belittling, intimidation, threatening harm
	Not allowing access to phone, transportation, mail, friends
	Provoking fear
Financial/material	Theft
	Manipulating finances
	Blocking access to money or property
	Extorting funds
	Failure to use elders' funds to meet their needs

FIGURE 30-12 Physical Indicators of Actual or Potential Elder Abuse/Neglect

General Appearance

Anxious, fearful, and passive

Poor eye contact

Looks to caregiver for answers

Poor hygiene and inappropriate dress

Underweight or malnourished

Physically handicapped

No glasses, false teeth, or hearing aid despite need

Skin

Contusions, abrasions, burns, and scars in various stages of healing

Decubitus ulcers, urine burns

Rope marks

Abdominal/Rectal

Distended

Internal bleeding

Fecal impactions

Musculoskeletal Fractures

Evidence of old, healed fractures

Current fractures and sprains

Limited range of motion

Contractures

Genital/Urinary

Vaginal lacerations, bruises, and infections

Urinary tract infections

Neurologic

Slurred speech

Confusion

From "Survivors of Family Violence," by J. C. Urbanic, 2000, in K. M. Fortinash and P. A. Holoday-Worret (Eds.), *Psychiatric Mental Health Nursing* (2nd ed., pp. 618–651), St. Louis: Mosby. Used with permission.

FIGURE 30-13 Assessing the Elder for Abuse

The following questions are suggestions for assessing abuse in an elder. The nurse might use these as a guide, but find her own words to access the information.

- Do you feel that you are imposing on others when you need assistance?
- Do you feel afraid to ask for help?
- Are you being supported in your efforts to get out to church, visit the senior center or friends?
- Have you ever been forced to sign documents or checks?
- Do you have concerns about your caretakers drinking or suspect they may be using drugs.
- Are you able to freely make phone calls, to have friends come to visit?
- Are you getting enough to eat and drink? Do you think that your meals are nutritious?
- Are there times where you're left alone for long periods of time?
- Has anyone threatened to harm you?
- Do you feel safe in your environment?
- Have you been hit or pushed, slapped or yelled at?
- Are you being called names, being put down, humiliated, or in other ways being talked to in such a way that you feel badly about yourself?

demonstrations can prevent passive neglect as well as reduce caregiver stress.

Nursing Intervention

Elder abuse victims are often reluctant to acknowledge the abuse. They may fear being moved to a nursing care home if authorities become involved. They may be ashamed that a child or spouse is abusing them, or they may fear retaliation from the perpetrator for reporting the violence. Abuse may also involve social isolation, and the elder may be unable to report what is happening. The fact that elders are adults with rights raises ethical issues that influence intervention strategies. The two guiding ethical principles of intervention in halting abusive acts are beneficence (to do good) and nonmaleficence (to do no harm). What the nurse determines as good (e.g., pushing for separation from the abuser or forcing institutionalization) may in fact be experienced as harmful by the elder.

Although reporting of elder abuse is mandatory in 42 states (Morris, 1998), the elder may refuse to cooperate with the process. Once the nurse has met the mandated legal obligation, the range of available interventions needs to be considered, including attempting to work with the caregiver to change any abusive behaviors. It may take considerable time, consistency, empathy, and patience to establish a trusting relationship with an elder abuse victim. The nurse needs to avoid any criticism of the elder or the caretaker, even when that person is abusive. Criticism may be viewed as abusive and may reinforce the elder's distrust of others.

Once trust has been established, the elder or the caretaker or both may open up to the nurse about the difficulties experienced and be receptive to additional help. The nurse may then become the liaison between social services and the family. The long-term goals of intervention are to stop the abuse and to help the family accept help and support, thus lowering the potential for future abuse. Not all families will respond to these efforts. In some cases, the only solution may be separation of the abuser and the victim. Most states have vulnerable elder protection laws specifically for elders with Alzheimer's or disabling infirmities.

A particular form of emotional abuse is **spiritual abuse.** This type of abuse is the "fear, stated or implied, that people are going to be punished in this life and/or tormented in hell-fire forever for failure to live life good enough to please god and earn admission to heaven" (Purcell, 1998, p. 227). An extreme form of spiritual abuse is **spiritual terrorism,** which may cause serious mental health problems. While spiritual abuse may be obvious or subtle, overt or covert, active or passive, spiritual terrorism is obvious, overt, and active. Abuse for most people is mild to severe. Spiritual terrorism "is characterized by literal theological interpretation emphasizing a strong dose of eternal hell-fire and damnation" (p. 228). An example would be the Spanish Inquisition, during which people were tortured to death to save their souls from damnation. The underlying cause is control; motivation by fear is at the heart of spiritual abuse.

One example of how spiritual abuse is harmful is the belief of many that one must not leave a marriage regardless of emotional, verbal, and/or physical abuse because one has a religious commitment to work out the problems within the marriage. When someone does leave, church members turn against the individual for leaving the marriage for reasons other than biblical reasons.

Discussing with clients about the positive image of God is necessary to promote spiritual health. Helping clients to reframe their image of God in a more positive way can facilitate their ability to find peace of mind.

HOMICIDE

The homicide rate in the United States is 10 times higher than that of many western European countries and thirty times higher than in Japan (Lamberg, 1998).

Although the United States continues to hold the lead as the most violent of industrialized countries in the world, the profile of violence has changed. Adolescents and young adults account for an increasing number of the victims and perpetrators of homicide (Christoffel, 2000). In fact, the United States also has the highest rate of childhood homicides among 26 industrialized countries (Christoffel, 2000). In the years spanning 1985–1994, the homicide rate for African American males aged 15–19 increased by 293%, while the homicide rates for white males in the same group rose by 214%. Homicide is now the leading cause of death among African American males aged 15–24, the second leading cause of death among white males aged 15–24, and the third leading cause of death in all children aged 5–14. Three-quarters of these homicides involve a firearm (Stanton, Baldwin,

& Rachuba, 1997), and according to a 1995 study, 1 out of 12 children now carry guns to school (Hennes, 1998).

Approximately one-third of women homicide victims are murdered by an intimate, husbands, or boyfriends. Three percent of male victims are killed by wives or girlfriends. In 1996 close to 1800 murders were attributed to intimates; nearly three out of four of these had a female victim (U.S. Department of Justice, 1998). Men most commonly murder a partner who is trying to leave the relationship. Women most frequently kill a partner in self-defense or in retribution for battering. Children under the age of 4 are most frequently killed by a family member or caretaker; older children are murdered primarily by acquaintances or strangers (U.S. Department of Justice, 1998).

MANDATED REPORTING OF VIOLENCE

Currently, 45 states and the District of Columbia have laws mandating that health care professionals and others report injuries resulting from crime, intentional violence, abuse, and injuries that involve weapons. These laws vary from state to state with regard to specific provisions such as the seriousness of the crime, the type of weapon involved, and what constitutes violence. Each community health nurse should obtain a copy of local reporting statutes.

Nurses are mandated reporters of suspected child abuse in all 50 states. Reports are made to the local Child Protective Services; failure to comply may result in a fine, arrest, and the possibility of civil action. Although health care professionals are protected against any liability resulting from a report made in good faith, most experience some apprehension about filing. The nurse may not be sure if a particular situation actually represents abuse or neglect. Child Protective Services is always willing to discuss the situation with the nurse to help determine whether it warrants reporting. It may be that not all cases reported will be investigated immediately because of the extensive number of child abuse cases handled. However, if problems continue to be reported, an investigation will become a priority. The child's safety and health are the nurse's primary concern. Reporting may be a life-saving measure.

Filing procedures and time lines vary from state to state. The nurse should be aware of the local and institutional procedure. Documentation is an important aspect of reporting. Charting should be chronological and in detail. Quote any important information given by the child or the parents and note any discrepancies between the history and the injury. See Cassidy (1999, pp. 668–669) for more specific details on documentation.

Most states now require health care professionals to report elder abuse. If abuse is suspected but there is not enough information to determine that it has occurred, the nurse should consult with the state agency responsible for elder abuse. The nurse will often be in the position of reporting *suspicions;* it is up to the state to investigate and determine if abuse has taken place. Elders capable of making informed decisions are free to decline any offered assistance providing they are not being coerced or threatened into refusing.

Controversy surrounding the idea of mandatory reporting of domestic violence stems from the fact that, although the goal of reporting is enhanced safety, that is not always the outcome. The risk of retaliation is high. Abusers continue to assault their partners through the period of prosecution. Even though mandatory reporting should shift the blame off of the victim, it frequently does not. Because many victims are afraid of worse treatment if the police are involved, there is the risk that if mandatory reporting becomes the norm, victims will simply stop seeking medical attention (or will be stopped by their batterers).

Clinicians may share the victim's concerns about reporting. Will the report result in protection for the woman or will it prompt the batterer to escalate his violence? Although this poses an ethical dilemma, nurses in some states are mandated reporters. It is important to know your state law with regard to domestic abuse (Valente, 2000).

LONG-TERM EFFECTS OF VIOLENCE

While immediate treatment is critical, the long-term effects of family violence must also be considered. One important disorder that appears following many kinds of violence is **posttraumatic stress disorder (PTSD).** This disorder affects individuals who have been "exposed to a traumatic event in which they or others were threatened with death or serious injury" (Fauman, 1994, p. 217). Symptoms include reexperiencing the trauma, avoiding stimuli associated with the trauma, numbing of general responsiveness, and persistent systems of arousal such as difficulty falling or staying asleep, irritability or outbursts of anger, difficulty concentrating, hypervigilance, and an exaggerated startle response. There is often a high risk of depression and suicide among those with PTSD.

Studies have shown the possibility of lasting changes in neurotransmitter function in adults and suggest that children may show similar changes. Initially, these functions were normal responses to prepare the body for self-protection. There is an increase in the output of adrenalin and noradrenalin and glucocorticoids. The output of serotonin is lowered. These changes are "thought to underlie behavioral symptoms of PTSD including difficulties with attention, concentration, and memory consolidation, greater irritability, exaggerated startle, and greater fluctuation in mood" (Graham-Bermann, 2001 p. 38).

Early neglect and abuse may impair the brain's limbic system. Children tend to shut down emotionally and have more difficulty forming and sustaining relationships at a time when these activities are a critical part of their development (Dahlberg & Potter, 2000).

Retrospective studies have shown that early physical abuse is associated with physically aggressive and violent behavior later in life. This violence includes adolescent violence, adult extrafamilial violence, physical abuse of one's children, and adult aggression toward dating partners and spouses (Rossman, 2001). Many children exhibit behavioral problems, sexualized behaviors, and self-esteem deficits. Both abuse and observation of parental abuse are linked to psychiatric symptoms, self-injurious behaviors, and poorer health in later life. While one cannot always be sure if child abuse is occurring along with domestic violence, it has been shown that families with identified spouse abuse were 4.9 times more likely to have an episode of child abuse (Toomey & Bernstein, 2001). Violent exposure may change how children use information as flexibly or completely as nonexposed peers. Learning tasks and following instructions can be more difficult. Earlier exposure to domestic violence and personal violence may interfere more extensively with the completion of developmental tasks.

Women who grew up with child abuse are more likely to abuse their children. Sexual abuse of the parent seems to have the strongest association with child abuse (Hall, Sachs, & Rayens, 1998; Toomey & Bernstein, 2001). They are also more at risk for alcohol and other drug abuse.

It is not only the victim who is affected. Nelson and Wampler (2000) noted that in marital couples where one had a history of childhood abuse, both partners were affected in that they both experienced lower relationship satisfaction and higher individual stress symptoms than couples where neither partner reports an abuse history. Pistorello and Follete (1998) found that many abused women have a guarded and vigilant approach to close interpersonal relationships, which frequently leads to issues in attaining an intimate connection with a partner as an adult. They also show a heightened need for control in the relationship.

One study reporting on psychopathology of child sexual abuse found that the percentage of women with lifetime depression was much higher than in the general population (39.3%–21.3%). They also reported the higher likelihood that adults who had been sexually abused as children were much more likely to have at least one of the major psychiatric disorders (mood, anxiety, or substance abuse disorder). The consequences tend to be more severe when the assault has been by a trusted acquaintance or relative than when perpetrated by a stranger (Molnar, Buka, & Kessler, 2001). Other disorders seen in children of battered women are eating disorders and substance abuse (Humphreys, 2001).

Impact of Violence on the Community

The consequences of family violence can also lead to family disintegration and economic disaster. Families may be separated by forced separation, divorce, or incarceration, with few resources to help them manage their lives. The community is economically impacted given the extent of legal, medical, social, and criminal justice services that must be used.

The effects of violence on a community is also an important consideration. One study indicated that the violence undermined the community's social functioning. People felt less free to move about and afraid of being on the streets. They worried about the intentions of their neighbors and retreated from the larger community group. The result was the presence of intergroup prejudice and the absence of common, unifying sites or symbols. Respondents on the study pointed out that "the cumulative effects of poverty, racism, and other forms of social injustice are not only potential causes of violence but forms of violence in and of themselves. Furthermore, all of these are problems that originate outside of the local community" (Fullilove, Heon, Jimenez, Parsons, Green, & Fullilove, 1998, p. 927).

PREVENTION

This chapter has covered issues such as child abuse, child sexual assault, domestic violence, rape, and elder abuse. It is clear that the ethic of violence may need to be examined to understand the amount of violence perpetrated by people of all walks of life. Regardless of the source of violence, however, the most powerful tool we have to combat it is prevention.

Primary Prevention

Violence prevention activities by community nurses may include but are not limited to political activism, networking, health promotion, education, counseling, and development of agency protocols. Cassidy (1999) emphasizes the importance of nurse advocacy, not only for each individual but also for the community at large. Advocating for the community is a political act as well as a caring act. Examples of advocacy actions are listed in Figure 30-14.

Health promotion activities for female clients should include groups or classes that (1) help them identify strengths and (2) encourage personal independence and assertive behaviors. Male clients may feel threatened by the changes taking place in society. Some men express anger that women are working in fields that were traditionally male and hold women responsible for their feelings of financial insecurity. Men or adolescent boys dealing with these issues may benefit from a progressive men's support group. Advocacy for school-based programs that teach age-appropriate assault prevention techniques helps to assure that children are learning methods to reduce their vulnerability to violence.

Anticipatory guidance can begin with individual interactions such as well-child checks. There is opportunity to talk about privacy, the right of the child to be examined with a trusted parent present, and the right to say no if someone tries to touch the child's genitals or touches the child in any other way that makes him or her uncomfortable.

Children who live in communities where they are exposed to daily violence need strong family support and community involvement to assist them in coping with and processing their realities. They also need to learn that violence is not the solution to problems. Evaluate the

---

REFLECTIVE THINKING

Mandatory Reporting

- Is it paternalistic to do something you consider in the client's best interest?
- If you report violence against the victim's wishes, are you putting that person in yet another situation of not being heard? Of disrespect?
- Will reporting undermine trust? Increase fear of health care providers?
- With whom can you consult about the situation before reporting?

FIGURE 30-14 Examples of Advocacy Action

- Offering community-based classes and support groups
- Speaking about violence at schools and civic groups
- Involvement in local activities that you perceive as important to reduce violence in the community
- Networking in the community to identify resources for clients who need counseling, education, and support around aggression issues
- Participating in advisory boards for rape crisis centers, shelters, antiviolence programs, and community alternatives to gang activity
- Developing assertiveness-training groups to provide an alternative to aggression
- Screening for drug and alcohol abuse and gang activity
- Establishing mentor programs to link teens with adult role models and support people
- Developing anticipatory guidance programs regarding developmental stages, to reduce parent frustrations concerning child behavior
- Establishing parenting groups
- Modeling effective adult–child communication skills in the community

family's method of conflict resolution. If families can learn and model nonviolent problem-solving methods, children will carry those lessons into the world each day.

Schools also play an important role in providing a curriculum that allows children to talk about the violence they are seeing and to learn alternative solutions. If schools in the community do not offer this, nurses can work with other community groups or existing programs. Churches, police departments, boys' and girls' clubs, and other youth-oriented programs can be approached if antiviolence programs, after-school recreational activities, and child care programs do not exist. Children also benefit emotionally and physically from martial arts training.

Some communities are recognizing the need to develop an integrated program in which a city's schools, churches, police, businesses, and youth organizations work closely together to develop programs for youth that emphasize prevention of crime and gang development.

In the past several years, and as recently as March 2001, we have witnessed children and adolescents gunning down their peers on school campuses. These incidents are extremely frightening and raise many questions about our culture and its impact on our children. An obvious theme for thought is gun control. Why are guns so readily available to children? Why do we need handguns? Is it safe to have guns in a home where there are children? Children are carrying guns and other weapons to school with increasing frequency (DuRaut et al., 1999). Research on violence among youth in the inner cities makes links to poverty, drugs, and despair. What will we discover about middle to upper class adolescents who open fire on their classmates? It is clear that violence prevention must begin at a very young age. Nurses can play a role by assessing risks in families and providing education. Does the family have guns in the house? Where are they kept? Where are the bullets? Do children play at the home of friends where weapons are accessible? Parents must be encouraged to think about these issues. How does the family handle anger? Are the children provided with problem-solving skills? Many children in this country also need a responsible caring adult who is paying attention to their feelings and their behaviors. Jane Gilgun, a professor of social work at the University of Minnesota, is a researcher in the area of violent behaviors. Figure 30-15 lists some of the behaviors Gilgun indicates are high risk for violent acting out.

Adolescent screening should explore family relationships, current relationships, history of violence including sexual violence, and dating violence. All teens should be asked what they know about sexual assault and relationship violence. Any misconceptions should be corrected. Explore what clients see as effective prevention and what kinds of warning signs they can identify with regard to

controlling or potentially assaultive people. Teens may benefit from assertion training.

Therapy or support groups aimed at assisting students with effective anger management might be appropriate. School nurses could screen adolescents for possible violent behaviors and set up classes and workshops to teach them how to handle conflict, frustration, and anger. Assertiveness-training, whether peer or counselor facilitated, decreases anger. One-third of schools provide expanded mental health services that include anger management classes and conflict resolution. The program also works with children who have witnessed or experienced violence (Lamberg, 1998b).

Children's exposure to media violence should be explored with parents and appropriate education provided. Discovering the family's philosophy regarding such issues as discipline, management of tantrums, and potty training is an important part of gathering a family history. Any tendency toward abusive parenting needs to be addressed and the family assisted in exploring alternative parenting techniques and nonviolent problem-solving methods. Families at risk such as teen parents; single-parent households; families with children who are physically, developmentally, or emotionally challenged; and alcohol- or drug-dependent families require frequent visits, careful evaluation, and parenting education. The nurse can assess strengths and weaknesses with the family and act

---

FIGURE 30-15 High-Risk Indicators for Violence

Attention should be paid to any of the following behaviors, the more risk factors the more serious the risk for violent acting out.

- Threats of violence particularly if the threat is repeated to various people
- Detailed description of how the violence will occur and to whom
- Violence writings such as stories or poems in conjunction with other risk factors
- A high stress event affecting the individual
- Preoccupation with violence: music, videos, movies, and books
- The means to commit the violence
- Being bullied or bullying others
- Feeling weak or powerless, attaching to others who are violent
- Family history of violence
- Connection to individuals who glorify violence

Adapted from *Detecting the Potential for Violence*, by J. F. Gilgun, 1999, Twin Cities: University of Minnesota, School of Social Work.

as a liaison to facilitate the assistance of appropriate organizations or support people.

The community health nurse should introduce the topic of violence as part of obtaining a complete history with all adults. Clients who give you a history of sleep disturbances, eating disorders, nightmares, alcohol or drug abuse, or self-abusive behaviors should be carefully and sensitively screened for a past or current history of sexual and physical abuse. The single most important thing that health care providers can do to prevent and reduce the amount and degree of violence is to ask about it (Cassidy, 1999).

Established protocols for dealing with the victims and perpetrators of violence should be part of every agency setting. These protocols should include a referral list of private and public community agencies that serve victims of violence.

Last, nurses must involve themselves in community mobilization to effect public policy aimed at the prevention and treatment of both victims and perpetrators. Such efforts as the First Star program (see Out of the Box) can only be successful when a multidisciplinary and intersectoral approach is taken. These complex issues cannot be solved quickly.

Secondary Prevention

Families using violence may be referred because abuse is suspected or has been confirmed or because a child is acting out violently at school. The nurse may identify symptoms of abuse when treating a family member in the clinical area. When abuse is suspected, intervention should take place as quickly as possible.

Out
of the Box

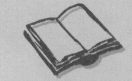

First Star

First Star was founded in 2000 by Peter Samuelson. It is a public policy initiative that has long-term goals of improving the lives of children in distress and preventing abuse in the future. Its mission is to "create new initiatives to strengthen existing laws and policies that improve the safety, health, and family life of America's children" (p. 31). First Star "seeks to improve the lives of children who suffer abuse, maltreatment, and neglect" (p. 31). The mission is implemented by:

- *Determining best practices for local, state, and federal government agencies and other organizations that impact children.*
- *Developing a state-by-state information database related to the safety and public health of children and to laws affecting them.*
- *Educating the public and specific groups about challenges facing children and how to help solve these problems.*
- *Advocating improved federal, state, and local laws and policies to enhance the lives of children.*

In process is a four-part program to evaluate and ensure basic civil rights for abused and neglected children in the United States. The program includes:

- *Research of the laws and conditions that affect the lives of children in the United States and provide an ever-updated database*
- *The First Star Institute (interdisciplinary study of laws affecting children and the psychology of children)*
- *Creating "accountability for official action or inaction with a focus on the elimination of laws that systematically deny a child the right to sue any state for misfeasance and that provide a shield of secrecy that is frequently misapplied to protect institutions and officials from accountability" (p. 32)*
- *Enhancing "public awareness of the plight of children, to explore the social dynamics in which abuse of children stimulates extreme concern yet historically results in very little progress or systemic improvements and . . . [creating] hopefulness about lasting solutions" (p. 32)*

First Star wants the support of the "home health care community to find creative ways of organizing and funding programs targeted to children who are victims of abuse, maltreatment, and neglect" (p. 32).

Source: Sams, D. (2001). First Star: A new approach to the fight against child abuse and neglect. Caring, 30(6), 30–32. ∎

When a family member has been physically injured or a child has acted out by running away, joining a gang, or assaulting another person or if sexual abuse has been diagnosed, an imbalance may exist between the problem and the family's available coping skills. The tension, discomfort, and anxiety resulting from the identified problem often motivate the family to seek or accept assistance and to participate in finding solutions. Crisis intervention methods are helpful at this time, as is establishment of a support network. The nurse will initially help family members identify what they individually understand about the problem and how they feel. Family members may, for instance, blame the victim for what has happened, alerting the nurse to belief systems that need to be addressed. Often in closed family systems, support networks are lacking and the nurse may need to work with the family to determine what agencies, family members, or friends would be accepted as a support system. Determining how the family has coped with past crises provides information about family strengths and helps the family identify or recall coping mechanisms that have served them before. Any healthy coping mechanisms, such as crying, expression of grief or sorrow, or comforting others in the family should be identified and supported by the nurse.

When the victim is a child and the nurse is in the position of filing the Child Protective Services (CPS) report, the family should be prepared for this event. Or the nurse may be working in conjunction with CPS. The crisis period is, by definition, approximately four to six weeks in length. Working with the family to establish goals and making any indicated referrals to family therapy, parenting classes, or other community support agencies should be completed as early in this cycle as possible to maximize openness in the family system.

In some cases a family member may have to be removed from the home. This person may be a sexually assaultive adult, although far too often it is the child victim who is removed to a foster home. If the nurse has the ability to maintain contact with that child, it is essential to help the child understand that removal from the home is not punishment. The community health nurse may be in a position to help other children in the family understand what has happened, to monitor the progress of short-term goals, and to work toward the prevention of any further abuse. These efforts should be coordinated with other agencies such as the legal system or social services.

It was mentioned earlier that abuse victims, especially sexual assault victims, are at high risk for suicidal behavior. If the child remains in the home, the nurse should be sure to ask about weapons in the home. Suicidal risk factors need to be carefully assessed. Other family members should be educated about warning signs for suicide and given information about appropriate community resources for family support. See Chapters 22 and 23 for a discussion of suicide.

Nurses should be aware of agencies, church groups, schools, and volunteer agencies in the community that work with gangs and should encourage teens who are drawn to gang activity to utilize these services. Early identification and acknowledgment of family problems in addition to working with the family to seek solutions can avert some of the drastic outcomes. Throughout this process, the nurse should remain open, direct, caring, flexible, and nonjudgmental. To achieve this stance, the nurse needs a personal support system in addition to good consultation.

REFLECTIVE THINKING

Is the Death Penalty the Solution to Violence?

Consider these facts:

- Of 38 death penalty states, 12 have no minimum age for imposing death.
- Since 1973, over 160 children have been sentenced to die.
- Five other countries execute juveniles: Iran, Nigeria, Pakistan, Saudi Arabia, and Yemen. We have more children scheduled for execution than any one of the five.
- Illinois executed 12 men on death row and exonerated 13 upon proof of innocence.
- Historically over 80% of individuals executed in the United States have been convicted of killing whites, though people of color comprise 50% of homicide victims.
- A 1991 Florida study showed that people who kill whites are three to four times more likely to get the death penalty than those who kill blacks.
- Death row inmates are 42% African American while African Americans make up 13% of the population.
- Ninety percent of individuals whom U.S. prosecutors seek to execute are African American or Mexican American.

Source: National Association of Criminal Defense Lawyers. *The death penalty is wrong.* [on-line]. Available: *www.NACDL.org.*

Tertiary Prevention

Tertiary prevention will involve working with families who have suffered the long-term consequences of violence. Examples include a family in which a parent or child has died as the result of violence; parents who have had children placed in foster homes; families in which a member has been incarcerated because of abuse; or a family with a child who is a runaway, a delinquent, sexually promiscuous, or substance addicted or has psychiatric problems related to abuse.

The nurse will be working with the family to maximize strengths, to heal from the trauma and loss, and to build support systems. Children and adolescents in families may need help with expressing their feelings about the violence that has altered the family, as well as their fears that the violence will be repeated. The family should be assessed for any remaining interactions that might be violent or frightening to any family member, including the use of violent language or aggressive nonverbal communication. Serious emotional effects in any family member call for appropriate referrals and follow-up.

Some male nurses have taken a proactive stance against violence and work with men who act out in violent ways. These nurses are in a position to educate men about their individual power to work against violence and the more subtle forms of approval of violence.

ISSUES AFFECTING THE NURSE

Working with clients who have been affected by violence is challenging for any helper, regardless of discipline. Nurses are well suited to address the needs of these clients by virtue of their focus on holistic care and advocacy. It is important, however, that they feel comfortable with their abilities and their support systems. Nursing education is a logical starting point for assuring that nurses are prepared to work in this arena, because contact with sexual assault survivors, abused and traumatized children, battered women, or neglected elders is inevitable.

Institutions need to provide clear protocols for dealing with community or family violence as well as clinical support and supervision for the nurses who are caring for the client or families affected by violence. Professional nursing organizations are in a position to set the tone for how nursing views violence and what the role of the professional nurse should be. Addressing these issues in publications, at conferences, and on a local level and taking a political stance are all ways of affirming nursing's central role in halting violence. This type of advocacy is also a way of supporting the individual nurse, who may at times feel isolated or afraid while dealing with some of these highly charged issues.

Dealing with violence—seeing its effects, hearing the painful stories, and caring for its victims—is emotionally challenging. Nurses are just as likely as their patients to have experienced physical, emotional, or sexual abuse. Recognizing this, Schroder and Weber (1998) developed a nonthreatening interactive workshop designed to educate health professionals about domestic violence. They comment that if a health care provider is currently or has been a victim of abuse, there is a good chance that denial will interfere with the ability to recognize a victim of domestic violence. Each nurse is called upon to examine individual judgments, control issues, codependency, and sometimes past and unresolved pain. This work is not something that should be done in isolation or silence: Clinical supervision is important.

Through all this, the nurse must attend to self-care, which means different things to different nurses. Some may find that they have unresolved issues that require therapy or codependent issues that need to be addressed. Others may need to increase their exercise in order to reduce their stress level or spend more time attending to spiritual life. Replenishing their own energy and spirit is crucial to maintaining good nursing care.

Men may have a difficult time with some of the information presented. Men are often the perpetrators of violence, and it may sometimes sound as if all men are being viewed as violent. All nurses have an obligation to not laugh at sexist, racist, or homophobic jokes; to eliminate demeaning language aimed at people of other races, religions, or sexual orientation; and to verbalize disapproval of abusive actions. These are all individual actions that will help to put an end to violence.

Leaders in health care, law enforcement, government, education, and religion are acknowledging the extent of the violence problem and are willing to take part in finding solutions. Domestic violence and sexual harassment are being debated in the open, increasing consciousness about the underpinnings of violence. Efforts are increasing to divert children from joining gangs and to find real solutions to gang violence. Gun control legislation is targeted at reducing the number of firearm-related homicides. Research efforts that address issues such as elder abuse, hate crimes, and the impact of violence on people of color may be crucial in the effort to halt violence.

Much may be learned from studying nonviolent cultures such as the Mbuti people, the Zuni Indians, and the Utku Eskimos (Campbell & Humphreys, 1984), in whose cultures children are not physically punished and are taught that jealousy and the use of force are unacceptable. In these cultures, competition is not valued, but gentleness and cooperation are, and caution, fear, and timidity are considered healthy traits.

These values are inherent in nursing. Nursing care has the potential to teach families and individuals that we all have the right and capability to live nonviolently. "Live the change you want for the world" (Mahatma Gandhi).

Perspectives...

EXTINGUISHING THE LIGHT

Heavy laden with chains
I cannot dance.
Movement unbearable
Mired in sorrow.

Wailing from within
Yet no cry escapes

Silent tears
As silent as the voices raised
Against rape

The silence is deafening.

I am alone.

In despair
I search the depths,
There is no reservoir
I crumble, broken

My spirit once bright with brilliant hues
Like fall spattered leaves once painted
Red and orange
Withers turns black
Dies

I free fall into oblivion
The dark I welcome
It meets me where I am.

Through the silence of my broken spirit
The moaning creeps grows louder.
The wails of my sisters and brothers assail me,
Ripping shard by shard the curtain
Of despair

Wailing . . .
Hope is an illusion

Wailing . . .
Oppression is reality

Wailing

20 years
200 years

2000 years of moans
Haunting cries
Muffled wails of defiled women and men
Generation by generation
Greeted with silence
1 heart breaking
2 hearts broken
Generations of hearts heavy with the dark memories

The heavens fill with their cries
The skies deluge with sorrowful weeping
The earth shivers with sorrow
The people turn away silently
Heavy laden with chains of impotent voice
I cannot dance

I am wounded
Struggling
I want to be deaf too
To the wailing
So like the masses.
But the moaning
The flow of tears
Unceasing
Finds me a river.
I have no strength to turn away.

Lights going out one by one
Ten by ten
Hundreds
Generation by generation
Innocence lost in bruised bodies
Broken children
Souls stolen in the night
In the daylight.

One more child moans in the darkness
One more light went out tonight.

—Pat Stewart (1995) Survivor

KEY CONCEPTS

◆ Violence may affect anyone regardless of race, culture, socioeconomic status, or educational background and is not limited to any particular country.

◆ Violence is a community and societal issue, not merely the problem of the individual victim.

◆ There is no one explanation for violence in any culture.

◆ Knowledge of existing theories and a broad political understanding can provide direction in the care of survivors of violence and in the development of effective prevention efforts.

◆ Guns and community violence are connected, although the management of guns in society is controversial.

◆ Community violence in the form of gangs has escalated in recent years.

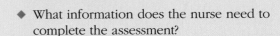

COMMUNITY NURSING VIEW

Child Protective Services has requested a public health nurse to visit the Miceli family. They have been notified by the family's nurse practitioner that the family has repeatedly failed to bring 20-month-old Celeste in for follow-up visits. The child has had a very serious candida diaper dermatitis that failed to respond to conservative treatment. The family repeatedly has not shown up for scheduled one-week follow-up visits; instead they returned two months later when the rash was once again to the point of bleeding and secondary infection. This pattern of behavior has gone on for eight months despite prevention education from the nurse practitioner and reminder calls to the family prior to scheduled visits. There has also been a concern about spousal abuse. The father, James, a 28-year-old part-time factory worker, is very controlling. He doesn't allow his wife, Marla, to drive or to go anywhere without him or one of her parents. The nurse practitioner reported an office visit to which Marla's father brought Celeste and Marla. James called during the visit and asked what time they had arrived and what time they would be leaving. During that same visit, Marla related that James told her he would not spend money on cloth diapers, as recommended, and thinks it's high time the baby started potty training.

Nursing Considerations

Assessment

◆ Are there risk factors for abuse? For neglect? If so, what are they?

◆ What information does the nurse need to complete the assessment?

Diagnosis

◆ What nursing diagnoses would be appropriate to this family?

Outcome Identification

◆ Given the diagnosis you have identified, what outcomes do you expect?

Planning/Interventions

◆ What levels of prevention need to be addressed?

◆ What areas of education will be needed by this family?

◆ What referral services might be useful for this family?

Evaluation

◆ What evaluation criteria will indicate if the interventions are effective?

◆ What should be done if interventions are ineffective?

◆ It is essential that nurses address their own biases regarding violence.

◆ Strategies for decreasing vulnerability to sexual assault should emphasize empowering behaviors as opposed to behaviors that restrict freedom.

◆ There are identifiable stages in the process of recovery from sexual assault.

◆ There are several forms of intimate-partner violence.

◆ Nurses can utilize the rape trauma syndrome model to assess clients and to determine appropriate interventions.

◆ Physical and behavioral clues can alert the nurse to the possibility of child abuse.

◆ The United States has the highest rate of homicide of any industrialized country.

◆ Nurses are mandated reporters for all aspects of family violence.

◆ Theories of learned helplessness and the cycle of violence in domestic abuse provide a framework for nursing interventions.

◆ Preventing caregiver burnout is a crucial aspect of preventing elder abuse.

◆ Assessing the potential for abuse is an important aspect of prevention.

◆ Asking clients about violence in their lives is one of the most important things the nurse can do.

◆ Violence has long-term effects on individuals and communities.

◆ Dealing with violence is emotionally challenging, and therefore replenishing one's own energy and spirit is crucial to maintaining good nursing care.

RESOURCES

Administration on Aging: www.aoa.dhls.gov
American Academy of Family Physicians: www.aafp.org
American Academy of Pediatrics: www.AAP.org
American Medical Association violence prevention:
    www.ama-assn.org
Center for the Study and Prevention of Violence:
    www.colorado.edu/cspv
Centers for Disease Control and Prevention: www.cdc.gov
Child Abuse Prevention Network: www.child-abuse.com
Elder abuse: www.webster.edu/~woolflm/abuse.html
Family Violence Prevention Fund:
    endabuse.org/programs/healthcare

Hate crimes: www.fbi.gov
Hate crimes initiatives: www.usdoj.gov
Medical termination of sexual assault: www.Pediatrics.org
Minnesota Center Against Violence and Abuse:
    www.mincava.umn.edu
National Association of Criminal Defense Lawyers:
    www.criminaljustice.org
National Library of Medicine: www.nlm.nih.gov
Nursing journals: www.nursingcenter.com
Sex offences and offenders: www.ojp.usdoj.gov/bjs/abstract
T.V. violence, Kansas State University: www.ksu.edu
Violence against women on-line resources: www.vaw.umn.edu

Chapter

31

SUBSTANCE ABUSE

Linda G. Dumas, RN, PhD, ANP
Mary Beatrice Hennessey Wohn, RN, MSN

I'd be so strung out . . . and I'd be shooting up and I'd be thinking, My god . . . I'm frying my brains . . . I don't want to fry my brains.

Personal communication with a formerly homeless and addicted woman talking of her response to a public service announcement that showed an egg with the message "This is your brain" and then showed an egg sizzling in a frying pan with the message "This is your brain on drugs."

COMPETENCIES

Upon completion of this chapter, the reader should be able to:

- Identify and define six substances commonly abused in the United States.

- Identify three populations at risk for substance abuse.

- Analyze common attitudes of nurses toward people who abuse substances.

- Discuss issues related to substance abuse at the primary, secondary, and tertiary levels of prevention.

- List settings where primary and secondary prevention can take place.

- Discuss the impact of managed care and cost cutting on tertiary-level intervention for people who abuse substances.

- Discuss differences between detoxification centers, transitional housing, and home care as referral resources for people who abuse substances.

- Discuss the many legal issues surrounding the treatment of substance abusers and substance abuse itself.

- Discuss the concept of caring as it might apply to the care of people who abuse alcohol, tobacco, and other drugs.

- Utilize electronic media for substance abuse information.

KEY TERMS

crack	freebase
crack babies	inhalant substances
cutting agents	needle and syringe
depressant	exchange programs
designer drugs	psychoactive
detoxification	substances
fetal alcohol syndrome	sedative

The vast majority of U.S. citizens use mind-altering substances. Alcohol, caffeine, nicotine, and prescribed and illicit drugs are a part of the American culture. A love-hate relationship is often apparent. Drugs have been taxed and studied, promoted and outlawed, controlled and extolled, used and abused. Health warning labels are legally mandated on tobacco and alcohol containers, and yet debate rages regarding the marketing of these products to youth (Difranza & Librett, 1999; Dority, 1997; Teinowitz, 1997).

The approaches of health care professionals to people who use and abuse various substances have been likewise ambivalent. Throughout history health providers have learned and relearned the same lessons: that addictions are both preventable and treatable. Interventions, however, are often ineffective because they are based on negative and inaccurate stereotypes (Sullivan, Handley, & Connors, 1994).

This chapter will discuss tobacco, alcohol, and other substance abuse from a community nursing perspective. Substance abuse has been studied from a number of different perspectives, and plans for treatment often reflect the perspective studied. For example, if substance abuse is viewed as strictly a pathophysiological problem, then a medical model would seem a reasonable treatment approach; whereas if it were seen as a behavioral problem, behavioral therapy techniques would seem a better option. This chapter takes an eclectic view of substance abuse. It recognizes that there are many different pathways to the addictions and many diverse and valid treatment approaches. Individual, family, and community dimensions are identified, with special attention to certain high-risk groups. Levels of prevention are addressed, and primary, secondary, and tertiary interventions are discussed.

A BRIEF HISTORY OF SUBSTANCE ABUSE IN THE UNITED STATES

Hewitt (1995) points out that there has been a historical inability to reach a national consensus about the role of alcohol in American society. At varying times over the past 150 years the excessive use of alcohol has been considered a sin, a crime, and a disease, and the excessive drinker a sinner, a criminal, and a victim. Alcohol was the first drug to be considered a problem in the United States, and the first attempt at controlling it took the form of an excise tax on whiskey. This law, passed in 1791, led to the so-called Whiskey Rebellion. Farmers who considered whiskey an economic necessity and a medium of exchange refused to pay the tax. President Washington called upon the militia of several states to enforce the law. This action was particularly significant as it was a test of the new federal government's ability to enforce its laws within a state (Witters & Venturelli, 1988).

Narcotic addiction first became a problem during the Civil War, when the hypodermic syringe was invented. Morphine was used widely for the treatment of pain and dysentery, and morphine addiction became known as "the Soldiers' disease" (Julien, 1985).

By the late 1800s, great strides relative to the conceptualization of alcoholism had been made. Addiction to alcohol was seen not only as a disease but also as an inherited disease with a progressive course (Palmer, 1996). The beliefs of the early founders of the Temperance Society were in harmony with those of Alcoholics Anonymous. By the turn of the century, however, the focus of the Temperance membership changed, and alcohol became a "demon." There was a campaign to rid society of alcohol, which in 1920 led to the ratification of the 18th Amendment to the U.S. Constitution, better known as prohibition. Prohibition overshadowed all the hard work that had been done to promote the concept of alcoholism as a disease. Interestingly, the 18th Amendment is the only amendment to the U.S. Constitution that has been repealed, another incidence of national ambivalence. The repeal occurred in 1933, and the disease concept was resurrected and expanded upon. Much of the later work on alcoholism as a disease was done in the 1950s at Yale, most notably by Jellinek (Levine, 1978).

In the late 1800s and early 1900s the use of cocaine reached epidemic proportions. Cocaine could be found in patent medicines, wine, and Coca-Cola. The Pure Food and Drug Act of 1906 was actually a labeling law aimed at controlling the patent medicine industry. This act required complete labeling of the contents in each container, specifically mentioning alcohol, morphine, opium, cocaine, heroin, and marijuana (Witters & Venturelli, 1988).

In the 1930s marijuana became the focus of concern. Newspaper and police reports associated crime with marijuana use, and the film *Reefer Madness* (now a cult classic) depicted high school use of marijuana as leading to murder, rape, prostitution, and madness (Ray, 1983). In 1937, concern about its effects led the federal government to classify marijuana as a schedule I substance (Gold, 1991). Under the Controlled Substances Act, the criteria by which a drug or substance is determined to be schedule I are: (1) It has a high potential for abuse; (2) it has no currently accepted medical use in treatment in the United States; and (3) there is a lack of accepted safety for its use under medical supervision (Lehne, 2000).

In the 1960s, the Vietnam War brought new patterns of drug use (McKim, 1986). The user tended to be better educated, and the drugs of choice were those that altered mood and consciousness. "Mind-expanding drugs" such as LSD became common. There was also an increase in heroin use. In the 1970s drugs were labeled by the government as "Public Enemy No. 1" (Ray, 1983).

The 1980s brought a resurgence in the popularity of cocaine. Chemists found a way to remove the impurities and the hydrochloride from the cocaine, thereby creating a smokable and much more potent product. Initially this process required the use of highly volatile products such as ether. It was later discovered that a relatively pure cocaine could be prepared using baking soda. This form, known as **crack** or **freebase** cocaine, delivers a potent but short-lived high followed by a longer depression. The availability of cocaine in freebase or crack form in-

creased. Crack cocaine is widely available, cheap, and highly addictive and therefore, in 2001, remains a serious problem (NIDA Infofax, 2001a).

In the 1980s, some high-profile people succumbed to drugs. The death of John Belushi from a "speedball" (a mixture of heroin and freebase cocaine) brought the method of "freebasing" to public awareness. The death of Len Bias, who was celebrating his selection to the Boston Celtics with what was reportedly his first use of cocaine, captured the attention of high school and college athletes. The death of Robert Kennedy's son David highlighted the fact that drugs can be devastating at all socioeconomic levels.

In the 1990s the use of marijuana made headlines (Buckley, 1996; Leo, 1996; Morganthau, 1997). More than two centuries after the Whiskey Rebellion the supremacy of federal law over states' rights was again being questioned. In late 1996, in what might someday be called "the marijuana rebellion," California and Arizona voters each approved propositions allowing prescription of marijuana for medical purposes (Buckley, 1996). This practice conflicts with federal law. In January of 1997 federal authorities warned physicians that they might face prosecution if they prescribe marijuana (Rogers, 1997). This debate continues into the 21st century. By the end of the decade, indicators for marijuana use reflected stabilization in most communities after the sharp rise in use from 1990 to 1998. Emergency rooms reported a decrease or stabilization of marijuana-related problems. Some large cities reported an increase in emergency room admissions where marijuana was the drug of abuse. Marijuana was the most likely illicit drug to be used in combination with other drugs of abuse such as Ecstasy and Vicodin, and there were reports of young marijuana users dipping joints in embalming fluid or codeine cough syrup (see http://www.Drugabuse.cov/infofax/nationaltrends.html. Marijuana was the most common drug reported used by male and female juveniles in 1999. Nearly half of males and 40% of females tested positive for marijuana. More American teens are experimenting with marijuana, while patterns of heavy drug use in the young have stabilized (Reuters, www.ABCnews.com., July 3, 2001).

On a positive note, the trend in marijuana use, both in America and globally, does not indicate that the use of marijuana leads to the use of heroin, cocaine, and other hard drugs. Marijuana use peaked at about 60% in the late 1990s, about 22% of high school seniors. Golub and Johnson note that the increase in marijuana use would be "good news" if it signals a "rejection of crack and heroin" (Reuters, 2001, p. 1).

In 2001, the Supreme Court heard the medical marijuana case. The argument positioned the federal government against many clients who were sick or dying of AIDS, cancer, and other end-of-life conditions. The court was "Openly skeptical" about the medical use of marijuana (http://www.infobeat.com/dgi-bin/WebObject).

The question at the center of the marijuana debate is the definition of addiction (Webber, 2001). When is a drug considered addictive? Is a drug considered an addiction when it changes the behavior of an animal or human? Does stopping marijuana use precipitate withdrawal symptoms, the hallmark of addiction? The argument involves two philosophically diverse groups: National Organization for the Reform of Marijuana Laws (NORML) argues that cannabis has been around for years and the evidence is not there to prove it is an addictive substance. On the other side of the argument are the folks who consider themselves marijuana addicts who belong to a 12-step program run by Marijuana Anonymous (http://www.marijuana-anonymous.org/).

Many groups continue to fight for the decriminalization of marijuana for medicinal use, such as treatment of cancer pain, treatment of glaucoma, and for multiple sclerosis (http://cbshealthwatch.medscape.com/cx/viewarticle/234198). The argument for medicinal use has strengthened the argument for legalization. Twenty-three states have laws that legalize marijuana for therapeutic use.

Another area of debate is the federally funded **needle and syringe exchange programs,** in which intravenous drug users can swap used needles and syringes for new ones (Chapman, 1997; Lurie & Drucker, 1997). Such programs started in Amsterdam in 1984 (van Ameijden, van den Hoek, & Coutinho, 1995) and the concept spread throughout the United Kingdom and to other European countries without opposition (Coutinho, 1995). Several studies in the Netherlands, Sweden, Australia, the United Kingdom, and the United States have demonstrated that needle and syringe exchange programs are effective in lowering the rates of needle sharing (Watters, Estilo, Clark, & Lorvick, 1994). The sharing of contaminated injection equipment is a major route for transmitting HIV. The Centers for Disease Control and Prevention (CDC) report that a little more than a third (35.3%) of reported AIDS cases are associated with intravenous drug abuse and that syringe exchange programs appear to be effective in preventing the transmission of infectious diseases (CDC, 2001).

Lurie and Drucker (1997) concluded that the absence of a needle exchange program in the United States has contributed to between 4000 and 10,000 cases of preventable HIV infection. Along with the costs in human suffering, they put the societal costs for treating the infections between a quarter and a half billion dollars. Needle and syringe exchange programs in the United States, however, continue to merit considerable opposition. Despite growing evidence to the contrary, there is concern that needle exchange programs will increase drug abuse.

Another issue for Americans relates to the relationship between syringe exchange programs (SEPs) and decriminalization of drugs. SEPs include HIV prevention education and a wide range of related public health services, including hepatitis prevention services for high-risk intravenous drug abusers (CDC, 2001). Many would argue that millions of dollars are spent in education programs for youth that have no evidence-based outcomes to document success or failure. The effectiveness is unknown (www.Economist.com). Advocates for alternative programs called "harm reduction programs" believe they have promise: SEPs, methadone programs, and prescription heroin are examples.

Health professionals need to consider the philosophy behind the SEPs and whether participation decreases incidence of HIV infection, AIDS, and hepatitis. They must be cognizant that a majority of participants in such programs are minority and low-income young adults. From a social perspective, can SEPs keep young men of color out of prison, lower the crime rates, and provide opportunities for better lives? Longitudinal studies are needed, but can the SEPs wait for the evidence before they are implemented?

Morbidity and Mortality

Morbidity and mortality patterns in the 1990s were characterized by the fact that most illnesses are social, behavioral, and environmental in origin. The addictions, AIDS, many cancers, liver disease, mental illness, cardiovascular disease, homicide, battering, motor vehicle accidents, birth defects, and work-related injuries are all examples of diseases with social or behavioral etiologies. Many of the events precipitating such problems are brought about by alcohol and drugs (Dumas, 1992a, 1992b; Frisch and Frisch, 1998; Hennessey, 1992; McKinlay, 1993). Morbidity and mortality profiles point to the fact that substance abuse is prevalent in American society (NIDA Infofax, 2001G). People with substance abuse and its related problems fill hospitals and home care caseloads.

SUBSTANCE ABUSE STATISTICS FOR THE 2000s

Tobacco use, substance abuse, and mental health are leading health indicators given in *Healthy People 2010*. [U.S. Department of Health and Human Services (USDHHS), 2000]. As leading indicators, they reflect the major public health concerns in the United States. They were selected for the quality of data that could be longitudinally measured and for their relevance as important public health problems. Underlying each indicator are disparities in race and in class *(Healthy People 2010)*. For the first time, *Healthy People 2010* has set the elimination rather than the decrease in health disparities as a goal for the nation (USDHHS, 2000a)!

Substance abuse statistics from the 1990s will influence trends in substance abuse through 2010. The Internet abounds with statistics and argument. The Substance Abuse and Mental Health Service Administration (SAMHSA) and its Office of Applied Studies (OAS) provide the most current national data on illicit drug use, alcohol, tobacco, drug-related emergency room encounters, and profiles of the U.S. substance abuse treatment system (SAMHSA 2001). Figure 31-1 provides the major SAMHSA OAS data collection systems for the United States, the District of Columbia, and Puerto Rico.

From 1994 to 1998, 77% of 12- to 17-year-olds reported being alcohol and drug-free during the previous month. Sixteen percent of adolescents reported alcohol as their drug of choice. There has been little variation in the use of alcohol since 1992 (USDHHS, 2000a, p. 33).

Among adolescents, 1998 data reported that 10% used illicit drugs in the past 30 days. Data reflect that adolescents are experimenting with a variety of drugs, including cocaine, crack, heroin, methamphetamines, and street drugs. There is a strong relationship between age at onset of use and strength of addiction (USDHHS, 2000a, p. 33).

In examining the results of the 1992 Institute for Social Research survey, the National Institute on Drug Abuse (NIDA) expressed concern in finding a decline in the perceived dangers of drug abuse as well as a decline in peer disapproval of drug use. It was feared that this softening of attitudes might presage an increase in drug abuse, and it appears that it did. The results of the 1994 survey showed a sharp increase in the use of marijuana, particularly by the younger groups interviewed.

The 1994 survey demonstrated that attitudes about drug use have continued to soften. Students now perceive less danger in the regular use of marijuana, in smoking one or more packs of cigarettes a day, or in trying cocaine (USDHHS, 1996). They also have less negative attitudes toward their peers who use tobacco and marijuana.

What are the reasons for this decreased negativity? Perhaps the youth of today find it harder to identify with Belushi, Bias, and Kennedy. Perhaps they do not have concrete examples on which to base their fears. Perhaps

the general public has become more complacent about drugs and has allowed the counterculture drug message to be stronger and louder than the voices against that message.

In summary, the NIDA fact sheets report that 14.8 million Americans were users of illicit drugs in 1999: 3.5 million people were dependent on drugs and 8.2 million were alcohol dependent (NIDA Infofax, 2001g). Indicators show a decreased use of crack cocaine, an increase in heroin and morphine, in particular among 18- to 25-year-olds, a leveling off of marijuana abuse after the end of the 1990s, a recent rise in the use of methamphetamines, in particular MDMA or "ecstasy," and an epidemic in the abuse of OxyContin clonazepam, Vicodin (hydrocodone), and Percocet (oxycodone). Hydrocodone appears to be the drug of choice for illicit drug users.

Nationwide trends are analyzed from a variety of sources, including emergency room data, medical examiner data, interviews and self-reporting, focus groups, and community-based sources. The Drug Abuse Warning Network (DAWN) report provides information about the impact of drug use on hospital emergency departments (DAWN ED) and in medical examiner offices in the United States (DAWN ME). It offers another dimension to the National Household Survey (NHS) prevalence data. (SAMHSA, 2001a).

THE NATURE OF ADDICTION

Despite years of study and debate, the nature of addiction, including the disease concept, continues to be controversial (Meyer, 1996). There are a number of theories: social, biological, psychological, behavioral, and cultural explanations for addictive behavior. Many different models for understanding the addictions have been proposed, and a variety of diagnostic tools have been developed. In 1994 the American Psychiatric Association published the fourth edition of its *Diagnostic and Statistical Manual* (DSM-IV). One interesting change from its previous edition is that in discussing substance abuse it dropped the term *psychoactive*. **Psychoactive substances** are drugs or chemicals that affect the mental state. Research has demonstrated that people who abuse substances not primarily characterized as psychoactive (e.g., steroids) can also meet diagnostic criteria for dependence (Lehner, 2000). The generic criteria for substance dependence as stated in DSM-IV are listed in Figure 31-2.

Alcoholism has been discussed as an inherited disease since the 1800s, but the first scientific evidence to support this theory did not come until the 1970s. In a classic 1973 study of twins, Goodwin and Winokur found that sons born to alcoholic fathers were three times more likely to become alcoholic than those of nonalcoholic fathers (Blum, Cull, Braverman, & Comings, 1996). Several

---

FIGURE 31-1 Electronic Databases

DAWN Drug Abuse Warning Network ED (Emergency departments; ME medical examiner offices)

MEDLINE

MEDSCAPE

MMMR of the CDC

NHS National Household Survey (out of SAMHSA)

NIDA National Institute of Drug Abuse

NIDC National Drug Intelligence Center

SAMHSA Substance Abuse and Mental Health Services Administration (Health and Human Services)

UN Web Site on Drugs: http://www.undcp.org/

FIGURE 31-2 Generic Criteria for Identification of Substance Dependence

A maladaptive pattern of substance use, leading to clinically significant impairment or distress, as manifested by three (or more) of the following, occurring at any time in the same 12-month period:

(1) tolerance, as defined by either of the following:

　(a) a need for markedly increased amounts of the substance to achieve intoxication or desired effect

　(b) markedly diminished effect with continued use of the same amount of the substance

(2) withdrawal, as manifested by either of the following:

　(a) the characteristic withdrawal syndrome for the substance (refer to Criteria A and B of the criteria sets for Withdrawal from the specific substances)

　(b) the same (or a closely related) substance is taken to relieve or avoid withdrawal symptoms

(3) the substance is often taken in larger amounts or over a longer period than was intended

(4) there is a persistent desire or unsuccessful efforts to cut down or control substance use

(5) a great deal of time is spent in activities necessary to obtain the substance (e.g., visiting multiple doctors or driving long distances), use the substance (e.g., chain-smoking), or recover from its effects

(6) important social, occupational, or recreational activities are given up or reduced because of substance use

(7) the substance use is continued despite knowledge of having a persistent or recurrent physical or psychological problem that is likely to have been caused or exacerbated by the substance (e.g., current cocaine use despite recognition of cocaine-induced depression, or continued drinking despite recognition that an ulcer was made worse by alcohol consumption)

Specify if:

With Physiological Dependence: evidence of tolerance or withdrawal (i.e., either item 1 or 2 is present)

Without Physiological Dependence: no evidence of tolerance or withdrawal (i.e., neither Item 1 nor 2 is present)

Course specifiers

Early Full Remission

Early Partial Remission

Sustained Full Remission

Sustained Partial Remission

On Agonist Therapy

In a Controlled Environment

Reprinted with permission from the *Diagnostic and Statistical Manual of Mental Disorders* (4th ed.), text revision, by American Psychiatric Association, 1994, Washington, DC: Author. Copyright 2000 by the American Psychiatric Association.

---

well-designed studies carried out in the 1990s confirm the earlier work, suggesting that unspecified genetic factors increase the risk of developing alcohol addiction (Meyer, 1996). Blum and colleagues (1996) propose that there is a common genetic basis involved in several disorders, including alcoholism, drug addiction, attention-deficit disorder, binge eating, and addictive gambling. They believe that there is an inborn chemical imbalance that alters the intercellular signaling in the brain's reward process; this alteration supplants a feeling of well-being with feelings of anxiety and anger and leads to a craving for a substance that could alleviate the negative feelings. They propose the term *reward deficiency syndrome* to describe this condition. Genetic research is ongoing and should continue to shed light on the nature of addiction.

EFFECTS OF SUBSTANCE ABUSE ON HEALTH

Substance abuse is associated with a wide range of health problems. Types of substances that are often abused include depressants, stimulants, hallucinogens, inhalants, marijuana, steroids, and prescription drugs. A **depressant** is an agent that depresses a body function or nerve activity. Included in this grouping are alcohol, barbiturates, and opiates (heroin). Stimulants are agents that temporarily increase functional activity. These include amphetamines, cocaine, caffeine, and tobacco. Hallucinogens cause the user to have hallucinations; LSD and some designer drugs are considered hallucinogens (Lehne, 2000).

The community health nurse who is aware of the associated health problems is in a better position to recognize when substance abuse might be a problem for a client. This section will review common health problems associated with the abuse of alcohol, heroin, tobacco, caffeine, marijuana, cocaine, methamphetamine, and other drugs of abuse.

Tobacco

Tobacco is considered a stimulant and is highly addictive. The user feels as if he or she performs better and is more alert. A decrease in appetite is experienced (Faltz, 1998). The connection between cigarette smoking and lung disease, particularly lung cancer, has been recognized since the 1950s. In 1989 the U.S. Surgeon General issued a report concluding that cigarettes and other forms of tobacco are addictive and that smoking is a major cause of stroke. Increasingly, studies are demonstrating the relationship of a wide range of illnesses to the use of tobacco in both smokable and smokeless forms, including lung cancer; cancers of the mouth, lips, esophagus, and larynx; emphysema; heart disease; stroke; and congestive heart failure. In addition, Ambrosone et al. (1996) demonstrated an increase in breast cancer related to past or present smoking in postmenopausal women who genetically cannot quickly metabolize certain carcinogenic chemicals. Each year in the United States, approximately 400,000 deaths result from cigarette smoking (CDC, 2000).

The population at highest risk for new smoking behaviors is children, in particular teenage girls (Dumas, 1992b). A lifetime of cigarette smoking will shorten a life expectancy by 10 years. Dumas (1992b) noted that 80% of lung cancers in women are caused by heavy smoking.

In March of 1997, the Liggett Group Inc., one of the country's leading cigarette makers, made national headlines by announcing at a news conference that smoking is addictive, that it causes cancer, and that tobacco marketing has been directed toward minors. The admission was made as part of a settlement in a law suit filed by 22 states accusing the tobacco industry of hiding knowledge of the adverse effects of tobacco use (Broder, 1997).

After an extensive review of the literature, the Agency for Health Care Policy and Research (AHCPA, 1996) issued guidelines to assist health care workers to convince smokers to quit. In the introduction the AHCPA states, "It is difficult to identify a condition in the United States that presents such a mix of lethality, prevalence, and neglect, and for which effective interventions are so readily available."

A CDC (2001) study notes that 16 million smokers try to stop smoking cigarettes for at least 24 hours each year.

Another two to three million want to stop but are unable to do so for even 24 hours. The good news is that 1.2 million smokers stop each year. There are 48 million adult smokers in the United States (CDC, 2001). The study correlated increased smoking cessation attempts with the availability of more pharmacological over-the-counter antismoking aids (CDC, 2001). Figure 31-3 indicates tobacco use statistics.

Another study noted that the value of cigarettes bought by young people in the 12- to 17-year-old age group range approximates $222 million in tax revenues and $480 million in tobacco industry products! The researchers suggest that the cigarette profits from young people could be used to enforce laws that prohibit the sale of cigarettes to the young (Difranza & Librett, 1999). The problem of tobacco use among the young is a major public health issue. Yet a 1999 study showed that over two-thirds of animated children's films featured tobacco or alcohol use in story plots. There were no associated clear messages in the films that pointed out the health consequences of tobacco use in the young. Another study determined that there were relationships, although not strong, between smoking and pulmonary metastasis from breast cancers in women. This is yet another indicator of the relationships between cigarettes, the lungs, and cancers (Murin & Inciardi, 2001).

On a more international note, a symposium called "Young Women and Tobacco: Hope for Tomorrow" focused

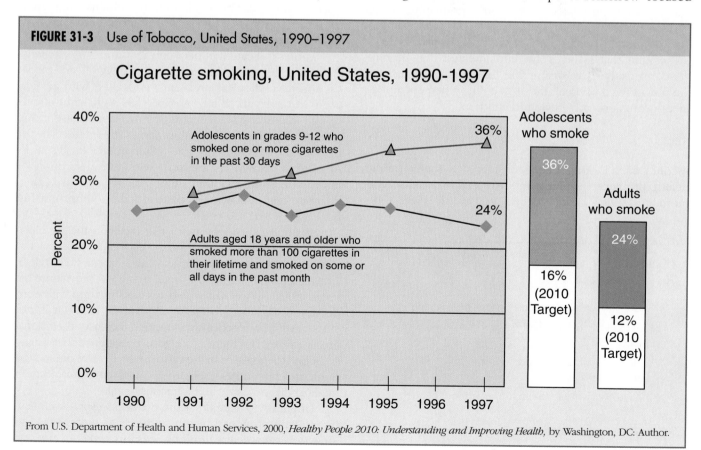

FIGURE 31-3 Use of Tobacco, United States, 1990–1997

Cigarette smoking, United States, 1990-1997

From U.S. Department of Health and Human Services, 2000, *Healthy People 2010: Understanding and Improving Health,* by Washington, DC: Author.

on community action and types of policy changes needed to stop the surge of young women and their relationship with tobacco. A trend has emerged in the United States, Canada, and most of the developed countries that females are smoking more than males. In developing countries, the smoking prevalence is rising, and in the United States and other developed countries, the rates are decreasing. Socioeconomic status and education are important predictors of smoking behaviors. In New Zealand and Australia as well as Canada, smoking prevalence is above 70% among the aborigines (Wilson, 2000, p. 2). Figure 31-4 summarizes some of the social, behavioral, and cultural themes that may influence young female smokers.

Margareta Haglund, president of the International Network of Women Against Tobacco, notes that in many European countries women have been ignored in national antismoking campaign (Wilson, 2000). She suggests the "slim" theme needs to be challenged and that soon in Europe the terms "slim" and "light" will be banned from cigarette advertising.

In the developing countries, for example in Latin America, the prevalence of smoking in young women is 22% and rapidly rising. In Brazil smoking has doubled over 15 years. Despite a media ban on tobacco advertising in Venezuela, 8 out of 10 students have been exposed to tobacco advertising. The next generation of women in developed and underdeveloped countries is at serious risk for smoking-related disease and premature death (Wilson, 2000).

Community health nurses have a role to play in making certain that policies are implemented that require gender-sensitive advertising and that tobacco industries are not allowed to break the 1998 court settlement agreement prohibiting advertising to children.

Alcohol

Alcoholism has long been considered a major public health problem, resulting in increased morbidity and mortality (Miller, Gold, Cocores, & Pottash, 1988; Califano, 1998). The use of moderate amounts of alcohol has been associated with a wide range of disorders that affect all body systems (USDHHS, 1990b). Alcohol is considered a depressant **(sedative)**. Alcohol is a small, water- and fat-soluble molecule that does not have to be broken down for absorption and easily reaches all areas of the body (Fishbein & Pease, 1996). Alcohol has the potential to cause great harm to all body tissues.

Alcohol exerts its effects both directly and indirectly. Harmful effects are due to the direct, irritating, and toxic effects of alcohol on the body, to the changes that take place during the metabolism of alcohol, to the aggravation of existing disease, to accidents while intoxicated, and to the irregular taking of prescribed treatments while intoxicated (Goroll, May, & Mulley, 2000). The user feels relaxed at first and experiences a decrease in inhibitions. As drinking continues, the user develops slurred speech and lack of physical coordination. Nausea and vomiting are common responses to extensive alcohol intake. Frequently, the user becomes very sleepy and depressed (Faltz, 1998).

The signs and symptoms of alcohol intoxication vary with the blood alcohol level and individual characteristics, including tolerance to the drug. Impairment increases directly with the level of alcohol in the blood, and an overdose of alcohol can lead to respiratory depression and death (Goroll et al., 2000). Withdrawal from alcohol can be dangerous. Symptoms range from mild discomfort to possibly fatal delirium tremens. High anxiety and sleep disturbances are common, and grand mal seizures frequently accompany withdrawal (Yost, 1996).

Studies indicate that between 25% and 50% of clients seen in general medical practice have significant physical and psychological problems associated with alcohol use (Goroll et. al., 2000). Alcohol has significant effects on the immune system secondary to liver disease, bone marrow depression, and malnutrition. These effects lower resistance to pneumonia and other infectious diseases. Alcohol is known to interfere with the absorption of many nutrients, including amino acids, glucose, zinc, thiamine, vitamin A, and folate, further compromising health (USDHHS, 1990a).

Alcohol consumption is a risk factor in the development of several types of cancers, especially those of the liver, esophagus, nasopharynx, and larynx (USDHHS, 1990a). Several studies indicate a higher prevalence of breast cancer in women who drink as compared with nondrinkers (Rosenberg, Metzger, & Palmer, 1993). It is not clear as yet how alcohol consumption increases the risk for breast cancer, but there is suggestive evidence that it may be linked to increases in the estrogen levels of women who drink (Reichman, 1994). Figure 31-5 illustrates the common medical diagnoses related to alcohol intake.

Liftik (1995) states that the prevalence of alcoholism in any type of mental health setting is as high as 30% to 70%. Persistent heavy drinking is associated with anxiety,

---

FIGURE 31-4 Women and Tobacco: Perceptions Thought to Influence Use

- Tobacco is a way to organize social relationships.
- Smoking is associated with an ability to control or enhance social situations.
- Smoking is associated with the suppression of negative emotions.
- Smoking is associated with themes of independence, rebellion.
- Smoking is associated with gender identity.

FIGURE 31-5   Common Alcohol-Related Diagnoses

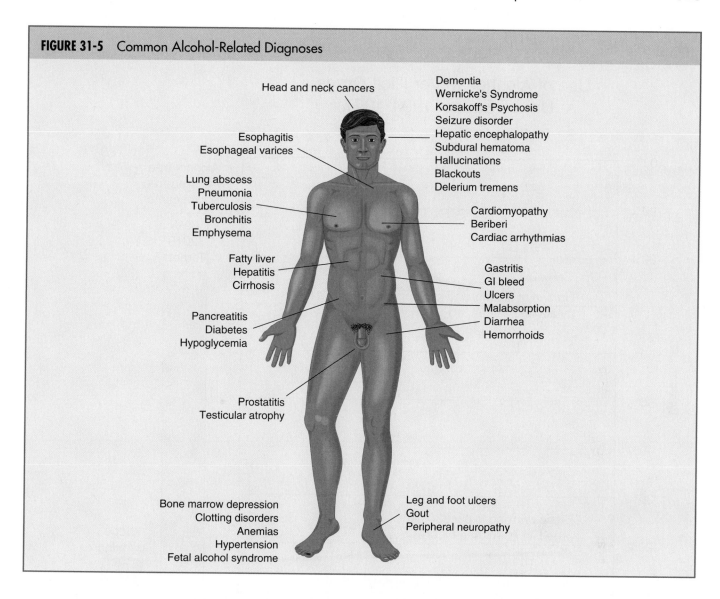

depression, psychosis, and cognitive deficits. Because treatment choices and outcomes differ, it is important to differentiate between primary psychiatric disorders and psychiatric symptoms that are secondary to alcohol intake or withdrawal. Secondary disorders will generally disappear with abstinence (Goroll et al., 1998).

An association between alcoholism and depression has long been recognized. Recent genetic research indicates that there is a commonality in the biochemical pathway of these two conditions. In an ongoing study, Nurnberger, et al. (2001) report that one or more genes on chromosome 1 may predispose some individuals to alcoholism and others to depression. In their study, the likelihood of major depression was found to be no higher in alcoholic subjects, as in non-alcoholic subjects, but depressive syndrome was significantly more common in the alcoholic subjects.

Depression can also be precipitated by the pharmacological effects of alcohol itself. Alcohol is a depressant drug. Its use is associated with several types of anemia

(Maruyama, Hirayama, Yamamoto, Koda, et al., 2001; Iwama, Iwase, Hayashi, Nakano, & Toyama, 1998; Davenport, 1996; Wheby, 1996). There is a decreased production of red blood cells in the bone marrow accompanied by an increased loss in the gastrointestinal tract, as well as decreased storage of iron, copper, and vitamin B_{12} in the liver. Depression is a common presenting complaint with anemia. Depression is also a common symptom of withdrawal, which decreases with abstinence from the drug. The grief reaction that an alcoholic experiences as he or she faces the prospect of life without alcohol is often profound. In each of these cases it is fruitless to treat the depression without addressing the underlying alcoholism.

Alcohol use is rising in adolescents, and it is the drug of choice in 15- to 17-year-olds. As the population ages, more older adults will be addicted to alcohol. Older adults are a population that has until recently not been targeted for education about alcohol abuse. See Figure 31-6 for projections about alcohol at 2010.

FIGURE 31-6 Use of Alcohol and/or Illicit Drugs, United States, 1994–1997

Use of Alcohol and/or Illicit Drugs, United States, 1994-1997

No use of alcohol or illicit drugs in past 30 days by adolescents (aged 12-17 years)

77%

Binge drinking in past 30 days (aged 18 years and older)

16%

Illicit drug use in past 30 days (aged 18 years and older)

6%

Alcohol-free and drug-free adolescents

89% (2010 Target)

77%

Binge drinking

16%

6% (2010 Target)

Illicit drug use

6%

3% (2010 Target)

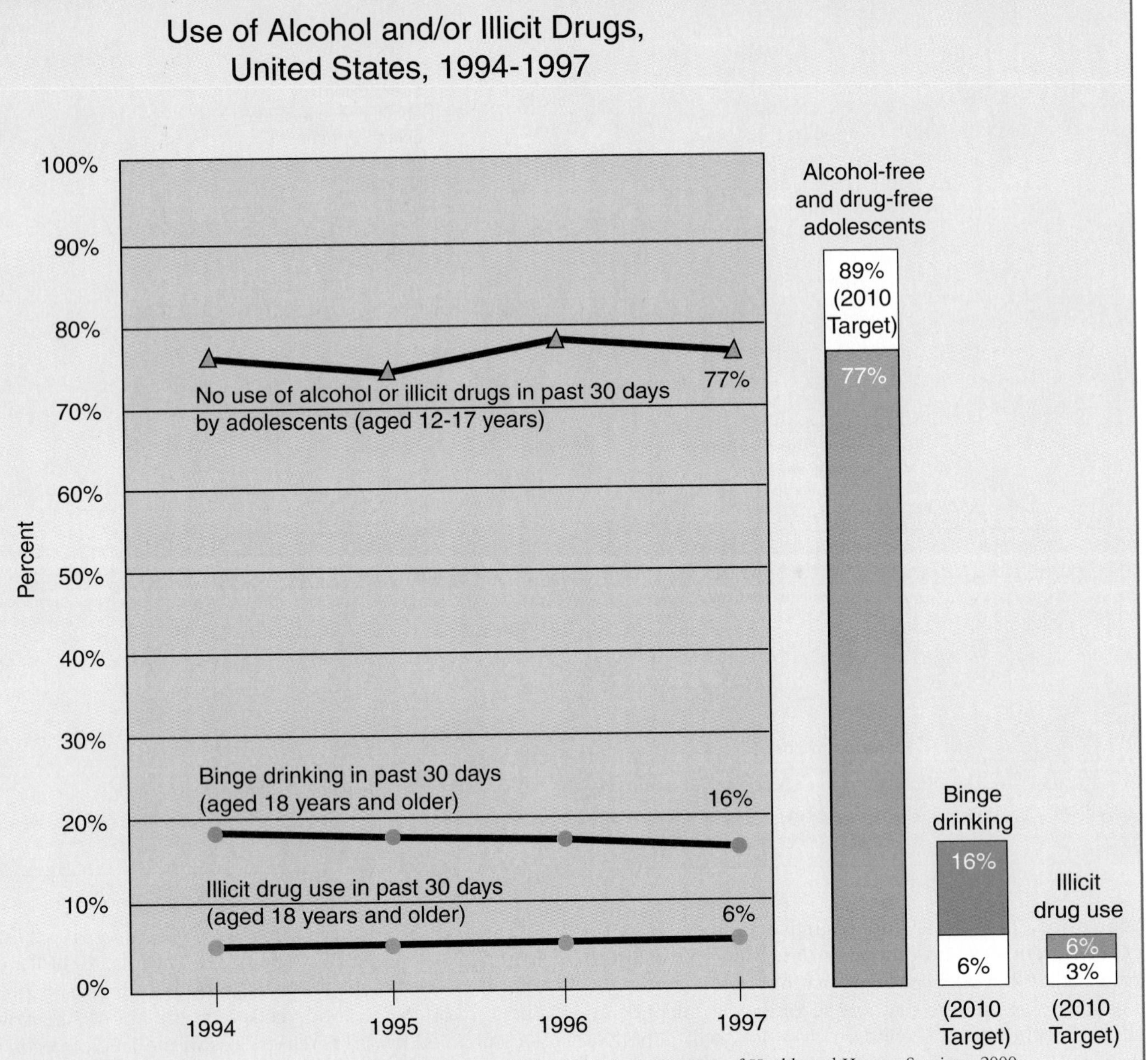

From *Healthy People 2010: Understanding and Improving Health,* by the U.S. Department of Health and Human Services, 2000, Washington, DC: Author.

Young people need to be targeted with education about legal, academic, and social consequences of drinking rather than the long-term health effects (Schwenk, 2000). Youths are rarely future oriented, and the legal ramifications of underage drinking will need to be one of the themes. National trends from the National Center for Health Statistics (NCHS) are consistent with other surveys that reflect a slowing or flat trend in the past few years. In 1999 fewer youths experienced binge drinking and heavy alcohol use. However, the number of drinkers under 21 in 1999 was 10.4 million to 6.8 million youths in-

dulging in binge drinking and 2.1 million were classified as heavy drinkers (SAMHSA, 2001). These are American adolescents 12 to 20 years of age.

In 1999, 105 million Americans 12 and older reported use of alcohol currently, 45 million engaged in binge drinking, and 12.5 million were classified as heavy drinkers (SAMHSA, 2001). It is important for the community nurse to consider the following relationships associated with alcohol. The role of alcohol abuse in the etiology of heroin-related deaths is being investigated; alcohol as a teratogen causing lasting birth defects and mental retardation is best known as fetal alcohol syndrome (FAS), and there are estimates of 12,000 new cases annually (Cramer & Davidhizar, 1999). There has been rather pallid response to the "panic" about FAS in the 1970s, and now there is a lack of adequate knowledge regarding FAS. When women do not know about the consequences of FAS, drinking behaviors bring about irreversible damage to many infants.

In the older adult, alcoholism can complicate symptoms of dementia and depression; the relationship between depression and alcoholism has been well documented. As the population ages, chronic drinking behaviors need to be identified early in the assessment phase. Hip fractures and other injuries are long-term consequences for elderly alcoholics and often lead to social isolation.

Alcohol is legal except for people under 21 years. Over 10 million children and adolescents drink alcohol. How do nurses better assess for alcohol abuse? Despite extensive use of illicit and prescription drugs in the United States, the most commonly used screens focus only on alcohol. The study by Brown, Leonard, Saunders, and Papasoiliotis (2001) describes a new screening test for two items: alcohol and other drug abuse.

The Two Item Conjoint Screen (TICS) was sensitive to polysubstance abuse disorders with 80% specificity and sensitivity (Brown et al., 2001). By adding the words "other drugs" or "drugs" in the two-question screen, alcohol or other drug problems such as those with marijuana or cocaine can be detected. The screen addresses the need for a broad scope of abused substances involving drugs other than alcohol.

Another brief test is the CAGE test. This test consists of the following four questions. In which the subject is asked to answer yes or no:

- Have you ever felt the need to **C**ut down on your drinking/drug use?
- Have you ever felt **A**nnoyed at criticisms of your drinking/drug use?
- Have you ever felt **G**uilty about something that's happened while drinking/using drugs?
- Have you ever felt the need for an **E**ye opener?

One yes response raises suspicions of alcohol/drug use problem. More than one is a strong indication that a problem exists (Coombs, 1997). Nurses across specialties need to be better educated in the importance of asking screening questions about substance abuse. Screening for more than one substance may be helpful.

Alcohol has also been implicated in the four leading causes of accidental death in the United States—motor vehicle accidents, falls, drownings, and fires. Automobile accidents are the leading cause of death between the ages of 15 and 24 and are a significant cause of death at all ages. An encouraging indication that prevention measures do work is found in the reduction in fatal automobile crashes since 1989. In 1989 alcohol related fatalities represented 49% of the total traffic fatalities for the year and in 1999 this was reduced to 38%. Possible reasons for the decrease are lowering of the legal blood alcohol levels and an increase in license revocation. Further diligence is needed as there is evidence that the trend is slowing down and perhaps reversing itself (NHTSA, 2001).

According to *Healthy People 2010* (USDHHS, 2000), the United States ranks first among industrialized nations in violent death rates. In the United States, suicide is the third leading cause of death between the ages of 15 and 24, and between 2 and 4 million people are physically battered each year by their partners. Alcohol and other substance abuse are consistently found to be associated with all forms of violence.

Another major concern is the use of alcohol during pregnancy resulting in fetal alcohol syndrome. This condition is characterized by low birth size and weight, developmental deficiencies, facial anomalies, cardiovascular defects, cognitive problems, hyperactivity, and learning difficulties. Because a safe level of drinking during pregnancy has not been established, it is generally recommended that a woman abstain from alcohol during pregnancy.

HEROIN

Heroin is considered a highly addictive opiate, a central nervous system (CNS) depressant. The estimated number of heroin users, which remained fixed at roughly 600,000 from the 1970s into the 1990s, almost quadrupled in the 1990s to an estimated 2.4 million users (NIDA, Infofax 2001b). Heroin is both physically and psychologically addicting and creates a strong craving in the user. Because tolerance to the effects of the drug develops quickly, increasing amounts are needed to achieve the desired effects (Fishbein & Pease, 1996). Euphoria is the initial response to the drug but then changes to drowsiness, reduced libido, difficulties with memory and concentration, and the absence of the sense of pain (Faltz, 1998).

Because heroin is an *illegal drug,* there is no quality control on its manufacture or sale. The strength of the drug and what is added to it (cutting agents) are unknown to the buyer. **Cutting agents** are substances added to street drugs to increase bulk (e.g., mannitol and starch), to mimic or enhance pharmacological effects (e.g., caffeine and lidocaine), or to combat side effects (e.g., vitamin C and/or dilantin). The contamination of heroin with cutting agents, the use of unsterile equipment, and combination with other drugs can lead to serious health consequences. An unsuspectedly pure batch often results in a number of overdoses, which can precipitate respiratory depression, coma, and possibly death (Ling & Wesson, 1990; USDHHS, 2000).

Buyers of street drugs can never be sure of what they are buying. In 1996, the health departments and poison control centers in four eastern U.S. cities reported at least 325 cases of overdoses requiring medical intervention for people who had used heroin bought on the street that had probably contained scopolamine, an anticholinergic drug. In one hospital in Baltimore, 22 patients who had reported taking heroin were treated; testing of a specimen identified scopolamine, quinine, and dextromethorphan but no heroin (CDC, 1996b).

Historically, heroin has been mainly administered by injection leading to extremely serious health threats. Unsterile intravenous injection can cause skin abscesses, inflammation of the veins, serum hepatitis, and subacute bacterial endocarditis. All of these have serious sequelae. Sharing of needles is a leading cause of HIV infection that leads to acquired immunodeficiency syndrome (AIDS). Figure 31-7 shows routes of administration of heroin.

There has been a shift in the populations who abuse heroin with the emergence of a more diverse group of users. The predominant users of heroin are adults over 30; however, there has been an increase in younger adults who use the drug. The drug trafficking of heroin is of global proportion, and the effects of its abuse are seen in developed and developing countries. The young

are attracted to heroin because it is cheap, the purity is high, and it can be sniffed or snorted, thus avoiding the dangers associated with injection. (NIDA, 2001b). Eighty-seven percent of the "new users" are under age 26, as compared to 1992, when it was 67%. In 1999 heroin was listed as the primary drug of abuse in treatment admissions in some of the largest American cities (NIDA, 2001b, p. 2).

Caffeine

The most ubiquitous and widely used psychoactive drug is caffeine. Caffeine, a stimulant, is found in coffee, tea, cocoa, soft drinks, and over-the-counter preparations. Over 80% of U.S. citizens consume it daily (Lamarine, 1994). The user feels stimulated with increased mental acuity and a sense that he or she can continue forever without becoming exhausted (Faltz, 1998). A 1994 study found evidence to support the existence of a caffeine dependence syndrome, which includes the development of tolerance to the effects, physical withdrawal, difficulty cutting down or controlling use, and continued use despite medical contraindications (Strain, Mumford, Silverman, & Griffiths, 1994).

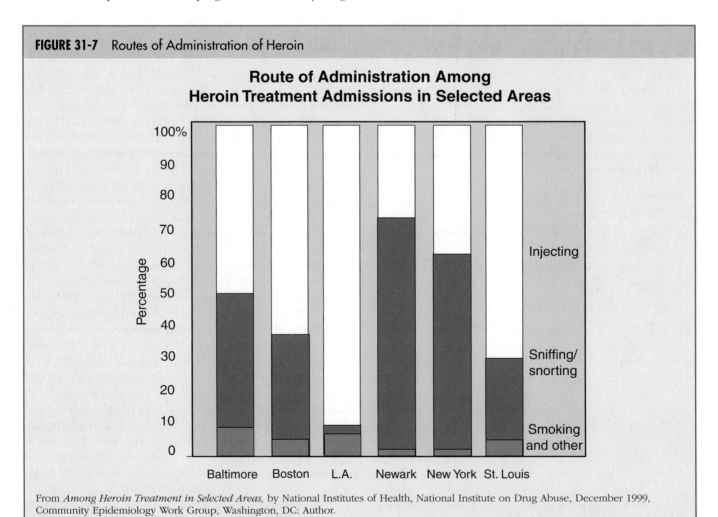

FIGURE 31-7 Routes of Administration of Heroin

From *Among Heroin Treatment in Selected Areas,* by National Institutes of Health, National Institute on Drug Abuse, December 1999, Community Epidemiology Work Group, Washington, DC: Author.

Caffeine continues to be studied in relation to a number of health problems. Among them are hypertension (Myers, 1988), cardiac arrhythmias (Myers, 1991), increased cholesterol (Pietinen, Geboers, & Kesteloot, 1988), heart disease (Klatsky, Friedman, & Armstrong, 1990), and malignancies (Rosenberg, 1990; Rosenberg, et al., 1993). Many studies have explored the relationships between caffeine and asthma. Caffeine is a weak bronchodilator and it may help asthmatic patients (Bara & Barley, 2001). See Figure 31-8 for a summary of the pharmacological effects of caffeine on the body's systems.

The point to be made about caffeine is it can be harmful and dangerous. Health teaching in the community setting relates to the use of restraint with caffeine consumption, especially for pregnant women, asthmatics on bronchodilators, and clients at risk for cardiac events and sequelae to worsening hypertension.

Marijuana

Marijuana has been both deified and vilified, often with more emotion on both sides than hard scientific data. There is, however, increasing evidence that it is both a physically harmful and addicting drug (Goroll et al., 2000). Use of the drug can lead to a sense of euphoria or depression and restlessness. The individual becomes relaxed and drowsy and experiences a heightened perception and awareness of color and sound. Time is distorted as are spatial perceptions. The user has poor coordination and often experiences a sense of weightlessness and tingling. Dry mouth, difficulty articulating words, and food cravings are other responses (Faltz, 1998). Tetrahydrocannabinol (THC) is the most psychologically active ingredient.

FIGURE 31-8 Pharmacological Effects of Caffeine

Central nervous system effects

- In low doses, decreases fatigue
- In high doses, insomnia, tremors, irritability

Cardiovascular effects

- High doses stimulate the heart
- High doses can lead to arrhythmias

Effects on the vasculature

- In central nervous system vasoconstrict
- In peripheral nervous system vasodilate

Effects on the respiratory system: bronchodilation

Renal effects: diuretic

Reproductive effects: in high doses can be teratogenic

Adapted from *Pharmacology for Nursing Care* (4th ed.), p. 362, by R. A. Lehne, 2000, Philadelphia, PA: Saunders.

Chronic use of marijuana can lead to cardiovascular, pulmonary, reproductive, and psychological problems (Goroll et al., 2000; NIDA Infofax, 2001f). Psychological effects include euphoria, distortions in space and time, paranoia, impairment in memory and concentration, and difficulties in abstraction (Goroll et al., 2000). In view of the increased usage of marijuana in the 8th- and 10th-grade groups (NIDA Infofax, 2001c), cognitive effects of the drug are of particular concern.

Withdrawal symptoms have been identified as irritability, nausea, weight loss, insomnia, and anxiety. According to Tierney (2000), the marijuana in use today is perhaps 30 times stronger than that cultivated in the 1960s.

Cocaine

Cocaine is a stimulant that is snorted or injected. Cocaine use can result in a number of physical problems that include inflammation of the nasal passages and damage to the nasal septum, hypertension, cardiac arrhythmias, heart attacks, seizures, strokes, and malnutrition (NIDA Infofax, 2001a). In addition, the person who injects the drug is exposed to all of the problems associated with unsterile intravenous injection. Chaisson et al. (1989) found that daily intravenous cocaine use significantly increased the risk of HIV infection, relative to use of heroin alone. Psychological problems include restlessness, irritability, depression, anxiety, and paranoia (Goroll et al., 2000; Tierney, 2000).

The process of "freeing" cocaine from its hydrochloride base is called freebasing. Smoking cocaine in freebase or crack form not only increases the euphoria but also increases the many associated dangers. The euphoria (or high) is rapid because the cocaine reaches the brain in seconds, but it is short-lived and lasts less than 15 minutes (Tierney, 2000). Crack is a short-acting, powerfully addictive drug that is often lethal. Crack cocaine constricts blood vessels and dangerously raises the blood pressure, possibly resulting in heart attack or stroke or severe respiratory problems (NIDA Infofax, 2001a; Tierney, 2000). The use of crack cocaine is responsible for a generation of young people who will live as cardiac cripples, with seriously damaged hearts and damaged lives.

Crack babies have physical problems and developmental delays due to their mother's prenatal use of cocaine. Crack babies have been found to have numerous problems including abnormal electroencephalograms (EEGs), an increased incidence of sudden infant death syndrome (SIDS), visual impairments, mental retardation, delayed development, and learning problems (Tierney, 2000). The children are prime subjects for abuse, because they tend to be tense infants and hyperactive children. This situation is compounded by the fact that the mother may continue her use of crack, which increases the potential for infant abuse and neglect.

As these children reach school age, they present tremendous challenges to their teachers and to school nurses. Sluder, Kinnison, and Cates (1996) have identified a complex range of cognitive, social, language, behavioral, and motor deficiencies characteristic of children who had prenatal drug exposure. School nurses need to be aware that the children might exhibit multiple disabilities and be prepared to work with the children, their teachers, and their parents. The school nurse should work with local and state agencies to develop resources to enhance the education and support of the children and their parents.

Cocaine was the drug of the 1980s and 1990s. It was used extensively during that time and this was reflected in its frequent depiction in television and movies. The highest rate of cocaine and crack use is among 18- to 25-year-old adults. Men use cocaine more than women with the highest use in African Americans (1.4%), followed by Hispanics (0.8%) and Caucasians (0.6%) [National Household Survey on Drug Abuse (NHSDA), 1997]. Illicit drug use in adults, which includes cocaine, rose from 14.7% in 1997 to 18.8% in 1999. Rates for other adult age groups have not changed. Adolescents continue to experiment with cocaine and crack inhalants and methamphetamines. The rate is down from the 1996–1997 high of 16% (USDHHS, 2000).

Studies support predictions that cocaine abuse may lead to strokes and mental deficits. In the 1980s cocaine-related strokes in young people became more prevalent, in particular after the use of crack cocaine (Stocker, 2001). In an NIDA-funded study in 1998 researchers Kaufman and Levin demonstrated that the vasoconstriction brought about by cocaine in the heart and vasculature happens in the brain also. Cocaine was found to have a cumulative effect on the brain's vasculature and an outcome can be stroke (Stocker, 2001). Mental deficits continue long after an individual has stopped using cocaine (NIDA, Infofax, 2001a). Cocaine abusers are at high risk for atherosclerosis; in summary, long-term use of cocaine or crack essentially changes the way the brain functions. Mental deficits can seriously interfere with work, family, and routine daily activities. Developmental delays are seen in cocaine and crack babies. Adults may be disinhibited and aggressive. Deficits must be identified and treatments modified to the deficit. Deleterious effects of cocaine use can also affect manual dexterity as well as cognitive skills (NIDA Infofax, 2001a). Community health nurses must be cognizant of the serious sequelae to cocaine and crack use. They are often the first health professionals to recognize the problem and facilitate interventions.

Finally, there is interesting clinical research being conducted around the use of acupuncture for the treatment of cocaine addiction (Margolin, 2000). Researchers considered clinical trials of 82 participants assigned randomly to one of three groups: auricular acupuncture, control acupuncture (acupuncture not thought to have treatment effect because of location), and relaxation. Findings provided support for the use of acupuncture for cocaine addiction. See Research Focus. Replication studies are pending; group and/or individual drug counseling will be used as random assignments in studying acupuncture. This research may herald the beginning of the use of alternative therapies and their combinations for cocaine and other illicit drug addictions. Cocaine and crack cocaine may be deadly addictions.

Methamphetamine

Methamphetamine is an amphetamine, a CNS stimulant manufactured chemically. Methamphetamine, variably known as "speed," "crank," and "go," has been a drug of abuse for many years. Its smokable form, usually referred to as "ice" or "crystal," has been available in the United States since the early 1980s (Beebe & Walley, 1995). In the 1990s it replaced cocaine as a drug of choice in some areas of the country, most notably in the West, South, and Midwest (NIDA Infofax, 2001e). The user experiences an initial euphoria followed by depression. The individual feels wide awake, has a decreased appetite, and experiences insomnia. With continued use, the user frequently becomes very suspicious of the actions of others, resulting in aggression (Faltz, 1998).

From 1991 to 1994, methamphetamine-related emergency department visits more than tripled, and methamphetamine-related deaths reported by medical examiners rose from 151 to 433 (CDC, 1995a). In view of the increased morbidity and mortality associated with the use of the drug, the Comprehensive Methamphetamine Control Act of 1996 was passed by Congress. This law increased the penalties for trafficking in methamphetamine and toughened the penalties for trafficking in the chemicals used to produce it.

Physical effects associated with methamphetamine abuse include weight loss, tachycardia, tachypnea, hyperthermia, insomnia, and muscle tremors (NIDA Infofax, 2001e; Volkow, 2001). In chronic users, the most common presentation is acute psychosis with auditory and visual hallucinations, aggressiveness, and extreme paranoia.

With the rise in amphetamine use in the 1980s and early 1990s and more rigorous control regulations, use of the drugs trended down in 1997 through early 1999, at which time there was a significant rise in Seattle, Denver, and Phoenix (NIDA Infofax, 2001e). Use of MDMA, or "Ecstasy," became more prevalent in 1999. In Boston, Ecstasy was the most frequently mentioned drug in telephone calls to the Poison Control Center in 2000 (NIDA Infofax, 2001e).

Ecstasy, or MDMA, is used in a variety of social settings leading to its association with "club drugs." Some interesting data showed that marijuana abuse in combi-

RESEARCH FOCUS

Acupuncture in Treatment of Cocaine Addiction

Study Problem/Purpose

This study was a randomized control trial to determine if the use of auricular acupuncture has any treatment effect on cocaine addiction.

Methods

Eighty-two dually addicted heroin and cocaine users being treated with methadone for their heroin addiction participated in this study. All were heavy users of cocaine. Participants were randomly assigned to one of three treatment groups: (a) auricular acupuncture (standard acupuncture); (b) control acupuncture (needles inserted into four ear points), not thought to have any treatment outcome; and (c) relaxation groups where commercially relaxing video imagery was shown to participants. Group sessions were provided five times a week for eight weeks. Urine was tested for cocaine three times a week.

Findings

Results showed that participants who received the auricular acupuncture were more likely to refrain from cocaine use compared to the control group through the course of the study. The use or nonuse of cocaine was documented by urine test. Additional findings showed that 58.8% of acupuncture participants remained free of cocaine during the last week of treatment compared to 23.5% of the control acupuncture group and 9.1% of the relaxation group.

Of the 82 participants who completed the study, 63% completed the eight-week trial. Of that 63%, 46% completed treatment auricular acupuncture, 63% completed the control acupuncture treatment, and 81% completed the relaxation control. Thus, despite the fewer total treatment weeks in the auricular acupuncture group, the participants were most likely to refrain from cocaine use during the study.

Implications

The study supported the use of acupuncture in cocaine addiction. Outcomes are preliminary, and further evidence is needed to support the hypothesis that acupuncture is an effective therapy for cocaine addicts. Research is also needed to provide evidence of acupuncture use as monotherapy or in combination with a western therapy.

Source: Margolin, A. (2000). A randomized controlled trial of auricular acupuncture for cocaine dependence. Arch. Intern. Med. 160, 2305–2312.

---

nation with MDMA increased from eight "mentions" (drug associated with emergency ward visits) in 1990 to 796 in 1999! (NIDA Infofax, 2001g). Marijuana loses its benign association when paired with MDMA.

In a recent study, the physical effects of the club drug Ecstasy, a methamphetamine, have been compared to dobutamine. Heart rate and blood pressure were increased significantly *without* an inotropic effect. It is another piece of evidence that methamphetamine can be very dangerous to an individual, in particular if the user is elderly or has a cardiac condition (Mendelson, 2000).

A second study provided evidence on the extent of damage that use of methamphetamines have on the brain (Volkow, 2000). Brain hypermetabolism was 14% higher in abusers compared to non–drug users. Such hypermetabolism is seen in brain disease states posttrauma or postradiation and can lead to very grave consequences. The population at greatest risk appears to be juveniles (NIDA Infofax, 2000e).

However, some new British research points to Ecstasy as a new clue for directions in the treatment for Parkinson's disease (PD). There is some evidence that patients with PD regain temporary control of their body after taking Ecstasy. While Ecstasy is really not an answer for PD, it does affect serotonin levels in the brain and may explain the reversal of rigidity and spasm after it has been taken (Nurses Medscape, 2001).

Properties of Sedatives, Narcotics, and Cocaine

Signs and symptoms of intoxication, overdose, and withdrawal from sedatives, narcotics, and cocaine are given in Table 31-1. The term *narcotic* has many definitions and has been commonly used to refer to a CNS depressant, or analgesic, or any drug that can lead to physical dependence (Lehne, 1995). Sedatives are included under the broad category of CNS depressants. Examples of narcotics are heroin, morphine, demerol, and Darvon. The

TABLE 31-1 Addictive Properties of Sedatives, Narcotics, and Cocaine

DRUG	ADDICTIVE PROPERTIES	USE INTOXICATION	OVERDOSE	WITHDRAWAL
Sedatives (alcohol, barbiturates)	Physically and psychologically addicting; tolerance	Relaxation; decreased inhibitions, judgment, reflexes; slurred speech, clumsiness, drowsiness, psychomotor retardation, labile mood	Sleepiness, shallow respiration, apnea, difficulty in arousal, decreased or absent response to painful stimuli, loss of deep tendon reflexes, cold clammy skin, dilated pupils, hypotension, coma and death	On a continuum: slight tremors → uncontrollable shaking; insomnia → total wakefulness; mild diaphoresis → drenching sweats; frequent dreams → vivid nightmares; nausea and vomiting dry heaves and total increased vital signs Convulsions possible
Narcotics	Physically and psychologically addicting; tolerance; craving	Euphoria, drowsiness, respiratory depression, constricted pupils, nausea, and insomnia	Slow and shallow breathing, pinpoint pupils, clammy skin, decreased consciousness, convulsions, coma, death	Watery eyes, runny nose, yawning, decreased appetite, tremors, panic, chills, sweating, nausea, muscle cramps, insomnia, increased vital signs
Cocaine	Strong psychological addiction; strong craving	Dilated pupils, increased vital signs, anorexia, insomnia, euphoria followed by letdown, dullness, tenseness, irritability; risk of seizures, heart and respiratory failure	Hyperthermia, panic attacks, seizures, arrhythmias, hypertension	Decreased energy, depression, fatigue, craving, insomnia, inability to feel pleasure

mildest form of CNS depression is sedation. At low doses sedatives diminish physical and mental responses but do not affect consciousness. Benzodiazepines and anxiolytics are newer terms for sedatives. Withdrawal from narcotics, although extremely uncomfortable to the client, poses less actual threat than withdrawal from sedatives such as alcohol or barbiturates (Julien, 1985). Heroin withdrawal is often described retrospectively by the client as a very bad case of the flu.

Other Drugs Misused and Abused

Several other substances are abused and misused, most notably steroids, inhalants, designer drugs, and prescription drugs.

Steroids

There has been an international rise in the use of anabolic steroids among adolescents and young adults. These drugs are used by young people, in particular for body building. The aim usually is high muscle development and to excel in sports in order to increase their self-esteem and popularity. Steroids are synthetic substances related to androgens. They are available only by prescription and are legally used to treat delayed growth and puberty, impotence, and wasting in AIDS and cancer clients (NIDA Notes, 2001, p. 1). Statistics indicate that use is highest among boys and men, but its use is rising in girls and young women. In the 1999 Monitoring the Future study, an NIDA-funded survey of drug abuse among adolescents, an estimated 2.7% of adolescents had taken anabolic steroids at least once. The prevalence of use in adolescents has risen approximately 50% since 1991 (NIDA Notes, 2001a, p. 1).

Methods of use are oral, injection, and transdermal. Steroids are prescribed very carefully because of their serious adverse effects. When taken illegally, the dosing may be up to 100 times greater than legal use (Webber, 2001). Athletes take steroids to build muscles and users self-titrate large doses. This practice is very dangerous. See Figure 31-9.

> ## FIGURE 31-9 Health Consequences of Steroid Abuse
>
> - Hormonal disruptions
> - Termination of growth among adolescents
> - Cardiovascular diseases
> - Liver diseases
> - Skin disorders, acne cysts
> - Infections such as endocarditis
> - Behavioral changes, depression, mood swings, fatigue
> - Anorexia and loss of sex drive when steroids are stopped
>
> From NIDA Notes, 2001.

In a Boston study on steroid abusers, research suggested that men who abused anabolic androgenic steroids went on to abuse opioids, heroin, and other prescription narcotics (Pope, 2001). Former steroid users abused opiates to calm steroid-induced mood swings, insomnia, and other CNS effects.

Steroids are used primarily by athletes in order to build muscle strength and to improve athletic prowess, but they bring with them physical and psychological risk. Associated risks include depression, aggressiveness, heart attacks and strokes, acne, hair loss, weakened tendons, breast development and testicular shrinkage in men, and facial hair, lowered voice, and irregular menstrual periods in women (NIDA Notes, 2001a). Symptoms of dependence on steroids consistent with DSM-IV criteria have been demonstrated, pointing to the need for an awareness of possible steroid dependence in clinical practice. DSM-IV includes anabolic steroids as a substance-related disorder (American Psychiatric Association, 1994).

Inhalants

The National Survey Results on Drug Use (USDHHS, 1994b) reported an increase in the use of **inhalant substances.** These volatile substances are purposely inhaled to produce intoxication. This group of drugs consists of gasoline, glues, paint thinners, cleaning fluids, aerosol propellants, lighter fluid, nitrous oxide, and ether, among others. The user experiences giddiness and euphoria. Inhalants are associated with a wide range of serious effects, including organic brain syndromes; pulmonary, liver, and kidney damage; and potentially fatal cardiac arrhythmias.

Hallucinogens and Designer Drugs

After a 15-year gradual decline, hallucinogens appear to be making a comeback. Lysergic acid diethylamide (LSD), a drug often associated with the 1960s, increasingly became a drug of the 1990s. The use of LSD by twelfth graders increased from 4.8% in 1988 to 6.8% in 1993, and at the same time there was a significant decline in the percentage of persons seeing a risk associated with taking LSD (USDHHS, 1994b).

Designer drugs is the name given to new drugs that are created by chemically altering known drugs. Several heroinlike drugs have been created, for example, by making chemical changes in demerol and fentanyl. Serious health risks have been associated with the use of designer drugs. The risks are dependent upon the ingredients in the drug and the conditions under which it was manufactured.

Prescription Drugs

The misuse of drugs that have been prescribed for a legitimate purpose is on the rise. Misuse might be accomplished by seeking prescriptions from several health care providers, by taking the drug in excess of the prescribed dose, or by forging or altering prescriptions. Large quantities of prescription drugs are diverted to the illicit drug market by use of fraudulent prescriptions.

The opioid oxycodone group is of particular concern. The OxyContin phenomenon is an example of the abuse of an opioid that is used to treat clients with severe pain. When used therapeutically, addiction to opioids is rare, and despite this knowledge, physicians and nurse practitioners prescribe in less than adequate doses because of fear of addiction. Clients rarely become addicted to the opioids and opioids are most successful in controlling severe, acute, or chronic pain.

A recent JAMA study (Joranson, Ruan, Gilson, & Dahl, 2000) examined data collection sources of the abuse of oxycodone and related opioids. The JAMA study reported a 23% use of oxycodone for medical purposes and no rise in illicit drug use. However, the Drug Abuse Warning Network (DAWN) data set noted significant rises between 1997 and 1999 of oxycodone "mentions" at autopsy and at emergency room visits (Marley, 2001).

OxyContin and heroin are both in the opioid family and therefore have similar effects. On the street, a bottle of 100 OxyContin tablets sells for $2000–$4000. In the pharmacy, the same bottle costs $400.00. OxyContin abusers chew, crush, snort, and inject the drug. With injection, there is rapid release and absorption (NIDA Infofax 2001b). There is also the risk of hepatitis B, C, and D. Illicit use of OxyContin is at an epidemic level. Other prescription drugs commonly associated with abuse are the benzodiazepines, in particular Ativan (lorazepam) and Valium (diazepam).

Although alcohol and the various other drugs are generally studied as separate entities, the common practice is to use two or more substances concomitantly. It is difficult enough to describe the effects of any psychoactive drug, because they vary depending upon experience with the drug, increasing and decreasing blood levels, intoxication, overdose, withdrawal, and so on. When a second or third drug is added with synergistic, additive, or antagonistic properties, the results are impossible to predict (Lehne, 2000).

LEGAL ISSUES

In discussions of addiction, the interface between medicine and the law is ambiguous. Drug addiction and alcoholism are highly correlated with crime and violence. The question of whether the addicted person is sick and should be treated in the health care system or is a criminal and is better dealt with by the law is a complicated debate. It covers many issues at many different levels.

One topic concerns the decriminalization of marijuana. Canada is the first country to have approved the medicinal use of marijuana. With a certificate from their doctor, patients who have a severe chronic condition such as cancer, HIV/AIDS, arthritis, or are terminally ill, are allowed to grow and smoke marijuana (Schiff, 2001). In the United States there are about eight states that permit the medical use of marijuana. This, however, remains contrary to federal law. As the present laws stand, a person who is sick and advised by a physician to take marijuana might be in compliance with state law and yet face federal penalties. Issues regarding the decriminalization of marijuana will continue to be played out. Should it be available only on the advice of a physician? Is enough known about its deleterious effects? Should it be sold like alcohol or tobacco?

The criminal offender is far more likely to have been drinking than under the influence of other drugs (NCADD, 1988). Between 1993 and 1998 there was an overall decrease in the incidence of violent crimes in the United States including those that were alcohol related. At the same time, surveys of violent offenders in State and Federal prisons and on probation revealed that 38% were drinking when they committed the crime for which they were incarcerated. More than 40% of murderers and nearly a half of those convicted of assault were drinking at the time of their offense (Greenfield & Henneberg, 2001). Abby and colleagues (2001) estimate that roughly 25% of American women have experienced sexual assault and that approximately one-half of the cases involved the consumption of alcohol by either perpetrator, victim or both.

The percentage of alcohol related traffic fatalities has also fallen over the past two decades. Increased education as well as tougher laws and more severe sanctions coincide with this decrease (Voas & Fisher, 2001). Alcohol impaired driving, however remains a major public health problem, killing more than 16,000 individuals in 1997 alone and injuring a million more. About three

in every ten Americans will be involved in an alcohol related automobile accident at some time during their life. In 1996, alcohol-related traffic deaths and injuries cost the nation $45 billion dollars in lost economic productivity and hospital and rehabilitation cost (USDHHS, 2000b).

Other legal issues include child abuse, possession of illicit substances, underage possession of alcohol and cigarettes, disorderly conduct, theft, the responsibility of both mother and father to an unborn child, juvenile delinquency, violation of restraining orders, and on and on. Most of these are not victimless crimes. Who should be treated? Who should be punished? What are the ramifications of these decisions? These are questions that must be considered by the community health nurse. Public health as well as individual health must be considered. Questions of policy must also be considered. Will supplying clean needles and syringes prevent the spread of AIDS or will it encourage the continued use of drugs? Will incarcerating drug-addicted pregnant women increase the chances of a healthy child or will it prevent addicted women from seeking prenatal care? Will denying disability benefits to individuals claiming disability due to drug or alcohol addiction provide needed incentive to sobriety or will it condemn people on the edge to the streets or to shelters? If the addictions are diseases, should the individual be held responsible for actions while intoxicated? Should there be mandatory drug testing in the workplace?

The nurse has many roles in this emotionally laden aspect of addiction. It is important for the nurse to have access to legal assistance through different agencies. Most communities have free attorneys or legal advice for women and elders who are in the midst of domestic violence. Other legal resources for clients can be found at shelters, hospitals, and welfare agencies. Some attorneys provide free assistance for people who are unable to hire their own legal representative. It is important for the community health nurse to act nonjudgmentally and guide clients to medical, legal, or mental health assistance in diverse settings. In order to do this well, the nurse becomes an advocate; the goal becomes treatment for an addiction. See Chapter 30 for more information regarding family and community violence.

NURSING CARE OF CLIENTS WHO ABUSE SUBSTANCES

Community health nurses are often the first to recognize the existence of a substance abuse problem. With knowledge of the addictions, nursing skills can be employed to help the client recognize and seek help for the problem. In their daily practice they continue to witness the ravages of substance abuse on urban men, women, and children. Nurses see too many addicted babies being born; too many youngsters suffering anomalies due to **fetal**

alcohol syndrome, caused by their mother's prenatal use of alcohol, struggling in school; too many young men and women showing early signs of HIV infection because they share needles; and too many stressed single mothers finding relief in drinking, smoking, snorting, and injecting drugs. Nurses also see increasing numbers of men and women in their middle years suffering the emotional and physical effects of chronic substance abuse.

The community health nurse sees firsthand that substance abuse problems are prevalent and costly. The cost is measured in dollars and, more importantly, by increases in violence, accidents, suicides, domestic abuse, physical problems, social and psychological problems, and premature death. Community health nurses are pivotal in identifying addictive behaviors and in decreasing their numerous associated problems (Talashek, Laina, Gerace, & Starr, 1994). Assessment and observation skills are employed to identify a problem, and a caring manner, good judgment, and effective communication skills influence the client's and the community's willingness to do something about it.

Effect of Attitudes on the Delivery of Care

Prior experiences, personal likes and dislikes, values, beliefs, family background, peer interests, education, and knowledge all affect the choices that people make and the way that they perceive others. The dictionary defines attitude as "a manner, disposition, feeling, position, etc. with regard to a person or thing" (Flexnor & Hauck, 1993, p.134). Nurses have varied feelings or attitudes with regard to working in different specialty areas.

The same dictionary further defines attitude as "a position or posture of the body appropriate to or expressive of an action, emotion, etc." (p. 134). A nurse wanting to work in psychiatry but assigned to a medical unit might well express displeasure in facial expression and body posture. It is important that nurses recognize ways that attitudes manifest themselves. Attitudes or feelings about particular clients or specific diagnoses are apparent in behavior as well as in speech. In communication, nonverbal content far outweighs the power of words in communicating a message. For the most part, however, people take responsibility only for what they put into words. It is not at all uncommon for a client to receive one message verbally and quite another nonverbally.

Most nurses have had prior experiences living with, working with, or caring for people addicted to alcohol and other drugs. These experiences, together with education, will determine how they react to the next client with the same diagnosis. Attitudes affect behavior, and some may produce more therapeutic outcomes than others. That does not mean that some attitudes are "good" and others are "bad"; in fact, labeling them as such tends to be countertherapeutic. Nurses must strive to examine

---

REFLECTIVE THINKING

Client Choices

It is your first day as a community health nurse and you have your choice of client assignments. Of the following choices, which would you be most apt to choose first, second, third, fourth, fifth, and sixth?

a. A 90-year-old man from a nursing home who has delirium

b. An 8-year-old boy who has Lyme disease

c. A 67-year-old woman who has been suicidal with alcoholic cirrhosis

d. A 22-year-old prenatal Spanish-speaking woman

e. A 26-year-old drug-addicted man with HIV infection

f. A 35-year-old client recovering from multiple trauma

- What influenced your decisions?
- Were they easy or hard to make?
- If you were assigned to your sixth choice, what would your feelings be about that assignment?
- How do you think those feelings might show in your behavior?
- Do you think that other members of your class would choose the same?

---

their own attitudes without labeling or judging. This examination may or may not result in change, but, at the very least, it should increase the nurse's awareness of nonverbal messages.

Attitudes toward people who use alcohol and other drugs tend to be inconsistent and conflicting. Although there is widespread acceptance that the addictions are treatable diseases, clients are often regarded as weakwilled, self-destructive people with little hope of change. This ingrained moralistic, pessimistic, and hopeless attitude, though often unrecognized by the nurse, affects all aspects of the nursing process. The nurse who has this attitude might be less apt to include questions regarding use and abuse in the assessment process and may miss obvious clues. If questions about substance abuse are included, they may be asked in a way that minimizes concern. This approach presents a problem, because early recognition, diagnosis, and prevention have the same value and benefits for the addictions as for other illnesses.

Some nurses view addictions as willful self-abuse or bad habits better treated by addiction specialists. These nurses might address the secondary problems created by the addiction without regard to the addiction itself. For example, a nurse who does not regard excessive drinking as a health issue might treat a client's high blood pressure, sleep disturbance, anxiety, or excessive bruising without considering the role that alcohol might be playing in causing those disorders. The planning of care becomes fragmented, and opportunities for education are lost.

Nurses must take a proactive stance in reducing the morbidity and mortality associated with the use of tobacco products. Strategies should be implemented to further reduce the availability and social acceptability of tobacco use in order to decrease the numbers of new users, particularly adolescents. Continued and increased education at all levels is necessary along with increased access to treatment programs. Perhaps in this endeavor nurses need to begin with themselves.

The Use of Labels

A nurse may insist that a client accept a label such as "alcoholic" or "addict" when the client is neither ready nor willing to do so. Clients as well as nurses have strong ideas about what an addicted person looks and acts like. It is often easy to exclude oneself from this description. "Uncle Joe was an alcoholic. He drank straight whiskey and was often disheveled and unemployed. I've been in the same job for several years and drink only martinis and manhattans. I therefore am not an alcoholic." This client might be willing to entertain the idea that an enlarged liver is related to alcohol intake. At the same time, the label "alcoholic" might be totally unacceptable. If a nurse attempts to apply such a label, credibility in the eyes of the client may be lost. Many clients are willing to consider that some of their problems may be related to their drinking or drug-taking practices and to seek intervention without ever accepting the diagnosis (Amodeo, 1995).

When a client is unwilling to accept the diagnosis of "alcoholic" or "drug addict," health care professionals may say that the client is "denying." Denial has long been considered a part of the addiction process. Wallace (1977) points out that diagnosing alcoholism is not easy and that professionals often have difficulty in agreeing as to how and why the diagnostic label should be applied. Wallace questions whether the clients should always be called "in denial" when they are unable to apply the label "alcoholic" to themselves.

Unrealistic Expectations

A nurse might feel that intervention that does not result in client sobriety is a failure. Evaluation of client outcome should be made from a realistic appraisal of the facts. For example, clients are often labeled treatment failures when they continue to drink or to take drugs after several trips to a detoxification facility. Detoxification, however, is exactly what the name implies, a process of safely removing toxic substances from the body. If this has been done, the intervention is a success regardless of the clients' subsequent behavior. A myriad of interventions might be necessary before sobriety is achieved. If the nurse honestly and skillfully treated the clients in accordance with a sound knowledge of the disease, neither credit nor blame is associated with treatment outcome.

Identifying Populations at Risk

High-risk or target populations for substance abuse cross all race, age, socioeconomic status, culture, and gender groups (NCHS, 1995). It is important to note that populations at risk vary by type of addiction and sequelae so that one does not assume that all clients will exhibit comparable behaviors or have similar health problems. Nurses may find it easier to think of populations at risk for alcoholism and the use of street drugs but more difficult to realize that substances such as nicotine, prescription drugs, and drugs that Americans use every day present serious problems for people in terms of lost productivity and disability.

All nurses need to have a good working knowledge of diverse populations at risk. Risk means that behaviors, social roles, genetic factors, health status, family history, gender, age, race, class, and occupation may, alone or together, increase one's vulnerability to addiction. Some

---

REFLECTIVE THINKING

The Homeless Shelter

You are beginning a community clinical rotation in an urban homeless shelter. You enter the shelter for the first time and see men lying drunk on the floor of the lobby. One man vomits and passes out.

- What immediately comes to mind when you see the men?
- Do you have biases? What are they? Are you making judgments on the basis of fact or emotion?
- How do you perceive the role of your classmates in helping you and themselves become more comfortable in the shelter setting?

populations are at higher risk than others to problems of substance abuse. Poverty, race, and other barriers to care are all important variables that contribute significantly to risk. The most pervasive of all risk factors is poverty. Poverty breeds despair and hopelessness, isolation, and anger. Any stressor, in particular an unremitting stressor such as poverty, can leave one at higher risk of substance abuse (Dumont, 1992).

Children and Youth

Children and youth are one of the more vulnerable populations at risk. Mother's use of drugs before the birth of a child can have a major impact on the health of that child. In addition to children who are born addicted or with FAS because of their mother's addiction, studies have shown that mothers who have been exposed to passive smoking in early pregnancy are at risk for small-for-gestational-age infants (Dejin-Karlsson, Hanson, Ostergren, Sjoberg, & Marsal, 1998). Also, the result of smoking mothers who breast feed is more nicotine in the infant's blood (Mascola, Vunakis, Tager, Speizer, & Hanrahan, 1998). Maternal substance use during pregnancy results in developmental disturbances in children. Faden and Graubard (2000) found that maternal drinking resulted in higher activity level, greater difficulty of management, tantrums, eating problems, and eating nonfood. Increased fearfulness, poorer motor skills, and shorter length of play were associated with maternal marijuana use. Maternal cigarette smoking during pregnancy results in less well developed language, higher activity level, greater difficulty of management, fearfulness, decreased ability to get along with peers, and increased tantrums.

The national trend has been a leveling or declining trend in illicit substance use, including marijuana and cigarette use, since 1997, after a period of significant increases in the early 1990 (SAMHSA, 2001). In 1998, the American Academy of Family Physicians estimated that about 3000 minors begin smoking each day in the United States, beginning between the sixth and ninth grades and addicted by age 20 (Miller, Gillesple, Billian, & Davel, 2001). In 2001, SAMHSA (2001) reports that that figure has declined by one-third.

Even with the leveling or declining trend, there continues to be a good deal of substance use and abuse among children and youth. Approximately 2.1 million youths aged 12–17 had used inhalants at some time in their lives as of 2000. This figure constituted 8.9% of youths (SAMHSA, 2001). Inhalants continue to be more prevalent among eighth graders at 17.9% in 2000 (NIDA Infofax, 2001a). The number of persons who used pain relievers nonmedically for the first time in 1999 was approximately 1.5 million. Youths aged 12–17 constitute the majority of this increase, from 78,000 initiates in 1985 to 722,000 in 2000.

The use of smokeless tobacco remains stable, as does the use of steroids and marijuana. Steroids is higher among males than females but is growing most rapidly among young women. Since 1991, there has been a 50% increase among 8th and 10th graders and 38% among 12th graders (NIDA Notes, 2001a). The use of alcohol has also remained stable. In one survey, 32.3% of 12th graders, 23.5% of 10th graders, and 8.3% of 8th graders reported having "been drunk" in the month prior to the survey (NIDA Infofax, 2001c). Although heroin use declined from 1.4% in 1999 to 1.1% in 2000, it rose (1.1 in 1999 to 1.5 in 2000) in 12th graders. While other opiates remained stable between 1999 and 2000, they are at their highest level since the survey began in 1991.

Rates of use of methamphetamine have remained stable and in 2000 were at 4.3% for 12th graders, 4% for 10th graders, and 2.5% of 8th graders (NIDA Infofax, 2001c). Although only a small percent of young people use heroin or cocaine, it must be remembered that use has sometimes begun by 8th grade (NIDA Infofax, 2001c). One drug that is on the increase is Ecstasy (MDMA). The heaviest use (5%) was reported between the ages of 18 and 25. From 1999 to 2000 the use of MDMA had increased for the second consecutive year (NIDA Infofax, 2001g).

Women

Women account for approximately one-third of the problem drinkers in the United States (NCADD, 2000). Important differences have been found in the effects of alcohol on women as compared to men and yet women have been under-represented in studies (Henderson, 2001).

Much of the early work on substance abuse was conducted exclusively with male subjects, and treatment programs were designed accordingly. Only relatively recently has research focused on the special needs of women. Many differences have emerged, and stereotypes have been challenged. When compared with men, women have different risk factors, different drinking and drug-taking patterns, different treatment needs, and different barriers to treatment.

Women who abuse substances are a diverse group, crossing racial, ethnic, and socioeconomic lines. Becker & Wolton-Moss (2001) report that heavy drinking among white women is more common than among African American or Latino women. Despite widely held stereotypes to the contrary, national survey data indicate that white women are significantly more apt to have used any illicit drug in their lifetime than African American or Latino women (USDHHS, 1994a). Despite this fact, women of color are much more likely to be tested for drug abuse than are white women and consequently are more apt to face criminal charges and child protection interventions (Maher, 1992).

Becker & Wolton-Moss (2001) identified major risk factors for women as childhood physical and sexual abuse, adult victimization by domestic violence, and a spouse or partner who abuses substances. Bean (1984) stresses the need for establishing an environment of safety in helping people to engage in alcoholism treatment. Women in abusive situations who feel threatened where they live will find it very difficult to engage in treatment.

There are important differences between the sexes with regard to alcohol. Women reach higher blood alcohol levels from drinking a given amount of alcohol than do men of comparable size. Women develop alcohol-related problems much earlier in their drinking careers than do men. Cirrhosis of the liver develops more quickly in an alcoholic woman, with an average of 13 years of drinking as compared with 22 years in a man.

Why do women suffer the effects of alcohol abuse differently than men? Data have shown that women have more physical and psychological problems from alcohol abuse than men. What is different is that women tend to hide or closet their alcoholism because of children, family, friends and the pressures of "social norms" (Fillmore et al., 1995; Thomasson, 1995).

In a 2001 study on gender difference in trauma patients, outcomes showed that males had higher rates of trauma related injuries than women. However, there were few differences between genders with respect to the severity of alcohol related symptoms. Women exhibited more evidence of alcohol-related physical and psychological harm (Gentillello et al., 2000). Other studies have suggested that ethanol pharmokinetics may be the reason women are more vulnerable to the ethanol toxicity than men (Thomasson, 1995).

The etiologies of why women are sicker with more liver dysfunction, psychological distress, and depression may rest with gender differences in kinetics and dynamics of the body and how it metabolizes ethanol. Whatever the etiology, it justifies the conviction held here that women must be included in clinical trials.

There is an increasing body of literature concerned with the relationship between the addictions and obstetric and gynecological problems, including damage to a developing fetus. Sexual dysfunction, infertility, miscarriage, and breast cancer have all been associated with heavy drinking. Substance abuse in women of childbearing age can have tragic consequences. Fetal alcohol syndrome (FAS) refers to a pattern of anomalies occurring in infants born to mothers who abused alcohol during pregnancy. Problems in the early years of life include prematurity, developmental delays, facial dysmorphia, neurological abnormalities, and mental retardation.

FAS and fetal alcohol effects (FAE) are caused from alcohol, which is a teratogen. A teratogen causes lasting birth defects to a fetus. FAS is one of the leading causes of mental retardation. FAS/FAE may also result in developmental delays and a wide array of behavioral and learning problems for the child. FAS/FAE ruin the lives of many children. It is estimated there are 12,000 new cases of FAS annually (Cramer & Davidhizar 1999).

FAS/FAE do not have to happen. They are preventable if pregnant women do not drink. School nurses, visiting nurses, public health nurses, and family nurse practitioners have compelling roles in decreasing the prevalence of the problem. Advocacy and education for the family, including the substance-abusing parent(s), are prerequisites for success in preventing FAS/FAE. Health providers and prospective parents need to be sensitized to the condition, its prevention, and its sequelae. Chaudhuri (2000) notes that there is no treatment of FAS in a child. Management by correction and rehabilitation is the only treatment available.

There is widespread intellectual acceptance of the addictions as treatable diseases, yet underneath the surface deeply ingrained, stereotypical beliefs can often be found. There is stigma associated with the addictions, and this is a particularly heavy burden for women. Women may tend to be judged by harsher standards than men. Rather than recognizing the primacy of the addiction, health care providers may focus on its consequences. "How can she do that to her children?" they may ask. The same question would sound heartless, even ludicrous, if the mother were suffering from multiple sclerosis or a brain tumor. Present controversy regarding mandatory testing of pregnant women, mandatory confinement of pregnant addicts during pregnancy, and criminalization of drug use by pregnant women add to the stigma (Finkelstein, 1994).

Perhaps because of the stigma and fear that their children will be taken away, women are slower to seek treatment for alcohol- and drug-related problems than are men. Often they seek help for associated depression or anxiety and are treated with psychotropic drugs that further compound their problems. Once the problem has been identified, the treatment plan often does not take into consideration the special needs of the woman.

Elders

Although problems with alcohol and other substance abuse are prevalent among the elderly, they tend to be underdiagnosed and sometimes ignored. In the overall population, substance abuse is more easily identified because people are active in work and family roles. In older adults, retirement changes some of these roles, and it is more difficult to identify the elderly substance abuser at home. Approximately 1%–3% of women and 12% of elderly men over 60 have severe problems relating to alcohol abuse (Ebersole & Hess, 1998). Providers, including physicians and nurses, do not routinely ask questions about alcohol and drugs in an assessment. The CAGE questionnaire or Two-Item Conjoint Screen, previously discussed, are brief and are a step forward in identifying elders with substance abuse problems.

Elderly alcoholic clients can be divided into two groups: those who developed alcoholism early in life and survived to old age and those who did not manifest symptoms until in their sixties or later. The latter group are often drinking in response to situational factors such as retirement, death of a spouse, loss of friends, loss of health, or other major life changes that accompany old age. Some may have been drinking the same amount for years with no problems, but changes related to aging and or the development of chronic illnesses now make this amount troublesome. Late-onset problem drinking is more prevalent in those who are wealthier and better educated. Fewer elderly women than men drink. Problems tend to develop at a later age for women but more often include the problematic use of prescribed psychoactive substances (Gomberg, 1995).

Aging modifies the rate of absorption, distribution, and excretion of drugs including alcohol (Lehne, 2000). Owing to decreased fluid volume in elders, blood alcohol content may reach higher levels. Older adults have more chronic illness and might be taking any number of prescription drugs. Alcohol interferes with at least one-half of the most commonly prescribed drugs (Hooyman & Kiyak, 1999).

Older adults who are drug abusers are commonly addicted to prescribed anxiolytics or they may misuse over-the-counter analgesics, coffee, and cigarettes (Ebersole & Hess, 1998). People over 65 use more over-the-counter medications than any other age group in the United States (National Guideline Clearinghouse, 2000). The elderly population will represent 21% of the U.S. population in 2040. The numbers of retired and aging men and women living alone will have major impact on our society. As the elderly bring their fortitude and wisdom to retirement, some will also bring loneliness, social isolation, and perhaps a history of substance abuse, including tobacco, alcohol, narcotics, and over-the-counter analgesics.

The effects of chronic drinking in the elderly can be profound. Associated illnesses include hypertension; cancers of the mouth, larynx, and esophagus (especially when combined with smoking); cirrhosis; and malnutrition. Falls are a major concern, because they often result in hip and other fractures.

The mixture of alcohol with various other drugs can present a risk. Tylenol, for example, when used with alcohol can increase the risk of liver damage. High doses of benzodiazepines with alcohol can cause death. The kinetics of aging leave the body more vulnerable to toxicity and intolerance. A Consensus Panel recommends that treatment settings for older adults who are withdrawing from prescription drugs or alcohol should (a) be age specific, (b) focus on coping with depression and loss, (c) focus on rebuilding formal and informal supports, and (d) provide counseling at a pace that is comfortable and age appropriate (National Guideline Clearing House, 2001).

Social isolation is both cause and effect of alcoholism in elders. Treatment approaches should include both education and the development of a social support network.

Gays, Lesbians, and Transgendered Persons

The issues for substance abuse in the gay, lesbian, and transgendered populations are as diverse as the demographics of the people who comprise them. Age and developmental stage are important parameters. The USDHHS Task Force on Youth Suicide (1989) estimated that gay youth accounted for 30% of completed suicides and that 40% of lesbian, gay, bisexual, or transgendered youths have attempted or thought about suicide. These are compelling statistics. Social isolation, stigma, and poor support systems cannot be separated from substance abuse, misuse, and less than optimal access to health services. The statistics may well be the tip of an iceberg. The prevalence of substance abuse in lesbian, gay, and transgender youth is linked with the stigma and pain that accompany a social identity that is not a societal norm. In one study, approximately 60% of gay young men met the criteria of substance misuse. They are more apt to use injectable drugs, use cocaine, smoke tobacco, drink alcohol, and have sexual relations before age 13 (Lee 2000). They are at highest risk for substance abuse.

Substance abuse in lesbian and gay adults presents differently. In the first edition of this text, alcohol-reporting rates for men and women were between 18 and 35 percent (Herber, Hunt and Dell 1994). More recent population-based surveys found little difference in drinking and substance abusing behaviors between heterosexual and gay men. Similarly, few differences were found between lesbian and nonlesbian women (Lee 2000).

Community health nurses can support gay, lesbian, and transexual clients by being advocates and ensuring better access to health care. Census surveys suggest that the population represents 2–10% of males in the United States and 1.4–7.5% of women. Advocacy assumes a knowledge base; nursing education must spend more time teaching students about the social and psychological concerns of gay, lesbian, and transgendered individuals. Evidence based research about social relationships, discrimination, substance abuse, and peer pressure is a mandate for nurses and other health providers.

Homeless and Mentally Ill Persons

The comorbidity of severe mental illness and alcohol and other drug disorders has been put as high as 50% in community mental health settings and is probably much higher among homeless people. Often, addiction treatment facilities exclude people with mental illness, and mental health facilities ignore or discriminate against people with addictions. Thus, the dually diagnosed client is left unserved.

Particularly vulnerable and at risk are homeless men and women with both substance abuse problems and mental illness. Overall, they have more trauma, physical illness, and legal problems than do other homeless people;

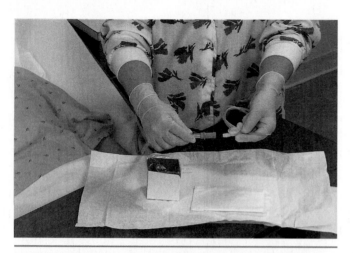

A substance-dependent health professional working with a client can be a lethal mix. If you suspect one of your colleagues to be abusing drugs or alcohol, it is your responsibility to report it. It may be a matter of life or death for the client as well as your colleague.

are more deficient in social and vocational skills; and are more apt to live on the streets than in shelters or other refuges for homeless people.

Those exhibiting symptoms of both substance abuse and mental illness are not a homogeneous group. Some with a primary mental illness use alcohol or other drugs to combat loneliness or to alleviate psychiatric symptoms. Others have a primary substance abuse problem and exhibit psychiatric symptoms secondary to drug use or withdrawal. A third group exhibits both disorders independent of each other. In any case, research has indicated that the most positive outcomes occur when the two problems are treated in an integrated manner.

Woody (1996) expresses concern about the lag that exists between present research and health policy. Often, addiction treatment is separated from medical, psychiatric, and other interventions, undermining the development of integrated treatment approaches. For more information regarding these subjects, see Chapters 29 and 33.

Nurses and Other Health Professionals

The American Nurses Association (ANA) estimates that from 6% to 8% of nurses use alcohol or other drugs to an extent sufficient to impair their professional performance (ANA 2001) and that 20% of all health professionals will become addicted over the lifetime of their careers (The impaired nurse, 2001, Hollerin & Rivellini, 2000). Substance abuse can have both personal and professional consequences. For example, according to the Chairman of the Connecticut State Board of Nursing, 80% of disciplinary cases brought before the board are related to substance abuse (Hollerin & Rivellini, 2000). Reasons often

cited for substance abuse in the helping professions are parental alcoholism, high stress, easy access to drugs, and an underlying belief that knowledge of the drug protects the user from succumbing to addiction.

Substance-abusing nurses and other health care professionals are often "protected" by misguided colleagues. Protecting them can be dangerous for both the impaired colleague and for clients. If impairment is suspected, colleagues need to report concerns to the supervisor, stating only the facts and not drawing conclusions. For example, "I am concerned about Miss Doe. She has missed three days of work in the past month and has returned late from lunch on four occasions in the last two weeks. She is usually well liked by the clients, but during this past week three clients complained of her being irritable and a fourth said she smelled alcohol on her breath. Yesterday, she fell asleep at the desk while writing her notes."

Some colleagues may interpret such a report as betrayal. This interpretation is rooted in the fundamental belief that substance abuse is a moral weakness or a crime, not an illness. Chemical addiction is a treatable illness and untreated can be dangerous. In one study, nearly 66% of chemically dependent nurses considered taking their lives as compared with less than 20% of nondependent nurses (Hughes & Smith, 1994). Helping a colleague to treatment for an addiction will not only protect client safety but could also save the life of the colleague. In some instances, the abuser self-reports. In any case, the consequences can be life-changing for the provider. For instance, the types of penalties in New York State include revocation or surrender of license, suspension, either actual or stayed probation, a fine, public service, and censure and reprimand (Laduke, 2000).

Employee assistance programs, programs associated with professional organizations, and programs of state licensure boards can be employed to assist the impaired professional.

THE GLOBALIZATION OF SUBSTANCE ABUSE

The measurement of global trends in drug use is difficult at best, and results may be less than accurate because the population is difficult to access, members self report, and reliability may be questionable. However, researchers have succeeded in pooling numbers and have standardized by region (UNDCP World Drug Report 2000). Table 31-2 shows the extent of drug abuse worldwide in the late 1990s.

Cannabis (marijuana) is the global drug of choice with 144 million users. Cannabis is followed by amphetamines and stimulants which are used by 28.7 million people worldwide. The total number of drug users is approximately 180 million people, which, as the table indicates, is 3 percent of world population. (UNDCP 2000). All of these estimates should be regarded with caution

TABLE 31-2 Global Extent of Drug Abuse in the Late 1990s

EXTENT OF DRUG ABUSE (ANNUAL PREVALENCE) IN THE LATE 1990S						
	ILLICIT DRUGS ALL	CANNABIS	AMPHETAMINE-TYPE STIMULANTS*	COCAINE	ALL OPIATES	HEROIN
GLOBAL (million people)	180	144.1	28.7	14	13.5	9.2
in % of global population	3.0%	2.4%	0.5%	0.2%	0.2%	0.15%
in % of global population age 15 and above	4.2%	3.4%	0.7%	0.3%	0.3%	0.22%

Amphetamines (methamphetamine and amphetamine) and substances of the ecstasy group.
Source: UNDCP, World Drug Report 2000.

because of the context (low income inner city communities are stereotypically associated more with illicit drug use than higher income communities, and because of the stigma and illegal nature of drug use, there are often built in biases in the criminal justice system and the helping professions. (UNDCP, 2000).

There are many positions on what should be done about the marketing and sale of drugs. What would decriminalization of drug use do to abusers in the United States and internationally? Like alcohol and tobacco, decriminalization of drugs such as cocaine and heroin would raise issues about who can distribute, distribution controls, restrictions around sale, and the application of quality controls.

Demographics indicate that illicit drug use has stabilized. The American market is the largest and Americans take more drugs per capita than counterparts in other countries. The following list contains some facts about drug use in America:

- Heavy drug use has stabilized since the 1980s.
- Use of cocaine and heroin has stabilized.
- Use of marijuana has increased.
- The average age of heroin addicts is rising.
- The crack epidemic has passed.
- Illicit drug use is increasing among the poor.

UNODCCP, 2001

This profile suggests that there are going to be more elderly addicts; the poor are increasingly victimized by the illicit drug market; young people have increasingly turned to marijuana; and the deadly epidemics of the 1980s have passed. "In America, tobacco kills proportionately more smokers than heroin kills its users and al-

cohol kills more drinkers than cocaine kills its devotees" (http://www. Economist.com). The marketing and distribution of illicit cannabis, cocaine, amphetamines, and heroin have brought the drug war to international proportions. The profits involved lead to widespread corruption, addiction, and ruined lives. The marketing of cigarettes to the young and the poor in Asia, Central America, and Europe is a practice for which all countries bear responsibility.

Is drug addiction a public health problem or is it a problem for the criminal justice system? In the United States, it is a crime. An alternative approach is found in Switzerland, where drug addiction is treated as a public health problem. The Swiss have a heroin maintenance program and cannabis is legal but regulated for personal use. The aim is to keep the users of 'soft drugs' like marijuana from moving into the ranks of hard-core abusers. There are fewer criminal records of young people and the young are kept out of the criminal justice system where criminalization may become a self-fulfilling prophecy for the young. Health care professionals need to arrive at their own conclusions while avoiding the imposition of judgment or bias on their patients (UNODCCP, 2001).

It is clear that illicit drug use has shifted to the world stage. The focus here has been on the marketing and distribution of illicit drugs, worldwide. There are also legalized drugs such as alcohol and tobacco, which are affecting global trends. The section on tobacco and women suggested the extent of harm to women worldwide by the marketing of acceptable drugs. Whether the drugs are legal or illegal, the corruption, greed, and ruined lives associated with their distribution is extensive. Community health nurses are in an optimal position to guide grass root action plans for community change.

Perspectives...

INSIGHTS OF A NURSE ON ALCOHOL ABUSE

My path to alcohol abuse began with binge drinking as a teenager. It progressed to more regular drinking as a young adult. Parties, liquor, music, and a general feeling of well-being came to be associated with scotch, cigarettes, and friends. It was difficult to feel good without the scotch. For years, it was "social drinking" and a lot of parties. It progressed to drinks at home, after work, alone. A drink before dinner, I would rationalize. Or two before dinner. It progressed to a pint of scotch each evening and commonly, a hangover each morning. It progressed to visiting different liquor stores each evening so that people would not know I was an alcoholic. I lived like that for 25 years. I worked, as a registered nurse; I was functional, and most people thought I just enjoyed a few drinks. I had car accidents and many "near misses." It was the '60s and '70s when cigarette smoking and heavy drinking were not only acceptable but the norm. One night, I went to dinner with friends, drank my usual, got into my car and ran into an unmarked police car. I was arrested for drunk driving with a blood alcohol level of 0.16. It was, as an officer pointed out, enough to cause a 180-pound man to pass out. I weighed 115 pounds. I went to court the next morning, was sentenced to a 60-day suspension of license and mandated to attend a three-month alcohol awareness program. I denied that I had a problem, but after three months of group work, I realized I had a big one. I was no longer drinking and driving. I was drinking and taking a cab. I realized that I was unable to stop drinking without professional help. Once I acknowledged that I had a problem, I moved slowly and sometimes painfully toward my goal—never another alcoholic drink for the rest of my life. I spent six months in an alcohol group, then two years with a support group that became my sustenance. I spent another year beginning the long road to making it on my own. It is now 15 years later and I have made it. I was one of the lucky ones. I didn't lose a job, hurt another in a motor vehicle accident, or hit the bottom. I am one of the lucky ones. I realize I can never become complacent about alcohol. I cannot stop drinking once I begin. Therefore, I will never drink again. Thank you, community support group, friends, and loved ones who helped me make it through a major life crisis. Recovery is hard work, and it never ends. Caring for others, being sober, and no longer struggling is a gift.

—Anonymous

LEVELS OF PREVENTION

In this chapter primary, secondary, and tertiary levels of prevention provide an organizing framework for a discussion of the prevention and treatment of substance abuse. However, the nursing process can be just as easily categorized by using terms such as health promotion, health maintenance, and health restoration. What is important is not the terms but the need for an organizing frame of reference in both community and hospital settings.

Primary Prevention

Drugs and alcohol are deeply rooted in our norms, our belief systems, and our customs. Preventing addiction, preventing a child from growing to become an adult with an addiction, means uprooting the societal beliefs about alcohol, about smoking, and about prescription and street drugs that are such an integral part of American life. This is no easy task.

Currently, funding priorities, provider roles, and health education models are shifting back to the neighborhoods and communities. Nurses are reclaiming the neighborhoods to practice the primary prevention they do so well (Portnoy & Dumas, 1994). Health providers and community members should meet in the community setting to mutually identify problems and define goals. If nurses are to be effective in teaching about drug and alcohol abuse, they must first assess the community's perception of the problem. Norms and belief systems must be discussed, particularly in relation to preventive care and the potential for some widely accepted behaviors to do great harm. This approach will require compromise, negotiation, and more acceptance of cultural diversity as related to drug and alcohol use.

A community is only as healthy as the people in its neighborhoods, and, although drug and alcohol abuse occur among all classes, the poor and disenfranchised suffer disproportionately from their effects (Dumas, 1992a). (See Chapter 32 for more information on poverty.) In assessing the community, the nurse must ask: Who are the highest-risk community groups? What kinds of treatments and outcomes are associated with different populations at risk? What happens to the poor, the disenfranchised, and the socially vulnerable substance abuser? What are public and private distinctions between access to care, utilization, and quality of services for substance abusers in the community? The answers to these questions will provide direction toward finding solutions to an escalating substance abuse problem. Nurses have a responsibility to teach, to promote health, and to advocate for the social change that will improve the quality of life for all citizens. The community nurse role is a challenge and presents an opportunity for nurses to make a difference.

Community Settings for Primary Prevention

There are many community settings where the nurse can teach about the prevention of alcohol, tobacco, and other drug abuse. The settings are as diverse as the nursing roles within them. The common bond shared by community health providers is the philosophy of care that is based on populations rather than individuals. Community settings include the neighborhood, the home, the school, the church, the workplace, the area council on aging, the community health center, the community youth center,

and the "streets" of the community. Community settings with populations at high risk for drug and alcohol problems are adult day health centers, shelters for homeless people, and the home. Table 31-3 lists community settings and typical health promotive nursing activities.

Home care is an ideal place to initiate health promotion instruction relating to substance abuse of all types. The visiting nurse, who is most often called upon to provide skilled nursing by a hospital or rehabilitation facility, can assess the client and family risk factors for substance abuse during early home visits and develop teaching plans accordingly. The public health nurse usually works out of a local health department or city hospital. Maternal-child health promotion efforts initiated by public health nurses are especially relevant to substance abuse education, because many women and their children are at high risk for problems. In visits to the home for maternal-child health promotion, the public health nurse is able to do informal teaching about abstinence or moderation with potentially addictive substances such as cigarettes, alcohol, and other drugs. Sharp assessment skills are required for all home visits, and there should be few differences between the goals of public health and visiting nurses in regard to substance abuse prevention.

Families need to be considered in primary prevention. It is important to help parents stay closely involved

---

TABLE 31-3 Community Settings and Health Promotion Activities

SETTING	HEALTH PROMOTION ACTIVITIES
School	Education on common addictive substances and the relationship between alcohol and violence
	Health teaching in the classroom on smoking behaviors, street drugs, substance abuse, and AIDS
	Student health fairs; visits to school by role models such as "Girl Power" promotion by Olympic champion Dominique Dawes
	Inclusion of parents, using PTA meetings as site for education
Workplace	Seminars on alcoholism
	Woman-to-woman discussion groups about high-risk behaviors, pregnancy, smoking cessation, fetal alcohol syndrome, HIV infection
	Education of men regarding the relationship between substance abuse and domestic violence
Clinic	
Outpatient	Health education related to primary illness and risk reduction
Community	Outreach and group work in elderly housing, schools, and throughout neighborhoods; target groups of all ages: children, elders, teens
Shelter	Health education groups; student-run projects
Home	Health promotion education; education about over-the-counter medication, drug schedule for pain
	Identification of high-risk individuals
	Assessment of risks to women and children; assessment of safety in home
Church	Narcotics Anonymous, Alcoholic Anonymous meetings on site; outreach, teen education
	Social activities without alcohol
Neighborhood	Outreach workers, discussion groups, family teaching
	Educating community activitists, leaders to carry on work after health providers leave
	Blood pressure screening; teaching relation of cardiovascular risk to drug abuse

with their children and their activities. They should know who their friends are. This closeness is particularly important in the preadolescent and adolescent years and is often more difficult to do as children become increasingly influenced by peer values. As the data demonstrate, children are exposed and can begin using drugs before the eighth grade—in some cases, much earlier (NIDA Infofax, 2001c).

Adult children should be cognizant of their parent's life situation, particularly after a spouse has died. Older adults are at risk for overmedicating prescription drugs and increasing their intake of alcohol.

As the community moves to the forefront of health delivery and as the concept of health promotion becomes more familiar to the public, broader goals emerge that address problems more difficult to solve. These are problems at the societal level, problems embedded in society and in our ways of life: for example, alcohol and smoking behaviors and the promotion of such behaviors by cigarette manufacturers and the media (McKinlay, 1974, 1993). The problem of FAS, the outcome of alcohol use in pregnancy which ruins the lives of many children, is 100% preventable (Weiner, Morse, & Garrido, 1989).

Of all the substances that are abused, tobacco is the most preventable. In most cases, if adolescents do not begin smoking by age 19, they are unlikely to ever smoke (Miller, et al, 2001). Therefore, it is important to develop smoking prevention programs in the lower grades. School nurses and teachers are key people who need to teach about the dangers of smoking to their classes. Nurses can also become politically active in working to ban smoking advertising aimed at the young. Vartiainen, Paavola, McAlister, and Puska (1998) noted that a school-based program combined with an intensive mass media component and adult antismoking program was most effective. One program that has been found effective is the Tar Wars Curriculum endorsed by the American Cancer Society and the American Lung Association. It is a prohealth tobacco education program and poster contest for fifth graders.

Secondary Prevention

Community health nurses work in a variety of settings with diverse clients. Clients with substance abuse problems are often evasive or ashamed of their problem or they are poor historians. Using effective assessment skills, the nurse can identify individuals with substance abuse problems as well as community factors that contribute to those problems.

Secondary prevention for families involves assisting family members to find ways to deal with a substance-abusing family member. Coping strategies range from assisting the member to accept treatment to helping the family to arrange for the person on drugs to leave the family home. In some situations, the family may have to relocate away from the substance-abusing member. These changes can be devastating for a family, and members

need the help of a support group or counselor to manage the drastic changes. Such groups as Alcoholics Anonymous can provide much needed support. Adult children can assist their parents to help them find a positive living situation and to make use of community resources as needed.

Assessment and Identification of Substance Abuse Problems

Assessment involves forming an alliance with the client and gathering information to determine the existence and extent of a problem. This process *precedes* diagnosis and intervention. To label a person or to offer solutions prematurely usually leads to a breakdown in communication (Hennessey, 1992).

Assessment is a mutual exploration involving the client, the nurse, the family, and other concerned individuals. It is important that the nurse work with the client as an ally. This approach involves treating the client with dignity, attending to the client's concerns, assessing for strengths as well as problem areas, and fostering an atmosphere that promotes mutual respect and the free expression of ideas and feelings.

Questions regarding drug and alcohol intake should be a part of every assessment interview. In order to elicit honest responses, the nurse should ask the questions in an open-ended, nonjudgmental, matter-of-fact manner (Liftik, 1995). Care should be taken not to jump to conclusions. The nurse is an explorer here, attempting to examine and understand the unknown, not a detective attempting to pin a diagnosis on a client.

Substance abuse problems are often manifested in several areas of a person's life. To get a clear and thorough picture, the nurse should not limit exploration to one area. For example, if physical findings indicate substance abuse, indicators should be sought in behavioral, occupational, legal, and social areas as well. Table 31-4 summarizes possible indicators of substance abuse.

Although there are often strong negative stereotypes about addicted people, there is no one clear picture. Addictions are prevalent in all strata of society; one addicted person can look quite different from another. There are few definitive diagnostic criteria.

Assessment should also include the client's perception of the problem and what steps, if any, have been taken to remedy the problem. Often, the client is aware that a problem exists and may have attempted to deal with it in the past, either alone or with help. What is now needed is a nonjudgmental person who is willing to listen as possible next steps are sorted out. Nurses may be surprised at how open and honest addicted people can be when the atmosphere for openness is created.

Assessment in the Workplace

The workplace is an important setting where an occupational health, public health, or visiting nurse can screen, identify, and participate in the treatment of people who

TABLE 31-4 Indications of Drug- or Alcohol-Related Problems

ENVIRONMENTAL	BEHAVIORAL	PHYSICAL	EMOTIONAL
Neglected children	Secretiveness	Unsteady gait	Personality change
Inadequate living facilities	Change in friends	Slurred speech	Moodiness
Frequent moves	Missed work or school	Odor of alcohol or inhalant on breath	Irritability
Unkempt house	Poor job or school performance	Constricted or dilated pupils	Anxiety
Poor personal hygiene	Frequent job changes	Needle or track marks	Attention deficit
Presence of empty bottles or drug paraphernalia	Failing grades	Runny nose or sniffling	Restlessness
Cigarette burns on furniture or rugs	Legal difficulties	Twitchiness or tremors	Euphoria
	Increase in accidents	Seizures	Depression
		Ecchymosis	Agitation
		Excoriation from picking or scratching	Paranoia
		Weight loss	
		Red eyes	

abuse alcohol, tobacco, and other drugs. In a time of managed care, it is becoming a setting of choice for insurers. Early identification and treatment contain costs by preventing outcomes of chronic alcoholism or drug abuse. In the work setting, more employee assistance programs are using routine or random testing and screening for a variety of drugs. Companies in the United States and worldwide can reap the rewards of employee assistance programs. Identification of people with substance abuse problems, however, presents challenges with respect to preserving anonymity while maximizing worker safety through treatment. Drug screening and HIV testing are understandably controversial as their use in the workplace increases.

Healthy People 2010 (USDHHS, 2000a) does not directly reference substance abuse as an important occupational health focus for the year 2000. It does, however, list HIV infection and AIDS as important areas of concern. There is a direct relationship between the use of intravenous drugs and HIV infection. In 1999, 18% of all AIDS cases were women, up from 6.7% in 1986. African-American women account for 61% of female HIV patients. In the U.S., AIDS was the fifth leading cause of death for all women aged 25–44 and the third leading cause of death for African-American women in this age group (Hader, Smith, Moore, & Holmberg, 2001). As the number of women in the work force increases, emphasis on identification and case finding of intravenous drug users and partners of intravenous drug users becomes imperative. Women at risk for HIV infection because they take intravenous drugs or have sex with infected partners are only one example of a target population in the workplace.

The increasing assimilation of women into the workforce has brought about considerable changes in women's workloads that may contribute to health problems and other negative consequences. An examination of three countries (U.S., Sweden, and the Netherlands) demonstrated that women contribute more effort to household chores and child care and less to the workplace than do men, resulting in increased and more diffusely distributed workloads (Hader, Smith, Moore, & Holmberg, 2001). Women are much more apt to drop out of the labor force for periods of time to raise children and to care for elderly parents. This fact, together with discrepancies in job opportunities and wages, leaves women less financially prepared for retirement and more vulnerable to poverty in old age (Warren, Rowlingson, and Whyly, 2001) The workplace, therefore, assumes a new significance as a site for primary and secondary prevention of diverse substance abuse problems in women. As the demographics of the workforce change, differences in values and beliefs and the cultural implications of teaching about safe sex, substance abuse, and AIDS will be a particular challenge to nurses. New program development is needed to target populations at risk, and language and cultural norms are important considerations in designing such programs. Employee assistance programs that focus on drug and alcohol abuse are best when tailored to the predominant risk group in the workplace.

The problem of FAS is also relevant at the level of secondary prevention. There is a scarcity of funded research for this preventable problem, and there are many alcoholic mothers who bear infants who qualify for the FAS diagnosis. Many children suffer from more subtle fetal alcohol effects (FAE) and because they do not display all of the classic signs of fetal alcohol syndrome, the cause of their problems are not identified. A better understanding of both FAS and FAE will help in the development of effective prevention strategies that identify and assist high risk women throughout pregnancy (Alcohol, Research and Health, 2000; Lewis, 1995). Public health attention has waned over the years, but the problem has not. It is important that nurses be adept at screening, case finding, and education in both adult and pediatric settings.

Screening, case finding, expert assessment skills, a non-judgmental attitude, and the ability to ask the right questions at the right time are important clinical skills for nurses in community settings. Using a brief questionnaire such as the CAGE (see p. 827) will help the community health nurse identify those pregnant women at risk for problem drinking.

Assessment in the Schools

The school is a primary care setting where nurses are redefining the problems, the work, and their roles. In Boston, a model of high school adolescent clinics is being tested in the inner city, with the goals of teaching conflict resolution and reducing substance abuse. Children in middle and high schools are at risk for addiction to alcohol, tobacco, and drugs. The direct relationship between violence and substance abuse is well documented (Hingson, Heeron, & Zakocs, 2001; Rodriquez & Brindis, 1995). Studies of homicide in the United States reveal that alcohol was present in the blood of victims in about one-half of all cases. Prothrow-Stith (1990, 1996) writes that the basic scenario for a homicide begins with two people of the same race who know each other. Add alcohol, a weapon, and an argument, and a situation emerges that "tough anticrime laws" can do little about. There is a direct relationship among alcohol, drugs, and violence for all Americans, but in particular for young people. Preventing the problem of substance abuse and emphasizing substance-free conflict assumes a growing importance for nurses in school settings.

Grade schools, middle schools, and high schools are excellent settings for primary prevention, but for many students secondary–prevention measures are indicated. In Boston, at the University of Massachusetts, community models are in place for senior nursing students to have a clinical experience in high schools, middle schools, and grade schools. The work is not easy, but the nurses and the students benefit from mutually rewarding relationships. Cardiopulmonary resuscitation, smoking, substance abuse, HIV/AIDS, and violence prevention are health-related topics that student nurses teach to inner city boys and girls. The outcomes have been positive, with students expressing more self-confidence and enthusiasm for learning. The school nurse model for baccalaureate registered nurse and non–registered nurse seniors is an exciting direction for community curricula (Igoe, 1994).

Assessment in the Home

The home is an important setting for secondary prevention such as screening and case finding. The home setting might be someone's apartment or house, a common living situation such as congregate housing, the community room in an elder housing complex, single-room occupancies, halfway houses, or quarterway houses.

Informal nursing clinics used to screen, advise, refer, and identify cases can also be used for health education. Informal education about addictive substances, about the more common substances that can harm such as cigarettes and over-the-counter medications, and the proper use of prescription drugs can take place here. Early referral can be made that will decrease the potential of substance abuse from social isolation, depression, and the loneliness of old age.

Visiting nursing is more formal, and clients are already in the system. They are being seen for a problem for which they have been referred to the home health agency. Whatever the reason the nurse is in the home,

---

✳ DECISION MAKING

Teaching Students about the Dangers of Smoking

You are a school nurse in an inner city high school. Over 60% of the students in this school smoke cigarettes. All are under 17 years old. When you discuss smoking in your health education class, the students respond to your discussion about the dangers of smoking with laughter and disregard for potential health problems.

◆ How do you proceed in getting a group of uninterested students to at least discuss smoking behaviors and the dangers of the habit?

◆ Would you present smoking as an addiction, a substance abuse similar to cocaine, marijuana, or alcohol abuse? Or would you present it as a public health issue?

◆ How do you respond in what seems to be a "no-win" situation in the short time you will have in the high school?

◆ What are the ethics that you might involve the students in discussing?

◆ What are the ethical issues involved with corporations that become "manufacturers of illness"?

the expert nurse will be able to make ongoing assessments of clients and their families at high risk for substance abuse. A comprehensive assessment tool should always have questions about substance abuse potential, drinking and smoking behaviors, and over-the-counter medications. In the home, clients feel safer, more in control, and less threatened when questions are asked that are troubling or compromising to their sense of integrity.

Tertiary Prevention

As health care organizations and insurers rein in costs, decreased reimbursement for interventions at the tertiary level are insufficient to meet the often complex care required by people who have social or behaviorally induced illnesses such as alcoholism or addiction. Tertiary care related to substance abuse includes treatment for liver failure from chronic alcoholism, the opportunistic infections of AIDS and intravenous drug abuse, the cardiomyopathies associated with cocaine abuse, and the emphysema and cancers due to cigarette smoking. Tertiary care addresses the malnutrition, the neurological damage, and the cardiovascular and pulmonary disabilities that emerge after years of self-neglect while on alcohol or other drugs. Also in tertiary care are people with organic brain disorders, cerebral vascular accidents, and disabilities related to falls, accidents, and violence. Many victims of FAS also need tertiary care for profound mental retardation.

Families who have been living with drug-abusing members, over time, develop many deficits in family functioning. The family may need encouragement to take advantage of services that are available to help them. Adult children of alcoholics or other drug abusers may be unaware of how their early drug experiences are influencing their present life in ways that prevent them from achieving their goals in life. The nurse can help the individual recognize the need for and to seek help.

One of the most devastating outcomes of chronic substance abuse in the family is to have that member either disappear or be found living on the streets. The family feels helpless to change the situation when the drug-abusing person refuses to be helped. The nurse can help by listening to the family discuss the problem and reinforce that they have done all they can and it is not their fault that the situation exists. In some instances, the substance abuser does reach out for help. The nurse can be influential in helping him or her to find a treatment program. Adult children may have to monitor a parent regarding medication intake. If the parent is ingesting alcohol, as well, there may be some disorientation and inaccurate drug taking. The nurse can provide resources for the family member for parental support and treatment.

At the tertiary level, options for a person with substance abuse problems include detoxification units, transitional or halfway houses, treatment in public and private hospitals, treatment in clinics and respite units for homeless people, and home care.

Detoxification Settings

A **detoxification** unit is generally where a chemically dependent person is sent to safely withdraw from alcohol or other drugs. Some detoxification centers are hospital based while others are free-standing, but all must have skilled nursing care to supervise potentially life-threatening withdrawal. In a detoxification center, the client's physical status is closely monitored and medications are administered to ensure a safe withdrawal and to minimize uncomfortable symptoms. If removal of toxic substances from the body is accomplished, the intervention is a success regardless of whether the individual returns to alcohol or other drug use. Some detoxification centers are combined with longer term treatment, usually 15–30 days. Facilities can be public or private, and there are significant distinctions between the two types. Private detoxification centers have quicker intake procedures, more options for longer stays, and more individualized, intensive therapy. Urban detoxification centers are usually full, and beds are frequently unavailable when the client is ready to seek treatment. Being able to pay makes a difference for people with substance abuse problems, just as it does for other high-risk populations in the United States.

Transitional Housing Programs

Transitional housing programs such as halfway houses are formal programs that are between detoxification and community reintegration for the substance abuser. They are structured programs with substance abuse counseling, relapse prevention work, life skills teaching, and health education. The transitional program affords more time in a protective environment for the recovering person. Medicaid will reimburse for most of the short-term programs, as will disability insurance. Medicare does not cover transitional programs.

Ideally, pregnant women in transition are referred to programs that are focused specifically on issues of women and children. Such programs can better address their individual issues with both substance abuse and their personal relationships.

Clients who are particularly at high risk are those with a dual diagnosis of Axis I and addiction. A new program that shows promise is the Recovery connection. See Out of the Box on next page.

Private Hospitals and Clinics

Private hospitals and clinics abound in the United States but must be paid for by the client or a private insurer. Private insurance coverage varies, but most policies will

Out
of the Box

The Recovery Connection

A new program in Boston focuses on a holistic and interdisciplinary model to break the cycle of chronic addiction in homeless men and women with dual diagnoses of Axis I and addiction. There are many interdisciplinary programs for substance abusers with most modeled on strong rules and regulations. In the Recovery Connection, traditional rules for participation such as abstinence are put in abeyance. The aim is to provide support to clients who, by their distressing socioeconomic and psychosocial circumstances, are often destined to fail. The system expects them to fail and the clients themselves expect to fail. Many addicted individuals "do not know how to handle success, joy or positive events in their lives. They may panic when things go WELL. They sabotage their programs and themselves because of the belief that they do not deserve to succeed" (comments by a shelter nurse).

The Recovery Connection has been funded to break rapid cycling through the addiction system by treating the clients in the shelter where they are known and have some connections through formal and informal relationships. This approach is called treatment-in-place. The place is a shelter, which is home to many homeless addicts, and although it is less than optimal as a home, it is the place where many homeless people feel most comfortable.

This program is unique because it treats the addict in a shelter and tolerates recidivism while the addict is in the program. The method of "cueing" or "coaching" is a technique to support addicted clients at an early stage in a recovery program. Clients are supported by coaching despite problems such as recidivism and "using." These behaviors would, in most recovery programs, mean immediate dismissal. In the Recovery Connection, multiple opportunities are created for clients to stay in the program and to succeed. Instead of being forced out of the program for unacceptable behaviors, clients see a series of rigorous consequences that have been put in place for those behaviors. Consequences range from addi-tional counseling, use of literature to develop insight into behavior, discussion groups, public apologies, and peer intervention.

The populations at risk are homeless men and women who have lived lives of poverty, anomie, despair, and a lack of hope. Many are young, urban, minority adults. Their lives have been characterized by violence associated with substance abuse and life on the streets. They are at risk for trauma, street violence, HIV infection, hepatitis C, and sexually transmitted diseases, and many are mentally ill. They may have trouble with literacy, writing, and basic math. They have no work skills. The plan is to accept directly into the program from an inpatient mental health facility. Because of this unique relationship between the shelter and mental health programs, the program presents an opportunity that would not typically be offered to mentally ill, addicted individuals.

The Model

- The population at risk—homeless, mentally ill, addicted men and women
- The program goal—to facilitate recovery with a structured in-shelter program with discharge to a transition house upon program completion
- Program design—based on the Alcoholics Anonymous/Narcotics Anonymous 12-step philosophy
- The method—collaborative interdisciplinary coaching and cueing activities
- Consequences that are supportive rather than punitive for inappropriate behaviors and recidivism
- Evaluation of outcomes—evidence-based: Does the "graduate" move forward to transitional housing and ongoing support or does the "graduate" return to addiction and the streets?
- Demographics of clients—race, age, gender, mental health history, physical illness, drugs of choice
- Referral sources
- Number who "graduate" from the program
- Longitudinal follow-up from graduation to transitional living—Did the model make a difference? ■

cover the cost for a detoxification unit or a private hospital. The federal and state third-party reimbursement programs, such as Medicare and Medicaid, will not. The Betty Ford Clinic is a well-known example of an expensive private clinic for substance abusers.

Clinics and Respite Units for Homeless People

Clinics for homeless people, often nurse managed, provide care for many indigent individuals who are suffering from the long-term effects of alcohol and other drug abuse. The individual often arrives at the clinic intoxicated and seeking help for a crisis situation, such as trauma, infection, or pain. To address more than the crisis presents a challenge to the nurse and can be a slow process. Many homeless, addicted people, because of previous negative experiences, distrust the formal health care system. They are reluctant to accept referrals. Because of active substance abuse, they miss appointments and their care is often episodic. Clinic nurses work to develop caring relationships that will enable clients to return to the clinic when they are not in crisis and to engage in active treatment. When trust is present, the client is also more apt to listen to and heed teaching regarding such things as not sharing needles and cleaning drug paraphernalia with bleach.

The Barbara McInnis House is an innovative program developed by the Health Care for the Homeless Project in Boston. The program addresses the needs of the many homeless and addicted people who are too sick and too weak to manage in the shelters but are not considered sick enough to be in the hospital. Under managed-care guidelines, many are discharged from the hospital to the street with complicated discharge instructions. The McInnis House gives the homeless person respite from the streets in a substance-free environment where help is available for medications, dressing changes, and other treatments.

Home Care

As clients are discharged from the hospital sooner and sicker, home care is an increasingly important community resource. Because home care is generally initiated by a referral system, it is often a setting for tertiary care.

Addicted women are a population at high risk in the home care setting. The care of addicted women and their children at home is complex and presents many challenges for the community health nurse. The nurse must balance being a support and a resource for the mother and child while, at the same time, providing structure and setting limits as needed. A woman who is actively abusing substances is generally in no condition to care for her children. Injury and neglect are common sequelae in these situations.

Dumas (1991) wrote of the tenuous relationship when caring for cocaine-addicted mothers and their chil-

---

✳ DECISION MAKING

Chronic Alcoholism and Hypertension

You are a home care nurse who admits a client to caseload. The client is a 68-year-old woman with acute and chronic alcoholism and hypertension. She is an active alcoholic and admits to drinking a half bottle of wine daily. Her blood pressure is 172/96. She has not taken her medication in three days. She lives alone in elderly housing. Evaluate the following decisions and give a rationale for your choice.

- ◆ You tell the client she needs detoxification and that you will see about having her admitted immediately to a unit.

- ◆ You assess the client's response to her alcoholism and evaluate her receptiveness to inpatient treatment. If she is not receptive, mandate an inhospital plan of care.

- ◆ You tell her she will need outside supports to assist her in a recovery. Review what some of these supports might be. Obtain a list of informal supports (friends and neighbors).

- ◆ You give her an extra dose of medicine because her blood pressure is high.

- ◆ You telephone the nurse practitioner or physician to collaborate on a plan of care for this client. Obtain a list of her formal professional supports.

- ◆ You refer her to Alcoholics Anonymous immediately.

---

dren. The visiting nurse must establish a primary and trusting relationship with the client and be skilled in both the art and science of nursing. Appointments must be kept, compliance evaluated, and expectations clearly articulated by the nurse.

> Effecting a balance between structure and flexibility with respect to nursing interventions is difficult at best, and the concept of "tough love" is an important one. Addicted individuals require a combination of structure, control, and compassion. Keeping these in balance is a difficult task that cannot be done alone. (p. 17)

Women and their children, in particular infants, are common populations at risk seen in the home. The women are increasingly being referred from hospitals after giving birth to premature, addicted, and overall high-risk infants. This is an excellent example of an opportunity for interdisciplinary collaboration. Nurses,

✳ DECISION MAKING

Client Needs and Managed Care

You are a nurse in a managed-care organization. You have an 18-year-old client who is an amphetamine addict. You realize he will need counseling and referral for his problem; he is becoming ill because of poor nutrition and his substance abuse.

Information indicates that he will be covered for three mental health visits and that he is not covered for any long-term stay in a detoxification facility. You realize that he is not going to do well attempting recovery on his own, without supports or structure. This is a dilemma that is becoming increasingly common in nursing practice.

◆ How do you resolve the disparity between what he needs and what his health plan will pay for?

◆ What approaches would you take to advocate for this client?

◆ What could you do within your organization with respect to making changes in what managed care will cover when problems are social and behavioral?

social workers, physicians, therapists, maternal-child workers, home health aides, and homemakers all have an important role to play in the client's recovery.

Mutual Support Groups

Alcoholics Anonymous (AA) and Narcotics Anonymous (NA) fellowships are informal community supports for individuals in recovery. They internalize a spiritual dimension wherein the fellowship becomes an integral part of the member's life. The support extends through all aspects of daily life. The 12-step program, the foundation of AA, takes members through the most difficult days of their lives. Narcotics Anonymous (NA) uses the same 12-step program as AA. They are counterpart programs for alcoholics and addicts. These are prototypes of self-help groups. Because of the anonymity implicit in the fellowship, there are few data that evaluate the effectiveness of AA and NA on recidivism rates. Despite the extensive development of treatment options for people suffering from addictions, Alcoholics Anonymous is the most widely accessed resource for people with alcohol problems and 12-step programs have been more effective than comparison programs in promoting abstinence (Humphreys, 1999).

In summary, there are diverse treatment modalities ranging from early detoxification programs to self-help groups in the community. The treatment modalities, much like the individuals who use them, take many different forms. Methods may be modified for some addicts depending on the program. In most programs, however, strict rules and structure, a limited setting, and an authoritarian environment are norm. Families may or may not be involved in the actual programs. Much depends on the relationship between the client and the family, as well as on the rules of the program with respect to family participation.

CARING AND CASE MANAGEMENT OF CLIENTS WHO ABUSE SUBSTANCES

The clinical care or case management of people who abuse substances presents difficulties under the best of circumstances. With the advent of managed care and changes in the health care system, several new problems have emerged. First, there are more cost constraints; many services relating to addiction and treatment are not covered, or are only partially covered, by third-party payors. Second, poverty, and in particular poverty among women and children, has become more of a stigma. Third, when health care is based on capitation, a predetermined cost per person, the human element is easily overlooked, as cost containment prevails. Managed care has changed the profile of health care delivery in the United States. Hospitals are downsizing; home care agencies are negotiating with insurers; and bureaucratic tasks have increased. There are escalating health care demands and fewer resources available to meet the demands. There is a lack of fit between available resources and the numbers of people who need them.

In the next decade, hospitals will be for the sickest, with increasing burdens put on home care. This trend will increase the difficulties in providing comprehensive care for addicted individuals. In the 1980s and early 1990s, the numbers of comprehensive substance abuse treatment centers increased with demonstrated success, but today they are reserved for the wealthy. Long-term care of the poor is for those with disease so advanced that it is unlikely that they will benefit from long-term intervention (Delbanco, 1996).

The clinical management of addicted people demands excellent medical surgical nursing skills, excellent assessment skills, a great deal of patience, a good sense of humor, and a strong sense of advocacy. It also requires a sound knowledge of community resources, admission procedures, and eligibility requirements for the different programs.

The concept of caring is an important component in working with people addicted to drugs and alcohol. Caring has traditionally been nurses' work, beginning with

COMMUNITY NURSING VIEW

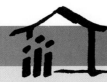

Ayla, a 34-year-old pregnant bank vice president, had recently separated from her husband of 10 years. She was first seen by the occupational health nurse at three months into her pregnancy with complaints of fatigue and poor weight gain. She had had no prenatal care. She admitted to depression over her recent separation and unplanned pregnancy. A drinking history revealed she had three or four scotches before dinner each evening and "a brandy" at bedtime. Weekends brought more drinking, and she admitted to "occasionally" going through a fifth of scotch on Saturdays and Sundays. "My drinking is not a problem. I'm just lonely and tired." She worked a five-day week and, in view of her risk, was offered a leave for the remainder of her pregnancy. She refused the leave and did not keep appointments with the occupational health nurse. She was seen again by the occupational health nurse at six months, when she went to the bank's health clinic with fatigue and headache. Her blood pressure was 170/90, heart rate 110 regular, respiratory rate 20, unlabored and lungs clear. She had a 1+ –2+ bilateral edema, and lung sounds were diminished but clear to auscultation. She appeared bloated, her fingers were swollen, and she had some red blotches on her face. She appeared sad and nervous. She had continued to smoke 10–12 cigarettes daily during her pregnancy, and despite efforts to improve her nutrition, her weight gain had been poor. She was depressed and anxious and admitted to a slight hangover on this particular day. "I am drinking more, but my pregnancy is almost over." She was referred to her obstetrician for immediate attention, and the nurse asked her to return later in the week for a blood pressure check and nutritional counseling. Ayla was also advised by the nurse to stop drinking for the remainder of her pregnancy. Ayla did not return to the clinic. The nurse did not seek her out at the work setting, and her obstetrician advised her to continue with monthly appointments and to stop drinking. Ayla said to a friend, "I go to the doctor each month and I'm trying to cut down on my drinking. I don't know what more they want from me. I just want my husband home again."

Ayla delivered a premature girl at 33 weeks, and head circumference was below normal. The infant was nervous and hypertonic. The infant had some respiratory distress and was placed in the intensive care nursery. She was discharged to home after two weeks. At six months, the baby was noted to have growth retardation and facial dysmorphia. She was diagnosed at six months with fetal alcohol syndrome. At this time, Ayla was hospitalized with a major depressive episode and the baby was placed in temporary foster care. The long-range plan was for Ayla and the baby to return home together to visiting nurse services and other community supports.

Nursing Considerations

Assessment

- At which time in Ayla's pregnancy would primary prevention have been optimal?
- What would be included in the preliminary assessment of Ayla?
- What is the prevailing female alcoholic stereotype that Ayla's case refutes?
- Distinguish questions related to primary, secondary, and tertiary prevention in the data collection.

Diagnosis

- List four nursing diagnoses for Ayla.

Outcome Identification

- Given the diagnosis you have identified, what outcomes do you expect?

Planning/Interventions

- What kinds of health promotion interventions would you plan for Ayla?
- What would you consider secondary prevention for Ayla?
- On what criteria will you base your nursing diagnoses?
- What kinds of skilled activities will you conduct for this dimension of care?
- How would you define tertiary prevention in this case?
- What would your nursing plan be, and how will the nursing process direct your plan?
- What would you have done differently if you had been Ayla's occupational health nurse?

(continues)

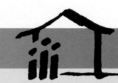

COMMUNITY NURSING VIEW (continued)

◆ Your tertiary level of prevention will involve both Ayla and her baby. What kind of plan for restoration of the health of both mother and infant will you delineate?◆
Which community facilities in your area will you use as resources when Ayla is back at home with her baby?

◆ What kinds of home health services will you suggest in your referral to the local visiting nurse association?

Evaluation

◆ How will success or failure at primary, secondary, and tertiary levels of prevention be evaluated?

◆ What would be the outcome of physical therapy for the infant?

Nightingale and moving forward to Wald. Caring characterizes the nursing role, and it is a component that medical students are learning in their curricula from nurses who have the greatest respect for its art.

Many of the populations at high risk for substance abuse and many of the people who abuse substances have social and economic issues that are profound. It hurts to look at them, it is frustrating to try to help them, and it is easy to shame them.

The concept of "disaffiliation" that Baum and Burnes (1993) emphasize in their book about homeless people also holds true for those addicted to alcohol and drugs. Community health nurses must be willing to help their clients bear the burden, to provide hope, to advocate for the future, and to listen, counsel, and assist them through the health care system with the goal of "reaffiliating" them.

Nurses have two very special gifts, a capacity to provide comfort and the knowledge to provide highly skilled clinical care. People who abuse substances have many needs, and the skilled nurse will be able to prioritize them with respect to what can and cannot be realistically accomplished.

KEY CONCEPTS

◆ The term *substance abuse* includes alcohol, tobacco, and other drug abuse.

◆ Substances frequently abused include alcohol, tobacco, marijuana, cocaine, methamphetamine, opiates, and prescription drugs.

◆ Alcoholism and drug addiction are "equal opportunity" addictions. They occur among all class, socioeconomic, gender, race, and culture groups.

◆ Women, elders, gays and lesbians, and persons who are homeless and mentally ill are at higher risk than others for the development of alcohol, tobacco, and other drug addiction.

◆ The upstream analogy invites diverse health providers to work at individual and societal levels to promote healthy behaviors and healthy lifestyles before illness occurs.

◆ Nurses need to be able to analyze their own attitudes toward people who abuse substances and to identify their preexisting biases and value judgments.

◆ Primary, secondary, and tertiary levels of prevention are an epidemiological method by which nurses can organize their approach to the problem of substance abuse.

◆ Cigarette smoking is an addictive behavior. The group at highest risk is adolescent girls.

◆ Poverty is a compelling risk factor for alcoholism and drug addiction.

◆ Education and guidance are interdisciplinary endeavors at all levels of prevention.

◆ Caring and clinical expertise are prerequisites for the practice of nursing with people addicted to alcohol, tobacco, and other drugs.

◆ Substance abuse in the United States is a part of an international perspective.

◆ Substance abuse in the United States is on a continuum defined by culture, economics, and stage of development.

RESOURCES

National Drug Intelligence Center: http://www.usdoj.gov/ndic
Oxycontin diversion and abuse:
http://www.usdoj.gov/ndic/pubs/651/abuse.htm

Chapter

32

POVERTY

June Hart Romeo, PhD, RN, NP-C

"Poverty—the most deadly and prevalent of all the diseases."

—Eugene O'Neill

COMPETENCIES

Upon completion of this chapter, the reader should be able to:

- Discuss different definitions of poverty.
- Examine the distribution of poverty in populations.
- Identify common health effects of poverty on individuals, families, and communities.
- Discuss at least three theories that explain poverty.
- Describe nursing intervention strategies with population aggregates who are poor.
- Discuss nurses' perceptions about poverty and the poor.
- Examine the various factors that influence poverty's impact on health.

KEY TERMS

culture-of-poverty	poverty
disenfranchised	poverty line/poverty threshold
feminization of poverty	
marginals	social class
marginalization	social class gradient
oppression	

According to the U.S. Census of 2000, more than 40 million Americans (about one in every seven persons) are living at or below the poverty line established by the federal government. The 2000 Bureau of the Census report showed that one in five households had difficulty meeting basic needs—everything from paying the utility bills to buying food for dinner. More than 43 million people in the United States, including 11 million children, have no health care insurance. Every month more than 100,000 people lose their health insurance. The World Health Organization (WHO) has found the quality of U.S. health care to rank 37th in the world, and the United States is the only advanced industrialized nation in the world without national health care (WHO, 1999b).

Persons, families, and aggregates living in poverty are at high risk for health problems. Persons in this population tend to use public health clinics and are in need of the services most often offered by nurses. This is a particularly challenging group for the community health nurse, due in part to lack of resources, lack of health insurance, and differences in priorities. The community health nurse can make a significant impact on the health of the poor.

The purpose of this chapter is to present the various dimensions of poverty and discuss the impact of poverty on health. The topic will be explored with a focus on families and aggregate populations.

WHO ARE THE POOR?

Who are the poor? Are they male or female? Children or the elderly? Are they the mentally ill or are they criminals? Are they just people who refuse to work? Or are they third-generation unmarried welfare mothers? All of us have preconceived notions about who they are. Here are some of the myths about the poor and some of the facts.

Myth 1: Most poor people are lazy. They are poor because they do not want to work.

In the United States, half the poor are either too old or too young to work. About 40% are under age 18, and another 10% are over age 65. About 30% of the poor who are of working age do work at least half the year (U.S. Bureau of the Census, 2000).

Myth 2: Most of the poor are Latinos or African Americans.

The poverty rates of Latinos and African Americans are much higher than that of whites; however, since there are so many more whites in the U.S. population, most poor people are white. Fifty-six percent of the poor are white, 21% are African American, and 19% are Latino (U.S. Bureau of the Census, 2000).

Myth 3: Most of the poor are single mothers and their children.

About 38% of the poor match this; however, 34% of the poor live in married-couple families. Twenty-two percent live alone, and 6% live in other settings (U.S. Bureau of the Census, 2000).

Myth 4: Most of the poor live in the inner city.

About 42% of the poor live in inner city areas, about 36% live in suburban areas, and 22% live in rural areas (U.S. Bureau of the Census, 2000).

Myth 5: The poor live on welfare.

Approximately half the income of poor adults comes from wages and pensions. About 25% comes from welfare, and about 22% from social security (U.S. Bureau of the Census, 2000).

DEFINITIONS OF POVERTY

Poverty can be defined as the lack of resources to meet basic needs, which include food, shelter, clothing, and health care. This definition, while describing poverty, is too general to use for determining eligibility for various types of assistance. It is, however, the definition that will

REFLECTIVE THINKING

Defining the Poor

Who are the poor? Are they male or female? Children or the elderly? Are they the mentally ill or are they criminals? Are they deadbeats who refuse to work? Or are they third-generation unmarried welfare mothers? All of us have preconceived notions about who they are, and they differ from person to person. Think about these statements. Do they reflect your notions? Why do you feel the way you do? Here are some of the myths about the poor and some of the facts.

✴ DECISION MAKING

Drawing the Poverty Line

Consider your own life. How much money would you have to make to consider yourself "not poor"? Would your income include enough money to take a vacation once a year? Would it include the cost of medication for hypertension or heart disease? Would it include presents for your children's birthdays? Would it include the cost of a winter coat or new shoes? Look through the rental property section of your local newspaper. How much does it cost to rent a modest apartment in a safe neighborhood? Could you live on $8501 comfortably? Work out a monthly budget and see just how far $8501 goes. Are you forced to make choices about what you will buy? Add into your budget the cost of two medications, one for hypertension that costs $65 per month and one for cardiovascular disease that costs $48 per month. Now what choices do you have to make? Consider what it must be like to be elderly, on a fixed income, and on four or five different medications.

If the decision were yours, how would you draw the poverty line? What flexibility would you build into it to ensure that it remained accurate across the country?

be used in this chapter. The U.S. government has established a measure called the **poverty line** (sometimes called the **poverty threshold**) for eligibility determination. This line determines who is and is not eligible for various government programs that offer assistance to the poor. The income established by the government for the poverty line in 2000 was $8501 for a single person of any age and of either sex. The poverty line for a family of four persons is $17,029. This definition is based on the assumption that families spend about one-third of their income on food. As you might think, this definition is unrealistic. The poverty line is consistent across the country and does not take into account differences in cost of living. How poverty is defined has serious consequences, since the government uses the poverty line to decide who will receive help and who will not (U.S. Bureau of the Census, 2000).

Now consider poverty in a relative sense. There is *absolute poverty* in the United States—a poverty due to a lack of basic necessities, which is life threatening. Thousands of homeless in the United States froze to death in the cold winter of 2000, and tens of thousands of people starved to death in the Third World countries during that same year. However, many of those considered poor by the material standards of the United States would not be considered poor if living under the same conditions in nations such as Chad, the Philippines, or India. In China, for example, in the 1990s a "highly paid" factory worker bringing home the equivalent of $112 a month in wages and living with other family members in a 600-square-foot apartment that has no hot water or refrigerator would not consider himself or herself to be poor by Chinese standards (Haub & Cornelius, 1999). The point is that poverty cannot simply be considered relative to the material existence of people throughout the world; in many important ways it is *relative to the so-*

ciety in which the poor find themselves. In large part, this is because the self-worth, the aspirations, and the expectations of people are shaped by the relative position of others in the society.

The contrasts of wealth and poverty are nowhere more striking than in many of the great cities of the United States, perhaps in New York City more than anywhere else. New York City is the financial capital of the nation and in some of its zip code areas we find an average income higher than anywhere else in the United States, and probably the world. But New York City also contains the greatest concentration of the nation's welfare recipients and poor. In 2000 it was estimated that each night more than 64,000 people in New York City had to sleep on the sidewalks, in parks, or over subway vents (U.S. Bureau of the Census, 2000).

Criticism of official poverty statistics include the obvious charge that poverty is underestimated in this country. Also, critics charge that a poverty line should consider the *relative* aspects of poverty. That is, because poverty is not only a material condition, we should consider poverty to exist when people are far below the average standard of living in the country. A relative poverty line could be drawn at about half of the average income of the population.

Absolute vs. Relative Poverty

You and a nursing colleague are working in a busy community health center that generally serves elders living on fixed incomes. One day an obviously very poor man comes to this clinic. He is very dirty, disheveled, and has several layers of very worn clothing on. He does not talk much but answers questions when asked for information. During your assessment, you find that he is having difficulty finding affordable housing and eats only every two to three days. Your colleague makes the comment, "If he thinks he has it so tough here, he should try living in Ethiopia." How would you respond? How does your colleague's statement fit in with the concepts of absolute versus relative poverty? Does the level of poverty in Ethiopia have any significance for this client?

DISTRIBUTION OF POVERTY

As stated previously, one in every seven Americans is living at or below the poverty line established by the federal government. One in five households had difficulty meeting basic needs—everything from paying the utility bills to buying food for dinner (U.S. Bureau of the Census, 2000).

In estimating the extent of poverty it is also useful to compare the existence of poverty across subcategories of the population. When this comparison is made, it is found that the chances of living in poverty are not randomly distributed in the society. Who is more likely to be poor—the elderly or the young? Approximately 11% of those aged 65 years and older are living in poverty, while 23% of those in the 18- to 64-year age range and 24% of those under 18 years of age are poor (U.S. Bureau of the Census, 2000). If we look at poverty rates by race and Hispanic origin, we see that the highest percentage of those living in poverty describe themselves as black (African American) or of mixed race (see Figure 32-1). Figure 32-2 gives the percentages of poverty-stricken

FIGURE 32-1 Poverty Rates by Age, 1999

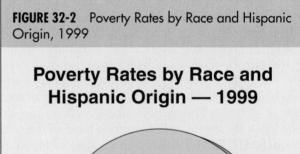

Poverty Rates by Age — 1999

☐ 65 years and over ☐ Under 18 years ☐ 18–64 years

From *Statistical Abstracts of the United States: The National Data Book,* by U.S. Bureau of the Census, 2000, Washington, DC: U.S. Government Printing Office.

FIGURE 32-2 Poverty Rates by Race and Hispanic Origin, 1999

Poverty Rates by Race and Hispanic Origin — 1999

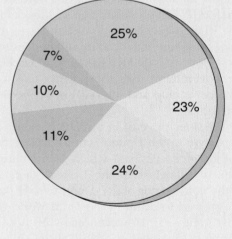

☐ Asian & Pacific Islander ☐ Black
☐ Hispanic ☐ White non-Hispanic
☐ White ☐ Other

Source: U.S. Census Bureau Current Population Survey, March 1999 and 2000.

From *Statistical Abstracts of the United States: The National Data Book,* by U.S. Bureau of the Census, 2000, Washington, DC: U.S. Government Printing Office.

FIGURE 32-3 Poverty Rates by Selected Characteristics: 1998 and 1999

Poverty Rates by Selected Characteristics: 1998 and 1999

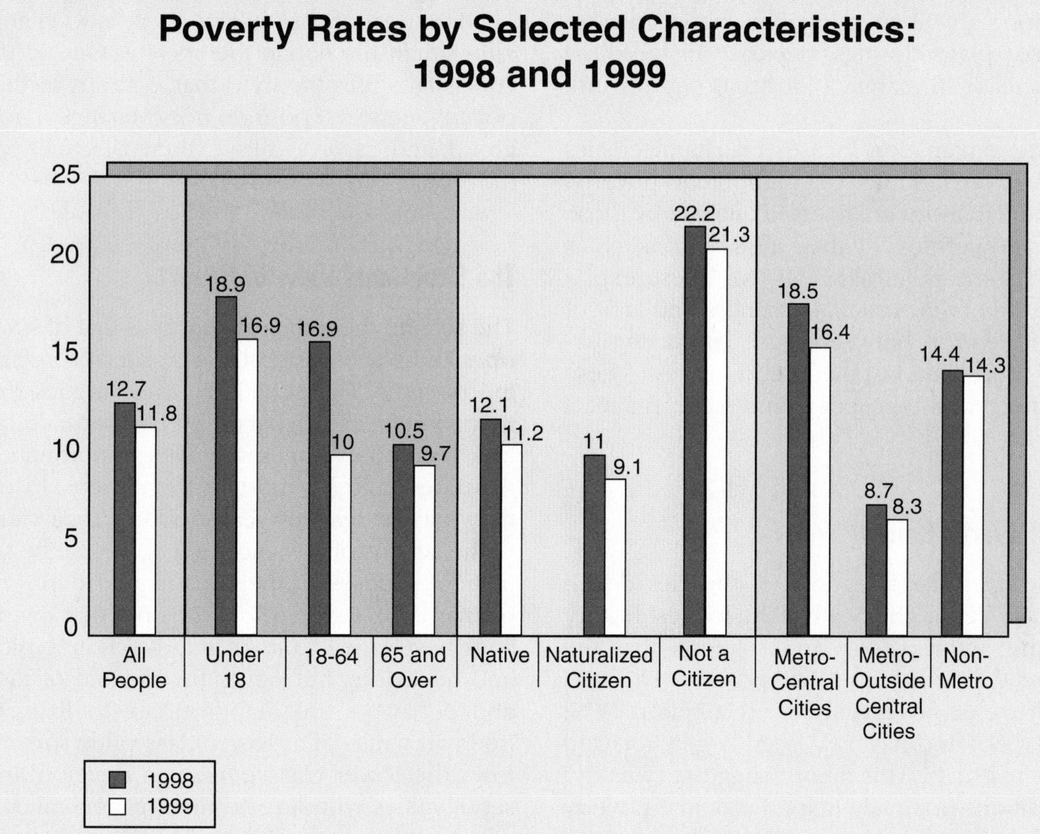

From *Statistical Abstracts of the United States: The National Data Book,* by U.S. Bureau of the Census, 2000, Washington, DC: U.S. Government Printing Office.

persons who describe themselves as members of each racial/ethnic category as asked by the U.S. Bureau of the Census (2000). Looking at these data, we can generalize that minorities, children, and female-headed households have a greater chance of being poor (see Figure 32-3).

Approximately 12% of the poor experience poverty for five years or longer (Rossi, 1989; U.S. Bureau of the

REFLECTIVE THINKING

Existence and Continuance of Poverty

Which do you think is more important in explaining the existence and continuance of poverty, the characteristics of the poor or the characteristics of the society? Can you focus on one of these without considering the others, or do you think they are intertwined?

Census, 2000). The majority of poor people do not like poverty and do what they can to *not* be poor. From one year to the next, the number of poor remains relatively stable. This means that while people are moving out of poverty, more are becoming poor every year.

Such a distribution of poverty raises questions about the nature of poverty. What characteristics increase a person's risk of poverty? More importantly, what is it about the nature of our society that helps produce greater poverty among some groups?

Reading the lay literature, one might think it is the characteristics of the poor themselves who have most often been held responsible. But the nature of class conflict in the U.S. system of social stratification suggests otherwise.

EXPLAINING POVERTY: MAJOR THEORIES OF POVERTY

Why are people poor? There are two major explanations that compete for attention. If examined from a sociological perspective, the focus would be on social structure.

This explanation emphasized features of society that deny some people access to education or to learning job skills. This focus emphasizes racial, ethnic, age, and gender discrimination as well as changes in the job market such as industrial plant closings, decrease in unskilled jobs, and an increase in marginal jobs that pay poverty wages.

A competing explanation focuses on characteristics of individuals who are assumed to contribute to poverty. Many of these explanations are rejected outright by those who make the study of poverty their life's work (such as sociologists and some political scientists). These explanations include stereotypes such as laziness and lack of intelligence. The tension between these competing explanations is of more than just theoretical interest. These explanations affect our perception and have practical consequences.

The Culture-of-Poverty Theory

There are basically three categories of theories developed to explain poverty. The first has the longest history in sociology and anthropology and suggests that the characteristics of the poor help cause poverty. This was termed the **culture-of-poverty** theory (Galbraith, 1979; Lewis, 1966a, 1966b) and has now been largely rejected by most recent research. This theory suggests (weakly) that social conditions originally helped produce poverty but, most importantly, this theory argues that poverty produces people with unique personal characteristics that in turn help ensure that the poor and their children remain poor. On a community level, there is said to be a lack of participation in the institutions of the wider society (except for contact with the criminal justice system and welfare institutions). On a family level, there is the absence of a long childhood, early initiation into sex, free unions or consensual marriages, a relatively high incidence of the abandonment of wives and children, and female-centered families. On an individual level, the poor are believed to have strong feelings of marginality, of helplessness, of dependence, and of inferiority. Other individual characteristics are believed to be a weak ego, lack of impulse control, a present-time orientation with relatively little ability to defer gratification and to plan for the future, a sense of fatalism, a value stress on male superiority, and a high tolerance for psychological pathology of all sorts. Social scientists have paid considerable attention to the "trait" of a present-time orientation, or an inability to delay gratification. This trait is said to be a coping mechanism, for example, because it would be psychologically damaging to continually worry about and plan for a future that holds no promise of a better life or more opportunities. In short, the poor must learn to live for today. This cultural trait is also seen as important in perpetuating poverty and preventing upward mo-

bility out of poverty because the poor learn not to delay gratification or plan for the future and are unable to take advantage of new opportunities.

The goal of this theory, then, is to change the poor rather than to change the society. One of the strongest criticisms of this theory is that, contrary to the culture-of-poverty view, the poor do not constitute a homogeneous group, and, as you will see, there is actually considerable movement out of poverty.

The Situational View of Poverty

The second theoretical category is that of *situational theories* and places more stress on social conditions as causing poverty. The situational view argues that the poor may sometimes behave differently *because* they are poor, lack secure jobs, or simply lack opportunities to live up to values held by most in the society. In other words, they may be reacting realistically to their situation. Many of the actions of low-income people can be seen as pragmatic responses to the stresses and deprivations of life (Gans, 1972; Lewis, 1967). It is not that low-income persons have failed to learn middle-class (typical) attitudes and behaviors, but rather that certain of these attitudes and behaviors are inappropriate to living in poverty. Rodman writes of a "lower class value stretch," which allows the lower class person to develop an alternative set of values without rejecting the general cultural norms of society (Rodman 1963). Socialization of the poor, according to this view, is not substantially different; the problem is that the conditions of lower income life are basically inconsistent with realization of the middle-class model. The poor do share many values with the dominant strata, but they must accept alternative ideals when the contradictions between cultural ideals and situational conditions are too sharp. For instance, the middle-class ideal of a traditional family structure (two parents) is still the dominant type among poor families but is more difficult to attain when the husband is unable to earn enough to support a family or when he is frequently unemployed. Although the conventional two-parent family is preferred, broken families may be more adaptive at certain stages in the lifetime of the adults: "Consensual unions provide a flexible adaptation that is functional under conditions in which fluctuating economic circumstances, actual or threatened incarceration, and other external conditions often make it advisable for cohabiting pairs to separate either temporarily or permanently and contract alternative unions, again either temporary or lasting" (Valentine, 1968, p. 107).

Many of the distinctive aspects of the low-income style of living are mere reflections of what one must do if one falls into poverty. The poor cannot save money because there is little money to save. They buy more expensive goods at neighborhood stores because transportation to faraway shopping centers is too costly or unavailable. They get forced into high-interest rates by loan sharks because banks will not offer them low-interest loans. They have a strong present orientation because they realistically surmise that the chances for substantial improvement of their socioeconomic status are not great or because they lack the resources to take needed actions to bring about improvement.

In general, this theory maintains that inequities in the opportunity structure constrain the behavior of the poor and that opening up the opportunity structure would allow the expression of underlying middle-class motivational and behavioral patterns (Davidson & Krackhardt, 1975). Without focusing on the overall system of inequality, the situational theory clearly takes the blame away from the poor person and places it on the pattern of opportunities. What is overlooked by the situational theory, however, is that better schools and job-training programs oriented toward the unskilled would help only a small percentage of the poor—not the aged, the low paid, the mentally ill, or the mothers.

The Conflict Theory of Poverty

Another theory is a *structural,* or *conflict,* view of poverty. This theory stresses the political and economic forces in the society that produce and maintain poverty (Mills, 1956; Dahrendorf, 1959; Collins, 1974; Schellenberg, 1996). Begin a structural level conflict view of poverty by considering the position of the poor in the occupational structure of society. The occupational structure is a situation of conflict and competition in the marketplace. Those with greater skills (skills that are in high demand and are relatively scarce) can demand and receive higher wages for their labor and maintain more secure jobs. The poor, of course, are at the bottom of the occupational structure. They have few skills, or only skills that can be easily learned by almost anyone (such as how to pick grapes or assemble a part on a gadget moving along on an assembly line).

Consider also the property structure. It is obvious that most poor and unskilled workers own little, and in most cases, no capital (such as owning a house, stocks, jewelry). This makes them dependent on others for their jobs and livelihood. Today, when the prospects for employment are reduced, as was with farm workers and coal miners, the poor are left with no resources.

Lastly, consider the authority structure in society. The poor are almost exclusively located at the bottom of the economic or occupational authority structures—where they are even subject to these authority structures through employment. They are among the unskilled laborers who give orders to no one; and when they do work, the poor are more likely to work in nonunion industries.

More importantly, the poor are found toward the bottom of the wider power structures of the society. Politically, the poor can be considered the most powerless of classes. The lower the position in the social system, the less likely people are to vote, contribute to political candidates, be represented by lobby organizations, or participate in voluntary organizations of the type that could represent the rights and interests of its members. When the poor have had influence, such political influence was often gained outside the normal channels of political influence—that is, through social movements and riots rather than traditional party politics. Because of their limited means of influence, the poor have usually won only small and often short-lasting concessions in the conflict over who gets what in society.

The Functionalist Theory of Poverty

In a nation as wealthy as the United States, the obvious question is why does pervasive poverty continue? Let us look at this from a functional theory point of view. Functional theorists would say that segments of our society *benefit* from the existence of the poor (Davis & Moore, 1945, 1953). There are a number of political, social, and economic functions that the poor perform for society. These include the following:

- The presence of the poor means that society's dirty work—physically dirty or dangerous, dead-end and underpaid, undignified and menial jobs—will be performed at low cost.

- Poverty creates jobs for occupations and professions that "service" the poor. It creates both legal employment (public health experts, social workers, community health nurses) and illegal jobs (drug dealers, prostitutes).

- The identification and punishment of the poor as deviants uphold the legitimacy of conventional social norms and "mainstream values" regarding hard work, thrift, and honesty.

- In our relatively hierarchical society, the existence of poor people guarantees the higher status of the more affluent.

- Due to the lack of political power, the poor often absorb the costs of social change. Under the policy of deinstitutionalization, mental patients released from long-term hospitals were "dumped" primarily into low-income communities and neighborhoods. Halfway houses for the rehabilitated substance abusers and the mentally ill are often rejected by more affluent communities and tend to end up in poorer neighborhoods.

By considering the above, it can be seen how functionalist theory demonstrates the "uses" of the poor to society.

SOCIAL INFLUENCES

The United States is a land of great contrasts. The wealthiest Americans, those in the top 1%, have approximately 95% of the total wealth of the other 99% of Americans (Beeghley, 2000). This staggering statistic has remained constant over the past five decades. The wealthiest Americans have vast resources available for their use, while those in the bottom 25% of the income bracket (those living *below* the poverty line) have almost none. Without resources it is difficult, if not impossible, to escape from poverty. Those living in poverty do not have the same choices open to them as do you and your classmates. To better understand this, one must understand the concepts of social class, marginalization, and oppression.

A **social class** is a group of people who rank closely to one another in wealth, power, and prestige. Standard definitions of social class include the upper class, into which a person is generally born, since it is very difficult, if not impossible, to move upward into this class. People in this class generally marry within their class. These are the people with wealth that places them within the upper 1% of the income bracket. Yet even in this highest of classes, there are two classes. There is a distinction between those with "old" money (inherited wealth) and those with "new" money (earned wealth, considered *nouveau riche*). The longer the wealth has been in the family, the more it adds to their prestige. Examples of families in the inherited wealth class include the Rockefellers, Vanderbilts, Mellons, Du Ponts, Chryslers, Fords, Morgans, and Nashes. While initially the wealth might have been earned, generations later it loses this "taint" and is considered inherited. Families in this class are generally philanthropic as well as rich and establish foundations and support charitable causes. Subsequent generations attend prestigious prep schools and universities, and heirs are likely to study business or law. These old-money families wield vast power and have extensive political connections to protect their huge economic empires.

Those at the lower end of the upper class 1% also possess vast sums of money and power, but it is new. Although these people have made fortunes in business, the stock market, inventions, entertainment, or sports, they have not attended the "right" schools and they lack the influential social networks that come with old money. One example of new money is Bill Gates, a cofounder of Microsoft Corporation. He is the wealthiest person in the world. His fortune of $70 billion continues to increase as his company develops new products. His home cost $50 million and he hung a $30 million painting in the living room. His fortune is so vast, that in 2000, when the Dow Jones Industrial Average dropped, Gates lost $35 billion (Domhoff, 1999).

Another example of vast wealth is that of John Castle, whose wealth came through banking and securities. He purchased John F. Kennedy's ocean-front estate in Palm Beach, Florida, then spent $11 million to remodel this 13,000-square-foot house, including adding bathrooms number 14 and 15. He has a nearby 10-acre ranch where his string of thoroughbred horses are housed. He also has a 45-foot custom-built yacht. He once boarded this yacht for an around-the-world trip, but he did not stay on board. He just joined the cruise from time to time while a full-time captain and crew kept the vessel sailing in the right direction. Whenever he felt like it, Castle would join the cruise for a few days, then fly back to the United States. He did this about a dozen times, flying 150,000 miles. When asked how much the custom-built yacht cost, Castle replied, "I don't want to know what anything costs. When you've got enough money, price doesn't make a difference. That's part of the freedom of being rich." Freedom indeed! Being rich also meant paying $1 million to charter a private jet to fly Spot, one of his horses, back and forth to the veterinarian. The cost of Spot's medical treatment was another $500,000 (Domhoff, 1999).

Sound like something out of science fiction? Yet there are other people who put John Castle to shame. Wayne Huizenga, the CEO of AutoNation, owns a 2000-acre country club with an 18-hole golf course, a 35,000-square-foot clubhouse, and 68 slips for sailing vessels. The club is so exclusive that its only members are Wayne Huizenga and his wife (Domhoff, 1999).

The upper middle class is the group most shaped by education. The majority of members of this class have a minimum of a baccalaureate degree, and many have postgraduate degrees in law, medicine, or business. They comprise about 15% of the population. The lower middle class, comprising about 32% of the population, have jobs in which they follow orders given by those who have upper middle class credentials. They tend to work in technical and lower level management. The distinction between lower middle class and the working class is slightly blurred. The working class, about 32% of the population, are relatively unskilled blue collar workers

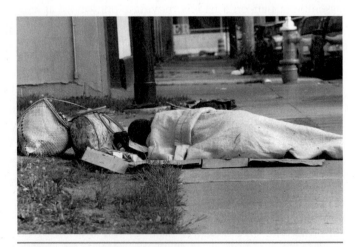

While some people live in great wealth, others are living on the street with no home. Copyright William C. Rieter. Used with permission.

(U.S. Bureau of Census, 2000). Compared with the lower middle class, they have less education and lower incomes. Their jobs are less secure, more routinized, and more closely supervised. One of their biggest fears is being laid off. With only a high school diploma, there is little hope of climbing up the social ladder. Job changes are usually lateral, so most concentrate on getting ahead by achieving seniority on the job rather than by changing jobs or type of work.

The working poor, approximately 16% of the population, are a relatively new class in the literature on poverty (U.S. Bureau of Census, 2000). These are persons who work in unskilled, low-paying, temporary, and seasonal jobs. Many are functionally illiterate and find it difficult to read want ads, figure out their pay stubs, and fill out a job application. Most are high school dropouts. They are not likely to vote. About 6 million of the working poor actually work full time but still must depend on assistance such as food stamps.

The underclass, previously termed "lower class," has a very limited chance of improving their status. Usually concentrated in the inner city, this group has little or no connection with the job market. Welfare, if available, coupled with food stamps and soup kitchens is their main support. About 4% of the population fall into this class (U.S. Bureau of Census, 2000). It is difficult, however, to count this group since many are homeless and therefore difficult to be "counted" by agencies such as the Census Bureau. Their presence on the streets bothers many people, who consider them "dirty, foul-smelling, and obnoxious." These are the fallout of the industrialization of our country. In another century, they would have found plentiful unskilled work as laborers on farms and in factories by ending horses and shoveling coal. In today's world of work, there is little such unskilled work available. For more information about the issues of the homeless, see Chapter 33.

Sandwiched in between the high earners in the professions and the technical workers are a group of middle-class workers often referred to as being in the "emerging professions." Emerging professions include teachers, middle-management administrators, and nurses. Money buys many essentials for upward mobility or maintenance of current status. It can buy more education, a place in a "better school," clothing appropriate for a job interview in a prestigious company, and a place where others with power and wealth congregate (such as a country club, professional organization, or better neighborhood).

These inequalities in class hierarchies lead to inequalities in power relationships, political interests, and economic policies that can interfere with health. One's chances of significantly effecting change in society increases proportionately to the resources one can command. Social structures, such as class and status, define how privilege, exploitation, and powerlessness are distributed among persons and groups in society. **Oppression** is a term used to indicate unequal power relations embedded in society. It is inherent in the social structuring of life, limitations and choices that are not equally experienced across groups. Oppressed persons are constrained in their quest for human potential.

In addition to the various social classes, there exists at the very bottom of the underclass a group of people called **marginals.** These people live on the margins, or edges, of society rather than in the mainstream. They are the people the system of labor cannot or will not use. **Marginalization** is perhaps the most dangerous form of oppression, in that a whole category of people is expelled from useful participation in social life and thus subjected to severe material deprivation and even extermination. This group is often referred to as being **disenfranchised.** This means that they do not have all the privileges and rights as do citizens in higher social classes. Those who live in poverty are often isolated in inner city neighborhoods or rural areas in which a middle or higher class person never travels. The marginalized generally include large numbers of homeless persons, persons with mental illness, the disabled, and the elderly and very young. These persons are often invisible in society. They have little voice and almost no power. They are unaware

---

REFLECTIVE THINKING

Experience of Being Poor

Consider, for a moment, being very poor. You have had to move four times in the past 10 months due to inability to pay the rent. You currently live in a three-room apartment and share a bathroom (which is on the next floor) with eight other families. It is often difficult to bathe, and your clothes are dirty since there is no washing machine. The laundromat is two miles away, a load of wash costs $5.00 to wash and dry, and it is difficult to haul all your laundry and two small children all that way. In this condition you would not make a good impression at a job interview for a fast-food worker, a housemaid, or a courier. You find it difficult to fill out a job application when you are not sure if your address will remain the same for more than a few weeks, and you have no phone number where you can be contacted. You can not even access benefits to which you are entitled if you do not have a stable address where a check can be mailed or a bank where you can cash it.

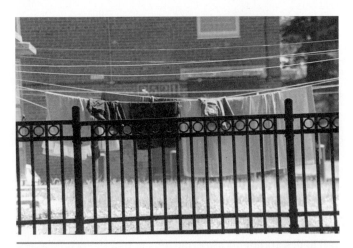

Having clotheslines on which to hang wash can be a luxury for some people. Copyright William C. Rieter. Used with permission.

of the alternatives to their current life and unconscious of their choices. These are the unempowered, the disenfranchised, and the marginalized.

CONSEQUENCES OF SOCIAL CLASS, OPPRESSION, AND DISENFRANCHISEMENT

Social class affects health, chances of living, and chances of dying. The empirical research demonstrates the following principle: The lower a person's social class, the more likely that individual is to die before the expected age. This holds true for all age groups. Infants born to the poor are more likely than those born in higher social classes to die during their first year of life. A larger proportion of the elderly poor die than do the more affluent elderly (Basch, 1999). Part of the reason for this diversity in death rates is unequal access to medical care. Consider the example of Terry.

Terry was a 21-year-old unemployed, uninsured man with Type I diabetes mellitus who lived in Somerville, Tennessee. One day he was found drenched in sweat by his neighbor, who immediately called an ambulance. Terry was rushed to the closest hospital where he had an outstanding bill of $9400. A notice had been posted in the emergency room alerting staff members about his debt in case Terry ever returned. However, on arrival to the emergency room, medical staff members judged Terry to be ill enough to require hospitalization. When the information of Terry's admission reached the hospital administration, Terry was already in bed in a hospital room. An administrator went to Terry's room, helped him to his feet, got him dressed, and escorted him to the parking lot. He was eventually found by neighbors under a tree in the lot and was taken home. He died 12 hours later.

Why was Terry denied medical treatment and his life cut short? *The fundamental reason is that in the United States health care is not a right of all citizens, but rather it is a commodity for sale.* This results in a two-tiered medical care system: superior care for those who can afford the cost and no care or inferior care for those who cannot. Unlike those in the middle and upper classes, those in the lower socioeconomic status groups in general do not have a personal physician. They usually spend hours waiting in overcrowded understaffed public health clinics.

Social class and income also affect mental health. Since the 1930s, research has found that the mental health of the lower classes is worse than that of the upper classes (Szaz, 1998). Consider the role of stress on mental health. The poor have less job security, fewer job opportunities, lower wages, more unpaid bills, more divorce, more alcoholism, greater vulnerability to crime, more physical illnesses, and more threat of eviction than do the middle and upper classes. People in the upper

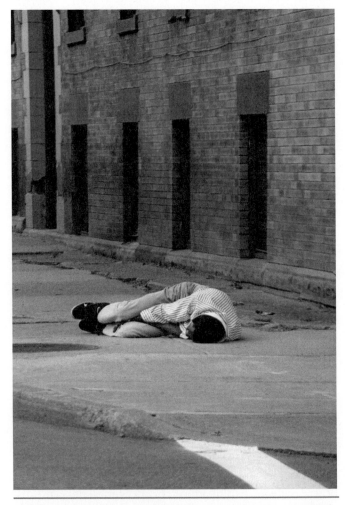

Some people have nowhere to go when they are sick. Copyright William C. Rieter. Used with permission.

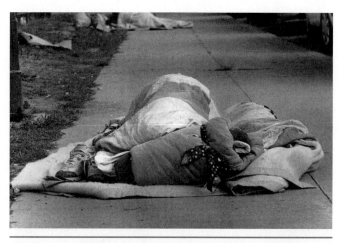

Sometimes a sudden life change can force a person to have no place for themselves and their possessions. Copyright William C. Rieter. Used with permission.

classes experience stress also, but in general, their resources are greater, offering them more coping mechanisms. Not only can they afford vacation, psychiatrists, and counseling, but their class position gives them greater control over their lives, which is key to good mental health.

It is well known that poverty and disease have a strong link and that the less money individuals have the more likely they are to be sick, to die young, and to die from disease that can be cured or treated (Basch, 1999). The lower the socioeconomic class, the less likely the individuals are to receive certain medication, certain surgeries, and certain medical therapies. The poorer persons are, the longer they will wait before needed surgery and/or therapy is offered. In the United States today, one in every six persons has no health insurance (U.S. Bureau of the Census, 2000).

CHILDREN AND POVERTY

Children are more likely to live in poverty than are adults. This fact holds true regardless of race or ethnicity, although poverty among Latino and African American children is greater than for other groups. Approximately 15 million

children are reared in poverty. That is, one in every five children lives in poverty. One in every six white children and one in every three Latino children are poor. *Forty-four percent of children in the United States live in or near poverty* (U.S. Bureau of Census, 2000). According to Daniel Moynihan, a sociologist and previous U.S. Senator, the cause of this staggering statistic is the breakdown of the traditional family unit (Henslin, 2000). In 1960, 1 in every 20 children was born to an unmarried woman. Today that figure is six times higher, and single women now account for one of three (32%) of all U.S. births. The relationship to social class is significant also, for only 6% of births occur in single women above the poverty line, while 44% of the births occur in single women below the poverty line (U.S. Bureau of the Census, 2000).

Regardless of the causes of child poverty, it is the consequences that we must be concerned about. Poor children are more likely to die before their first birthday, go hungry, become malnourished, develop more slowly, and have more health problems. They are also more likely to drop out of school, engage in criminal activities, and have children while in their teens. All of these factors perpetuate the cycle of poverty.

It has also been demonstrated empirically that children living in poverty have a higher incidence of asthma. Poverty contributes to the etiology, exacerbation, recognition, and management of asthma. Children living in poverty suffer more asthma attacks and have a greater number of emergency room visits for asthma. It is thought that the housing conditions of the poor (dirt and dust, poor ventilation, rats and rat droppings, and cockroaches) contribute to the illness. The literature acknowledges the effect of low income and low educational and occupational levels on infant mortality, low birthweight, and birth defects (Basch, 1999).

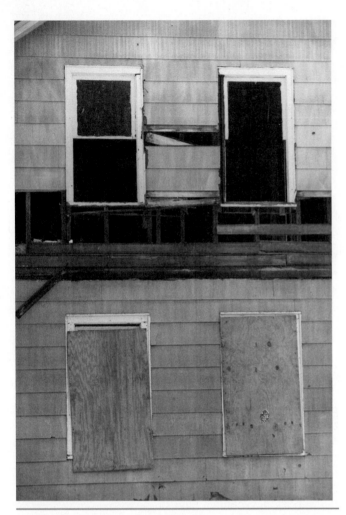

People living in poverty sometimes have only abandoned property in which to live. Copyright William C. Rieter. Used with permission.

On a global level, children born into poverty in countries less industrialized than the United States suffer horribly. Take, for example, the children in the slums of Brazil, where poverty is such a problem that children (and adults) swarm over the garbage dumps to try to find enough decaying food to stay alive. The owners of these dumps hire armed guards to keep the poor out so they can sell the garbage for pig food. Poor children scavenging in the dumps are killed routinely. Each year, the Brazilian police and death squads murder about 2000 children. Some associations of shop owners even put hit men on retainer and auction victims off to the lowest bidder. The going rate is half a month's salary—figured at the low Brazilian minimum wage. Many homeless children roam the streets. They will do anything for any price to survive. These children are part of the so-called dangerous classes who threaten the status quo. The "respectable" classes see these children as nothing but trouble; they are bad for business,

as customers feel uncomfortable or intimidated when they see a group of begging children in front of stores. With no social institutions to care for these children, one solution is to kill them (Basch, 1999; Huggins, 1993; Muraskin, 1998). As noted by sociologist Martha Huggins (1993), murder sends a clear message—especially if it is accompanied by ritual torture—gouging out the eyes, ripping open the chest, cutting off the genitals, raping the girls, and burning the victim's body.

THE FEMINIZATION OF POVERTY

Since World War II, an increasing proportion of the poor in the United States have been women. Many of these women are divorced or unmarried mothers. Approximately two out of every three persons considered poor by the federal government are women. Female householders accounted for approximately 26% of the nation's poor in 1956. By 1999, this figure had risen to almost 60% (Basch, 1999). This trend is known as the **feminization of poverty** and is evident not only in the United States but throughout the world. A major factor in the feminization of poverty has been the increase in families with women as single heads of the household (see Figure 32-4). In 1998 approximately 13% of all people in the United States lived in poverty, compared to 33% of households headed by single mothers (U.S. Bureau of Census, 2000). Sociologists trace this higher rate of poverty among women to three factors: the difficulty in finding affordable child care, sexual harassment, and sex discrimination in the labor market.

During the past 20 years, female-headed families have become an increasing proportion of the low-income population not only in the United States but also in Canada, throughout Europe, and in developing countries. This trend is also similar in the three countries with the most advanced legislation on behalf of women: Israel, Sweden, and Russia. In these countries there are national health care programs, housing subsidies, and other forms of government assistance, yet the feminization of poverty persists.

In every society in the world, gender is a basis for social stratification. Gender is seldom the sole basis for stratifying people, but gender cuts across all systems of social stratification. As discussed above, people are sorted into categories and given different access to the good things available in their society. Apparently these distinctions generally favor males. It is remarkable, for example, that in every society of the world, men's earnings are higher than women's. Of the 885 million adults in the world who are illiterate, two-thirds are women, and of the 13 million school-age children who receive no education, two-thirds are girls (Henslin 2000).

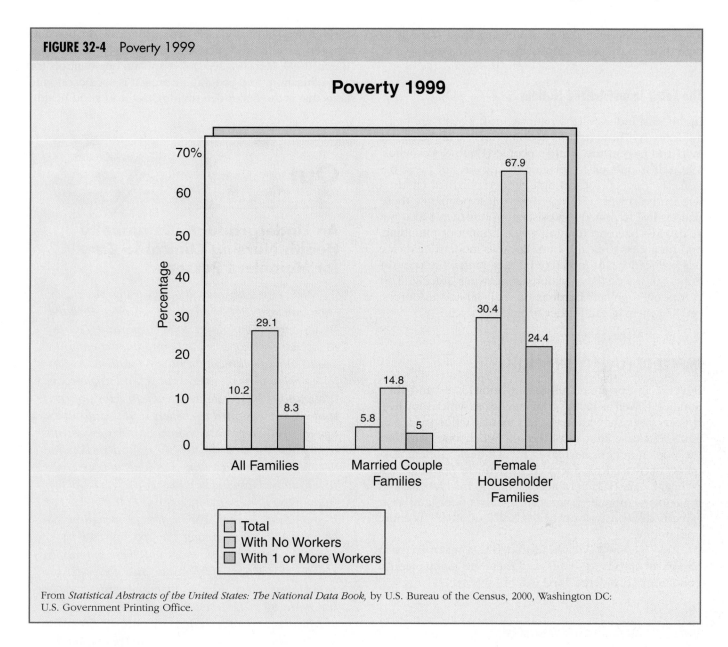

FIGURE 32-4 Poverty 1999

Poverty 1999

Percentage

All Families: Total 10.2, With No Workers 29.1, With 1 or More Workers 8.3

Married Couple Families: Total 5.8, With No Workers 14.8, With 1 or More Workers 5

Female Householder Families: Total 30.4, With No Workers 67.9, With 1 or More Workers 24.4

- ☐ Total
- ☐ With No Workers
- ☐ With 1 or More Workers

From *Statistical Abstracts of the United States: The National Data Book,* by U.S. Bureau of the Census, 2000, Washington DC: U.S. Government Printing Office.

GLOBAL POVERTY

Just as people within a nation are stratified by power, prestige, and property, so are the world's nations. Nations, generally classified as First, Second, or Third World, might better be described as "most industrialized," "industrializing," and "least industrialized" (Henslin, 2000).

The Most Industrialized Nations

The most industrialized nations are the United States, Canada, Great Britain, France, Germany, Switzerland, and the other industrialized nations of western Europe—Japan, Australia, and New Zealand. Although one sees systemic economic variations, these nations are capitalistic. Although these nations have only 16% of the world's people, they have 31% of the earth's land (Haub & Cor-

nelius, 1999). Their wealth is so enormous that even their poor live better and longer lives than do the average citizens of the least industrialized nations.

The Industrializing Nations

This group includes most of the former Soviet Union and its former satellites in eastern Europe. These nations account for 20% of the earth's land and 16% of its people (Haub & Cornelius, 1999). Most inhabitants of these nations have much lower incomes and standards of living than people who live in the most industrialized nations. Most, however, are better off than members of the least industrialized. For example, on such measures as access to electricity, indoor plumbing, automobiles, telephones, and even food, citizens of the industrializing nations rank lower than those in the most industrialized but higher than those in the least industrialized.

The Least Industrialized Nations

In the least industrialized nations, most people are peasant farmers. These nations account for 49% of the earth's land and 68% of the world's people (Haub & Cornelius, 1999). It is difficult to imagine the poverty of these nations. In Angola, for example, undernourished children live in the sewers (McNeil 1999). Most people of these nations live in poverty, subsisting on less than $1000 per year. Most have no running water, no indoor plumbing, and no access to health care. Because modern medicine has reduced infant mortality but not births, the population of most of these nations is growing quickly. This places even greater burdens on their limited resources, causing them to fall further behind each year.

IMPACT OF POVERTY ON HEALTH

Poverty has profound effects on individuals and their families as well as on the communities in which they live. Poverty coexists with many factors that influence a person's and/or community's health. When one considers the poor nutrition, decreased mental health, unemployment, decreased productivity, inadequate housing, lack of health care or lack of accessibility to health care, and high infant mortality, one can readily understand how poverty takes its toll on health and can affect an entire community.

Low income has been identified as a major factor in almost all chronic diseases, and there are many medical conditions considered "diseases of poverty."

Increased Morbidity and Mortality

In 1978, the WHO, in the Alma-Ata Declaration, spelled out the dependence of human health on social and economic development and noted that adequate living conditions are necessary for health. During the 1980s, the number of persons in the world who were living in extreme poverty increased. Currently, extreme poverty afflicts more than 20% of the world's population (Basch, 1999). A recent report from WHO states that up to 43% of children in the developing nations have stunted growth due to malnutrition. There is an annual toll of more than 12 million deaths in children under age 5 that are attributable to the effects of poverty. In the least developed countries, the average life expectancy is 43 years. In the most developed countries it is 78 years. Nurses and other professionals are committed to reducing the higher risk of illness and death due to poverty. It is known that as socioeconomic status improves, so does health. The causal factors of this correlation continue to be investigated, but

research and statistics clearly demonstrate the relationship between poverty and increased morbidity and mortality (Basch, 1999; Henslin, 2000). Even when one controls for race, education, and geographic area, it is socioeconomic status that is the major determining factor in good health.

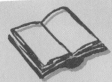

Out of the Box

An Undergraduate Community Health Nursing Clinical to Care for Homeless Persons

At the Intercollegiate College of Nursing/Washington State University State College of Nursing in Spokane, Washington, Drs. Zana Rae Higgs and Dianne Kinzel have developed an undergraduate community health nursing clinical for nursing students to care for homeless persons, the very poor, and single-room occupancy (SRO) hotel residents. In teams of two, students are assigned to shelters and social service agencies that serve these populations. Arrangements were made for students to have front-door keys for SRO hotels to permit willing residents to have visits. In addition to making home visits, each team of two students set up a miniclinic at one of the shelters or a community agency. The Bridgewalk program is a coordinated effort among the Spokane Neighborhood Action Homeless Program, the Community Health Association of Spokane, and the Veterans Homeless Project. The team makes trips weekly (or more often if needed) to sites under bridges/ overpasses and other known camps of homeless persons and nonshelter sites which are frequented by homeless persons. A nurse from the Spokane Regional Health District's Needle Exchange Program often joins the group. A team goes out in the early morning and also in the early evening. Known all over the city, they are recognized and greeted during their weekly walks. These walks are well publicized so that the poor and homeless know when to expect the nursing students, the police know they are "walking," and the people in general have come to look for them. Faculty are available by pager or cell phone and make periodic visits to the sites. This is an excellent example of the true art and essence of caring in community health nursing and client advocacy in practice (Higgs & Kinzel, 2001). ■

The poor have higher rates of infant and maternal mortality, diabetes (particularly Type 2 diabetes), cardiovascular disease, HIV, tuberculosis, and cancer. Other variables related to poverty that increase poor health include low occupational status, lack of education and educational opportunities, jobs with low control, cultural health beliefs, social isolation, poor nutrition, and poor housing. Inadequate housing contributes to poor health through lack of heat and/or electricity, inadequate refrigeration for food, and lack of security from violence and crime. Toxic waste storage facilities are more often located in poor neighborhoods than in more affluent neighborhoods.

Poverty and Health

The number of persons living in extreme poverty in the United States has been increasing over the past decade. *Almost 45% of all poor persons have incomes of less than half of the poverty line* (National Coalition for the Homeless, 2000). Persons living in poverty have higher rates of chronic illness, higher infant morbidity and mortality, shorter life expectancy, more complex health problems, and more significant complications resulting from chronic disease. Very often, these poor outcomes are the direct result of barriers to health care access. Barriers may be physical, such as no health care facility or clinic in a geographic location or lack of transportation. Barriers may also result from lack of health insurance and income inadequate to pay for health care and inconvenient clinic hours. Or, barriers may be more subtle, such as negative attitudes on the part of health care workers, language difficulties, and low self-esteem. Hospitalization rates for the poor are more than three times greater than those for the more affluent.

DIFFERENCES IN HEALTH CARE BETWEEN SOCIOECONOMIC GROUPS

Social class and income affect our chances of living and dying. The principle is simple: The lower a person's income and, therefore, social class, the more likely that individual is to die before the expected age. This principle holds true for all ages. Infants born to the poor are more likely to die before their first birthday, and a larger proportion of elders who are poor die each year than do wealthy elders. The distribution of disease and health care is also affected by income in many instances.

Coronary Artery Disease

Both race and poverty are associated with the use of diagnostic cardiac catheterization and coronary revascularization during treatment of acute myocardial infarction. The *Cooperative Cardiovascular Project* was designed to measure inconsistencies in treatment for acute myocar-

dial infarction among Medicare beneficiaries. In this study, demographic analysis demonstrated that among a population of 169,079 clients who were considered candidates for one or more of four therapeutic treatment modalities (based on current American College of Cardiology and American Heart Association guidelines), black, poor, and female patients were less likely to be offered reperfusion therapy, yet white, male, nonpoor patients were offered reperfusion (Rathore et al., 2000). Research has shown that poverty has been associated with diminished use of cardiac procedures in the treatment of acute myocardial infarction and with a lower quality of care among Medicare beneficiaries in the treatment of other conditions (Chandra, Ziegelstein, & Rogers, 1998; Broyles, McCauley, & Baird-Holmes, 1999). It has been demonstrated that poor Medicare clients hospitalized with acute myocardial infarction had worse processes of care and greater instability at discharge (Broyles et al., 1999). Studies suggest poverty is associated with less optimal medical treatment of myocardial infarction (Broyles et al., 1999; Chandra et al., 1998; Schulman, Berlin, & Harless, 1999). Decreased use of myocardial infarction therapies among poor clients is difficult to explain. While deductibles or copayments required of Medicare beneficiaries might account for variation in the use of high-cost outpatient procedures, it is unlikely that they would influence the use of low-cost medical therapies once a client is admitted. Since hospitals receive a standard Diagnosis Related Group (DRG) payment of Medicare clients with acute myocardial infarction, there should be no financial incentive to withhold therapy, specific to poor clients, once clients have been hospitalized. Adjustment for race, sex, physician specialty, geographic location, and hospital characteristics indicate that undertreatment of the poor is not attributable to confounding demographic or system factors.

In evaluating consistency in waiting time for cardiac surgery, it has been shown that poor clients wait an average of three weeks longer for surgery than those considered nonpoor (Manson-Siddle & Robinson, 1998) and that this is consistent around the world. Social call differences in mortality from coronary heart disease have widened over the past three decades. Despite being at greater risk of developing coronary heart disease and dying from it, clients in lower socioeconomic groups are less likely to be investigated once the disease develops and are less likely to be referred for cardiac surgery thereafter, even if good candidates. Mortality and morbidity rates from coronary heart disease show a **social class gradient,** with more deprived groups experiencing a greater burden of disease. In men, it has been demonstrated that the mortality from coronary heart disease is 40% higher in laborers than in white-collar workers.

Although social inequalities in coronary heart disease have been found in most countries, they vary in magnitude. The United Kingdom, for instance, has a much higher social class gradient that does Sweden, even though both have nationalized health care. The overall mortality from coronary heart disease has declined worldwide over the past three decades. This decline, however, has been greater in the most affluent groups. As a result, the social class gradient in such mortality has increased. Despite being more likely to develop coronary heart disease and die from it, clients in lower socioeconomic groups are less likely to be investigated with angiography once the disease develops and are less likely to be referred for coronary artery bypass grafting.

Type 2 Diabetes Mellitus

Research has demonstrated that adults in lower socioeconomic groups who have Type 2 diabetes mellitus have poor glycemic control and greater morbidity and mortality than their more affluent counterparts (Baumer, Hunt, & Shield, 1998; Chaturvedi, Jarrett, Shipley, & Fuller, 1998; Robinson, Lloyd, & Stevens, 1998). There have also been reports of an increased prevalence in Type 2 diabetes mellitus (but not Type 1) in areas of social deprivation (Broyles et al., 1999). Data from these studies confirm a strong correlation between social deprivation and the prevalence of Type 2 diabetes mellitus. Low socioeconomic status is known to be associated with a variety of markers of poor health, including overall all-cause mortality. Mortality in diabetes is similarly adversely affected by lower socioeconomic status, which may be related to increased rates of cardiovascular risk factors. The data, unfortunately, do not give clues as to why Type 2 diabetes mellitus should be overrepresented in social deprived areas, and further work to clarify this is needed. The studies reviewed above did not have diabetic populations with a higher percentage of elderly. Interestingly, a study from the United Kingdom showed a positive relationship between glucose intolerance and the blue-collar and working classes which was independent of age and measures of adiposity such as body mass index and waist-hip ratio (Chaturvedi et al., 1998).

HIV Infection

There is a large and increasing number of poor and homeless people with health problems related to HIV infection. HIV and AIDS are leading causes of premature mortality, and the relation between indicators of low socioeconomic status and HIV-associated mortality is of growing concern. If class differences are important in determining the outcome of HIV infections, this will become increasingly critical as the HIV/AIDS epidemic shifts toward the more socially and economically disadvantaged. Prospective studies of HIV-positive clients have concentrated on pathophysiological, clinical, and viral markers as predictors of rapid disease progression. Recently, studies have also taken into account the association between socioeconomic status and survival in HIV-positive persons. One such study (Broyles et al., 1999) occurred within a universal health care system which provided physician services, hospital stays, and HIV-related drugs at no charge to study participants. This study showed that low-income men were significantly younger at date of infection than were high-income men. The data analysis demonstrated a statistically significant association between high income and longer survival, even when controlling for age. This mortality risk was 60% higher in the low-income group than in the high income group and persisted even after adjustment for CD4 count, use of anti-retroviral therapies, *Pneumocystis carinii* pneumonia (PCP) prophylaxis, and year of infection. All subjects had standard follow-up care and management of HIV-related problems from a selected group of physicians. All physicians had substantial expertise in the treatment of HIV-related disease and practiced in conjunction with a major HIV referral center. Study subjects were covered by the Canadian universal health insurance system, which funds all physician, hospital, diagnostic, and medication costs through direct reimbursement to the provider. For more information about HIV/AIDS, see Chapter 26.

Cancer Survival

Cancer survival has been clearly linked to socioeconomic status, and thousands of cancer deaths could be avoided if all clients shared survival rates of the most affluent (Basch, 1999). It is believed by some that much of this disparity is due to differences in availability and use of screening and preventive services. The American Cancer Society (ACS) estimates that it would be possible to increase the cancer cure rate from roughly 50% to 75% just by getting people to take advantage of early detection procedures that already exist. The ACS estimates that poor clients, irrespective of race, have a 10%–15% lower five-year survival rate than middle-class and affluent Americans. Late diagnosis is believed to be responsible for at least one-half of the difference in survival among the poor (Basch, 1999).

Poverty is also associated with diminished access to health care and an increased incidence of cancer. In a study in which mammography targeted poor and underserved women in low-socioeconomic areas, differences were found between poor white and poor black women's use of this screening which could not be explained by health insurance coverage, usual source of health care, metropolitan status, or region of residence (Makuc, Breen, & Freid, 1999). For uninsured individuals, diagnosis and treatment of cancer can be a financial disaster and often inaccessible. Studies have shown that African American poor women attending urban public health clinics are not offered mammography, breast examination, or cervical cancer screening appropriately or on a regular basis (Broyles et al., 1999). Other studies show that physicians are less likely to recommend preventive services to low-socioeconomic-status clients in general (Amarasingham, Spalding, & Anderson, 2000). Even when low cost or free outpatient services are found, treatment can result in expensive inpatient care for unpredictable complications. Clients must generally purchase drugs from local pharmacies that may not be able to dispense on credit or on a billed basis. Patient assistance funds available through pharmaceutical companies are often cumbersome or require advance payment with future reimbursement. Even when some or all of the treatment is covered, clients must pay out-of-pocket expenses for transportation, child care, homemaker services, nonprescription medications, orphan drugs, and lost wages. Low-income clients can spend more than half of their income on cancer and its treatment if they are under 65 years of age, have an income of less than $20,000 per year, and are in the hospital for more than two days in a six-month period. For more information about cancer as a chronic illness, see Chapter 27.

COMMUNITY HEALTH NURSING ROLE

The community health nurse (CHN) is in an excellent position to impact the health and health care of the poor in significant ways. By being in the neighborhood, clients come to know the CHN and have the opportunity to develop trust that clients in other types of clinics and agencies do not have. When working with very poor clients, primary-, secondary-, and tertiary-prevention strategies take on new meanings.

Primary Prevention

Primary prevention encompasses actions that will prevent the initial occurrence of disease or injury. When assessing very poor clients, it is important to determine what their health priorities are rather than what you believe them to be. Often the CHN will find that food and shelter are high on the list. As has been discussed previously, the poor are at higher risks for many diseases. Primary-prevention strategies the CHN might consider would be encouraging clients to get the influenza vaccine and pneumovax at younger ages than might normally be done. Immunizations in general should be emphasized as a high priority. As discussed earlier in this chapter, children living in poverty are at higher risk for disease and for complications of disease. There are many programs that offer immunizations free or at low cost. The CHN should familiarize himself or herself with these programs in his or her geographic area, so as to be able to counsel and refer clients appropriately. Also, simple things such as teaching clients who live in cold climates to wear two pair of socks in the winter, instead of one, will help prevent frostbite, skin breakdown, and infections.

Many people remain poor because they have never learned to read. This deficit prevents the attainment of education and higher paying jobs. The CHN can help to facilitate the development of literacy programs for both children and adults. With greater reading skills, many families can improve their economic situation.

Secondary Prevention

Skin ulcerations and infections can contribute to a poor state of health, especially in clients who may suffer from poor nutrition as well. Teaching clients how to care for their skin under less than ideal conditions (such as having no running water, heat, or soap) will also help prevent minor skin conditions from becoming grossly infected or spreading to systemic infection.

Many poor women care more about where their next meal is coming from than they do about screening mammography and Pap smears. It is imperative for the CHN to educate poor clients on the importance of screening and to assist clients to prioritize their own screening needs. Screening for hypertension, for example, or for body infestations, depression, and malnutrition may be seen as more immediately useful to the very poor than are testicular self-examination and smoking cessation.

Walking through a client's home and offering assistance in improving safety are also within the purvue of the CHN, as is helping clients to find adequate and

RESEARCH FOCUS

Caring on the Ragged Edge: Nursing Persons Who Are Disenfranchised

Study Problem/Purpose

What is it like to care for people who are outside the mainstream of society? The purpose of this study was to bring to reflective awareness the unique nature of caring for disenfranchised and often outcast clients—those who have been thrust beyond the walls of community—and to learn anew the world of caring. Using concepts from theories of caring as the theoretical underpinning, the investigator affirmed the intrinsic value of all persons and identified caring as a reciprocal process of learning from one another. The investigator sought information on the lived experience of those nurses whose work it is to care for the disenfranchised.

Methods

Nursing leaders identified seven nurses who maintain compassionate and effective relationships with disenfranchised patient populations. The nurses practiced in a variety of settings, including community health, school nursing, mental health, and health promotion. Interviews were recorded by extensive handwritten fieldnotes and concurrently recorded by audiotape. The three questions that guided the interview were: (1) What is it like to care for persons for whom the mainstream often does not care? (2) Would you tell me about one or two experiences of caring for marginalized people that have special meaning for you? (3) What is the meaning of caring for the patient population you serve?

Using M. Ray's phenomenological approach to the study of the lived experience of caring, interview dialogues proceeded using a clue- and cue-taking process after the initial question (Ray, 1991). Answers were transcribed into text and analyzed for themes, meta-phors, and metaphors that capture the essence of caring on the ragged edge.

Findings

Twenty-five narratives were transcribed and encoded. The analyses revealed the oppression experienced by vulnerable populations, as seen by the nurses caring for them, and the fact that this group seldom rises up against the oppressive structures. Also revealed was the concept that this should not stop the wise nurse from understanding the nature of power structures that deprive human beings of sustenance, rights, and dignity. The author/investigator concludes by saying that, as nurses, we should challenge those oppressive structures through civic involvement on both the personal and professional levels. Major themes also included fear and silencing which kept nurses from "rising up" at all levels of organization and community.

Implications

These data suggest that nurses often are in a position to provide care to those considered outside the mainstream of society. The community health nurse is in a particularly sensitive position to observe oppressive situations under which his or her clients suffer. Poverty itself is oppressive, as are the social structures that support its existence and continuance. To those living in poverty and on the "ragged edge," the community health nurse may provide the only link to the mainstream community and be the only one to provide unconditional caring. Power is born when caring others value another and believe in human potential.

Source: Zerwekh, J. V. (2000). Caring on the ragged edge: Nursing persons who are disenfranchised. Advances in Nursing Science, 22(4), 47–61.

---

appropriate storage for medications, insulin needles, and supplies. In homes infested with insects or rodents, finding appropriate medication storage may be a challenge.

Many families need help in finding and using community resources. The nurse needs to be an advocate for families so that they become connected with appropriate agencies and services. They need to become acquainted with such services as well baby clinics, meal sites, programs that provide clothing and funds for emergencies as well as the governmental agencies that provide aid to families in need.

Tertiary Prevention

Assisting a client to use a sterile or clean technique when no running water is available can be challenging. Teaching basic rehabilitation activities for clients restricted by foot ulcers, severe peripheral vascular disease, and arthri-

Perspectives...

DOWN AND OUT IN NEW YORK CITY: A PARTICIPANT OBSERVATION STUDY

As a nurse practitioner whose practice consists mainly of the very poor and marginalized, I wanted to see what it was like to be a member of this group and be in need of health care. One always hears of all the free or low-cost clinics and programs for the poor, but I wondered what it would be like to try to access them. I wanted to know what barriers there were and whether they were obvious or subtle.

To obtain this information, I dressed as a person in extreme poverty, used my research funds to go to New York City, and for four days attempted to access the clinics described as offering services for the poor. Using a fictitious name, I presented at four separate clinics with a chief complaint of a headache that worsened over several days and included blurred vision. A condition not requiring diagnostic tools such as radiographs and blood work was chosen in order not to divert scarce resources from those who actually needed them.

I was laughed at by a receptionist in one setting (the receptionist laughed and stated to a co-worker, "she probably fell down when she was drunk and can't remember").

At the clinics for the homeless and poor, my questions about length of wait time went unanswered in three of the four settings. In three of the four settings the history and physical examination were cursory. Treatment was offered at one of three centers, consisting of one acetaminophen. Three of the centers offered no information regarding signs/symptoms to look for or reasons to return. The fourth clinic, which was actually a mobile van that moved to various locations around the city, kept the long line of waiting clients (we lined up outside in the cold) informed of how much longer the wait would be. The nurse at this facility introduced herself and offered several openings for me to discuss health problems of a sensitive nature, such as violence, abuse, and rape. This clinic also offered a list of other resources and everyone I spoke with asked me if I was "safe." I was told by the nurse that there were things she could offer me that might help if I felt I was not safe and that I could return at any time to request them.

My findings demonstrated health care for the poor is often based on the following assumptions:

- The poor and marginalized often bring on their own health problems due to their behavior.
- The poor and marginalized do not have feelings and cannot hear rude remarks.
- The poor and marginalized must wait indefinite periods of time before receiving care.
- Attempting to access health care when part of a marginalized population can be a very humiliating experience.
- In spite of the barriers, there are committed nurses and health care workers who demonstrate concern for the marginalized and consider them as fellow human beings.

This experience has significant implications for nursing. The poor and marginalized may feel "unwelcome" at clinics set up to provide care for them. They are often treated in a manner that is humiliating. Nurses working in settings that provide care for these populations should remember that each person, no matter how "disgusting" he or she appears, is someone's father, wife, or mother and deserves to be treated as such. So, next time you are tired and weary from an exceptionally long day that was filled with sick and disgruntled patients with more unmet needs than you can list and you cannot wait to get home, but you notice one more needy and dirty person in the waiting room, before you get angry and tell her to come back tomorrow, remember, it might be *me,* collecting more data.

—June Hart Romeo, PhD, RN, NP-C

tis could be a major tertiary strategy for the CHN. Often, the very poor live in places that do not have elevators, handrails, and other assistive devises. An elderly person with arthritis or another of the conditions listed previously and whose mobility is restricted by the condition will need assistance in finding alternative ways to cope with normal activities of daily living. The CHN can do a walk-through of the home and look for safety hazards as well as offer suggestions on suitable arrangements of furniture to make it easier for the client to get around.

There are many homeless programs that provide services for job skill development and other rehabilitation services to facilitate a move to permanent housing. Alcohol and other drug programs are an important resource for many people living in poverty. The nurse can help the individual and family to connect to a resource and also be a

COMMUNITY NURSING VIEW

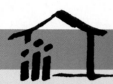

Mr. Alvaro, a 59-year-old male, presents to your community health clinic. He lives approximately 120 miles away and rides the free "vets van" provided by his local VFW association. Mr. Alvaro has a history of poorly controlled type 2 diabetes mellitus, retinopathy, peripheral neuropathies so severe that he cannot feel the floor with his feet, autonomic neuropathies that cause a chronic persistent diarrhea unamenable to medication other than codeine, and albuminuria. His IQ is in the mid-eighties. His blood glucose consistently runs in the low 200s and he has recently been started on insulin. He says he can inject it, but sometimes does not want to "stick" himself with the needle so he squirts the insulin in his hands and rubs it into his scalp. You tell him it is not absorbed through the scalp, and he replies that since you are "only a nurse," you do not know *everything,* and maybe it will be absorbed if he does it long enough.

You notice he is not wearing socks, even though it is winter. You discuss with him the need to wear socks and prevent foot injuries since he has diabetes. As he gets up to sit on the examination table, he trips and loses control of his bowels. As you assist him in getting cleaned up, you notice he is not wearing underwear either. Later on, the van driver tells you that Mr. Alvaro is so poor he lives in a trailer in a cornfield on someone's farm and has no running water, no electricity, no phone, and no heat. He lives with his daughter who had "brain fever" as a child and was never able to go to school.

Nursing Considerations

Assessment

◆ What information about Mr. Alvaro do you consider most important to you as a nurse?

◆ What additional information do you need?

◆ What are Mr. Alvaro's major problems?

◆ Which problems do you think are outside your scope of practice?

Diagnosis

◆ What are some possible nursing diagnoses?

◆ How would you prioritize Mr. Alvaro's problems?

◆ What are your greatest concerns about Mr. Alvaro's health at this time?

Outcome Identification

◆ Given your diagnoses, what outcomes would you like to see in Mr. Alvaro?

◆ Realistically, what outcomes do you think you can expect in this client?

Planning/Interventions

◆ How would you get Mr. Alvaro involved in his treatment?

◆ What would you include in your short-term plan of care?

◆ What are some realistic nursing interventions for Mr. Alvaro?

◆ In spite of the geographic distance, are there any community resources you might be able to offer him?

Evaluation

◆ How will you evaluate Mr. Alvaro's progress?

◆ Over what time period will your evaluation take place?

---

part of planning projects to develop more such resources. Most communities have too few to meet client needs.

An aspect of nursing practice important at all levels of prevention is that of caring. As nurses, some of the "services" most valued by disenfranchised clients are such things as treating them with respect, demonstrating empathy, and showing confidence. It takes courage to work with disenfranchised groups as well as high levels of skills and knowledge. This group is one of the most challenging a CHN may work with in his or her

nursing career but also one that will teach the nurse much about the art of nursing. Working with this type of population requires the ability to integrate one's work with other disciplines, to utilize community services, and to seek out new ways of meeting client needs. It is important for the CHN to develop working partnerships with other health professionals in order to best meet clients' needs. See the Research Focus for a more in-depth discussion of the value of caring in working with the disenfranchised.

KEY CONCEPTS

- ◆ Poverty is not necessarily the fault of the poor, but rather of the society.

- ◆ The number of persons living in poverty is increasing steadily, and the income gap between the poor and nonpoor is also widening.

- ◆ The poor are a very diverse group. They are individuals who are in a situation but still have feelings, problems, and needs, just like everyone else.

- ◆ The poor tend to be sicker and have less control over their health than do the nonpoor.

- ◆ Health problems of particular concern to the poor include diseases of childhood, malnutrition, cardiovascular disease, diseases of dirt (such as asthma, lice, infestations), HIV infection, tuberculosis, psychiatric disorders, and trauma.

- ◆ The poor have limited access to the health care system and lack basic resources.

- ◆ Basic nursing care can offer significant help to the poor.

- ◆ The community health nurse can be a particularly appropriate advocate for patients living in poverty and to effect change in the health care system.

RESOURCES

Center on Hunger and Poverty: nutrition.tufts.edu
Child Poverty News is From the National Center for Children in Poverty: www.cpmcnet.columbia.edu/dept/nccp
Joint Center for Poverty Research: www.jcpr.org
Poverty and Race Research Action Council (PRRAC): www.prrac.org
Poverty and Sustainable Livelihoods: www.undp.org
U.S. Bureau of the Census: www.census.gov

Chapter

33

HOMELESSNESS

Mary Beatrice Hennessey Wohn, RN, MSN

We all deserve the basics of life. Nobody should be allowed to freeze to death, to starve to death. What we need most of all is acceptance and love.

—*Herlihy-Starr*

COMPETENCIES

Upon completion of this chapter the reader should be able to:

- Discuss the history and present scope of homelessness in the United States.
- Discuss at least four factors that could increase a person's risk of becoming homeless.
- Identify two ways that private groups and two ways that public agencies have attempted to deal with the problem of homelessness.
- Describe the pioneering role that nurses have played in bringing health care to the homeless people.
- List and examine the features of homelessness that lead to poor health.
- Discuss five health problems that pose a particular threat to homeless people.
- Describe intervention strategies at each level of prevention.

KEY TERMS

compliance	noncompliance
deinstitutionalization	panhandling
guest	shelters
homelessness	soup kitchens
meal sites	

Over the past two decades, the number of homeless men, women, and children has increased dramatically, to perhaps as many as 3 million people. Economic, political and sociological factors have contributed to this increase. Private sector and public sector agencies have combined forces to seek innovative ways to deal with the problem. Homeless people tend to have more health problems than the general population and, once ill, to have difficulties managing their health problems.

Nurses have been at the forefront in bringing health care to homeless people. By employing strategies at the primary, secondary and tertiary levels of prevention, the community health nurse can continue to have a powerful impact in increasing access to care and improving the general health of homeless people.

The Pine Street Inn shelter, I don't believe it! Isn't that some flophouse for drunks? Did the school run out of hospitals to send us to? I know one thing, I'm not going there. I'll quit school first.

That was the reaction of one nursing student to her community/mental health assignment in 1979. It was typical of the reactions of students assigned to a 250-bed shelter for homeless men in downtown Boston. The students were to spend a semester at a volunteer nurses' clinic established at the shelter seven years earlier. Very little had been written about homelessness. The problem had yet to attract the attention of the media or social activists.

I've done Public Health Nursing but never in a shelter. I couldn't believe I had to go to Pine Street. The first day I had my mother-in-law on the cell phone. I was so scared. I told her to stay on the phone while I walked from my car into the building. I had to walk right by some homeless people.

That was the reaction of a nursing student in 2001 on the first day of her rotation at the Pine Street Inn, which now houses more than a thousand men and women in its various programs. Much has been written about homelessness and the problem has certainly received the attention of the media and social activists; yet misconceptions and stereotypes persist.

Homelessness is a complex and controversial issue. Discussions regarding definition, accurate census, causes and solutions often lead to heated debate.

There is no agreement on definition of **homelessness.** Some include only the people who are living on the streets and in emergency shelters. Others include people living in abandoned buildings, in camping areas, and in single-room occupancy (SRO) hotels. Still others include people believed to be on the verge of homelessness because they have doubled up with families or friends in overcrowded apartments.

Different methods of counting homeless people yield vastly different results. The two most common methods are point-in-time counts and period-prevalence counts. Point-in-time counts attempt to count all of the people who are literally homeless on a given day or during a given week. This method yields numbers between 500,000 and 750,000 people (Wright, Rubin, & Devine, 1998). Period-prevalence counts look at the number of people who have experienced homelessness over a given period of time. This method has yielded numbers as high as 12 million people (National Coalition for the Homeless [NCH], 1999b).

The lack of an agreed upon definition, as well as the difficulties in counting an often transient population and differences in methodology, has led to widely varying estimates of the numbers of homeless people. Despite the disagreement on the actual number, however, all sources seem to agree that the number is too high and is rising.

The debate becomes even more heated when the causes of homelessness are discussed. Wright et al. (1998) view poverty and the lack of affordable housing as precursors, setting the stage for the most vulnerable citizens to become homeless. Baum and Burnes (1993) think this stance homogenizes a disparate population, confuses poverty with disabling conditions, and leads to the inaccurate conclusion that a single solution is sufficient to solve the problem.

Other causes often cited and debated include employment issues, increased cost of living, inadequate minimum wage, lack of access to adequate health insurance and health care, decreased public assistance, domestic violence, mental illness, alcoholism, and drug addiction. Dail (2000) points out that most of these causes are directly related to poverty.

It is not the purpose of this chapter to solve or even take sides in these debates. The interested student can find many compelling arguments for conflicting viewpoints in the literature. The main focus of this chapter is on the health care needs of homeless populations and the role of the community health nurse in meeting those needs. The chapter begins with a brief review of the history of homelessness, discusses its impact on individuals, families, and communities, and describes private and public responses to the problem.

HISTORICAL DEVELOPMENT OF HOMELESSNESS

In the 1950s and 1960s, the idea of large numbers of people in the United States with no permanent address, huddled in doorways, living in shantytowns or squatter settlements, begging on the streets, and searching garbage for sustenance was unthinkable. These were things that people did in developing countries, in famine- and drought-ravaged Africa, in overcrowded India, in poverty-stricken South America. Such problems, it was believed, could not exist in affluent, industrialized societies.

However, there have been homeless people in the United States throughout its history. The numbers have fluctuated in response to economic and political events. Interestingly, early efforts to deal with the problem were aimed, mainly, at providing institutional care for the mentally ill (Jones, 1983). In the first half of the 20th century, the Great Depression and the world wars added numbers to the homeless ranks.

In 1963 the Mental Retardation and Community Mental Health Center Construction Act was passed. This led to large-scale **deinstitutionalization** of patients in state mental hospitals (Torrey, 1998). Supervised living arrangements and follow-up treatment were to be arranged within the community for the discharged patients released. Because community-based resources were never adequate to meet their needs, many of the deinstitutionalized people found themselves with no place to go. Concurrently, the decriminalization of alcoholism and public drunkenness left on the streets many chronic alcoholics who might have previously spent the night in jail cells.

The 1970s trend toward urban renewal led to displacement of many poor families and a sharp decline in available SRO dwellings. During the 1970s and 1980s it is estimated that approximately 1 million SRO units were lost. Gentrification throughout the 1980s and 1990s resulted in a further decrease in housing for the most impoverished. Older inner city housing units were bought up by the affluent and renovated into posh, expensive living quarters (Wright et al., 1998). A dramatic rise in unemployment to 9.7% in 1982, coupled with a decrease in unemployment benefits, increased the number of families living below the poverty line (Burt, 1992). Other major factors such as increased rents and decreased federal funds to build and/or rehabilitate low-income housing further reduced the housing supply and placed decent, affordable housing out of the reach of many (Kozol, 1988).

Recent Developments and Scope of the Problem

During the 1980s, the problem of homelessness burst upon the public awareness. For example, the subject heading "Homeless Persons" is not found in the *Cumulated Index Medicus* until 1986, but in that year alone there are 39 citations under that title. As both advocates and government agencies reported an increase in numbers, the visibility of homelessness also increased.

Harrington (1962), in his classic work *The Other America: Poverty in the United States,* spoke of "the invisible poor." He described the poor as being segregated from the rest of the populace, in both urban neighborhoods and rural settings. He warned that urban renewal would force poor people into slums and that poverty, lack of education, and lack of medical care would force people from their rural homes into the cities, where they would become misfits. He expressed concern that the poor's lack of visibility kept them out of public awareness and therefore off the public agenda.

By contrast, some of today's homeless people make themselves quite visible in urban settings. They can be seen **panhandling,** or begging on city streets. Some wear signs saying such things as "Help the homeless" or "I am a father of two. I work for food." They might approach cars at stoplights, wipe the windshield, and ask for a handout. The visible homeless, although a small sample, often shape the public perception of the whole population.

Careful studies of the homeless population have always revealed diversity. The stereotypes, which reflect only the most visible, have never presented a true picture of the population and have often interfered with efforts to help. The generic term *homeless* implies that the individuals in this group have more in common than they actually do. This perception is especially so today, as families with young children, the majority headed by women, constitute 36% of the overall number, and evidence indicates that this number is increasing. The U.S. Conference of Mayors (2000) reports a 17% increase in requests for shelter by homeless families with 74% of the surveyed cities reporting an increase. Wright et al. (1998)

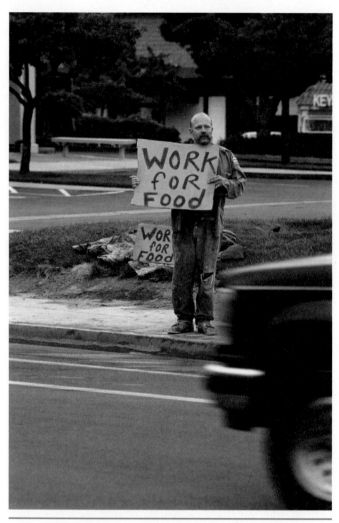

The visible homeless shape the public perception of the homeless; however, the homeless population includes diverse types of people and circumstances.
Courtesy of Photodisc.

point out that, although homelessness is not new, there has been a dramatic change in the population. Many of today's homeless people are young and relatively well educated; they are dominated by racial and ethnic minorities and include large numbers of homeless women, children, and families.

In a 25-city survey, the U.S. Conference of Mayors (2000) reported that single men accounted for 44% of the homeless population; families with children 36%; single women 13%; and unaccompanied youth 7%. Also, 50% of the homeless population was reported to be black, 35% white, 12% Hispanic, 2% Native Americans, and 1% Asians (Figure 33-1). Ringwalt, Green, Robertson, and McPheeters (1998) found that 5% of youth aged 12–17 were homeless for at least one night of the past year.

According to the NCH (1999f), veterans are overrepresented in the homeless population. It reports that 40% of homeless men are veterans as compared to 34% in the general population. It describes the homeless veterans more likely to be white, better educated, and previously or currently married than are homeless nonveterans. In addition, 1.6% of homeless veterans are female. In 2000, the U.S. Conference of Mayors, in its survey of 25 cities, found 15% of the urban homeless population to be veterans. (U.S. Conference of Mayors, 2000).

Etiology

The origins of the current homelessness situation are complex. Economic, social, personal, and political influences all contribute to this growing crisis.

Economic Influences

Throughout the years, persons who study homelessness and those who work with homeless people have linked

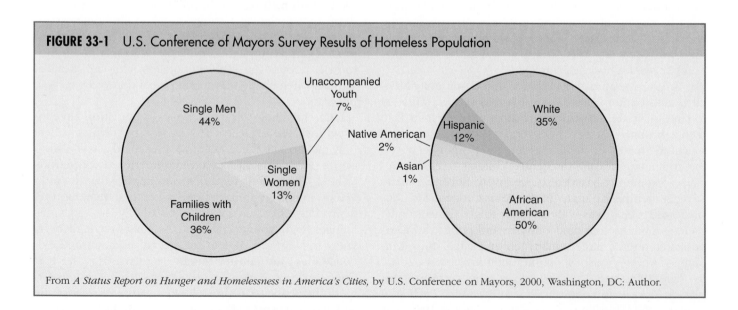

FIGURE 33-1 U.S. Conference of Mayors Survey Results of Homeless Population

From *A Status Report on Hunger and Homelessness in America's Cities,* by U.S. Conference on Mayors, 2000, Washington, DC: Author.

the problem with the economy. Today, despite a healthy economy, many U.S. citizens are unable to afford housing. Nearly 1% of the U.S. population, 2.3 million individuals, are likely to experience a spell of homelessness at least once during a year. Housing costs are on the rise while extreme poverty and other vulnerabilities are a fact of life for millions of people. (Millions still face homelessness in a booming economy, 2000.) Lack of affordable housing is the main factor identified by the U.S. Conference of Mayors (2000). Other factors identified are low-paying jobs, substance abuse, and mental illness, coupled with the lack of needed services, domestic violence, and changes and cuts in public assistance.

The NCH cites two trends as largely responsible for the increase in homelessness: the lack of affordable rental housing and the growing increase in poverty (NCH, 1999). Although latest U.S. Bureau of the Census statistics (2000) show an across-the-board decline in poverty levels, children and female-headed households continue to be overrepresented. Bassuk, Weinreb, Buckner, Browne, Salomon, and Bassuk (1996) report that in 1993 nearly 36% of all families headed by women were living under the federally established poverty level. This was even higher for black and Latino female-headed families, with rates of 49.9% and 52.6%, respectively. Children make up 26% of the total population and 38% of the poor. In 1993 the top 20% of U.S. households received 48.9% of the aggregate income while the bottom 20% received only 3.6%. Despite the strong economic growth in the United States, the disparity continued to grow. In the late 1990s the average income of U.S. families in the top 20% was more than 10 times that of families in the lower 20%. During the last two decades, the income for the top 20% grew in all but three states with an average growth exceeding $34,000, while the income for the poorest 5% actually declined in 18 states (see Figure 33-2). Changes were attributed to globalization, the decline of manufacturing jobs, and the expansion of low-wage service jobs, immigration, the lower real value of the minimum wage, and fewer and weaker unions ("State income inequality," 2000; "From welfare to worsefare," 2000).

The Personal Responsibility and Work Act passed by Congress in August of 1996 replaced the federal welfare system by shifting the responsibility for administration to the states (Katz, 1996). States are awarded block grants and, with some federal guidelines, decide who receives benefits. The act limits recipients to five years of eligibility and requires that they find work within two years. These changes have brought about a dramatic drop in welfare caseloads. Early findings, however, show that despite the fact that many former welfare recipients have jobs, their income is often less than it was before the reforms were enacted. Most of the new jobs pay well below the poverty line. The number of those receiving food stamps went down 33% while the requests for food from **soup kitchens** (a place where food is offered either free

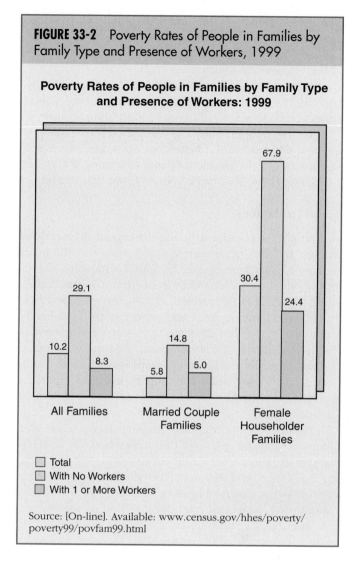

FIGURE 33-2   Poverty Rates of People in Families by Family Type and Presence of Workers, 1999

Poverty Rates of People in Families by Family Type and Presence of Workers: 1999

Source: [On-line]. Available: www.census.gov/hhes/poverty/poverty99/povfam99.html

or at greatly reduced price to those in need) and food banks increased 18% ("From welfare to worsefare," 2000; U.S. Conference of Mayors, 2000). Many lose health insurance despite continued eligibility. In 1997, 675,000 people, including 400,000 children, lost health insurance as a result of welfare reform (NCH, 1999d).

Also affected by economic changes are many elderly men and women who, despite what had appeared to be adequate planning, find themselves on a fixed income that is insufficient to meet even their most basic needs for food and shelter. Some manage to stay in their homes, stretching their meager pension money by using soup kitchens and elderly meal sites. Others end up in shelters. These forms of support are discussed in detail later in this chapter.

Many people now in the shelter system are eligible for some sort of economic relief from sources such as Temporary Assistance to Needy Families (TANF), Social Security, the Veterans' Administration, Workers' Compensation. Often they are unaware of their eligibility status.

Even when they have the knowledge, the nature of their disability or the powerlessness inherent in being homeless, or both, may make it difficult, if not impossible, to obtain services on their own.

Some observers believe that the economics of homelessness has been overplayed and that a focus on economics leads to a new, but equally inaccurate, stereotype of homeless people. They express concern that this perspective will lead to the belief that housing alone is sufficient to solve the problem (Baum & Burnes, 1993). For a full discussion of issues of poverty, see Chapter 32.

Social Influences

The family as a social unit has undergone tremendous change and has become less stable (Bassuk, Rubin, & Lauriat, 1986). Changes date back to the Industrial Revolution, which brought a shift from rural to urban living. Often a nuclear family moved, leaving the extended family behind, changing roles and expectations of all family members. In the last 25 years, the role of women has changed dramatically; women are now able to make choices regarding education, employment, and childbearing. It is now quite common to have both parents working, and children are often left in the care of outside agencies.

Attitudes regarding sex and marriage have also changed, and the marriage union has become less stable. There is more sexual freedom outside of marriage for both men and women, and divorce is no longer viewed as the catastrophe it once was. This is not necessarily true, however, for poor families, as the disruption of family ties and the experience of divorce can be quite catastrophic. One result is an increase in single-parent homeless families. McMurray (1990) states that most studies fail to recognize the impact of family dissolution on homelessness. The loss of extended family and community support has had an especially strong impact on single mothers. Studies have demonstrated that homeless mothers experienced significantly more stressors than their domiciled counterparts (Gorzka, 1999; Wagner & Menke, 1991). Low wages, lack of affordable housing, inadequate child support and child care options, inadequate health care, and the threat of violence all add to the problems of the homeless mother (Polakow, 1998). It is estimated that more than half of families become homeless because the mother is fleeing domestic violence.

Personal Influences

Individual circumstances and personal characteristics place some people at a higher risk of becoming homeless. Most notable among these are the presence of physical and/or mental disability and addiction to drugs or alcohol. These factors will be examined more closely in the section on health issues of homeless people. Other factors include poverty, family violence, the availability of personal supports, educational level, and marketable skills.

Political Influences

Examples of how political policy can affect the numbers of homeless people and their access to health care can be seen at all levels of government. The allocation of funds and the rules and restrictions regarding their use determine who will be helped and how. Initially, much of the aid at all levels was aimed at emergency intervention without attention to the complex and diverse needs of the population or to their need for permanent housing.

At the local level, examples can be seen in zoning legislation. These laws often prohibit transitional housing or remove the incentives for developing low-cost residential housing.

An example at the state level can be seen in the laws regarding the care of the mentally ill, which have resulted in many psychotic individuals being left on the streets to fend for themselves. Another example at the state level is the enactment of the Welfare Reform Bill. As previously discussed under economic influences, the individual states now have broader rights in determining who will receive benefits.

REFLECTIVE THINKING

Homelessness

Imagine that this happened to you.

You are a new graduate nurse who, having difficulty finding a full-time job, found a part-time job on a medical-surgical unit of a local hospital. This is your first nursing job and it pays well but has no fringe benefits. A few weeks ago you moved into a very nice apartment. While moving some boxes into your new apartment, you severely injured your back. It will be well over a year before you will be able to work again. You have no health insurance.

- Will you be able to continue to afford the rather high rent on your apartment? Do you have savings or other assets to support you for a while? Do you have family or friends who will support you? For how long?
- Who is going to pay your extensive medical bills?
- What benefits might be available to you?

Numerous examples of public policy that may have exacerbated homelessness have been cited at the federal level. Kozol (1988) asserts that during the early 1980s "the White House cut virtually all federal funds to build or rehabilitate low-income housing. Federal support for low-income housing dropped from $28 billion to $9 billion between 1981 and 1986" (p. 13). Redburn and Buss (1986) suggest that the reduction of federal social welfare spending, together with stricter eligibility requirements for benefits during the Reagan years, is another explanation for the rise of homelessness. Another example at the federal level can be seen in income tax laws that provide loopholes for the rich while putting a heavier tax burden on those with less money. There has been a decline in public assistance in recent years. The Personal Responsibility and Work Opportunity Reconciliation Act of 1996 replaced the Aid to Families with Dependent Children (AFDC) program with a block grant program called Temporary Assistance to Needy Families (TANF). TANF benefits and food stamps combined are below the poverty level and in every state the median TANF benefit for a family of three is approximately one-third of the poverty level (NCH, 1999d).

IMPACT OF HOMELESSNESS

Homelessness has profound effects on the individual, the family, and the community. Community health nurses need to understand these effects before they can devise meaningful interventions.

Impact on the Individual

Being homeless is devastating to the individual. A sense of powerlessness and low self-esteem are reinforced time and again throughout the day. Misunderstood, feared, ridiculed, avoided and stereotyped, the homeless suffer

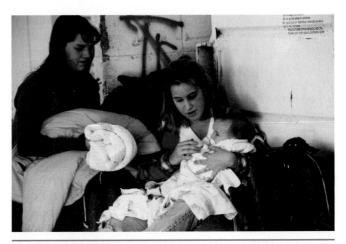

The faces of homelessness. Courtesy of Photodisc.

a continual barrage of assaults to their sense of self. The feeling of worthlessness that low self-esteem generates can block motivation to find employment, housing, and other essential needs (DiBlasio & Belcher, 1993). Sleeping in a different place every night, often with no choice as to where or with whom, leads to disorientation and dissociation. The longer the person is on the street, the more difficult it is to become domiciled again. The individual is trapped in a vicious circle. A person needs income in order to afford a place to live, but the lack of a fixed address limits employment opportunities and, in many cases, excludes the person from benefits.

In *Travels with Lisbeth,* Eighner (1993) describes three years of living on the streets, traveling between Texas and California with his dog Lisbeth. He describes his experiences of searching through dumpsters and finding places to sleep as well as his interactions with dogcatchers, police, and doctors. His firsthand stories are vivid and articulate. Despite his often humorous accounts, he describes most days on the streets as consisting of unrelenting boredom. Lack of direction and the absence of progress, he states, make time nearly meaningless.

Impact on the Family

Homeless families are relatively new in the modern era of homelessness. In *Rachel and Her Children,* Kozol (1988) vividly portrays the plight of the homeless family, documenting the effects of living in welfare hotels, constantly moving, losing neighborhood connections, frequently changing schools, and so on. At the National Symposium on Homelessness, Rosenheck, Bassuk, and Salomon (1999) discuss the effect of homelessness on the family. The average family consists of a single mother in her late twenties with two young children and an income significantly below the federal poverty level. Most have lost their housing because of lack of money or are fleeing a violent situation. Studies of homeless mothers have

DECISION MAKING

Factors of Homelessness

List the factors that have led to the increasing numbers of homeless people in the United States over the past twenty-five years.

◆ Take any one of the identified factors and discuss, in retrospect, how community health nurses might have intervened to lessen the impact of this particular factor.

◆ What actions can community health nurses take at the present time to lessen the impact of this particular factor?

demonstrated an extremely high rate of domestic violence. In one study as many as 92% had experienced severe sexual and/or physical abuse. They have generally moved three to five times prior to becoming homeless, often living in substandard housing or doubling up with relatives or friends. They arrive at a shelter feeling frightened, depressed, and out of control. While it provides them refuge from the street, the shelter can bring on added stress. Overcrowded conditions and parenting in public can further rob the mother of a sense of autonomy or personal control. Some shelters require that the mother relinquish responsibility for setting rules for their own children and follow shelter-imposed rules and curfews. The parent-child relationship can suffer under these conditions. Homeless mothers experience depression at twice the level of the general population, and in one study (Bassuk et al., 1996) nearly one-third had attempted suicide before age 18.

Polikow (1998), using vivid examples from her own caseload, portrays the lives and daily experiences of school-aged children, whom she refers to as "discards of the post-modern 1990s." Most often living with a single mother and one or two siblings, homeless children are subject to frequent changes in school, sometimes as many as four or five in a single school year. They are often viewed as an extra unwelcome burden by teachers and are taunted and victimized by classmates. They are called names such as "shelter rat" or "garbage picker." Under such conditions, it is hard to make friends and next to impossible to do school studies.

An area yet to be studied is the impact on the family when one of its members becomes homeless. Parents, spouses, and children of homeless people have often tried in vain to seek help for a homeless family member. There is a stigma attached to alcoholism, addiction, and psychiatric problems. When homelessness is added to one of these conditions, it is very difficult for family members to seek and receive support.

Homeless Elders

Although elders now make up a smaller percentage of the homeless population, the actual number of homeless individuals aged 50 and over has increased. Because of the tight housing market and the aging of the baby boomers, it is expected that their numbers will continue to rise. For many homeless elders the shelters are a formidable place, often crowded with young intoxicated individuals. Studies have demonstrated that the elderly are more prone to victimization and are also more apt to be ignored by the police. Many feel particularly vulnerable in the shelters and prefer to sleep on the street. Their lives are often further complicated by chronic illness, difficulty in ambulating, psychiatric illness, cognitive disorders, decreased hearing, diminished eyesight, and poor dentition (NCH, 1999g).

Impact on the Community

Homelessness is a community problem. Communities suffer when so many of the members are suffering. Unfortunately many members of the community refuse to recognize and take responsibility for the problem. This disregard for homeless people and their problems can be seen in the language people use, often referring to the homeless as "those people." It can be seen in the so-called NIMBY (Not In My Back Yard) syndrome. "I think its wonderful that somebody wants to help 'them' but there are children in this neighborhood. Put 'those people' somewhere else."

HEALTH PROBLEMS COMMON IN HOMELESS POPULATIONS

Homeless people are subject to the same illnesses and medical conditions found in the general population. However, as with all economically depressed groups, they tend to be sicker and to have more health management difficulties. Small problems left untreated tend to become major.

Following are examples of health problems commonly encountered in homeless populations. Prior to the discussion of each health problem, a vignette presents a real-life example. Although mainly discussed as discrete entities, several of these conditions more often occur concurrently. Where applicable, the health problems will be discussed in relation to the national health objectives identified by *Healthy People 2010* (USDHHS, 2000).

Nutritional Deficiencies

The outreach van stopped in the alleyway. It was late in the shift, and supplies had dwindled. Two men got up from where they were huddled at a heating grate; two others joined them from a nearby doorway. Together they timidly approached the van. "Whatcha got to eat?" asked one. Looking over the diminished supplies and seeing only instant soup and peanut butter and jelly sandwiches, the worker answered, "I'm afraid we're down to the daily special, soup du jour, and peanut butter sandwiches prepared with essence of grape jelly." The man grinned and replied, "Say, that special wouldn't come with coffee, would it?"

Nutritional deficiencies underlie many of the health problems found in homeless populations. In *Healthy People 2010* (USDHHS, 2000), concern is expressed regarding the nutritional status of homeless people and limited available data. Silliman, Yamanoha, and Morrissey (1998), citing several studies, conclude that homeless people are at nutritional risk. Their study, conducted in

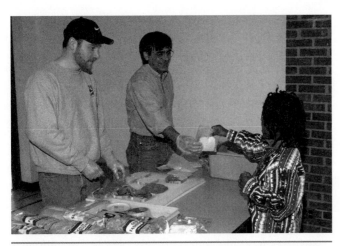

Attempts to provide a well-balanced diet do not necessarily meet the special needs of a significant number of poor homeless people.

northern California, found that homeless people living in rural areas were even more at risk for malnutrition than their urban counterparts. Because homeless people depend on handouts, it is extremely difficult, even for those so inclined, to obtain a well-balanced diet. Poor nutrition leads to apathy and decreased energy, further compounding the problem. Alcoholism and the use of street drugs or prescription drugs can lead to vitamin deficiencies, which in turn decrease healing ability and temperature control (Strasser, Damrosch & Gaines, 1991).

Even when attempts are made to provide a well-balanced diet, the special needs of a significant number of homeless people are not met. The elderly, individuals with poor dentition, growing children, and those on therapeutic diets are particularly affected. McMurray-Avila (1998) cites malnutrition, exposure to the elements, violence, lack of facilities to maintain personal hygiene, fatigue, and increased exposure to communicable diseases as factors leading to significantly higher rates of ill health in homeless persons as compared to those with stable housing. These factors are even more pronounced in the unsheltered homeless population.

Peripheral Vascular Disease

The clinic nurse was surprised when she saw Henry's foot. She had been treating him off and on for years, and his foot looked better than usual. The edema and hyperpigmentation were still present, but the ulcer over his ankle looked smaller with no sign of infection. He told her that he had just been discharged from a three-month stay in a veterans' hospital. Later in the day she happened to see him sitting on a park bench, shoes and socks wet and muddy, with his three heavy bags next to him.

Homeless people are frequently afflicted by leg ulcers, peripheral vascular disease, and cellulitis which could lead to limb-threatening and life-threatening infections (O'Connell, 1999). The lifestyles of homeless people tend to compound the problem. They rarely have a place to sit down with their feet elevated during the day. Venous return is hampered when they spend a great deal of time on their feet or sitting on park benches with their feet down. Some homeless people sleep in an upright position. They are exposed to all extremes of weather.

Homeless people often have no change of socks and wear ill-fitting shoes, increasing the chance that their skin will break down. This situation frequently leads to infections, as their surroundings are often unsanitary and they lack the facilities to maintain hygiene. Poor nutrition hampers their healing abilities. Even feet that are not compromised by peripheral vascular disease break down and become macerated when a person wears the same damp socks for days.

Chronic Conditions

Dolores had been admitted to the hospital several times for the treatment of metastatic cancer and had received both chemotherapy and radiation. The hospital stays seemed to do her good. Upon leaving she would appear rested and better nourished, only to return two to four weeks later, cachectic, exhausted and, twice, with pneumonia. She explained that she was a single parent of four girls, ages 2 to 10. Her sister-in-law would care for the children while she was in the hospital but felt that this was Dolores's responsibility once she was discharged. Concerned that Dolores did not keep an arranged appointment, the nurse decided to make a home visit. The address in the chart turned out to be that of the sister-in-law. From there the nurse was directed to an abandoned, unheated building where Dolores and her four children illegally occupied an apartment. The apartment was furnished only with mattresses on the floor. In the bathtub, there were signs of a fire, which Dolores said she lit to keep warm on really cold nights.

Dolores and her children would not be included in a census of the homeless. Indeed, she did not consider herself homeless. Her story illustrates the need to be thorough in assessment and the importance of considering homelessness in after-care planning.

Comparing data from homeless clients with national statistics, homeless people suffer from most chronic physical disorders at an elevated rate (McMurray, Gelberg & Breakey, 1999; Wright, 1990). This statement is supported by the NCH (1999), who note that homeless people have extremely high rates of both chronic and acute health problems. Chronic medical conditions commonly encountered include diabetes, heart disease, respiratory disorders, seizure disorders, hypertension and malignancies. See Chapter 27 for more information on chronic illness. The control of these conditions, difficult under the best of circumstances, presents a major challenge to homeless people. Since there is no place to store medications, they are often lost or stolen. There is no safe place for diabetics to keep insulin, syringes and needles. Concern about where to spend the night takes precedence over keeping medical appointments. The stress of having no fixed address exacerbates many chronic conditions. Living in crowded, often smoke-filled shelters, having no place to rest or to wash, and lacking a balanced diet all compound the problem. The loneliness and humiliation of being homeless, the lack of self-esteem, and the lack of a supportive person who cares often rob the homeless individual of the motivation to maintain health.

HIV/AIDS Infections

Margaret had been diagnosed with AIDS and wanted to find a place to live other than the shelter. She was asked what she found most difficult about living in the shelter with an HIV infection. She answered, "I guess I should say that I catch every little bug that comes through, or that I get real tired during the day and there's no place to lie down, or that it's real hard to stay sober here, but you know, I really think the hardest part is not having a private bathroom when I get diarrhea real bad."

Recent reports in the literature (Song, 1999; Smereck & Hockman, 1998; St. Lawrence & Brasfield, 1995) support the observations of shelter workers that there is a large and increasing number of homeless people with problems related to the human immunodeficiency virus (HIV). Song (1999) reports that of the 400,000–600,000 individuals estimated to be living with AIDS, approximately one-third to one-half are either homeless or at imminent risk to become so. In a study of risk factors for death conducted in Boston (Lebow, Bierer, O'Connell, Orav, & Brennan, 1998), the strongest predictor of death was a diagnosis of AIDS. Also significantly increasing the risk of mortality was HIV infection, both symptomatic and asymptomatic. Significant differences were found in a retrospective study in which homeless individuals with HIV were compared with housed persons (Lebow et al., 1995). The homeless group were more apt to be African American or Latino, more likely to have intravenous drug use as a risk factor, and at greater risk of opportunistic infection.

Many persons with HIV infections find themselves with no place to go except a shelter. AIDS and AIDS-related illnesses present major management difficulties in this setting. Sharing dormitory and living space, often with hundreds of others, puts a person with a compro-

mised immune system at high risk for tuberculosis and other communicable diseases. Spending the day with companions who are actively using alcohol and other drugs increases the likelihood that the HIV-infected person will do likewise. When intoxicated, a person is highly likely to share needles and engage in unsafe sexual practices. *Healthy People 2010* (USDHHS, 2000) addresses the need to enhance prevention strategies for populations at particular high risk such as injection drug users, homeless persons, runaway youth, mentally ill persons, and incarcerated persons. Encouraging safer injecting practices, promoting safer sexual behavior, and increasing knowledge of HIV status are prevention measures mentioned.

Nurses working with homeless people can intervene by assisting clients to find help for their addiction problems, encouraging the provision of HIV counseling and testing in shelter clinics, offering information regarding safe sexual practices and providing condoms, educating clients regarding the dangers of sharing needles and other paraphernalia (works), providing bleach and teaching how to disinfect the works, and providing information regarding needle exchange programs.

The prevalence of HIV infection and the existence of risk factors have been examined in detail in certain subgroups. Several authors have examined runaway youth and other adolescents living on the streets (DeMatteo et al., 1999; Walters, 1999; Whitbeck & Hoyt, 1999; MacDonald, Fisher, Wells, Doherty, & Bowie, 1994). Often dire circumstances in the home precede life in the streets. These circumstances include extreme poverty, violence, drug and alcohol abuse, rejection, physical abuse, and sexual abuse. The stress of being on the streets, lack of self-esteem, immaturity, exploitation, and sexual abuse put the youth at high risk for HIV infection. There is a high incidence of risky behavior, including intravenous drug abuse, sharing needles, prostitution, anal intercourse, unprotected sex, and sex with multiple partners. Walters (1999) reported that for some homeless youth testing HIV positive was perceived as advantageous in procuring basic needs such as food and shelter.

Another identified group at high risk for HIV infection is homeless women. A study by Fisher, Hovell, Hofstetter, and Hough (1995) found long-term homeless women to be at particularly high risk for battery, rape, mental distress and lack of a supportive network. Domestic violence is cited as a major cause of homelessness for women. Once a woman becomes homeless, factors associated with survival on the streets increase the risk for HIV infections. A woman might trade sex for money or team up with a male protector, often an IV drug abuser. Fear for safety, the use of drugs, and perceived dependency upon the male increase the difficulties in negotiating for safer sex. *Healthy People 2010* (USDHHS, 2000) addresses the difficulties experienced by women, particularly young females having intercourse with older males. Intimidation and threats of mistrust by their partners make it very difficult to discuss condom use. Programs aimed at developing effective negotiating skills are identified as a critical element of increased condom use.

The results of these and other studies point out the need for community health nurses to develop population-specific education and intervention strategies. For more information on HIV/AIDS see Chapter 26.

Other Infectious Diseases

Bob is a chronic alcoholic who lives on the streets. He hasn't been feeling very well lately. He has lost weight, and he often wakes up coughing at night. He finds it hard to get back to sleep because, for some reason, he has been perspiring a lot and his clothes have been soaking wet. He did have a Mantoux test for TB but was on a bender when he was due back to have it read. That was three weeks ago.

In 1989 the Centers for Disease Control and Prevention (CDC) announced the goal of eliminating tuberculosis (TB) from the United States by the year 2010 (CDC, 1994). From 1953 through 1984 the number of reported cases of TB in the United States declined by an average of almost 5% per year (CDC, 1992). From 1985 through 1993 the number of new cases increased by 14%, with a high of 10.5 per 100,000 population in 1992. The increase was attributed to at least four factors: the association of TB with the HIV epidemic; immigration from countries where TB is common; the transmission of TB in congregate settings (such as shelters for homeless people); and a deterioration of the health care infrastructure (CDC, 1994). Further complicating the problem was the concurrent increase in the incidence of multidrug-resistant TB, most commonly found among patients infected with HIV (CDC, 1993). There has been a steady decline in tuberculosis cases since 1993 with a rate of 5.8 per 100,000 population reported in 2000 (CDC, 2001). An objective of *Healthy People 2010* (USDHHS, 2000) is to reduce the incidence of tuberculosis to 1.0 per 100,000. See Chapter 27 for more information about TB.

The control and management of infectious diseases among homeless people present a major challenge. Crowded living conditions, poor nutrition, substance abuse, stress and chronic medical problems put them at high risk. Influenza and tuberculosis can spread quickly in a shelter setting. Case finding is difficult in a population that is often transient and distrustful of the health care system. Routine surveillance for tuberculosis using a Mantoux test requires that the person return to have the test read. When positive sputum is found, it might be difficult to locate a person who has no fixed address. By the time the client is located, he may have stayed at several different shelters, exposing an unknown number of people to the illness.

Case management of tuberculosis infection presents another series of challenges. It is hard to take medications for six months to a year, especially since the medications have side effects and can interfere with drinking. Clients are more apt to reveal contacts to a person whom they trust. They are also more apt to follow through on treatment when it is explained by a nurse who is a trusted friend, rather than by an impersonal member of the health establishment.

An objective of *Healthy People 2010* (USDHHS, 2000) is "to increase to at least 90% the proportion of people found to have tuberculosis infection who completed courses of preventive therapy." This would be an increase from 74% reported in 1996. Taking medications might not be a high priority to homeless people, especially when they are not feeling sick. McGinnis (1995) reports that preventive therapy for TB can be successfully delivered to a mobile, homeless population using a case management model together with an incentive program. She has found the most success using cash as an incentive, paying clients for each week of directly observed therapy. When the incentive is coupled with sensitive nursing care that respects the client's right to make decisions, the likelihood of completing the course of therapy is greatly increased.

Thermatoregulatory Disorders

Bill was telling the story from his hospital bed. "Me'n Jimmy were out, you know. We'd had a few pops and were real glad we'd managed to get ahold of a bottle of port. It was real cold I guess, but the port warmed us up good. We had one of them army blankets and we went over to the grate at the library. It didn't seem all that cold really, except for the wind. I managed to get to sleep pretty quick. Next thing I know, some security guard's waking me up and there's red flashing lights and stuff. I tried to get up but it was like my legs weren't there. I found out later that Jimmy bought it. I guess I'm lucky just to have frostbite."

Hypothermia is not only a problem of extreme cold. It can occur in temperatures as high as 59°F–64°F, especially if the person is not sheltered or is inadequately dressed. Wind and water immersion magnify the effect. The CDC (2000b) identifies risk factors for death by hypothermia as older age, lack of adequate housing, homelessness, mental impairment, drug overdosage, and alcohol impairment with contributing factors of malnutrition, lack of fitness, severe illness, and drug use and/or abuse. It puts mortality estimates at 75%–90% for those with hypothermia and underlying disease as compared to less than 10% for those with hypothermia alone.

Homeless people have little protection from the weather and often are victims of hypothermia and frostbite. They are apt to be wet from the rain, over- or under-dressed, and unprotected from the wind. Alcohol, commonly used to fend off the cold, does just the opposite. Although it gives a subjective feeling of warmth, it produces peripheral vasodilation, resulting in more rapid heat loss. Alcohol and drugs dull the perception of cold. The presence of dampness or wind hastens the development of hypothermia.

A homeless person wearing or carrying a heavy coat on a warm spring day might be viewed as "crazy" by a passerby. With no place to store the coat, the person has little choice but to carry or wear it. That same coat might be a lifesaver during the night when the wind picks up and the temperature drops into the forties. Burns suffered from fires, started in an effort to keep warm, are a secondary problem related to the cold weather. Dangers during the warm weather are heat exhaustion, heat stroke, and dehydration.

Infestations

The student nurse was taking care of Joe, a long-term guest at the shelter. Diagnosed as a paranoid schizophrenic, Joe referred to himself as "a State Kid." This reference dated back to his early days in a state hospital for mentally ill children. Indeed, Joe had never lived independently, moving directly from a state hospital into the shelter. As she took his blood pressure, the student noticed something move on his head. Looking more closely, she noticed a small grayish white bug moving through his hair. The skin around the base of his neck was reddened, and there were dandruff-like nits clinging to the shafts of his hair. Suspecting that Joe had lice, but never having seen them before, the student asked her instructor for confirmation. Hearing the question, Joe became quite upset, stating emphatically that "lice do not grow on cultured hair."

Lice and scabies have been around since antiquity, are distributed worldwide, and continue to this day. There are about 300 million cases of scabies in the world each year and hundreds of millions of cases of pediculosis worldwide (Chosidow, 2000). Most especially affected are school children, nursing home residents, homeless populations, hospital personnel, and individuals who are immunocompromised.

Crowded living conditions, sleeping close together for warmth and comfort, infrequent laundering of clothing, sharing clothing and bedding, poor hygiene, embarrassment about seeking help, and difficulty locating and treating contacts all contribute to a high incidence of lice and scabies in the homeless population. Infestations present a major management problem and often go untreated and unnoticed until secondary infections are apparent. Louse-borne infectious diseases are on the rise. Lice carry the organism *Bartonella quintana,* the cause of trench fever, first recognized during World War I. Infestations can result in endocarditis and bacteremia (Chosidow, 2000; O'Connell, 1999). Chosidow (2000) cautions about the unrestrained use of over-the-counter products to treat infestations. With no safeguards to prevent indiscriminate use, there is greater risk that resistance may develop.

Alcoholism and Other Substance Abuse

The shelter nurse treated Danny's foot, noting some new signs of infection at the amputation site where he had lost three toes to frostbite. Seeing his bloated face and puffy eyes, she thought, how pathetic he looks. She had first met him 25 years earlier. He had been a handsome, young man. Drinking heavily and depressed, he had slit his wrists and was admitted to the psychiatric unit where she worked. Before discharge he was told that he was an alcoholic and that there was little that the professionals could do for him until he "reached bottom" and found some motivation. It was up to him. Looking at him now, it is hard to believe that he is only 45. He appears to be in his sixties. Clearly, he has reached bottom. Now the professionals are busy treating young men in their twenties, while they can be helped, before they lose everything.

Danny's story is typical of many of the middle-aged alcoholics dependent on the shelter system. The treatment of alcoholism has changed dramatically over the past 25 years. Previously it was thought that the individual had to lose everything in order to be engaged in treatment. Now it is believed that the sooner treatment is begun, the better the prognosis. The instillation of hope is considered the cornerstone of successful treatment of alcoholism. Danny and others like him have been given a consistent message of hopelessness.

The middle-aged and older alcoholic men have been joined by a younger group of alcoholic and polydrug abusers. Because they are homeless, alienated from their families, do not have cars, and work mainly at day labor, they are deprived of the traditional means of accessing care. Due to their impoverished state, they are also more likely to share needles, putting them at a high risk of exposure to AIDS.

The extent of alcoholism and substance abuse in the homeless populations reported in the literature varies greatly, depending on research methods and locus of study. There is no generally accepted number with respect to prevalence (NCH, 1999c). Examination of several studies reveals that about a half of the homeless people studied have at some time in their lives had a diagnosable substance abuse disorder. A history of alcohol abuse occurred in almost half of homeless single adults and a history of drug abuse in approximately one-third (McMurray-Avila, Gelberg, & Breakey, 1999).

The combination of poverty and substance abuse put individuals at particular risk of homelessness. This risk is even more so for the dually diagnosed or those with concurrent physical disorders. In the past many urban alcoholic men lived in the SRO units which were lost to gentrification, condominium conversion, and abandonment in the 1970s and 1980s. In 1996 President Clinton signed into law (P.L. 104-126) legislation that denied Supplemental Security Income (SSI) and Social Security Disability (SSD) to individuals whose addictions were considered to be contributing factors to their disability status. For many individuals this loss meant the difference between being housed and being homeless. Because of the link between SSI and Medicaid in most states, the loss of SSI also meant the loss of health coverage. The impact of these changes was studied by examining the impact on individuals served nationwide by Health Care for the Homeless (HCH). Of a total of 3648 homeless people interviewed, 193 (5.6%) had lost their SSI or SSD benefits in the 12 months prior to the survey. Fifty-two percent of this group reported that the loss was related to the new law. Three-quarters of the individuals who had been paying for their own housing prior to losing benefits lost their housing. Of the 193 individuals, 51 were enrolled in treatment programs at the time that benefits ended and 15 (29.4%) of them were required to leave their program (SSI and SSD Benefits termination, 1999).

Two of the objectives of *Healthy People 2010* (US-DHHS, 2000) address reducing the treatment gap for illicit drug use and for alcohol problems. Homeless people face numerous barriers to treatment and recovery. They include lack of insurance, long waiting lists for addiction treatment, lack of a fixed address to obtain notification of acceptance into a program, lack of transportation, and lack of documentation. In February 2001 *Health Care for the Homeless Mobilizer* (2001) announced that after several years of advocacy the National Health Care for the Homeless Council and the National Coalition for the Homeless secured from Congress a $10 million appropriation for a new targeted homeless addiction services program. Hopefully programs will be developed to reduce the treatment gap for homeless individuals. For more information about substance abuse, see Chapter 31.

Mental Illness

Rita is an intelligent, articulate woman. She functioned quite well in a responsible position until an automobile accident left her disfigured and her sister dead. Now years after the accident, she resides at the shelter. Her disfigured appearance, her biting sarcasm, and her aloof manner present a formidable picture. She has never had a psychiatric hospitaliza-

tion and refuses suggestions that she seek outpatient counseling. She was evaluated by psychiatry during an inpatient stay for kidney stones and was given the diagnosis of chronic paranoid schizophrenia.

Lately she has had problems with nocturnal incontinence. She describes this as a terrible laundry problem. "I don't know what they are doing with the laundry" she says, "but every morning when I wake up, the sheets are wet from my hips to my knees." The staff noticed that her clothes were stained during a recent bout of diarrhea. When they

Perspectives...

INSIGHTS OF A HOMELESS PERSON

Helen was in the shelter for eight months before finding suitable housing. She is now taking classes at a local college and plans to pursue a career in nursing. In discussing her experience, she talked about how angry labels and stereotypes make her. "Like when I was in the shelter I often wondered if I was losing my mind. I saw friends who had been pretty normal begin to act real bizarre . . . but I could understand it. It made sense. Like one woman who didn't like staying at the shelter because her old man would know where to find her. She'd stay outside. I had to stay outside a few times and its hard to sleep. If you stay in a public place where it's safe, the police are apt to tell you to move, but you really can't sleep anyplace. Things get stolen or you could get beaten or raped so you're always sleeping with one eye open. I mean they talk about people getting psychotic from spending time in intensive care units, but they're not labeled crazy for the rest of their lives. Even if you stay in the shelter, it's usually a different bed every night and different people (who knows what they're going to do?) next to you. And then the way you dress, like it's mainly donated clothing that might not fit or the colors don't go together and you have to carry your stuff because there's no place to store it. I can remember looking in the mirror one time and thinking, Oh my god, am I a bag lady? Am I really crazy?

It took me a while after I got my own place to get my confidence and self-esteem back. A lot of the women in the shelter aren't crazy. They're incredibly strong. I'd like to see some of the people who label them "crazy" live with the stressors that they live with."

—Anonymous

approached her, she looked at them sternly and stated, "I don't understand why some people find it necessary to deposit their excrement at my anus."

There appears to be a general consensus that approximately one-third of the adult homeless population suffer from a major psychiatric disorder, including schizophrenia and affective disorders (McMurray-Avila et al., 1999). Most studies report a larger percentage of homeless women than men suffering from psychiatric illnesses. Approximately 20%–25% of the single, adult homeless population suffer from severe and persistent mental illness (Koegal, Burnham, & Baumohl, 1996). This is significantly higher than in the general population.

Advocates who witnessed the increasing numbers of homeless mentally ill during the 1970s and early 1980s, and who struggle now to find adequate care for severely mentally ill clients, point to changes in the mental health system as a major cause of the problem. They believe that many of the present shelter guests would previously have occupied state psychiatric hospital beds. Now, deinstitutionalized, or never institutionalized, they are left to fend for themselves on the streets. The adverse effects of stress on health in general and mental health in particular are addressed in *Healthy People 2010* (USDHHS, 2000). A goal is to decrease the proportion of homeless adults aged 18 and over who have serious mental illness to 19% from a baseline of 25% in 1996.

There is discussion in the literature as to whether mental illness is a cause or an effect of homelessness. Client insights mirror this dichotomy (see Perspectives). The NCH (1999a) does not believe that deinstitutionalization caused the increase in the numbers of homeless people but it does state that premature and unplanned discharges brought about by managed-care arrangements may be contributing to the continued presence of seriously mentally ill in the population. Although there is a disproportionate number of mentally ill people in the homeless population, they represent only 5% of the nation's mentally ill. Mentally ill individuals are homeless for the same reasons as other homeless people—poverty, inadequate housing, minimal supports and inadequate health care.

Regardless of whether mental illness is the cause or effect of homelessness, the mentally ill are a particularly vulnerable group. Frightened, paranoid, withdrawn, and haunted by voices, they struggle to protect their fragile egos. They tend to be distrustful of the formal service system. Often not street-smart, they are ridiculed and victimized by others. Many mental health professionals prefer not to work with the chronically mentally ill. Homeless chronic patients present even more challenges. They tend to be transient and are inconsistent in keeping appointments. Many do not take prescribed medications. Some express the feeling that taking medication causes them to decrease vigilance and thus become more vulnerable. The work can be painstaking and slow, and the rewards are difficult to measure. Efforts to help must include measures that address the homeless-

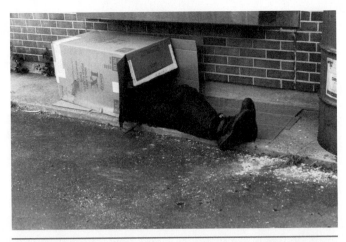

Without shelter, homeless people often find unique and creative ways of protecting themselves from the elements, possibly putting them at even greater risk from predators.

ness. McMurray-Avila et al. (1999) stress the importance of patients having access to a full range of services, including diagnosis and treatment planning, medication management, hospitalization, counseling and supportive therapy, rehabilitation and social skills training, income support, housing, and case management. Chinman, Rosenheck, and Lam (2000) demonstrated the value of relationship in the case management of homeless clients. In a study of 2798 clients, those who reported a high alliance with their case managers had significantly fewer days of homelessness. Another group of homeless mentally ill are those suffering from organic brain syndrome. Due to disorientation and memory impairment, they often have difficulty negotiating the shelter system. They are often also prey to violence.

Trauma

Jerry, an elderly man, limped into the shelter. He was covered with blood. He pleaded with shelter staff to go help his friend Scotty. "He's hurt awful bad," he said. "I can't wake him up." Both men were returning to the shelter and had taken a short cut through an empty lot. They were approached by seven boys, roughly 12 to 14 years old. "Get out of here," the boys said. "We might want to play baseball here tomorrow and we don't want you messing the place up." The boys then proceeded to trip, kick, stone, and beat the men with baseball bats. Scotty had a fractured skull and a broken hip. Jerry had a fractured wrist, several broken ribs and facial lacerations.

Homeless people are particularly vulnerable to injury, accident, and assault. Life on the streets is dangerous and trauma is a frequent occurrence. Elderly men and women are prey to young thugs, who beat them for their possessions or because of some warped sense of entitlement. As reported in the section on HIV, domestic violence is a major cause of homelessness for women, and long-term homeless women are at particular high risk for battery and rape (Fisher et al., 1995). Seizures, falls when intoxicated, fights, and burns account for more incidents of trauma.

Often, treatment of trauma is delayed. A homeless person who is lying on the street due to trauma is often seen as drunk and is ignored. There is a reluctance on the part of many street people to go to the hospital for x-rays or stitches when they believe that they will be kept waiting for a long time. Negative experiences at the hospital in the past keep many people from seeking prompt treatment.

In 1998, only five states had emergency medical services and trauma systems linking prehospital, hospital, and rehabilitation services in order to prevent trauma deaths and long-term disability. An objective of *Healthy People 2010* (USDHHS, 2000) is to increase those services to 50 states. Reducing the delay in receiving services and coordinating the services received could go a long way toward reducing death and disability in homeless populations.

Buhrich, Hodder, and Teesson (2000) report an almost universal experience of trauma among homeless men and women in Sydney, Australia. In their study all women and over 90% of the men reported at least one event of trauma in their life. Fifty-eight percent suffered serious physical assault and 55% witnessed someone being badly injured or killed. Half of the women and 10% of the men reported being raped.

Childhood Illnesses

The 8-year-old girl was lying on a bench outside of a shelter with her head in her sister's lap. She had just vomited and complained that her stomach hurt. She wanted nothing to do with the student nurse who had come from the nurses' clinic at the mother's request. "Why won't you let the nurse see you?" the mother asked. "I don't want to," the girl answered. "I don't feel good and I want to go home." "Yes," replied the mother, "but where's that?" "I don't know," answered the girl, "all I know is that I want to go there."

Homelessness has a severe effect on the physical health and mental well-being of children. When compared with their house counterparts, homeless children experience poorer health, more depression, anxiety and behavioral problems, more developmental delays, and poorer academic achievement. Many families leaving welfare as a result of reform also lose health insurance, despite continued Medicaid eligibility. One study showed that 400,000 children lost health insurance in 1997 as a result of welfare reform (NCH, 1999).

In New York City 38% of the children in the city's shelters have asthma. This is four times the rate of other children in the city and six times the rate nationwide. In addition, 27% of the homeless children were diagnosed

---

DECISION MAKING

Assessment of School Children

You are a school nurse in an elementary school. A teacher tells you that she has a student who comes to school every day without a lunch. She is usually dirty and wears ill-fitting shoes. She seems listless and appears severely underweight. She usually has not done her homework. Her attendance is poor. The teacher wants you to talk to the child and find out what is wrong.

◆ From the description of this child, what signs might suggest that this child is homeless?

◆ What would be your first step in addressing the teacher's concerns.

◆ What interventions would you suggest?

---

with otitis media, as compared with 18% nationally. Recurrent otitis media can lead to hearing loss, speech language delay, and decreased attention span. Past studies have attributed developmental delays in homeless children to the stress of homelessness and maternal depression. Unmet health care needs might also be contributing factors (Redlener & Johnson, 1999).

There are inadequate resources to meet the needs of homeless children. According to *Healthy People 2000* (USDHHS, 1990) 40% of battered women and children were turned away from emergency shelter in 1987 owing to lack of space. The goal was to reduce that to less than 10% by the year 2000; however, according to *Healthy People 2010* (USDHHS, 2000), there has been no reported movement in this direction.

With the frequent moves to which homeless families are subjected and the constant stress under which the parents operate, it is not surprising that preventive health measures take a low priority and that health care is crisis oriented and episodic. For example, seventy-seven percent of all New York two year olds have received their proper immunizations as opposed to only 39% of homeless two to three year olds (Redlener & Johnson, 1999).

INTERNATIONAL PERSPECTIVES

Other industrialized countries have also reported an increase in homelessness. Across the European Union some 3 million people are homeless while another 15 million live in substandard or overcrowded dwellings. The European Observatory on Homelessness, an agency of the European Federation of National Organizations Working with the Homeless (FEANTSA), has conducted research to assess the problem of homelessness across its 15 member states. Homelessness appears to be growing in most of the states and reasons given parallel those in the United States. More people are living as single adults, marriages are less stable, and life expectancy has been extended, putting increased demands on the stock of available housing. A growing number of people are living in poverty. Social welfare benefits have been limited and there is a decline in public housing. Particularly vulnerable groups are identified as youth, those with mental illness and/or addiction problems, women, and single mothers with children (Parmentier, 1998). Sleegers (2000) compared homelessness in Amsterdam with that in New York City. There are more people homeless in Amsterdam today than 15 years ago. However, as the Netherlands is a welfare state and more than half of the housing is public, the increase there is not due to lack of housing. It was attributed to a growing number of people who were no longer able to function independently, most notably, the mentally ill, who would have been hospitalized 20 years ago, and older long-term heroin abusers.

In Finland, during the past decade, great strides were made toward a national goal of eliminating homelessness. The number of homeless people was halved from 20,000 in the mid-1980s to 10,000 in 1998. A strong political commitment was backed up with the necessary financial resources. Affordable housing was made available and

needed support provided to vulnerable individuals. In the capital city of Helsinki, where half of the nation's homeless people live, they were able to reduce shelter beds from 2000 to 900. In 1995 the Finnish Constitution was amended to include the right to a home. Priorities, however, have now shifted, and the National Housing Board and the National Board of Welfare have been abolished. Advocates are concerned that the hard-won achievements will be undone if new resources are not found (Finland, 1998).

In 1986 there were virtually no people living on the streets in Japan. In 1996, according to government statistics, there are 3300 homeless people in Tokyo. Social workers say the number is closer to 10,000. The economic recession and the decay of the family as a unit are cited as precipitants (Kakuchi, 1996).

The fastest growing segment of the homeless population in Canada is street youth, aged 12–25. It is estimated that there are over 50,000 youth living on the streets in Canada. The most commonly cited reason for leaving home was negative family environment. Ayerst (1999) found Canada's street youth to have higher rates of stress and depression than their housed counterparts and more apt to engage in acts of self-harm and to use drugs and alcohol. See Research Focus.

RESEARCH FOCUS

Depression and Stress in Street Youth

Study Problem/Purpose

This study explored the depression levels and coping methods of 27 youths living on the streets in Canada. Results were compared with a control group of an equal number of nonrunaway peers. The study was conducted to increase understanding of the effects of homelessness on youth in order to guide professionals to develop more effective interventions.

Methods

A questionnaire consisting of six sections (demographics, depression, self-esteem, coping methods, family background, and stress) was administered to random samples of street youths and housed high school students. Depression, self-esteem, and life stress were evaluated using standardized scales. Evaluation of the other factors is discussed.

Findings

The street youths had a significantly higher mean level of depression with the most commonly cited reasons:

money, shelter, food, family stress, and separation from friends. Street youths had a significantly higher current stress level than the nonrunaway group and reported even higher stress when living at home. The street youths generally employed less positive coping mechanisms and were more apt to engage in drug and alcohol use and self-harm. The author cautions regarding the interpretation of coping mechanisms because some of those considered maladaptive might actually serve an adaptive purpose for a child living on the street.

Implications

The article points out the necessity to evaluate homeless youths for depression, levels of stress, and danger of self-harm. Care must be taken to explore the youths' total situation when examining coping mechanisms. By first understanding the purpose of the coping mechanism, the youths might be helped to develop less harmful techniques.

Source: Ayerst, S. L. (1999). Depression and stress in street youth. Adolescence, 34 (135), 567–575.

RESPONSES TO THE PROBLEM

Both public and private organizations and agencies are developing programs to help homeless people. The community health nurse needs to be aware of both types of programs and how they can be used individually and collectively to meet the needs of the homeless population.

Responses from the Private Sector

Until the 1960s, much of the help that homeless people received was carried out by volunteer civic and church groups who founded shelters and soup kitchens. Some were small independent efforts; others, such as the Salvation Army, had a national network (Bogue, 1963).

Shelters

Shelters vary greatly from one to another. They range from those that supply only a place to get in out of the weather to those that deliver a wide range of services, including meals, individual counseling, advocacy, health services, day programs, employment training, and rehabilitative facilities. Some shelter providers believe that the provision of a wide range of services legitimizes shelters

as an acceptable alternative care system for the homeless and that this type of shelter takes the pressure off other agencies to recognize and work with homeless people. Others think that unless the shelters provide the services, homeless people will go without.

Shelters also vary in terms of who is eligible to receive their services. Some may screen by age, sex, diagnosis, or behavior. Some of this screening is clearly spelled out in written policy, and some is done by more subtle means. Shelter **guests** themselves often have a good feel for who is and who is not welcome at the various shelters. Rules and requirements also vary, making some shelters more or less acceptable to individual guests.

Some shelters are specialized, set up to deal with specific problems. One example is shelters for battered women, where women seeking refuge from an abusive situation can find protection and support for themselves and their children.

Soup Kitchens and Outreach Vans

Food services to homeless people are also provided in a variety of ways, and many are specialized to meet the needs of certain groups. Soup kitchens are places where food is offered either free or at a greatly reduced price. These services often provide emotional as well as physical nourishment. Soup kitchens and outreach vans try to meet the needs of homeless people where they live or where they congregate. Soup and a sandwich are generally served by a person who knows and cares about the individual being served. **Meal sites** might cater to a specific population, such as the elderly or women, by offering meals at greatly reduced prices. Being allowed to help with the preparation and serving the meals family style often help a homeless person to feel that this is more than just a handout.

Day Programs

Some sites combine luncheon services with a wide range of social, recreational, and health services. Many shelters close their doors during the daytime. Day programs fill the gap and provide much needed services for many.

Responses from the Public Sector

As the homeless population increased in the 1980s, it became apparent to the private sector groups that their efforts were no longer sufficient to meet the growing demand for services. Much of the early lobbying for increased public awareness and government response was the result of the work done by grass-roots organizers.

In the mid 1980s, the Robert Wood Johnson Foundation, in partnership with the Pew Charitable Trusts, provided seed money to 19 major cities to help deal with homelessness. The program was cosponsored by the U.S. Conference of Mayors. The purposes of the grants were

---

REFLECTIVE THINKING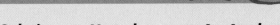

Solutions to Homelessness: An Analogy

A woman with a severe circulatory disorder developed a blister on her left foot; without treatment, the blister became an ulcer. The ulcer frightened her so much that she ignored it, hoping it would just go away. When it didn't, she put a Band-Aid on it. Seeing no improvement, she became increasingly angry and upset. She continued to add Band-Aids until osteomyelitis developed. Her pain was so severe that by the time it became necessary, she readily agreed to amputation.

- Can you see an analogy between this story and society's manner of dealing with homelessness?
- Can you identify "Band-Aid solutions" that have been used to deal with community problems in your neighborhood?
- What strategies might be helpful to move beyond the "Band-Aid solutions?"

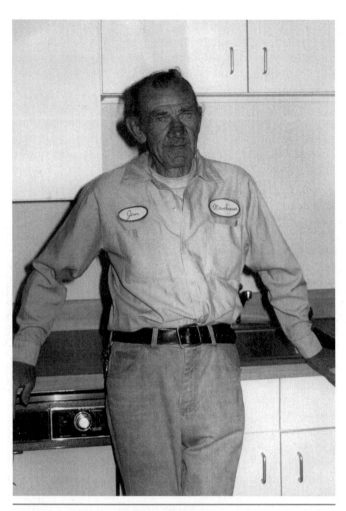

An 86-year-old man who has lived for many years in a shelter for homeless people proudly stands in the kitchen he keeps clean at a meal site for the elderly.
Courtesy of gentleman pictured.

to develop programs to meet the basic health care needs of homeless people, to improve their access to care and benefits, and to encourage citywide involvement and response. The money was earmarked to be spent in direct care to homeless people with the expectation that services would continue, supported by public funding, when private grant monies ran out. In the first four years of this program, primary care, assessment, and referral services were provided to more than 200,000 homeless persons, and all funded cities found the resources to continue after foundation funding had ended (Somers, et al., 1990).

Local Programs

Many local municipalities have now become active in providing shelter services for their homeless citizens. Both state and local funds are being used to support them. It is becoming increasingly common to have health clinics at these sites.

State Programs

Response to the crisis at the state level has varied considerably from state to state and over time. This response can be witnessed in the enactment of the welfare reform legislation which gives the states, with some federal guidelines, broad authority to decide how these funds will be spent. The legislation includes both rewards and penalties to encourage states to place people in jobs, giving the states an incentive to inflate their success in order to qualify for federal bonuses (Zuckerman, 2000a). The result has been a large decrease in the number of families dependent on welfare and an increase in work and/or dependence on others. In fact, by June 1999, the number of people on welfare fell 49% from their high of 5 million families in 1994 (Council of State Governments, 2000). This fact, for many, gave credence to the anecdotal stories in the media regarding "welfare queens" and others who cheated the system. There is a need to be cautious, however, in evaluating the success of welfare solely on the evidence of decreasing numbers.

Zuckerman (2000b) points out that decisions regarding welfare reform had little to do with research, although statistics were used. Studies on the effects of the law are showing that many of the mothers who have left welfare are doing poorly and the number of children living at less than half of the poverty level has increased. She questions whether this new research will be used to influence welfare policies in the future. She also expresses concern that policy changes will now be even more difficult to enact and evaluate because decisions are being made in 50 different states rather than by the federal government.

The National Campaign for Jobs and Income Support is a newly formed coalition of grass-roots organizations in 40 states that have united to advance progressive antipoverty policies at state and national levels. It addresses the issue of welfare reform and the need to evaluate its effectiveness by a reduction in poverty rather than by a reduction in caseloads. It expresses concern that since states are allowed to keep the money they do not spend on poor families, there is a strong incentive to discourage people from accessing assistance. It released a report showing that states were accumulating unspent TANF money, money it believes should be put into programs to help the needy. It names states which have diverted funds meant for needy families to cover other fiscal priorities. It would like Congress to establish greater accountability and performance measures as a condition of TANF grants when the law comes up for reauthorization in 2002 (*Poverty amidst plenty,* 2001).

Because there is a variation from state to state and over time, it is important for nurses to familiarize themselves with the laws and social policies of their particular state and how these affect both the numbers of homeless people and their access to services.

Federal Programs

The federal government has responded to the homeless crisis through a number of agencies. The Federal Emergency Management Agency provided funding for increased shelter and meals. The Department of Defense made certain military facilities available to the homeless, paid for the necessary renovation, and donated blankets and cots to shelters. The Department of Agriculture is responsible for the Women, Infants and Children (WIC) program. This program provides shelter and nutritional assistance to families in need.

The Stewart B. McKinney Homeless Assistance Act was passed in 1987 to provide assistance to homeless people with handicaps. This law, which focuses on vulnerable populations, was designed to organize, coordinate, and enhance federal support to homeless individuals. Among other things, it has provided grant money aimed at developing and supporting a required set of mental health services for mentally ill persons who are homeless or at risk to become so (Mauch & Mulkern, 1992). In 1994 the Department of Housing and Urban Development (HUD) changed the process by which McKinney Homeless Assistance funds were awarded, requiring that applicants demonstrate a plan of continuing care and include input from community stakeholders. The change was made to encourage system integration and to provide a comprehensive view that addresses clients needs from emergency shelter through transitional programs to permanent housing (Dennis, Cocozza, & Steadman, 1999). Shelter Plus Care, another HUD program, provides housing subsidies linked to treatment and case management. The Center for Mental Health Services (Substance Abuse and Mental Health Services Administration) funded the Projects for Assistance in Transition from Homelessness (PATH) Program, which has been successful in moving some patients from homelessness to supportive housing.

NURSING CARE OF HOMELESS PEOPLE

In *Healthy People 2010: National Health Promotion and Disease Prevention Objectives* (USDHHS, 2000), a number of major health problems have been identified and objectives set which call for interventions at the primary, secondary, and tertiary levels of prevention. The focus is not only on personal health but also on targeted populations considered at risk. An emphasis is put on improving access to appropriate preventive care and addresses concern that "major changes in the structure of the U.S. health care system, including the increasing influence of market forces, changes in payment and delivery systems, and welfare reform, have significant implications for vulnerable and at-risk populations" (USDHHS, 2000, Chapter 1).

Nurses have been at the forefront in recognizing the difficulties that homeless people experience in obtaining health care and in developing innovative ways to improve their access to care. Lenehan, McInnis, O'Donnell, & Hennessey (1985) describe the experiences of a group of nurses who, in 1972, brought nursing care to the Pine Street Inn, a large shelter for homeless men in downtown Boston. As emergency room nurses, they had treated guests from the nearby shelter. Often the men arrived intoxicated, disheveled, and unruly. They came to the emergency room for routine care. They returned a few nights later in worse shape, with dirty, unchanged bandages and unfilled prescriptions. It would have been easy to dismiss them as noncompliant and uncaring.

Instead, the nurses embarked on a 30-day experiment to meet the men on their own turf. They brought some supplies and used an office in the shelter. Timidly at first, and at times defensively, the men entered the nurses' clinic. They found that this group of health care professionals was different. They did not present themselves as all-knowing. In fact, in this setting, the nurses were more nervous and less sure of themselves than the men. They were willing to listen and learn from the men. There was communication and caring that had not been felt in the hustle-bustle of the emergency room. The men felt accepted and cared for, even when they did not keep appointments or follow advice. Clinic schedules were arranged for the convenience of the clients rather than the other way around. An attitude of acceptance and consultation helped the client to feel like a partner with the nurse rather than a passive recipient of health care and advice. The nurses' "experimental clinic" continues to this day and has become a national model for health care for the homeless. In the summer of 1995, the Pine Street Inn Clinics, which now number four, were highlighted in *Reflections,* a publication of Sigma Theta Tau, Int., the International Nursing Honor Society. Using basic nursing skills, clinic nurses handled more than 132,000 visits in 1994 (Goldsmith, 1995). They were licensed by the Massachusetts Department of Public Health as a freestanding nurses' clinic in 1996. Several such clinics have since been described in the literature.

There are many advantages to having a nurses' clinic in a shelter for the homeless. With daily contact, the nurse becomes a trusted ally and is able to practice in a preventive role before a crisis develops. Being familiar with a client's baseline health status, the nurse recognizes health threats in the early stages and has concrete data to assist the client in understanding and accepting any need for further intervention. A nurse-managed clinic is cost effective, stresses prevention, and reduces the use of emergency rooms for nonemergency situations. Being in the shelter also allows the nurse to observe trends, recognize environmental hazards, and serve as a role model to other shelter staff.

Nurses practicing in a shelter often experience firsthand the barriers that homeless people encounter in their attempts to obtain health care. For many homeless people health care is not a priority. Making sure of a bed for the night, getting food, finishing a bottle, getting a fix, or working in day labor might all take precedence. Many deny there is a problem despite clear evidence to the contrary. Some avoid seeking help in hospital and social service institutions for fear of the authorities they might encounter, such as officials from the Immigration and Naturalization Services, police, and child protection agencies. Others are embarrassed by their homeless state, their poor hygiene, and the fact that they have delayed seeking help. Often this is fueled by negative experiences with care providers in the past when they felt labeled or demeaned because of their homeless status, their diagnosis, or their ethnic or cultural origin. For many inability to speak English presents a major barrier. Lack of insurance and inability to pay for services is an obstacle to others. This is often complicated by lack of identification papers for those who have had their IDs misplaced or stolen or those who are undocumented aliens.

Even when they do seek help, displacement from their neighborhood of origin and frequent moves lead to fragmentation of care and diminish the chance of forming a relationship with an on-going care provider. They find themselves again and again answering the same painful questions, some embarrassing and difficult to talk about, as they watch warily, steeling themselves for signs of judgment. They are often poor self-advocates, unable to articulate their situation, and only the presenting problem is attended to with no attention to the underlying causes.

Follow-up presents another series of challenges. They might not understand follow-up instructions or after-care plans due to limited fluency in English or inability to read English. Even when the follow-up plan is understood, it might be impossible to follow while living on the street or in a shelter. Therapeutic diets are not available. Money is often not available to purchase needed medicines or equipment, nor is transportation to the hospital for diagnostic testing and follow-up appointments. The lack of a fixed address or phone number where the individual can be reached makes it impossible to receive reminders of appointments or notification of changes. When they do not return for appointments, they are labeled "uncooperative" or "noncompliant," further alienating them from supportive care.

Fergusen and Ragosta (1998) discuss another type of barrier which occurs when care is episodic and uncoordinated. Using a case example, they discuss the risk of mortality in a group of particularly vulnerable homeless individuals who die despite numerous hospital visits, diagnostic procedures, and excellent care at several agencies. This group has a shared collection of traits that they propose be labeled the HARM (Homeless at Risk of Mortality) syndrome. The traits are chronic organic brain syndrome related to long-term substance abuse, out-of-control social behavior, multiple injuries, prior documented concern regarding mental status and/or competency, inability to recognize dangerous situations, gradual loss of

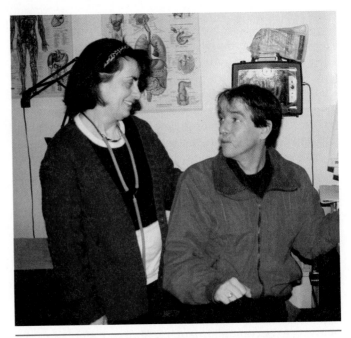

The caring relationship is apparent in this interchange between a nurse and a client in a nurses' clinic located in a shelter for homeless people.
Courtesy of Pat O'Conner.

social supports, and massive treatment resistance. They propose and describe a proactive, multidisciplinary, integrated approach to identifying persons at risk and ensuring quality rehabilitative services.

Nurses working in the shelter serve as teachers to other health care providers regarding the needs of homeless people. As advocates and teachers, they facilitate access to needed services for this often-underserved population.

The Nurse's Role in Prevention

Early nursing efforts targeting homeless populations describe secondary and tertiary intervention (which was often crisis driven) delivered mainly to middle-aged, white, alcoholic men (Lenehan et al., 1985). As the population of homeless people increased and became more diverse, the role of community health nurses expanded. They now care for homeless people across the life span and from diverse cultural, ethnic, and minority groups. Primary prevention strategies are often the focus of intervention.

Working in clinics, meal sites, outreach vans, and other places where homeless people congregate, the community health nurse often has the first and most consistent professional contact with a homeless client. Responsibilities include relationship building; triage; first-aid; ongoing treatments; monitoring of health status, medication, and therapeutic diets; health education and referral; and liaison with other health care providers. Relationship building and maintenance of self-esteem are important aspects at all levels of prevention. If a person is treated with dignity and respect, there is a much better chance that advice will be heeded, prescribed treatments followed, and return appointments kept. Efforts are made to plan care *with* rather than *for* the client, so that care plans are tailored to fit the needs and the resources of the individual.

A number of factors can lead to the breakdown of physical and mental health in homeless people. These include (but are not limited to) stress, exposure to extremes of temperature, sleep deprivation, crowded living conditions, inadequate facilities to maintain personal hygiene, poor nutrition, inadequate clothing, and ill-fitting shoes. Following are some examples of how nurses can intervene at each level of prevention in order to eliminate or minimize these risks.

Primary Prevention

In primary prevention, efforts are aimed both at preventing people from becoming homeless and at preventing morbidity in those who are. An assessment of the community will give a picture of the extent of homelessness, a determination of contributing factors, and available resources. The assessment will help the community health nurse plan where efforts will be most effective. Recognizing a client at risk and bolstering available supports might help to maintain a client in the community. Counseling and support services to homeless mothers and homeless pregnant women should help to prevent second generation homelessness.

Valued and trusted by the community, the nurse's participation in neighborhood associations, on community boards, and in the political process can have a powerful impact on public policy. This involvement will take on particular importance as changes in the welfare regulations are enacted. There are many caring people at neighborhood, state, and federal levels who are influencing policy without understanding the full impact of the policies on human lives. Unlike the nurses, they rarely get close enough to hear the human cries of pain and suffering. Community health nurses must make those cries real to them. At the same time, community health nurses must learn to describe their observations with specific, systematic data reports, lest they be dismissed as "anecdotal."

Once a person becomes homeless, the community health nurse can be a positive influence in the promotion and maintenance of health. Examples include working to insure safe and sanitary living quarters, the availability of a nutritionally sound diet, adequate ventilation, and the administration of vaccines against influenza and pneumonia. Educational programs can be developed regarding specific health threats. One example is programs to prevent acquired immunodeficiency syndrome (AIDS), including safer sexual practices, distribution of condoms, and cleansing of intravenous drug needles. Pamphlets and other educational materials developed must be geared to the understanding of the client with attention paid to possible language barriers, cultural practices and illiteracy.

Secondary Prevention

Efforts at the secondary level are aimed at early detection and prevention of disability. Routine screening of shelter staff and guests for tuberculosis and administration of appropriate prophylactic medications are excellent examples of secondary prevention. Other examples include blood pressure screening; teaching breast self-examination, early detection of skin, head and neck, prostate, and other cancers; early detection and treatment of diabetes; treatment of wounds, blisters, and cuts before infection sets in; and monitoring prescribed treatments and medications.

Nurses need to be aware of shelter rules and policies that affect the health of the guests. Shelter rules should be flexible enough to allow guests with health problems, such as high blood pressure, fevers, or casts, to stay inside on those days when the weather poses a threat.

Many of the conditions from which homeless people suffer are stigmatizing conditions, as is homelessness itself. The nurse's sensitivity to the client's feelings helps to facilitate trust, allowing the client to give a more complete history. Together they can then develop a care plan that is feasible. Visiting local facilities for the care of homeless people will give the community health nurse a better picture of the day-to-day situation that a homeless person faces. Networking with shelter clinics offers a better understanding of what can and what cannot be accomplished there. See Out of the Box for an example of a secondary-prevention program.

Tertiary Prevention

Early case finding and treatment of chronic illness in the homeless population can minimize disability. Discharge planning that recognizes the limited resources of homeless clients can result in the development of realistic aftercare plans leading to healthier practices.

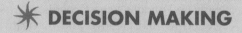

✳ DECISION MAKING

Communication with Homeless People

Accompany a homeless, poorly dressed, and/or intoxicated individual to a health care setting. Pay attention to both verbal and nonverbal messages that are given. Are the messages congruent? Discuss with classmates how verbal and nonverbal communication facilitated or interfered with the care of the client.

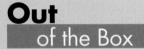

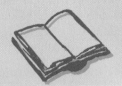

Nursing Careers for the Homeless: A Curriculum for Success

A comprehensive academic and social strategy program was designed to assist homeless individuals who have an interest in and aptitude for nursing to achieve careers in nursing. A three-month preadmission readiness program focuses on socialization to nursing, building self-esteem, academic achievement, and career exploration. The second phase includes academic, social, financial support, as well as assistance with job placement and follow-up. Ninety-six students have been enrolled since 1994 and 73% have graduated. Despite the many obstacles faced by homeless people, many can move beyond homelessness with support and encouragement. ∎

—*Powell, Lee, Nichols,*
Kamara & Sawyer, 1999

Agencies often have subtle, and some not so subtle, ways of treating a homeless person as a second-class citizen. Agency expectation that the homeless client will not follow through on a treatment plan often becomes a self-fulfilling prophecy. Rehabilitation hospitals often choose who will receive their services (and who will not) on the basis of the availability of home support. Homeless people with an acute flare-up of a chronic illness should be admitted to the hospital sooner and discharged later than patients with homes. The opposite is often done. The community health nurse's involvement in discharge planning and in educating other health care providers might help to minimize the many barriers that a homeless person faces in order to maintain an optimal level of health.

Much progress has been made in the intervention and treatment of early and middle-stage alcoholics. Nursing research is needed to find creative and innovative ways of helping the homeless alcoholic, who is often a late-stage, chronically ill individual.

Nursing Theories

Working as a nurse with homeless people is enjoyable and rewarding. It can also be challenging, frustrating, draining, difficult, and exciting. The nurses who pioneered the role at the Pine Street Inn in Boston in 1972

were visionaries. They saw themselves as primarily responsible to their clients and set up a framework based on caring and mutual respect.

They recognized the importance of relationship. They understood that success would depend not so much on what they knew as on the attitude that they conveyed. Foot soaks became a hallmark of their clinic. What better way to demonstrate caring than to soak and massage tired and aching feet? The words **compliance,** meaning a disposition or tendency to yield to others, and **noncompliance,** meaning failure to yield or obey, became taboo. The nurses realized that people might make unhealthy decisions for a variety of reasons. Sometimes there was simply no real opportunity to do otherwise. When the difficulty appeared to be a lack of knowledge, an attempt was made to create an atmosphere where clients could learn about their health condition and options for treatment (Lenehan et al., 1985).

It is easy to picture Virginia Henderson (1966) working in a clinic for the homeless. Her book, *The Nature of Nursing,* could serve as a guide to nurses working with homeless people. In it she states:

> The nurse who sees herself as reinforcing the [client] when he lacks will, knowledge, or strength will make an effort to know him, understand him, "get inside his skin," . . . this process of putting oneself in another's place is always difficult and only relatively successful. It requires a listening ear and constant observation and interpretation of non-verbal behavior. It also demands of the nurse self-understanding and the recognition of emotions that block her concentration on the patient's need and helpful responses to these needs. It calls for a willingness on the nurse's part to selectively express what she is feeling and thinking so that a *mutual* understanding may develop between nurse and patient. (p. 24)

Watson (1985) explores the role of human-to-human caring and its incorporation into the nursing process. She views caring as an essential part of nursing and recognizes the challenge of maintaining its importance in an increasingly technological world. Her thoughtful and scholarly work affirms and validates the work being done in shelter nursing clinics.

ADDITIONAL ISSUES IN CARING FOR HOMELESS PEOPLE

Several factors to be considered by the community health nurse in assessing and planning care for homeless clients have been discussed. However, the above-mentioned health problems rarely occur in isolation. As stated earlier, several health problems may be present in the same individual, each having an effect on the course and treatment of the others.

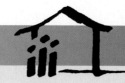

COMMUNITY NURSING VIEW

It was shortly after midnight when the outreach van stopped at the doorway of an abandoned building. A man huddled in the corner, clutching a bottle of vodka. As she approached him, the nurse noticed that his left leg was noticeably larger than the right and that the pants leg was stained with drainage.

The man gave his name as Richard Polk. In answer to the nurse's concern, he said he had been in the hospital for the leg but had signed out. He refused to allow the nurse to look at the leg or to take his temperature. When she reached to touch his forehead, he pulled back with a frightened expression and said, "You weren't in 'Nam lady. What do you think it was like watching my best friend get his head blown off? They're all around, you know. They're up in the trees now." He looked around as if expecting gunfire at any moment.

He became increasingly agitated when the nurse suggested that he be seen at the hospital. He appeared to be responding to internal stimuli and muttered about his combat experiences in Vietnam. He refused to go anywhere until he finished his bottle. The van returned at 4 A.M. The bottle was empty. The man, now quite intoxicated, refused to accept any help. There was fresh, foul smelling drainage on the pants leg.

When they returned to the shelter, the nurse found a chart for Mr. Polk in the clinic. It had limited information. He had been seen in the clinic a week earlier for a draining infected wound on his left leg. His temperature was 99.4°F, and the area surrounding the wound was reddened and warm to the touch. There was a moderate amount of serosanguineous drainage on the dressing. There was mention that he had signed out of the hospital three days earlier. The only personal information that he had given was his birth date (July 23, 1962) and that he was allergic to Trilafon, Artane, and Lithium.

Nursing Considerations

Assessment

- Are there any inconsistencies in the information that is presented?
- Is any information presented that would make the nurse think that Mr. Polk has a major psychiatric illness?
- What additional information is needed?
- What are Mr. Polk's strengths?

Diagnosis

- What could be possible nursing diagnoses?
- Prioritize his problems.
- Would Mr. Polk be considered a danger to himself?

Outcome Identification

- Given your diagnoses, what outcomes could you expect to achieve?

Planning/Interventions

- How could the nurse engage Mr. Polk in treatment?
- Are there any commitment laws in your state that could be used to bring Mr. Polk into treatment against his will?

Evaluation

- What would determine Mr. Polk's progress in meeting his goals of treatment?

There are several other important considerations not discussed in this chapter or mentioned only briefly. They include cultural and religious differences, sexual orientation, legal status, criminal record, language barriers, and literacy. Each can have a powerful impact on a client's ability to accept care and follow through on a treatment plan. It is important that community health nurses be thorough in their assessments so that care plans are both acceptable and feasible.

The problem of homelessness is complex and defies simplistic solutions. Where does the nurse begin? A homeless woman answered the question this way:

Try not to look at homelessness as a massive social, political, or public health problem. That view is discouraging. Look at it instead as a problem involving people; individual people. If each person did something to help one homeless person, the problem wouldn't be so big. When I say help, I don't mean take somebody home or buy them a meal or even give them a quarter when they're begging on the street. I mean something as simple as looking a person straight in the eye and saying, "I'm sorry, but I can't help you out today." (Anonymous, personal communication)

KEY CONCEPTS

- Homelessness is not a new phenomenon in the United States.

- Since the early 1980s, the number of homeless men, women, and children has been increasing at an alarming rate, with estimates now ranging up to 3 million people.

- Homeless individuals are a diverse group. The term *homelessness* should not imply that individuals in this group have anything more in common than the lack of a fixed address.

- Responses to the problem began with grass-roots organizers and private agencies but now come from local, state, and federal government as well.

- Nurses were the first professionals to bring health care to homeless people.

- Nurses, working within the scope of basic nursing practice, can do a great deal for homeless people.

- Homeless people tend to be sicker, have more stress and have fewer supports than domiciled individuals.

- Health problems of particular concern include nutritional disorders, peripheral vascular disease, infectious diseases including HIV infections, infestations, substance abuse, psychiatric disorders and trauma.

- People without homes have limited access to the health care system and lack the necessary resources to follow a regimen of care.

- Intervention is most effective when nursing care plans are developed *with* rather than *for* the client, and the highest priority is given to the client's concerns.

- The community health nurse is in a position to intervene at all levels of prevention.

RESOURCES

Coalition on Human Needs: http://www.chn.org/homeless
Homelessness: http://www.welfareinfo.org/homeless.htm
National Coalition for Homeless Veterans: http://www.nchv.org
National Coalition for the Homeless: http://nationalhomeless.org
National Health Care for the Homeless Council:
    http://www.nhchc.org
Urban Institute: www.urban.org

Marshelle Thobaben, RN, C, MS, APNP, FNP, PHN
Patricia Biteman, RN, MSN

MAKING THE CONNECTION

Chapter 26 Communicable Diseases

A good fit of illness proves the value of health; real danger tries one's mettle; and self-sacrifice sweetens character. Let no one who sincerely desires to help the work in this way, delay going through any fear; for the worth of life lies in the experiences that fill it, and this is one which cannot be forgotten.

—Louisa May Alcott, 1863, p. 139

COMPETENCIES

Upon completion of this chapter, the reader should be able to:

- Discuss the history of rural health.
- Compare and contrast the various definitions of *rural.*
- Identify rural and frontier values.
- Examine the health status of rural residents.
- Discuss the factors that influence the rural health care delivery system.
- Discuss key legislation and programs affecting rural health.
- Identify alternatives available to the rural community for providing rural health care.
- Discuss the various roles community health nurses play in rural communities.

KEY TERMS

frontier area

metropolitan (metro) areas (MAs)

migrant farm worker

nonmetropolitan (nonmetro) areas

rural areas

rural health clinics

rural nursing

seasonal farm worker

telehealth

Urban Cluster (UC)

urbanized area (UA)

Rural community health nurses are an integral part of a community's health and have potential power in influencing local health policy. They play more than one role in clients' lives, which increases the potential for continuity of care. In the absence of a health center, it is the community health nurses who respond to people's concerns about cholesterol, diabetes, immunizations, and birth control, as well as medical issues. This chapter provides a historical overview of rural health and discusses definitions, legislation, health problems of rural residents, and rural community health nursing roles.

HISTORICAL OVERVIEW OF RURAL HEALTH

The 1800 census counted 5,308,000 citizens; 92.6% were rural residents and only 3.8% were living in urban areas (Grun, 1991). The care of the ill in both rural and urban areas fell to wives, mothers, and daughters. Women traded remedies handed down by their mothers and cared for the sick, with the doctor making occasional house calls with his black bag. All that was known about medicine was contained in the black bag that the doctor carried.

The first hospital in the United States was founded in Philadelphia in 1752 by Benjamin Franklin; hospitals were basically established to accommodate persons whose homes could not provide the most routine nursing care (Sharpe, 1980, p. 10). Hospitals were places of pestilence and isolation; people were admitted when there was no other alternative.

In 1841 the first wagon train left for California, opening the West to new settlers. The settlement of new territories moved nursing care farther away from hospitals and into remote outposts.

Life expectancy in the United States was 40 years in 1850. The advent of preventive medicine and pasteurization, bacteriology, and immunization did much to increase longevity over the next 100 years.

The Civil War raged from 1861 to 1865. More hospitals were built to care for wounded soldiers. Dorothea Dix supervised the training of the first 100 nurses and continued to recruit more. Louisa May Alcott was one of those temporary nurses. She was a nurse in a field hospital during the Civil War, caring for the sick and injured with scarce resources in an alternative setting. She became a nurse out of her desire to do something as the great battles were fought. Many of the first rural nurses began their practice following the same inner drive.

In the last quarter of the 19th century, the hospital became the center of medical care because of the development of new technology. Surgical, x-ray, and laboratory facilities combined with long-term nursing care made the hospital a better place to recover. The size of houses decreased, and families began living in apartments to be closer to new jobs; business and industries grew.

As the cities and hospitals grew, the distance between rural communities also grew. In the 1885 census, 64.9% of the country was rural and 35.1% was urban. Farming community residents found the transportation to large hospitals difficult. Health in the rural communities declined.

In 1908 Lillian Wald determined there was a need for organized rural nursing service. The Visiting Nurse Department was started in 1909 by the Metropolitan Life Insurance Company to furnish nursing services to Manhattan. The service expanded to other policyholders, and by 1912 there were 589 Metropolitan Life nursing centers in the Northeast. Wald continued to present the plight of isolated communities, believing that mobile nurses could reduce the rate of mortality from childbirth and infant diseases. She was instrumental in persuading the American Red Cross to establish the rural nursing service in 1912. The name was later changed to the Town and Country Nursing Service. The ranks were too small to make a big impact. The nurses reported diseases, quarantined contagious persons, cared for the acutely ill, and delivered babies. In place of adequate medical supplies, the rural nurse improvised, a characteristic that remains constant today (Bushy, 1991).

The 1920 census was the first to show growth in urban areas surpassing that of rural areas. Then 48% of the population was rural while 51.2% was urban. Mary Breckinridge founded the Frontier Nursing Service in 1925 in Leslie County, Kentucky. The nurses worked primarily as midwives and reduced the rate of stillbirths by one-third. They also offered care for infants and children. Well-child visits were augmented with lessons about diet, sanitation, and cleanliness. The rural nurses also gave inoculations against typhoid, diphtheria, and smallpox.

Two world wars increased the population in cities as the demand for industrialization grew. Women worked as nurses or teachers or in factories. The wars resulted in the growth of hospitals as technology improved. Soon, hospitals were the centers of medicine and teaching. Development continued until medical costs skyrocketed in the 1970s, resulting in federal controls in the form of Medicare and Medicaid. Reimbursement declined, and the rural hospitals were the first to close during the 1980s.

The advent of hospital reform, managed care, and reduced hospital stays has precipitated a growth in rural home health nursing care that will continue into the 21st century. Nurses working for a licensed agency make home visits to follow up on treatments started in acute-care centers. Despite the passage of more than 70 years, rural nurses are still required to be experienced generalists, with a high level of resourcefulness. The future of rural nursing will rely on telehealth technology. Telehealth will be discussed later in this chapter.

DEFINITIONS OF *RURAL*

Community health nurses need to be aware of the diverse definitions of *rural* and of the diversity of rural populations. Rural areas are often thought of as either be-

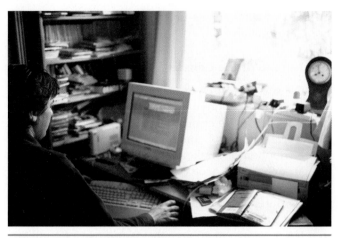

The rural population is changing with the influx of people who can use the computer to telecommute.
(Photo courtesy of PhotoDisc)

ing the Western frontier or farmlands. People imagine farms with acres of land separating farms, with rural towns located sporadically and the population as consisting of pioneers, hunters, trappers, ranchers, and Native Americans. However, rural populations include members of every cultural and ethnic group and cross all economic boundaries. They consist of retired persons, artists, small-business owners, writers, and others who can use the computer to extend their work desk.

There is no agreement among health professionals or policymakers on a single definition that best describes rural areas. The same geographic area could be considered rural by one definition and metropolitan by another. How rural is defined can have impact on any change in public policy, including receiving federal funding and identifying health care shortage areas (Ricketts, Johnson-Webb, & Taylor, 1998).

The U.S. rural areas vary along a continuum from frontier to urbanlike. A **frontier area's** greatest defining characteristic is its isolation, having fewer than six or seven persons per square mile. The frontier areas are characterized by considerable distance from central places, poor access to market areas, and people's relative isolation from each other in large geographic areas. There are 26 states with frontier areas. The states that have more than 15% of their population in frontier counties and with a total frontier population of greater than 250,000 are Wyoming (18 counties, 246,156 population), Alaska (21 counties), Montana (47 counties), South Dakota (37 counties), and Idaho (22 counties) (Zelarney & Ciarlo, 2000).

Federal Agencies' Definitions

The U.S. Bureau of the Census, the U.S. Office of Management and Budget (USOMB), and the U.S. Department of Agriculture (USDA) provide the three most common federal definitions of rural. They define rural

---

REFLECTIVE THINKING

Your Image of Rural

- When you think about clients living in rural areas, what thoughts come to mind?
- How old are they?
- Where do they live? What does their home look like? How do they make a living?
- What are their health care problems? Where do they get their health care?

in terms of rural versus urban and metropolitan versus nonmetropolitan.

U.S. Bureau of the Census

The Census Bureau collects, analyzes, and disseminates statistical data on population and the economy. These data are used to determine eligibility for reimbursement of government funds, funding for research projects, and the distribution of public monies.

An **urbanized area (UA)** consists of densely settled territory that contains 50,000 or more people. The U.S. Census Bureau delineates UAs to provide a better separation of urban and rural territory. At least 35,000 people in a UA must live in an area that is not part of a military reservation (U.S. Bureau of the Census, 2001b).

The U.S. Census Bureau introduced the **Urban Cluster (UC)** for Census 2000 to provide a more consistent and accurate measure of the population concentration in and around places. It consists of densely settled territory that has at least 2500 people but fewer than 50,000 people (U.S. Bureau of the Census, 2001b).

Rural area consists of all territory, population, and housing units located outside of UAs and UCs (U.S. Bureau of the Census, 2001b). Approximately one-fourth of all U.S. citizens live in rural areas, according to the U.S. Bureau of the Census (Bushy, 2000).

U.S. Office of Management and Budget

The predominant mission of the USOMB is to assist the president in overseeing the preparation of the federal budget and to supervise its administration in executive branch agencies. It classifies counties as either **metropolitan areas** (MA) or **nonmetropolitan areas.** The MA classification is a statistical standard developed for use by federal agencies in the production, analysis, and publication of data. In 1999, about $86 billion in tax incentives and $141 billion in federal monies were designated to provide direct health care services, promote disease prevention, conduct and support research, and help train the nation's health care work force. The activities of the USOMB and distribution of federal resources have allowed progress to be made in decreasing infant mortality, extending life expectancy, and reducing the fatality among persons with HIV/AIDS [U.S. Executive Office of the President (USEOP), 1998].

The MA designation includes the following considerations:

- Each MA must contain either at least one city with 50,000 or more residents or a Bureau of the Census defined urbanized area with a total MA population of at least 100,000 (75,000 in New England).

- Each MA must include the county in which the central city is located (the central county) and additional contiguous counties (fringe counties) if

they are economically and socially integrated with the central county. The county or counties that include a MA and any outlying counties that are part of the same large market area with a specific level of commuting to the central county for work and commercial activity are called metropolitan (metro). Metropolitan areas in New England are composed of cities and towns rather than whole counties (U.S. Bureau of the Census, 2001).

- All counties not classified as metropolitan are by definition nonmetropolitan (nonmetro); they have boundaries outside of metro areas and have no cities with as many as 50,000 residents (USDA, 2001).

According to the U.S. Bureau of the Census (2000), 225,981,679 residents live inside metropolitan areas and 55,440,227 residents live outside metropolitan areas. Figure 34-1 illustrates the continued decrease in growth rates for nonmetropolitan counties. Racial and ethnic minorities constituted 15.2%–18% of all rural residents in

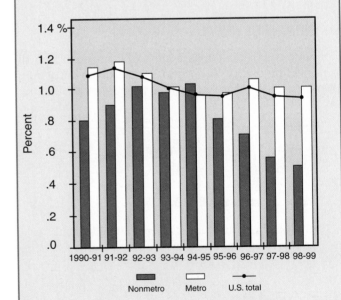

FIGURE 34-1 Population Decline for Nonmetropolitan Areas

Annual population growth rates for metro counties, nonmetro counties, and the Nation, 1990–1999

The pace of nonmetro population growth in 1998–1999 continues the slowdown that began after 1994–1995

From *Rural Population and Migration: Rural Population Change,* by U.S. Department of Agriculture, Economic Research Service (ERS), 2000, [On-line]. Available: http://www.ers.usda.gov/briefing/Population/popchange.

TABLE 34-1 The Race of Residents in Nonmetropolitan Areas*

RACE	PERCENTAGE OF RESIDENTS	NUMBER OF RESIDENTS
African America	8.6	4,764,919
American Indian or Alaska	1.9	1,054,824
Native		
Asian	0.8	416,888
Asian Indian	0.1	53,218
Chinese	0.1	56,714
Filipino	0.2	101,229
Japanese	0.1	71,789
Korean	0.1	42,029
Vietnamese	0.1	28,266
Other Asian	0.1	63,643
Hispanic or Latino (of any race)	5.6	3,131,876
Mexican	3.8	2,132,552
Puerto Rican	0.2	125,015
Cuban	0.1	36,161
Other Hispanic or Latino	1.5	838,178
Native Hawaiian and other Pacific Islander	0.1	59,820
Native Hawaiian	0.1	37,782
Guamanian or Chamorro	—	5,856
Samoan	—	5,620
Other Pacific Islander	—	10,562
White	84.8	46,991,330
Some other race	2.4	1,316,884
Two or more races	1.5	835,562

The numbers may add to more than the total population and the percentages may add to more than 100% because individuals may report more than one race.

From U.S. Bureau of the Census. (2001). Profile of general demographic characteristics: 2000 census of population and housing, United States. [On-line]. Available: http://blue.census.gov/Press-Release/www/2001/2khus.pdf.

2001. Table 34-1 provides the data on the race of the residents living outside metropolitan areas.

U.S. Department of Agriculture

The USDA economic research agency, the Economic Research Service (ERS), has a classification system of non-metro counties, known as ERS typology. This system is widely used by researchers, policy analysts, and public officials as a source of information about the economic and social diversity characterizing rural U.S. areas. The classification system is based on 2288 U.S. counties designed as nonmetropolitan (nonmetro) in 1993. The typology consists of 11 types of nonmetro counties classified into one of six nonoverlapping economic types (farming, mining, manufacturing, government, services, and nonspecialized). It also classifies counties into five overlapping rural policy-relevant types (retirement destination, federal lands, persistent poverty, commuting, and transfer-dependent) (USDA, 2000b). Tables 34-2 and 34-3 are examples of the ERS typology.

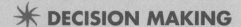

✳ DECISION MAKING

Defining Rurality

You are conducting a research study analyzing the rate of alcoholism among the adolescent and adult residents in a particular rural area.

◆ What criteria would you include in your definition of rural?

◆ How would you decide the criteria?

The ERS typology indicates the diversity and wide range of economic activities—from manufacturing to recreational services—in rural (nonmetro) areas. The rural economies have shifted from being dependent on farming, forestry, and mining to experiencing a striking diversity of economic activities. Nonmetro areas vary

TABLE 34-2 Nonmetro Counties Based on Economy Types

TYPE	LOCATION	POPULATION SHIFT	ECONOMIC BASE
Farming dependent (556 counties)	Concentrated in the Midwest	Declined through outmigration	Economic decline; they lost 111,000 farming jobs
Mining dependent (146 counties)	Mostly located in South or West; distinct specialization in different types of mining activities, including coal, gas, oil, and metals	Declined through outmigration	Economic decline with a 27% loss of jobs
Manufacturing dependent (506 counties)	Often located contiguous to a metro area; exhibit a more urban orientation; located mainly in the southeast	More densely populated than other types	Economy grew slightly
Government dependent (244 counties)	Scattered across the nation; specialize in federal, state, and local government activities	Grew	Economy grew with an overall gain of 433,000 new jobs
Services dependent (323 counties)	Fairly evenly distributed across the country with a slightly higher representation in the west; service-sector jobs, which include centers for trade and services, consumer service centers for residential areas, and centers of specialized services such as recreation.	Grew significantly	Economy grew with a 24% growth in earnings
Nonspecialized (484 counties)	Large majority are in the south; did not qualify for one of the activities such as construction, forestry, or fisheries	No data	Reflected both strong and weak economies; two-thirds experienced growth

From U.S. Department of Agriculture, Economic Research Service (ERS). (2000). Measuring rurality: What is rural? *[On-line]. Available: http://www.ers.usda.gov/Briefing/Rurality/whatisrural.*

dramatically in their health needs. Strategies to address problems in each area must fit the community. The role of the community health nurse is to match the health needs of the nonmetro community with the potential available funds for state, county, and federal programs.

RURAL AND FRONTIER VALUES

There are many advantages to living in rural areas, which is summed up by the term *quality of life.* Rural areas have environmental beauty and purity, with some areas having mountains, rivers, and forests and others farmlands. They have clean air and water and are close access to outdoor activities and sports such as hiking, fishing, hunting. They have affordable housing, plenty of parking, no traffic jams, low crime rates, and solitude when one wants it. They have a sense of "community,"

where the church and community are the centers for socialization. They are more family oriented, where residents are related or acquainted, with extended kinships. They know their local government leadership and have access to them. They often have informal social/professional interactions. There is a perception of a more relaxed pace of life. The move to rural areas was popular in the 1990s. Professionals looking for a better place to raise children, quieter neighborhoods, and acreage for leisure pursuits chose to leave the urban areas. Improved technology made the world more accessible through better telenetting.

There is a tendency for rural residents to be independent, self-reliant, conservative, religious, work-oriented, individualist, fatalistic, and distrusting of outsiders, including new health care providers. Weinert and Burman (1999) use the Sampler Quilt as a metaphor for defining rural populations. Each block of the Sampler

TABLE 34-3   Nonmetro Counties Based on Policy Criteria

TYPE	LOCATION	ECONOMY
Retirement-destination (190 counties)	Fifteen percent or greater increase in population aged 60 and above; over 80% are in the south or west, most prevalently in Florida and the southwest	Served as recreational or resort sites; 60% of these counties had job growth faster than the national average
Federal lands (270 counties)	Seventy-six percent of these counties are in the western states and are federally owned; had larger land areas and are more sparsely populated than all-nonmetro counties; on average, grew faster than all-nonmetro counties	Approximately 70% of the jobs were in services or government sectors, reflecting the recreational use and land management function of the group, strong growth in service sector jobs
Commuting (381 counties)	A majority are in the south, where counties have smaller land areas and are more apt to adjoin metro areas than all-nonmetro counties	Economies shaped by workers commuting to jobs in other counties; the level of economic activity within the local economies was less than in all-nonmetro counties
Persistent poverty (504 counties)	Eighty-five percent of these counties are located in the south	A distinguishing feature is a disproportionate number of economically at-risk people including minorities, female-headed households, high school dropouts, and disabled persons; unemployment was considerably higher and incomes considerably lower than in all-nonmetro counties
Transfer dependent (381 counties)	Economies were heavily based on unearned income from government transfer payments, including Social Security, unemployment insurance, Medicare, Medicaid, food stamps, government pensions, and welfare benefits; the large majority are in the southern states; they are sparsely populated and usually remote from metro areas; about three-fifths of these counties were also in the persistent poverty category	They include a large number of elderly; overall economies grew more slowly with real earnings declining by 9%

From *U.S. Department of Agriculture, Economic Research Service (ERS). (2000).* Measuring rurality: What is rural? [*On-line*]. *Available: http://www.ers.usda.gov/Briefing/Rurality/whatisrural.*

Quilt is made from different fabric and stitched in a different pattern. When the quilt is finished, it reveals a complete project, a blend of fabric and design unique to the quilt itself. Rural and urban areas are mixtures of persons, resources, and economics. Each community is unique to itself, rural or urban. The authors suggest avoiding generalizations about rural and urban values. They are as diverse as the persons who live there.

Many residents view health as synonymous with being productive and able to work. Their attitudes, values, and health beliefs affect their utilization of the health care system and may prevent them from timely entry into the health care system if they have an illness or a condition, such as pregnancy, that they consider normal. They are more likely to obtain help through the informal system of family and neighbors than through any formal health care system [American Nurses Association (ANA), 1996; Davis & Magilvy, 2000].

Lee (1993) writes that health behaviors are the result of values learned during childhood. In farming and

 DECISION MAKING

Understanding Differences in Rural Communities' Values

You are organizing a preventive health care program on hypertension for the Iroquois Native Americans of the rural northeast and the Vietnamese immigrants of rural western Kansas.

◆ How would your programs compare? What would be the similarities? The differences?

ranching environments, children grow up with values of productivity, industriousness, role performance, and independence. If they do not complete their tasks, no one is there to take the responsibility for them. In rural families, it is the women's role to care for the family's health.

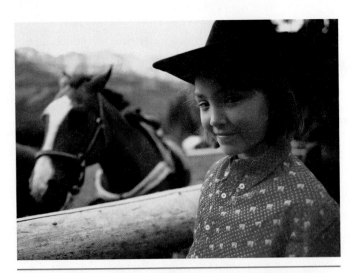

Rural children are more likely to be uninsured than urban children because their parents are self-employed and are unable to attain or afford health insurance. (Photo courtesy of PhotoDisc)

Women take care of colds, flu symptoms, and cuts and abrasions. They determine when outside assistance will be sought. They attempt to care for the husbands' health but are often restricted by the work season (p. 25).

Community health nurses need to consider the values of rural communities and their residents when planning preventive health care and providing clients direct nursing care. Unless they do, it is likely that they will be distrusted by their clients and their services will not be accepted in the community (ANA, 1996; Weinert & Burman, 1999).

HEALTH STATUS OF RURAL RESIDENTS

This section includes the types of rural health issues related to children, people who have mental health problems, farm workers, and Native Americans.

Rural residents in general have poorer health than urban residents. Adults in rural areas are more than 36% more likely to report their health as fair or poor than in urban areas (*Healthy People 2010*; USDHHS, 2000b). The barriers include lack of transportation, unpredictable and demanding work schedules that conflict with clinic hours, lack of health care providers, distrust of providers, language barriers, and the tangle of managed care.

Rural Children

The health status of rural and migrant children is affected by poverty and the associated challenges created by a marginal socioeconomic status. Rural children are more likely than urban children to be uninsured; rural residents are likely to be self-employed and without comprehensive health care coverage because of the high cost. Rural children with treatable problems often cannot

access primary care services and thus are likely to develop an acute illness. The Colorado Migrant Health Program (1998) has established a list of factors related to poverty and poor access to health care. Many of these factors could be prevented with better childhood health care. Some of these factors are dental disease, hearing impairment resulting from untreated otitis media, poor immunization status, absent prenatal care, and high-risk pregnancies.

Only 33% of migrant women receive prenatal care during the first trimester of pregnancy. Infant mortality is twice the national average. Gwyther and Jenkins (1998) cite farm injuries, chemical exposure, infectious diseases, and poor nutrition as additional problems common in the children of migrant and seasonal farm workers.

Research to identify problems specific to rural clusters must be done. Based on this data, community health nurses can improve the physical well-being of rural children by developing a comprehensive preventive health care plan. It can include such activities as screening programs, mobile clinics, and health education presentations.

Nonmetro Elderly

One-quarter of the elderly population live in nonmetro areas and have characteristics and needs that differ from the metro elderly. The rural elderly are a diverse group. Their environment varies from clusters of educated, wealthy retirees to uneducated older populations in remote rural areas. Older persons in good health and highly educated will be in a position to better avail themselves of available programs and services (Rogers, 1999). The elderly have a higher percentage of chronic diseases. According to the Centers for Disease Control and Prevention (CDC), 46.7% of the rural adult population have chronic conditions compared to 39.2% in the metropolitan areas (USDHHS, 2000b). Davis and Magilvy (2000) suggest that rural older adults found the formal health care system too complex and confusing, particularly as the complexity of health problems increased. The nonmetro elderly poor are apt to be less healthy than their wealthier counterparts because they have less access to support services, good housing, adequate nutrition, and transportation.

Community health nurses can reach the nonmetro elderly by documenting the need for services and establishing clinics in churches, grange halls, or mobile units that make frequent rounds of the outlying areas. Nurses are also needed to help the elderly decipher complex information and provide assistance through the maze of the health care system (Davis & Magilvy, 2000).

Mental Health

Rural areas in general tend to be economically unstable, and that instability may have an impact on the mental health of residents because they work continuously for very little gain. High rates of unemployment, isolation, and severe economic difficulties increase the incidence of mental illness. Chronic stress experienced by rural families in farming, mining, forestry, and fishing-dependent economies takes its toll. The resulting depression, anxiety, or substance abuse requires attention which is often more difficult to get than in urban areas. Isolation results in long trips for people to receive treatment for mental health problems. Transportation can be an obstacle for them to receive care, because they do not have private transportation and inexpensive public transportation is not available. Poverty is a factor in the mental health of rural residents because it is persistent and involves complex social, psychological, and cultural problems. Mental health services for inpatient mental health services, suicide prevention, crisis intervention, support groups, and individual services rely on a large volume of cases or donations from nonprofit foundations to support their existence. The volume of clients needed to support such services is often not available in rural areas. Recent changes in the health care system (including managed care) that emphasize cost containment could further imperil access to mental health services for people in rural and frontier areas. There is concern that, in the effort to trim the health care costs, rural mental health services could continue to suffer disproportionately (National Institute of Mental Health [NIMH], 2000).

Rural residents are unlikely to be offered a full array of behavioral health services. Community health nurses may be the only resource available for mentally ill and substance abuse clients in rural areas. This lack of services is particularly problematic when nurses have clients who need inpatient treatment, such as a client who is suicidal. The community health nurse must work closely with other professionals and the client's informal network of family and friends to try to provide the type of care a client may need [National Rural Health Association (NRHA), 1999b].

Farm Workers

The majority of the nation's most dangerous occupations are located in rural areas. Agricultural occupations including farming, ranching, and commercial fishing are among the most hazardous occupations, with the death rate approximately four times that of all other industries combined. In 1997, there were 705 incidences of fatal injuries and 50,544 incidences of nonfatal injuries on U.S. farms. In terms of injuries per farm, operators and family members were killed at a rate of 0.27 per 1000 farms and were injured at a rate of 11.4 per 1000 farms. In comparison, hired laborers were killed at a rate of 0.30 per 1000 farms reporting hired labor expenditures and injured at a rate of 44.2 per 1000 farms reporting hired labor expenditures (USDA, 2000d). Approximately

32,800 agricultural-related injuries occurred to children or adolescents under the age of 20 who lived on, worked on, or visited a farm operation in 1998 (NASS, 1999). The injuries occurred at a rate of 1.7 injuries per every 100 farms. The majority of these injuries happened to male youth (NASS, 1999).

Hired labor is an important part of the U.S. farm production process. Federal laws and regulations have been enacted to govern farm workers' working conditions, employment, taxes, and wages. Examples of such laws are the Fair Labor Standards Act of 1938 (FLSA), which contains provisions and standards on minimum wages, maximum hours allowable without overtime pay, child labor, and recordkeeping. The Occupational Safety and Health Act of 1970 (OSHA) focuses on assuring safe and healthful working conditions for working adults and contains standards affecting several aspects of the agricultural workplace. Its provisions cover standards for temporary labor camps, field sanitation, hazardous substances, cadmium usage, and logging operations. Farm employers that do not employ 11 or more employees on at least one day are exempt from all OSHA provisions, except for the temporary labor camp provision. The Federal Insecticide, Fungicide, and Rodenticide Act of 1947 (FIFRA) sets an overall risk-benefit standard for pesticide registration, requiring that all pesticides perform their intended function when used according to labeling instructions without imposing unreasonable risks of adverse effects on human health or the environment. The Environmental Protection Agency (EPA) requires the certification of all pesticide applicators and their employees who will be applying pesticides.

It may be possible to reduce the risk of occupational injuries through regulation, engineering, education, or a combination of these methods. However, farm machinery's longevity outlasts many safety devices and safety innovations take years to become widely used. Developing effective farm safety education programs requires the cooperation of all parties involved in farming—operators, family members, farm workers, manufacturers, researchers, and farm safety specialists (Runyan, 1998). Community health nurses can help reduce high-risk, nonfatal agricultural injuries by the application of primary preventive nursing approaches. Farmers and farm workers receive little formal safety training, and they often work alone and far from assistance should an injury occur (Runyan, 1998). Community health nurses can use preventive techniques such as preventive programs in English and Spanish on potential human errors that contribute to injuries, handling emergencies, and safety around farm animals and equipment. They can also do screenings for agricultural work-related injuries, stress reduction techniques, and counseling.

Figure 34-2 provides a summary of the health care problems experienced with the rural population, and Table 34-4 offers a typology for health care needs of communities.

- Almost one in three rural adults are in poor to fair health and have at least one major chronic illness.

- Higher rates of occupational injuries and traumatic injuries occur in rural areas than in urban areas; clients face worse outcomes and higher risks of death than urban clients because of transportation problems and lack of advanced life support training for emergency medical personnel.

- Rural hospitals and other health care resources are unavailable, and clients lack choices; rural hospitals are shifting rapidly toward outpatient services and show a decline in admissions and lengths of stay compared with urban hospitals.

- Primary care nurses and other primary health care providers are in short supply or unavailable.

- Adequate treatment for alcoholism and drug abuse is lacking because of a scarcity of mental health professionals.

- A high proportion of rural residents have no comprehensive health insurance coverage.

Adapted from Factors *Affecting Children's Health: A Rural Profile* 1(2), by Center for Health Policy (CHPa), 1997.

Migrant and Seasonal Farm Workers

A **migrant farm worker** is a person employed in agricultural work of a seasonal or other temporary nature who is required to be absent overnight from his or her permanent place of residence. A **seasonal farm worker** is a person employed in agricultural work of a seasonal or other temporary nature who is not required to be absent overnight from his or her permanent place of residence. The actual size of the racially and culturally diverse migrant and seasonal farm worker labor force is difficult to determine. The U.S. Public Health Service estimates 3.5 million migrant and seasonal farm workers in the United States [Migrant Clinician Network (MCN), 2001]. Data on farm workers is hard to collect. They often do not have a fixed address and work intermittently in various occupations during a year. Many live in rural remote areas and half are here without permits. In addition, they have limited English-speaking abilities and low educational levels and are distrustful of government agencies or agents such as census enumerators (Bugarin & Elias, 1998).

The labor force is a diverse one, and its composition varies from region to region. It is estimated that 85% of all migrant workers are minorities, of whom most are Hispanic (including Mexican American, Puerto Ricans, Cubans, and workers from Mexico and Central and South America). The migrant population also includes Black Americans, Jamaicans, Haitians, Laotians, Thais, and other racial and ethnic minorities. Therefore, the farm workers' cultures are as varied as they are. They bring their own culture (National Center for Farmworkers Health [NCFH], 2001b). Historically, the migrant stream has been described by three geographic locations. These are the East Coast Migrant Stream, the Midwest Migrant Stream, and the West Coast Migrant Stream. Migrant families often migrate together to maximize their income. Some families settle in a town to seek better educational or work opportunities. See Table 34-5 for a description of the three migrant stream patterns (CDC, 1992).

Seventy-seven percent of all farm workers in 1997–1998 were Mexican born. Their average age was 31, and 80% of farm workers were men. Spanish was the

TABLE 34-4 Typology for Health Care Needs of Communities

TYPE OF COMMUNITY	POPULATION SHIFT	NEEDED HEALTH CARE SERVICES
Aging counties	Fairly recently low fertility rates; existing population is aging	Increased demand for services for the elderly
Previous out-migration counties	Young people have migrated out in past decades, leaving a smaller number of older adults needing health care. As a result of normal reproduction rates, a mostly young adult population now exists.	Increased demand for obstetric and pediatric services
Boom counties	Substantial in-migration of young adults, both single and with families	Need for obstetric, pediatric, emergency, and substance abuse services
Retirement counties	Gradual influx of elderly residents	Need for health services for the elderly and health services providers

Adapted from **Rural Frontier Nursing: The Challenge to Grow** *(pp. 7–8), by American Nurses Association, 1996, Washington, DC: Author.*

RESEARCH FOCUS

Quiet Pride: The Experience of Chronic Illness by Rural Older Adults

Study Problem/Purpose

The purpose of this descriptive ethnographic study was to explore how chronic illness is experienced and managed by rural Hispanic and non-Hispanic older adults and their families and to identify how the health care system and community facilitate or inhibit the ability to manage chronic illness in a changing health care environment.

Methods

Audiotaped interviews from 42 Hispanic and white, non-Hispanic participants, participant observations, examination of documents and artifacts, and photography in rural Colorado provided data for the study. Participants were interviewed in their homes several times over a one-year period.

Findings

The study revealed that living with chronic illness was a proactive, reciprocal learning process shaped by interrelationships in the context of multiple, diverse communities. Participants expressed living with chronic illness as a quiet pride on the journey toward living a meaningful life.

Implications

Findings provide an understanding of relationships that constitute the experience of elders living with chronic illness in rural communities. Viewing life as meaningful in the context of a broader understanding of health and well-being is important for nursing practice and future models of care.

Source: Davis, R., & Magilvy, J. (2000). Quiet Pride: The experience of chronic illness by rural older adults. Journal of Nursing Scholarship, 32(4), 385-390.

TABLE 34-5 Migrant Travel Patterns

MIGRANT STREAM	CULTURAL GROUP	HOME BASE
East Coast	Hispanic, primarily Mexican Americans, Mexicans, Central American refugees, and Puerto Ricans; others include African Americans, Haitians, and Appalachian Caucasians	Primary home base is southern Florida; reside in ethnically homogeneous labor camps, including family unit housing or single-sex barracks; during harvest season, farm workers may change camps or move to a new location
Midwest	Mexican Americans, southeast Asians	Primary home base is southern Texas; work crops there before moving up into the midwestern states; may also move to East and West Coast migrant streams; family unit travels "upstream" from the home base in groups with children and other relatives; live primarily in labor camps
West Coast	Mexican Americans, African Americans, non-Hispanic Caucasians, and an increasing number of southeast Asians	Primary home base is southern California; stream runs north through Idaho, Oregon, and Washington; primary individual family, some males from Mexico; live in migrant camps when they leave their home base

From "Prevention and Control of Tuberculosis in Migrant Farm Workers: Recommendations of the Advisory Council for the Elimination of Tuberculosis," by Centers for Disease Control and Prevention, 1992, Morbidity and Mortality Weekly Reports, June 6.

---

predominant language of farm workers (84%) followed by English (12%). The remaining 4% reported native languages such as Tagalog, Ilocano, Creole, and Mixtec. Only one-tenth of foreign-born farm workers spoke or read English fluently. The median highest education was sixth grade with only 15% completing 12 years or more. Migrant workers are hired by agricultural farmers or employees and by farm labor contractors. The contractors act as intermediaries between the farmers and field hands. Several states are heavily involved with the farm worker movement. Crops relying on migrants for production/ picking are fruits and nuts, vegetables, and field crops such as strawberries and artichokes. The median wage is between $7500 and $9999 (USDL, 2000).

Housing

Housing for migrant farm workers is scarce. Private housing is not subject to federal regulation. The housing that is available is often substandard (unsanitary, lacks safe drinking water and bathing or laundry facilities) and expensive. Workers face barriers in obtaining housing in local private housing markets because not enough rental units are available or rental units are unavailable to migrant farm workers because they cannot provide deposits or make long-term rental commitments.

Migrant farm worker employers recognize that the lack of housing is a serious problem, but they face several disincentives to providing housing. Employers traditionally met the need through the establishment of labor camps, but construction and maintenance was expensive, and the enforcement of housing standards has created a trend toward discontinuing providing housing. As a result, migrant farm workers often share a small, grower-provided room with several other people.

Migrant workers stay in residential neighborhoods, relying on relatives and friends when they can. It is not unusual to have three or four families per house with seven or eight people to a room. Four to 10 persons can rent a garage for several hundred dollars a month. Migrants also pack into trailers, tool sheds, caves, fields, and parking lots.

Some states are more active in providing assistance for the development of migrant housing. Florida, for example, has a program that provides mortgages for the construction or substantial rehabilitation of rental housing that is affordable to very low income tenants (NCFH, 2001a).

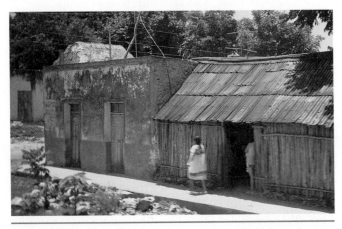

Migrant workers often live in substandard housing.
Photo courtesy of Elmer Cooper.

Health Problems

The federal migrant health care program spends $65 million a year and provides more than 100 clinics across the United States, but this is not enough to meet the needs of the migrant workers and their families. Mobile units are effective means for community health nurses to reach these isolated and transient clients, but few health centers have the resources to establish mobile programs. Most migrant and seasonal farm workers make annual incomes well below the federal poverty rate. Rarely do they have access to disability benefits or occupational rehabilitation. Many who have paid into Social Security have difficulty proving their claim for benefits. Insurance coverage for seasonal workers is usually nonexistent, leaving only the choice of waiting until a condition needs to be seen in the emergency room. In addition, migrant workers often face linguistic, cultural, financial, immigration, educational, and other barriers that also make it difficult for them to obtain needed health care services (ANA, 1996; Health Resources and Services Administration [HRSA], 1998; NCFH, 2001a).

Migrant and seasonal farm workers are at greater risk and have more complex health problems than the general population because of poverty, malnutrition, infectious diseases, exposure to pesticides, and substandard housing. Acute and chronic respiratory distress due to conditions such as grain fever syndrome, asthma, allergic alveolitis, and chronic bronchitis from occupational exposure to grain dust have been reported. Exposure to pesticides increases the risk of cancer, dermatologic conditions, and chronic ailments. Refer to Table 34-6.

Farm workers suffer from the highest rate of toxic chemical injuries of any group of workers in the U.S. Thousands of pesticides are registered with the EPA and currently in use in the U.S. fields. Three hundred and fifty are registered for use on food crops. At least 101 are probable or possible human carcinogens. In addition to cancer, pesticide exposure has been linked to brain damage, hormone disruption, and birth defects. Both OSHA and the EPA have laws which apply to pesticides, but the agricultural industry has convinced lawmakers to exclude farm workers from federal and state labor legislation and has pressured for weak or nonexistent enforcement of the limited legal rights afforded farm workers. From 1991 to 1996, the California Environmental Protection Agency's Department of Pesticide Regulation (DPR) reported 3991 cases of occupational poisonings by agricultural pesticides, an average of 665 cases per year. The majority of poisonings occur when farm workers are doing fieldwork such as picking, field packing, weeding, and irrigating. Exposure also occurs when swimming or bathing in drain or irrigation ditches. Poor housing and lack of water means a worker is not bathing immediately after exposure, which leads to pro-

TABLE 34-6 Examples of Occupational Hazards for Migrant and Seasonal Farm Workers

OCCUPATIONAL HAZARD	HEALTH PROBLEMS
Farm work	Low back pain, disc disease, arthritis, sprains, carpal tunnel syndrome, lacerations, soft tissue trauma, eye injuries
Toxic chemicals	Pesticide-related dermatitis and conjunctivitis; effects associated with chronic low-level pesticide exposure: headaches, blurred vision, malaise, anxiety, unknown risk for cancer, birth defects
Pterygium	Chronic eye exposure to wind and sun (secondary to)

From Colorado AHEC Program Internet Page, *1997.*

longed contact with toxic substances (Reeves, Schafer, Hallward, & Katten, 1999).

The transient nature of migrant and seasonal farm work makes it difficult for community health nurses to monitor these clients and for clients to obtain adequate treatment. This characteristic of migrant workers is particularly difficult for health care professionals working with clients who have contracted a communicable disease. The most recent study about migrant workers and tuberculosis (TB) states that migrant and seasonal farm workers are approximately six times more likely to develop TB than the general population of employed adults (CDC, 1992). Rural nurses caring for clients who are suspected to have or are diagnosed with TB face challenges in helping their clients obtain adequate care. It is the primary health care provider's responsibility to immediately notify the public health department when they know or suspect that their clients have TB. Notification permits public health officials to examine contacts and initiate other health department diagnostic, preventive, or client management services. Rural public health nurses should help ensure that the following services are available to clients and their family or other contacts (CDC, 1992):

- Detection, diagnosis, appropriate treatment, and monitoring for those who have TB

- Contact investigation and preventive therapy for those exposed to infectious clients, including widespread tuberculin test screening for workers and family screening

Migrants who are placed on antituberculosis treatment or preventive therapy should be given records they can take with them when they move, to indicate their current treatment and diagnostic status. Special care should be taken to instruct them on how to take their medications and how and where to get additional medication and medical care at their new destination. Out-of-state communications regarding TB care should be routed through state health departments to ensure that the information is transmitted appropriately and that necessary follow-up is initiated (CDC, 1992). For more information regarding TB see Chapter 26.

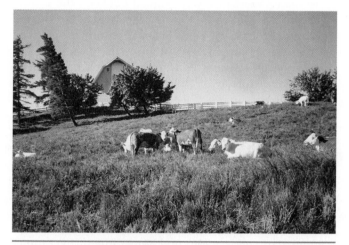

The community health nurse must always consider the values of the community when planning care.

To follow TB clients and provide continuity of care, The Binational Migrant Tuberculoses Referral and Tracking Network Project (TB Net) has been used. Enrolled clients receive a Portable Patient Tuberculosis Record which fits in their wallet and contains pertinent treatment and laboratory information. Clients can present their TB card to any clinic they visit. Providers contact the registry for more detailed information and are responsible to return fax the most current data to the centralized registry (Dougherty, 1996). Considering the difficulties encountered with TB detection, treatment, and follow-up, one can only gasp when confronted with the potential of HIV/AIDS. Fifty percent of farm workers are single males traveling throughout the United States living 10 to a room. The only available health care is emergency room coverage. HIV/AIDS requires intensive medical treatment.

The majority of migrant and seasonal workers are Latino, and diabetes is a particular problem with the Latino community. The CDC established the National Hispanic/Latino Diabetes Initiative for Action in 1995. In 1994, the American Diabetes Association established the Diabetes Assistance & Resources (DAR) program, a nationwide, community-based program to increase diabetes awareness in the Latino community about the seriousness of the disease. It is known that farm workers have more clinic visits for diabetes than for other health problems, and it remains to be studied how complex the problem is in the workforce (D'Arrigo & Keegan, 2000).

Native Americans and Alaska Natives

The Indian Health Service (IHS) is the major federal health care provider to the Native American and Alaska Native people. The original inhabitants of North America are citizens both of their tribes and of the United States. More than 350 treaties were signed between the United States and the Native American tribes between 1784 and 1800. On the basis of treaty rights, the Native American people participate in federal financial programs and other services, such as education and health care. The IHS and the Bureau of Indian Affairs (BIA) administer services under the umbrella of the USDHHS.

The IHS provides health services to approximately 1.5 million American Indians and Alaska Natives who belong to more than 550 federally recognized tribes in 35 states (USDHHS, 2001a). The health status of Native Americans and Alaska Natives is not equal with the general U.S. population. Poor nutrition, unsafe water supplies, and inadequate waste disposal facilities have resulted in greater incidence of illness in the Native American population. Many reservations and Native American communities are located in isolated areas without accessible health care, including a lack of maternal and child health care and other types of preventive health care. The leading cause of death for children and young adults is accidents (USDHHS, 2001a). The leading causes of death for the adult Native American population are (USDHHS, 2001b):

- Diseases of the heart
- Malignant neoplasms
- Accidents
- Diabetes mellitus
- Chronic liver disease and cirrhosis

The IHS has worked with the Public Health Service to improve the health of the Native Americans. Preventive health services are provided by clinical staff at IHS and tribal facilities and by community health personnel working directly with the Native American community. Among the IHS programs that have been designed to reduce mortality and raise life expectancy are the Diabetes Program, the Mental Health Program, the Community Representative Program, the Dental Program, the Accident and Injury Reduction Program, and The Native American Cardiology Program. This major initiative was developed to provide direct cardiovascular care to Native Americans at reservation clinics (USDHHS, 2001a). Community health nurses who are not Native American, however, need to appreciate the difference between Western medicine and Native American healing practices. They work on reservations in the capacity of health educators, substance abuse counselors, and safety program advisors. They will need to recognize that a dual health care system exists and to learn to work cooperatively with tribal healers.

FACTORS INFLUENCING THE RURAL HEALTH CARE DELIVERY SYSTEM

Factors that have affected the delivery of health care in rural areas include the reorganization of health care delivery systems; the availability, accessibility, and acceptability of health care services; and the poverty level of some rural residents.

Availability, Accessibility, and Acceptability of Health Care

One of the great flaws of the present system of medical care is that it is not available to all segments of the population. Medical services must be available, accessible, and acceptable to clients when they decide to seek care. Availability is the existence of essential services and the necessary personnel to provide essential services. Accessibility implies that the client has access to as well as the ability to purchase needed services. Appropriateness and acceptability means that a service is offered in a manner that is congruent with the values of a target population (Bushy, 2000).

Since the 1950s, the traditional method of rural health care delivery has revolved around a hospital with a laboratory for fluid and tissue examination, x-ray capabilities, surgical suites, and an emergency room. A physician needed the support of a hospital to better care for clients. The rural hospital was the center for trauma triage and acute exacerbation of asthma, diabetes, epilepsy, and other chronic conditions. The management of health care has changed in the past decade. Programs have been excised and personnel decreased in efforts to cut costs. Rural hospitals are struggling to keep doors open in the face of competition, accelerating capital and technical requirements, decreased population base, depressed economies, disproportionate rates of uninsurance and poor insurance, and changing federal reimbursement (Hagopian & Hart, 2001). Those that depend on Medicare clients for the majority of their revenue may need to change the type of services offered to benefit from *the Medicare, Medicaid, and SCHIP Balanced Budget Refinement Act of 1999* (BBRA of 1999). For rural hospitals to survive, they will need to expand outpatient services, embrace telemedicine and telehealth initiatives, and seek alternative funding sources (Robinson, Savage, & Grant, 2001).

The federal government has designated areas with a shortage of health care practitioners as Health Professional Shortage Areas (HPSAs), which qualifies them for federal grant dollars. Additionally, National Health Serve Corps (NHSC) offers scholarships or loan repayments in exchange for a period of service at HPSA sites. In 1997 a new nationwide limited-service rural hospital project entitled the Medicare Rural Hospital Flexibility Program (called FLEX program) was created by Congress under the Balanced Budget Act, which established a permanent hospital payment classification certified for Medicare reimbursement called critical access hospitals (CAHs). In order to qualify as a CAH, a hospital must maintain no more than 15 acute-care beds and up to 10 swing beds, keep clients hospitalized on average no more than 96 hours, and provide 24-hour emergency care. As of December 1999, over 100 CAHs have been designated (Henderson & Coopey, 2000).

Poverty of Rural Areas

The demographics of rural populations have led to higher health care costs. This is due to an older population that tends to use more health care services; more widespread poverty and uninsured residents than in urban areas; employers that are less likely than urban employers to offer private health insurance; and the health status of rural residents that is frequently poorer than their urban counterparts [Rural Policy Research Institute (RPRI), 2000].

The number and percentage of U.S. citizens without health insurance continues to increase. Recent U.S. Census Bureau figures indicate that 43.2 million citizens (16.1% of the population) lack health insurance, with rural and frontier residents being more severely affected. Despite having a higher percentage of people 65 and older who qualify for Medicare (18% rural vs. 15% in urban areas), rural America still has a 20% higher rate of uninsurance than its urban counterpart. This higher percentage of uninsurance and underinsurance is a result of having a higher percentage of people who are self-employed, work for small businesses, do seasonal work, or fail to apply for Medicaid (NRHA, 1999a).

The available income for the poor must be spent on necessities such as food, heat, and clothing. Few poor families have enough money to pay cash at the doctor's office or at the prescription counter. Some physicians will not accept the indigent as clients.

LEGISLATION AND PROGRAMS AFFECTING RURAL HEALTH

The last 30 years have been marked with an increase in legislation and public programs aimed at protecting rural health care and improving the status of farm workers.

Examples of *Healthy People 2010* (USDHHS, 2000b) goals and objectives specific to rural life include:

- Access to Quality Health Services: *Goal:* Improve access to comprehensive, high-quality health care services. *Objective: 1-11.* Increase the proportion of persons who have access to rapidly responding prehospital emergency medical services. According to *Healthy People 2010: Objectives for Improving Health,* in rural areas, the capability is defined as an interval of less than 10 minutes from the time an emergency call is placed to arrival on the scene for at least 80% of EMS responses.

- Cancer: *Goal:* Reduce the number of new cancer cases as well as the illness, disability, and death caused by cancer. *Objectives: 3-9.* Increase the proportion of persons who use at least one of the following protective measures that may reduce the risk of skin cancer: avoid the sun between 10 A.M. and 4 P.M., wear sun-protective clothing when exposed to sunlight, use sunscreen with a sun-protective factor (SPF) of 15 or higher, and avoid artificial sources of ultraviolet light.

- Environmental Health: *Goal:* Promote health for all through a healthy environment. *Objective: 8-13.* Reduce pesticide exposures that result in visits to a health care facility. Pesticide exposures include those involving disinfectants, fungicides, herbicides, insecticides, moth repellants, and rodenticides, as defined by the EPA.

- Occupational Safety and Health: *Goal:* Promote the health and safety of people at work through prevention and early intervention. *Objective: 20-8.* Reduce occupational skin diseases or disorders among full-time workers.

Rural Occupational Health and Safety

The Occupational Safety and Health Act of 1970 was enacted "to assure so far as possible every working man and woman in the Nation safe and healthful working conditions and to preserve our human resources" (OSHA, 2001). It established the Occupational Safety and Health Administration (OSHA) and the National Institute for Occupational Safety and Health (NIOSH) as two distinct agencies with separate responsibilities. OSHA is in the U.S. Department of Labor and is responsible for creating and enforcing workplace safety and health regulations. NIOSH is in the U.S. Department of Health and Human Services and is a research agency. They often work together toward the common goal of protecting worker safety and health (OSHA, 2001).

NIOSH is the federal agency responsible for conducting research and making recommendations for the prevention of work-related disease and injury. The institute is part of the Centers for Disease Control and

Prevention (CDC). NIOSH is responsible for conducting research on the full scope of occupational disease and injury, ranging from lung disease in miners to carpal tunnel syndrome in computer users. NIOSH is a diverse organization made up of employees representing a wide range of disciplines including industrial hygiene, nursing, epidemiology, engineering, medicine, and statistics. NIOSH has developed an extensive agricultural safety and health program to address the high risks of injuries and illnesses experienced by workers and families in agriculture (NIOSH, 2001).

The Migrant and Seasonal Agricultural Worker Protection Act

The Migrant and Seasonal Agricultural Worker Protection Act (MSPA), passed in 1983, was designed to provide migrant and seasonal farm workers with specific rights. It gave them protection concerning pay, working conditions, and work-related conditions. It requires farm labor contractors to register with the U.S. Department of Labor and to assure necessary protections for farm workers, agricultural associations, and agricultural employers. A major requirement of employers and contractors under the MSPA is to provide workers with a statement of the conditions of their employment. This law requires that each farm labor contractor, agricultural employer, and agricultural association that recruits any migrant or day-haul worker must provide the following information in writing to each worker:

- Place of employment
- Wage rates to be paid
- Crops and kinds of activities in which the worker is to be employed
- Period of employment
- Transportation, housing, and any other employee benefits to be provided and any costs to be charged to workers
- Existence of any strike, work stoppage, slowdown or interruption of operations by employees at the place of employment
- Whether anyone is paid a commission for items that may be sold to workers while they are employed

The same information must be provided in writing to any seasonal worker, but only if requested. The information must be provided in the language common to the farm worker if they are not fluent in English as necessary and reasonable (USDA, 2001).

The Office of Rural Health Policy

The Office of Rural Health Policy (ORHP), authorized by Congress in December 1987, promotes better health care service in rural America. The ORHP works both within government, at federal, state, and local levels, and with the private sector—with associations, foundations, providers, and community leaders—to seek solutions to rural health care problems. It is responsible for policy advocacy and information development.

ORHP responsibilities include the following:

- Express the views of rural constituencies within the federal government; advise the Secretary of Health and Human Services on the rural impact of the department's policies and regulations.
- Promote **rural health clinics**—clinics that are certified under a federal law to provide care in underserved areas and therefore receive cost-based Medicare and Medicaid reimbursements. In part, because of these efforts, the rural health clinic program has grown dramatically in recent years.
- Provide staff support to the National Advisory Committee on Rural Health. This committee is an 18-member citizens' panel of nationally recognized rural health experts. It was chartered in 1987 to advise the Secretary of Health and Human Services on ways to address health care problems in rural America.
- Promote federal, state, and local cooperation by supporting and working with state offices of rural health. ORHP promotes state and local empowerment to meet rural health needs in several ways: by supporting state offices of rural health; by encouraging the formation of state rural health associations; and by working with a variety of state agencies to improve rural health.

The ORHP administers programs designed to support the direct delivery of services in rural areas by offering competitive grants that promote institutional partnerships that will leverage scarce local resources. The Rural Health Services Outreach Grants may be used for a variety of health or educational services. The types of projects have ranged from creating hospice care, training paramedics, providing community health education, and offering prenatal care (ORHP, 2000).

Congress expanded the rural outreach program in 1997 to include network development grants. These grants are designed for organizations that want to establish formal, vertically integrated (three or more organizations that collectively provide a range of primary and acute-care services) health care services in rural communities. This could include an acute-care facility, a physician group practice, and a home health agency. Rural telemedicine grants are given to increase access to quality care services in underserved rural communities using telecommunications and information technology. Examples include radiology, dermatology, cardiology, orthopedics, gynecology, and mental health care. It is designed to reduce the isolation of rural providers and foster integrated health care delivery systems through network development (ORHP, 2000). Community Health Centers and Migrant Health Clinics is a $1 billion federal grant program that supports community-run health centers in medically underserved areas. It is made up of public or nonprofit providers that offer a specified array of primary care services, including transportation and translation (ORHP, 2000).

The Health Professions Education Programs, under Title VII of the Public Health Services Act, administers $300 million in annual grant dollars for professional education. It administers the Interdisciplinary Rural Training grants, which promote rural health care practice by supporting interdisciplinary training at rural sites, and the Area Health Education Center (AHEC) program, which helps train medical and health professional students in rural areas (ORHP, 2000).

Rural Information Center Health Service

The ORHP initiated a national Rural Information Center Health Service (RICHS) that provides a toll-free line accessible to rural residents throughout the nation. It provides customized assistance to individuals seeking rural health information, searches databases on requested topics, and distributes monographs available from other government offices and agencies to organizations and experts in the field. It posts on its Web site rural health information on funding resources, upcoming conferences, publications, full-text documents, and links to other relevant sites on the World Wide Web.

The National Rural Recruitment and Retention Network

The ORHP supported the development of the National Rural Recruitment and Retention Network to improve the recruitment and retention of health professionals in rural areas. It consists of 45 state-based organizations committed to assisting health professionals to locate suitable practices in rural and frontier areas throughout the country. They have information regarding rural practice sites in their respective states and will assist health professionals and their families to identify the resources necessary to meet their personal and professional needs [National Rural Recruitment and Retention Network (NRRRN), 2001].

ALTERNATIVES TO IMPROVE RURAL HEALTH CARE

Recent advances in technology and the restructuring of health care delivery have improved the outlook for rural health services. See Out of the Box.

Telehealth

Telehealth is the most recent addition in the available improvements for rural health. It is the practice of health care delivery, diagnosis, consultation, treatment, transfer

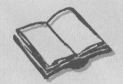

Out
of the Box

Sharing Secrets

"Telecommunication promises to be a viable alternative for supportive interventions in rural areas" (Smith & Weinert, 2000, p. 645). The old party line telephones of 50 years ago have given way to computer networks as a way to communicate with a friend, expand education, and link health care providers or conduct business. Recently computers have been instrumental in providing the necessary components of therapeutic support groups. Women in rural areas have been able to utilize networks to give and receive social support to other women with chronic diseases, cancer, and diabetes. The flexibility of asynchronous but interactive communication plays an important role in the information sharing. This method of sharing secrets appeals to women as the computer mailbox can be accessed at any time. Questions about dry skin, diet, and even sexuality can be asked and answered with complete confidentiality. ∎

Source: Smith, L., & Weinert, C. (2000). Telecommunication support for rural women with diabetes. Diabetes Educator, 26(4), 645–655.

of medical data, and education using interactive audio, video, and data communications. The Office for the Advancement of Telehealth (OAT) reported that 30% of rural hospitals use telemedicine to deliver patient care. Teleradiology is the most prevalent. A survey by the Association of Telemedicine Service Providers estimated that the number of teleconsultations in 1998 had grown to more than 58,000. Consultation from rural areas to urban medical centers regarding cardiology, orthopedics, dermatology, and mental health will soon be followed by consults about management of chronic illness, emergency triage, surgical follow-up, correctional facility care and home health care. Telehealth has often been used to provide a link to primary care services in outlying areas where only a physician assistant or nurse practitioner is available (Telehealth, 1999). Today a client may have an x-ray taken in the local rural health clinic and read by a radiologist at a medical center or home office. Clinical information is shared using available technologies, including electronic mail, the transmission of still images via facsimile, or full interactive video conferencing. Community health nurses can use telehealth to monitor the

REFLECTIVE THINKING

Use of Telehealth

How would you react to a diagnosis given to you by a practitioner reading an x-ray study that had been taken by you at the local rural clinic but read from a computer terminal an eight-hour drive away?

- Would you feel confident in the diagnosis?
- Would you feel that the process is impersonal?

health status of their clients, to transfer client electronic medical records, to assist in diagnosis for clients, and to consult with other professionals. It is a resource for community health nurses for interactive continuing education, and an electronic library.

Emergency Medical Services

Since the late 1960s when civilian emergency medical service (EMS) was first conceptualized and implemented, it has become institutionalized throughout the United States at the intersection of the public safety and the medical care systems. The EMS system is initiated by calling for emergency help or medical assistance, and most citizens expect to immediately receive life-saving medical advice from trained dispatchers, while paramedics and an ambulance race to their aid. EMS is particularly critical to rural and frontier residents because they experience disproportionate levels of serious injuries and their distance from traditional health resources increases the morbidity and mortality associated with trauma and medical emergencies. In many rural and frontier communities, however, these expectations are not met because of long distances, poor roads, difficult terrains, severe climate conditions, lack of or limited telephone service, inadequate public education, organizational instability, underfinancing, inadequate access to training and medical direction, a lack of volunteers willing to commit to the considerable demands of emergency response, and insufficient infrastructure resources to support advanced emergency call systems or reliable radio communications systems between the field and base hospitals (NRHA, 2000).

All emergency personnel answering calls should have training in EMS techniques so that critical first-aid and medical advice can be given to callers before the emergency responders arrive. Dispatch centers should be considered as partners vin implementing triage systems to direct clients to the appropriate level and

source of health care service. In the traditional EMS system, clients in rural and frontier settings often are transported long distances to health care facilities that are not closely affiliated with local health care resources. In some cases, this practice is appropriate because some clients, particularly a severely injured trauma client, may require sophisticated tertiary care. However, far too often this long-distance transportation simply reflects the traditional separation of the EMS service from local primary care providers, public health, and social service agencies that might be able to deal effectively with the needs of the client. It is essential to the health of rural and frontier communities that the EMS system be integrated into a health care system that is cooperative, shares limited health care resources, provides a broad education to the EMS providers, recognizes innovative methods of health care delivery, and is appropriately reimbursed (NRHA, 2000).

Rural Health Clinics

Passage of the federal Rural Health Clinic Services Act of 1977 (P.L. 95-120) provided for establishment of rural health clinics in underserved areas. It also established reimbursement of a fixed price per encounter to clinics. This law increased flexibility and allowed practitioners to see clients in clinics, homes, extended-care facilities, or other settings. Individual states govern the scope of practice of the rural health clinic and its providers. State regulation allows the community to consider its needs and the needs of its diverse population.

THE NURSE'S ROLE IN RURAL COMMUNITY HEALTH NURSING PRACTICE

Bigbee (1993) defines **rural nursing** as the practice of professional nursing within the physical and sociocultural context of sparsely populated communities that involves continual interaction of the rural environment, the nurse, and her practice. It has a rich heritage, especially in rural community health and maternal child health (pp. 131–132).

In 1989 the Rural Nurse Organization was formed. Its official journal is the *Online Journal of Rural Nursing and Health Care*. The International Federation for Rural and Remote Nurses (IFRRN) is a federation of nurses that represents rural nurses worldwide. Currently established, the IFRRN is the world's first and widest reaching international organization for rural and remote nurses.

To meet the health needs of communities, rural community health nurses need to be trained in working with persons from various cultural backgrounds, practicing disease prevention and health promotion in community-based settings, and working in teams with other professionals (Sternas, O'Hare, Lehman, & Milligan, 1999). The

National Institute for Occupational Safety and Health (NIOSH), through its 16 university-based Education and Research Centers (ERCs), supports academic degree programs and research training opportunities in the core areas of industrial hygiene, occupational health nursing, occupational medicine, and occupational safety, plus specialized areas relevant to the occupational safety and health field. Additionally, NIOSH supports ERC short-term continuing education (CE) programs for occupational safety and health professionals and others with worker safety and health responsibilities (NIOSH, 2001).

Rural Nursing

The ANA (1996) cited the following characteristics of rural/frontier nurses:

- Their roles require them to be expert generalists because of the diverse skills they need to work with clients across the life span and with diverse health conditions.

- They need to be independent and self-reliant since they make on-site decisions in clinical settings (homes and rural health clinics) that can be at some distance from support.

- They have community ties and relationships that provide for close client contact and potential for continuity of care, unless they are a newcomer and then will have to gain the trust of the community.

- Social and professional roles intertwine so that inadvertent breaches of confidentiality are a concern.

- They have a positive community visibility that has been linked to professional pride, self-esteem, and a potential role in shaping health policy at the community health agency and community level (ANA, 1996).

Rural community health nurses work in diverse communities that have clients with a variety of health care needs. They are an integral part of a community's health. They are resource persons and role models. Rural health nurses can assess the health needs of the client, family, and community by evaluating their health practices and providing primary care. They can provide counseling, health education, and advocacy services. They need electronic access to the latest nursing, medical, and psychiatric health information to keep up to date in their profession (ANA, 1996).

They need to be resourceful in meeting the preventive and treatment needs of the population, who are often geographically isolated, relatively older, poorer, and less insured. They need to be familiar with their community's resources, and work collaboratively with other health and social service professionals. They will need to prioritize their scarce health resources on the basis of the needs of the populations they serve. They need to be involved in planning, implementing, and coordinating community health programs and services. They may find information from Table 34-3 useful as they begin their planning for the health needs of their communities (ANA, 1996).

Professional-Community-Client Partnerships

The *Healthy People 2010* initiatives are centered on a commitment to collaboration among diverse constituencies so that everyone feels a sense of ownership in the plan. Community health nurses need to identify and work with all entities that influence community health—from other government agencies to businesses to not-for-profit organizations to the general citizenry. Addressing the challenge of health improvement is a shared responsibility that requires the active participation and leadership of the federal government, states, local governments, policymakers, health care providers, professionals, business executives, educators, community leaders, and the public itself.

According to the RPRI (2000), the average rural resident has little idea how important the health sector is to the rural economy. It is needed for business and industrial growth, to attract retirees, and for jobs (RPRI, 2000).

The National Rural Health Association provides a set of principles, based on rural health services research and on the experiences of rural communities, that is correlated with community success in sustaining rural health care systems. The principles include:

- Well-informed community providers and residents who have access to relevant, practical information and successful rural models and who are knowledgeable about state and federal policies that affect rural health services.

- A bold vision of the desired local services and broad communitywide support for and participation in the work to sustain local health services and a willingness to take risks on behalf of their vision.

- Effective local health care leadership and system control of the elements of the delivery system—institutions such as hospitals and long-term care facilities, provider practices, and health care dollars.

- A high level of teamwork, respect, and collaboration among community providers and openness to partnerships and affiliations with other regional providers and with value-compatible urban providers (NRHA, 1998).

Rural hospital closures, difficulty in recruiting physicians, and the ability to establish rural centers of health have stimulated thought on methods aimed at improving

Perspectives...

INSIGHTS OF A RURAL COMMUNITY HEALTH NURSE

When I first began working in a rural community, it was easy to be so burdened with tasks and paperwork that I missed knowing the clients I was serving. As a rural community health nurse, I learned quickly that I needed to have insight into my own culture and the cultures of my clients. I assumed that clients had the same values and background that I had. As I gained more experience, I began to imagine that each client was surrounded by an invisible ring of light that reflected his or her inner life. The ring of light contains cultural practices, religious beliefs, habits, lifestyles, pride, dreams, and hopes. I realized that I could not fully assess clients without first recognizing that the halo exists and that I could not completely care for clients without incorporating it into my interventions. I also learned not to be judgmental and to be extremely careful not to breach client confidentiality, since I saw my clients in more than one role. The grocery clerk from the nearest supermarket was Friday night's alcohol poisoning admission and my referral for substance abuse counseling. The pitcher on my son's baseball team was admitted to the emergency room with bruises; the admitting nurse had to report the father for possible child abuse, and the case was referred to me for follow-up. Community health nurses need to learn as much as possible about their own cultures to understand the basis of their beliefs, to learn about the cultures of the clients they serve, to be nonjudgmental, and to be extremely confidential about their clients' problems. This knowledge will give them a basis for beginning to become compassionate community health nurses.

—Anonymous

rural health. Partnership interventions among community agencies and health and social service professionals are a recent strategy to reduce health risks and to improve rural health services. Community assessment program planning and evaluation were discussed in Chapters 15 and 16 and provide foundational knowledge for community health nurses who wish to participate in partnership interventions for solving community problems. Leaders are needed who have these collaborative skills and who are able to work in partnership with others.

Sensitivity to the rural community's values and lifestyles among the partners is essential to successful outcomes.

A community partnership begins with the identification of a problem area—immunization, cancer screening, or better nutrition, for example. Once an area of need has been identified, the community health nurses gather data to better assess the strengths and weaknesses of the community targeted. Analysis of the data in the community committee format allows sharing of the information and results in setting goals. A task force consisting of a community health officer, community health nurses, and members of the community must then decide what actions need to be taken.

Community health nurses working in a partnership can help beat the barriers in providing clients continuity of care. Client care requirements are complex, regulations are constricting, and reimbursable options for noninstitutional care can be limiting. Acute-care discharge planners need to create collaborative partnerships with other health care providers, such as home health agencies. These partnerships provide for clinical efficiencies and cost avoidance opportunities and are a win-win-win situation for all involved. Additionally, the benefit of partnership is increased accuracy in the level of care and services planned for clients posttransition from acute care (Austin, 1999).

The Health Care Strategic Change Initiative (SCI) of the National Rural Development Partnership (NRDP) is a national network of rural health care leaders and advocates who work through State Rural Development Councils (SRDCs) and with other rural constituents to create opportunities for creative partnerships to improve the health of rural citizens. Its goals are to identify issues and trends in health care that have an impact on rural America and to collect, compile, analyze, and disseminate information about rural health legislation, innovative programming, and other important issues to work to ensure the health care concerns of rural communities are communicated to national, state, and local leaders. Additional goals include providing a forum for idea exchange and opportunities for creative partnerships between SRDCs and other partners (e.g., state offices of rural health, state rural health associations, state hospital associations, and health professional schools) and improving the health and well-being of America's rural communities (NRDP, 2001).

Community-oriented primary health care (COPHC) is an effective model for delivery of primary health care based on the epidemiologically assessed needs of the population. It requires that the health team and the responsible agencies or institutions take upon themselves responsibility for the provision of care in relation to these measured needs of all those persons entitled to the service. The COPHC is an interdisciplinary model which blends primary care, public health, and prevention services (COPC, 1998).

COMMUNITY NURSING VIEW

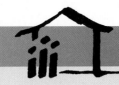

David, a three-year old Native American, was brought to a tribal health center with symptoms of fever, malaise, nausea, abdominal discomfort, and loss of appetite. He appears jaundiced. He lives with his extended family on a large rural Native American reservation. He attends a tribal preschool during the day. David and his family attended the annual salmon festival one week prior to his clinic visit. He was diagnosed with hepatitis A.

Nursing Considerations

Assessment

◆ What other assessment data need to be obtained?

◆ What cultural beliefs would need to be considered?

◆ What issues need to be explored with David? With his family? With the community?

Diagnosis

◆ What nursing diagnoses are appropriate to this client? Family? Community?

◆ What is the priority of his diagnoses?

Outcome Identification

◆ Are David and his contacts successfully identified and treated for hepatitis A?

◆ Do David, his family, and the community (preschool, etc.) understand the risks of hepatitis A and how to prevent it in the future?

◆ Are David, his family, and the community satisfied with the nursing services they received?

Planning/Interventions

◆ How would a contract be developed with this family?

◆ How will the nurse explain the concept of communicable disease to the family?

◆ What teaching with the family would be initiated?

◆ How will the nurse explain to the family that this situation cannot be kept confidential?

◆ How will the nurse explain to the family the need to investigate possible contacts?

◆ What kind of plan would be developed to investigate possible contacts in a rural area?

◆ What referrals would be made to other agencies? Why?

◆ Is it a requirement to report this case to the local health authority? Why or why not?

Evaluation

◆ What will the nurse do if the family or community is noncompliant or misunderstands how to care for David and themselves?

◆ How will the nurse know when to terminate visits with this family?

A primary care case management (PCCM) provider is a provider (usually a physician, physician group practice, or entity employing or having other arrangements with such physicians, nurse practitioners, nurse midwives, or physician assistants) who contracts to locate, coordinate, and monitor covered primary care (and sometimes additional services) (HCFA, 2000). Medicare contracting managed-care plans are required to provide their Medicare enrollees those services that are covered under Medicare and available to other fee-for-service Medicare beneficiaries residing in the geographic area covered by the plan (HCFA, 1999).

Rural community health nurses are in an excellent position to contribute to the research agenda and to improve the quality of care for their clients and the community. Areas of concern are maintaining access to quality health care services and developing a sustainable delivery system. They must be a part of the national, statewide, and local coalition building and information sharing to rebuild or improve their community's health care systems. They need to form recruitment networks to draw interested nurses and other health care practitioners to their communities.

 KEY CONCEPTS

◆ Rural health nursing has had a diverse history, with nurses working in the battlefields, small hospitals, clinics, and currently through telecommunications.

◆ Rurality is a complex concept that is defined by different standards by different federal agencies and researchers.

◆ Rural counties are diverse both economically and by policy types.

◆ Rural and urban residents' differences are due to demographic or socioeconomic composition of the areas in which they live, not necessarily their values.

◆ Rural minorities are at risk for health problems because of the nature of their work, lifestyles, and lack of adequate health care resources.

◆ Owing to the nature of their jobs, migrant and seasonal farm workers are exposed to many potential health problems and often only have intermittent follow-up care.

◆ Federal legislation affects the availability of health programs to rural residents.

◆ Regional health networks such as telehealth and emergency medical services are an alternative for providing health care to rural communities.

◆ Rural community health nurses must be expert generalists, independent, and self-reliant.

◆ Rural community health nurses see clients in professional as well as social roles, so confidentiality must be closely guarded.

RESOURCES

National Association for Rural Mental Health: www.narmh.org

National Organization of State Offices of Rural Health: www.ruralcenter.org/nosorh

National Rural Health Association: www.nrharural.org

National Rural Health Resource Center: www.ruralcenter.org/nrhrc

National Rural Health Services Research Database: www.muskie.usm.maine.edu/research

National Rural Recruitment and Retention Network: www.3rnet.org

North Carolina Rural Health Research Center: www.shepscenter.unc.edu

Office for the Advancement of Telehealth (HRSA): http://telehealth.hrsa.gov

Office of Rural Health Policy (HRSA): http://www.ruralhealth.hrsa.gov

Project HOPE Walsh Center for Rural Health Analysis: www.projhope.org/CHA

Rural Health Policy Research Institute (RUPRI): www.rupri.org

Rural Information Center Health Service (RICHS): www.nal.usda.gov/ric/richs

Rural Nurse Organization: http://www.rno.org

Rural PSYCH_Resource Center for Rural Behavioral Health: www.apa.org/rural

WWAMI Rural Health Research Center: www.fammed.washington.edu/wamirhrc

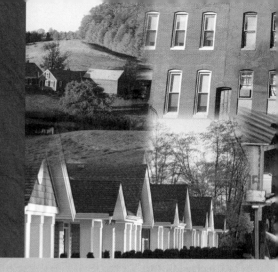

APPENDIX A
Community Resources

U.S. HEALTH-RELATED ORGANIZATIONS—GENERAL

American Health Care Association (AHCA)
1201 L Street, NW
Washington, DC 20005
(202) 842-4444
http://www.ahca.org

American Health Foundation
201 East 42nd Street 675
New York, NY 10017
(212) 953-1982
http://www.ahf.org

American Public Health Association (APHA)
800 I Street Northwest
Washington, DC 20001
(202) 777-APHA
http://www.apha.org

Department of Health and Human Services
200 Independence Avenue, SW
Washington, DC 20201
(877) 696-6775
http://www.os.dhhs.gov

Division for Vital Records and Health Statistics
Michigan Department of Public Health
P.O. Box 30721
Lansing, MI 48909
(517) 335-8666
http://www.mdch.state.mi.us

Food and Drug Administration
5600 Fishers Lane
Rockville, Maryland 20857
(888) 463-6332
http://www.fda.gov

W.K. Kellogg Foundation
One Michigan Avenue East
Battle Creek, Michigan 49017-4058
(616) 968-1611
http://www.wkkf.org

Rockefeller Foundation
420 Fifth Avenue
New York, NY 10018-2702
(212) 852-8483
http://www.rockfound.org

U.S. HEALTH-RELATED ORGANIZATIONS—SPECIFIC

Aging

Alliance for Retired Americans
888 16th St. NW
Washington, DC 20006
(888) 373-6497
http://www.retiredamericans.org

American Association of Homes & Services for the Aging
2519 Connecticut Ave. NW
Washington, DC 20008
(202) 783-2242
http://www.aahsa.org

American Association of Retired Persons
601 E. St., NW
Washington, DC 20049
(800) 424-3410
http://www.aarp.org

American Geriatrics Society
Empire State Building
350 Fifth Avenue, Suite 801,
New York, NY 10018
(212) 308-1414
http://www.americangeriatrics.org

American Society on Aging
833 Market Street, Suite 511
San Francisco, CA 94103
(415) 974-9600
http://www.asaging.org

Gray Panthers
733 15th Street, NW, Suite 437
Washington, DC 20005
(800) 280-5362 or (202) 737-6637
http://www.graypanthers.org

Health Promotion Institute
c/o National Council on Aging
400 3rd St. SW, Suite 200
Washington, DC 20024
(202) 479-1200
http://www.ncoa.org

National Council on the Aging
409 3rd Street, SW
Washington, DC 20024
(202) 479-1200
http://www.ncoa.org

Child Health

American School Health Association
7263 State Route 43
P.O. Box 708
Kent, OH 44240
(330) 678-1601
http://www.ashaweb.org

Learning Disabilities Association of America
4156 Library Road
Pittsburgh, PA 15234-1349
(412) 341-1515
http://www.ldanatl.com

National Information Center for Children and Youth with Disabilities
P.O. Box 1492
Washington, DC 20013
(800) 695-0285
http://www.nichcy.org

National Institute of Child Health and Human Development
Bldg 31, Room 2A32, MSC 2425
31 Center Drive
Bethesda, MD 20892-2425
(800) 370-2943
http://www.nichd.nih.gov

Death and Dying

Children's Hospice International
901 North Pitt St., Suite 230
Alexandria, VA 22314
(703) 684-0330, (800) 2-4-CHILD
http://www.chionline.org

The National Hospice and Palliative Care Organization
1700 Diagonal Road, Suite 625
Alexandria, VA 22314
(703) 837-1500
http://www.nhpco.org

Dental Health and Treatment

American Dental Association
211 East Chicago Avenue
Chicago, IL 60611
(312) 440-2500
http://www.ada.org

Disabilities (General)

March of Dimes Birth Defects Foundation
1275 Mamaroneck Avenue
White Plains, NY 10605
(888) 663-4637
http://www.modimes.org

National Organization on Disability
910 16th Street, NW, Room 600
Washington, DC 20006
(202) 293-5960
http://www.nod.org

National Parent Network on Disabilities (NPND)
1130 17th St. NW, Suite 400
Washington, DC 20036
(202) 463-2299
http://www.npnd.org

Society for Accessible Travel & Hospitality (SATH)
347 Fifth Ave., Suite 610
New York, NY 10016
(212) 447-7284
http://www.sath.org

Disabilities (Mental)

Association for Children and Adults with Learning Disabilities
4900 Girard Road
Pittsburgh, PA 15227
(412) 881-2263
http://www.acldonline.org

Association for Retarded Citizens, National Headquarters Office
1010 Wayne Ave., Suite 650
Silver Spring, MD 20910
(301) 565-3842
http://www.thearc.org

Autism Society for America
7910 Woodmont Avenue, Suite 300
Bethesda, MD 20814-3067
(800) 657-0881
(800) 3AUTISM, (301) 657-0881
http://www.autism-society.org

National Association for Down's Syndrome
P.O. Box 4542
Oak Park, IL 60522
(630) 325-9112
http://www.nads.org

National Center for Learning Disabilities
381 Park Avenue South, Suite 1401
New York, NY 10016
(888) 575-7373
http://www.ncld.org

Stuttering Foundation of America
3100 Walnut Grove Road, Suite 603
P.O. Box 11749
Memphis, TN 38111-0749
(800) 992-9392
http://www.stuttersfa.org

Disabilities (Physical)

Alexander Graham Bell Association for the Deaf
3417 Volta Place, NW
Washington, DC 20007-2778
(202) 337-5220
http://www.agbell.org

American Foundation for the Blind, Headquarters
11 Penn Plaza, Suite 300
New York, NY 10001
(212) 502-7600
http://www.afb.org

Association for Education and Rehabilitation of the Blind & Visually Impaired
4600 Duke Street, #430
P.O. Box 22397
Alexandria, VA 22304
(703) 823-9690
http://www.aerbvi.org

Braille Institute
741 North Vermont Avenue
Los Angeles, CA 90029
(323) 663-1111
http://www.brailleinstitute.org

National Center on Physical Activity and Disability (NCPAD)
1640 W. Roosevelt Road
Chicago, IL 60608-6904
(800) 900-8086
http://www.uic.edu/orgs/ncpad

Winners on Wheels
2842 Business Park Avenue
Fresno, CA 93727
(800) WOWTALK
http://www.wowusa.com

Disaster Care

American Red Cross
P.O. Box 37243
Washington, DC 20013
(800) 435-7669
http://www.redcross.org

The Salvation Army
615 Slaters Lane
P.O. Box 269
Alexandria, VA 22313
(703) 684-5500
http://www.salvationarmy.org

Disease/Disorder Prevention and Research

Alzheimer's Association National Office
919 North Michigan Avenue
Suite 1100
Chicago, IL 60611-1676
(800) 272-3900 or (312) 335-8700
http:www.alz.org

American Cancer Society, Inc.
1599 Clifton Rd. NE
Atlanta, GA 30329
(800) 227-2345
http://www.cancer.org

American Diabetes Association National Service Center
1701 North Beauregard Street
Alexandria, VA 22311
(800) 342-2383
http://www.diabetes.org/ada

American Epilepsy Society
342 North Main Street
West Hartford, CT 06117-2507
(860) 586-7505
http://www.aesnet.org

American Heart Association, Inc. (AHA)
7272 Greenville Avenue
Dallas, TX 75231
(800) AHA-USA1
http://www.americanheart.org

American Liver Foundation
75 Maiden Lane
Suite 603
New York, NY 10038
(800) 465-4837
http://www.liverfoundation.org

American Lung Association
1740 Broadway
New York, NY 10019
(212) 315-8700
http://www.lungusa.org

American Parkinson Disease Association
1250 Hylan Blvd. Ste 4B
Staten Island, NY 10305
(800) 223-2732
http://www.apdaparkinson.com

Arthritis Foundation
1330 West Peachtree St.
Atlanta, GA 30309
(404) 872-7100
http://www.arthritis.org

Asthma and Allergy Foundation of America (AAFA)
1233 20th Street, NW
Suite 402
Washington, DC 20036
(800) 727-8462 or (202) 462-7643
http://www.aafa.org

Centers for Disease Control and Prevention (CDC)
1600 Clifton Road, NE
Atlanta, GA 30333
(800) 311-3435
http://www.cdc.gov

Hepatitis Foundation International
30 Sunrise Terrace
Cedar Grove, NJ 07009-1423
(973) 239-1035 or (800) 891-0707
http://www.hepfi.org

Huntington's Disease Society of America
158 West 29th Street, 7th Floor
New York, NY 10001-5300
(800) 345-hdsa
http://www.hdsa.org

Juvenile Diabetes Foundation International
120 Wall St.
New York, NY 10005
(800) 533-CURE
http://www.jdf.org

Leukemia & Lymphoma Society, Inc.
1311 Mamaroneck Ave.
White Plains, NY 10605
(914) 949-5213
http://www.leukemia-lymphoma.org

Living Bank
4545 Post Oak Place Drive
Houston, TX 77027
(713) 528-2971 or (800) 528-2971
http://www.livingbank.org

Lupus Foundation of America
1300 Piccard Drive
Suite 200
Rockville, MD 20850-4303
(301) 670-9292 or (800) 558-0121
http://www.lupus.org

Mended Hearts, Inc.
c/o American Heart Association
7272 Greenville Ave.
Dallas, TX 75231
(419) 472-4351
http://www.mendedhearts100.com

Multiple Sclerosis Association of America
706 Haddonfield Road
Cherry Hill, NJ 08002
(800) 532-7667
http://www.msaa.com

Muscular Dystrophy Association
3300 E. Sunrise Drive
Tucson, AZ 85718
(800) 572-1717
http://www.mdausa.org

Myasthenia Gravis Foundation of America
5841 Cedar Lake Road
Suite 204
Minneapolis, MN 55416
(800) 541-5454 or (952) 545-9438
http://www.myasthenia.org

National Cancer Institute
Building 31, Room 10A 31
31 Center Drive, MSC 2580
Bethesda, MD 20892-2580
(301) 435-3848 or (800) 422-6237
http://www.nci.nih.gov

National Hemophilia Foundation
116 West 32nd Street, 11th Floor
New York, NY 10001
(212) 328-3700 or (800) 42HANDI
http://www.hemophilia.org

National Institute of Neurological Disorders and Stroke (NINDS)
Neuroscience Center—Division of Extramural Research
6001 Executive Boulevard
Suite 3309
Bethesda, MD 20892-9531
(301) 496-9746 or (800) 352-9424
http://www.ninds.nih.gov

National Kidney Foundation, Inc.
30 East 33rd St., Suite 1100
New York, NY 10016
(800) 622-9010
http://www.kidney.org

National Organization for Rare Disorders, Inc.
P.O. Box 8923
New Fairfield, CT 06812-8923
(203) 746-6518 or (800) 999-6673
http://www.rarediseases.org

National Osteoporosis Foundation
1232 22nd Street NW
Washington, DC 20037-1292
(202) 223-2226
http://www.nof.org

National Tay-Sachs & Allied Diseases Association
2001 Beacon St., Suite 204
Brighton, MA 02135
(800) 906-8723
http://www.ntsad.org

United Cerebral Palsy/ New York City
Mktg Dept.
80 Maiden Lane, 8th floor
NY, NY 10038
(800) GIVEUCP or (212) 683-6700 x212
http://www.ucpnyc.org

Ethnic Health

Asian & Pacific Islander American Health Forum
942 Market Street, Suite 200
San Francisco, CA 94102
(415) 954-9988; and
440 1st Street NW
Suite 430
Washington, DC 20001
(202) 624-0007
http://www.apiahf.org

Indian Health Services
5300 Homestead Road, NE
Albuquerque, NM 87110
(505) 248-4115
http://www.ihs.gov

National Indian Health Board
1385 So. Colorado Blvd, Suite A-707
Denver, CO 80222
(303) 759-3075
http://www.nihb.org

Fitness

Aerobics and Fitness Association of America
15250 Ventura Boulevard
Suite 200
Sherman Oaks, CA 91403-3297
(877) 968-7263
http://www.afaa.com

American Alliance for Health, Physical Education, Recreation & Dance
1900 Association Drive
Reston, Virginia 20191-1598
(800) 213-7193
http://www.aahperd.org

National Association for Health & Fitness
401 W. Michigan St.
Indianapolis, IN 46202-3233
(317) 955-0957
http://www.physicalfitness.org

Health Care Delivery

Agency for Healthcare Research and Quality
2101 E. Jefferson St., Suite 501
Rockville, MD 20852
(301) 594-1364
http://www.ahcpr.gov

Health Care Financing Administration (HCFA)
Centers for Medicare & Medicaid Services
7500 Security Boulevard
Baltimore, MD 21244-1850
(410) 786-3000
http://www.hcfa.hhs.gov

National Association for Home Care
228 Seventh Street, SE
Washington, DC 20003
(202) 547-7424
http://www.nahc.org

Injury Treatment and Prevention

Agency for Toxic Substances and Disease Registry (ATSDR)
1600 Clifton Rd., NE
Mail Stop E-28
Atlanta, GA 30333
(404) 498-0004 or (888) 422-8737
http://www.atsdr.cdc.gov

American Association of Poison Control Centers
3201 New Mexico Avenue, Suite 310
Washington, DC 20016
(202) 362-7217
http://www.aapcc.org

American Burn Association (ABA)
625 N. Michigan Ave., Ste 1530
Chicago, IL 60611
(312) 642-9260 or (800) 548-2876
http://www.ameriburn.org

Consumer Product Safety Commission
4330 East-West Highway
Bethesda, MD 20814-4408
(301) 504-0990
http://www.cpsc.gov

National Safety Council
1121 Spring Lake Drive
Itasca, IL 60143-3201
(630) 285-1121
http://www.nsc.org

Maternal/Child Health

Administration for Children and Families
U.S. Department of Health and Human Services
200 Independence Ave. SW
Washington, DC 20201
(202) 619-0257 or (877) 696-6775
http://www.hhs.gov

American Society for Reproductive Medicine
1209 Montgomery Highway
Birmingham, AL 35216-2809
(205) 978-5000
http://www.ASRM.org

International Childbirth Education Association
P.O. Box 20048
Minneapolis, MN 55420
(952) 854-8660
http://www.ICEA.org

La Leche League International
1400 N. Meacham Rd.
Schaumburg, IL 60173
(847) 519-7730
http://www.lalecheleague.org

Maternal and Child Health Bureau
Health Resources and Services Administration, HHS
Parklawn Building Room 18-05
5600 Fishers Lane
Rockville, MD 20857
(301) 443-2250
http://www.mchb.hrsa.gov

National Association of Childbearing Centers
3123 Gottschall Road
Perkiomenville, PA 18074-9546
(215) 234-8068
http://www.birthcenters.org

National Sudden Infant Death Syndrome Foundation
8200 Professional Plaza, Suite 104
Landover, MD 20785
(800) 221-SIDS
http://www.sidsalliance.org

Planned Parenthood Federation of America
810 Seventh Street
New York, NY 10019
(212) 541-7800
http://www.plannedparenthood.org

Mental Illness

American Association of Suicidology
4201 Connecticut Avenue, NW
Suite 408
Washington, DC 20008
(202) 237-2280
http://www.suicidology.org

National Hotline Network: 800-SUICIDE

American Counseling Association
5999 Stevenson Ave.
Alexandria, VA 22304-3300
(800) 347-6647
http://www.counseling.org

National Alliance for the Mentally Ill (NAMI)
Colonial Place Three
2107 Wilson Blvd., Suite 300
Arlington, VA 22201
(800) 950-6264
http://www.nami.org

National Mental Health Association
1021 Prince Street
Alexandria, VA 22314-2971
(703) 684-7722
http://www.nmha.org

Migrant Health

Migrant Clinicians Network
P.O. Box 164285
1001 Land Creek Cove
Austin, TX 78716
(512) 327-2017
http://www.migrantclinician.org

National Center for Farmworker Health, Inc.
1770 FM 967
Buda, TX 78610
(512) 312-2700
http://www.ncfh.org

Nursing Organizations

American Association of Occupational Health Nurses, Inc. (AAOHN)
2920 Brandywine Road, Suite 100
Atlanta, GA 30341
(770) 455-7757
http://www.aaohn.org

American Nurses Association (ANA)
600 Maryland Avenue, SW
Suite 100 W.
Washington, DC 20024-2571
(800) 274-4ANA
http://www.nursingworld.org

Hospice and Palliative Nurses Association
Penn Center West One, Suite 229
Pittsburg, PA 15276
(412) 787-9301
http://www.hpna.org

International Association of School Nurses
P.O. Box 1300
Scarborough, ME 04070-1300
(207) 883-2117 or (877) 627-6476
http://www.nasn.org

National Nurses Society on Addictions (NNSA)
1500 Sunday Dr., Suite 102
Raleigh, NC 27607
(919) 783-5871
http://www.intnsa.org

Nurse Healers-Professional Associates, Inc. (NH-PA)
3760 South Highland Drive
Suite 429
Salt Lake City, UT 84106
(801) 273-3399
http://www.therapeutic-touch.org

Visiting Nurse Associations of America
11 Beacon Street, Suite 910
Boston, MA 02108
(617) 523-4042
http://www.vnaa.org

Nutritional Health

National Dairy Council
Contact local Dairy Council
http://www.Nationaldairycouncil.org

Society for Nutrition Education
N. Meridian, Suite 200
Indianapolis, IN 46260
(800) 235-6690
http://www.sne.org

Occupational and Environmental Health

The EnviroLink Network
5801 Beacon St., Suite 2
Pittsburgh, PA 15217
(412) 689-6400
http://www.envirolink.netforchange.com

Extension Toxicology Network (EXTOXNET)
University of Davis
Davis, CA 95616-8588
(916) 752-2936
http://www.ace.ace.orst.edu/info/extoxnet/ghindex.html

Job Accommodation Network
West Virginia University
P.O. Box 6080
Morgantown, WV 26506-6080
(800) 526-7234
www.jan.wvu.edu

National Coalition Against the Misuse of Pesticides (NCAMP)
701 E Street, SE, Suite 200
Washington, DC 20003
(202) 543-5450
http://www.beyondpesticides.org

National Environmental Health Association
720 South Colorado Boulevard
Suite 970-S
Denver, CO 80246-1925
(303) 756-9090
http://www.neha.org

National Institute for Occupational Safety and Health (NIOSH)
Hubert H. Humphrey Building
200 Independence Avenue, SW
Room 715H
Washington, DC 20201
(800) 35-NIOSH
http://www.cdc.gov/niosh/homepage.html

Occupational Safety and Health Administration (OSHA)
U.S. Department of Labor
200 Constitution Avenue, NW
Room 3647
Washington, DC 20210
Office of Information and Consumer Affairs:
(202) 693-2400
Office of Statistics: (202) 219-6463
http://www.osha.gov

Pesticide Education Center
P.O. Box 420870
San Francisco, CA 94142-0870
(415) 391-8511
http://www.igc.apc.org/pesticides

Society for Occupational and Environmental Health
6278 Old McLean Village Drive
McLean, VA 22101
(703) 556-9222
http://www.soeh.org

U.S. Environmental Protection Agency (EPA)
1200 Pennsylvania Ave. NW
Washington, DC 20460
Contact specific regions
http://www.epa.gov

Rural Health

National Association of Rural Health Clinics
426 C Street, NE
Washington, DC 20002
(202) 543-0348
http://www.narhc.org

National Association for Rural Mental Health
3700 W. Division Street, Suite 105
St. Cloud, MN 56301
(320) 202-1820
http://www.narmh.org

National Organization of State Offices of Rural Health
Office of Community and Rural Health
P.O. Box 47834
Olympia, WA 98504-7834
(360) 705-6762
http://www.ruralcenter.org/nosorh

National Rural Health Association (NRHA)
1 West Armour Boulevard, Suite 203
Kansas City, MO 64111-2087
(816) 756-3140
http://www.nrharural.org

Rural Information Center Health Service (RICHS)
National Agricultural Library
Room 304, 11301 Baltimore Avenue
Beltsville, MD 20705-2351
(800) 633-7701; (301) 504-5547
http://www.nal.usda.gov/ric/richs

Sexual Health

American Association of Sex Educators, Counselors and Therapists (AASECT)
P.O. Box 5488
Richmond, VA 23220-0488
State offices listed on the Internet
http://www.AASECT.org

The Society for the Scientific Study of Sexuality
P.O. Box 416
Allentown, PA 18105-0416
(610) 530-2483
http://www.sexscience.org

Substance Abuse/Addictions

AL-ANON and ALATEEN Family Group Headquarters, Inc.
1600 Corporate Landing Parkway
Virginia Beach, VA 23454
No telephone contact
http://www.al-anon.org

Alcoholics Anonymous World Services
P.O. Box 459
Grand Central Station
New York, NY 10163
http://www.Alcoholics-anonymous.org

Alcohol and Drug Problems Association of North America, Inc.
307 North Main Street
St. Charles, MO 63301
(314) 589-6702
http://www.adpana.com

National Committee for the Prevention of Alcoholism and Drug Dependency
12501 Old Columbia Pike
Silver Springs, MD 20904
(301) 680-6719
http://www.odphp.osophs.dhhs.gov

National Council on Alcoholism and Drug Dependence, Inc. (NCADD)
20 Exchange Place, Suite 2902
New York, NY 10005
(212) 269-7797
http://www.ncadd.org

Wellness

National Wellness Institute
1300 College Court
P.O. Box 827
Stevens Point, WI 54481-0827
(715) 342-2969
http://www.nationalwellness.org

Wellness Councils of America
President: 9802 Nicholas Street
Suite 315
Omaha, NE 68114
(402) 827-3590
http://www.welcoa.org

Women's Health

National Women's Health Resource Center
5255 Loughboro Road, NM
Washington, DC 20016
(877) 986-9472
http://www.healthywomen.org

Nursing Network on Violence Against Women
PMB165, 1801 H St.
Modesto, CA 95354-1215
(888) 909-9993
http://www.nnvawi.org

CANADIAN HEALTH-RELATED ORGANIZATIONS-GENERAL

(List compiled by Tania Nahulak, Judy Seguin, Cindy Zachow, and Chantelle Grahma, who were nursing students at Okanagan University College, Kelowna, British Columbia, when the list was compiled.)

Canadian Medical Association
1867 Alta Vista Drive
Ottawa, Ontario K1G 3Y6
(613) 731-9331 or (800) 457-4205
http://www.cma.ca

Canadian Public Health Association
1565 Carling Avenue, Suite 400
Ottawa, Ontario K1Z 8R1
(613) 725-3769
http://www.cpha.ca

David Foster Foundation Society
3795 Carey Road
Victoria, British Columbia V8Z 6T8
(250) 475-1223
http://www.davidfosterfoundation.org

Health Canada (General Inquiries)
A.L. 090 0C2
Ottawa, Ontario K1A 0K9
(613) 957-2991
http://www.hc-sc.gc.ca

Statistics Canada
National Capital Region Statistics Canada
R.H. Coats Building, Lobby
Holland Avenue
Ottawa, Ontario K1A 0T6
(800) 263-1136
http://www.statcan.ca/start.html

CANADIAN HEALTH-RELATED ORGANIZATIONS-SPECIFIC

Aging

The Canadian Association on Gerontology
100 – 824 Meath Street
Ottawa, Ontario K1Z 6E8
(613) 728-9347
http://www.cagacg.org

Health Canada's Division of Aging and Seniors
Population Health Dictorate, Health Canada
Address Locator: 1908A1
(613) 952-7606
http://www.hc-sc.gc.ca

Alternative Medicine

Acupuncture Foundation of Canada Institute
2131 Lawrence Avenue East
Suite 204
Scarborough, Ontario M1R 5G4
(416) 752-3988
http://www.afcinstitute.com

Canadian Association for Music Therapy
Wilfrid Laurier University
Waterloo, Ontario, N2L 3C5
(519) 884-1970 ext. 6828 or
 (800) 996-CAMT
http://www.musictherapy.ca

Child Health

Canadian Child Care Federation
201-383 Parkdale Ave. Suite 201
Ottawa, Ontario K1Y 4R4
(800) 858-1412
http://www.cfc_efc.ca/cccf

Canadian Foundation for the Study of Infant Deaths
586 Eglinton Ave. East, Suite 308
Toronto, Ontario, M4P 1P2
(800) END-SIDS or (416) 488-3260
http://www.sidscanada.org

Canadian Institute of Child Health
384 Bank Street, Suite 300
Ottawa, Ontario, K2P 1Y4
(613) 230-8838
http://www.cich.ca

Kids Help Phone/Jeunesse J'Ecoute
439 University Avenue, Suite 300
Toronto, Ontario M5G 1Y8
(416) 586-5437
http://www.kidshelp.sympatico.ca

Community Care

Canadian Association for Community Care
45 Rideau Street, Suite 701
Ottawa, Ontario, K1N 5W8
(613) 241-7510
http://www.cace-acssc.com

Death and Dying

The Canadian Hospice Palliative Care Association
43 Bruyère Street, Suite 131C
Ottawa, Ontario K1N 5C8
(800) 668-2785
http://www.cpca.net

Dying with Dignity
155 Eglinton Avenue East, Suite 705
Toronto, Ontario M4P 1G8
(800) 495-6156
http://www.web.apc.org/dwd

Dental Health and Treatment

Canadian Dental Association
1815 Alta Vista Drive
Ottawa, Ontario K1G 3Y6
(613) 532-1770
http://www.cda-adc.ca

Disabilities (General)

Active Living Alliance for Canadians with a Disability
720 Belfast Road, Suite 104
Ottawa, Ontario K1G 0Z5
(613) 244-0052
(800) 771-0663
http://www.ala.ca

Canadian Abilities Foundation
489 College Street, Suite 501
Toronto, Ontario M6G 1A5
(416) 923-1885
http://www.enablelink.org

Neil Squire Foundation—National Office
2250 Boundary Road, Suite 220
Burnaby, British Columbia V5M 3Z3
(604) 473-9363
http://www.neilsquire.ca

Disabilities (Physical)

Association for the Neurologically Disabled of Canada (ANDC)
59 Clement Road
Etobicoke, Ontario N9R 1Y5
(800) 561-1497
http://www.and.ca

Canadian Association of the Deaf
251 Bank Street, Suite 203
Ottawa, Ontario K2P 1X3
(613) 565-2882
http://www.cad.ca

Canadian Association for People Who Stutter (CAPS)
P.O. Box 440
Montreal, Quebec H4A 3P8
(888) 788-8837
http://www.webcon.net/~caps

Canadian Down Syndrome Society
811 14 Street, NW
Calgary, Alberta T2N 2A4
(403) 270-8500
http://www.cdss.ca

Canadian Foundation for Physically Disabled Persons
731 Runnymede Road
Toronto, Ontario M6N 3V7
(416) 760-7351
http://www3.sympatico.ca/whynot

Canadian Hard of Hearing Association
2435 Holly Lane, Suite 205
Ottawa, Ontario K1V 7P2
(613) 526-1584
(800) 263-8068
http://www.netfx.ca/chha-nc

Canadian National Institute for the Blind-Toronto
1929 Bayview Avenue
Toronto, Ontario M4G 3E8
(416) 486-2500
http://www.cnib.ca

Canadian Paraplegic Association-National
1101 prom. Prince of Wales Drive
Suite 230
Ottawa, Ontario K2C 3W7
(613) 723-1033
(800) 720-4933
http://www.canparaplegic.org national

Canadian Spinal Research Organization
120 Newkirk Road, Unit 2
Richmond Hill, Ontario L4C 9S7
(905) 508-4000
http://www.csro.com

Easter Seals/March of Dimes National Council
90 Eglinton Avenue East
Suite 511
Toronto, Ontario M4P 2Y3
(416) 932-8382
http://www.esmodnc.org

Learning Disabilities Association of Canada
323 Chapel Street, Suite 200
Ottawa, Ontario K1N 7Z2
(613) 238-5721
http://www.ldac-taac.ca

Disaster Care

Canadian Red Cross—National Office
170 Metcalf Street
Ottawa, Ontario K2P 2P2
(613) 740-1900
http://www.redcross.ca

Disease/Disorder Prevention and Research

Asthma Society of Canada
130 Bridgeland Ave., Suite 425
Toronto, Canada M6A 1Z4
(416) 787-4050 or (800) 787-3880
http://www.asthmasociety.com

Autism Society of Canada
P.O. Box 65
Orangeville, Ontario L9W
(519) 942-8720
http://www.autismsocietycanada.ca

Autism Treatment Services of Canada
404 94th Avenue SE
Calgary, Alberta T2J 0E8
(403) 253-6961
http://www.autism.ca

Breast Cancer Society of Canada
401 St. Clair St.
Point Edward, Ontario N7V 1P2
(519) 336-0746 or (800) 567-8767
http://www.bcsc.ca

Canadian Cancer Society (National Office)
10 Alcorn Ave., Suite 200
Toronto, Ontario M4V 3B1
(416) 961-7223
http://www.cancer.ca

Canadian Cardiovascular Society
222 Queen St., Suite 1403
Ottawa, Ontario K1P 5V9
(613) 569-3407
http://www.ccs.ca

Canadian Diabetes Association
15 Toronto St., Suite 800
Toronto, Ontario M5C 2E3
(416) 363-3373 or (800) 226-8464
http://www.diabetes.ca

Canadian Cystic Fibrosis Foundation
1992 Yonge St, Suite 207
Toronto, Ontario M45 1Z7
(416) 932-3900
http://www.cysticfibrosis.ca

Canadian Hemophilia Society
625 President Kennedy Ave.
Suite 1210
Montreal, Quebec H3A 1K2
(800) 668-2686 or (514) 848-0503
http://www.hemophilia.ca

Canadian Infectious Disease Society
2197 Riverside Dr., Suite 504
Ottawa, Ontario K1H 7X3
(613) 260-3233
http://www.cids.medical.org

Canadian Lung Association
3 Raymond St., Suite 300
Ottawa, Ontario K1R 1A3
(613) 569-6411
http://www.lung.ca

Childhood Cancer Foundation-Candlelighters Canada
55 Eglinton Ave. East, Suite 401
Toronto, Ontario M4P 1G8
(416) 489-6440 or (800) 363-1062
http://www.candlelighters.ca

Crohn's and Colitis Foundation of Canada
60 St. Clair Ave East, Suite 600
Toronto, Ontario M4T 1N5
(416) 920-5035
http://www.ccfc.ca

Heart and Stroke Foundation of Canada
222 Queen St., Suite 1402
Ottawa, Ontario K1P 5V9
(613) 569-4361
http://www2.heartandstroke.ca

Kidney Foundation of Canada
5165 Sherbrooke St. West, Suite 300
Montreal, Quebec H4A 1T6
(514) 369-4806 or (800) 361-7494
http://www.kidney.ca

Multiple Sclerosis Society of Canada
250 Bloor St. East, Suite 1000
Toronto, Ontario M4W 3P9
(416) 922-6065
http://www.mssociety.ca

Parkinson Society Canada
4211 Yonge St., Suite 316
Toronto, Ontario M2P 2A9
(416) 227-9700 or (800) 565-3000
http://www.parkinson.ca

Sleep/Wake Disorders Canada
3080 Yonge St., Suite 5055
Toronto, Ontario M4N 3N1
(418) 483-9654
http://www.swdca.org

Spina Bifida and Hydrocephalus Association of Canada
167 Lombard Ave., #167
Winnipeg, Manitoba R3B 0T6
(204) 925-3650
http://www.sbhac.ca

Family Health

Canadian Association of Family Resource Programs
331 Cooper St., Suite 707
Ottawa, Ontario K2P 0G5
(613) 237-7667
http://www.frp.ca

One Parent Families Association of Canada
1099 Kingston Rd., Suite 222
Pickering, Ontario L1V 1B5
(905) 831-7098
http://www.geocities/opfaca

Fitness

Canadian Fitness and Lifestyle Research Institute
185 Somerset St. West, Suite 201
Ottawa, Ontario K2P 0J2
(613) 233-5528
http://www.cflri.ca

Health Care Delivery

Canadian Institute for Health Information
377 Dalhousie St., Suite 200
Ottawa, Ontario K1N 9N8
(613) 241-7860
http://www.cihi.ca

Canadian Institute for Health Promotion Research
University of British Columbia, Institute of Health Promotion Research
Library Processing Centre
2206 East Mall, Rm 324
Vancouver, British Columbia V6T 1Z3
(604) 822-2258
http://www.ihpr.ubc.ca

Injury Treatment and Prevention

Canadian Collaborating Centres for Injury Prevention and Control, Health Canada
AL 0900 C2
Ottawa, Canada K1A 0K9
(613) 957-2991
http://www.hc-sc.gc.ca

MADD Canada
6507 C Mississauga Rd.
Mississauga, Ontario L5N 1A6
(905) 813-6233 or (800) 665-6233
http://www.madd.ca

War Amps of Canada
2827 Riverside Dr.
Ottawa, Ontario K1V 0C4
(613) 731-3821 or (800) 465-2677
http://www.waramps.ca

Maternal and Child Health

Canadian Institute of Child Health
384 Bank St., Suite 300
Ottawa, Canada K2P 1Y4
(613) 230-8838
http://www.cich.ca

Planned Parenthood Federation of Canada
1 Nicholas St., Suite 430
Ottawa, Ontario
http://www.ppfc.ca

Mental Health

Alzheimer Society of Canada
20 Eglinton Ave. W., Suite 1200
Toronto, Ontario M4R 1K8
(416) 488-8772 or (800) 616-8816
(valid only in Canada)
http://www.alzheimer.ca

Canadian Association for Suicide Prevention
c/o The Support Network
11456 Jasper Ave. #301
Edmonton, Alberta T5K 0M1
(780) 482-0198
http://www.suicideprevention.ca

Canadian Mental Health Association (National)
2160 Yonge St.
Toronto, Ontario M4S 2Z3
(416) 484-7750
http://www.cmha.ca

National Clearing House on Family Violence, Health Canada
Healthy Communities Division, Centre for Healthy Human Development

Health Canada
Jeanne Mance Bldg., Tunney's Pasture
Ottawa, Ontario L1A 1B4
(613) 957-2938
http://www.hc-sc.gc.ca/hppb/familyviolence

Schizophrenia Society of Canada
75 The Donway West, Suite 814
Don Mills, Ontario M3C 2E9
(416) 445-8204
http://www.schizophrenia.ca

Nutritional Health

National Institute of Nutrition
265 Carling Ave.,
Suite 302
Ottawa, Ontario K1S 2E1
(613) 235-3355
http://www.nin.ca

Nursing Organizations

Canadian Nurses Organization
50 Driveway
Ottawa, Ontario K2P 1E2
(613) 237-2133 or (800) 361-8404
http://www.cna-nurses.ca

Canadian Nursing Students' Association
350 Albert St., Suite 325
Ottawa, Ontario K1R 1B1
(613) 563-1236
http://www.aeic.ca

Occupational and Environmental Health

Canada Safety Council
1020 Thomas Spratt Place
Ottawa, Ontario K1G 5L5
(613) 739-1535
http://www.safety-council.org

Canadian Centre for Occupational Health and Safety
250 Main St. East
Hamilton, Ontario L8N 1H6
(905) 572-4400 or (800) 263-8466
(in Canada)
http://www.ccohs.ca

Canadian Standards Association
178 Rexdale Blvd.
Rexdale, Ontario M9W 1R3
(416) 747-4000
http:www.css.info.com/info/csa

Sexual Health

Sex Information and Education Council of Canada
850 Coxwell Ave.
Toronto, Ontario M4C 5R1
(416) 466-5304
http://www.sieccan.org

Substance Abuse/Addictions

Canadian Centre on Substance Abuse
75 Albert St., Suite 300
Ottawa, Ontario K1P 5E7

(613) 235-4048
http://www.ccsa.ca

Responsible Gambling Council
505 Consumers Rd., Suite 801
Toronto, Ontario M2J 4V8
(416) 499-9800
http://www.cfcg.org

Canadian Foundation for Drug Policy
70 MacDonald St.
Ottawa, Ontario K2P 1H6
(613) 236-1027
http://www.cfdp.ca

Women's Health

Canadian Women's Health Network
419 Graham Ave., Suite 203
Winnipeg, Manitoba R3C 0M3
(204) 942-5500
http://www.cwhn.ca

National Network on Environments and Women's Health
c/o Centre for Health Studies
York University
4700 Keele St.
Toronto, Ontario M3J 1P3
(416) 736-2100
http://www.yorku.ca

AUSTRALIAN HEALTH-RELATED ORGANIZATIONS

Australian Centre for Development and Innovation in Health (unit of the Australian Institute for Primary Care)
La Trobe University, Faculty of Health Sciences
Melbourne, Victoria 3086
(03) 9479-3700
http://www.latrobe.edu.au/aipc/cdih

Australian Complementary Health Association
247 Flinders Lane
Melbourne, Victoria 3000
(03) 9650-5327
http://www.vicnet.net.au

Australian Department of Health and Aging
GPO Box 9848
Canberra, ACT 2601
(02) 6289-1555
http://www.health.gov.au

Australian Institute of Health and Welfare
6A Traeger Court
Fern Hill Park
Bruce, ACT 2617
(02) 6244-1000
http://www.aihw.gov.au

Mental Health Council of Australia
P.O. Box 174
Deakin West, ACT 2600

(02) 6285-3100
http://www.mhca.com.au

National Centre for Epidemiology and Population Health
The Australian National University
Canberra, ACT 0200
(02) 6125-2378
http://www.nceph.anu.edu.au

Public Health Association of Australia, Inc.
20 Napier Close, Unit 2
Deakin, ACT 2600
(02) 6285-2373
http://www.pha.org.au

INTERNATIONAL HEALTH-RELATED ORGANIZATIONS

European Society for Quality in Health Care
c/o European Organization for Quality (EQA)/ESQH
Rue du Luxembourg 3BE
1000 Brussel, Belgium
(Ph.): 0032-2-5010735
http://www.esqh.net

Global Health Council
1701 K St. NW, Suite 600
Washington, DC 20006-1503
(202) 833-5900
http://www.globalhealth.org

International Council of Nurses
3, Place Jean-Marteau
1201 Geneva, Switzerland
41 (22) 908-01-00
http://www.icn.ch

International Healthy Cities Foundation
One Kaiser Plaza, Suite 1930
Oakland, California 94612
(510) 271-2660
http://www.oneworld.org/cities

International Society for Quality Health Care
St. Vincent's Hospital
41 Victoria Parade
Fitzroy, Victoria, Australia 3065
61 3 9417 6971
http://www.isqua.org.au

Pan American Health Organization
Regional Office of WHO
525 Twenty-Third St. NW
Washington, D.C. 20037
(202) 974-3000
http://www.paho.org

World Federation for Mental Health
1021 Prince St.
Alexandria, Virginia, 22314-2971
FAX (703) 519-7648
www.wfmh.org

World Health Organization
Avenue Appia 20
1211 Geneva 27
Switzerland
(00 41 22) 791-21-11
www.who.org

APPENDIX B

The Friedman Family Assessment Model (Short Form)

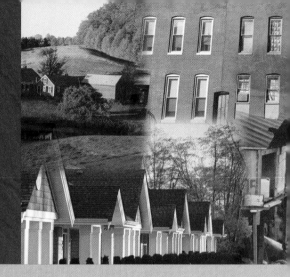

Before using the following guidelines in completing family assessments, two words of caution: first, not all areas included will be germane for each of the families visited. The guidelines are comprehensive and allow depth when probing is necessary. The student should not feel that every subarea needs to be covered when the broad area of inquiry poses no problems to the family or concern to the health worker. Second, by virtue of the interdependence of the family system, one will find unavoidable redundancy. For the sake of efficiency, the assessor should try not to repeat data, but to refer the reader back to sections where this information has already been described.

IDENTIFYING DATA

1. **Family Name**
2. **Address and Phone**
3. **Family Composition**
   See Table B-1.
4. **Type of Family Form**
5. **Cultural (Ethnic) Background**
6. **Religious Identification**
7. **Social Class Status**
8. **Family's Recreational or Leisure Time Activities**

DEVELOPMENTAL STAGE AND HISTORY OF FAMILY

9. **Family's Present Developmental Stage**
10. **Extent of Family Developmental Tasks Fulfillment**
11. **Nuclear Family History**
12. **History of Family of Origin of Both Parents**

ENVIRONMENTAL DATA

13. **Characteristics of Home**
14. **Characteristics of Neighborhood and Larger Community**
15. **Family's Geographical Mobility**
16. **Family's Associations and Transactions with Community**
17. **Family's Social Support System or Network**
    Ecomap
    Family genogram

FAMILY STRUCTURE

18. **Communication Patterns**

    Extent of Functional and Dysfunctional Communication (types of recurring patterns)
    Extent of Emotional (Affective) Messages and How Expressed
    Characteristics of Communication within Family Subsystems
    Extent of Congruent and Incongruent Messages
    Types of Dysfunctional Communication Processes Seen in Family
    Areas of Open and Closed Communication
    Familial and Contextual Variables Affecting Communication

19. **Power Structure**

    Power Outcomes
    Decision-Making Process
    Power Bases
    Variables Affecting Family Power
    Overall Family System and Subsystem Power (Family power continuum placement)

20. **Role Structure**

    Formal Role Structure
    Informal Role Structure
    Analysis of Role Models (optional)
    Variables Affecting Role Structure

21. **Family Values**

    Compare the family with American or family's reference group values and/or identify important family values and their importance (priority) in family.
    Congruence between the Family's Values and Values of the Family's Reference Group or Wider Community
    Congruence between the Family's Values and Family Members' Values
    Variables Influencing Family Values
    Values Consciously or Unconsciously Held
    Presence of Value Conflicts in Family
    Effect of the Above Values and Value Conflicts on Health Status of Family

TABLE B-1 Family Composition Form					
NAME (LAST, FIRST)	**GENDER**	**RELATIONSHIP**	**DATE/PLACE OF BIRTH**	**OCCUPATION**	**EDUCATION**
1. (Father)					
2. (Mother)					
3. (Oldest child)					
4.					
5.					
6.					
7.					
8.					

FAMILY FUNCTIONS

22. **Affective Function**

   Family Need—Response Patterns
   Mutual Nurturance, Closeness, and Identification
      Family attachment diagram
   Separateness and Connectedness

23. **Socialization Function**

   Family Child-Rearing Practices
   Adaptability of Child-Rearing Practices for Family Form and Family's Situation
   Who Is (are) Socializing Agent(s) for Child(ren)?
   Value of Children in Family
   Cultural Beliefs That Influence Family's Child-Rearing Patterns
   Social Class Influence on Child-Rearing Patterns
   Estimation about Whether Family Is at Risk for Child-Rearing Problems and If So, Indication of High-Risk Factors
   Adequacy of Home Environment for Children's Needs to Play

24. **Health Care Function**

   Family's Health Beliefs, Values, and Behaviors
   Family's Definitions of Health—Illness and Their Level of Knowledge
   Family's Perceived Health Status and Illness Susceptibility
   Family's Dietary Practices

      Adequacy of family diet (recommended three-day food history record)

      Function of mealtimes and attitudes toward food and mealtimes

      Shopping (and planning) practices

      Person(s) responsible for planning, shopping, and preparation of meals

   Sleep and Rest Habits
   Physical Activity and Recreation Practices (not covered earlier)
   Family's Drug Habits
   Family's Role in Self-Care Practices
   Medically Based Preventive Measures (physicals, eye and hearing tests, and immunizations)
   Dental Health Practices
   Family Health History (both general and specific diseases—environmentally and genetically related)
   Health Care Services Received
   Feelings and Perceptions Regarding Health Services
   Emergency Health Services
   Source of Payments for Health and Other Services
   Logistics of Receiving Care

FAMILY STRESS AND COPING

25. **Short- and Long-Term Familial Stressors and Strengths**

26. **Extent of Family's Ability to Respond, Based on Objective Appraisal of Stress-Producing Situations**

27. **Coping Strategies Utilized (present/past)**

   Differences in Family Members' Ways of Coping
   Family's Inner Coping Strategies
   Family's External Coping Strategies

28. **Dysfunctional Adaptive Strategies Utilized (present/past; extent of usage)**

From: Family Nursing: Theory and Practice *(4 ed.), by M. M. Friedman, 1998, East Norwalk, CT: Appleton & Lange. Copyright 1998 by Appleton & Lange. Used with permission.*

This appendix lists the broad content areas recommended for family assessment. In-depth discussion of each of these content areas and related theoretical and research foundations, as well as relevant diagnoses and intervention guidelines, are included in the original source.

APPENDIX C
Functional Assessments:
Instrumental Activities of Daily Living (IADLs) and Physical Self-Maintenance Activities

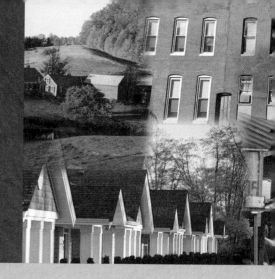

I. Instrumental Activities of Daily Living
A. Ability to use telephone
1. Operates telephone independently—looks up and dials numbers
2. Dials a few well-known numbers
3. Answers phone but does not dial or use touch tone
4. Does not use telephone at all

B. Housekeeping
1. Maintains house independently or with occasional assistance for "heavy work"
2. Performs light tasks such as bedmaking and dishwashing
3. Performs light daily tasks but cannot maintain adequate level of cleanliness
4. Needs assistance with all home maintenance tasks
5. Does not participate in any tasks

C. Laundry
1. Does personal laundry completely
2. Launders small items such as socks and stockings
3. All laundry must be done by others

D. Mode of transportation
1. Independently drives own car or uses public transportation
2. Arranges own travel via taxi or special transportation services, but does not use public transportation and does not drive
3. Travels on public transportation when assisted or with others
4. Travel limited to taxi or auto with assistance
5. Does not travel at all

E. Responsibility for medications
1. Takes medication in correct dosages at correct time independently
2. Takes medication if medication is prepared in advance in separate doses
3. Not capable of dispensing own medications

F. Ability to handle finances
1. Independently manages finances—writes checks, pays bills, keeps track of income
2. Manages own finances with assistance
3. Not capable of managing own finances

G. Shopping
1. Does all of the shopping independently
2. Shops for small purchases independently
3. Not able to go shopping without assistance
4. Unable to shop for any purchase

H. Food preparation
1. Able to prepare and serve food without assistance
2. Prepares adequate meals if supplied with food
3. Able to heat and serve prepared meals
4. Unable to prepare and serve meals

Adapted from "Assessment of Older People: Self-Maintaining and Instrumental Activities of Daily Living" by M. Lawton and E. Brody, 1969, The Gerontologist, 9, *pp. 179–186.*

II. Physical Self-Maintenance Activities
A. Feeding
1. Eats without assistance
2. Eats with minor assistance at meal times and helps in cleaning up
3. Feeds self with moderate assistance
4. Requires extensive assistance—all meals
5. Does not feed self at all and resists efforts of others to feed him/her

B. Toilet
1. Cares for self completely, no incontinence
2. Needs to be reminded or needs help in cleaning self
3. Soils the bed while asleep—more than once a week
4. Soils clothing while awake—more than once a week
5. No control of bladder/bowel

C. Grooming (hair, nails, hands, face)
1. Able to care for self
2. Occasional minor assistance needed (e.g., with shaving)
3. Moderate and regular assistance needed

4. Needs total grooming care, but accepts some
5. Actively negates efforts of others to maintain grooming

D. Bathing
1. Bathes self without help
2. Bathes self with help into and out of tub or shower
3. Can wash face and hands only
4. Does not wash self but is cooperative
5. Does not try to wash self and resists efforts of others to help

E. Dressing
1. Dresses, undresses, and selects clothes from wardrobe
2. Dresses and undresses with minor assistance
3. Needs moderate assistance in dressing or selection of clothes

4. Needs major assistance
5. Completely unable to dress self and resists efforts of others to help

F. Ambulation
1. Ambulates about grounds or city without assistance
2. Ambulates within residence or nearby
3. Ambulates with assistance of
   a. another person
   b. a railing
   c. cane
   d. walker
   e. wheelchair
4. Sits unsupported in chair or wheelchair but cannot propel self
5. Bedridden more than half the time

APPENDIX D

Community Assessment Guide: The Place, the People, and the Social System

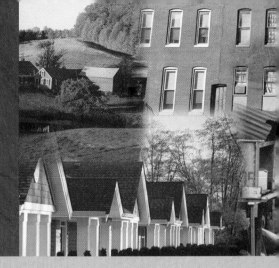

The community health assessment guide is a tool that guides the community health nurse in the systematic collection of data about the characteristics of an identified community and the formulation of community health diagnoses about the community's assets and health problems and concerns. The guide provides a method for assessing relevant community parameters and identifies categories and subcategories that provide direction for the organization of data in a meaningful way.

Community _____   Date _____

I. Overview
   A. Description of the community
      1. History
      2. Type of community: urban, suburban, rural

II. The Community As a Place
   A. Description: general identifying data
      1. Location
      2. Topography
      3. Climate
   B. Boundaries, area in square miles
   C. Environment
      1. Sanitation: water supply, sewage, garbage, trash
      2. Pollutants, toxic substances, animal reservoirs or vectors, flora and fauna
      3. Air quality: color, odor, particulates
      4. Food supply: sources, preparation
   D. Housing
      1. Types of housing (public and private)
      2. Condition of housing
      3. Percent owned, rented
      4. Housing for special populations
         a. Near homeless
         b. Homeless
         c. Frail elders
   E. Leading industries and occupations

III. The People of the Community
   A. Population profile
      1. Total population for ____ (year of last census)
      2. Population density
      3. Population changes in past 10 years
      4. Population per square mile
      5. Mobility
      6. Types of families
   B. Vital and demographic population characteristics
      1. Age distribution
      2. Sex distribution
      3. Race distribution
      4. Ethnic group composition and distribution
      5. Socioeconomic status
         a. Income of family
         b. Major occupations
         c. Estimated level of unemployment
         d. Percent below poverty level
         e. Percent retired
      6. Educational level
      7. Religious distribution
      8. Marriage and divorce rates
      9. Birth and death rates
   C. Leading causes of morbidity
      1. Incidence rates (specific diseases)
      2. Prevalence rates (specific diseases)
   D. Mortality characteristics
      1. Crude death rate
      2. Age-specific death rate
      3. Infant mortality rate
      4. Maternal mortality rate
      5. Leading causes of death

IV. The Community As a Social System
   A. Government and leadership
      1. Type of government (mayor, city manager, board of supervisors)
      2. City offices (location, hours, services, access)
   B. Education
      1. Public educational facilities
      2. Private educational facilities
      3. Libraries
      4. Services for special populations
         a. Pregnant teens
         b. Adults with special problems
         c. Children and adults who are developmentally disabled
         d. Children and adults who are blind and/or deaf

C. Transportation
   1. Transport systems: bus, suburban train, private auto, air, streetcar, other
   2. Transportation provisions for special populations
      a. Elders
      b. Homeless/near homeless
      c. Adults with disabilities
D. Communication resources
   1. Newspapers
   2. Radio stations
   3. Television
   4. Key community leaders and/or decision makers
   5. Internet Web sites
   6. Other
E. Religious resources
   1. Churches and other religious facilities
   2. Community programs and services (e.g., health ministries, parish nursing)
   3. Major religious leaders
F. Recreation resources
   1. Public and private facilities
   2. Programs for special population groups
      a. People with disabilities
      b. Elders
      c. Blind and deaf
      d. Other
G. Community safety (protection)
   1. Fire protection (describe)
   2. Police protection, including county detention facilities (describe)
   3. Disaster preparation
H. Stores and shops
   1. Types and location
   2. Access
I. Community health facilities and resources (see Section V)

V. **Community Health Facilities and Resources**
(Resource access, availability, eligibility)
   A. Health systems
      1. Hospitals (type and services rendered): acute care facilities—emergency medical, surgical, intensive care, psychiatric
      2. Rehabilitation health care facilities: physical conditions, alcoholism, and substance abuse
      3. Home health services: hospice and home health agencies
      4. Long-term care facilities (e.g., skilled nursing facilities)
      5. Respite care services for special population groups
      6. Ambulatory services
         a. Hospital ambulatory clinics
         b. Public health service clinics

   c. Nursing centers
   d. Community mental health centers
   e. Crisis clinics
   f. Community health centers
      7. Special health services for targeted populations
         a. Preschool
         b. School age
         c. Adult or young adult
         d. Adults and children with handicaps (e.g., regional centers for developmentally disabled)
      8. Other
         a. School health services
         b. Occupational health services
   B. Public health and social services
      1. Health departments (various programs)
      2. Social services
         a. Department of social services
            (1) County level—location of suboffices
            (2) Official (public) social services, major programs (e.g., adult services, children's services, Welfare to Work)—eligibility, services rendered, location
         b. Social Security (USA)
            (1) Location and program availability
            (2) Eligibility
   C. Voluntary health organizations
      1. Cancer Society
      2. Heart Association
      3. Red Cross
      4. Women's shelter
      5. Suicide prevention
      6. Rape crisis centers
      7. Family service agency
      8. Catholic Charities
      9. Alzheimer's Association
     10. Lung Association
     11. Diabetes Association
   D. Health-related planning groups
      1. Area Agency on Aging
      2. Senior coordinating councils
      3. High-risk infant coordinating councils
      4. Healthy Communities Coordinating Teams
      5. Multipurpose agencies
      6. Teen violence prevention planning teams

VI. **Summary**
   A. What are the major assets of the community and from whose perspective—health care provider's, community members', etc.?
      1. The place
      2. The people
      3. The resources (availability, accessibility, acceptability; public and private)

B. What are the major health problems/needs?
1. The place
2. The people
3. The resources (availability, accessibility, acceptability; public and private)

C. Identify and propose the contributions of nurses, other health care providers, community leaders, community residents, etc., to the solutions
D. Which of the health problems/needs should be given priority—first, second, and third? Why?

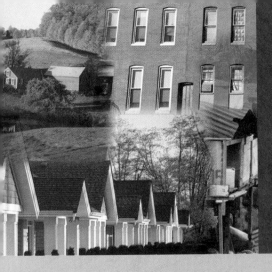

APPENDIX E
Environmental Assessment:
Home Safety for Disabled or Older Adults

The Environmental Assessment guide is a tool that assists the community health nurse in the systematic collection of data about the home safety of disabled or older adults. It provides a way to assess the home for actual or potential safety hazards.

I. Entrance and Exit Areas

A. Is the housing on the ground level?   ____ Yes   ____ No

     1. If **no,** is there an elevator?   ____ Yes   ____ No

        Stairs?   ____ Yes   ____ No

     2. If there are stairs, how many?   _____

B. Can the client get to and from the entrance easily?   ____ Yes   ____ No

C. Are there any problems outside the house/apartment (e.g., steep path, lack of handrails on stairs)?   ____ Yes   ____ No

     1. If **yes,** please describe _____

     _____

     _____

II. Living Area

A. What type of heating is there? (Circle all that apply.)

     1. Gas

     2. Electric

     3. Wood

     4. Central heating

     5. Space heater(s)

B. Is the heating system clean and operable?   ____ Yes   ____ No

C. Are electrical cords well away from rugs and out of walkways?   ____ Yes   ____ No

D. Are there any scatter (throw) rugs on the floor?   ____ Yes   ____ No

E. If there are stairs, are they well lit?   ____ Yes   ____ No

F. Are all chairs and sofas at a safe height for getting up and down?   ____ Yes   ____ No

G. Is lighting adequate for walking?   ____ Yes   ____ No

H. Is the furniture arranged for safety?   ____ Yes   ____ No

I. Do the windows close completely?   ____ Yes   ____ No

III. Kitchen Area

A. Is the kitchen easy to get to for the person?   ____ Yes   ____ No

B. Are the appliances in good operating condition?   ____ Yes   ____ No

C. Are sharp items placed safely in storage areas?   ____ Yes   ____ No

D. Are poisonous and toxic items stored safely?   ____ Yes   ____ No

E. Are the stove and cooking area free from grease and dust? ____ Yes ____ No

F. Are the foods stored properly? ____ Yes ____ No

G. Are the following facilities accessible?

    1. Refrigerator ____ Yes ____ No

    2. Sink ____ Yes ____ No

    3. Kitchen faucets ____ Yes ____ No

    4. Stove ____ Yes ____ No

    5. Cupboard ____ Yes ____ No

    6. Kitchen counters ____ Yes ____ No

IV. Bathroom Area

A. Is the toilet easily accessible? ____ Yes ____ No

B. Are bathing facilities easily accessible? ____ Yes ____ No

C. Are the bathing facilities safe? ____ Yes ____ No

D. Are there railings or grab bars in the tub or shower area? ____ Yes ____ No

    1. If there are railings or bars, are they secure and strong? ____ Yes ____ No

E. Are there any visible electrical cords? ____ Yes ____ No

    1. If **yes,** are they a safe distance from water? ____ Yes ____ No

F. Is the floor nonskid? ____ Yes ____ No

G. Is the bathtub or shower nonskid? ____ Yes ____ No

V. Other Areas

A. Are there fire escape plans? ____ Yes ____ No

B. Is there a fire alarm that can be heard by the person? ____ Yes ____ No

C. Does the person know where the nearest fire alarm is? ____ Yes ____ No

D. Are all flammable items stored safely away from the heat? ____ Yes ____ No

E. Can the phone(s) be easily reached in an emergency? ____ Yes ____ No

F. Are emergency numbers visible and easily accessible? ____ Yes ____ No

Safety Checklist

1. Insufficient heating/cooking ____ Yes ____ No ____ Needs Action

2. Improper storage of poisonous and toxic items ____ Yes ____ No ____ Needs Action

3. Improper food storage ____ Yes ____ No ____ Needs Action

4. Insufficient/improper cooking facilities ____ Yes ____ No ____ Needs Action

5. Railings or grab bars absent ____ Yes ____ No ____ Needs Action

6. Elevators broken ____ Yes ____ No ____ Needs Action

7. Unsafe toilets ____ Yes ____ No ____ Needs Action

Environmental Summary: _____

_____

_____

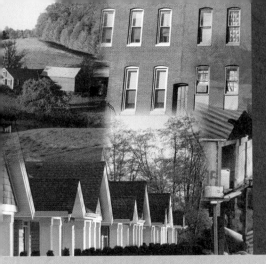

The Service Satisfaction Questionnaire is a tool that can be used to collect data regarding client perceptions of the nursing care received. The collection of this information is an important part of the outcome measurement process. Service satisfaction questionnaires should be administered to clients on a regular basis, with response data analyzed in order to provide information that will assist in quality improvement.

Introduction

We would like your opinion on the nature of our community health nursing services. Your opinions are very important to us, and we thank you for your help. We want to provide our clients with the best community health nursing services possible. We ask these questions so that we may develop services that will be helpful to all of our clients. The information you provide is considered confidential. Your decision whether to complete this questionnaire will not affect your future relations with our nursing program. Your completion of this questionnaire indicates that you have given your consent to do so, having read the information provided above. Thank you.

Instructions: Please check your response to each of the questions below.

1. **When you first met the nurse, how well did she/he explain the reason for the visits with you?**
   - _____ Very well
   - _____ Well
   - _____ Moderately
   - _____ Poorly
   - _____ Very poorly

2. **Did the nurse involve you in planning for your health care?**
   - _____ Yes
   - _____ No

3. **How would you evaluate the nursing care and services you receive/have received?**
   - _____ Excellent
   - _____ Good
   - _____ Average
   - _____ Poor
   - _____ Very poor

4. **Did you feel that you could talk to the nurse about concerns or questions you had regarding your health and health care?**
   - _____ Yes
   - _____ No

5. **Did the nurse encourage you to ask questions about your health conditions and concerns?**
   - _____ Yes
   - _____ No

6. **Overall, how satisfied were you with the way information about your health condition was discussed with you?**
   - _____ Very satisfied
   - _____ Satisfied
   - _____ Neutral
   - _____ Dissatisfied
   - _____ Very dissatisfied

7. **Overall, how would you rate the respect and courtesy the nurse from (the agency's name) has shown to you?**

____ Excellent

____ Good

____ Average

____ Poor

____ Very poor

8. **How much do you think you have been assisted by your visit(s) with the nurse?**

____ A great deal

____ Quite a bit

____ Somewhat

____ A little

____ Not at all

____ Not sure

9. **Do you think that additional health-related services should be provided by the nurse?**

____ Yes

____ No

____ Not sure

If you answered **yes** to question 9, what services would you recommend? _____

_____

10. **Do you have any suggestions for ways that we could improve our nursing service to you? If yes, please comment.** _____

_____

_____

Background Information

1. **What is your age?**

____ 19 years or younger

____ 20–29

____ 30–39

____ 40–49

____ 50–59

____ 60–69

____ 70–79

____ 80+

2. **What is your gender?**

____ Male

____ Female

3. **What is your marital status?**

____ Married

____ Single

____ Divorced

____ Widowed

____ Separated

4. **What is your ethnic origin?**

____ Asian/Pacific Islander

____ African American

____ Latino

____ Mixed race

Please indicate origins _____

____ Native American/Alaskan

____ Caucasian

____ Other

Please indicate _____

____ Decline to state

5. **What is your current family composition?**

____ Single-parent/female

____ Single-parent/male

____ Two parents with children

____ Single person

____ Two adults with no children

____ Extended family (e.g., aunt, grandmother living with you)

____ Other (please specify: _____)

Thank you for taking the time to complete this questionnaire. We appreciate your assistance.

acculturation The process by which new members of a culture learn its ways and become part of that culture.

achieved role Role activities that are not ordinarily assigned but are earned.

acquaintance rape Rape by an individual known to the victim.

acquired immunity Immunity conferred by the transfer of antibodies from mother to child via the placenta or breastfeeding.

active immunity Immunity developed by introducing an infectious agent or vaccine into the host.

active listening Carefully listening to another and reflecting back content and meaning to check for accuracy and facilitate further exploration.

activity center A place where persons needing extensive or pervasive supports can be taught self-care, social skills, homemaking, and leisure activities skills.

acupoints Abbreviated term for *acupuncture point*. An energetic pore in skin through which subtle energy from the surrounding environment is carried throughout the body via the meridians, supplying nutritive chi energy to the deeper organs, blood vessels, and nervous system.

acupressure A system of applying pressure with the thumbs to acupoints along the meridians rather than inserting needles as in acupuncture.

acupuncture Ancient practice of inserting needles into the acupoints to treat disease or relieve pain by harmonizing and balancing chi.

advanced-practice nurse A nurse with masters- or doctoral-level education in any aspect of clinical nursing practice.

advocacy role Nursing role involving acting or speaking for someone who may be unable to act or speak for him- or herself.

advocate A person who speaks or acts for an individual or group of individuals who may be unable to speak for themselves.

aerobic conditioning Use of an exercise program planned to improve cardiorespiratory fitness; such a program requires a consistent supply of oxygen to the tissues over a sustained period of time. Conditioning requires steady, continuous movement, producing an increased, sustained heart rate equal to 60%–85% of the person's maximum possible heart rate. Examples are vigorous walking, running, swimming, cycling, rowing, and cross-country skiing.

affective function A family function that provides affirmation, support, and respect for one another.

affective learning objectives Learning objectives set by the nurse educator that describe attitude changes the client will attain to meet the educational goal.

ageism Any attitude or action constituting discrimination against an individual because of age.

agent A causative factor, such as a biological or chemical agent that must be present (or absent) in the environment for disease occurrence in a susceptible host.

aggregate Identification of a group of individuals who share a common concern.

airborne transmission Microorganisms suspended in the air spread to a suitable port of entry.

allopathic Practices derived from scientific models and technology.

alternative therapies/health care A term used to categorize integrative therapies used in place of scientifically recognized medical care and treatment.

amended A parliamentary or constitutional document (e.g., a bill) that is different from the original.

analytic epidemiological studies Study designs that examine groups of individuals in order to make comparisons and associations and to determine causal relationships; also known as *cohort, cross-sectional,* and *case-control studies*.

andragogy Adult learning which addresses the learner's need to be a part of the process rather than a passive recipient.

anorexia nervosa A psychophysiological disorder, usually occurring in teenage women, characterized by an abnormal fear of becoming obese, a distorted self-image, a persistent aversion to food, and severe weight loss.

approach strategy Strategy used by an individual that signifies an effort to confront the challenges of a chronic illness.

Asperger's disorder Severe and sustained impairment in social interaction with restrictive, repetitive patterns of behavior, although there are no delays in curiosity, language, or cognitive and skills acquisitions.

assessment The systematic collection of data to assist in identifying the health status, assets, health needs and problems, and available resources of the community.

assets assessment Part of the planning process whereby health care professionals identify the resources and strengths of the client or community.

assimilated family style A family acculturative style where there is full assimilation to the host culture.

assurance The role of a public agency in ensuring that high-priority personal and communitywide health services are available.

attack rate The number of cases of disease in a specific population divided by the total population at risk for a limited time period, usually expressed as a percentage.

attention-deficit/hyperactivity disorder A neurobiologically based disability characterized by hyperactivity, impulsiveness, and inattentiveness.

attributable risk percentage (AR%) A statistical measure that estimates the number of cases of a disease attributable to the exposure of interest.

author The legislator who submits a bill in the legislative process.

autistic disorder Markedly abnormal or impaired development in social interaction and communication and a markedly restricted repertoire of activity and interests, generally without a period of normal development.

autistic spectrum disorders A group of closely related life-long developmental disabilities including autistic disorder, Asperger's disorder, and pervasive developmental disorder, not otherwise specified.

autonomy The principle of respect for persons that is based on the recognition of humans as unconditionally worthy agents, regardless of any special characteristics, conditions, or circumstances. Involves self-determination and the right to make choices for oneself.

battered women Women who are in physically and/or emotionally abusive relationships with their spouses or partners in which battering is ongoing.

batterer One who beats or strikes another person.

beauty The quality of being aesthetically pleasing to the senses; the harmonious experience of color, sound, form, order, fragrance, taste, and texture.

behavior modification The changing of behavior by manipulating environmental stimuli.

behavioral learning objectives Learning objectives set by the nurse educator that describe the behaviors or actions the client will perform to meet the educational goal. Behavioral learning objectives specify the activity in which the client will engage, the circumstances under which the activity will be performed, and how the nurse and client will know when learning has been achieved.

beneficence The ethical principle of doing or promoting good that requires abstention from injuring others and promotion of the legitimate interests of others primarily by preventing or avoiding possible harm.

best interest judgment A proxy decision made on behalf of another based on what is thought to be in the best interest of the other in the circumstances and on what a reasonable person would decide in the given situation.

bias An error in the study design caused by the tendency of researchers to expect certain conclusions on the basis of their own personal beliefs that results in incorrect conclusions regarding the association between potential risk factors and disease occurrence.

bicultural A person who holds two distinctly different cultures, lifestyles, or sets of values in equal or nearly equal proportions.

bioaccumulative Accumulation over time of certain materials in the environment, due to inability to go through the natural process of decay; applies to products such as plastics.

biodiversity The variety of life that now exists; vital to maintaining ecological balance.

biofeedback training A technique of learning to control certain emotional states, such as anxiety, by training oneself, with the aid of electronic devices, to modify involuntary body functions, such as blood pressure or heartbeat.

biographical disruption The change in people's self-image, relationships, and life plans that can accompany chronic illness.

biographical work The work that a chronically ill person does to adjust to living with the impact of chronic illness on identity, body, and sense of time.

biological mother A woman who gives birth to and raises her own children.

biometrics The application of statistical methods to biological facts.

biomonitoring The use of biological data to determine the extent of toxic substances in the human body.

biopersistent The quality of not decaying and continuing to exist for many years; usually applies to synthetic materials.

biotechnology The use of scientific techniques, including genetic engineering, to create, improve, or modify plants, animals, and microorganisms.

bioterrorism The intentional use of infectious agents as weapons by terrorists to further personal or political agendas.

biracial A person who is born of two distinctly different races and cultures.

blended (or binuclear) family The combination of two divorced families via remarriage.

block nursing Links registered nurses to individuals and families in their neighborhoods who may need nursing services, support services, and other resources to promote their optimal health.

bonadaptation Successful adaptation whereby the family is able to stabilize itself in a growth-producing way.

boundary An abstract demarcation line composed of family rules that separates the focal system from its environment; may be more or less open.

bulimia nervosa An eating disorder in which one alternates between abnormal craving for and aversion to food; characterized by episodes of excessive food intake followed by periods of fasting and self-induced vomiting or diarrhea.

cachexia Weight loss, wasting of muscle, loss of appetite, general debility that can occur during a chronic disease.

capacity building A technique that enhances community development through a focus on the whole community or with particular population groups that address both social isolation and poverty.

capitation A health insurance payment mechanism wherein a fixed amount is paid per person to cover health care services received or needed for a specific period of time.

caregiver A person, usually a family member, who has the primary responsibility to care for at least one dependent member of the family.

caring Those assistive, enabling, supportive, or facilitative behaviors toward or for another individual or group to promote health, prevent disease, and facilitate healing.

carrier A host that harbors an infectious agent without noticeable signs of disease or infection. The carrier state can exist while the host is healthy or during a specific time period in the natural history of the disease, when infection is not apparent. The carrier state can be of long or short duration.

case-control study An analytic epidemiological study design that assembles study groups after a disease has occurred; also called a *retrospective study*.

case fatality rate Deaths from a specific disease calculated by dividing the number of deaths from a specific disease in a given time period by the number of persons diagnosed with the disease.

case management Coordinating and allocating services for clients to enhance continuity and appropriateness of care developed in response to client needs and problems.

case reports Client (case) history studies used in epidemiological descriptive studies.

case series A compilation of case reports.

cause-specific death rate Number of deaths from a specific cause; expressed as a number per 100,000 population.

centering Finding within oneself a sense of inner being that is quiet and at peace, where one feels integrated and focused.

Centers for Disease Control and Prevention (CDC) An agency of the U.S. Department of Health and Human Services, whose mission is to promote health and quality of life by preventing and controlling disease, injury, and disability.

cerebral palsy A group of disorders characterized by abnormal control of movement and posture, secondary to a static encephalopathy occurring prenatally, perinatally, or in early childhood.

chakra One of the seven main energy centers in the human body which transforms higher frequency subtle energies into chemical, hormonal, and cellular changes in the body.

chaotic family Crisis-prone family whose members rebound from one crisis to another

chemical agents Poisons and allergens.

chemical terrorism The intentional use of chemicals as weapons by terrorists to further personal or political agendas.

chi (qi, ki) A form of vital energy, sometimes described as a life force, that is believed to control the functioning of the human body, according to traditional Chinese medicine. Chi is believed to flow through the body along invisible channels. Illness occurs when there is an imbalance or obstruction of *chi*.

child abuse Physical or mental injury, sexual abuse or exploitation, negligent treatment, or maltreatment of a child by a person who is responsible for the child's welfare.

child neglect The failure of a family to provide a child with basic needs of food, clothing, shelter, supervision, education, emotional affection, stimulation, or health care.

childhood disintegrative disorder Marked regression in multiple areas of functioning following a period of at least two years of apparently normal development. Behavior generally is similar to those with autistic disorder.

chronic disease A long-term physiological or psychological disorder.

chronic illness A social phenomenon that accompanies a disease that cannot be cured and extends over a period of time.

circular questioning Questions that are neutral, accepting, and exploratory and are used to expose patterns that connect persons, objects, actions, perceptions, ideas, feelings, events, beliefs, and context.

circumplex model of marital and family systems A map of types of marriages and family system attributes that mediate or buffer stressors and demand; illustrates the types of balanced and unbalanced relationships.

clarity Clarity in communication occurs when the verbal and nonverbal communication say the same thing so that the message is clear to the receiver.

client centered All communication in a helping relationship is client centered since the goal is the well-being of the client.

client cost sharing Requirement that the client pay for a portion of the health care received.

clinical nurse specialist An expert practitioner with graduate preparation in a nursing specialty.

clinical supervision The process by which one nurse confers with another (usually more advanced) for the purpose of consultation regarding the nursing care of a client or clients.

closed questions Questions that limit or restrict clients' responses to specific information and can usually be answered with one word or a short phrase; used to gather very specific information.

coalition A collective that is characterized as a temporary alliance of diverse members who come together for joint action in support of a shared goal.

cognitive learning objectives Learning objectives set by the nurse educator that describe how the knowledge gained by the client will be revealed.

cognitive organization The person's intellectual grasp of the material.

cohort study An analytic epidemiological study design that assembles study groups before disease occurrence to observe and compare the rates of a health outcome over time; also called a *prospective study*.

collaborate To work with others to achieve common goals in a collegial manner.

collaborator An approach to interpreting in which the interpreter and nurse function as colleagues and engage in interaction with the client as appropriate to the situation.

collective A group that is brought together to pursue an agreed-upon goal, action, or set of actions.

communicable disease A disease in a susceptible host that is caused by a potentially harmful infectious organism or its toxic products; spread by direct or indirect contact with an infectious agent (human, animal, or inanimate reservoir).

communication The process of sharing information using a common set of rules.

community A group of people sharing common interests, needs, resources, and environment; an interrelating and interacting group of people with shared needs and interests.

community assessment The process of critically examining the characteristics, resources, and needs of a community in collaboration with that community, in order to develop strategies to improve the health and quality of life of the community.

community-based nursing The practice in nursing which focuses on the provision of personal care to individuals and families in the community.

community capacity The strengths, resources, and problem-solving abilities of a community.

community competence The ability of a community to collaborate in identifying its problems and in effectively planning responses to those problems.

community health Meeting collective needs by identifying problems and supporting community participation in the process within the community and society.

community health nurse generalist The community health nurse prepared at the baccalaureate level. The focus of practice is individuals and families within a community context, with the primary responsibility being the population as a whole.

community health nurse specialist The community health nurse prepared at the master's or doctoral level. Focus of practice for the master's-prepared nurse is the health of populations; the doctoral-prepared nurse focuses on population health, health policy, and research.

community health nursing Synthesis of nursing and public health practice applied to promoting, protecting, and preserving the health of populations.

community of interest A group of people who share values, beliefs, or interests on a particular issue.

community nursing centers Nurse-managed settings established in underserved areas, where clients can receive monitoring, screening, treatment, and a variety of nursing services.

community organization A multifaceted theoretical approach intended to create change at the community level; models include community development, social action, and social planning.

community-oriented nursing practice Provision of health care focused on the assessment of major health and environmental problems, health surveillance, and monitoring of population health status.

community participation The active involvement of community members in assessing, planning, implementing, and evaluating health programs.

comparative need Need determined on the basis of comparison with another similar area, group, or person.

compassion A quality of presence with another; an entering into the experience of the other; a sensitivity to pain and suffering of others.

complementary and alternative medicine (CAM) The practice, education, and research of the medically unrecognized therapies.

complementary health care services The use of integrative therapies and treatment unrecognized by conventional scientific medicine in addition to conventional medical care to promote health and healing.

compliance A disposition or tendency to yield to others; submissiveness.

concept An abstract version of the real world or of a concrete idea.

conflict A difference between two or more persons when they hold seemingly incompatible ideas, interests, or values; can be spoken or unspoken.

conflict management Efforts to work together while at the same time recognizing and accepting the conflicts inherent in the relationships involved.

conflict resolution Methods to resolve conflicts by expressing concerns and differences of opinion until clarity and resolution are achieved.

consciousness In the person-environment relationship, the organizing factor commonly experienced as awareness, thoughts, emotions, beliefs, and perceptions; the totality of thoughts, feelings, images, and impressions that shape our reality of person-environment processes.

consultant One who provides clients with professional advice, services, or information to assist them in making informed decisions.

contact A person who because of exposure to an infectious agent or environment has the potential for developing an infectious disease.

contacting phase Encompasses the antecedent event (when the nurse becomes aware of an individual or family who is identified as desiring or needing a visit) and the going-to-see phase (when the nurse journeys to the home and gains information about the neighborhood and the family's place in it).

content-oriented groups Those groups whose purpose and focus are to meet certain goals or perform specific tasks.

contexts The places or settings where community health nursing services are provided.

contextual family structure The dimension of the family that includes ethnicity, race, social class, religion, and the environment.

contextual stimuli In Roy's theory, all factors other than focal stimuli that contribute to adaptive behavior.

contextualism Understanding the individual in the context of the family and the family in the context of the culture.

continuity Reflects connectedness of thought and coherence in the flow of language; thought is easy to follow and understand, and the client's concerns are carried through the interaction.

continuum of care The succession of services needed by the individual as he or she moves from one life stage to another.

contract In the health care setting, a working agreement that is not legally binding between two or more parties; promotes self-care and facilitates a family focus on health needs.

coordination The efficient management and delivery of services without gaps and overlaps.

copayment Cost-sharing arrangement whereby the person who is insured pays a specified charge.

coping A strategy developed by people to enable them to live with illness.

correctional health nursing A branch of professional nursing that provides nursing services to clients in correctional facilities.

correlational study A descriptive epidemiological study design used to compare aggregate populations for potential exposures of disease.

cost analysis of health programs An evaluation of the costs of a program in relation to health outcomes; requires consideration of the values and needs that gave rise to the program, the short- and long-term outcomes, and the human and material dimensions.

counseling Assisting clients in the use of problem-solving processes to decide on the course of action most appropriate for them.

crack A freebase form of cocaine formed by mixing cocaine with baking soda and water and separating it from its hydrochloride base, making it usable for smoking.

crack babies Babies with physical problems and developmental delays secondary to the mother's prenatal use of cocaine.

created environment In the Neuman systems model, a protective, unconsciously derived environment that exists for all clients and acts as an intrapersonal protective shield against the reality of the environment.

critical thinking Use of logic/analytical and intuitive/creative approaches to solving problems; involves looking at a situation from multiple perspectives.

cross-sectional survey A descriptive epidemiological study design that uses a representative sample of the population to collect information on current health status, personal characteristics, and potential risk factors or exposures at one point in time.

cultural assessment The collection, verification, and organization of data about the beliefs, values, and health care practices that clients share or have shared with others of the same culture.

cultural compatibility The hypothesis that assessment and intervention outcomes in the care of multicultural groups are enhanced when racial and ethnic barriers between client and nurse are erased.

cultural competence Represents a level of skill development by which one is able to work effectively with those from various cultures; skills are learned through using a conscious process of creating awareness of one's existence, sensations, thoughts, and environment in order to understand oneself and to accept cultural variations.

culturally diverse care The great variability in nursing approaches needed to give culturally appropriate care to a rapidly changing, heterogeneous client population.

cultural diversity The great variety of cultural values, beliefs, and behavior; a term used to reflect appreciation for the richness of human experience in these areas.

cultural sensitivity Awareness of the nurse that cultural variables may affect assessment and treatment outcomes.

cultural values Values that are desirable or preferred ways of acting or knowing something that over time are reinforced and sustained by the culture and ultimately govern one's action or decisions.

culture The values, beliefs, norms, and practices of a particular group that are learned and shared and that guide thought, decisions, and actions in a patterned way.

culture bound Being limited to one's own view of reality and, therefore, unable to accept or even consider the views of another culture.

culture of poverty A theory that has now been largely rejected by most recent research. This theory weakly suggests that social conditions originally helped produce poverty, but most importantly, this theory argues that poverty produces people with unique personal characteristics that in turn help ensure that the poor, and their children, remain poor.

curing Elimination of the signs and symptoms of disease.

cutting agents Substances added to street drugs to increase bulk (e.g., mannitol and starch), to mimic or enhance pharmacological effects (e.g., caffeine and lidocaine), or to combat side effects (e.g., vitamin C and dilantin).

date rape Rape by an individual the victim is dating.

decision making The process of "gaining the assent and commitment of family members to carry out a course of action or to maintain the status quo (Friedman, 1992).

deep relaxation A positively perceived state or response in which a person feels psychological or physiological relief of tension or strain. Relaxation can be present or absent throughout the body, affecting visceral functions, skeletal muscle activity, and cerebral activities such as thoughts, perceptions, and emotional states.

deinstitutionalization The phenomenon of shifting the population experiencing major psychiatric disorders from large inpatient institutions to community-based care.

demography The statistical science or study of populations, related to age-specific categories, birth and death rates, marital status, and ethnicity.

deontology The ethical theory according to which actions are inherently right or wrong independent of the consequences; based on the morality of the action itself.

depressants An agent that depresses a body function or nerve activity.

descriptive epidemiological studies Epidemiological study designs that contribute to the description of a disease or condition by examining the essential features of person, place, and time.

designer drugs Analogues of known drugs created for their psychoactive properties.

determinants of health Factors that influence the risk for health outcomes.

detoxification The process of removing toxins from the body.

developmental approach to care A method of encouraging development and skill acquisition based on present developmental level rather than chronological age.

developmental assessment Observation and assessment of a child's skills in physical, social, and mental domains compared with established age-related norms.

developmental assessment tools Tools used by nurses and other care providers to assess developmental progress of children; observation and interviewing are used and the results recorded; the resulting record provides a measure of how the child is developing in different areas and serves as a tool that can be used in teaching parents how to determine potential readiness.

developmental disorder A severe, chronic condition attributable to mental or physical impairment, or both, manifested before age 22 and likely to continue indefinitely, resulting in substantial limitations in three or more areas, including self-care, receptive and expressive language, and learning, and requiring a combination and sequence of special, interdisciplinary, or generic care, treatment, or other

services, individually planned and coordinated, required for an extended period or throughout life.

developmental model of services Programs of care and instruction designed to promote skill acquisition to the highest level possible, regardless of age or severity of handicap.

developmental tasks The work that each family must complete at each stage of development before movement to the next stage is possible.

developmental theory Theory that families evolve through typical developmental stages during the life cycle; each stage is characterized by specific issues and tasks; also called the *life cycle approach*.

diagnosis-related group (DRG) System of classification for cost of inpatient services based on diagnosis, age, sex, and presence of complications.

differentiation A living system's capability to advance to a higher order of complexity and organization.

dimensions of environment The nature of and relationship among the various aspects of environment within the whole.

direct transmission Immediate transfer of disease from infected host to susceptible host.

directive approach The nurse defines the nature of the client's problem and prescribes appropriate solutions, providing specific, concrete information needed for problem solving.

disability Results from impairment and is a restriction on lack of ability to perform an activity in a manner or within a range considered normal.

disability-adjusted life year (DALY) An internationally standardized measure that expresses years of life lost to premature death and years lived with a disability of specified severity and duration.

disease frequency Occurrence of disease as measured by various rates such as morbidity rate.

disease/injury prevention Those activities or actions that seek to protect clients from potential or actual health threats and related harmful consequences.

disenfranchised A group of people who do not have all the privileges and rights as do citizens in higher social class.

disengaged family Family that is distanced or totally cut off from family relationships.

domestic violence A broad term encompassing a spectrum of violence within a family. It may (and usually

does) refer to a husband battering his wife but more broadly addresses any intrafamilial violence such as elder or child abuse.

downstream thinking A microscopic focus that by nature is characterized primarily by short-term individual-based interventions.

early intervention Services to infants and young children and their families designed to promote health, development, and family functioning. Services are interdisciplinary and individually designed.

ecological approach Incorporation of developmental, systems, and situational perspectives to understand the family within the multiperson environmental system within which the family is enmeshed; encompasses the following subsystems, the totality of which makes up the ecosystem: microsystem, mesosystem, exosystem, and macrosystem.

ecological balance The complex relationships among living things and between a specific organism and its environment.

ecological system The interrelationship between living things and their environment.

ecology The study of relations and interactions among all organisms within the total environment; in community health, the individual's interaction with his or her social, cultural, and physical environments.

ecomap A visual overview of the complex ecological system of the family, showing the family's organizational patterns and relationships.

economic function Maintenance of economic survival in society.

economic policy Course of action intended to influence or control the behavior of an economy.

economics Social science concerned with the ways that society allocates scarce resources (commonly known as goods and services) in the most cost-efficient way.

ecosystem The relationships and interactions among all subsystems, including microsystem, mesosystem, exosystem, and macrosystem.

educator role Nursing role that involves assisting others to gain knowledge, skills, or characteristics needed for living a healthy life.

ego One of Freud's three main theoretical elements (with id and superego) of the mental mechanism; its function is to mediate between the demands of the other two, serving as compromiser, adapter, and executor.

ego integrity versus despair Erikson's final conflict of development wherein the adult must accept his life as inevitable or, in failing this task, feel futility and hopelessness.

elder abuse A form of violence against older adults; may include physical abuse, neglect, intimidation, cruel punishment, financial abuse, abandonment, isolation, or other treatment resulting in physical harm or mental suffering; the deprivation by a custodian of goods or services necessary to avoid physical harm or mental suffering.

emerging diseases New, reemerging, or drug-resistant infections whose incidence in humans has increased within the past two decades or whose incidence threatens to increase in the near future.

emotional abuse Verbal or behavioral actions that diminish another's self-worth and self-esteem so that he or she feels uncared for, inept, and worthless.

empathy Understanding the subjective world of the other and then communicating that understanding.

employee assistance programs (EAPs) Company-provided programs such as counseling, chemical rehabilitation, or stress management that are helpful in supporting workers' attempts at maintaining or restoring productivity.

empowerment The process whereby individuals feel increasingly in control of their own affairs.

empowerment education A particular approach to community education that is based on Freire's ideas and makes use of active learning methods to engage clients in determining their own needs and priorities.

empty nest syndrome Parents' response to children's leaving home, leaving the parents as a couple again.

enculturation The process of acquiring knowledge and internalizing values and attitudes about a culture.

endemic The constant presence of an infectious agent or disease within a defined geographic area.

energy In the Neuman systems model, an innately or genetically acquired primary and basic power resource for the client as a system; a resource for system empowerment toward achievement of the highest level of wellness; the force needed to meet the demands for system integrity.

energy field The whole of a person's being as reflected in one's presence via observation, sensation, or intuition.

enmeshed family Family in which individual needs are sacrificed for the group.

enthusiasm Teaching behavior characterized by interest in and excitement about the subject being taught.

entropy Tending toward maximum disorder and disintegration; occurs when a system is either too open or too closed, causing family dysfunction.

entry phase Second phase of home visit, which moves from the going-to-see phase to the seeing phase.

environment Internal and external factors that constitute the context for agent-host interactions; the aspect of existence perceived outside the self; this perception changes with alterations in awareness and expansion of consciousness; one of the concepts of the nursing metaparadigm.

environmental hazards Those aspects of the environment that present real or potential danger to the human being, usually categorized as chemical, physical, mechanical, or psychosocial.

environmental health Those aspects of human health, disease, and injury that are determined or influenced by factors in the environment. This includes the study of both the direct pathological effects of various chemical, physical, and biological agents as well as the effects on health of the broad physical and social environment.

environmental justice The fair treatment and meaningful involvement of all people regardless of race, ethnicity, income, national origin, or educational level with respect to the development, implementation, and enforcement of environmental laws, regulation, and policies.

epidemic A number of cases of an infectious agent or disease (outbreak) clearly in excess of the normally expected frequency of that disease in that population.

epidemiology An applied science that studies the distribution and determinants of health-related states or events in populations.

epilepsy A condition characterized by repeated abnormal electrical discharges from neurons in the cortex of the brain resulting in loss of consciousness, behavior changes, involuntary movements, altered muscle tone, or abnormal sensory phenomena.

epistemologic Pertaining to the nature and foundations of knowledge.

equifinality The quality of there being a characteristic final state regardless of initial state. For instance, people tend to develop habitual ways of behaving and communicating so that whatever the topic, their way of dealing with it will be the same.

equilibrium Self-regulation, or adaptation that results from a dynamic balance or steady state.

equipotentiality The quality of different end states being possible from the same initial conditions.

era A period or stage of development in Levinson's theory of development, which is divided into early adulthood, middle adulthood, and late adulthood.

eradication Via the extermination of infectious agents, irreversible termination of the ability to transmit infection after the successful global eradication of infection.

ergonomics The study of the relationship between individuals and their work or working environment, especially with regard to fitting jobs to the needs and abilities of workers.

ethics The study of the nature and justification of principles that guide human behaviors and are applied to special areas in which moral problems arise.

ethnicity A group whose members share a common social and cultural heritage passed on to successive generations, such that members feel a bond or sense of identity with one another.

ethnocentrism The belief that one's own lifeway is the "right" way or is at least better than another.

exosystem The major institutions of the society.

expressed need Demand for services demonstrated by action: for example, putting a name on a waiting list.

expressive functions The affective dimension of the family.

extended family Traditionally, those members of the nuclear family and other blood-related persons, usually the family of origin (grandparents, aunts, uncles, cousins), called "kin"; more recently, people who identify themselves as "family" but are not necessarily related by blood or through adoption.

external family structure The dimension of the family structure that includes extended family and the larger systems of the community.

failure to thrive (FTT) Lack of adequate growth in the absence of an organic defect during the first year of life; those infants falling below the 3rd percentile on growth charts are evaluated for either insufficient contact with the mother or lack of stimulation.

false-negative test A screening test result that is negative when the individual actually has the disease of interest.

false-positive test A screening test result that is positive when the individual does not have the disease of interest.

family A social context of two or more people characterized by mutual attachment, caring, long-term commitment, and responsibility to provide individual growth, supportive relationships, health of members and of the unit, and maintenance of the organization and system during constant individual, family, and societal change.

family acculturative styles Ways in which the family can be understood as a cultural system; include the integrated bicultural, marginalized, traditional-oriented, nonresistive, assimilated, and separatist family styles.

family as client The family considered as a set of interacting parts; assessment of the dynamics among these parts renders the whole family the client.

family as context The family considered as the context within which individuals are assessed; emphasis is placed primarily on the individual, keeping in mind that she or he is part of a larger system.

family-centered nursing practice Set of principles that help the nurse address the important health issues of families and individual family members; views the family as the basic unit of care.

family cohesion Emotional bonding among family members.

family communication Transactional process whereby meanings are created and shared with others; in the Circumplex Model, considered a facilitating dimension.

family flexibility Amount of change in the family's leadership, role relationships, and relationship rules.

family functions The ways that families meet the needs of individuals and purposes of the broader society.

family health tree A genogram that includes the family health history.

family interactional theories Those theories that focus on the ways that family members relate to the family and on internal family dynamics.

family myths Longstanding family beliefs that shape family members' interactions with one another and with the outside world; unchallenged by family members, who distort their perceptions if necessary to keep the myths secure.

family networks Patterns of communication that families develop in order to deal with the needs of family living, specifically needs of regulating time and space, sharing resources, and organizing activities.

family of origin (or **orientation**) The family unit into which a person is born.

family process Interactions between family members whereby they accomplish their instrumental and expressive tasks.

family of procreation The family created for the purpose of raising children.

family roles Repetitive patterns of behavior by which family members fulfill family functions.

family strengths Characteristics that contribute to family unity and solidarity in order to manage the family's life successfully and to foster health and healing.

family structure The family's role structure, value systems, communication processes, and power structure.

family systems theories Those theories that emerge from sociology and psychology and are related to general systems theory, structural-functional approaches, and developmental theory but tend to focus on ways to change "dysfunctional" families.

family values Principles, standards, or qualities that family members believe to be worthwhile and hold dear.

fecal/oral transmission Transmission of an infectious agent directly via the hands or other objects that are contaminated with an infectious organism from human or animal feces and then placed in the mouth.

feedback The process of providing a circular information loop so that the system can receive and respond to its own output. A self-corrective process whereby the system adjusts both internally and externally. Feedback can be negative or positive. Positive feedback refers to input that is returned to the system as information that moves the system toward change. Negative feedback promotes equilibrium and stability, not change.

fee-for-service Method of paying health care providers for service or treatment, wherein a provider bills for each client encounter or service rendered and identified by a claim for payment.

feelings reflection A statement on the part of the listener that reflects feelings expressed by the speaker as heard by the listener.

felt need Those needs which people say they need.

feminization of poverty A trend evident in the U.S. and throughout the world since World War II. In this trend, an increasing portion of the poor have been women. Many are divorced or unmarried mothers.

fetal alcohol syndrome A pattern of anomalies occurring in infants born to mothers who abused alcohol during pregnancy.

fidelity The principle of promise keeping; the duty to keep one's promise or word.

finance controls Cost control strategy that attempts to limit the flow of funds into public or private health care insurance plans.

financing Amount of dollars that flow from payors to an insurance plan, either private or governmental.

first-order change Change in the degree of family functioning but not in the family system.

flow and transformation The process whereby input travels through the system in its original state or transformed so that the system can use it.

focal stimuli In Roy's theory, factors that precipitate an adaptive response.

focal system The particular system under study.

folk health system The cultural health care practices used by people in addition to or in place of those used in the professional health care system.

forensic nursing The field of nursing involving legal, civil, and human rights of victims and perpetrators of violent crime involving death and injury.

formal roles Roles explicitly assigned to family members as needed to keep the family functioning.

formal teaching Prearranged, planned teaching.

formative evaluation An ongoing evaluation that provides information regarding program performance "along the way"; permits improvements while programming is happening.

freebase A homemade refining process by which cocaine hydrochloride (HCl) is chemically "freed" from its HCl base to form a less stable but more potent drug.

frontier area An area that has fewer than 6 or 7 persons per square mile.

general systems theory The theory that the whole of any system is more than the sum of its parts, such that the whole can be understood only by study of the entire system in all its aspects; theory that describes the ways that units interact with larger and smaller units; used to explain the way that the family interacts with its members and with society.

generation gap Conflict between parents and adolescents.

generativity versus stagnation Erikson's middle-adult conflict wherein one seeks productivity as opposed to self-indulgence that leads to personal impoverishment.

genogram A graph outlining a family's history over a period of time, usually over three generations.

gentrification To convert an aging area in a city into a more affluent middle-class neighborhood by remodeling dwellings, resulting in increased property values and displacement of the poor.

global burden of disease (GBD) A method of measurement of health status in a population that quantifies not only the number of deaths but also the impact of premature death and disability on a population.

gross domestic product (GDP) All the goods and services produced for domestic use by a nation in one year.

growth Increase in body size or changes in structure, function, and complexity of body cell content and metabolic and biochemical processes up to the point of maturity.

guest A homeless person being housed temporarily in a hotel, shelter, boarding house, or the like.

guided imagery An imaging process wherein the guide tells the person or group of persons what to imagine and how to progress through the exercise, leaving the individuals to respond silently in their own ways; used to facilitate inner healing processes.

handicap Disadvantage resulting from impairment and disability.

healer One who facilitates the healing process by using a therapy intended to balance and harmonize the human energy field.

healing A process of moving toward fulfillment of one's highest potential; involves integration of body, emotions, mind, and spirit.

healing environment An environmental state that supports natural healing processes of the person and/or family and is characterized by caring, safety, nurturance, order, and beauty.

healing practices Practices intended to facilitate integration of one's whole self and relationships.

health Within the person-environment process, a state of well-being that is dependent on the nature of relationships within the system; one of the concepts of nursing's metaparadigm.

health balance The state of well-being resulting from the harmonious interaction of body, mind, spirit, and environment.

health behaviors Those behaviors exhibited by persons that affect their health either constructively or destructively; may be consciously selected, although unconscious needs may thwart the person's ability to carry out conscious intentions.

health care function The provision of physical necessities to keep the family healthy; health care and health practices that influence the family's health status.

health care policy Those public policies related to health and health services; actions taken by a government concerning health.

health determinant A factor that helps to either create or diminish health.

health education Learning experiences designed to facilitate self-awareness, provide information, and support change through the teaching process for the purpose of promoting health.

health maintenance organization (HMO) A health care organization formed within certain areas that emphasizes prevention, wellness, and coordination of primary care in an effort to decrease utilization of high-cost, high-tech, acute-care services; an organization or set of related entities organized for the purpose of providing health benefits to an enrolled population for a predetermined fixed periodic amount to be paid by the purchaser (e.g., government, employer, individual). There are four general models of HMOs: staff, medical groups, independent practice associations, and networks.

health potential The ability to cope with environmental changes.

health promotion Activities or interventions that identify the risk factors related to disease; the lifestyle changes related to disease prevention; the process of enabling individuals and communities to increase their control over and improve their health; these activities or strategies are directed toward developing the resources of clients to maintain or enhance their physical, social, emotional, and spiritual well-being.

health protection Those activities designed to maintain the current level of health, actively prevent disease, detect disease early, thwart disease processes, or maintain functioning within the constraints of disease.

health risk communication Informing people about environmental health hazards and health risks.

healthy public policy Health policies that focus on local and global health problems and incorporate input from stakeholders and various perspectives.

helicy A Rogerian concept that the human-environment interrelationship is characterized by a "continuous innovative, unpredictable, increasing diversity of human and environmental field patterns." The word *helicy* refers to the spiral shape of a helix.

hierarchy of systems The level of influence of one system with respect to another. The closer the supra- or subsystem to the focal system, the greater the influence.

historical religion A religion that has formed over the past few thousand years and has a written history of actual events and sacred texts to guide the followers.

holism The belief that living beings are interacting wholes who are more than the mere sum of their parts.

holistic healing therapies Noninvasive therapies used to stimulate healing of the whole person by integrating body, mind, and spirit.

hologram A three-dimensional image produced by an interference pattern of light (as laser light). Each individual part of the interference pattern contains the entire image. The entire image is revealed when the interference pattern is exposed to coherent light of the proper frequency.

home health nursing Skilled nursing and other related services provided to individuals and families in their places of residence for the purpose of promoting, maintaining, or restoring health.

homelessness Residing with relatives, living on the streets, or living in shelters during difficult times.

homeopathy A system of medical treatment based on the theory of treating certain diseases with very small doses of drugs that, in a healthy person in large doses, would produce symptoms like those of the disease.

homogeneity A situation in which all persons from a particular ethnic group or culture share the same beliefs, values, and behaviors.

horizontal transmission Transfer of disease or antibodies from person to person.

hospice A coordinated program of supportive, palliative services for terminally ill clients and their families.

host A person or living species capable of being infected.

house of origin The part of the legislature (Senate, House, Assembly) to which a bill is first introduced by its author; the author's house.

human aggregate dimension That aspect of environment comprising the set of characteristics that apply to the group of persons within the environment.

human development The patterned, orderly, lifelong changes in structure, thought, and behavior that evolve as a result of physical and mental capacity, experiences, and learning; the result of an integration of environmental, cultural, and psychological forces within the human being.

human energy field pattern A term used by Rogers to indicate the irreducible, indivisible, multidimensional nature of a person's energy field which is identified by pattern and manifests characteristics specific to the whole and cannot be predicted from knowledge of the parts.

human responses The various ways human beings respond to environment; a significant aspect for assessment in the person-environment interrelationship.

id One of Freud's three main theoretical elements (with ego and superego) of the mental mechanism; the part of personality design that contains the unconscious and instinct.

idiopathic failure to thrive Lack of adequate growth wherein the infant falls below the 3rd percentile of growth, in the face of adequate parenting skills, good maternal-child attachment, and no apparent organic cause for the lack of growth.

imagery A quasi-perceptual event of which we are self-consciously aware and which exists in the absence of stimuli that produce genuine sensory or perceptual counterparts. This event is a mental representation of reality, or fantasy. Imagery encompasses all five modes of perception (visual, auditory, kinesthetic, olfactory, and gustatory).

immunity An acquired resistance to specific diseases.

impairment Abnormality of body structure and appearance or disturbance of organs or systems resulting from any cause.

incest The crime of sexual relations between persons related by blood, especially between parents and children or brother and sister.

incidence The frequency of new cases of a health outcome in a specified population during a given time period.

incidence rate The rate of new cases of a condition or disease in a population in a specified time period; provides an estimate of the condition/disease risk in that population.

inclusion Requiring children with disabilities to have the most contact possible with children who do not have disabilities.

incrementalism The creation of public policy through individual steps that come together to form a certain direction, such as enacting separate laws relating to a common concept.

indemnity insurance Insurance benefits provided in cash that utilize a payment method to the beneficiary rather than in services (service benefits); fee-for-service.

indicator A particular type of performance measurement used in quality improvement.

indirect transmission Transfer of a disease by way of human host having contact with vehicles that support and transport the infectious agent.

industrial hygiene That science and art devoted to the anticipation, recognition, evaluation, and control of those environmental factors or stresses in or from the workplace that may cause sickness, impaired health and well-being, or significant discomfort and inefficiency among workers or among citizens of the community.

infant mortality rate The number of deaths of infants under 1 year of age in a year divided by the number of live births in the same year per 1000 live births; a measure of local, state, and national health status.

infectious agents Bacteria, fungi, viruses, metazoa, and protozoa.

inflation Rise in the general level of prices; an increase in the amount of money in circulation, resulting in a sudden fall in the value of money and an increase in prices.

informal roles Covert roles that meet the emotional needs of the individual and/or maintain the family equilibrium.

informal teaching Spontaneous teaching that takes advantage of a teachable moment without prior planning.

inhalant substance A volatile substance purposely inhaled to produce intoxication.

inner aspect of aging One's relationship to oneself and contentment with aging.

input Energy, matter, and information that the system must receive and process in order to survive.

insider's perspective A person's lived experience.

instrumental function The activities that assist individuals in the management of their lives, such as cooking, housekeeping, paying bills, shopping, and doing laundry (activities of daily living).

integrality A Rogerian concept that the human-environment interrelationship is characterized by a "continuous mutual human field and environmental field process"; that the human field pattern is inseparable from that of the environmental field.

integrated bicultural family style A family acculturative style in which the elements of both cultures are integrated, resulting in a balanced acceptance of two or more cultures.

integrative models of health Those models that address a broad range of biological, emotional, mental, social, and spiritual factors.

integrative therapies Therapies used with the intention of stimulating healing processes by harmonizing and balancing body, emotions, mind, and spirit.

Interactive Guided Imagery A therapeutic process developed and taught by Bresler and Rossman in which the provider provides the structure for the imagery process and the client guides the experience by using images that emerge from the subconscious during an altered state induced by deep relaxation. The client plans for follow-up and further intervention with the provider.

interdisciplinary services Diagnostic, developmental, educational, or other services provided by members of different disciplines functioning as a team.

intergovernmental organizations Those organizations that deal with health concerns on an ongoing basis and collaborate with national governments, private foundations, and other efforts to improve health: e.g., the World Health Organization.

internal dimension That aspect of environment commonly referred to as aspects of the person; physical body composition, biochemistry, genetics, attitudes, beliefs, and life experience.

internal family structure The dimension of family structure that includes family composition, gender, rank order, subsystems, and boundaries.

International Council of Nurses (ICN) An international organization that represents 112 national nursing organizations as members, with as many as 1 million nurses; it is the primary organization to promote the advancement of nurses.

interpenetrating processes The theory that nothing is whole in itself and that everything exists throughout the whole of everything else.

interpersonal systems Those systems or patterns that involve more than one person in an exchange of energy, such as in communication.

intersectoral collaboration Coordinated action by sectors of a community from governmental officials to grass-roots community organizations to plan and implement health care strategies.

intervention study Epidemiological study design that is experimental in nature and used to test a hypothesis about a cause-and-effect relationship.

intimacy versus isolation Erikson's task of young adults whereby the individual develops close relationships with others or suffers loneliness and isolation.

intrapersonal systems Those aspects of ourselves that we experience within ourselves, such as thoughts, beliefs, feelings, and attitudes; significant for both the nurse and client because they influence the nature of our relationships as well as our behavior.

investigator role The investigative role of the nurse involved in assessment of the environment and in data gathering; formulating a nursing diagnosis related to the community environment is inherent in the role.

ionizing radiation Radiation resulting from energy transferred through electromagnetic waves or subatomic particles; causes a variety of health effects as it passes through human tissue.

Jin Shin Jyutsu A touch therapy developed and taught by Mary Burmeister, similar in nature to acupressure, in which the nurse or provider holds "safety energy locks" along flows of energy to balance and harmonize the energy field.

justice The principle of fairness that is served when an individual is given that which he or she is due, owed, deserves, or can legitimately claim.

Ki See *chi*.

killed A slang expression referring to a bill's defeat.

Krieger-Kunz method of Therapeutic Touch The method of Therapeutic Touch developed for nursing practice by Dolores Krieger and Dora Kunz since the early 1970s; a specific technique and a body of research and literature involving this technique.

lacto-ovovegan diet A vegetarian diet that includes both dairy products and eggs.

lactovegan diet A vegetarian diet that includes dairy products but no eggs.

leading health indicators Ten major health concerns identified in *Healthy People 2010* documents on the basis of their ability to motivate action, availability of data to measure progress, and their importance as public health issues.

learned helplessness Decreasing motivation to respond to abusive treatment secondary to chronic feelings of helplessness and inability to control certain outcomes.

learning process A process involving the whole person and reflected in a change of behavior; involves cognitive, affective, and psychomotor components.

legitimate power The shared agreement among family members to designate a person to be the leader and to make the decisions.

levels of prevention A three-level model of intervention (primary, secondary, tertiary) used in the epidemiological approach, designed to prevent or to halt or reverse the process of pathological change as early as possible in order to prevent damage.

lobby The act of influencing legislators to take certain positions on prospective bills or issues.

locus of control The perception regarding source of control in one's life; internal locus of control is the perception that the person is in control, whereas external locus of control is the perception that outside influences are in control.

lose-win approach A destructive approach to conflict resolution whereby, regardless of his or her own needs, one person gives in to another person by being nonassertive and nonresponsible.

low birthweight (LBW) Neonate weight of less than 2500 grams resulting from prematurity or being small for gestational age.

macroeconomics Subscience focusing on the aggregate performance of all markets in a market system and on the choices made by that large market system.

macrosystem The institutional patterns of the culture.

mainstreaming The philosophy and activities associated with providing services to persons with disabilities in community settings, especially in school programs, to promote their fullest participation with those who have no disabilities.

maladaptation Unsuccessful adaptation wherein the results are a more chaotic state, sacrificed family growth and development, and markedly lowered overall sense of well-being, trust, and sense of order and coherence in the family.

male climacteric A feeling of anxiety over signs of aging in late-middle-aged men.

managed care A health service payment or delivery arrangement wherein the health plan attempts to control or coordinate use of services by its enrolled members in order to contain expenditures, improve quality, or both; arrangements usually involve a defined delivery system with providers who have some form of contractual arrangement with the plan.

managed-care organization An entity that integrates financing and management and the delivery of health care services to an enrolled population.

managed competition An approach to health system reform wherein health plans compete to provide health insurance coverage for enrollees; relies on market incentives (namely more subscribers and revenue) to encourage health care plans to keep down the cost of care; typically, enrollees sign up with a purchasing entity that purchases the services of competing health plans, offering enrollees a choice of the contracting health plans; purchasing strategy aimed at obtaining maximum value for employers and consumers; rewards suppliers who do the most efficient job of providing health care services that improve quality, cut costs, and satisfy customers.

marginalization The most dangerous form of oppression, a whole category of people who are expelled from useful participation in social life and thus subjected to severe material deprivation and even extermination.

marginalized family style A family acculturative style in which there is loss of identity with both the traditional culture and the majority culture.

marginals A group of people that live on the margins, or the edges of society rather than in the mainstream.

market system Mechanism whereby society allocates scarce resources.

maternal mortality rate Deaths of mothers at time of birth, expressed as a number per 100,000 live births.

maturation The emergence of genetic potential for changes in form, structure, complexity, integration, organization, and function, both physically and mentally.

maturity A state of complete growth or development that promotes physical and psychological well-being.

McMaster model of family functioning Describes a set of positive characteristics of a healthy family; focuses on the following six dimensions: problem solving, communication, role function, affective responsiveness, affective involvement, and behavior control.

meal site A place where meals are offered to a specific population such as the elderly or homeless, or usually at a greatly reduced cost.

meanings reflection A statement by the listener that reflects meanings and facts apparent in something expressed by the speaker, allowing for further exploration and clarification.

measures of association Statistical analysis methods used to investigate the relationship between two or more variables or events.

Medicaid A health program that is funded by federal and state taxes and pays for the health care of low-income persons.

medical assistive device An appliance that replaces or augments inadequate body functions necessary to sustain life.

Medicare Part A Government-run hospital insurance plan that helps pay for hospital, home health, skilled nursing facility, and hospice care for elderly and some disabled persons; financed primarily by payroll taxes paid by workers and employers.

Medicare Part B Government-run insurance plan that pays for physician, outpatient hospital, and other services for the aged and disabled; financed primarily by transfers from the general fund (tax revenues) of the U.S. Treasury and by monthly premiums paid by beneficiaries.

menopause Cessation of menstruation, or female climacteric.

Mental hygiene movement Founded in 1909, later renamed the Mental Health Association, it is the leading voluntary citizens organization in mental health. It emphasizes education and public awareness techniques to promote prevention and effective treatment.

mental retardation Significantly sub-average intellectual functioning existing with related limitations in adaptive skills such as communication, self-direction, self-care, social skills, health, academics, or work, with onset before age 18.

meridians A microtubular channel which carries a subtle nutritive energy (chi) to the various organs, nerves, and blood vessels.

mesosystem The interrelationships of the major settings of a person's life.

metropolitan (metro) area (MA) An area containing core counties with one or more central cities of at least 50,000 residents or with a Census Bureau–defined urban area (a total metro area population of 100,000 or more).

microeconomics Subscience focusing on the individual markets that make up the market systems and on the choices made by small economic units such as individual consumers and individual firms.

microsystem The immediate setting within which a person fulfills his or her roles.

midlife crisis The period of middle adulthood when the individual confronts his or her aging process.

midrange groups Those groups that focus on both content or tasks and process.

migrant farm worker A person employed in agricultural work of a seasonal or other temporary nature who is required to be absent overnight from his or her permanent place of residence.

minority The label applied to race, ethnicity, religion, occupation, gender, or sexual orientation; implies less in number than the general population or having characteristics perceived as undesirable by those in power.

mode of transmission The mechanism by which an infectious agent is transferred from an infected host to an uninfected host.

model A representation of perceived reality.

moral agency The ability to act according to moral standards.

moral obligation Duty to act in a particular way in response to ethical and moral norms.

morbidity rate A disease rate, specifically prevalence and incidence rates of diseases in a total population at risk in a specified time period.

morphogenesis A natural tendency of a normal social organization to grow.

morphostasis A balance between stability and a tendency to grow.

mortality rate The number of deaths from all causes divided by the total population at a particular time and place.

multidisciplinary team A group of health care professionals from diverse fields who work in a coordinated fashion toward a common goal.

mutation An anomaly in the genetic makeup of an organism; responsible for antibiotic resistance.

natural history of a disease The course that a disease would take from onset to resolution without intervention by humans.

natural immunity Immunity conferred when the host acquires an infection and develops antibodies that protect against subsequent infection.

needle and syringe exchange programs Programs in which intravenous drug users can exchange used needles and syringes for new ones; developed to help prevent the spread of HIV/AIDS.

needs assessment The systematic appraisal of the type, depth, and nature of health needs and problems as perceived by clients, health providers, or both, in a given community.

negentropy Tending toward maximum order; appropriate balance between openness and closedness is maintained.

negotiation A set of strategies for resolution of conflict between individuals and groups in which there are mutually acceptable tradeoffs; a set of highly complex communication skills that offers opportunity for all concerned to win.

network therapy An approach directed toward changing a family network that is reinforcing a dysfunctional stalemate.

neurotransmitter Nervous system chemicals that facilitate the transmission of impulses across the synapses between neurons.

newborn screening State programs providing blood tests on newborns to detect treatable conditions such as phenylketonuria, hypothyroidism, and galactosemia.

NIMBYism (Not in my back yard) A psychological reaction predicated on fear of what someone with a mental illness might do to harm others in their neighborhoods.

noncompliance Failure to yield or obey. A term often used in a negative way to describe a client's failure to follow the treatment regimen prescribed by health care professionals.

nondirective approach Clients are encouraged to seek solutions to their own problems and express thoughts and feelings as the nurses facilitate this exploration by asking open questions.

nonlegitimate power Characterized by domination or exploitation that suggests power against another's will.

nonmaleficence The principle of doing no harm.

nonmetropolitan areas Areas outside the boundaries of metropolitan areas that do not have a city of at least 50,000 residents.

nonorganic failure to thrive (NFTT) Lack of adequate growth wherein the infant falls below the 3rd percentile on the growth charts and there is no physical cause for the lack of growth; usually accompanies inadequate parenting skills or lack of parental attachment to the child.

nonverbal behaviors Those behaviors that communicate attitudes, meaning, or content to another, either intentionally or unintentionally, through gestures or other body language.

normalization A principle of service to people with disabilities, particularly mental retardation, that requires culturally appropriate methods and services to be provided in culturally appropriate settings so the individual may participate in community life as fully as possible.

normalizing A coping strategy used by people to control the impact of chronic illness on their lives.

normative need Need identified as such by professional opinion.

nosocomial infection An infection that develops in a health care setting and that was not present in the client at the time of admission.

nuclear family Husband, wife, and their children (natural, adopted, or both).

nurturance Things the environment provides that support health and healing, such as nutritious food, shelter, supplies, and respectful touch; also, the act of providing these things.

nutritive elements Substances such as vitamins or proteins that, if excessive or deficient, act as an agent of disease.

observational studies Nonexperimental studies that describe, compare, and explain disease occurrence.

occupational/environmental health nursing Specialty nursing practice that provides health care services to workers and worker populations.

odds ratio A statistical measure of association reflecting the ratio of two odds reflecting the relative risk (RR) when the specific risk of disease of both the exposed and the unexposed groups is low. Calculated when incidence rates are unavailable.

official international health organizations Agencies throughout the world that participate in collaborative arrangements via official governmental structure.

open questions Questions that do not restrict the client's responses but are instead intended to solicit the client's views, opinions, thoughts, and feelings; a means of getting clients to freely disclose information pertinent to their health.

open systems Those systems, such as human beings, that exist in interrela-

tionship with their environment, taking in and assimilating energy and eliminating waste.

openness/closedness Extent to which a system permits or screens out input, or new information.

operant conditioning The concept of seeking to discover what elicits a particular behavior and what subsequently reinforces it.

oppression A term used to indicate unequal power relations embedded in society.

order That element of the environment constituting methodical and harmonious arrangement of things.

organic failure to thrive (OFTT) Lack of adequate growth wherein the infant falls below the 3rd percentile on the growth charts and the cause is a physical condition.

organizational dimension That aspect of environment related to how time, space, and things are structured.

orthomolecular therapies Use of chemicals such as magnesium, melatonin, and megavitamins to treat diseases.

osteopathy System of medical practice based on the theory that diseases are due chiefly to a loss of structural integrity.

Outcome and Assessment Information Set (OASIS) Federally mandated requirement for all home health agencies whose purpose is to measure outcomes for outcome-based quality improvement.

outcome evaluation An assessment of change in a client's health status resulting from program implementation and whether this change was the intended result; requires selection of indicators sensitive to the program activities.

outer (or social) aspect of aging One's relationship with society as one ages.

out-of-pocket expenses Expenses not covered by a health care plan and, therefore, borne by the person.

output The result of the system's processing of input.

ovovegan diet A vegetarian diet that includes eggs but no dairy products.

palliative Serving to alleviate without curing; nursing actions that reduce or lessen pain or other symptoms for terminally ill clients.

Pan American Health Organization (PAHO) A health organization that focuses its efforts on the Americas; its major functions are to identify public health factors that are related to health and to distribute public health data that include epidemiological information, information about the health sys-

tems within the countries, and various environmental issues.

pandemic A worldwide outbreak of an epidemic disease.

panhandling Begging, especially on the streets.

paradigm A worldview or perspective of the universe and how it came to be and how it functions.

paradigm shift The idea that the Western world is shifting its mechanical worldview to a more holistic worldview.

parish nursing A community health nursing role in which a church or religious group provides services that promote health and facilitate healing to its members; a subspecialty of community health nursing that provides noninvasive health care services to the members of faith congregations.

partner abuse Physical, emotional, or sexual abuse perpetrated by one partner in an intimate relationship against the other. This term is inclusive of same-sex partners, unmarried heterosexual partners, and unmarried heterosexual men who are abused by female partners.

partnership The shared participation and agreement between a client and the nurse regarding the mutual identification of needs and resources, development of a plan, decisions regarding division of responsibilities, setting time limits, evaluation, and renegotiation; a relationship between individuals, groups, or organizations wherein the different participants in the relationship work together to achieve shared goals.

pathogenicity The ability or power of an infectious agent to produce disease.

patriarchy A male-dominated system in which males hold the majority of power; government rule, or domination, by men.

pattern appraisal The term used in Rogerian nursing theory to address what is generally called *health assessment,* because organizational patterns of the human-environment interrelationship determine health in this philosophy or conceptual model for nursing practice.

patterns Family behaviors, beliefs, and values that together make up the uniqueness that is the family; ways of behaving, feeling, believing, choosing, valuing, and perceiving that form a picture of the person-environment interrelationship.

pedagogy Teacher-directed education.

performance improvement An approach that focuses on a continuous effort to strive to improve the service through a process of action planning.

performance knowledge A quality management approach that addresses knowledge of clients, scope of services, identification and prioritization of services, standards that address structure/process outcomes, and the development of organization-specific performance standards.

performance measurement Use of indicators that enable health care organizations to measure outcomes as a function of individual and organizational performance.

person-environment interrelationship The whole of the interpenetrating, inseparable process that makes up the person and environment.

pervasive developmental disorder, not otherwise specified Characteristic of pervasive developmental disorders but that do not meet the diagnostic criteria for pervasive developmental disorder: schizophrenia, schizotypal personality disorder, or avoidant personality disorder. Includes "atypical autism."

pervasive developmental disorders Characterized by severe and pervasive impairment in several areas of development, particularly social and communications skills and restricted, stereotyped behaviors, interests, and activities.

philanthropic foundations Organizations that use funds from private endowments to support health-related projects.

physical agents Agents of disease that must be present or absent for a problem to occur. Examples include radiation, excessive sun exposure, mechanical agents.

physical dimension That aspect of environmental structures constituting the physical things we need for survival and safety, such as architecture, cleanliness, air, soil, water, food, and clothing.

physical environment The dwelling and the conditions both inside and outside.

plumbism A neurological condition caused by lead poisoning in children and that may be reversed in the early stages of the condition.

point of prevalence The total number of persons with a disease at a specific point of time.

policy Governmental practice that guides and directs action in all spheres of social interaction such as national defense policy, environmental policy, economic policy, and health care policy.

policy development Provision of leadership in developing comprehensive public health policies, including the use of scientific knowledge in decision making about policy.

policy framework The policies in place that determine how the organizational framework is structured to meet the needs of society and individuals within that society.

political action/political activism Activities and/or strategies involved in influencing the political process.

politics A process by which one influences the decisions of others and exerts control over situations and events.

population approach (population-focused health care) An element of health promotion whereby focus is on communities or aggregates.

population-focused practice Health care approach based on the notion that understanding the population's health is critical; focus is on diagnosing the population's health needs and assets and formulating interventions at the population level.

posttraumatic stress disorder An important disorder that appears following many kinds of violence. This disorder affects individuals who have been exposed to a traumatic event in which they or others were threatened with death or serious injury. Symptoms include reexperiencing the trauma, avoiding stimuli associated with the trauma, and numbing or general responsiveness, irritability or outbursts of anger, difficulty concentrating, hypervigilance, an exaggerated startle response. There is often a high risk of depression and suicide among those with this disorder.

poverty The lack of resources to meet basic needs which include food, shelter, clothing, and health care.

poverty line A measure established by the U.S. government which is sometimes called the poverty threshold for eligibility determination. This line determines who is and is not eligible for various government programs that offer assistance to the poor.

power Actual or potential ability of individual family members to change the behavior of other family members; also called *influence* and *dominance*; control or command over others; the ability to do or act; achievement of the desired result.

power bases Sources from which a family's power is derived.

power outcomes The final decision made, including who ultimately has control of the situation.

power processes Processes used in arriving at family decisions; also called *decision-making processes*.

power resources A person's physical, psychological, and social strengths.

powerlessness A sense of lack of control over the outcomes of one's life.

PRECEDE-PROCEED model A health promotion planning framework useful in applying the epidemiological approach to community health planning.

preexisting condition A health problem that was diagnosed or treated before an insurance policy was issued.

preferred-provider organization (PPO) A managed-care health plan that contracts with networks or panels of providers to furnish services; providers are paid on a negotiated-fee schedule. Unlike HMOs, PPOs do not provide the services themselves. Enrollees are offered a financial incentive to use providers on the preferred list, but they may use nonnetwork providers as well.

pregnancy-induced hypertension (PIH) Formerly known as toxemia; a condition of pregnancy that may cause physical harm to the mother and the fetus; characterized by hypertension, proteinuria, and edema; common among adolescents.

pregnancy outcome Health status of mother and infant at birth.

prenatal diagnosis Examination of the fetus by fetoscopy, amniocentesis, chorionic villus biopsy, ultrasound, or x-ray to detect abnormality.

prenatal risk assessment An assessment of a pregnant female for factors that may affect pregnancy outcome.

presbycusis Loss of hearing associated with aging.

presbyopia Farsightedness resulting from age-related changes in the elasticity of the lens of the eye.

prevalence The number of existing cases of a health outcome in a specified population at a designated place and time.

prevalence rate A proportion or percentage of a disease or condition in a population at any given time.

prevention Activities designed to intervene in the course of a disease or health-related conditions before pathology occurs (primary prevention); to detect and treat a disease early (secondary prevention); and to limit a disability or associated conditions (tertiary prevention).

prevention trials An epidemiological intervention study design used to compare measures or interventions aimed at the prevention of disease.

primal religion Those religions that have existed through oral tradition in tribal circumstances for as long as human beings have lived on the earth.

primary health care A model for health care that emphasizes equity, accessibility (close to home), full participation by communities, acceptable and affordable technology, intersectoral collaboration, and care that is health promotive and disease preventive; based on practical, scientifically sound and socially acceptable methods and technology made universally accessible to individuals and families in the community and at a level the country can afford to maintain at every stage of development in the spirit of self-reliance and self-determination. The activities deemed necessary to meet the Health for All objectives.

primary prevention Activities designed to promote health and prevent disease processes or injuries.

principled negotiation Decision making based on the merits of an issue rather than on taking positions and trying to get the other party to come to our own position.

principlism System of theory and practice whereby ethical decisions in health care are made exclusively via the formal application of ethical principles.

private organizations Privately owned organizations that provide financial and technical assistance for health care, employment, and access.

private voluntary organizations Organizations that provide different health care assistance programs; may be either religious or secular groups.

process evaluation An assessment of how well program activities are carried out; an account of that which actually happened or is happening in the program; involves interpretation of program outcomes in relation to process evaluation.

process-oriented groups Those groups that focus on relating and getting along with people.

program A service designed to produce particular results.

program evaluation The process of inquiry to assess the performance of a program, to determine whether a service is needed, likely to be used, and actually assists clients.

program implementation The process of putting into action the program plan.

program planning The process of identifying the situation, deciding on a more desirable situation, and designing actions to create the desirable situation.

programming Processes that when carried out together produce a program and the desired results; involves assessment, planning, implementation, evaluation, and sequential and iterative work.

programming models Representations of approaches to programming that offer explanations of the processes involved and, therefore, guide the programmer.

project team Group of people who conduct a community assessment; responsible for development of a research plan and time frame and for collection and analysis of information already available.

promotional indicators A measure of positive growth or enhanced functioning of a child, youth, family, or community.

prospective study An epidemiological study design that assembles study groups before disease occurrence.

pseudomutuality Long-term dysfunctional adaptive strategy that maintains family homeostasis at the expense of meeting the family's affective function.

psychoactive Substances, drugs, or chemicals that affect mental state.

psychoanalysis A treatment technique that uses free association and the interpretation of dreams to trace emotions and behaviors to repressed drives and instincts. By being made aware of the existence, origins, and inappropriate expression of these unconscious processes, the clients can eliminate or diminish the undesirable effects; a theory of psychology and a system of psychotherapy, developed by Freud.

psychological environment Developmental stages, family dynamics, and emotional strengths.

psychomotor learning objectives Learning objectives set by the nurse educator that describe what skills the client will be able to perform to meet the educational goal.

psychoneuroimmunology Study of the communication and interactions among the psyche, the nervous system, the immune system, the endocrine system, and other body systems via informational substances such as neuropeptides, hormones, and neurotransmitters.

psychotherapy The process of addressing symptom relief, resolution of problems, or personal growth through interacting in a prescribed way with a therapist.

public health Organized community efforts designed to protect health, promote health, and prevent disease.

public health nursing The field of nursing that synthesizes the public health, social, and nursing sciences to promote and protect the health of individuals, families, and communities.

quality assurance The accountability of the provider to deliver quality care.

quality improvement The process of attaining a higher level of performance or quality that is superior to previous levels and the actual attainment of that quality level.

quantum mechanics That branch of physics concerned with the energetic characteristics of matter at the subatomic level.

quantum theory The branch of physics which studies the energetic characteristics of matter at the subatomic level, supporting the position that subatomic particles have no meaningful trajectory, only constant and unpredictable motion; there is no certainty that matter exists, only "tendencies to exist."

qi See *chi.*

race Biological characteristics such as skin color and bone structure that are genetically transmitted from one generation to another.

rape Sexual contact occurring without the victim's consent, involving the use or threat of force and sexual penetration of the victim's vagina, mouth, or rectum.

rationing Limits placed on health care; including implicit rationing, which limits the capacity of the system and uses consumer triaging as a method of determining who will be served, and explicit rationing, whereby price and ability to pay are used to control costs.

reference group A group of others undergoing role transition.

regulatory finance controls Cost controls restricting the amount of state and federal tax revenues deposited into programs that fund health care programs such as Medicare and Medicaid.

reimbursement Flow of dollars from the insurance company to providers or hospitals.

reimbursement controls Cost control strategies including price and utilization controls and patient cost sharing.

relative risk An epidemiological measure of association that indicates the likelihood that an exposed group will develop a disease or condition relative to those not exposed.

relaxation response An alert, hypometabolic state of decreased sympathetic nervous system arousal that may be achieved in several ways, including breathing exercises, relaxation and imagery exercises, biofeedback, and prayer. This response increases the sense of mental and physical well-being.

religions A specific belief system regarding divine and superhuman power and involving a code of ethics and philosophical assumptions that lead to certain rituals, worship, and conduct by believers.

repetitive-motion injuries (RMIs) Injuries that occur over time (and usually on the job) as a result of repetitively performing the same motion.

reproductive function Ensures the continuity of both the family and society.

reservoir Any host or environment where an infectious agent normally lives and multiplies.

residual stimuli In Roy's theory, factors that may affect behavior but for which the effects are not validated.

Resiliency model of family stress, adjustment, and adaptation Emphasizes family adaptation and includes family types and levels of vulnerability.

resonancy A Rogerian concept that the human-environment interrelationship is characterized by a "continuous change from lower to higher frequency wave patterns in human and environmental fields." The word *resonance* refers to the effect produced when the vibration frequency of one body is greatly amplified by reinforcing vibrations at the same frequency from another body.

respect Trust that a person is capable of and has potential for learning and healing and can benefit from a caring environment.

retrospective study An epidemiological study design that assembles study groups after disease occurrence.

Rhett's disorder Following normal perinatal development, between 5 and 48 months head growth diminishes; purposeful hand skills are lost to stereotyped hand-wringing and washing movements. Problems with coordination of gait and trunk develop along with severe impairment of language and psychomotor skills. Reported only in females.

risk The probability that an event, outcome, disease, or condition will develop in a specified time period.

risk factors Precursors to disease that increase one's risk of the disease (e.g., demographic variables, certain health practices, family history of disease, and certain physiological changes).

role ambiguity Vague, ill-defined, or unclear role demands.

role conflict Result of contradictory or incompatible role expectations regarding one's role.

role incompetence Subjective feelings that may result when one's resources are inadequate to meet the demands of a role.

role modeling The process of enacting a role that others can observe and emulate.

role overload Having insufficient time to carry out all expected role functions.

role rehearsal The internal preparation and overt practice of new role behaviors.

role strain Emotional discomfort caused by a sense of conflicting role expectations, a lack of clear role expectations, inability to accomplish what is expected in the role within the time allotted, and/or perception of inadequate skills to meet role expectations.

role transition A process of learning new role behaviors, reviewing previously learned material, and mediating conflicts between different role expectations.

rules Characteristic relationship patterns within which a system operates; express the values of the system and the roles appropriate to behavior within the system; distinguish the system from other systems and, therefore, from the system boundaries; explicit or implicit regulations regarding what is acceptable or unacceptable to which the family is expected to adhere.

rural area An area with fewer than 2,500 residents and open territories.

rural health clinics Clinics that are certified under federal law to provide care in underserved areas within sparsely populated areas.

rural nursing The practice of professional nursing within the physical and sociocultural context of sparsely populated communities that involves continual interaction of the rural environment, the nurse, and the nurse's practice.

safety That component of environment that protects and keeps a person secure, unharmed, and free from danger.

safety energy locks In Jin Shin Jyutsu, those points along the energy pathways that are held by the practitioner to open up and balance the energy flow.

school nursing A branch of community health nursing that seeks to identify or prevent school health problems and intervene to remedy or reduce these problems.

seasonal farm worker A person employed in agricultural work of a seasonal or temporary nature who is not required to be absent overnight from his or her permanent place of residence.

secondary prevention Actions taken for the purpose of detecting disease in the early stages before there are clinically evident signs and symptoms present; early diagnosis and treatment.

secondhand smoke Tobacco smoke inhaled indirectly, from the environment; exposure determined by cotinine (the chemical metabolized by the body from nicotine) blood levels.

sedative A depressant drug that produces soothing or relaxing effects at lower doses and induces sleep at higher doses.

self-care An individual's acts and decisions to sustain life, health, well-being, and safety in the environment; personal health care performed by the client, often in collaboration with health care providers.

self-determination The right and responsibility of one to decide and direct one's choices.

self-efficacy The power to produce effects and intended results on one's own health and in one's own life.

self-esteem Feelings about oneself and how one measures up to that which one expects. People with high self-esteem see themselves as measuring up to their expectations for themselves; conversely, people with low self-esteem recognize a great disparity between who they actually are and their expectations of who they should be.

sensitivity The probability that an individual who has the disease of interest will have a positive screening test result.

separatist family style A family acculturative style in which the family does not feel comfortable assimilating and actively opposes doing so.

shamans Individuals of ancient tradition known to have various supernatural power, which include the practice of magic and medicine. In addition, these persons were known as priests, mystics, and poets, combating not only disease, but demons and the power of evil. Shamanism is a religious phenomenon of many indigenous cultures throughout the world.

sheltered employment A work center where supports are available and individual productivity may be set at noncompetitive levels.

shelters Facilities established to assist homeless people. Services offered vary from those that simply provide a place to get in out of the weather to those that offer a wide range of services. Some are specialized to deal with specific populations such as runaway youth and battered women.

Sigma Theta Tau, International An international honor society of nursing whose purpose is to promote excellence in nursing education, practice, and research.

small-group residence A facility licensed to provide housing, food, and programs to no more than 15 clients.

social capital Economic resources that can be accessed through social networks.

social class A group of people who rank closely to one another in wealth, power and prestige.

social class gradient More deprived groups who experience a greater burden of disease.

social dimension The aspect or dimension of environment provided by that aspect comprising social relationships, connection, and support.

social environment Religion, race, culture, social class, economic status, and external resources such as school, church, and health resources.

social justice The entitlement of all persons to basic necessities, such as adequate income and health protection, and the acceptance of collective action and obligation to make such possible.

social support A perceived sense of support from a complex network of interpersonal ties and from backup support systems for nurturance.

social systems Those systems that involve groups of different sizes and populations and their organizational processes and patterns of energy. Communication within and among these systems is a significant aspect of community health nursing, and the nurse with communication skills applicable to a variety of social systems can be influential in the community.

soup kitchen A place where food is offered either free or at greatly reduced price to individuals in need.

specificity The probability that an individual who does not have the disease of interest will have a negative screening test result.

spiritual abuse Instilled fear of being punished in this life or the next for failing to live a life good enough to please God or gain admittance to heaven.

spiritual assessment The collection, verification, and organization of data regarding the client's beliefs and feelings about such things as the meaning of life, love, hope, forgiveness, and life

after death, as well as the client's degree of connectedness to self, others, and a larger purpose in life. Spirituality refers to a sense of oneness with all of creation and of humanity and to the search for and discovery of life meaning and purpose.

spiritual terrorism An extreme form of spiritual abuse that is obvious, overt, and active.

spirituality The human belief system pertaining to humankind's innermost concerns and values, ultimately affecting behavior, relationship to the world, and relationship to God.

sponsor An individual or group who conceives of and may draft a bill to be presented in the legislature by a legislator.

spousal abuse Physical, emotional, or sexual abuse perpetrated by either a husband or a wife against the marriage partner; marital rape.

status epilepticus A medical emergency characterized by continuous seizures occurring without interruptions.

steering committee Group of people from outside the project team who oversee the project, providing outside advice and ensuring that the project achieves its goals.

stereotyping Assuming that all people of a cultural, racial, or ethnic group are alike and share the same values or beliefs.

stigma The disgrace or reproach experienced by mentally ill people and their families. In general, it can be assigned to anyone who is perceived by others to be in a discredited position.

story telling The sharing of stories between people, sometimes from one's life and sometimes in the form of parables, myths, and metaphors. Life meanings change as stories are shared in different life contexts.

strategic planning Increasing effectiveness by first identifying goals and then by determining how best to achieve them; used in educational activities such as teaching and public speaking.

stress Both a response and a stimulus as well as the interaction of person and environment; the response to stress is a critical determinant in health and illness.

stress response The nonspecific response of the body to any demand, which Selye called the general adaptation response.

stressors Environmental pressures that trigger the stress response.

structural evaluation The assessment of resources used in a program.

structural-functional framework Framework focusing on interaction of

the family and its internal-external environment; deemphasizes the importance of growth, change, and disequilibrium of a family over time.

structure building The period of development in young adulthood when the person fashions a lifestyle.

subenvironments An idea similar to dimensions of environment; used for the sake of analysis and assessment of environments.

substituted judgment A proxy decision for another based on an understanding of what the other would decide were that person able to decide on his or her own behalf.

subsystems The smaller units or systems of which a larger unit or system consists.

summative evaluation The retrospective assessment of how well a program performed up to the point of evaluation; a method used to assess program outcomes.

summative reflection The nurse sums up a conversation so that there is an understanding of what has been accomplished so far, clarifying and bringing closure to a meeting or discussion.

superego One of Freud's three main theoretical elements (with id and ego) of the mental mechanism; the part of the personality structure associated with ethics, standards, and self-criticism, formed by identification with important persons, especially parents, early in life.

Superfund site A hazardous waste site designated by the U.S. Environmental Protection Agency as being a threat to human health.

supported employment A job coach or other support ensures success at a competitive job.

suprasystem The larger system of which smaller systems are a part.

surrogate mother A woman who, for someone other than herself, carries a child conceived from an egg not necessarily her own.

surveillance The systematic collection and evaluation of all aspects of disease occurrence and spread, resulting in information that may be useful in the control of the disease.

sustainable development Growth and development within a society that is intended to meet the needs of the present without compromising the ability of future generations to meet their own needs.

sustainable environment An environment in which health is maintained for future generations.

system A goal-directed unit made up of interdependent, interacting parts that endure over a period of time. According to Rogers, the parts are interpenetrating processes within the larger system throughout the whole.

teaching Helping another gain knowledge, understanding, and/or skills by instructing, demonstrating, or guiding the learning process in some way.

teaching/learning process The teacher-learner interaction wherein each participant communicates information, emotions, perceptions, and attitudes to the other.

technology assisted Dependent upon a device that substitutes for a body function.

telecommunications The use of wire, radio, optical, or other electromagnetic channels to transmit or receive signals for voice, data, and video communications by e-mail, computer conferencing, long-distance blackboards, and bulletin board systems.

telehealth Use of telecommunications to deliver health care services and to provide health care professionals and consumers access to medical information.

telehome health Adjunct to home visits where technology is installed in a client's home and the nurse is able to monitor care and observe and interact with the client from the agency home base.

telenursing A form of telehealth in which nursing practice is delivered via telecommunications, using technologies such as telephones, computers, and interactive transmissions of voice, data, and video.

teleology The ethical theory that determines rightness or wrongness solely on the basis of an estimate of the probable outcome; a theory of purpose, ends, goals, or final causes.

teratogenic effects The disruption of normal fetal development by an agent such as a drug or substance, affecting the genetic structure of the fetus and causing malformations.

termination phase The third phase of the home visit; the nurse summarizes accomplishments, discusses plans for the next visit, discusses referrals, and prepares documentation for the visit as prescribed by the agency for which the nurse is working.

terrorism Violence or threat of violence to produce fear and coerce or intimidate governments or societies in the pursuit of political, religious, or ideological goals.

terrorist A violent person prepared to use and committed to using force to attain goals.

tertiary prevention The treatment, care, and rehabilitation of people who have acquired acute or chronic disease, with the goal of limiting disability and minimizing the extent and severity of health problems.

testimony Communicating to a committee or the legislature evidence in support of a fact, statement, or bill.

therapeutic communication Communication that helps the client cope with stress, get along with other people, adapt to situations that cannot be changed, and overcome emotional and mental blocks that prevent evolution of one's potential as a human being.

therapeutic landscapes Those changing places, settings, situations, locales, and milieus that encompass the physical, psychological, and social environments associated with treatment or healing; these places often have a reputation for achieving physical, mental, and spiritual healing.

Therapeutic Touch (TT) A holistic therapy whereby there is a consciously directed manipulation of energy; the practitioner uses the hands to facilitate the healing process.

therapeutic trials An epidemiological intervention study design used to compare measures or interventions aimed at therapeutic benefits.

third-party payor Entity other than the provider or consumer that is responsible for total or partial payment of health care costs.

total quality management/continuous quality improvement Management philosophy that emphasizes the processes and principles that address the goal of continuous improvement of quality.

touch therapy One of multiple energy-releasing and balancing modalities that use the hands to promote health and facilitate healing in the receiver or client.

toxicology The science or study of poisons.

traditional family Usually children, a legal marriage, blood kinship bonds, and a lifestyle that has its genesis in the family.

traditional indicators Measures of reduction or elimination of diseases or dysfunctional or at-risk behaviors and conditions.

traditional-oriented nonresistive style A family acculturative style that is composed of first-generation parents and children who are traditionally oriented and have had little exposure to the host country.

transactional field theory Theory that views the individual in the context of his or her transactional field, which is composed of all aspects of that individual's life.

transcultural nursing A client-nurse relationship wherein the parties are from different cultures; the nurse works within the cultural framework of the client as well as within the health care system of which the nurse is a part.

transition A coordinated set of activities for a student, designed within an outcome-oriented process, that promotes movement from school to postschool activities, including post–secondary education, vocational training, integrated employment, continuing and adult education, adult services, independent living, or community participation.

trigger lock A lock that fits into a gun trigger so that the gun cannot be fired until the lock is unlocked.

uncertainty The inability to make meaning of or predict life events.

unintentional injury Accidental injury, a major health problem for children and the leading cause of death and disability in children under the age of 14.

United Nations Children's Emergency Fund (UNICEF) International organization that was originally formed to assist the children who lived in European war countries but currently has a worldwide focus.

universalistic argument The position stating that effective assessment and intervention outcomes can be similar across multicultural groups independent of client-nurse racial/ethnic differences or similarities and proposes that what is relevant in the care of multicultural groups is evidence that the nurse displays both cultural sensitivity and cultural competence.

upstream thinking Identifying and modifying those economic, political, and environmental variables that are contributing factors to poor health worldwide.

urban areas (ua) Consist of densely settled territories that contain 50,000 or more people.

urban cluster (uc) Densely settled territory that has at least 2,500 people but fewer than 50,000 people.

usual and customary reimbursement Arrangement whereby the provider agrees to accept a predetermined level of reimbursement for service.

utilitarianism The ethical theory used to determine whether actions are wrong or right depending on their outcomes, the utility of an action being based on whether that action brings about a greater number of good consequences as opposed to evil consequences and, by extension, greater good than evil in the world as a whole; one type of teleology.

utilization controls Cost control strategy aimed at the supply side of the health care market, whereby a provider is evaluated against other providers who supply similar services so as to determine cost of care in relation to quality and outcomes.

vector An agent that actively carries a germ to a susceptible host.

vegans Vegetarians who eat no meat, eggs, or dairy products.

veracity The principle of truth telling; the duty to tell the truth.

vertical transmission Disease or antibody transfer from mother to child.

very low birthweight Neonate weight of 1500 grams or less.

veto Power of a chief executive to reject bills passed by the legislature.

virulence An agent's degree of pathogenicity, or ability to invade and harm the host.

visualization In the imagery process, the use of visual pictures in the mind as opposed to hearing, smell, touch, taste, and movement.

vital statistics Systematically tabulated data on vital events such as births, deaths, marriages, divorces, adoptions, annulments, separations, and health events that are based on registration of these events.

warmth Conveying to others that you like to be with them and that you accept them as they are; extending warmth enhances closeness and makes the nurse more approachable from the perspective of both clients and colleagues.

wellness Moving toward the fulfillment of one's potential as a human being; physically, emotionally, mentally, and spiritually; a dynamic state of health wherein individuals, families, and population groups progress to a higher level of functioning.

wider family Relationships that emerge from lifestyle and are voluntary and independent of necessary biological or kin connections; participants may or may not share a common dwelling.

wife abuse Physical, emotional, or sexual abuse perpetrated by a husband against his wife.

windshield survey Observation of a community while driving a car or riding public transportation in order to collect data for a community assessment.

win-lose approach A destructive form of conflict resolution whereby, without regard for the concerns and wishes of the other person, one person gets what he or she wants by "bulldozing" the other person; an aggressive and nonresponsible approach.

win-win approach A constructive form of conflict resolution whereby, via assertiveness and responsibility, both parties gain something and are happy with the outcome.

World Bank Places major emphasis on assisting countries where economic development is needed.

World Health Organization A major intergovernmental organization that deals with health concerns at the international level.

yang In Chinese philosophy, the active, positive, masculine force or principle in the universe; source of light and heat; it is always complementary to and contrasted with yin.

yin In Chinese philosophy, the passive, negative, feminine force or principle in the universe; it is always complementary to and contrasted with yang.

zoonosis An infection that can be transmitted from animals to humans.

CHAPTER 1: CARING IN COMMUNITY HEALTH NURSING

American Nurses Association. (1980). *A conceptual model of community health nursing* (ANA Pub. No. Ch-10). Kansas City, MO: Author.

American Public Health Association. (1981). *The definition and role of public health nursing practice in the delivery of health care: A statement of the public health nursing section.* Washington, DC: Author.

American Public Health Association, Public Health Nursing Section. (1996). *The definition and role of public health nursing—A statement of the Public Health Nursing Section.* Washington, DC: Author.

Association of Community Health Nursing Educators, Task Force on Basic Community Health Nursing Education. (1990). *Essentials of baccalaureate nursing education for entry level community health nursing practice.* Louisville, KY: Author.

Benner, P., & Wrubel, J. (1989). *The primacy of caring: Stress and coping in health and illness.* Menlo Park, CA: Addison-Wesley.

Boykin, A., & Schoenhofer, S. (1993). *Nursing as caring: A model for transforming practice.* New York: National League for Nursing Press.

Breslow, L. (1990). A health promotion primer for the 1990s. *Health Affairs, 9*(2), 6–21.

Callahan, D. (1990). *What kind of life: Limits of medical progress.* New York: Simon & Schuster.

Dossey, B. M. (Ed.) (1997). *Core curriculum for holistic nursing.* Gaithersburg, MD: Aspen.

Engebretson, J. (2000). Caring presence: A case study. *International Journal for Human Caring, 4*(2), 33–39.

Fawcett, J. (1995). *Analysis and evaluation of conceptual models of nursing* (3rd ed.). Philadelphia: F. A. Davis.

Freeman, R. B. (1963). *Public health nursing practice* (3rd ed.). Philadelphia: W. B. Saunders.

Freudenberg, N. (2000). Time for a national agenda to improve the health of urban populations. *American Journal of Public Health, 90*(6), 835–840.

Fry, S. T. (1991). A theory of caring: Pitfalls and promises. In D. A. Gaut &

M. M. Leininger (Eds.), *Caring: The compassionate healer* (pp. 161–172). New York: National League for Nursing.

Fry, S. T. (1993). The ethic of care: Nursing's excellence for a troubled world. In D. A. Gaut (Ed.), *A global agenda for caring* (p. 30). New York: National League for Nursing.

Gadow, S. A. (1980). Existential advocacy: Philosophical foundation of nursing. In S. Spicker & S. Gadow (Eds.), *Nursing images and ideals: Opening dialogue with the humanities* (pp. 79–101). New York: Springer Publishing.

Gadow, S. A. (1985). Nurse and patient: The caring relationship. In A. Bishop & J. R. Scudder (Eds.), *Caring, curing, coping: Nurse, physician, patient relationships* (pp. 31–43). Birmingham, AL: University of Alabama.

Gaut, D. A. (1981). Conceptual analysis of caring: Research method. In M. Leininger (Ed.), *Caring: An essential human need* (pp. 17–24). Thorofare, NJ: Charles B. Slack.

Gaut, D. A. (1989). A philosophic orientation to caring research. In M. M. Leininger (Ed.), *Care: The essence of nursing and health* (pp. 17–25). Detroit, MI: Wayne State University Press.

Gaut, D. A. (Ed.). (1992). *The presence of caring in nursing.* New York: National League for Nursing Press.

Gaut, D. A. (1993). A vision of wholeness for nursing. *Journal of Holistic Nursing, 11*(2), 164–171.

Gaylin, W. (1976). *Caring.* New York: Avon.

Gebbie, K. M., & Hwang, I. (2000). Preparing currently employed public health nurses for changes in the health system. *American Journal of Public Health, 9*(5), 716–721.

Gilligan, C. (1977). In a different voice: Women's conceptions of self and of morality. *Harvard Educational Review, 47,* 481–517.

Hanlon, J., & Pickett, G. (1984). *Public health: Administration and practice* (8th ed.). St. Louis, MO: Times Mirror/Mosby.

Henderson, V. (1993). Health is everybody's business. In M. Styles & P. Moccia (Eds.), *On nursing: A literary celebration, an anthology* (pp. 38–42). New York: National League for Nursing.

Institute of Medicine, Committee for the Study of the Future of Public Health. (1988). *The future of public health.* Washington, DC: National Academy Press.

Ippolito-Shepherd, J., & Cerqueria, M. T. (2000). Global conference on health promotion. In *International Health Section, Fall 2000.* Washington, DC: American Public Health Association.

Kickbusch, I. (1989). The new public health orientation for the city. In *WHO Healthy Cities Papers No. 4.* (pp. 43–54). Copenhagen, Denmark: FADL Publishers.

Lakomy, J. M. (1993). The interdisciplinary meanings of human caring. In D. A. Gaut (Ed.), *A global agenda for caring* (pp. 181–189). New York: National League for Nursing.

Larson, P. L. (1986). Cancer nurses perceptions of caring. *Cancer Nursing, 9*(2), 86–91.

Leavell, H. R., & Clark, E. G. (1958). *Preventive medicine for the doctor in his community.* New York: McGraw-Hill.

Leininger, M. (1977). The phenomenon of caring: Caring—The essence and central focus of nursing. *Nursing Research Report, 12*(1), 2–14.

Leininger, M. M. (1991). *Culture care diversity and universality: A theory of nursing.* New York: National League for Nursing.

Leininger, M. M. (Ed.). (1984). *Care: The essence of nursing and health.* Thorofare, NJ: Charles B. Slack.

Mayeroff, M. (1971). *On caring.* New York: Harper & Row.

McKinlay, J. B. (1979). A case for refocusing upstream: The political economy of illness. In E. G. Jaco (Ed.), *Patients, physicians, and illness* (3rd ed., pp. 9–25). New York: Free Press.

Morse, J. M., Bottorff, J., Neander, W., & Solberg, S. (1999). Comparative analysis of conceptualizations and theories of caring. *Image: Journal of Nursing Scholarship, 23*(2), 119–126.

Nijuis, H. G. (1989). Contemporary municipal health departments in the Netherlands: A proposed potential for new public health. In World Health Organization, The new public health in an urban context: Paradoxes and solutions, *WHO Healthy Cities Papers No. 4* (pp. 17–39). Copenhagen, Denmark: FADL Publishers.

Noack, H. (1987). Concepts of health and health promotion. In T. Abelin, Z. J. Brzezinski, & V. D. L. Carstairs (Eds.), *Health promotion and protection* (WHO Regional Publications, European series 22). Copenhagen, Denmark: World Health Organization and the International Epidemiological Association.

Noddings, N. (1984). *Caring: A feminine approach to ethics and moral education*. Berkeley, CA: University of California Press.

Ottawa Charter for Health Promotion. (1987). *Health Promotion, 1*(4), iii.

Patterson, J., & Zderad, L. (1976). *Humanistic nursing*. New York: John Wiley & Sons.

Pellegrino, E. (1985). The caring ethic: The relation of physician to patient. In A. H. Bishop & J. R. Scudder (Eds.), *Caring, curing, coping: Nurse, physician, patient relationships* (pp. 8–30). Birmingham, AL: University of Alabama Press.

Pender, N. (1996). *Health promotion in nursing practice* (3rd ed.). Stamford, CT: Appleton & Lange.

Pickett, G., & Hanlon, J. (1990). *Public health administration and practice*. St. Louis, MO: Times Mirror/Mosby College Publishing.

Public Health Functions Steering Committee. (1994). *Public health in America*. U.S. Public Health Service. [On-line]. Available: http://www.health.gov/phfunctions/public.htm.

Ray, M. (1981). A philosophical analysis of caring within nursing. In M. Leininger (Ed.), *Caring: An essential human need* (pp. 25–36). Thorofare, NJ: Charles B. Slack.

Ray, M. (1987). Health care economics and human caring in nursing: Why the moral conflict must be resolved. *Family and Community Health, 10,* 35–43.

Ray, M. A. (1999). The future of caring in the challenging health care environment. *International Journal for Human Caring, 3*(1), 7–11.

Roach, M. S. (1989). *The human act of caring: A blueprint for the health professions*. Ottawa, Canada: Canadian Hospital Association.

Roach, M. S. (1991). The call to consciousness: Compassion in today's health world. In D. A. Gaut & M. M. Leininger (Eds.), *Caring: The compassionate healer* (pp. 7–17). New York: National League for Nursing.

Rodriquez-Garcia, R., & Akhter, M. (2000). Human rights: The foundation of public health practice. *American Journal of Public Health, 90*(5), 693–694.

Salmon, M. E. (1993). Public health policy forum: Public health nursing—The opportunity of a century. *American Journal of Public Health, 12*(83), 1674–1675.

Shugars, D. A., O'Neil, E. H., & Bader, J. D. (Eds.). (1991). *Healthy America: Practitioners for 2005*. Durham, NC: The Pew Health Professionals Commission.

Snyder, M., Brandt, C. L., & Tseng, Y. (2000). Measuring intervention outcomes: Impact of nurse characteristics. *International Journal for Human Caring, 4*(1), 36–42.

Snyder, M., & Lindquist, R. (1998). *Complementary/alternative therapies in nursing* (3rd ed.). New York: Springer.

U.S. Department of Health and Human Services. (1991). *Healthy people 2000: National health promotion and disease prevention objectives*. Rockville, MD: Author.

Wald, L. D. (1971). *The house on Henry Street*. New York: Dover Publications.

Watson, J. (1985). *Nursing: Human science and human care: A theory of nursing*. Norwalk, CT: Appleton-Century-Crofts.

Watson, J. M. (1988). New dimensions of human caring theory. *Nursing Science Quarterly, 1*(4), 175–181.

Williams, C. A. (2000). Community-oriented population-focused practice: The foundation of specialization in public health nursing. In M. Stanhope & J. Lancaster (Eds.), *Community and public health nursing* (5th ed., pp. 3–19). St. Louis, MO: Mosby.

World Health Organization. (1974). *Chronicle of WHO, 1,* 1–2.

World Health Organization. (1988a). A guide to assessing healthy cities. In *WHO Healthy Cities Papers No. 3.* Copenhagen, Denmark: FADL Publishers.

World Health Organization. (1988b). Promoting health in the urban context. In *WHO Healthy Cities Papers No. 1.* Copenhagen, Denmark: FADL Publishers.

World Health Organization. (1989). The new public health in an urban context: Paradoxes and solutions. In *WHO Healthy Cities Papers No. 4.* Copenhagen, Denmark: FADL Publishers.

World Health Organization. (1998a). *Health for all: Origins and mandate, special publication: The world health report: Life in the 21st century—vision for all.* Geneva, Switzerland: Author.

World Health Organization. (1998b). *Health for all in the 21st Century.* Geneva, Switzerland: Author.

World Health Organization, Regional Office for Europe. (1984). *Health promotion: A discussion document on the concepts and principles.* Copenhagen, Denmark: WHO Europe, FADL Publishers.

Zerwekh, J. V. (1993). Commentary: Going to the people—Public health nursing today and tomorrow. *American Journal of Public Health, 83*(12), 1676–1678.

CHAPTER 2: HISTORICAL DEVELOPMENT OF COMMUNITY HEALTH NURSING

Allen, C. E. (1991). Holistic concepts and the professionalism of public health nursing. *Public Health Nursing, 8*(2), 74–80.

American Public Health Association. (1993). *A century of caring: A celebration of public health nursing in the United States, 1893–1993*. Washington, DC: USPHS Division of Nursing.

Anderson, C. L., Morton, R. F., & Green, L. W. (1978). *Community health* (3rd ed.). St. Louis, MO: Mosby.

Ashton, J. (1992). *Healthy cities*. Buckingham, England: Open University Press.

Basch, P. F. (1990). *Textbook of international health*. New York: Oxford University Press.

Booth, R. (1989). Summary. *Journal of Professional Nursing, 5*(5), 271–272.

Brainard, A. M. (1985). *The evolution of public health nursing*. New York: Garland. [Reprinted from Brainard, A. M. (1922). *The evolution of public health nursing*. Philadelphia: W. B. Saunders.]

Browne, H. (1966). A tribute to Mary Breckinridge. *Nursing Outlook, 14,* 5.

Brundtland, G. R. (1999). *Message from the Director-General. World health report 1999: Making a difference*. Geneva, Switzerland: World Health Organization.

Buhler-Wilkerson, K. (1985). Public health nursing: In sickness or health. *American Journal of Public Health, 75,* 1155–1161.

Bullough, V., Church, O. M., & Stern, A. (1988). *American nursing: A bibliographic dictionary*. New York: Garland Publishing.

Cassedy, J. H. (1962). Hygeia: A midvictorian dream of a city of health. *Journal of the History of Medicine, 17*(2), 217–228.

Chadwick, H. D. (1937). The diseases of the inhabitants of the Commonwealth. *New England Journal of Medicine, 216,* 8.

Cohen, I. B. (1984). Florence Nightingale. *Scientific American, 250*(3), 128–137.

Deloughery, G. L. (1977). *History and trends of professional nursing* (8th ed.). St. Louis, MO: Mosby.

Dock, L. L., & Stewart, I. M. (1925). *A short history of nursing: From the earliest time to the present day*. New York: G. P. Putnam.

Dock, L. L., & Stewart, I. M. (1938). *A short history of nursing* (4th ed.). New York: Putnam.

Dolan, J. (1978). *History of nursing*. Philadelphia: Saunders.

Donahue, M. P. (1991). Why nursing history? *Journal of Professional Nursing, 7*(2), 77.

Duhl, L. (1992). Healthy cities: Myth or reality. In J. Ashton (Ed.), *Healthy cities* (pp. 15–21). Buckingham, England: Open University Press.

Duhl, L., & Hancock, T. (1988). Community self-evaluation: A guide to assessing healthy cities. In *Healthy Cities Papers*. Copenhagen, Denmark: FADL Publishers.

Fagin, C. (1978). Primary care as an academic discipline. *Nursing Outlook, 26,* 750–753.

Fee, E. (1991). The origins and development of public health in the United States. In W. Holland, R. Detels, & G. Knox (Eds.), *Oxford textbook of public health* (2nd ed., pp. 3–22). Oxford, England: Oxford University Press.

Finer, S. E. (1952). *The life and times of Sir Edwin Chadwick*. London: Methuen.

Ford, L. C., & Silver, H. K. (1967). The expanded role of the nurse in child care. *Nursing Outlook, 15*(9), 43–45.

Freeman, R. (1964). *Public health nursing practice* (3rd ed.). Philadelphia: W. B. Saunders.

Friedman, E. (1990). Troubled past of an invisible profession. *Journal of American Medical Association, 264,* 2851–2855, 2958.

Frontier Nursing Service. (1999). *Today, yesterday, tomorrow: A demonstration in family centered primary health care*. Wendover, KY: Frontier Nursing Service.

Gardner, M. S. (1919). *Public health nursing*. New York: Macmillan.

Gardner, M. S. (1952). *Public health nursing* (3rd ed.). New York: Macmillan.

Ginzberg, E. (1985). *American medicine: The power shifts*. Totowa, NJ: Rowman & Allanheld.

Goldwater, M., & Zusy, M. (1990). *Prescription for nurses effective political action*. Philadelphia: Mosby.

Goodnow, M. (1933). *Outlines of nursing history*. Philadelphia: W. B. Saunders.

Green, L. W. (1996). Commentary. In U.S. Department of Health and Human Services, Public Health Service, *Healthy People 2000: Midcourse review and 1995 revisions*. Sudbury, MA: Jones & Bartlett.

Grier, B., & Grier, M. (1978). Contributions of the passionate statistician. *Research in Nursing and Health, 1,* 103–109.

Hamilton, D. (1989). The cost of caring: The Metropolitan Life Insurance company's visiting nurse service, 1909–1953. *Bulletin of the History of Medicine, 63,* 414–434.

Hanlon, J. (1964). *Principles of public health administration*. St. Louis, MO: Mosby.

Hanlon, J., & Pickett, G. (1984). *Public health: Administration and practice* (8th ed.). St. Louis, MO: Times Mirror/Mosby.

Harding, H. O. (1926). Health opportunities in Harlem. *Opportunity: Journal of Negro Life, 4,* 386–387.

Haupt, A. C. (1953). Forty years of teamwork in public health nursing. *American Journal of Nursing, 53,* 81–84.

Health Targets and Implementation Committee. (1988). *Health for all Australians: Report to the Australian Health Ministers' Advisory Council and the Australian Health Ministers' Conference,* Canberra, Australia: Australian Government Publishing Service.

Igoe, J. B. (1980). Changing patterns in school health nursing. *Nursing Outlook, 28,* 486–492.

Institute of Medicine. (1988). *The future of public health*. Washington, DC: National Academy of Science.

Jensen, D. M. (1959). *History and trends of professional nursing* (4th ed.). St. Louis, MO: Mosby.

Kalisch, P. L., & Kalisch, B. J. (1982). *Politics of nursing*. Philadelphia: J. B. Lippincott.

Kalisch, P. L., & Kalisch, B. J. (1995). *The advance of American nursing* (3rd ed.). Philadelphia: J. B. Lippincott.

Kaufman, M., Hawkins, J. W., Higgins, L. P., & Friedman, A. H. (1988). *Dictionary of American nursing bibliography*. Westport, CT: Greenwood Press.

Keeling, A., & Ramos, C. (1995). The role of nursing history in preparing nursing for the future. *N & HC: Perspectives on Community, 16*(1), 30–34.

Kelly, L. Y. (1971). *Dimensions of professional nursing* (4th ed.). New York: Macmillan.

Kelly, L. Y. (1981). *Dimensions of professional nursing* (5th ed.). New York: Macmillan.

Kelly, L. Y. (1991). *Dimensions of professional nursing* (6th ed.). New York: Pergamon Press.

Kiernan, F. (1952). *Citizens on the march: History of the New York Tuberculosis and Health Association*. New York: New York Tuberculosis and Health Association.

Lamont, L., & Lees, P. (1994). Practicing community health nursing in the context of primary health care. In C. Cooney (Ed.), *Primary health care: The way to the future* (pp. 313–329). Sydney, Australia: Prentice Hall.

Lancaster, J. (1996). History of community health and community health nursing. In M. Stanhope & J. Lancaster (Eds.), *Community health nursing: Process and practice for promoting health* (4th ed., pp. 3–19). St. Louis, MO: Mosby.

Maynard, T. (1939). *The apostle of charity: The life of St. Vincent de Paul*. New York: Dial Press.

McKeown, T. (1976). *The role of medicine—Dream, mirage, or nemesis*. London: Nuffield Provincial Hospitals Trust.

McNeil, E. E. (1967). *Transition in public health nursing*. John Sundwall lecture. University of Michigan, February 27.

Mosley, M. O. (1995). Mabel K. Staupers: A pioneer in professional nursing. *N & HC: Perspectives on Community, 16*(1), 12–17.

National Organization of Public Health Nursing. (1944). Approval of Skidmore College of Nursing as preparing students for public health nursing. *Public Health Nursing, 36,* 371.

Nightingale, F (1867). Letter to the editor, Macmillan magazine as cited in M. Styles & P. Moccial. (1993). *On nursing: A literary celebration.* New York: National League for Nursing.

Nightingale, F. (1969). *Notes on nursing: What it is and what it is not.* New York: Dover. (Original work published in 1859.)

Novak, J. C. (1988). The social mandate and historical bases for nursing's role in health promotion. *Journal of Professional Nursing, 4*(2), 80–87.

Osofsky, G. (1966). *Harlem tragedy: An emergency slum. Harlem: The making of a ghetto.* New York: Harper and Row.

Pan American Health Organization, World Health Organization (2001). *128th Session of the Executive Committee: Health, drinking water, and sanitation in sustainable human development* (CE128/13). Washington, DC: World Health Organization.

Pickett, G., & Hanlon, R. (1990). *Public health administration and practice* (9th ed.). St. Louis, MO: Times Mirror/ Mosby.

Public Health Service. (1958). *General organization, functions, procedures, and forms.* Washington, DC: U.S. Government Printing Office.

Roberts, D. E., & Heinrich, J. (1985). Public health nursing comes of age. *American Journal of Public Health, 75*(10), 1162–1172.

Roberts, M. M. (1954). *American nursing, history and interpretation.* New York: Macmillan.

Rodgers, B. L. (1989). Concepts, analysis and the development of nursing knowledge: The evolutionary cycle. *Journal of Advanced Nursing, 14.*

Rosen, G. (1958). *A history of public health.* New York: MD Publications.

Ruth, M. V., & Partridge, K. B. (1978). Differences in perceptions of education and practice. *Nursing Outlook, 26,* 622–628.

Smillie, W. G. (1952). *Preventive medicine and public health* (2nd ed.). New York: Macmillan.

Styles, M. (1992). Commentary: Nightingale: The enduring symbol. In *Nightingale, notes on nursing* (commemorative edition). Philadelphia: J. B. Lippincott.

Tinkham, C. W., & Voorhies, E. F. (1977). *Community health nursing: Evolution and practice.* New York: Appleton-Century-Crofts.

U.S. Department of Health and Human Services. (1990). *Healthy people 2000: National health promotion and disease prevention objectives. Summary report.* Washington, DC: Author.

U.S. Department of Health and Human Services. (2000). *Healthy people 2010: Understanding and improving health.* Washington, DC: U.S. Government Printing Office.

U.S. Public Health Service, Division of Nursing. (1993). *A century of caring: A celebration of public health nursing in the United States, 1893–1993.* Washington, DC: U.S. Government Printing Office.

Wald, L. (1971). *The house on Henry Street.* New York: Dover. (Reprinted from 1915 edition, New York: Henry Holt & Co.)

Walker, L., & Avant, K. (1995). *Strategies for theory construction in nursing* (3rd ed.). Norwalk, CT: Appleton & Lange.

Waters, Y. (1912). *Visiting nursing in the United States.* New York: Charities Publication Committee, The Russell Sage Foundation.

Wilde, M. H. (1997). The caring connection in nursing: A concept analysis. *International Journal for Human Caring, 1*(1), 18–24.

Winslow, E. E. (1923). *The evolution and significance of the modern public health campaign.* New Haven, CT: Yale University Press.

World Health Organization. (2000). *The WHO report 2000—Health systems: Improving performance.* Geneva, Switzerland: Author.

World Health Organization, Regional Office for Europe. (1985). *Targets for health for all.* Copenhagen, Denmark: Author.

World Health Organization, Regional Office for Europe. (1991). *Targets for health for all.* Copenhagen, Denmark: Author.

CHAPTER 3: NATIONAL AND INTERNATIONAL HEALTH PERSPECTIVES

American Public Health Association (2000a). *The nation's health: WHO calls for global agenda for the disabled.* Washington, DC: Author.

American Public Health Association (2000b). *The nation's health: Global AIDS deaths reach record high of 2.6 million.* Washington, DC: Author.

Anderson, C. M. (1996). Women for women's health: Uganda. *Nursing Outlook, 44,* 141.

Annan, K. A., Johnston, D. J., Kohler, H., & Wolfensohn, J. D. (2000). *Foreword: 2000: A better world for all.* New York: International Monetary Fund, Organization for Economic Co-operation and Development, United Nations, and World Bank.

Blane, D. (1995). Editorial: Social determinants of health-socioeconomic status, social class and ethnicity. *American Journal of Public Health, 85*(7), 903–904.

Brockherhoff, M. P. (2000). An urbanizing world. *Population Bulletin, 55*(3), 3–44.

Brodney, K., & Dobkin, J. (1991). Resurgent tuberculosis in New York City: Human immunodeficiency virus, homelessness, and the decline of tuberculosis control programs. *American Review of Respiratory Disease, 144,* 745–749.

Brundtland, G. H. (2000). Editorial: Mental health in the 21st century. *Bulletin of the World Health Organization: The International Journal of Public Health, 78*(4), 411.

Centers for Disease Control and Prevention. (1988). Tuberculosis, final data—United States, 1986. *Morbidity and Mortality Weekly Report, 36,* 817–820.

Centers for Disease Control and Prevention. (1993). *AIDS: An expanding tragedy. The final report of the National Commission on AIDS.* Rockville, MD: Centers for Disease Control and Prevention National AIDS Clearing House.

Centers for Disease Control and Prevention. (1995). Tuberculosis morbidity—United States, 1994. *Morbidity and Mortality Weekly Report, 44,* 387–389.

Dreher, M. (1996). Nursing: A cultural phenomenon. *Reflections: Sigma Theta Tau, International, 22*(4), 4.

Dubos, R., & Dubos, J. (1952). *The white plague: Tuberculosis, man, and society,* Boston, MA: Little, Brown, & Co.

Duhl, L., & Drake, J. (1995). Healthy cities: A systemic view of health. *Current Issues in Public Health, 1,* 105–109.

Fee, F. (1987). *Disease and discovery: A history of the Johns Hopkins School of Hygiene and Public Health, 1916–1939.* Baltimore, MD: Johns Hopkins University Press.

Fleming, P. L., Wortley, P. M., Karon, J. M., DeCork, K. M., & Janssen, R. S. (2000). Tracing the HIV epidemic: Current issues, future challenges. *American Journal of Public Health, 90*(7), 1037–1041.

Foege, W. H., Rosenberg, M. L., & Mercy, J. A. (1995). Public health and violence prevention. *Current Issues in Public Health, 1*(1), 2–9.

Friedan, T. R. (1994). Tuberculosis control and social changes. *American Journal of Public Health, 84*(11), 1721–1723.

Hamburg, M. A. (1995). Tuberculosis and its control in the 1990s. *Current Issues in Public Health, 1*(2), 49–54.

Hancock, T., & Garrett, M. (1995). Beyond medicine: Health challenges and strategies in the 21st century. *Futures, 27*(9/10), 935–951.

Heggenhougen, H. K. (1995). The world mental health report. *Current Issues in Public Health, 1*(6), 267–271.

Heiby, J. R. (1998). Quality improvement and the integrated management of childhood illnesses: Lessons from developed countries. *Quality Improvement, 24*(5), 264.

Johns Hopkins University, Population Information Program. (2000). Population and the environment: The global challenge. *Population Reports.* Baltimore, MD: Johns Hopkins School of Public Health, Population Information Program. [On-line]. Available: www.jhuccp.org.

Johns Hopkins University, Population Information Program. (2001). Population growth and urbanization: Cities at the forefront. Preview edition. *Population Reports.* Baltimore, MD: Johns Hopkins, School of Public Health, Population Information Program. [On-line]. Available: www.jhuccp.org.

Kickbusch, I. (1989). The new public health orientation for the city. In *WHO Healthy Cities Papers, The new public health in an urban context: Paradoxes and solutions* (pp. 43–54). Copenhagen, Denmark: FADL Publishers.

Lee, P. R., & Estes, C. L. (1994). *The nation's health* (4th ed.). Boston: Jones & Bartlett.

MacDorman, M. F., & Rosenberg, H. M. (1993). Trends in infant mortality by cause of death and other characteristics. In *Vital Health Statistics* (pp. 93–185). Washington, DC: U.S. Public Health Service.

McKeown, T. (1978). Determinants of health. In P. R. Lee & C. L. Estes (Eds.). (1994). *The nation's health* (4th ed., pp. 6–13). Boston: Jones & Bartlett.

Melse, J. M., Essink-Bot, M., Kramers, P. G., & Hoeymans, N. (2000). A national burden of disease calculation: Dutch disability-adjusted life-years. *American Journal of Public Health, 90*(8), 1241–1247.

Morabia, A. (2000). Worldwide surveillance of risk factors to promote global health. *American Journal of Public Health, 90*(1), 22–24.

Murray, C. J., & Lopez, A. D. (1996). *Summary: The global burden of disease, global burden of disease and injury series.* Cambridge, MA: Harvard School of Public Health on behalf of the World Health Organization and the World Bank, Harvard University Press.

Murray, C. J., & Lopez, A. D. (2000). *Progress and directions in refining the global burden of disease approach: A response to Williams.* Discussion paper from global programme on evidence for health policy. Geneva, Switzerland: World Health Organization.

National Center for Health Statistics. (1992). *Health, United States 1981–1991, and Prevention Profile,* (Publication No. PHS 92-1232). Hyattsville, MD: U.S. Department of Health and Human Services.

Nijhuis, H. G. (1989). Contemporary municipal health departments in the Netherlands: A proposed potential for new public health. In *WHO Healthy Cities Papers, The new public health in an urban context: Paradoxes and solutions* (pp. 17–39). Copenhagen, Denmark: FADL Publishers.

Pew Environmental Health Commission. (2000). *Attack asthma: Why America needs a public health defense system to battle environmental threats.* Baltimore, MD: Author.

Porter-O'Grady, T. (1995). Introduction. In A. Boykin (Ed.), *Power, politics, & public policy: A matter of caring.* (p. xvii). New York: National League for Nursing Press.

Ramos, M. (1997). Caring for patients, profession, and world: The social activism of Lavinia Lloyd Dock. *International Journal for Human Caring, 1*(1), 12–17.

Rice, D. (1994). Health status and national priority. In P. R. Lee & C. L.

Estes, (Eds.), *The nation's health* (4th ed.). Boston, MA: Jones & Bartlett.

Rosenberg, M. L., & Fenley, M. A. (1990). *Violence in America: A public health approach.* New York: Oxford University Press.

Singh, G. P., & Yu, W. (1995). Infant mortality in the United States: Trends, differentials and projections, 1950 through 2010. *American Journal of Public Health, 85*(7), 957–964.

United Nations, Organization for Economic Co-operation and Development, International Monetary Fund, & World Bank. (2000b). *2000: A better world for all.* Washington, DC: Communication Development and London: Grundy & Northedge.

United Nations, World Health Organization, & Pan American Health Organization. (2000a). *Provisional Report: HIV and AIDS in the Americas: An epidemic with many faces.* [On-line]. Available: www.paho.org.

United Nations Population Division. (2000c). *World urbanization prospects: The 1999 revision.* New York: Author.

United Nations Population Division. (2001). *World population prospects: The 2000 revision—Highlights.* New York: Author.

U.S. Department of Health and Human Services. (1993). *Healthy people 2000 review, 1992.* Hyattsville, MD: Author.

U.S. Department of Health and Human Services. (1996). *Healthy people 2000: Midcourse review and 1995 revisions.* Sudbury, MA: Jones & Bartlett.

U.S. Department of Health and Human Services, Centers for Disease Control and Prevention. (2000a). *CDC Update: A glance at the epidemic.* Atlanta, GA: Author.

U.S. Department of Health and Human Services. (2000b). *Healthy people 2010: Understanding and improving health.* Washington, DC: U.S. Government Printing Office.

Upadhuay, U. D., & Robey, B. (1999). Why family planning matters. In *Population Reports, Series J* (9). Baltimore: Johns Hopkins University, School of Public Health, Population Information Program, 32.

Wilson, M. E. (1995). Anticipating new diseases. *Current Issues in Public Health, 1*(2), 90–95.

World Bank. (1993). *World development report 1993: Investing in health.* New York: Oxford University Press.

World Health Organization. (1991). *Statistics annuals 1990–1991*. Geneva, Switzerland: Author.

World Health Organization. (1998). *Fifty facts from the World Health Report 1998: Global health situations and trends 1955–2025*. Geneva, Switzerland: Author.

World Health Organization. (1999a). *Report on infectious diseases: Removing obstacles to healthy development*. Geneva, Switzerland: Author.

World Health Organization. (1999b). *World health report 1999*. Geneva, Switzerland: Author.

World Health Organization. (2000a). *Setting the WHO agenda for mental health. Bulletin of the World Health Organization, 78*(4), 500–514.

World Health Organization Fact Sheet. (2000b). *Tuberculosis F-S 104*. [On-line]. Available: www.who.int/inf-fs/fact104.

World Health Organization Fact Sheet. (2000c). *HIV, TB, and malaria—Three major infectious disease threats, Back 001*. [On-line]. Available: www.who.int/inf-fs/en/back001.

World Health Organization. (2001a). *Global health issues: 107th Session of WHOs Executive Board*. Press Release WHO/03-2001. [On-line]. Available: www.who.int/inf-pr-2001/en/pr2001.

World Health Organization. (2001b). *WHO launches mental health 2001 campaign*. Press Release WHO/01. [On-line]. Available: www.who.int/inf-pr-2001.

World Health Organization. (2001c). *WHO opens office in Lyon (France) to help developing countries detect and control epidemics and emerging diseases*. Press Release WHO/06-2001. [On-line]. Available: www.who.int/inf-pr-2001.

Worldwatch Institute. (2000). *Obesity epidemic threatens health in exercise-deprived societies: Worldwatch Issue Alert*. [On-line]. Available: www.worldwatch.org/chairman/issue.

CHAPTER 4: HEALTH CARE DELIVERY IN THE UNITED STATES

American Nurses Association. (1993). *Nursing's agenda for reform*. Washington, DC: American Nurses Publishing.

American Nursing Home Association. (1970–1971). *Nursing home fact book 3*. Washington, DC.

American Nursing Home Association (1993). *Nursing home fact book*. Washington, DC: Author.

Association of State and Territorial Health Officials. (1994). *Public health and prevention are essential to health care reform*. Washinton, DC: Author

Aydellotte, M. K., Barger, S. E., Branstetter, E., Fehring, R. J., Lindgren, K., Lundeen, S., & Riesch, S. K. (1987). *The nursing center: Concept and design*. Kansas City, MO: American Nurses Association.

De Law, N., Greenberg, G., & Kinchen, K. A. (1992). Layman's guide to the U.S. health care system. *Health Care Financing Review, 14*(1), 151–169.

Dieckmann, J. (2000). History of public health and public and community health nursing. In M. Stanhope & J. Lancaster. *Community and public health nursing* (5th ed.) (pp. 20–41). St. Louis, MO: Mosby.

Eisenberg, D. M., Kessler, R. C., Foster, C., Norlock, F. E., Calkins, D. R., & Delbanco, T. L. (1993). Unconventional medicine in the United States: Prevalence, costs, and patterns of use. *New England Journal of Medicine, 328*, 246–252.

Elazar, D. (1966). *American federalism: A view from the states*. New York: Crowell.

Ellencweig, A. Y., & Yoshpe, R. B. (1984). Definition of public health. *Public Health Review, 12*, 65–78.

Employee Benefit Research Institute. (2000). *Sources of health insurance and characteristics of the uninsured*. Washington, DC.: Author.

Fogel, B. S., Brock, D., Goldscheider, F., & Royall, D. (1994). *Cognitive dysfunction and the need for long-term care: Implications for public policy*. Washington, DC: Public Policy Institute, AARP.

Glass, L. (1989). The historic origin of nursing centers. In *Nursing centers: Meeting the demand for quality health care* (pp. 21–23). New York: National League for Nursing.

Holahan, J., Zuckerman, S., Evans, A., & Rangarajan, S. (1998). Medicaid managed care in thirteen states. *Health Affairs, 17*(1), 43–63.

Institute of Medicine, Committee for the Study of the Future of Public Health. (1988). *The future of public health*. Washington, DC: National Academy Press.

Institute of Medicine (1996). *Healthy communities: New partnerships for health*. Washington, DC: National Academy Press.

Institute of Medicine (1997). *Improving health in the community: A role for performance monitoring*. Washington, DC: National Academy Press.

Judy, R., & D'Amico, C. (1997). *Work force 2020*. Indianapolis, IN: Hudson Institute.

Koop, C. E. (1991). *Koop*. New York: Random House.

Kopf, E. W. (1991). Florence Nightingale as statistician. In B. W. Spradley (Ed.), *Readings in community health nursing* (4th ed., pp. 274–285). Philadelphia: J.B. Lippincott Co.

Kuhn, T. (1986). *The structure of scientific revolutions*. New York: New American Libraries.

Letsch, S. (1993). National health care spending in 1991. *Health Affairs, 12*(1), 94–110.

Levit, K., Sowan, C., Lazenby, H., Sensenig, A., McDonnell, P., Stiller, J., Martin, A., & the Health Accounts Team. (2000). Health spending in 1998: Signals of change. *Health Affairs, 19*(1), 124–132.

Lockhart, C. (1992). *Influences on the healthcare system*. Tempe, AZ: C. Lockhart Associates.

Lockhart, C. (1994). Community nursing centers: An analysis of status and needs. In B. Murphy (Ed.), *Nursing centers: The time is now* (pp. 2–18). New York: National League for Nursing.

Manning, M. (1984). *The hospice alternative: Living with dying*. London: Souvenir Press.

Marion, L. N. (1996). *Nursing's vision for primary health care in the 21st century*. Washington, DC: American Nurses Association.

Morgan, P. A. (1986). Developing a free-standing ambulatory surgery center. *The College Review,* Fall.

Mundinger, M. O. (1983). *Home care controversy: Too little, too late, too costly*. Rockville, MD: Aspen Systems Corporation.

Oermann, M. H., & Templin, T. (2000). Important attributes of quality health care: Consumer perspectives. *Journal of Nursing Scholarship, 32*(2).

Priester, R. (1992). *Taking values seriously: A values framework for the U.S. health care system*. Minneapolis, MN: Center for Biomedical Ethics, University of Minnesota.

Rakich, J. S., Longest, B. B., & Darr, K. (1992). *Managing health services organizations (3rd ed.). Baltimore, MD: Health Professions Press.

Riesch, S. K. (1990). *A review of the state of the art of research on nursing centers*. In *Differentiating nursing practice: Into the twenty-first century* (pp. 91–104). From proceedings of the 18th annual Conference of the American Academy of Nursing. Washington, DC: American Academy of Nursing.

Safriet, B. J. (1992). Health care dollars and regulatory sense: The role of advanced practice nursing. *Yale Journal of Regulation, 9*(2), 417–488.

Sharp, N. (1992). Community nursing centers: Coming of age. *Nursing Management, 23*(8), 18–20.

Shi, L., & Singh, D. A. (2000). *Delivering health care in America: A systems approach*. Gaithersburg, MD: Aspen Publishers.

Stryker, R. (1988). Historical obstacles to management of nursing homes. In G. K. Gordon & R. Stryker (Eds.), *Creative long-term care administration* (2nd ed., pp. 6–7). Springfield, IL: Charles C. Thomas.

U.S. Bureau of the Census (2000). *Statistical abstracts of the United States*. Washington, DC: U.S. Government Printing Office.

U.S. Department of Health and Human Services. (1991). *Healthy People 2000: National health promotion and disease prevention objectives* (DHHS Publication No. [PHS]91-50212). Washington, DC: Author.

U.S. Department of Health and Human Services. (2000). *Healthy people 2010: Understanding and improving health*. Washington, DC: U. S. Government Printing Office.

Webster's New World Collegiate Dictionary. (1999). New York: Macmillan.

Williams, S. J., & Torrens, P. R. (Eds.). (1999). *Introduction to health services* (5th ed.). Clifton Park, NY: Delmar Learning.

World Health Organization. (1978). *Primary health care*. Geneva, Switzerland: Author.

CHAPTER 5: HEALTH CARE SYSTEMS IN THE WORLD

American Public Health Association. (1997). *The nation's health (6)*, 24.

Ashton, J., & Seymour, H. (1988). *The new public health*. Philadelphia: Open University.

Basch, P. F. (1990). *Textbook of international health*. New York: Oxford University Press.

Berman, P. (1996). Health sector reform: A worldwide perspective. *Current Issues in Public Health, 2*(1), 34–38.

Bloom, A. L. (2000). *Health reform in Australia and New Zealand*. South Melbourne, Australia: Oxford University Press.

Brundtland, G. R. (2000). *Fifth global conference on health promotion, June 5, 2000*. [On-line]. Available: http://www.who.int/director-general/ speeches/2000/200065-mexico.

Brundtland, G. K. (2001). *Message from the Director-General, The world health report 2000—Health systems: Improving performance*. Geneva, Switzerland: World Health Organization.

Commonwealth Department of Health, Housing, and Community Services. (1992). *Annual report 91–92: Statistical supplement*. Canberra: Australian Government Printing Office.

Commonwealth Department of Human Services and Health. (1995). *Department of Human Services and Health: Statistical overview 1993–1994*. Canberra: Australian Government Printing Service.

Curtis, S., Petukrova, N., & Taketr, A. (1995). Health care reforms in Russia: The example of St. Petersburg. *Social Science and Medicine 40*(6), 755–765.

Dreher, M. C. (1997). Creating a multitude of opportunities for nurses to interact: Global sharing among nurses. *Reflections, 23*(2), 5.

Duckett, S. (1995). The council of Australian government's agenda—A Commonwealth perspective. In *Health and Community Services Conference Proceedings, Planning for change*. Melbourne, Victoria, Australia: Department of Health and Community Services.

Global Health Council. (2000). *2000 Annual Report*. [On-line]. Available: www. globalhealth.org/view_top. php3.

Global Health Council. (2001). *About the global health council*. [On-line]. Available: www.globalhealth.org/ view_top.php3.

Health System and Policy Division, Health Canada. (1999). *Canada's health care system*. Ottawa, Canada: Health Canada.

International Council of Nurses. (2000). *Nursing and development: Position Statement*. Geneva, Switzerland: Author.

International Council of Nurses. (2001). *About the International Council of Nurses*. Geneva, Switzerland: Author.

Katz, M. F., & Kreuter, M. W. (1997). Community assessment and empowerment. In E. D. Schutchfield & W. C. Keck (Eds.), *Principles of public health practice*. Clifton Park, NY: Delmar Learning.

Lasker, R. D., & the Committee on Medicine and Public Health. (1997). *Medicine and public health: The power of collaboration*. New York: New York Academy of Medicine.

Lin, V., & King, C. (2000). Intergovernmental reforms in public health. In A. L. Bloom (Ed.), *Health reform in Australia and New Zealand*. South Melbourne, Australia: Oxford University Press.

McElmurry, B. J., & Keeney, G. B. (1999). Primary health care. In J. J. Fitzpatrick (Ed.), *Annual review of nursing research* (Vol. 17). New York: Springer.

Messias, D. K. (2001). Globalization, nursing, and health for all. *Journal of Nursing Scholarship, 33*(1), 9–11.

Miotto Wright, M., Godue, C., Manfredi, M., & Korniewicz, D. M. (1998). Nursing education and international health in the United States, Latin America, and the Caribbean. *Image: Journal of Nursing Scholarship, 30*(1), 31–36.

Murray, C. (2000). *In Press Release, World Health Report 2000: World Health Organization assesses the world's health systems*. [On-line] www.who.int/whr/2000/en/press.

Pan American Health Organization. (2001). *Press release: New Caribbean plan to prevent HIV/AIDS launched*. [On-line]. Available: http://www. paho.org/press-010214.

Perfiljeva, G. (1997). Progress in Russia: Working together for change. *Reflections, 23*(2), 8–9.

Pike, S. (1995). Health promotion now: The development of policy. In S. Pike & D. Forster (Eds.), *Health promotion for all (27–38)*. Edinburgh: Churchill Livingstone.

Pike, S., & Forster, D. (1995). *Health promotion for all*. Edinburgh: Churchill Livingstone.

Podger, A., & Hagan, P. (2000). Reforming the Australian health care system: The role of government. In A. L. Bloom (Ed.), *Health reform in Australia and New Zealand*. South Melbourne, Australia: Oxford University Press.

Quinn, S. (1981). *What about me? Caring for the carers.* Geneva, Switzerland: International Council of Nurses.

Roach, M. S. (1995). The dominant paradigm of the modern world. In A. Boykin (Ed.), *Power, politics, and public policy: A matter of caring* (pp. 3–10). New York: National League for Nursing.

Ross Kerr, J. C. (1997). The Canadian health care system: Overview and issues. In J. C. McCloskey & H. Grace (Eds.), *Current issues in nursing* (5th ed., pp. 460–466). St. Louis, MO: C. V. Mosby.

Salmon, M. E. (1998). Guest editorial—The future of public health nursing: A state of mind. Washington, DC: American Public Health Association, *Public Health Nursing Section Newsletter, 3.*

Smith, L. S. (1997). Nursing in Russia: Impact of recent political changes. In J. C. McCloskey & H. Grace (Eds.), *Current issues in nursing* (5th ed., pp. 686–694). St. Louis, MO: C. V. Mosby.

Somjen, A. (2000). Distinguishing features of reform in Australia and New Zealand. In A. L. Bloom (Ed.), *Health reform in Australia and New Zealand.* South Melbourne, Australia: Oxford University Press.

United Kingdom Department of Health. (2000). *The new National Health Service: Executive factsheet.* [On-line]. Available: http://www.doh.gov.uk/nhspack.htm.

World Health Organization. (1978). *Alma Ata 1978: Primary health care.* Geneva, Switzerland: Author.

World Health Organization. (1986). *The Ottawa charter for health promotion.* Geneva, Switzerland: Author.

World Health Organization. (1993). *Health for all targets: The health policy for Europe* (updated ed.). Copenhagen: WHO, Regional Office for Europe.

World Health Organization. (1999). *World health report—1999: Making a difference.* Geneva, Switzerland: Author.

World Health Organization. (2000). *World health report 2000—Health systems: Improving performance.* Geneva, Switzerland: Author.

World Health Organization. (2001a). *Press release WHO/06: WHO opens an office in Lyon (France) to help developing countries detect and control epidemics and emerging diseases.*

[On-line]. Available: http://www.who.int/inf-pr-2001.

World Health Organization. (2001b). *Press release WHO/18: As burden of mental disorders looms large, countries report lack of mental health programmes.* [On-line]. Available: http:who.int/inf-pr-2001/en/pr2001.

Wright, M. M., Godue, C., Manfredi, M., & Korniewicz, D. (1998). Nursing education and international health in the United States, Latin America, and the Caribbean. *Image: The Journal of Nursing Scholarship, 30*(1), pp. 31–36.

Zamurs, A. (1995). Service development in the new environment. In *Health and Community Services Conference Proceedings, Planning for change* (pp. 21–24). Melbourne, Australia: Health and Community Services.

CHAPTER 6: HEALTH CARE ECONOMICS

Abel-Smith, B. (1992). Cost containment and new priorities in the European community. *The Milbank Quarterly, 70*(3), 393–415.

Agency for Health Care Policy and Research. (1996–1998, 2000). *Medical expenditures panel survey.* Rockville, MD: U.S. Public Health Service.

American Nurses Association. (1995). *Agenda for health care reform.* Washington, DC: Author.

America's bubble economy. (1998, April 18). *The Economist, 347*(8064), 4, 19–22.

Barker, J. A. (1992). *Paradigms: The business of discovering the future.* New York: Harper Press.

Berrand, N. L., & Schroeder, S. A. (1994). Lessons from the states. *Inquiry, 31*(1), 10–13.

Bodenheimer, T. S., & Grumbach, K. (1998). *Understanding health policy: A clinical approach.* Stamford, CT: Appleton & Lange.

Brooten, D. (1994). A randomized trial of early hospital discharge and home follow-up of women who have unplanned cesarean section. *Obstetrics and Gynecology, 84,* 832–834.

Centers for Disease Control and Prevention. (2001). *National Vital Statistics Report, 48*(18).

Centers for Medicare & Medicaid Services. (2002). *Medicare and you.* Baltimore, MD: Author. Retrieved from http://www.medicare.gov.

Congressional Budget Office. (1993, March). *Analysis of president's budgetary proposals.* Washington, DC: Author.

Congressional Budget Office. (1995, September). *Analysis of the administration health proposal.* Washington, DC: Author.

Crow, G. L. (2001). Caring and professional practice settings: The impact of technology, change, and efficiency. *Nursing Administration Quarterly, 25*(3), 15–23.

Davis, K. (1994). Availability of medical care and its financing. In P. Lee & C. Estes (Eds.), *The nation's health* (4th ed., pp. 296–302). Boston: Jones & Bartlett.

Duffy, J. (1993). *Economics.* Lincoln, NE: Cliff.

Enthoven, A. C. (1993). The history and principles of managed competition. *Health Affairs, 12,* 24–48.

Enthoven, A. C. (1994). Why not the Clinton health plan? *Inquiry, 31*(2), 129–136.

Enthoven, A. C. (1996, April). Driving down costs while maintaining quality. *Kaiser Permanente Teleconference.* Oakland, CA.

Enthoven, A. C., & Kronick R. (1994). Universal health insurance through incentive programs. In P. Lee & C. Estes (Eds.). *The nation's health* (4th ed., pp. 284–291). Boston: Jones & Bartlett.

Finkler, S. A., & Kovner, C. T. (2000). *Financial management for nurse managers and executives* (3rd ed.). Philadelphia: Saunders.

Fry, S. T. (1994). *Ethics in nursing practice: A guide to ethical decision making.* Geneva, Switzerland: International Council of Nurses.

Health Care Financing Administration. (1996, March 11), [On-line]. Available: www.hcfa.gov.

Health Care Financing Administration. (1997a, January 27). *Medicare Bulletin,* Washington, DC: Author.

Health Care Financing Administration. (1997b, April 21). *Medical Expenditures Panel Survey.* Washington, DC: Author.

Health Care Financing Administration. (1998a, January). *Medicare Bulletin.* Washington, DC: Author.

Health Care Financing Administration. (1998b, April). *Medicaid Bulletin.* Washington, DC: Author.

Health Care Financing Administration. (1999). *Medicaid Bulletin.* Washington, DC: Author.

Health Care Financing Administration, Office of the Actuary. (2000a). *National health expenditures aggregate, per capita, percent distribution, and annual percent change by source of funds: Calendar years 1960–2000* [On-line]. Available: http://www. hcfa.gov/stats/nhe-oact/tables/ nhegdp00.csv.

Health Care Financing Administration, Office of the Actuary. (2000b). *National health expenditures by type of service and source of funds: Calendar years 1960–2000* [On-line]. Available: http://www.hcfa.gov/stats/ nhe-oact/tables/nhe00.csv.

Health Care Financing Administration. (2000c). *Medical expenditure panel survey.* Washington, DC: Author.

Health Care Financing Administration, Office of the Actuary. (2001a, January). Tables 1, 2, 4, 5.

Health Care Financing Administration. (2001b, January). *Medicare Bulletin.* Washington, DC: Author.

Health Care Financing Administration. (2001c, January). *Medicaid Bulletin.* Washington, DC: Author.

Heshmat, S. (2001). *An overview of managerial economics in the health care system.* Clifton Park, NY: Delmar Learning.

Iglehart, J. K. (1994). The American health care system: Managed care. In P. Lee & C. Estes (Eds.), *The nation's health* (4th ed., pp. 231–233). Boston: Jones & Barlett.

Institute of Medicine. (1996). *Using performance monitoring to improve community health: Conceptual framework and community experience.* Washington, DC: Author.

Kronick, R. (1993). Perspectives: Design issues in managed care. *Health Affairs* (Suppl. 12), 87–98.

Lamm, R. D. (1994). The brave new world of health care. In P. Lee & C. Estes (Eds.), *The nation's health* (4th ed., p. 152). Boston: Jones & Bartlett.

Lee, P. R., & Estes, C. L. (1994). *The nation's health* (4th ed.). Boston: Jones & Bartlett.

Leininger, M. M. (Ed.). (1981). *Caring: An essential human need.* Thorofare, NJ: Charles B. Slack. (Reprinted in 1988 by Wayne State University Press, Detroit, MI.)

Levit, K. R., Olin, G. L., & Letsch, S. W. (1992). American health insurance coverage, 1980–91. *Health Affairs, 14*(1), 31–57.

Litman, T. J. (1994). Government and health: The political aspects of health

care: A sociopolitical overview. In P. Lee & C. Estes (Eds.), *The nation's health* (4th ed., pp. 107–120). Boston: Jones & Bartlett.

Lundberg, G. D. (1994). National health care reform: The aura of inevitability intensifies. In P. Lee & C. Estes (Eds.), *The nation's health* (4th ed., pp. 238–244). Boston: Jones & Bartlett.

Mechanic, D. (1994). Managed care: Rhetoric and realities. *Inquiry, 31*(2), 124–128.

New York Times, July 2, 2001, page C1.

Patients or profits. (1998, March 7). *The Economist, 346*(8058), 6, 23–24.

Prospective Payment Assessment Commission. (1997). *Medicare and the American health care system. Report to the Congress. June 1997.* Washington, DC: Author.

Reinhardt, U. E. (1993). Reorganizing the financial flows in U.S. health care delivery. *Health Affairs, 12,* 172–193.

Senior Rx: Immediate helping hand. (2001, January 29). *The Washington Post,* p. A12.

Staines, V. S. (1993). Impact of managed care on national health spending. *Health Affairs, 12* (Suppl. 3), 248–257.

U.S. Census Bureau. (1997, November 10). *Insured and uninsured U.S. citizens.* Washington, DC: U.S. Government Printing Office.

U.S. Census Bureau. (1998). *Health insurance coverage: 1998* [On-line]. Available: http://www.census.gov/ hhes/hlthins/hlthin98.html.

U.S. Census Bureau. (1999). *Health insurance coverage: 1999* [On-line]. Available: http://www.census.gov/ hhes/hlthins/hlthin99/hlt99asc.html.

U.S. Census Bureau. (2000). *Statistical abstracts of the United States.* Tables 172, 174, 177.

U.S. Office of Management and Budget. (2001). *A blueprint for new beginnings: A responsible budget for America's priorities* [On-line]. Available: http://www.whitehouse.gov/ news/usbudget/blueprint/budtoc.html.

U.S. Office of Management and Budget. (2002). Table 12-1: Federal resources in support of health. *Budget of the United States Government, Fiscal Year 2002* [On-line]. Available: http://www.whitehouse.gov/omb/ budget/fy2002/budget.html.

Walsey, T. P. (1992). *What has government done to our health care?* New York: Cato Institute.

Wessels, W. J. (1993). *Economics.* New York: Barron's Business Review Press.

White House Fact Sheet. (1998, April 6). *The health of America.* Washington, DC: U.S. Government Printing Office.

Wilber, K. (1996). *A brief history of everything.* Boston: Shambhala.

Wilson, E. O. (1998). *Consilience: The unity of knowledge.* New York: Knopf.

World Health Organization. (1998, October 1). *World health report.* Geneva, Switzerland: Author.

World Health Organization. (2000). *World health report and statistics.* Geneva, Switzerland: Author.

CHAPTER 7: PHILOSOPHICAL AND ETHICAL PERSPECTIVES

Aiken, T. D., & Catalano, J. T. (1994). *Legal, ethical, and political issues in nursing.* Philadelphia: F. A. Davis.

American Health Consultants. (1994). The new face of bioethics: County ethics committee reviews health and social service decisions. *Medical Ethics Advisor, 10*(9), 114–115.

American Nurses Association. (1985). *Code for nurses, with interpretive statements.* Kansas City, MO: Author.

Annas, G. J. (1978). Patient's rights movement. In W. T. Reich (Ed.), *Encyclopedia of bioethics,* (Vol. 3). New York: Free Press.

Beauchamp, D. (2001). Public health as social justice. In W. Teays & L. Purdy (Eds.), *Bioethics, justice, and health care* (pp. 20–23). Belmont, CA: Wadsworth.

Beauchamp, T. L., & Childress, J. F. (1994). *Principles of biomedical ethics* (4th ed.). New York: Oxford University Press.

Beauchamp, T. L., & Walters, L. R. (1994). *Contemporary issues in bioethics* (4th ed.). Belmont, CA: Wadsworth.

Beauchamp, T. L., & Walters, L. R. (1999). *Contemporary issues in bioethics* (5th ed.). Belmont, CA: Wadsworth.

Benjamin, M., & Curtis, J. (1992). *Ethics in nursing* (3rd ed.). New York: Oxford University Press.

Burkhardt, M. A., & Nathaniel, A. K. (1998). *Ethics and issues in contemporary nursing.* Clifton Park, NY: Delmar Learning.

Christoffel, T. H. (2001). The right to care. In W. Teays & L. Purdy (Eds.), *Bioethics, justice, and health care* (pp. 112–117). Belmont, CA: Wadsworth.

Collopy, B., Dubler, N., & Zuckerman, C. (1990). The ethics of home care: Autonomy and accommodation. *Hastings Center Report, 20*(2, Special Suppl.), 1–16.

Daniels, N. (1979). Rights to health care and distributive justice: Programmed worries. *Journal of Medical Philosophy, 4,* 174–191.

Darragh, M., & McCarrick, P. M. (2000). Public health ethics: Health by the numbers. *Kennedy Institute of Ethics Journal, 8*(3), 339–358.

DeLaune, S., & Ladner, P. (1998). *Fundamentals of nursing: Standards and practices.* Clifton Park, NY: Delmar Learning.

Devetere, R. J. (2000). *Practical decision making in health care ethics.* Washington, DC: Georgetown University.

DuBose, E. R., Hamel, R., & O'Connell, L. J. (Eds.). (1994). *A matter of principles? Ferment in U.S. bioethics.* Valley Forge, PA: Trinity.

Fadiman, A. (1997). *The spirit catches you and you fall down.* New York: Farrar, Straus and Giroux.

Fazzone, P. A., Barloon, L. F., McConnell, S. J., & Chitty, J. A. (2000). Personal safety, violence, and home health. *Public Health Nursing, 17*(1), 43–52.

Gastmans, C., Dierckx de Casterle, B., & Schotsmans, P. (1998). Nursing considered as moral practice: A philosophical-ethical interpretation of nursing. *Kennedy Institute of Ethics Journal, 8*(1), 43–69.

Gudorf, C. E. (1994). A feminist critique of biomedical principlism. In E. R. DuBose, R. Hamel, & L. J. O'Connell (Eds.), *A matter of principles? Ferment in U.S. bioethics* (pp. 164–181). Valley Forge, PA: Trinity.

Higgs, Z. R., Bayne, T., & Murphy, D. (2001). Health care access: A consumer perspective. *Public Health Nursing, 18*(1), 3–12.

Husted, G. L., & Husted, J. H. (1995). *Ethical decision making in nursing* (2nd ed.). St. Louis, MO: Mosby Yearbook.

International Council of Nurses. (1973). *ICN code for nurses: Ethical concepts applied to nursing.* Geneva, Switzerland: Imprimeries Populaires.

Joint Commission on Accreditation of Healthcare Organizations. (1990). *1991 Joint Commission accreditation manual for hospitals,* Vol. 1: *Standards.* Oakbrook Terrace, IL: Author.

Joint Commission on Accreditation of Healthcare Organizations. (1994). *Joint Commission 1995 accreditation manual for hospitals.* Vol. 1: *Standards.* Oakbrook Terrace, IL: Author.

Joint Commission on Accreditation of Healthcare Organizations. (1996). *Joint Commission 1996 accreditation manual for hospitals,* Vol. 1: *Standards.* Oakbrook Terrace, IL: Author.

Joint Commission on Accreditation of Healthcare Organizations. (2000). *Comprehensive accreditation manual for hospitals: The official handbook.* Oakbrook, IL: Joint Commission Resources.

Kuehl, K. S., Shapiro, S., & Sivasubramanian, K. N. (1992). Should a school honor a student's DNR order? Case history of S. A. *Kennedy Institute of Ethics Journal, 2*(1), 1–3.

Ladd, R. E., Pasquerella, L., & Smith, S. (2000). What to do when the end is near: Issues in home health care nursing. *Public Health Nursing, 17*(2), 103–110.

Leddy, S., & Pepper, J. M. (1998). *Conceptual bases of professional nursing* (4th ed.). Philadelphia: J. B. Lippincott.

Leininger, M. M. (1990) *Ethical and moral dimensions of care.* Detroit, MI: Wayne State University.

Magilvy, J. K., & Congdon, J. A. G. (2000). The crisis nature of health care transitions for rural older adults. *Public Health Nursing, 17*(5), 336–345.

Manning, R. C. (1992). *Speaking from the heart: A feminist perspective on ethics.* Lanham, MD: Rowman & Littlefield.

Mason, L. (1995). The Denver community bioethics committee: Healthcare decisions in adult protection and long-term care settings. *Healthcare Ethics Committee Forum, 7*(5), 284–289.

Mitchell, C. (1990). Ethical dilemmas. *Critical Care Nursing Clinics of North America, 2*(3), 427–430.

Monagle, J. F., & Thomasma, D. C. (1998). *Health care ethics: Critical issues for the 21st century.* Gaithersburg, MD: Aspen.

Munson, R. (2000). *Intervention and reflection: Basic issues in medical ethics* (6th ed.). Belmont, CA: Wadsworth.

National Commission for the Protection of Human Subjects of Biomedical and Behavioral Research. (1978). Washington, DC: U.S. Department of Health, Education, and Welfare.

Pence, G. E. (1990). The Baby Doe Case. In *Classic cases in medical ethics* (pp. 136–163). New York: McGraw-Hill.

President's Commission. (1983). *Deciding to forego life-sustaining treatment: Ethical, medical and legal issues in treatment decisions.* Washington, DC: U.S. Government Printing Office.

Ross, J. W., Glaser, J. W., Rasinski-Gregory, D., McIver, Gibson, J., & Bayley, C. (1993). *Health care ethics committees: The next generation.* Chicago, IL: American Hospital Association.

Scofield, G. R. (1992). A lawyer responds: A student's right to forgo CPR. *Kennedy Institute of Ethics Journal, 2*(1), 4–12.

Sherwin, S. (1992). *No longer patient: Feminist ethics and health care.* Philadelphia: Temple University.

Smith, D. H., & Veatch, R. M. (Eds.). (1987). *Guidelines on the termination of life-sustaining treatment and the care of the dying: A report by the Hastings Center.* Bloomington, IN: Indiana University.

Strike, K. A. (1992). An educator responds: A school's interest in denying the request. *Kennedy Institute of Ethics Journal, 2*(1), 19–23.

Taylor, C. R. (1998). Reflections on "Nursing considered as moral practice." *Kennedy Institute of Ethics Journal, 8*(1), 71–82.

Teays, W., & Purdy, L. (2001). *Bioethics, justice, and health care.* Belmont, CA: Wadsworth.

Walker, N. U. (1993). Keeping moral space open: New images of ethics consulting. *Hastings Center Report, 23*(2), 33–40.

Younger, S. J. (1992). A physician/ethicist responds: A student's rights are not so simple. *Kennedy Institute of Ethics Journal, 2*(1), 13–18.

CHAPTER 8: SPIRITUAL AND CULTURAL PERSPECTIVES

Adair, M. (1984). *Working inside out: Tools for change.* Oakland, CA: Wingbow.

Andrews, M. (1999a). Theoretical foundations in transcultural nursing. In M. Andrews & J. Boyle (Eds.), *Transcultural concepts in nursing care* (3rd ed. Philadelphia: J. B. Lippincott, pp. 3–22.

Andrews, M. (1999b). Culture and nutrition. In M. Andrews & J. Boyle (Eds.), *Transcultural concepts in nursing care* (3rd ed., pp. 341–377). Philadelphia: J. B. Lippincott.

Andrews, M. (1999c). Transcultural perspectives in the nursing care of children. In M. Andrews & J. Boyle (Eds.), *Transcultural concepts in nursing care* (3rd ed., pp. 107–159). Philadelphia: J. B. Lippincott.

Andrews, M. & Boyle, J. (1999). Andrews/Boyle transcultural nursing assessment guide. In M. Andrews & J. Boyle (Eds.), *Transcultural concepts in nursing care* (3rd ed., pp. 308–337). Philadelphia: J. B. Lippincott.

Andrews, M., & Herberg, P. (1999). Transcultural nursing care. In M. Andrews & J. Boyle (Eds.), *Transcultural concepts in nursing care* (3rd ed., pp. 23–77). Philadelphia: J. B. Lippincott.

Arrien, A. (1993). *The four-fold way: Walking the paths of the warrior, teacher, healer, and visionary.* San Francisco: Harper.

Azzam, A. (1964). *The eternal message of Muhammad.* New York: New American Library.

Barrington, R. (1997). *Repatterning an urban Indian clinic through Rogerian Nursing Science and caring framework.* Unpublished paper presented at the regional meeting of the Society of Rogerian Scholars, San Diego, CA.

Boyle, J. (1999). Culture family and community. In M. Andrews & J. Boyle (Eds.), *Transcultural concepts in nursing care* (2nd ed., pp. 308–337). Philadelphia: J. B. Lippincott.

Burkhardt, M., & Nagai-Jacobson, M. (2000). Spirituality and health. In B. Dossey, L. Keegan, & C. Guzzetta (Eds.), *Holistic nursing: A handbook for practice* (3rd ed., pp. 91–121). Gaithersburg, MD: Aspen.

Campinha-Bacote, J. (1998). *The process of cultural competence in the delivery of healthcare services: A culturally competent model of care.* Cincinnati, OH: Transcultural C.A.R.E. Associates.

Canda, E., & Furman, L. (1999). *Spiritual diversity in social work practice: The heart of helping.* New York: The Free Press.

Complete works of Swami Vivekananda. (1989). Calcutta, India: Advaita Ashrama.

Dana, R. (1993). *Multicultural assessment perspectives for professional psychology.* Boston: Allyn & Bacon.

Dossey, B. & Guzzetta, C. (2000). Holistic nursing practice. In B. Dossey, L. Keegan, & C. Guzzetta (Eds.), *Holistic nursing: A handbook for practice* (3rd ed., pp. 5–33). Gaithersburg, MD: Aspen.

Frankl, V. (1959). *Man's search for meaning.* New York: Pocket Books.

Giger, J. M., & Davidhizar, R. E. (1999). *Transcultural nursing: Assessment and intervention* (2nd ed). St. Louis, MO: Mosby Year-Book.

Govier, I. (2000). Spiritual care in nursing: A systematic approach. *Nursing Standard, 14*(17), 32–36.

Grossman, D. (1994, July). Enhancing your "cultural competence." *American Journal of Nursing,* 58–62.

Heinberg, R. (1989). *Memories and visions of paradise: Exploring the universal myth of a golden age.* Los Angeles: Jeremy P. Tarcher.

Hover-Kramer, D. (2000). Relationships. In B. Dossey, L. Keegan, & C. Guzzetta (Eds.), *Holistic nursing: A handbook for practice* (3rd ed., pp. 639–660). Gaithersburg, MD: Aspen.

Isaia, D., Parker, V., & Murrow, E. (1999). Spiritual well-being among older adults. *Journal of Gerontological Nursing, 25*(8), 16–21.

Kunz, D. (1992). Video II: The method. In J. Quinn (Producer), *Therapeutic touch: Healing through human energy fields* (videotape series). New York: National League for Nursing.

Lauderdale, J. (1999). Childbearing and transcultural nursing care issues. In M. Andrews & J. Boyle (Eds.), *Transcultural concepts in nursing care* (3rd ed., pp. 81–106). Philadelphia: J. B. Lippincott.

Leininger, M. (1978). *Transcultural nursing: Concepts, theories, and practices.* New York: John Wiley.

Leininger, M. (1984). Care: The essence of nursing and health. In M. Leininger (Ed.), *Care: The essence of nursing and health.* Thorofare, NJ: Slack.

Leininger, M. (1991). The theory of culture care diversity and universality. In M. Leininger (Ed.), *Culture care diversity and universality: A theory of nursing* (pp. 5–68). New York: National League for Nursing.

Lustig, M. & Koester, J. (1999). *Intercultural competence: Interpersonal communication across cultures* (3rd ed). New York: Addison Wesley Longman.

Maslow, A. (1968). *Toward a psychology of being* (2nd ed.). New York: Van Nostrand.

McKenna, M. (1999). Caring for the older adult client. Nursing challenges in a changing context. In M. Andrews & J. Boyle (Eds). *Transcultural concepts in nursing care* (3rd ed., pp. 189–220). Philadelphia: J.B. Lippincott.

Miller, W., & Thoresen, C. (1999). Spirituality and health. In W. Miller (Ed.), *Integrating spirituality into treatment: Resources for practitioners.* Washington, DC: American Psychological Association.

Mitchell, S. (1991). *The Gospel according to Jesus.* New York: Harper Collins.

Nasr, S. (1975). *Islam and the plight of modern man.* London: Longman.

Neuman, B. (1995). *The Neuman systems model* (3rd ed.). Norwalk, CT: Appleton & Lange.

Newman, M. (1994). *Health as expanding consciousness* (2nd ed.). New York: National League for Nursing.

North American Nursing Diagnosis Association. (1999). *Nursing diagnosis: Definitions and classification.* Philadelphia: Author.

Paniagua, F. (1998). Cross-cultural guidelines in family therapy practice. *Family Journal of Counseling and Therapy for Couples and Families, 4,* 127–138.

Pender, N. J. (1996). *Health promotion in nursing practice* (3rd ed.). Stamford, CT: Appleton & Lange.

Purnell, L., & Paulanka, B. (1998). *Transcultural health care: A culturally competent approach.* Philadelphia: F. A. Davis.

Rankin, S., & Stallings, K. (2001). *Patient education: Principles and practice* (4th ed.). Philadelphia: J. B. Lippincott.

Rogers, M. E. (1990). Nursing: Science of unitary, irreducible, human beings: Update 1990. In E. A. M. Barrett (Ed.), *Visions of Rogers' science-based nursing.* New York: National League for Nursing.

Schubert, P. (1989). Mutual connectedness: Holistic nursing practice under varying conditions of intimacy. Ph.D. dissertation, University of California, San Francisco, 1989. *Dissertation Abstracts International, 50,* 4987B.

Schubert, P., & Lionberger, H. (1995). Mutual connectedness: A study of client-nurse interaction using the

Grounded Theory method. *Journal of Holistic Nursing, 13*(2), 102–116.

Smith, H. (1991). *The world's religions: Our great wisdom traditions.* San Francisco: Harper.

Spector, R. (1996). *Cultural diversity in health and illness* (4th ed.). Stamford, CT: Appleton & Lange.

Steinberg, M. (1974). *Basic Judaism.* New York: Harcourt, Brace & World.

Stevens Barnum, B. (1996). *Spirituality in nursing: From traditional to New Age.* New York: Springer.

Touba, N. (1995). *Female genital mutilation: A call for global action.* New York: Women, Ink.

Tharp, R. (1991). Cultural diversity and treatment of children. *Journal of Consulting and Clinical Psychology, 59,* 799–812.

Travelbee, J. (1971). *Interpersonal aspects of nursing* (2nd. ed.). Philadelphia: Davis.

Viswananda (1938/1992). Unity of religions. In Ramakrishna Mission Institute of Culture (1992), *The religions of the world. Proceedings of the Sri Ramakrishna centenary parliament of religions 1 March–8 March, 1937* (pp. 235–237). Calcutta: The Ramakrishna Mission Institute of Culture.

Watson, J. (1988). *Nursing: Human science and human care: A theory of nursing.* New York: National League for Nursing.

CHAPTER 9: ENVIRONMENTAL PERSPECTIVES

Ader, R., Felten, D., & Cohen, N. (Eds.). (2000). *Psychoneurology* (3rd ed.). Washington, DC: Academic Press.

Agency for Toxic Substances and Disease Registry, Centers for Disease Control and Prevention, National Institutes of Health. (2000). *Healthy People 2010: Environmental health.* Washington, DC: United States Department of Health and Human Services. [On-line]. Available: www. health.gov/healthypeople/Document/ HTML/Volume1/08Environmental.htm.

American Nurses Association (1995). *Nursing: A social policy statement.* Kansas City, MO: Author.

Apperson, M. (2001). Records point to trouble. *The news & advance.* [On-line]. Available: www.healthyschools.org.

Bohm, D. (1980). *Wholeness and the implicate order.* London: Rutledge & Kegan Paul.

Brink, S. & Zeesman, A. (1997). *Measuring social well-being: An index of social health for Canada.* [On-line]. Available: www.hrdc-rhc.gc.ca/ streatpol/art/publications/research/ abr-97-9e.shtml.

Bureau of Labor Statistics. (2000). Work injuries and illnesses. *Department of Labor News.* Washington, DC: Department of Labor.

California Public Health Foundation (1992). *Kids and the environment: Toxic hazards. A course on pediatric environmental health.* Berkeley, CA: Author.

Center for Bioethics. (1992). *Taking values seriously: A values framework for the U.S. health care system.* Minneapolis, MN: University of Minnesota.

Centers for Disease Control and Prevention. (2000). *Healthy people 2010: Occupational safety and health.* Washington, DC: United States Department of Health and Human Services.

Centers for Disease Control and Prevention, National Center for Health Statistics. (1998–1999). *Healthy People 2000 Review.* In USDHHS, *Healthy People 2010.* Washington, DC: USDHHS.

Chia, S., Chia, H., & Tan, J. (2000). Prevalence of headache among handheld cellular telephone users in Singapore: A community study. *Environmental Health Perspectives, 108*(11), 1059–1062.

Colodzin, B. (1993). Respect and "real work." *Noetic Sciences Review, 25,* 30–31.

Dass, R. (1993). Compassion: The delicate balance. In R. Walsh & F. Vaughan (Eds.), *Paths beyond ego: The transpersonal vision* (pp. 234–236). Los Angeles: Jeremy P. Tarcher/Perigee.

Environmental Protection Agency. (1998). *Final guidance for incorporating environmental justice concerns in EPA's NEPA compliance analysis.* Washington, DC: U.S. Government Printing Office.

Frumkin, H., & Walker, D. (1997). Minority workers and communities. In J. M. Last (Ed.), *Public health and preventive medicine* (14th ed.). Norwalk, CT: Appleton-Century-Crofts.

Herbert, N. (1987). *Quantum reality: Beyond the new physics.* Garden City, NY: Anchor.

Institute of Medicine. (1995). *Nursing, health, and the environment.* Washington, DC: National Academy Press.

Institute of Medicine. (1999). *Toward environmental justice; research, education, and healthy policy needs.* Washington, DC: National Academy Press.

Jackson, R. (1998). *Statement of Richard Jackson, Director, National Center for Environmental Health Centers for Disease Control and Prevention, Department of Health and Human Services before the Subcommittee on Labor, Health and Human Services, and Education Committee on Appropriations, U.S. Senate on June 1, 1998.* [On-line]. Available: http://www. cdc.gov/ncidod/diseases/jackson.htm.

Josten, L., Clarke, P., Ostwald, S., Stoskopf, C., & Shannon, M. (1995). Public health nursing education: Back to the future for public health sciences. *Family and Community Health, 18*(1), 36–48.

Kim, H. S. (1983). *The nature of theoretical thinking.* East Norwalk, CT: Appleton-Century-Crofts.

Koplan, J. (1999). Foreward: Framework for program evaluation in public health. *MMWR 48*(RR11), 1.90. [On-line]. Available: www.cdc.gov/mmwr/ preview/mmwrhtml/rr4811al.htm.

Koplan, J. (2001). *Building infrastructure to protect the public's health. A public health training network broadcast sponsored by the Association of State and Territorial Health Officials in partnership with USDHHS, CDC, HRSA, and FDA.* [On-line]. Available: www.cdc.gov.

Lum, M. (1995). Environmental public health: Future direction, future skills. *Family and Community Health, 18*(1), 24–35.

Maslow, A. (1962). Health as transcendence of the environment. *Journal of Humanistic Psychology, 9*(1), 12–20.

McDade, J., & Franz, D. (1998). Bioterrorism as a public health threat. *Emerging Infectious Diseases, 4*(3). [On-line]. Available: http://www.cdc. gov/ncidod/eid/vol4no3/mcdade.htm.

McPhaul, K. (website coordinator). *Environmental health definitions and principles.* EnviRN, University of Maryland, School of Nursing. [On-line]. Available: www.envirn. umaryland.edu/basic.htm.

Miringoff, M., & Miringoff, M. L. (1999). *The social health of the nation: How is America really doing?* Tarrytown, NY: Oxford University Press.

Moos, R. (1979). Social-ecological perspectives on health. In G. Stone, F. Cohen, & N. Adler (Eds.), *Health psy-*

chology: A handbook. San Francisco: Jossey-Bass.

National Institute of Environmental Health Sciences. (2000). Good science for good decisions; Introduction. *NIEHS: Strategic Plan 2000* (March 2000). [On-line]. Available: www.niehs.nih.gov/external/plan2000/goodsci.htm.

Neufeld, A., & Harrison, M. (1990). The development of nursing diagnoses for aggregates and groups. *Public Health Nursing, 7*(4), 251–252.

Neufer, L. (1994). The role of the community health nurse in environmental health. *Public Health Nursing, 11*(3), 155–162.

Neuman, B. (1995). *The Neuman systems model* (3rd ed.) Norwalk, CT: Appleton & Lange.

Newman, M. (1994). *Health as expanding consciousness* (2nd ed.). St. Louis: C.V. Mosby.

Nightingale, F. (1860/1969). *Notes on nursing.* New York: Dover.

Phillips, L., (1995). Chattanooga Creed: Case study of the public health nursing role in environmental health. *Public Health Nursing, 12*(5), 335–340.

Powers, A. (1988). Social networks, social support, and elderly institutionalized people. *Advances in Nursing Science, 10*(2), 40–58.

Public Health Service. (1994). *Public health in America.* Washington, DC: Author.

Puntillo, K. (1992). *A model of environment.* Unpublished paper for class syllabus. Rohnert Park, CA: Sonoma State University.

Raven, P. (1998). *Nature and human society: The quest for a sustainable world (2000).* Washington, DC: National Academy Press.

Rogers, M. (1990). Nursing: Science of unitary, irreducible, human beings: Update 1990. In E. A. M. Barrett (Ed.), *Visions of Rogers' science-based nursing.* New York: National League for Nursing.

Rowe, J., & Kahn, R. (1998). *Successful aging.* New York: Dell.

Salmon, M. (1995). Public health policy: Creating a healthy future for the American public. *Family and Community Health, 18*(1), 1–11.

Schubert, P. (1989). Mutual connectedness: Holistic nursing practice under varying conditions of intimacy. Ph. D. dissertation, University of California, San Francisco, 1989. *Dissertation Abstracts International, 50,* 4987B.

Schubert, P., & Lionberger, H. (1995). Mutual connectedness: A study of client-nurse interaction using the Grounded Theory method. *Journal of Holistic Nursing, 13*(2), 102–116.

Sorrell, J. M. (1994). Remembrance of things past through writing: Esthetic patterns of knowing in nursing. *Advances in Nursing Science, 17*(1), 60–70.

United States Department of Health and Human Services. (2000). *Healthy people 2010: Understanding and improving health.* Washington, DC: Author.

U.S. Department of Health and Human Services. (2000b). *Healthy People 2010: Understanding and improving health.* Washington, DC: Author.

U.S. Department of Health and Human Services. (1997). *Healthy People 2000: Progress review.* Washington, DC: Author.

von Bertalanffy, L. (1968). *General systems theory.* New York: George Braziller.

Weiss, G., & Lonquist, L. (1999). *The sociology of health, healing, and illness* (3rd ed.). Upper Saddle River, NJ: Prentice-Hall.

Whitehead, A. (1969). *Process and reality: An essay in cosmology.* New York: Free Press.

Williams, C. (1995). Beyond the Institute of Medicine report: A critical analysis and public health forecast. *Family and Community Health, 18*(1), 12–23.

World Health Organization (1974). *Chronicle of WHO, 1,* 1–2.

World Health Organization (1997). *Indicators for policy and decision making in environmental health (Draft).* Geneva, Switzerland: Author.

CHAPTER 10: CARING COMMUNICATION AND CLIENT TEACHING/LEARNING

American Nurses' Association. (1995). *What you need to know about today's workplace: A survival guide for the workplace.* Washington, DC: Author.

American Nurses Association. (1997). Telehealth: A tool for nursing practice. *Nursing Trends and Issues, 2*(4), 1–7.

Anderson, K. N., Anderson, L. E., & Glanze, W. D. (Eds.). (1998) *Mosby's medical, nursing and allied health dictionary* (5th ed.). (1998). St. Louis, MO: Mosby.

Andrews, M. A., & Boyle, J. S. (1999). *Transcultural concepts in nursing care* (3rd ed.). Philadelphia: J. B. Lippincott.

Arnold, E., & Boggs, K. (1999). *Interpersonal relationships* (3rd ed.). Philadelphia: W.B. Saunders.

Balzer-Riley, J. (2000). *Communication in nursing* (4th ed.). St. Louis, MO: Mosby.

Boyd, M. D., Graham, B. A., Gleit, C. J., & Whitman, N. I. (1998). Health teaching in nursing practice. In M. D. Boyd, B. A. Graham, C. J. Gleit, & N. I. Whitman (Eds.), *Health teaching in nursing practice: A professional model* (3rd ed., pp. 3–20). Stamford, CT: Appleton & Lange.

Boyd, M. D. (1998). Strategies for effective teaching. In M. D. Boyd, B. A. Graham, C. J. Gleit, & N. I. Whitman (Eds.), *Health teaching in nursing practice: A professional model* (3rd ed., pp. 201–228). Stamford, CT: Appleton & Lange.

Buber, M. (1958). *I and thou.* New York: Charles Scribner.

Carpenito, L. J. (1997). *Handbook of nursing diagnosis* (7th ed.). Philadelphia: J. B. Lippincott.

Cushnie, P. (1988). Conflict: Developing resolution skills. *American Operating Room Nurses Journal, 47*(3), 732–742.

Deep, S., & Sussman, L. (1996). *Yes you can!* Reading, MA: Addison-Wesley.

Doak, L. G., Doak, C. C., & Root, J. H. (1996). *Teaching patients with low literacy skills.* Philadelphia: J. B. Lippincott.

Egan, G. (1982). *The skilled helper: Model, skills and methods for effective helping* (2nd ed.). Monterey, CA: Brooks/Cole Publishing.

Fisher, E. (1999, March–April). Low literacy levels in adults: Implications for patient education. *Journal of Continuing Education in Nursing, 30*(2), 56–61.

Freire, P. (1983). *Education for critical consciousness* (2nd ed.). New York: Continuum Press.

French, K. S., & Larrabee, J. H. (1999). Relationships among educational material readability, client literacy, perceived beneficence, and perceived quality. *Journal of Nursing Care Quality, 13*(6), 68–82.

Giger, J. N., & Davidhizar, R. E. (1999). *Transcultural nursing: Assessment and intervention* (3rd ed.). St. Louis, MO: Mosby.

Gleit, C. J. (1998). Theories of learning. In M. D. Boyd, B. A. Graham, C. J.

Gleit, & N. I. Whitman (Eds.), *Health teaching in nursing practice: A professional model* (3rd ed., pp. 65–98). Stamford, CT: Appleton & Lange.

Gordon, T. (1970). *Parent effectiveness training: The "no-lose" program for raising responsible children.* New York: Peter H. Wyden.

Graham, B. A., & Gleit, C. J. (1998). Teaching in selected settings. In M. D. Boyd, B. A. Graham, C. J. Gleit, & N. I. Whitman (Eds.), *Health teaching in nursing practice: A professional model* (3rd ed.). Stamford, CT: Appleton & Lange.

Kelly, M. L., & Fitzsimons, V. M. (2000). *Understanding cultural diversity: Culture, curriculum, and community in nursing.* Boston: Jones & Bartlett.

Kilmann, R., & Thomas, K. W. (1975). Interpersonal conflict-handling behavior as reflections of Jungian personality. *Psychological Reports, 37,* 971–980.

King, I. (1981). *A theory for nursing: Systems, concepts, process.* New York: John Wiley & Sons.

Kinsella, A. (1998). *Home healthcare, wired and ready for telemedicine . . . the second generation.* Sunriver, OR: Information for Tomorrow.

Klemm, P., Reppert, K., & Visich, L. (1998). A nontraditional cancer support group: The Internet. *Computers in Nursing, 16*(1), 31–36.

Knowles, M. (1990). *The adult learner* (4th ed.). Houston, TX: Gulf.

Knowles, M., Holton, E., & Swanson, R. A. (1998). *The adult learner: The definitive classic in adult education and human development* (5th ed.). Houston, TX: Gulf.

Krieger, D. (1993). *Accepting your power to heal: The personal practice of Therapeutic Touch.* Sante Fe, NM: Bear.

Loomis, M. (1979). *Group process for nurses.* St. Louis, MO: Mosby.

Marquis, B. L., & Huston, C. J. (2000). *Leadership roles and management functions in nursing: Theory and application* (3rd ed.). Philadelphia: J. B. Lippincott.

Miller, B., & Bodie, M. (1994). Determination of reading comprehension level for effective patient health education materials. *Nursing Research, 43*(2), 118–119.

Northouse, L. L., & Northouse, P. G. (1998). *Health communication: Strategies for health professionals* (3rd ed.). Stamford, CT: Appleton & Lange.

Orlando, I. (1961). *The dynamic nurse-patient relationship.* New York: G. P. Putnam's Sons.

Orlando, I. (1972). *The discipline and teaching of nursing process.* New York: G. P. Putnam's Sons.

Peplau, H. E. (1952). *Interpersonal relations in nursing.* New York: G. P. Putnam's Sons.

Peplau, H. E. (1960). Talking with patients. *American Journal of Nursing, 60,* 964.

Rankin, S. H., & Stallings, K. D. (2001). *Patient education: Principles, and practice* (4th ed.). Philadelphia: J. B. Lippincott.

Robinson, T., Patrick, K., Eng, T., & Gustafson, D. (1998). An evidence-based approach to interactive health communication: A challenge to medicine in the information age. *Journal of the American Medical Association, 280*(14), 1264–1269.

Rogers, C. R. (1951). *Client-centered therapy.* Boston: Houghton Mifflin.

Rogers, C. R. (1972). The process of the basic encounter group. In R. Diedrich & H. A. Dye (Eds.), *Group procedures, purposes, processes and outcomes.* Boston: Houghton Mifflin.

Rogers, M. E. (1990). Nursing: Science of unitary, irreducible, human beings: Update 1990. In E. A. Manhart Barrett (Ed.), *Visions of Rogers' science-based nursing.* New York: National League for Nursing.

Schubert, P. E. (1989). Mutual connectedness: Holistic nursing practice under varying conditions of intimacy. *Dissertation Abstracts International, 50,* 4987B.

Schubert, P. E., & Lionberger, H. J. (1995). Mutual connectedness: A study of client-nurse interaction using the grounded theory method. *Journal of Holistic Nursing, 13,* 102–116.

Skiba, D. J., & Barton, A. J. (2000). Health-oriented telecommunications. In M. J. Ball, K. J. Hannah, S. K. Newbold, & J. V. Douglas (Eds.), *Nursing informatics: Where caring and technology meet* (3rd ed.). New York: Springer-Verlag.

Stuart, G. & Laraia, M. (1997). *Stuart & Sundeen's principles and practice of psychiatric nursing.* St. Louis, MO: Mosby.

Travelbee, J. (1963). What do we mean by rapport? *American Journal of Nursing, 63,* 70–72.

Travelbee, J. (1964). What is wrong with sympathy? *American Journal of Nursing, 64,* 68–71.

Travelbee, J. (1971). *Interpersonal aspects of nursing* (2nd ed.). Philadelphia: F. A. Davis.

Truax, C., & Carkhuff, R. (1967). *Toward effective counseling and psychotherapy: Training and practice.* Chicago: Aldine.

Tubbs, S., & Moss, S. (2000). *Human communication* (8th ed.). Boston: McGraw-Hill.

Tuckman, B. (1965). Developmental sequences in small groups. *Psychological Bulletin, 63*(6), 384–399.

U.S. Department of Health and Human Services. *Healthy people 2010: Understanding and improving health.* Washington, DC: U.S. Government Printing Office, 2000.

Velsor-Friedrich, B. (2000, February). Healthy People 2000/2010: Health appraisal of the nation and future objectives, *Journal of Pediatric Nursing, 15*(1), 47–48.

Walker, M. A., & Harris, G. L. (1995). *Negotiation: Six steps to success.* Upper Saddle River, NJ: Bantam Books.

Wallerstein, N. & Bernstein, E. (1988). Empowerment education: Freire's ideas adapted to health education. *Health Education Quarterly, 15,* 379–394.

Whitman, N. I. (1998). Assessment of the learner. In M. D. Boyd, B. A. Graham, C. J. Gleit, & M. D. Boyd (Eds.), *Health teaching in nursing practice: A professional model* (3rd ed.). Stamford, CT: Appleton & Lange.

Yalom, I. (1975). *The theory and practice of group psychotherapy* (2nd ed.). New York: Basic Books.

Yalom, I. (1983). *Inpatient group psychotherapy.* New York: Basic Books.

Zarefsky, D. (1999). *Public speaking: Strategies for success* (2nd ed.). Boston: Allyn & Bacon

CHAPTER 11: HEALTH PROMOTION AND DISEASE PREVENTION PERSPECTIVES

American Nurses' Association (1987). *The nursing center: Concept and design.* Kansas City, MO: Author

Becker, M. H. (1974). *The Health Belief Model and personal health behavior.* Thorofare, NJ: Charles B. Slack.

Beddome, G. (1995). Community-as-client assessment: A Neuman-based guide for education and practice. In B. Neuman (Ed.), *The Neuman Systems Model* (3rd ed., pp. 567–580). Norwalk, CT: Appleton & Lange.

Donatelle, R. J., Davis, L. G., Hoover, C. F., & Harding, A. (1998). *Access to health* (8th ed.). Englewood Cliffs, NJ: Prentice-Hall.

Dunst, C., Trivette, C. & Deal, A. (Eds.). (1994). *Supporting and strengthening families: Methods, strategies and practices.* Cambridge, MA: Brookline.

Edelman, C., & Mandle, C. (1998). *Health promotion throughout the lifespan* (4th ed.). St. Louis: Mosby.

Environmental Protection Agency. (2000). *Health problems pesticides may pose.* [On-line]. Available: http://www.epa.gov/pesticides/food/risks.htm.

Fielding, J. (1999). The future of health promotion. In J. Rippe (Ed.), *Lifestyle medicine* (pp. 939–944). Malden, MA: Blackwell Science.

Friedman, H., Thomas, W., Klein, A., & Friedman, L. (1996). *Psychoneuroimmunology.* Boca Raton, FL: CRC Press.

Gullette, E., & Blumenthal, J. (1999). Psychosocial considerations in coronary heart disease: Implications for rehabilitation. In J. Rippe (Ed.), *Lifestyle medicine* (pp. 789–800). Malden, MA: Blackwell Science.

Hardman, J., Limbrid, L., Molinoff, P., Rudden, R., & Goodman-Gilman, A. (1996). *Goodman & Gilman's pharmaceutical basis of therapeutics* (9th ed., pp. 554–559). New York: McGraw-Hill Health Profession Division.

Lepler, S., Rosenkrantz, R., Diehl, D., Koser, G. (Draft, May 1999). *Promotion indicators for children and families: A concept paper.* Paper submitted by the Family Resource Coalition of America at a Symposium on Promotional Indicators May 11–12, 1999, Minneapolis, MN.

Lindsley, G., & Stephenson, L. (1999). Sleep, health, and well-being. In J. Rippe (Ed.), *Lifestyle medicine* (pp. 1226–1241). Malden, MA: Blackwell Science.

Lino, M., Basiotis, P., Anand, R. K., & Variyam, J. (1998, August). The diet quality of Americans. *Nutrition Insights.* USDA Center for Nutrition Policy and Promotion. [On-line]. Available: http://www.usda.gov/cnpp.

National Institute of Neurological Disorders and Stroke/National Institutes of Health. (2000). *Brain basics: Understanding sleep.* [On-line]. Available: http://www.ninds.nih.gov/health_and_medical/pubs/understanding_sleep_brain_basic_htm.

National Mental Health Association (2001). *Leading the way for America's mental health. Stress—coping with everyday problems.* [On-line]. Available: http://www.nmha.org/infoctr/factsheets/41.cfm.

National Sleep Foundation. (2000). *When you can't sleep: The ABCs of ZZZs.* Adapted by the National Institute of Neurological Disorders and Stroke. [On-line]. Available: http://www.ninds.nih.gov/health_and_medical/pubs/understanding_sleep_brain_basic_htm.

Neuman, B. (1990). Health as a continuum based on the Neuman Systems Model. *Nursing Science Quarterly, 3* (3) pp. 129–135.

Neuman, B. (1995). *The Neuman Systems Model* (3rd ed.). Norwalk, CT: Appleton & Lange.

Newman, M. (1994). *Health as expanding consciousness* (2nd ed.). New York: National League for Nursing.

O'Donnell, M. (1999). The impact on health of workplace health promotion programs and the methodologic quality of the research literature. In J. Rippe (Ed.), *Lifestyle medicine* (pp. 920–927). Malden, MA: Blackwell Science.

Old Ways Preservation and Trust. (1999–2001). *The traditional healthy vegetarian diet pyramid.* [On-line]. Available: http://oldwayspt.org/html/p_veg2.htm.

Pender, N. J. (1996). *Health promotion in nursing practice* (3rd ed.). Stamford, CT: Appleton & Lange.

Pender, N. J., Murdaugh, C., & Parsons, M. (2002). *Health promotion in nursing practice* (4th ed.) Upper Saddle River, NJ: Prentice-Hall.

Plotnikoff, N., & Faith, R. (1998). *Stress and immunity.* Boca Raton, FL: CRC Press.

Rankin, S., & Stallings, K. (2001). *Patient education: Principles and practice* (4th ed.). Philadelphia: J. B. Lippincott Williams & Wilkins.

Rew, L. (2000). Self-reflection: Consulting the truth within. In B. Dossey, L. Keegan, & C. Guzzeta (Eds.), *Holistic nursing: A handbook for practice* (3rd ed., pp. 407–424). Gaithersburg, MD: Aspen.

Rogers, M. (1990). Nursing: Science of unitary, irreducible human beings: Update 1990. In E. A. M. Barrett (Ed.), *Visions of Rogers' science-based nursing,* New York: National League for Nursing.

Rose, B., & Keegan, L. (2000). Exercise and movement. In B. Dossey, L. Keegan, & C. Guzzeta (Eds.), *Holistic nursing: A handbook for practice* (3rd ed., pp. 453–468). Gaithersburg, MD: Aspen.

Rosenstock, I. (1966). Why people use health services. *Millbank Memorial Fund Quarterly, 44,* 99–127.

Ryan, R., & Travis, J. (1981). *Wellness workbook* (2nd ed.). Berkeley, CA: Ten Speed Press.

Schubert, P. (1989). Mutual connectedness: Holistic nursing practice under varying conditions of intimacy. *Dissertation Abstracts International, 50,* 1987B.

Schubert, P., & Lionberger, H. (1995). Mutual connectedness: A study of client-nurse interaction using the grounded theory method. *Journal of Holistic Nursing, 13*(2), 102–116.

Thibodeaux, G., & Patton, L. (1997). *The human body in health and disease* (2nd ed.). St. Louis, MO: Mosby.

U.S. Department of Agriculture. (1999, August). *Biotechnology.* [On-line]. Available: http://www.usda.gov/news/releases/1999/07/0285.

U.S. Department of Agriculture/Department of Health and Human Services. (2000a). *Nutrition and your health: Dietary guidelines for Americans* (5th ed.). Washington, DC: Author.

U.S. Department of Health and Human Services. (1980). *Promoting health/preventing disease.* Washington, DC: Author.

U.S. Department of Health and Human Services. (1990). *Healthy People 2000: National health promotion and disease prevention objectives.* Washington, DC: Author.

U.S. Department of Health and Human Services. (1996). *Physical activity and health: A report of the Surgeon General.* Atlanta, GA: U.S. Department of Health and Human Services, Centers for Disease Control and Prevention, National Center for Chronic Disease Prevention and Health Promotion.

U.S. Department of Health and Human Services. (2000). *Healthy People 2010: Understanding and improving health.* Washington, DC: Author.

U.S. Food and Drug Administration/Center for Food Safety and Applied Nutrition (2001, January). *CFSAN 2001 program priorities.* [On-line].

Available: http://vm.cfsan.fda.gov/ ~dms/cfsan101.html.

U.S. Food and Drug Administration/ Center for Nutrition Policy and Promotion. (1998). *The healthy eating index (HEI)*. [On-line]. Available: http://www.nal.usda.gov/fnic/HEI/ execsum.html.

Velicer, W. F., Prochaska, J. O., Fava, J. L., Norman, G. J., & Redding, C. A. (1998). Smoking cessation and stress management: Applications of the Transtheoretical Model of behavior change. *Homeostasis, 38,* 216–233.

Wilson, M. (1999). Health promotion in the workplace. In J. M. Rippe (Ed.), *Lifestyle medicine* (pp. 901–911). Malden, MA: Blackwell Science.

World Health Organization. (1981). *Global strategy for health for all by the year 2000.* Geneva, Switzerland: Author.

World Health Organization. (1986). Ottawa Charter for Health Promotion. *Health Promotion, 1*(4), iii.

CHAPTER 12: INTEGRATIVE HEALTH CARE PERSPECTIVES

Anselmo, J., & Kolkmeier, L. (2000). Relaxation: The first step to restore, renew, and self-heal. In B. Dossey, L. Keegan, & C. Guzetta (Eds.). *Holistic nursing: A handbook for practice* (3rd ed., pp. 497–535). Gaithersburg, MD: Aspen.

Astin, J. (1998). Why patients use alternative medicine. *Journal of the American Medical Association, 279,* 1548–1553.

Benson, H. (1975). *The relaxation response.* New York: William Morrow.

Bohm, D. (1980). *Wholeness and the implicate order.* London: Routledge & Kegan Paul.

Burmeister, M. (1980). *Introducing Jin Shin Jyutsu Is, Book I.* Scottsdale, AZ: Jin Shin Jyutsu.

Burmeister, M. (1981). *Introducing Jin Shin Jyutsu Is, Book II.* Scottsdale, AZ: Jin Shin Jyutsu.

Burmeister, M. (1994). *Text 1.* Scottsdale, AZ: Jin Shin Jyutsu.

Capra, F. (1977). *The Tao of physics.* New York: Bantam.

Clark, C. (2000). *Integrating complementary health procedures into practice.* New York: Springer.

Cugelman, A. (1998). Therapeutic Touch: An extension of professional skills. *Journal of CANNT, 8,* 30–32.

Dossey, B., & Keegan, L. (2000). Self-assessments: Facilitating healing in self and others. In B. Dossey, L. Keegan, & C. Guzzetta (Eds.), *Holistic nursing: A handbook for practice* (3rd ed., pp. 361–373). Gaithersburg, MD: Aspen.

Egan, E. (1998). Therapeutic Touch. In M. Snyder & R. Lindquist (Eds.), *Complementary/alternative in nursing* (3rd ed., pp. 49–62). New York: Springer.

Eisenberg, D., Davis, R., Ettner, S., Appel, S., Wilkey, S., Rompay, M., & Kessler, R. (1998). Trends in alternative medicine use in the United States, 1990–1997. *Journal of the American Medical Association, 280,* 1569–1575.

Gordon, A., Merenstein, J. H., D'Amico, F., & Hudgens, D. (1998). The effects of Therapeutic Touch on patients with osteoarthritis of the knee. *Journal of Family Practice, 47*(4), 271–277.

Graham, H. (1999). *Complementary therapies in context: The psychology of healing.* Philadelphia: Jessica Kingsley.

Hatcher, T. (2001). The proverbial herb. *American Journal of Nursing, 101*(2), 36–43.

Herbert, N. (1987). *Quantum reality: Beyond the new physics.* Garden City, NY: Anchor.

Hover-Kramer, D. (1993). *Healing touch: A resource for health care professionals.* Clifton Park, NY: Delmar Learning.

Hunt, V. (1995). *Infinite mind: The science of human vibrations.* Malibu, CA: Malibu Publishing.

Ireland, M. (1998). Therapeutic Touch with HIV-infected children: A pilot study. *Journal of the Association of Nurses AIDS Care, 9*(4), 68–77.

Jonsen, A. (1998). *Clinical ethics* (4th ed.). New York: MacMillan.

Keegan, L. (1994). *The nurse as healer.* Clifton Park, NY: Delmar Learning.

Keegan, L. (2000). Holistic ethics. In B. Dossey, L. Keegan, & C. Guzzetta (Eds.), *Holistic nursing: A handbook for practice* (3rd ed., pp. 159–168). Gaithersburg, MD: Aspen.

Krieger, D. (1979). *The Therapeutic Touch: How to use your hands to help or to heal.* New York: Prentice-Hall.

Krieger, D. (1993). *Accepting your power to heal: The personal practice of Therapeutic Touch.* Santa Fe: Bear.

Lionberger, H. (1985). An interpretive study of nurses' practice of Therapeutic Touch. *Dissertation Abstracts International, 46,* 2624B.

Merriam-Webster's collegiate dictionary. (Undated). [On-line]. Available: http://www.m-w.com.cgi-bin/dictionary.

Motoyama, H. (1986). Before polarization current and the acupuncture meridians. *Journal of Holistic Medicine, 8,* 1–2.

National Center for Complementary and Alternative Medicine. (1999). *Acupuncture information and resources.* [On-line]. Available: http://nccam. nih.gov/nccam/fcp/factsheets/ acupuncture.

National Center for Complementary and Alternative Medicine. (2000a). *Statement by Stephen E. Straus, M.D., Director, National Center for Complementary and Alternative Medicine before the Senate Appropriations Subcommittee on Labor, HHS, Education, and Related Agencies.* [On-line]. Available: http://nccam.nih.gov/ ne/senate.

National Center for Complementary and Alternative Medicine. (2000b). *Major domains of complementary and alternative medicine: For consumers and practitioners.* [On-line]. Available: http://nccam.nih.gov/nccam/ fcp/classify.

National Center for Complementary and Alternative Medicine. (2001a). *What is complementary and alternative medicine?* [On-line]. Available: http:// nccam.nih.gov/nccam/fep/faq/index.

National Center for Complementary and Alternative Medicine. (2001b). *Report: "Can alternative medicine be integrated into mainstream care?"* Conference January 23–24, 2001, London, England. Sponsored by NC-CAM and the Royal College of Physicians. [On-line]. Available: http:// nccam.nih.gov/ne/meeting_012301.

National Center for Complementary and Alternative Medicine. (2001c). *About NCCAM: General information.* [On-line]. Available: http://nccam.nih.gov/ nccam/an/general.

National Center for Complementary and Alternative Medicine. (2001d). *Fiscal year 2002 budget request.* [On-line]. Available: http://nccam.nih.gov/ne/ testimony/may2001.

National Center for Complementary and Alternative Medicine. (2001e). *Approaching complementary and alter-*

native therapies. [On-line]. Available: http://nccam.nih.gov/nccam/fcp/faq/considercam.

Newman, M. A. (1994). *Health as expanding consciousness* (2nd ed.). New York: National League for Nursing.

Nurse Healers — Professional Associates (NH-PA). (1992). *Therapeutic Touch teaching guidelines: Beginner's level Krieger/Kunz method.* New York: Author.

Nurse Healers — Professional Associates (NH-PA). (1994). *Therapeutic Touch teaching guidelines: Intermediate Level Krieger/Kunz method.* Allison Park, PA: Author.

Nurse Healers — Professional Associates, International (NH-PAI). (1998). *Basic assumptions underlying Therapeutic Touch practice. Nurse Healers-Professional Associates International (NH-PAI) Basic Core Curriculum* (p. 201). Salt Lake City, UT: Author.

Patel, M. (1987). Evaluation of holistic medicine. *Social Science and Medicine, 24*(2), 174.

Pelletier, K. (2000). *The best alternative medicine: What works? What does not?* New York: Simon & Schuster.

Pribram, K. (1971). *Languages of the brain.* New York: Prentice-Hall.

Prigogine, I., & Stengers, I. (1984). *Order out of chaos.* Boulder, CO: Shambhala.

Quinn, J. (1992). Therapeutic Touch: Healing through human energy fields. In *Video I: Theory and research.* New York: National League for Nursing.

Quinn, J. (2000). Transpersonal human caring and healing. In B. Dossey, L. Keegan, & C. Guzzetta (Eds.), *Holistic nursing: A handbook for practice* (3rd ed., pp. 37–47.) Gaithersburg, MD: Aspen.

Quinn, J. M., & Strelkauskas, A. J. (1993). Psychoimmunologic effects of Therapeutic Touch on practitioners and recently bereaved recipients: A pilot study. *Advances in Nursing Science, 15*(4), 13–26.

Rama, S. (1978). *Living with the Himalayan masters.* Honesdale, PA: Himalayan International Institute.

Rawnsley, M. (1985). HEALTH: A Rogerian perspective. *Journal of Holistic Nursing, 3*(1), 25–29.

Rew, L. (1996). *Nurse as healer: Awareness in healing* (L. Keegan, Series Ed.). Clifton Park, NY: Delmar Learning.

Rogers, M. E. (1970). *An introduction to the theoretical basis of nursing.* Philadelphia: F. A. Davis.

Rogers, M. E. (1980). Nursing: A science of unitary man. In J. P. Riehl & C. Roy (Eds.), *Conceptual models for nursing practice* (2nd ed., pp. 329–337). New York: Appleton-Century-Crofts.

Rogers, M. E. (1981). Science of unitary man: A paradigm for nursing. In G. E. Laskar (Ed.), *Applied systems and cybernetics (Vol. IV).* New York: Pergamon.

Rogers, M. E. (1983). Science of unitary human beings: A paradigm for nursing. In I. W. Clements & F. B. Roberts (Eds.), *Family health: A theoretical approach to nursing care* (pp. 219–227). New York: John Wiley & Sons.

Rogers, M. E. (1985). A paradigm for nursing. In R. Wood & J. Kekhababh (Eds.), *Examining the cultural implications of Martha E. Rogers' science of unitary human beings* (pp. 13–23). Lecompton, KS: Wood-Kekhababh Associates.

Rogers, M. E. (1986). Science of unitary human beings. In V. Malinski (Ed.), *Explorations on Martha Rogers' science of unitary human beings* (pp. 3–8). Norwalk, CT: Appleton-Century-Crofts.

Rogers, M. E. (1987). Rogers science of unitary human beings. In R. Parse (Ed.), *Nursing science: Major paradigms, theories, and critiques* (pp. 139–146). Philadelphia: W. B. Saunders.

Rogers, M. E. (1990). Nursing: Science of unitary, irreducible, human beings: Update 1990. In E. A. M. Barrett (Ed.), *Visions of Rogers' science-based nursing.* New York: National League for Nursing.

Rossman, M. (1993). *Mind/body medicine: How to use your mind for better health.* New York: Consumer Reports Books.

Rossman, M., & Bresler, D. (1994). *Interactive Guided Imagery^{SM}: Clinical techniques for brief therapy and health psychology: A training workbook* (5th ed.). Mill Valley, CA: Academy for Guided Imagery.

Rossman, M., & Bresler, D. (2001). *What is Interactive Guided Imagery^{SM}?* [On-line]. Available: www.interactiveimagery.com/index_ie.

Schaub, B., & Dossey, B. (2000). Imagery: Awakening the inner body. In *Holistic nursing: A handbook for*

practice (3rd ed., pp. 749–772). Gaithersburg, MD: Aspen.

Schubert, P. (1989). Mutual connectedness: Holistic nursing practice under varying conditions of intimacy. *Dissertation Abstracts International, 50,* 4987B.

Schubert, P., & Lionberger, H. (1995). Mutual connectedness: A study of client-nurse interaction using the grounded theory method. *Journal of Holistic Nursing, 13*(2), 102–116.

Slater, V. (2000). Energetic healing. In B. Dossey, L. Keegan, & C. Guzzetta (Eds.), *Holistic nursing: A handbook for practice* (3rd ed.). Gaithersburg, MD: Aspen.

Spiegel, D., Stroud, P., & Fyfe, A. (1998). Complementary medicine. *Western Journal of Medicine, 168,* 241–247.

Sugarman, J., & Burk, L. (1998). Physicians' ethical obligations regarding alternative medicine. *Journal of the American Medical Association 280,* 1623–1625.

Tedeschi, M. (2000). *Essential anatomy: For healing and martial arts.* New York: Weatherhill.

Turner, J., Clark, A., Gauthier, D., & Williams, M. (1998). The effect of Therapeutic Touch on pain and anxiety in burn patients. *Journal of Advanced Nursing, 28*(1), 10–20.

University of Colorado Health Sciences Center. (1994). *University of Colorado Report on Touch Therapy.* Department of Medicine. Denver, CO: Author.

Wirth, D. (1990). The effects of non-contact Therapeutic Touch on the healing rate of full thickness dermal wounds. *Subtle Energies, 1*(1), 1–20.

Zahourek, R. (1988). *Relaxation and imagery: Tools for therapeutic communication and intervention.* Philadelphia: W. B. Saunders.

Zukav, G. (1979). *The dancing Wu Li masters: On overview of the new physics.* New York: William Morrow.

CHAPTER 13: POPULATION-FOCUSED PRACTICE

American Public Health Association, Public Health Nursing Section. (1996). *The definition and role of public health nursing—A statement of the APHA Public Health Nursing Section* (pp. 1–4). Washington, DC: American Public Health Association.

Anderson, I. (1996). Aboriginal well-being. In C. Grbich (Ed.), *Health in*

Australia: Sociological concepts and issues. Australia: Prentice-Hall.

Ashton, J., & Seymour, H. (1988). *The new public health*. Philadelphia: Open University Press, Milton Keynes.

Bastian, H. (1989). A guide to WHO and "WHO speak." *Consumer Health Forum, 9,* 15.

Baum, F., Fry, D., & Lennie, I. (Eds.). (1992). *Community health policy and practice in Australia,* Sydney: Pluto Press.

Beck, U. (1989). On the way to the industrial risk-society: Outline of an argument. *Thesis Eleven, 23,* 86–105.

Black, D., Townsend, P., & Davidson, N. (1982). Great Britain: Working group on inequalities in health. In *Inequalities in Health: The Black Report*. Harmondsworth: Penguin.

Blane, D. (1987). The value of labour-power and health. In G. Scambler (Ed.), *Sociological theory and medical sociology*. London: Tavistock Publications.

Brown, L., Donovan, J., & Islip, R. (1988). *A guidebook for leaders of new parents' groups*. Paper presented at the AECA 18th National Conference, Canberra, Australia.

Cheek, J., & Willis, E. (1998). Health risk analysis and sociomedical technologies of the self—Private health insurance gets into health promotion. *Australian Journal of Social Issues, 33*(12), 119–132.

Collier, P. (1998). *Social capital and poverty: Social capital initiative*. Working Paper No. 4. New York: The World Bank: Social Development Family Environmentally and Socially Sustainable Development Network.

Department of Family and Community Services. (2000). *Stronger families and communities strategy*. Canberra: Australian Government Printers.

Fifth global conference on health promotion, homepage conference report. (2001, February 8). [Online]. Available: http://www.who.int/conference/products/conferencereport.htm.

Foley, M., & Edwards, B. (1999). Is it time to disinvest in social capital? *Journal of Public Policy, 19*(2), 141–173.

Foucault, M. (1980). *Power/Knowledge: Selected interviews and other writings, 1972–1977*. (C. Gordon, trans.). Brighton: Harvester Press.

Friedman, J. (1992). *Empowerment: The politics of alternative development*. Cambridge, MA: Blackwell.

Gardner, H. (1992). *Health policy: Development, implementation, and evaluation in Australia*. Melbourne: Churchill Livingstone.

Hawe, P., Degeling, D., Hall, J., & Brierley, A. (1990). *Evaluating health promotion*. New South Wales: MacLerman & Petty.

Institute of Medicine, Committee for the Study of the Future of Public Health. (1988). *The future of public health*. Washington, DC: National Academy Press.

Jackson, T., Mitchel, S., & Wright, M. (1989). The community development continuum. *Community Health Studies, 13*(1).

Keck, C. W., & Scutchfield, E. D. (1997). The future of public health. In F. D. Scutchfield & C. W. Keck (Eds.), *Principles of public health practice*. Clifton Park, NY: Delmar Learning.

Labonte, R. (1990). Heart health inequalities in Canada: Models, theory and planning. *Health Promotion International, 7*(2), 119–128.

Lord, J., & McKillop, F. (1990, Fall). A study of personal empowerment: Implications for health promotion. *Health Promotion*.

Lundberg O. (1991). Causal explanations for class inequalities in health—An empirical analysis. *Social Science and Medicine, 32*(4), 385–393.

Marmot, M., & Thorell, T. (1988). Social class and cardiovascular disease: The contribution of work. *International Journal of Health Services, 18*(4), 659j–674.

McKeown, T. (1962). Reasons for the decline of mortality in England and Wales during the nineteenth century. *Population Studies, 16*(2), 94–122.

McKnight, J. (1986). *The need for oldness*. Paper presented at the Center on Aging, McGraw Medical Center, Northwestern University, Evanston, IL.

McPherson, P. (1992). Health for all Australians. In Heather Gardner (Ed.), *Health policy: Development, implementation and evaluation in Australia* (p. 120). Melbourne: Churchill Livingstone.

Mosely, H. (1988). Is there a middle way? Categorical programmes for primary health care. *Social Science and Medicine, 26*(9), 907–908.

National Association for County Health Officials. (1994). *Blueprint for a healthy community: A guide for local health departments*. Washington, DC: Author.

National Centre for Epidemiology and Population Health. (1991). *The role of primary health care in health promotion in Australia*. Commonwealth Department of Health, Housing and Community Services and National Better Health Program. Canberra, Australia: Author.

Newell, K. (1988). Selective primary health care: The counter revolution. *Social Science and Medicine, 26*(9), 903–906.

North, F., Syme, L., Feeney, A., Shipley, M., & Marmot, M. (1996). Psychological work environment and sickness absence among British civil servants: The Whitehall 11 study. *American Journal of Public Health, 86*(3), 332–340.

Peterson, A. (1994 June) Community development and health promotion: Empowerment or regulation? *Australian Journal of Public Health, 18*(2), 213–217.

Powles, J., & Salzberg, M. (1989). Work, class or life-style? Explaining inequalities in health. In G. Lupton & J. Najman (Eds.), *Sociology of health and illness: Australian readings* (pp. 135–168). South Melbourne: MacMillan.

Raeburn, J., & Rootman, I. (1998). *People-centered health promotion*. Brisbane, Australia: John Wiley & Sons.

Rappaport, J., (1987). Terms of empowerment/exemplars of prevention: Towards a theory for community psychology. *Journal of Community Psychology, 15,* 2.

Russell, G., Barclay, L., Edgecombe, G., Donovan, J., Habib, G., Callaghan, H., & Pawson, Q. (1999). *Fitting fathers into families: Men and the fatherhood role in contemporary Australia*. Report for Department of Family and Community Services, Media & Publications Unit. Canberra, ACT: Commonwealth Department of Family and Community Services.

Scheyner, S., Landefeld, J. S., & Sandifer, F. H. (1981). Biomedical research and illness: 1900–1979. *Millbank Memorial Fund Quarterly/Health and Society, 59*(1).

Stacey, M. (1988). Strengthening communities. *Health Promotion, 2*(4), 321.

Syme, S. L. (1989). Control and health: A personal perspective. In A. Steptoe & A. Appels (Eds.), *Stress, personal control, and health*. Chichester: Wiley.

Telleen, S., Herzog A., & Kilbane, T. (1989, July). Impact of a family support program on mothers' social support and parenting stress. *American Journal of Orthopsychiatry, 59*(3) 410–419.

U.S. Department of Health and Human Services. (2000, November). *Healthy people 2010: Understanding and improving health* (2nd ed.). Washington, DC: U.S. Government Printing Office.

Vagero, D. (1991). Inequalities in health: Some theoretical and empirical problems. *Social Science and Medicine, 32*(4), 367–371.

Walsh, J. (1988). Selectivity within primary health care. *Social Science and Medicine, 26*(9), 899–902.

Warren, K. S. (1988). The evolution of selective primary health care. *Social Science and Medicine, 26*(9), 891–898.

Washington State Department of Health. (1994). *Public health improvement plan.* Olympia, WA: Author.

Williams, C. A. (1996). Community-based population-focused practice: The foundation of specialization in public health nursing. In M. Stanhope & J. Lancaster, *Community health nursing: Promoting health of aggregates, families, and individuals* (pp. 21–33). St. Louis, MO: Mosby.

Willis, E. (1990). *Advanced nursing studies 3.* Adelaide, Australia: The Flinders University of South Australia, Master of Nursing, School of Nursing.

Willis, K. (1999). Compromise, country women, and cancer: Women's health policy in Australia. *Annual Review of Health Social Science, 9,* 51–60.

Wisner, B. (1988). GOBI versus PHC? Some dangers of selective primary health care. *Social Science and Medicine, 26*(9), 963–969.

World Health Organization, *Jakarta Declaration on Health Promotion into the 21st Century.* (2001, February 8). [On-line]. Available: http://www.who.int/dsa/cat95/zjak.htm.

World Health Organization. (1978a). *Declaration of Alma Ata.* Geneva, Switzerland: Author.

World Health Organization. (1978b). *Primary health care: Report of the international conference on primary health care.* Geneva, Switzerland: Author.

World Health Organization. (1986). *Ottawa Charter for Health Promotion.* Ottawa, Canada: Author.

World Health Organization. (1993). *Implementation of the global strategy*

for health for all: Second evaluation. Eighth report on the world health situation, Vol. 1. Global Review. Geneva, Switzerland: Author.

World Health Organization & Commonwealth Department of Community Services and Health. (1988). *Proceedings of the Second International Conference of Health Promotion,* April 5–9. Adelaide, Australia: World Health Organization, p. 2.

World Health Organization, Regional Office for Europe. (1985). *Primary health care in industrialised countries.* Report of 1983 Conference in Bordeaux on Primary Health Care in Industrialised Countries, Euro Reports and Studies #95. Copenhagen, Denmark: Author.

World Health Report press release. (2001, February 8). [On-line]. Available: http://www.who.int/whr/2000/en/pressrelease.htm.

CHAPTER 14: EPIDEMIOLOGY

Diez-Roux, A. V. (1998). Bringing context back into epidemiology: Variables and fallacies in multilevel analysis. *American Journal of Public Health, 88*(2), 216.

Freeman, R. (1963). *Public health nursing practice* (3rd ed.). Philadelphia: W. B. Saunders.

Friedman, G. (1987). *Primer of epidemiology.* New York: McGraw-Hill.

Green, L. (1996). *Community health.* St. Louis, MO: Times Mirror/Mosby.

Green, L., & Kreuter, M. (1991). *Health promotion planning: An educational and environmental approach.* Mountain View: Mayfield Publishing.

Greenberg, R., Daniels, S. R., Flanders, W. D., Eley, J. W., & Boring III, J. R. (1996). *Medical epidemiology* (2nd ed.). Stamford, CT: Appleton & Lange.

Hennekens, C., & Buring, J. (1987). *Epidemiology in medicine.* Boston: Little, Brown, and Company.

Last, J. (1995). *Dictionary of epidemiology.* New York: Oxford University Press.

Lilienfeld, D., & Stolley, P. (1994). *Foundations of epidemiology.* New York: Oxford University Press.

Morton, R., Hebel, J., & McCarter, R. (1996). *A study guide to epidemiology and biostatistics.* Gaithersburg, MD: Aspen Publishers.

Nurses' Health Study Newsletter (2000, June). Boston, MA.: Channing Laboratory.

Teutsch, S., Churchill, R., & Elliott, R. (1994). *Principles and practice of public health surveillance,* New York: Oxford University Press.

U.S. Department of Health and Human Services. (1990). *Healthy people 2000.* Washington, DC: Author.

U.S. Department of Health and Human Services. (2000). *Healthy People 2010.* Washington, DC: U.S. Government Printing Office.

CHAPTER 15: ASSESSING THE COMMUNITY

Alexander, J. W. (2001). Community service now and in the future. In N.P. Chaska (Ed.), *The nursing profession, tomorrow and beyond* (pp. 547–559). Thousand Oaks, CA. Sage Publications.

American Public Health Association, (1991). *Healthy communities 2000 model standards: Guidelines for community attainment of the year 2000 national health objectives.* Washington, DC: Author.

Anderson, E., & McFarlane, J. (1988). *Community as client: Application of the nursing process.* Philadelphia: J. B. Lippincott.

Association of State and Territorial Directors of Nursing. (2000). *Public health nursing, a partner for healthy populations.* Washington, DC: American Nurses Publishing.

Aller, J. (1988). *Exploring legislative arrangements for promoting primary health care in Australia.* Adelaide, Australia: Social Health Branch, South Australian Health Commission.

Barton, J. A., Smith, M. C., Brown, N. J., & Supples, J. M. (1993). Methodological issues in a team approach to community health needs assessment. *Nursing Outlook, 41*(6).

Baum, F. (1992). Researching community health: Evaluation and needs assessment that makes an impact. In F. Baum, D. Fry, & I. Lennie (Eds.), *Community health: Policy and practice in Australia.* Sydney, Australia: Pluto Press in association with Australian Community Health Association.

Baum, F. E. (1995). Researching public health: Behind the qualitative-quantitative debate. *Social Science and Medicine, 40*(4), 459–468.

Baum, F. E., & Cooke, R. D. (1988). Community-health needs assessment:

Use of the Nottingham health profile in an Australian study. *Medical Journal of Australia, 150,* 581–590.

Becker, M. H. (1986). The tyranny of health promotion. *Public Health Review, 14* 15–25.

Berry, M., Doherty, A., Hope, A., Sixsmith, J., & Kelleher, C. (2000). A community needs assessment for rural mental health promotion. *Health Education Research, 15,* 293–304.

Billings, J. R., & Cowley, S. (1995). Approaches to community needs assessment: A literature review. *Journal of Advanced Nursing, 22,* 721–730.

Bowling, A. (1992). *"Local voices" in purchasing health care: An exploratory exercise in public consultation in priority setting.* London: Needs Assessment Unit. St. Bartholomew's Hospital Medical College.

Bradshaw, J. (1972, March 30). The concept of social need. *New Society,* 640–643.

Brady, J.C. & Brady, D.F. (2000). The trashing of the Rockaways by city and state. *The World & I: The Magazine For Lifelong Learners, 1*(5), 304–315.

Brennan, A. (1992). The Altona Clean Air Project. *Health Issues, 32,* 18–20.

Brown, V. (1985). Towards an epidemiology of health: A basis for planning community health programs. *Health Policy, 4,* 331–340.

Bryson, L., & Mowbray, M. (1981). "Community": The spray-on solution, *Australian Journal of Social Issues, 16*(4), 255–267.

Caretto, V. A., & McCormick, C. S. (1991). Community as client: A hands-on experience for baccalaureate nursing students. *Journal of Community Health Nursing, 8*(5), 179–189.

Chalmers, K., & Kristajanson, L. (1989). The theoretical basis for nursing at the community level: A comparison of three models. *Journal of Advanced Nursing, 14,* 569–574.

Chu, C. (1994). Assessing community needs and integrated environmental impact assessment. In C. Chu & R. Simpson (Eds.), *Ecological public health: From vision to practice.* Nathan, Queensland: Institute of Applied Environmental Research, Griffith University and Ontario, Centre for Health Promotion, University of Toronto.

Clark, D. B. (1973). The concept of community: A re-examination. *Sociological Review, 21*(3), 397–415.

Cooney, C. (1994). Community assessment: A vital component of Primary Health Care Objectives. In C. Cooney (Ed.), *Primary health care: The way to the future,* Sydney, Australia: Prentice-Hall.

Davis, R. (2000). Holographic community: Reconceptualizing the meaning of community in an era of health care reforms. *Nursing Outlook, 48,* 294–301.

Denham, A., Quinn, S. C., & Gamble, D. (1998). Community organizing for health promotion in the rural south: An exploration of community competence. Community interventions. *Family and Community Health, 21,* 1–21.

Department of Health. (1998). *Report of the national task force on suicide.* Dublin: Stationery Office.

Development of healthy people 2010 objectives. (2000). [On-line]. Available: http://EDAVIS@OSOPHS/DHHS.gov.

Eng, E., & Parker, E. (1994). Measuring community competence in the Mississippi Delta: The interface between program evaluation and empowerment. *Health Education Quarterly, 21*(2), 199–220.

Eng, E., Salmon, M. E., & Mullan, F. (1992). Community empowerment: The critical base for primary health care. *Family and Community Health, 15*(1), 1–12.

Epp. J. (1986). *Achieving health for all: A Framework for health promotion.* Ottawa. Canada: National Health and Welfare.

Ewles, L., & Simnett, I. (1992). *Promoting health: A practical guide.* London: Scutari Press.

Flower, J. (1994, May/June). A worldwide movement for health. *Health Care Forum Journal,* pp. 48–53.

Forster, J. L., Murray, D. M., Wolfson, M., Blaine, T. M., Wagenaar, A. C., & Hennrikus, D. J. (1998). The effects of community policies to reduce youth access to tobacco. *American Journal of Public Health, 88*(4), 1193–1198.

Gilmore, G. D., Campbell, M. D., & Becker, B. (1989). *Needs assessment strategies for health education and health promotion.* Indianapolis, IN: Benchmark Press.

Green, L. W., & Kreuter, M. W. (1991). *Health promotion planning: An educational and environmental approach.* Mountain View: Mayfield.

Hancock, T., & Duhl, L. (1985). *World Health Organization Healthy Cities Project: Promoting health in the urban context.* Copenhagen, Denmark: The WHO Healthy Cities Project Office, FADL Publishers.

Hawe, P. (1994). Capturing the meaning of "community" in community intervention evaluation: Some contributions from community psychology. *Health Promotion International, 9*(3), 199–210.

Hawe, P., Degeling, D., & Hall, J. (1990). *Evaluating health promotion: A health worker's guide.* Sydney, Australia: MacLennan and Petty.

Health Targets and Implementation Committee. (1988). *Health for All Australians.* Canberra, Australia: Australian Government Publishing Service.

Healthy people 2010. (2000). [On-line]. Available: http:www.health.gov/healthypeople/document/HTML/volume/intro.htm.

Institute of Medicine. (1988). *The future of public health.* Washington, DC: National Academy Press.

Kang, R. (1995). Building community capacity for health promotion: A challenge for public health nurses. *Public Health Nursing, 12*(5), 312–318.

Koerner, J. (2001). Nightingale II, nursing in the new millenium. In N. P. Chaska (Ed.), *The nursing profession: Tomorrow and beyond* (pp. 17–24). Thousand Oaks, CA: Sage Publications.

Kreuter, M. W. (1984). Health promotion: The role of public health in the community for free exchange. *Health Promotions Monographs, 4.* New York: Columbia University, Center for Health Promotion.

Kuehnert, P. L. (1995). The interactive and organizational model of community as client: A model for public health nursing practice. *Public Health Nursing, 12*(1), 9–17.

Labonte, R. (1994). Health promotion and empowerment: Reflections on professional practice. *Health Education Quarterly, 21*(2), 253–268.

Living at home/block nurse program, Inc. (1994). *How to start the living at home/block nurse program in your community.*

McBride, T. (1988). Poverty action in a community health center. *Health Issues, September* (15), 24–27.

McKenzie, J. F., & Jurs, J. L. (1993). *Planning, implementing, and evaluating health programs: A primer.* New York: Macmillan.

Mendieta, C. (1999). *The heart of the community: NEST: A working model of community-based long term care for elders*. San Francisco, CA: Neighborhood Elders Support Team, U.S. Agency on Aging.

Minkler, M. (1994). Ten commitments for community health education. *Health Education Research, 9*(4), 527–534.

Murphy, B., Cockburn, J., & Murphy, M. (1992). Focus groups in health research. *Health Promotion Journal of Australia, 2*(2), 37–40.

Murray, C. J., & Lopez, A. D. (1996). *Summary: The Global Burden of Disease and Inquiry Series*. Cambridge, MA: The Harvard School of Public Health on behalf of the World Health Organization and the World Bank. Harvard University Press.

Ong, B. N., Humphris, G., Annett, H., & Rifkin, S. (1991). Rapid appraisal in an urban setting, an example from the developed world. *Social Science and Medicine, 32*(8), 909–915.

Patrick, D. L. (1986). Measurement of health and quality of life. In D. L. Patrick & G. Scambler (Eds.), *Sociology as applied to medicine*. London: Bailliere Tindall.

Peckham, S., & Spanton, J. (1994). Community development approaches to health needs assessment. *Health Visitor, 67*(4), 124–125.

Reininger, B., Dinh-Zarr, T., Sinicrope, P. S., & Martin, D. W. (1999). Dimensions of participation and leadership: Implications for community-based health promotion for youth. *Family and Community Health, 22*(2), 72–82.

Rissel, C. (1991). The tyranny of needs assessment in health. *Evaluation Journal of Australia, 3*(1), 26–31.

Rissel, C. (1996). A communitarian correction for health outcomes in New South Wales? *Australian Journal of Primary Health—Interchange, 2*(2), 36–45.

Rorden, J. W., & McLennan, J. (1992). *Community health nursing: Theory and practice*. Sydney, Australia: Harcourt Brace.

Ruffing-Rahal, M. A. (1987). Resident/provider contrasts in community health priorities. *Public Health Nursing, 4*(4), 242–246.

Russell, C. K., Gregory, D. M., Wotton, D., Mordoch, E., & Counts, M. M. (1996). ACTION: Application and extension of the GENESIS community analysis model. *Public Health Nursing, 13*(3), 187–194.

Ryan, W. (1976). *Blaming the victim*. New York: Vintage Books.

Shields, L., & Lindsey, E. (1998). Community health promotion nursing practice. *Advances in Nursing Science, 20*(23), 1.

Shuster, G. F., & Goeppinger, J. (1996). Community as client: Using the nursing process to promote health. In M. Stanhope & J. Lancaster (Eds.), *Community health nursing: Process and practice for promoting health* (4th ed., pp. 289–314) St. Louis, MO: C. V. Mosby.

Southern Community Health Research Unit. (1991). *Planning healthy communities: A guide to community needs assessment*. Bedford Park, South Australia: Southern Community Health Research Unit.

Stalker, K. (1993). The best laid plans . . . gang aft agley? Assessing population needs in Scotland. *Health and Social Care, 2*, 1–9.

Stanhope, M. & Knollmueller, R. (2000). *Handbook of community based and home health nursing process* (3rd ed.). St. Louis, MO: Mosby.

Stevens, P. E. (1996). Focus groups: Collecting aggregate-level data to understand community health phenomena. *Public Health Nursing, 13*(3), 170–176.

Twelvetrees, A. (1987). *Community work*. London: Macmillan.

U.S. Department of Health and Human Services. (1991). *Healthy people 2000: National health promotion and disease prevention objectives*. Washington, DC: Author.

Van de Ven, A. H., & Delbecq. A. L. (1972). The nominal group process as a research instrument for exploratory health studies. *American Journal of Public Health, 62*, 337–342.

Wass, A. (1994). *Promoting health: The primary health care approach*. Sydney: Harcourt Brace and Company.

World Health Organization. (1978). The Declaration of Alma-Ata. Re-produced in *World Health*. 1988. August/September, pp. 16–17.

World Health Organization, Health and Welfare Canada, Canadian Public Health Association. (1986). *Ottawa Charter for Health Promotion*. Copenhagen, Denmark: FADL Publishers.

CHAPTER 16: PROGRAM PLANNING, IMPLEMENTATION, AND EVALUATION

Armstrong, P., Armstrong, H., Bourgeault, I., Choiniere, J. Mykhalovskiy, E., & White, J. (2000). *Heal thyself: Managing health care reform*. Aurora, Ontario, Canada: Garamond.

Attridge, C., Budgen, C., Hilton, A., McDavid, J. Molzahn, A., & Purkis, M. E. (1997). The Comox Valley nursing centre demonstration project: How did it work? *Canadian Nurse, 93*(2), 34–38.

Bassett-Smith, J. (2001). *Women with breast cancer and their living in and through discourses: A feminist post modern study*. Unpublished doctoral dissertation, University of Victoria, B. C., Canada.

Bateson, M. C. (1990). *Composing a life*. New York: Penguin Books.

Baum, F., & Saunders, D. (1995). Can health promotion & primary health care achieve Health for All without a return to their more radical agenda? *Health Promotion International, 10*(2), 149–160.

Bent, K. (1993). Perspectives on critical and feminist theory in developing nursing praxis. *Journal of Professional Nursing, 9*(5), 296–303.

Borich, G. D., & Jemelka, R. P. (1982). *Programs and systems: An evaluation perspective*. New York: Academic Press.

Bracht, N. (Ed.). (1990). *Health promotion at the community level*. Newbury Park, CA: Sage.

Bracht, N., & Kingsbury, L. (1990) Community organization principles in health promotion: A five stage model. In N. Bracht (Ed.), *Health promotion at the community level* (pp. 66–89). Newbury Park, CA: Sage.

British Columbia Ministry of Health. (1989). *Healthy communities: The process*. Victoria, B.C.: Author.

Budgen, C. M. (1987). Modeling: A method for program development. *Journal of Nursing Administration, 17*(12), 19–25.

Budgen, C., & Bates, M. (1996). *Campus Health Services project evaluation report*. Kelowna, B.C. Canada: Okanagan University College, Department of Nursing.

Buresh, B., & Gordon, S. (2000). *From silence to voice*. Ottawa, Ontario: Canadian Nurses Association.

Butler, M., & Marquis, S. (1998). *Pregnancy outreach programs qualitative evaluation: A pilot project*. Ottawa, Canada: Health Canada.

Butterfield, P. G. (1990). Thinking upstream: Nurturing a conceptual understanding of the societal context of health behavior. *Advances in Nursing Science, 12*(2), 1–8.

Canadian Nurses Association. (1997). *Code of ethics*. Ottawa, Canada: Author.

Canadian Public Health Association. (2000). *An ounce of prevention: Strengthening the balance in health care reform*. Ottawa, Canada: Author.

Chalmers, K., & Bramadat, I. (1996). Community development: Theoretical and practical issues for community health nursing in Canada. *Journal of Advanced Nursing, 24*, 719–726.

Chinn, P. (2001), *Peace and power: Building communities for the future* (5th ed.). New York: National League for Nursing.

Clarke, H., & Mass, H. (1998). Comox Valley Nursing Centre: From collaboration to empowerment. *Public Health Nursing, 15*(3), 216–224.

Covey, S., Merrill, A., & Merrill, R. (1997). *First things first every day: Because where you're headed is more important than how fast you're going*. New York: Simon & Schuster.

Delbecq, A. (1983). The nominal group technique for understanding the qualitative dimensions of client needs. In R. Bell (Ed.), *Assessing health and human service needs* (pp. 191–209). New York: Human Sciences.

Dignan, M. B., & Carr, P. A. (1992). *Program planning for health education and promotion* (2nd ed.). Philadelphia: Lea & Febiger.

Donabedian, A. (1996). The quality of care: How can it be assessed? In J. Schmele (Ed.), *Quality management in nursing and health care*. Clifton Park, NY: Delmar Learning.

Drevdahl, D. (1995). Coming to voice: The power of emancipatory community interventions. *Advances in Nursing Science, 18*(2), 13–24.

Eisler, R. (2000). *Tomorrow's children: A blueprint for partnership education in the 21st century*. Boulder, CO: Westview.

Eng, E., Salmon, M. E., & Mullan, F. (1992). Community empowerment: The critical base for primary health care. *Family Community Health, 15*(1), 1–12.

English, J. (2000). Community development. In M. Stewart (Ed.), *Community nursing: Promoting Canadians' health* (2nd ed., pp. 403–419). Toronto, Canada: W. B. Saunders.

Evans, R., Barer, M., & Marmor, T. (Eds.). (1994). *Why are some people healthy and others not? The determinants of the health of populations*. New York: Aldine de Gruyter.

Federal, Provincial and Territorial Advisory Committee on Population Health. (1999). *Toward a healthy future: Second report on the health of Canadians*. Ottawa: Health Canada.

Fletcher, M. (2001). The Manitoba pediatric cardiac surgery inquest report. *Canadian Nurse, 97*(2), 14–16.

Frank, J. W. (1995). Why "population health"? *Canadian Journal of Public Health, 86*(3), 162–164.

Freire, P. (1970/1993). *Pedagogy of the oppressed* (20th ed.). New York: Continuum.

Frohlich, K., & Potvin, L. (1999). Collective lifestyles as a target for health promotion. *Canadian Journal of Public Health. 90*(Suppl. 1), S11–13.

Fuller, C. (1998). *Caring for profit: How corporations are taking over Canada's health care system*. Vancouver, Canada: New Star.

Gadow, S. (1996) Ethical narratives in practice. *Nursing Science Quarterly, 9*(1), 8–9.

Green, L., & Kreuter, M. (1993). Are community organization and health promotion one process or two? Commentary. *American Journal of Health Promotion, 7*(3), 221.

Green, L., & Kreuter, M. (1999). *Health promotion planning: An educational and ecological approach*. Mountain View, CA: Mayfield.

Green, L., Richard, L., & Potvin, L. (1996). Ecological foundations of health promotion. *American Journal of Health Promotion, 10*(4), 270–281.

Hamilton, N., & Bhatti, T. (1996). *Population health promotion: An integrated model of population health and health promotion*. Ottawa, Canada: Health Promotion Development Division.

Hancock, T. (1993). Health, human development & the community ecosystem: Three ecological models. *Health Promotion International, 8*(1), 41–47.

Hancock, T. (1999). Future directions in population health. *Canadian Journal of Public Health, 90*(Suppl. 1), S68–70.

Hancock, T., Labonte, R., & Edwards, R. (1999). Indicators that count! Measuring population health at the community level. *Canadian Journal of Public Health, 90*(Suppl. 1), S22–26.

Hartrick, G. (2000). Developing health promoting practice with families: One pedagogical experience. *Journal of Advanced Nursing, 17*(3), 27–34.

Hartrick, G. (2001). Beyond interpersonal interactions: The significance of relationship in health promoting practice. In L. Young & V. Hayes (Eds.), *Transforming health promotion practice: Concepts, issues and applications*. Philadelphia: F. A. Davis.

Hilton, A., Budgen, C., Molzahn, A., & Attridge, C. (2001). Developing and testing instruments to measure client outcomes at the Comox Valley Nursing Centre. *Journal of Public Health Nursing*.

Hutchison, R. R., & Quartaro, E. G. (1995). High-risk vulnerable population and volunteers: A model of education and service collaboration. *Journal of Community Health Nursing, 12*(2), 111–119.

Johns, C. (1999). Reflection as empowerment. *Nursing Inquiry, 6*, 241–249.

Kaluzney, A., & Veney, J. (1999). Evaluating health care programs and services. In S. Williams & P. Torrens (Eds.), *Introduction to health services*. New York: Wiley.

Keating, D., & Hertzman, C. (1999). *Developmental health and the wealth of nations*. New York: Guilford.

Kendall, J. (1992). Fighting back: Promoting emancipatory nursing actions. *Advances in Nursing Science, 15*(2), 1–15.

Labonte, R. (1993). Health promotion & empowerment frameworks: Practice frameworks. *Issues in Health Promotion, Series 3*. Toronto, Canada: University of Toronto.

Labonte, R. (1998). Healthy public policy and the World Trade Organization: A proposal for an international health presence in future world trade/investment talks. *Health Promotion International, 13*(3), 245–256.

Labonte, R. (1999). Health promotion in the near future: Remembrances of activism past. *Health Education Journal, 58*, 365–367.

Labonte, R., Feather, J., & Hills, M. (1999). Story/dialogue method for health promotion. *Health Education Research, 14*(1), 39–50.

Leonard, V. W. (1991). A Heideggerian phenomenologic perspective on the concept of the person. *Advances in Nursing Science, 11*(4), 40–55.

Lindsey, E., Sheilds, L., & Stajduhar, K. (1999). Creating effective partnerships: Relating community development to participatory research.

Journal of Advanced Nursing, 29, 1238–1245.

Marlatt, G., & George, W. (1998). Relapse prevention and the maintenance of optimal health. In S. A. Shumaker, E. Schron, J. Ockene, & W. McBee (Eds.), *The handbook of health behavior change* (2nd ed., pp. 33–58). New York: Springer.

Marlatt, G., & George, W. (Eds.). (1985). *Relapse prevention.* New York: Guilford Press.

McKenzie, J. F., & Smeltzer, J. (2001). *Planning, implementing, and evaluating health promotion programs: A primer* (3rd ed.). Boston: Allyn & Bacon.

McKnight, J. (2001). *Community capacity: People, place, technology.* Workshop on community development at Vernon, B.C., Canada: Vernon School District.

McKnight, J., & Kretzmann, J. (1992). Mapping community capacity. *New Designs, Winter,* 9–15.

McMurray, A. (1999). *Community health and wellness: A socioecological approach.* New York: Mosby.

Minkler, M. (1990). Improving health through community organization. In K. Glanz, F. M. Lewis, & B. K. Rimer (Eds.), *Health behavior and health education* (pp. 257–285). San Francisco, CA: Jossey Bass.

Minkler, M. (1999). Personal responsibility for health? A review of the arguments at the century's end. *Health Education & Behavior, 26*(1), 121–140.

Mullet, J. (1995). *Program performance evaluation framework for Regional Health Boards and Community Health Councils.* Unpublished paper, Ministry of Health, Victoria, B. C.

Munroe, V. (2000). Immunization blitz reaches Canada's poorest neighbourhood. *Canadian Nurse, 96*(1), 16.

Nicoll, L. (2001). *Nurses' guide to the Internet* (3rd ed.). Philadelphia: J. B. Lippincott.

Perlmutter, F., & Cnaan, R. (1999). Community development as a public sector agenda. *Journal of Community Practice, 6*(4), 57–77.

Pirie, P. (1990). Evaluating health promotion programs: Basic questions and approaches. In N. Bracht (Ed.), *Health promotion at the community level* (pp. 201–208). Newbury Park, CA: Sage.

Pratt, L. (1997). RN with a cause. *Chatelaine, September,* 76–81. Toronto, Canada: Maclean-Hunter.

Prochaska, J., Johnson, S., & Lee, P. (1998). The transtheoretical model of behavior change. In S. A. Shumaker, E. Schron, J. Ockene, & W. McBee (Eds.), *The handbook of health behavior change* (2nd ed., pp. 59–84). New York: Springer.

Prochaska, J., Norcross, J., & Diclemente, C. (1994). *Changing for good.* New York: Avon.

Provincial Health Officer. (2000). *A report on the health of British Columbians: Annual report 1999.* Victoria, BC, Canada: Ministry of Health.

Rissel, C. (1994). Empowerment: The holy grail of health promotion? *Health Promotion International, 9*(1), 39–47.

Ritchie, J. (1997). Happenings: The national forum on health. *Canadian Journal of Nursing Research, 29*(2), 119–128.

Roberts, S. J. (1983). Oppressed group behavior: Implications for nursing. *Advances in Nursing Science, 5*(4), 21–30.

Rogers, E. (1998). *Diffusion of innovations* (4th ed.). New York: Free Press.

Rossi, P., & Freeman, H. (1999). *Evaluation: A systematic approach.* Beverly Hills, CA: Sage.

Schroeder, C., & Gadow, S. (2000). An advocacy approach to ethics and community health. In E. Anderson & J. McFarlane (Eds.), *Community as partner* (3rd ed., pp. 78–91). Philadelphia: J. B. Lippincott.

Shediac-Rizkallah, M., & Bone, L. (1998). Planning for the sustainability of community-based health programs: Conceptual frameworks and future directions for research, practice and policy. *Health Education Research, 13*(1), 87–108.

Sheilds, L., & Lindsey, E. (1998). Community health promotion nursing practice. *Advances in Nursing Science, 20*(4), 23–36.

Skelton, R. (1994). Nursing and empowerment: Concepts and strategies. *Journal of Advanced Nursing, 19,* 415–423.

Smith, G. (1997). *Shaping the future health system through community based approaches.* Keynote presentation at the 21st Quadrennial International Congress of Nurses, Vancouver, BC, Canada.

Smith, M. (1998) Empowerment evaluation: Theoretical and methodological considerations. *Evaluation and Program Planning, 21,* 255–261.

Steckler, A., Orville, K., Eng, E., & Dawson, L. (1992). Summary of a formative evaluation of PATCH. *Journal of Health Education, 23*(3), 174–178.

Steingraber, S. (1997). *Living downstream: An ecologist's look at cancer & the environment.* Menlo Park, CA: Addison-Wesley.

Steuart, G. W. (1959/1993). The importance of programme planning. *Health Education Quarterly* (Suppl.), S21–27.

Stevens, P. (1989). A critical reconceptualization of the environment in nursing. *Advances in Nursing Science, 11*(4), 56–68.

Stewart, M. J. (Ed.). (2000). *Community nursing: Promoting Canadian's health* (2nd ed.), Toronto, Canada: W. B. Saunders.

Tang, S., & Anderson, J. (1999). Human agency and the process of healing: Lessons learned from women living with a chronic illness—'re-writing the expert'. *Nursing Inquiry, 6,* 83–93.

U.S. Department of Health and Human Services. (2000). *Healthy People 2010: Understanding and improving health.* Washington, DC: U.S. Government Printing Office.

United Way. (1996). *Measuring program outcomes: A practical approach.* Item #0989. Alexandria, VA: Author.

Van Norstrand, C. H. (1993). *Gender responsible leadership: Detecting bias implementing interventions.* Newbury Park, CA: Sage.

Wallerstein, N. (1992). Powerlessness, empowerment, and health: Implications for health promotion. *Journal of Health Promotion, 6*(3), 197–205.

Wallerstein, N., & Bernstein, E. (1988). Empowerment education: Freire's ideas adapted to health education. *Health Education Quarterly, 15*(4), 379–394.

Wolton, K., Amit, H., Kalma, S., Hillman, L., Hillman, D., & Cosway, N. (1995, January). *Basic concepts of international health.* Module. Ottawa, Canada: Canadian University Consortium for Health in Development.

Wong-Rieger, D., & David, L. (1995). Using program logic models to plan and evaluate education and prevention programs. In A. Love (Ed.), *Evaluation methods sourcebook II* (pp. 120–135). Ottawa, Canada: Canadian Evaluation Society.

World Health Organization. (1978). *Alma-Alta 1978. Report of the international* conference on primary health care. Geneva, Switzerland: Author.

World Health Organization. (1986). *Ottawa Charter for Health Promotion.* Ottawa, Canada: Canadian Public Health Association.

World Health Organization. (1997). *The Jakarta Declaration on Health Promotion into the 21st Century.* Geneva: Author.

World Health Organization. (1998). *Population health-putting concepts into action: A final report.* Geneva, Switzerland: Author.

World Health Organization European Working Group. (1998). Health promotion evaluation: Recommendations to policymakers. *Health Promotion, 34*(4), III–VIII.

Zerwekh, J. (1992). The practice of empowerment and coercion by expert public health nurses. *Image, 24*(2), 101–105.

CHAPTER 17: QUALITY MANAGEMENT

American Nurses Association (1982). *A conceptual model of community health nursing.* Kansas City, MO: Author.

American Public Health Association (1996). *The definition and role of public health nursing in the delivery of health care: A statement of the Public Health Nursing Section.* Washington, DC: Author.

Association of Community Health Nursing Educators. (1991a). *Essential components of masters level practice in community health nursing.* Lexington, KY: Author.

Association of Community Health Nursing Educators. (1991b). *Essentials of baccalaureate education.* Louisville, KY: Author.

Association of Community Health Nursing Educators. (1993). *Perspectives on doctoral education in community health nursing.* Lexington, KY: Author.

Berwick, D.M. (1989). Continuous improvement as an ideal in health care. *New England Journal of Medicine,* 320, 53.

Crosby, P. B (1979). *Quality is free.* New York: New American Library.

Davis, E. R. (1994). Total quality management for home care. Gaithersburg, MD: Aspen.

Deming, W. E. (1986). *Out of the crisis.* Cambridge, MA: Massachusetts Institute of Technology, Center for Advanced Engineering Study.

Dingman, S. K., Williams, M., Fosbinder, D., & Warnick, M. (1999). Implementing a caring model to improve patient satisfaction. *The Journal of Nursing Administration,* 29 (12), 30–37.

Donabedian, A. (1981). *Explorations in quality assessment and monitoring* (Vol. 2). Ann Arbor, MI: Health Administration Press.

Donabedian, A. (1985). *Explorations in quality assessment and monitoring* (Vol. 3). Ann Arbor, MI: Health Administration Press.

Donabedian, A. (1990). The seven pillars of quality. *Archives of Pathological Laboratory Medicine, 114,* 1115.

Durch, J., Bailey, L. A., & Stotto, M. A. (Eds.). (1997). *Improving health in the community: A role for performance monitoring.* Washington, DC: National Academy Press.

European Society for Quality in Health Care. (2001). *ESQH Constitution.* [On-line]. Available: www.esgh.net/constitution.htm.

Green, E. (1997). In J. M. Katz & E. Green. *Managing quality: A system-wide performance management in health care.* (pp. 257). St. Louis, MO: Mosby.

International Society for Quality in Health Care (2001). *About ISQua.* [On-line]. Available: www.isqua.org.au.

JCAHO (1994). *Lexicon dictionary of health care terms, organizations, and acronyms for the era of reform.* Chicago, IL: Author.

Juran, J. M. (1988). *Juran's quality control handbook* (4th ed.). New York: McGraw-Hill.

Katz, J. M., & Green, E. (1997). *Managing quality: A guide to system wide performance management in health care* (2nd ed.). St. Louis, MO: Mosby.

Lalonde, B. (1988). Assuring the quality home care via the assessment of client outcomes. *Caring, 7*(1), 20.

Lohr, K. N. (Ed.). (1990). *Medicare: A strategy for quality assurance* (Vol. 1). Washington, DC: National Academy Press.

Lynn, M. R., & McMillan, B. J. (1999). Do nurses know what patients think is important in nursing care? *Journal of Nursing Care Quality, 13*(5), 65–74.

Maloney, K., & Chaiken, B. P. (1999). An overview of outcomes research and measurement. *Journal of Health Care Quality,* 1–12. [On-line]. Available: www.allenpress.com/ihq/084.

McLaughlin, C. P., & Kaluzny, A. D. (1994). Defining total quality management/continuous quality improvement. In C. P. McLaughlin & A. D. Kaluzny (Eds.), *Continuous quality improvement in health care: Theory implementation and applications.* Gaithersburg, MD: Aspen.

National Association for Healthcare Quality. (2001). *About NAHQ.* [Online]. Available: www.nahq.orq.

Oermann, M. H., & Templin, T. (2000). Important attributes of quality health care: Consumer perspectives. *Journal of Nursing Scholarship, 32*(2), 167–172.

Oermann, M. H., Weglarz, C., & Templin, T. (1999). Veterans' views of quality nursing care. *Veterans' Health System Journal, 4*(12), 33–36.

Walton, M. (1986). *The Deming management method.* New York: Putnam.

Wold, J. L. (2000). Quality management. In M. Stanhope & J. Lancaster (Eds.), *Community and public health nursing* (5th ed.). St. Louis, MO: Mosby.

Young, G. (1998). The privatization of quality assurance in health care. In P. K. Halverson, A. D. Kaluzny & C. P. McLaughlin. *Managed care and public health.* Gaithersberg, MD: Aspen.

CHAPTER 18: POWER, POLITICS, AND PUBLIC POLICY

Ackoff, R. L. (1974). *Redesigning the future: A systems approach to societal problems.* New York: Wiley.

American Association of Colleges of Nursing. (1998). *Essentials of baccalaureate nursing education for professional nursing practice.* Washington, DC: Author.

American Nurses Association. (1980). *Social policy statement.* Kansas City, MO: Author.

American Nurses Association. (1991). *Nursing's agenda for health care reform.* Kansas City, MO: Author.

American Nurses Association. (1995). *Social policy statement.* Washington, DC: Author.

American Nurses Association. (1996). *Successes and challenges in the federal legislative arena.* ANA Policy Series. Washington, DC: Author.

American Nurses Association. (1999). *Scope and standards of public health nursing practice.* Washington, DC: Author.

Association of Community Health Nurse Educators. (2000). *Essentials of baccalaureate nursing education for entry level community health nursing practice*. Louisville, KY: Author.

Backer, B. A. (1993). Lillian Wald: Connecting caring with activism. *Nursing and Health Care, 14*(3), 128.

Bavier, A. (1995). Where research and practice meet—Opportunities at the Agency for Health Care Policy and Research. *Nursing Policy Forum, 1*(4), 21.

Blyth, M., & Evans, N. (2000). Fighting for the family. *Ladies Home Journal. 117*(11), 130–138.

Brown, S. (1996). Incorporating political socialization theory into baccalaureate nursing education. *Nursing Outlook, 44*(3), 3.

Caterinicchio, M. J. (1995). AACN Perspective, Redefining nursing in the midst of health care reform. *Nursing Policy Forum, 1*(1), 9.

Centers for Disease Control and Prevention, Division on Tuberculosis Elimination, National Center for HIV, STD, and TB Prevention. (2000). *Tuberculosis in the United States National Surveillance System: Highlights from 1999*. Atlanta, GA: Author.

Chaffee, M. (1996). The nurse in Washington internship (NIWI). *Nursing Policy Forum, 2*(1), 24.

Cohen, S. S., Mason, D. J., Korner, C., Leavitt, J. K., Pulcini, J., & Sochalski. J. (1996). Stages of nursing's political development: Where we've been and where we ought to go, *Nursing Outlook, 44*(6), 259–266.

Conger, C. O., & Johnson, P. J. (2000). Politics and nursing: Integrating political involvement and nursing education. *Nurse Educator, 25*(2), 99–103.

Constantino, J. N. (2000). Breaking the cycle of violence. *Healthline, 19*(1), 10–11.

Deans, B. (2001, April 23). Summit ends with free trade agreement. *Austin American Statesman,* p. A1.

Dunn, W. N. (1994). *Public policy analysis: An introduction* (2nd ed.). Englewood Cliffs, NJ: Prentice-Hall.

Fielding, J., & Ulene, V. (2000, March 27). Our health. TB remains persistent problem in the U.S. *Los Angeles Times* (Health), p. S3.

Freed, L. (1996). *Political action handbook for nurses*. Santa Rosa, CA: Professor Publishing.

Hall-Long, B. A. (1995). Nursing's past, present, and future political experiences. *Nursing and Health Care: Perspectives on Community, 16*(1), 27.

Hopkins, G. (2000). School violence: Have we learned our lesson? *Vibrant Life, 16*(5), 34–37.

Jennings, C. (1995). The time is now. *Nursing Policy Forum, 1*(1), 5.

Keane, C. R., Lave, J. R., Ricci, E. M., & LaVallee, C. P. (1999). The impact of a children's health insurance program by age. *Pediatrics, 104*(5), 1051–1058.

Kelly, T. (2000, November 27). In the fight against TB, hope for an invisible weapon. *New York Times* (Metropolitan Desk), Section B3, p3.

Lescavage N. (1995). Nurses make your presence felt: Taking off the rose colored glasses. *Nursing Policy Forum, 1*(1), 18–21.

Livsey, K. (1995). AAOHN Perspective—Leaders in workplace health and safety. *Nursing Policy Forum, 1*(1), 14.

Loquist, R. S. (1999). Regulation: Parallel and powerful. In J. A. Milstead (Ed.), *Health policy and politics. A nurses guide* (pp. 105–146). Gaithersberg, MD: Aspen.

MacPherson, K. I. (1987). Health care policy, values, and nursing. *Advances in Nursing Science, 9*(3), 1–11.

Mason, D. J., Talbott, S. W., and Leavitt, J. K., (Eds.). (1993). *Policy and politics for nurses: Action and change in the workplace, government organization and community* (2nd ed.). Philadelphia: W. B. Saunders.

Mason, D. J., Talbott, S. W., & Leavitt, J. K. (Eds.). (1998). *Policy and politics for nurses: Action and change in the workplace, government, organization, and community* (3rd ed.). Philadelphia: W. B. Saunders.

Milio, N. (1981). *Promoting health through public policy*. Philadelphia: F. A. Davis.

Milstead, J. A. (1999). *Health policy and politics: A nurses guide*. Gaithersburg, MD: Aspen.

Olds, D. L., Eckenrode, J., Henderson, C., Kitzman, H., Powers, J., Cole, R., Sidora, K., Morris, P., Pettit, L., & Luckey, D. (1997). Long-term effects of home visitation on maternal life course and child abuse and neglect: Fifteen-year follow-up of a randomized trial. *Journal of the American Medical Association, 278,* 637–643.

Porter-O'Grady, T. (1994). Building partnerships in health care: Creating whole systems change. *Nursing and Health Care, 15*(1), 38.

Roberts, L. (2000). The comeback plague: Once nearly conquered, TB is rebounding in menacing new strains. *U.S. News and World Report, 128*(12), 50–51.

Ruben, D. (2000). The presidential election: Who will you vote for? *Parenting, 14*(8), 144–146.

Simon, R. (2000, September 4). Rollin' on the river Gore's making waves, but who are these "working families"? *U.S. News and World Report,* pp. 12–14.

Stanhope, M., & Lancaster, J. (1996). *Community health nursing: Promoting health of aggregates, families and individuals* (4th ed.). St. Louis, MO: Mosby.

Swan, S. (1995). AONE Perspective-meeting the needs of the future. *Nursing Policy Forum, 1*(1), 11.

Towers, J. (1995). AANP Perspectives—Nurse practitioners and health policy. *Nursing Policy Forum, 1*(1), 13.

Tri-Council for Nursing. (1991). *Nursing's agenda for health care reform*. Washington, DC: American Nurses Association.

U.S. Department of Health and Human Services. (1995). *Healthy people 2000: Midcourse review and 1995 revision*. Sudbury, MA: Jones & Barlett.

U.S. Department of Health and Human Services. (2000). *Healthy People 2010, Understanding and improving health*. Washington, DC: U.S. Government Printing Office.

U.S. Department of Health and Human Services, Office of Disease Prevention and Health Promotion, Office of Public Health and Science (2001). *Healthy people in healthy communities: A community planning guide using Healthy People 2010*. [Online]. Available: www.health.gov/healthypeople/Publications/HealthyCommunities2001.

Weis, D. (1995). Challenging our values—Directing health care reform. *Nursing Policy Forum, 1*(1), 26.

Williams, A. (1993). Community health learning experiences and political activism: A model for baccalaureate curriculum revolution content. *Journal of Nursing Education, 32*(8), 353.

CHAPTER 19: VARIED ROLES OF COMMUNITY HEALTH NURSING

American Hospital Association (AHA). (2000). *Consumers rights,* p4.

American Nurses Association. (1987). *Standards and scope of hospice nursing practice*. Kansas City, MO: Author.

Association of State and Territorial Directors of Nursing. (2000). Public health nursing: A partner for healthy populations. Washington, DC, American Nurses Publishing.

Beecroft, P. (1997). CNS' role in health care. *Clinical nurse specialist.* Philadelphia: Williams & Wilkins.

Burns, N., Garret, J., & Grove, S. (2000). *The practice of nursing research.* St. Louis, MO: Mosby.

Case Management Society of America. (1994). Cited in Bechtel, et al. Case managing from other cultures. The *Journal of Care Management,* 4, October 1998. p 88.

Chen, F., Leahy, M., McMahon, B., Mirch, M., & Devinney, D. (1999). Foundational knowledge and major practice domains of case management. *Journal of Case Management,* 5(1), 10–15.

Clark, M. J. (1999). *Nursing in the community* (3rd ed.). Stamford, CT: Appleton & Lange.

Cohen, E., & Cesta, T. (1997). *Nursing case management: From concept to evaluation* (2nd ed.). St. Louis, MO: Mosby.

Flarey, D. L. (1995). *Redesigning nursing care delivery: Transforming our future.* Philadelphia: J. B. Lippincott.

Gray, M. (2001). Advanced practice roles in nursing. In N. Task (Ed.), *The nursing profession tomorrow and beyond.* Thousand Oaks, CA: Sage Publications.

Heider, J. (1985). The ripple effect. In J. Heider (Ed.), *The tao of leadership* (p. 107). Atlanta, GA: Humanics New Age.

Kane, R. A. (1990). What is case management anyway? In R. A. Kane, K. Urv-Wong, & C. King (Eds.), *Case management: What is it anyway?* (pp. 1–17). Minneapolis, MN: University of Minnesota Long-Term Care DECISIONS Resource Center.

Klainberg, M., Holzemer, S., Leonard, M., & Arnold, J. (1998). *Community health nursing: An alliance for health.* New York: McGraw-Hill.

Koniak-Griffin, D., Anderson, N., Verzemnieks, I., & Brecht, M. (2000). A public health early intervention program for adolescent mothers: Outcomes from pregnancy through 6 weeks postpartum. *Nursing Research,* 49, 130–132.

Kosik, S. H. (1972). Patient advocacy or fighting the system? *American Journal of Nursing,* 72, 695–698.

Kuehnert, P. L. (1991). The public health policy advocate: Fostering the health

of communities. *Clinical Nurse Specialist,* 5, 5–10.

Leddy, S., & Pepper, J. M. (1998). Conceptual basis of professional nursing (4th ed.). Philadelphia: J. B. Lippincott.

LoBiondo-Wood, G., & Haber, J. (1994). *Nursing research: Methods, critical appraisal, and utilization.* St. Louis, MO: Mosby.

Mayeroff, M. (1971). *On caring.* New York: Harper & Row.

Mullahy, C. (1999). Case manager: An ethnically responsible solution. *Journal of Case Management,* 10(5), 59–62.

Powell, S. K. (1996). *Nursing case management: A practical guide to success in managed care.* Philadelphia: Lippincott-Raven.

Rankin, S. H., & Stallings, K. D. (1996). *Patient education: Issues, principles, practices* (3rd ed.). Philadelphia: J. B. Lippincott.

Redford, L. (2001). Case management: The wave of the future. *Journal of Case Management,* 1, 5–8.

Redman, B. (2001). *The practice of patient education* (9th ed.). St. Louis, MO: Mosby.

Shi, L., & Singh, D. (1998). *Delivering health care in America: A systems approach.* Gaithersberg, MD: Aspen.

Shelov, S. P. (1994). Editorial: The children's agenda for the 1990s and beyond. *American Journal of Public Health,* 84, 1066–1067.

Spearman, L., Daugherty, J., & Reign, B. (2000). Patient teaching to promote behavioral change. *Nursing Outlook,* 48, 281–287.

U.S. Department of Health and Human Services. (2000). *Healthy people 2010.* Washington, DC: Author.

Wolfe, G. (1998). Cost savings and case management. *Journal of Case Management,* 4(4), 87–91.

Spradley, B. W., & Allender, J. A. (1996). *Community health nursing: Concepts and practice* (4th ed.). Philadelphia: J. B. Lippincott.

CHAPTER 20: PRACTICE SPECIALTIES FOR COMMUITY HEALTH NURSING

American Nurses Association. (1994). *Fact sheet: Violence and mental illness.* Washington, DC: American Psychiatric Association.

American Nurses Association. (1995). *Scope and standards of practice in correctional facilities.* Washington, DC: American Nurses Publishing.

American Nurses Association. (1998). *Position statements: Nurses' participation in capital punishment.* Washington, DC: American Nurses Publishing.

American Nurses Association. (1999). *Scope and standards of public health nursing practice.* Washington, DC: American Nurses Publishing.

American Association of Occupational Health Nurses. (1999). *Competencies and performance criteria in occupational and environmental health.* Atlanta, GA: American Association of Occupational Health Nurses, Inc.

American Association of Occupational Health Nurses. (2001). *AAOHN position statement.* Jan. Inc., 49(1).

Armer, F., Humbles, P. (1995, March/April). Parish nursing: Extending health care to African Americans. *Nursing and Health Care Perspectives on Community,* 16, 120–122.

Association of State and Territorial Directors of Nursing. (2000). *Public health nursing: A partner for healthy population.* Washington, DC: American Nurses Publishing.

Ayer, T. (2000, February). Redesigning for success: Managing the prospective payment system. *Home Care Provider,* 5.

Beecroft, P. (1997). Clinical nurse specialists future role in health care. *Clinical Nurse Specialist.*

Burns, N., & Grove, S. (2000). *The practice of nursing research* (4th ed.). Philadelphia: W. B. Saunders.

California Association of Home Health Agencies (2000, February). *Home care facts and statistics.* Sacramento, CA: Author.

Clark, M. J. (1998). Nursing in the community (3rd. ed.). Stamford, CT: Appleton-Lange.

Health Ministries Association. (1998). *Scope and standards of parish nursing practice.* Washington, DC: American Nurses Publishing.

Home health nursing standards of care. (1999). Washington, DC: American Nurses Publishing.

Hospice and Palliative Nurses Association. (2000). *Scope and standards of parish nursing practice.* Dubuque, IA: Kendall/Hunt Publishing.

International Association of Forensic Nurses. (1997). *Scope and standards of forensic nursing practice.* Washington, DC: American Nurses Publishing.

Jamieson, M. K. (1990). Block nursing: Practicing autonomous nursing in the community. *Nurse Health Care,* 11(5), 250.

Josten, L., Clarke, P., Oswold, S. S., Stoskopf, S., & Morrow, S. (1995). Healthy America: Practitioners for 2005. *Family and Community Health, 18*(1), 36–48.

Kelly, R. (2001, June). Benefits improvement and protection act should help home care. *Home Health Provider, 18,* 97.

Konik-Griffin, D., Anderson, N., Vezzemnicks, I., & Brecht, M. L. (2000, May/June). A public health nursing early intervention program for adolescent mothers. Outcomes from pregnancy through 6 weeks postpartum. *Nursing Research 49*(30), 130–138.

Leddy, S., & Pepper, J. M. (1998). *Conceptual basis of professional nursing* (4th ed.). Philadelphia: J. B. Lippincott.

Lowry, R., Cohen, H., Modzelesdki, K., Kann, L., Collins, J., & Kolbe, H. (1999, November). Issues in school health. *Journal of School Health, 69*(7), 347–354.

Lynch, V. (1999, March). The new detectives: Forensic nurses advance health and justice. *Nurseweek, 17*(4).

Marks, R. (2001, June). Home health care, ethics, and the family. *Home Health Provider, 76,* 77.

Mendietta, C. (1999). *The health of the community; NEST; A working model of community-based long term care for elders. Neighborhood elder support team.* U.S. Agency on Aging Award #90.

National Mental Health Association. (1995). *National mental health association position statement: Violence in America.* [On-line]. Available: http://www.mhsource.com/hy/vvmi.html.

National Association of School Nurses. (1998) *Standards of professional school nursing practice.* Scarbnough, ME: Author.

Nativid, D. (2000, July/August). Robots and nurses. *Nursing Outlook, 48*(4), 149.

Nurses's handbook of alternative and complementary therapies. (1998). Springhouse, PA: Springhouse Publishers.

Peternely-Taylor, C. A., & Huff, A. G. (1997). Forensic psychiatric nursing. In B. S. Johnson (Ed.), *Adaptation and growth: Psychiatric nursing* (4th ed.). Philadelphia: Lippincott-Raven.

Quad Council of Public Health Nursing Organizations. (1999). *Scope and standards of public health nursing.* Washington, DC: American Nurses Publishing.

Reincow, K., & Allenworth, D. (1996). Conducting a comprehensive school health program. *School Health, 66,* 59.

Reinhard, S. C., et al. (1996). Promoting healthy communities through neighborhood nursing. *Nursing Outlook, 44*(5), 223.

Rich, A. (1999). *Midnight salvaged 1995–1998.* New York: W. W. Norton.

Schank, M., Weiss, S., & Matheus, R. (1996). Parish nursing: Ministry of healing. *Geriatric Nursing, 17,* 11–13.

State of California. (1997). *Healthy families: Conference report summary on AB1126 and SB903.* Sacramento, CA: State of California.

Tyrrell, A., & Eyles, P. (1999, October). Health promotion in elementary schools: A newsletter as one strategy. *Journal of School Health, 69*(8), 341–343.

Warhole, M. (1998). Health care technology issues in home care. *Home Care Provider, 5,* 3.

Wieck, L. (2000, January/February). A vision for nursing: The future revisited. *Nursing Outlook, 48*(1).

Williams, C. (2000). Forward. In M. Stanhope & J. Lancaster (Eds.), *Community and public health nursing.* St. Louis, MO: Mosby.

Wurzbad, S. (1999, March/April). Managed care: More conflict for primary health nursing. *Nursing Outlook, 47*(2).

CHAPTER 21: THE HOME VISIT

Byrd, M. E. (1995a). A concept analysis of home visiting. *Public Health Nursing, 12,* 83–89.

Byrd, M. E. (1995b). The home visiting process in the contexts of the voluntary vs. required visit: Examples from fieldwork. *Public Health Nursing, 12,* 196–202.

Byrd, M. E. (1998). Long-term maternal-child home visiting. *Public Health Nursing, 15,* 235–242.

Dansky, K. H., Bowles, K. H., & Palmer, L. (1999). How telehomecare affects patients. *Caring Magazine, 18*(8) 10–14.

D'Avanzo, C. E., Frye, B., & Froman, R. (1994). Stress in Cambodian refugee families. *Image: Journal of Nursing Scholarship, 26,* 100–105.

Davis, L. L. (1998). Telephone-based interventions with family caregivers: A feasibility study. *Journal of Family Nursing, 4,* 255–270.

Dimmick, S. L., Mustaleski, C., Burgiss, S. G., & Welsh, T. (2000). A case study of benefits & potential savings in rural home telemedicine. *Home Healthcare Nurse, 18,* 125–135.

Durkin, N., & Wilson, C. (1999). Simple steps to keep yourself safe. *Home Healthcare Nurse, 17,* 430–435.

Fazzone, P. A., Barloon, L. F., McConnell, S. J., & Chitty, J. A. (2000). Personal safety, violence, and home health. *Public Health Nursing, 17,* 43–52.

Hanks, C. A., & Smith, J. (1999). Implementing nurse home visitation programs. *Public Health Nursing, 16,* 235–245.

Hayes, R. P., Duffey, E. B., Dunbar, J., Wages, J. W., & Holbrook, S. E. (1998). Staff perceptions of emergency and home-care telemedicine. *Journal of Telemedicine and Telecare, 4,* 101–107. As cited in S. L. Dimmick, C. Mustaleski, S. B. Burgiss, & T. Welsh (2000). A case study of benefits and potential savings in rural home telemedicine. *Home Healthcare Nurse, 18,* 125–135.

Janosik, E. H. (1994). *Crisis counseling: A contemporary approach* (2nd ed.). Boston: Jones and Bartlett.

Kleinberg, K. (2001). Technologies to enable home care. *Caring, 20*(1), 36–37.

Kosier, B., Erb, G., Berman, A. J., & Burke, K. (2000). *Fundamentals of nursing: Concepts, process, and practice* (6th ed.). Upper Saddle River, NJ: Prentice-Hall.

Kristjanson, L. J., & Chalmers, K. I. (1999). Preventive work with families: Issues facing public health nurses. In G. D. Wegner & R. J. Alexander (Eds.), *Reading in family nursing* (2nd ed., pp. 361–372). Philadelphia: J. B. Lippincott.

Monks, K. M. (2000). *Pocket guide to home health care.* Philadelphia: W. B. Saunders.

Murray, R. B., & Zentner, J. P. (2001). *Health promotion strategies throughout the life span* (7th ed.). Upper Saddle River, NJ: Prentice-Hall.

National vital statistics system. (1998). [On-line]. Available: http://www.health.gov/healthypeople/document/html/objectives/15-27.htm.

Rice, R. (1995). *Manual of home health nursing procedures.* St. Louis, MO: Mosby Year-Book.

Rice, R. (1998). Home visit safety. *Home Healthcare Nurse, 16,* 241–242.

Rice, R. (2000). Handbook of home health nursing procedures (2nd ed.). St. Louis, MO: Mosby.

Riley, B. J. (2000). *Communications in nursing* (4th ed.). St. Louis, MO: Mosby.

Ruskin, J. (1865). Sesame and lilies, of kings treasures; of queen's gardens. Section 68. As quoted in J. Bartlett, *Bartlett's Familiar Quotations* (13th and centennial ed.). Boston: Little Brown & Co.

Shaul, M. P. (2000). What you should know before embarking on tele-home health: Lessons learned from a pilot study. *Home Healthcare Nurse, 18,* 470–475.

Sperling, R. L. (1998). What's this OASIS, anyway? *Home Healthcare Nurse, 16* 373–374.

Sperling, R. L. (1999). How OASIS relates to the Medicare 485. *Home Healthcare Nurse, 17,* 82–85.

Thomas, R. B., Barnard, K. E., & Sumners, G. A. (1993). Family nursing diagnosis as a framework for family assessment. In S. L. Feetham, S. B. Meister, J. M. Bell, & C. L. Gilliss (Eds.), *The nursing of families* (pp. 127–136). Newbury Park, CA: Sage.

Welsh, (2000). A case study of benefits and potential savings in rural home telemedicine. *Home Healthcare Nurse, 18,* 125–135.

Wright, L. M., & Leahey, M. W. (2000). *Nurses and families: A guide to family assessment and intervention* (3rd ed.). Philadelphia: F. A. Davis.

Zerwekh, J. P. (1992). Laying the groundwork for family self-help. Locating families, building trust, and building strength. *Public Health Nursing, 9*(1), 15–21.

Zerwekh, J. P. (1991). A family caregiving model for public health nursing. *Nursing Outlook, 39,* 213–217.

Zerwekh, J. V. (1997). Making the connection during home visits: Narratives of expert nurses. *International Journal for Human Caring, 1*(1), 25–29.

CHAPTER 22: CARE OF INFANTS, CHILDREN, AND ADOLESCENTS

American Academy of Pediatrics. (1998, November 2.). *Smaller than average infants at greater risk for chronic disease later in life.* Press release. [On-line]. Available: www.aap.org/advocacy/archives/novsml.htm.

American Academy of Pediatrics Committee on Adolescence. (2000, April). Suicide and suicide attempts in adolescents. *Pediatrics, 104*(4), 871–874.

American Academy of Pediatrics Committee on Injury and Poison Prevention. (2000, April). *Pediatrics. 105* (5), 888–895.

American Dental Association. (2001, July). *Frequently asked questions: gum disease (periodontal disease)* [On-line]. Available: http://www.ada.org/public/faq/gums.html.

American Psychiatric Association. (1994). *Diagnostic and statistical manual of mental disorders* (4th ed.). Washington, DC: Author.

American Psychiatric Association. (2000, January). Disease definition, epidemiology, and natural history." In *practice guideline for the treatment of patients with eating disorders* [On-line]. Available: http://www.psych.org/clin_res/guide.bk42301.cfm.

Anderson, R., Crespo, C., Bartlett, S., Cheskin, L, & Pratt, M. (1998, March). Relationship of physical activity and television with body weight and level of fatness among children. *Journal of the American Medical Association, 279*(12), 938–942.

Barber, B. (1994). Cultural, family, and personal contexts of parent-adolescent conflict. *Journal of Marriage and the Family, 56,* 375–386.

Beard, J. (2000). Iron requirements in adolescent females. *Journal of Nutrition, 130,* 440S–442S.

Behrman, R., & Kliegman, B. (1998). *Nelson essentials of pediatrics* (3rd ed.). Philadelphia: W. B. Saunders.

Berkey, C., Rockett, H., Field, A., Gillman, M., Frazier, A., Carmargo, C., & Colditz, G. (2000). Activity, dietary intake, and weight changes in a longitudinal study of preadolescent and adolescent boys and girls. *Pediatrics, 105*(4), 56.

Birch, L., & Fisher, J. (1998). Development of eating behaviors among children and adolescents. *Pediatrics, 101*(3), 539–549.

Bolger, & Scarr, S. (1995). Not so far from home: How family characteristics predict child care quality. *Early Development and Parenting, 4*(3), 103–112.

Borowsky, I. (2000). Attention deficit/hyperactivity disorder. In C. Berkowitz (Ed.), *Pediatrics: A primary care approach* (2nd ed., pp. 469–473). Philadelphia: W. B. Saunders.

Bronner, Y. L. (1996). Nutritional status outcomes for children: Ethnic, cultural and environmental contexts. *Journal of the American Dietetic Association, 96*(9) 891–903.

Brooks-Gunn, J., & Duncan, G. (1997, Summer/Fall). The effects of poverty on children. *The Future of Children: Children and Poverty, 7*(2), 55–71.

Centers for Disease Control and Prevention. (1994b). *Summary of 1991 report: Preventing lead poisoning in young children.* Washington, DC: Author.

Centers for Disease Control and Prevention. (1997). Update: Blood lead levels—United States, 1991–1994. *Morbidity and Mortality Weekly Report, 46,* 141–146. (Erratum, 1997, *MMWR, 46,* 607.)

Centers for Disease Control and Prevention. (2000a, June 9). *Youth risk behavior surveillance survey—U.S.—1999. Morbidity and Mortality Weekly Report, 49*(SS05), 1–96.

Centers for Disease Control and Prevention. (2000b, October 13). *Facts about: youth tobacco surveillance United States, 1998–1999.* Press release.

Centers for Disease Control and Prevention. (2000c). Recommendations for blood lead screening of young children enrolled in Medicaid: Targeting a group at high risk. *Morbidity and Mortality Weekly Report, 49,* RR-14.

Centers for Disease Control and Prevention. (2000d). *HIV/AIDS Surveillance Report U.S. HIV and AIDS cases reported through June 2000.* Vol. 12, No. 1.

Centers for Disease Control and Prevention. (2000e). *Male and female reported HIV in adolescents (13–19) and adults (20–24), reported by sex and age at diagnosis, reported in 1999.* [On-line]. Available: www.cdc.gov/hiv/graphics/images/1265/1265.pdf.

Centers for Disease Control and Prevention. (2001). Division of HIV/AIDS Prevention. *Basic statistics—international statistics.*

Children's Defense Fund. (2000a, Fall). *Comprehensive immigrant outreach through building community partnerships. Sign them up!* [On-line]. Available: www.childrensdefense.org.

Children's Defense Fund. (2000b). *Key facts: Children's health coverage in 1999.* [On-line]. Available: www.childrensdefense.org.

Clemen-Stone, S., Eigsti, D., & McGuire, S. (1998). *Comprehensive family and community health nursing* (5th ed.). St. Louis, MO: Mosby-Year Book.

Cole, T. J. (1991). Weight-stature indices to measure underweight, overweight, and obesity. In J. H. Himes (Ed.), *Anthropometric assessment of nutritional status* (pp. 83–111). New York: Wiley Liss.

Committee on Dietary Allowances, Food and Nutrition Board, National Research Council. (1989). *Recommended dietary allowances* (10th ed.). Washington, DC: National Academy Press.

Committee on Nutrition. (1999). Calcium requirements of infants, children, and adolescents. *American Academy of Pediatrics, 104*(5), 1152–1157.

Conrad, N. (1991). Where do they turn? Social support systems of suicidal high school adolescents. *Journal of Psychosocial Nursing, 29*(3), 14–20.

Danielson, R. (1998). Adolescent violence in America. *Clinician Reviews, 8*(5), 167–184.

Davis, J., & Sherer, K. (1994). Applied nutrition and diet therapy for nurses (2nd ed., pp. 520–539, 545–559). Philadelphia: W. B. Saunders.

Dietz, W. H. (1998). Health consequences of obesity in youth: Childhood predictors of adult disease. *Pediatrics 101*(3), 518–525.

Domel, S. B., Thomson, W. O., Davis, H. C., Baranowski, T., Leonard, S. B., & Baranowski, J. (1996). Psychosocial predictors of fruit and vegetable consumption among elementary school children. *Health Education Research, 11,* 299–308.

Dryfoos, J. (1998). *Safe passage: Making it through adolescence in a risky society.* New York: Oxford University Press.

DuRant, R., Treiber, F., Goodman, E., & Woods, E. (1996) Intentions to use violence among young adolescents. *Pediatrics, 98*(6), 1104–1108.

Duvall, E., & Miller, B. (1984). *Marriage and family development* (6th ed.). New York: Harper & Row.

Dworetzky, J. (1995). *Human development: A lifespan approach* (6th ed.). St. Paul, MN: West Publishing.

Edelman, M. (1997). New CDF report on state of America's children finds child well-being lagging despite economic recovery. In *Children's Defense Fund. The state of America's children yearbook 1997.* Washington, DC: Children's Defense Fund.

Edelstein, C. K. (1989). Early clues to anorexia and bulimia. *Patient Care, 23*(13), 155–175.

Escobedo, L., Chorba, J., & Waxweiler, R. (1995). Patterns of alcohol use and the risk of drinking and driving among U.S. high school students. *American Journal of Public Health, 85,* 976–978.

Food Research and Action Center (1998). *Fact sheet on hunger in the United States.* Washington, DC: Author.

Friedman, M. (1998). *Family nursing: Research, theory and practice* (4th ed.). Stamford, CT: Appleton & Lange.

Fritz, T., & Barbie, M. (1993). What are the warning signs for suicidal adolescents? *Journal of Psychosocial Nursing, 32*(2), 37–40.

Gavagen, T., & Brodyaga, L. (1996, March 1). Medical care for immigrants and refugees. *American Family Physician.*

Gill, C. (1995). Protecting our children: Where have we gone and where should we go from here? *Journal of Psychosocial Nursing, 33*(3), 31–35.

Grover, G. (2000). Dental care. In C. Berkowitz (Ed.), *Pediatrics: A primary care approach* (2nd ed.). Philadelphia: W. B. Saunders.

Hanson, S. (2001). *Family health care nursing: Theory, practice, and research* (2nd ed.). Philadelphia: F. A. Davis.

Hewell, S., & Andrews, J. (1996). Contraceptive use among female adolescents. *Clinical Nursing Research, 5*(3), 356–363.

Hill, J., & Trowbridge, F. (1998). Childhood obesity: Future directions and research priorities. *Pediatrics, 101*(3), 570–574.

Himes, J. H., & Dietz, W. H. (1994). Guidelines for overweight in adolescent preventive services: Recommendations from an expert committee. The Expert Committee on Clinical Guidelines for Overweight in Adolescent Preventive Services. *American Journal of Clinical Nutrition, 32,* 607–629.

Institute of Medicine. (1995). *Nursing, health, and the environment.* Washington, DC: National Academy Press.

Irwin, C. (1993). Topical areas of interest for promoting health: From the perspective of the physician. In S. Millstein, A. Petersen, & E. Nightengale (Eds.), *Promoting the health of adolescents: New directions for the twenty-first century* (pp. 328–332). New York: Oxford University Press.

Jacobson, L., & Wilkenson, C. (1994). Review of teenage health: Time for a new direction. *British Journal of General Practice, 44,* 313–424.

Johnson, S. L., & Birch, L. L. (1994). Parent's and children's adiposity and eating style. *Pediatrics, 94,* 653–661.

Kafka, R., & London, P. (1991, Fall). Communication in relationships and adolescent substance use: The influence of parents and friends. *Adolescence, 26*(103), 587–597.

Kennedy, E., & Powell, R. (1997). Changing eating patterns of American children: A view from 1996. *Journal of the American College on Nutrition 16,* 524–529.

Lewis, C., Battisich, V., & Schaps, E. (1990). School-based primary prevention: What is an effective program? *New Directions for Child Development, 50,* 35–39.

Lutz, C., & Przytulski, K. (1997). *Nutrition and diet therapy* (2nd ed.). Philadelphia: F. A. Davis.

Mannuzza, K., & Klein, R. (2000, July). Long term prognosis in attention-deficit/hyperactivity disorder. *Child and Adolescent Psychiatric Clinics of North America, 3*(9), 711–726.

McLoyd, V. (1998). Socioeconomic disadvantage and child development. *American Psychologist, 53*(2), 185–204.

Mercugliano, M. (1999, October). What is attention-deficit/hyperactivity disorder? *Pediatric Clinics of North America, 46*(5), 831–843.

Montemayor, R. (1983). Parents and adolescents in conflict: All families some of the time and some families most of the time. *Journal of Early Adolescence, 3,* 83–103.

Murray, R., & Zentner, J. (2001). *Health assessment and promotion strategies throughout the lifespan* (7th ed.). Upper Saddle River, NJ: Prentice-Hall.

National Center for Injury Prevention and Control. (1997). *Fact sheet: Childhood injury.* Atlanta, GA: Division of Unintentional Injury Prevention.

National Center for Health Statistics. (1999). *Health; United States 1999.* Hyattsville, MD: U.S. Department of Health and Human Services.

National SAFE KIDS Campaign. (n.d.). *Injury fact sheet: Trends in unintentional childhood injury prevention* [electronic version]. Washington, DC: Author.

Nelson, J. (1997). *Positive discipline.* New York: Ballantine.

Paule, M. G., Rowland, A. S., Ferguson, S. A., Chelonis, J. J., Tannock, R. S., Wanson, J. M., & Castellanos, F. X. (2000). Attention deficit/hyperactivity disorder: Characteristics, interventions and models. *Neurotoxicol Teratology, 22*(5), 631–651.

Pillitteri, A. (1999). *Maternal and child health nursing: Care of the childbearing and childrearing family* (3rd ed.). Philadelphia: J. B. Lippincott.

Popper, C. W. (2000, July). Pharmacologic alternatives to psychostimulants for the treatment of attention-deficit/hyperactivity disorder. *Child and Adolescent Psychiatric Clinics of North America, 9*(3), 605–646, viii.

Potts, N., & Mandleco, B. (2002). *Pediatric nursing: Caring for children and their families.* Clifton Park, NY: Delmar Learning.

Rosenbaum, M., & Leibel, R. L. (1998). The physiology of body weight regulation: Relevance to the etiology of obesity in children. *Pediatrics, 101,* 525–539.

Scarr, S. (1998). American child care today. *American Psychologist, 53*(2), 95–108.

School lunch program-fact sheet. [On-line]. Available: www.fns.usda.gov/cnd/Lunch/AboutLunch/faqs.htm.

Schubert, P., & Lionberger, H. (1995). Mutual connectedness: A study of client-nurse interaction using the Grounded Theory method. *Journal of Holistic Nursing, 13*(2), 102–116.

Sniffen, M. (1998, April 13). Gangs, violence rising in schools (Associated Press). *Record, 13,* A-5.

Stanfield, P. (1997). *Nutrition and diet therapy: Self instructional modules* (3rd ed.). Boston: Jones and Bartlett.

Steiner, H. (1998, April). Anorexia nervosa and bulimia in children and adolescents: A review of the past 10 years. *Journal of the American Academy of Child and Adolescent Psychiatry.* [On-line]. Available: www.findarticles.com.

Strasburger, V., & Donnerstein, E. (1999, January). Children, adolescents, and the media: Issues and solutions. *Pediatrics, 103*(1), 129–139.

Strauss, R., & Knight, J. (1999). Influence of the home environment on the development of obesity in children. *Pediatrics, 106*(6), 85.

Townsend, C., & Roth, R. (2000). *Nutrition and diet therapy* (7th ed.). Clifton Park, NY: Delmar Learning.

Troiano, R. P., & Flegal, K. M. (1998). Overweight children and adolescents: Description, epidemiology, and demographics. *Pediatrics, 101*(3), 497–504.

Troiano, R. P., Flegal, K. M., Kuczmarski, R. J., Campbell, S. M., & Johnson, C. L. (1995). Overweight prevalence and trends for children and adolescents: The National Health and Nutrition Examination Surveys, 1963 to 1991. *Archives of Pediatric Adolescent Medicine, 149,* 1085–1091.

Turner, J., & Helms, D. (1995). *Lifespan development* (5th ed.). New York: Holt, Rinehart & Winston.

U.S. Department of Education. (1997, November). *Parents Guide to the Internet.* Washington, DC: Author. [On-line]. Available: http://www.ed.gov/pubs/parents/internet.

U.S. Department of Health and Human Services. (1997). Guidelines for school and community programs to promote lifelong physical activity among young people. *Morbidity and Mortality Weekly Report, 46,* 1–36.

U.S. Department of Health and Human Services. (2000a). *Healthy people 2010: National health promotion and disease prevention objectives:* Washington, DC: Author.

U.S. Department of Health and Human Services. (2000b, April 10). HHS reports new child abuse and neglect statistics. *HHS News.*

U.S. Department of Health and Human Services. (2001, February 2). *The state of children's health insurance program (SCHIP).* HHS Fact Sheet. [On-line]. Available: www.hhs.gov.news/press/2001pres/01fsschip.html.

Ventura, S. J., Peters, K. D., Martin, J. A., & Maurer, J. D. (1997). Births and deaths: United States 1996. *Monthly Vital Statistics Report, 46*(1), Suppl. 2.

Waller, G. (1998). Perceived control in eating disorders: Relationship with reported sexual abuse. *International Journal of Eating Disorders, 23*(2), 213–216.

Webster, D., Gainer, P., & Champion, H. (1995). Weapon carrying among inner-city junior high students: Defensive behavior vs. aggressive delinquency. *American Journal of Public Health, 85,* 1604–1608.

Whitney, E., & Rolfes, S. (1996). *Understanding nutrition* (7th ed.). St. Paul, MN: West.

Williams, J. O., Achterberg, C., & Sylvester, G. P. (1995). Targeting marketing of food products to ethnic minority youths. In C. L. Willams & S. Y. Kimm (Eds.), *Prevention and treatment of childhood obesity* (107–114). Ann, NY: Academy Science.

World Health Organization. (1995). *World Health Statistics Annual, 1994.* Geneva, Switzerland: Author.

Young, S. (2000, June). ADHD children grown up: An empirical review. *Counselling Psychology Quarterly, 13*(2), 191–200.

CHAPTER 23: CARE OF YOUNG, MIDDLE, AND OLDER ADULTS

Abaya, C. (2001). *The sandwich generation.* [On-line]. Available: http://members.aol.com/sandwichgen.

Albery, I. P., Gossop, M., & Strang, J. (1998). Illicit drugs and driving: A review of epidemiological, behavioral and psychological correlates. *Journal of Substance Misuse for Nursing, Health and Social Care, 3*(3), 140–149.

American Psychiatric Association. (2000). *Diagnostic and statistical manual of mental disorders* (4th edition text revision). Washington, DC: Author.

Andrews, M., & Boyle, J. (1999). *Transcultural concepts in nursing care* (3rd ed.). Philadelphia: J. B. Lippincott.

Anglin, L. T. (1994). Historical perspectives: Influences of the past. In J. Zerwekh & J. C. Claborn (Eds.), *Nursing today* (pp. 29–49). Philadelphia: W. B. Saunders.

Banani, S. (1987). Life's rainbow. In S. Martz (Ed.), *When I am an old woman I shall wear purple* (p. 181). Manhattan Beach, CA: Papier-Mache Press.

Bee, H. (1998). *Life span development* (2nd ed.). New York: Longman.

Bellis, M. A., Hale, G., Bennett, A., Chaudry, M., & Kilgoyle, M. (2000). Tbeza uncovered: Changes in substance use and sexual behavior amongst young people visiting an international night-life resort. *International Journal of Drug Policy, 11*(3), 235–244.

Blasinsky, M. (1998). Family dynamics: Influencing care of the older adult. *Activities, Adaptation and Aging, 4,* 65–72.

Butler, R. N. (1963). The life review: An interpretation of reminiscence in the aged. *Psychiatry, 26,* 65–75.

Cancian, M., & Meyer, D. R. (2000). Work after welfare: Women's work-effort, occupation, and economic well-being. *Social Work Research, 24*(2), 69–86.

Carpenito, L. J. (1999). *Nursing care plans and documentation* (3rd ed.). Philadelphia: J. B. Lippincott.

Centers for Disease Control and Prevention. (1999). National Center for Health Statistics. [On-line]. Available: www.cdc.gov/nchs/fastats/pdf.

Centers for Disease Control and Prevention. (2000a). National Center for HIV, STD and TB Prevention, Divisions of HIV/AIDS Prevention. *Survey Report, 12*(1).

Centers for Disease Control and Prevention. (2000b). [On-line]. Available: www.cdc.gov/nccdphp/drb.

Cerwonka, E. R., Isbell, T. R., & Hansen, C. E. (2000). Psychosocial factors as predictors of unsafe sexual practices among young adults. *AIDS Education and Prevention, 12*(2), 141–153.

Cumella, S., Grattan, E., & Vostanis, P. (1998). The mental health of children in homeless families and their contact with health, education, and social services. *Health and Social Care in the Community, 6*(5), 331–342.

Dolcini, M. M., & Catania, J. A. (2000). Psychosocial profiles of women with risky sexual partners: The National AIDS Behavioral Surveys (NABS). *AIDS and Behavior, 4*(3), 297–308.

Donnelly, J., Hollenbeck, W., Eadie, C., Duncan, D. F., & Eburne, N. (2000). College students' distorted perceptions of drug dangers: Overestimation and underestimation of licit and illicit drugs. *International Electronic Journal of Health Education, 3*(4), 272–277.

Ebersole, P., & Hess, P. (1998). *Toward healthy aging: Human needs and nursing response* (5th ed.). St Louis, MO: Mosby.

Erikson, E. H. (1963). *Childhood and society* (2nd ed.), New York: W. W. Norton.

Feigelman, W., Gorman, B. S., & Lee, J. A. (1998). Binge drinkers, illicit drug users and polydrug users: An epidemiological study of American collegians. *Journal of Alcohol and Drug Education, 44*(1), 47–69.

Fuller, G. F. (2000). Falls in the elderly. *American Family Physician, 61,* 2159–2168, 2173–2174.

Fullilove, M. T., Green, L., & Fullilove, R. E. (1999). Building momentum: An ethnographic study of inner-city redevelopment. *American Journal of Public Health, 89*(6), 840–844.

Gambassi, G. (1998). Systematic assessment of geriatric drug use via epidemiology. *Journal of the American Medical Association.* [On-line]. Available: www.psarising.com/medicalpike/paintuntreated.htm.

Haemmerlie, F. M., Montgomery, R. L., & Crowell, S. L. (1999). Alcohol abuse by university students and its relationship to sociomoral reasoning. *Journal of Alcohol and Drug Education, 44*(2), 29–43.

Henderson, B. E., Bernstein, L., & Ross, R. K. (1999). Adolescent and young adult genital cancer. *Cancer Medicine.* [On-line]. Available: www.cancernetwork.com.

Hicks, T. J. (1999). Spirituality and the elderly: Nursing implications with nursing home residents. *Geriatric Nursing: American Journal of Care for the Aging, 20*(3), 144–146.

John D. and Catherine T. MacArthur Foundation Research Network on Successful Midlife Development. (2001, April 28). *Midlife research* [On-line]. Available: http://midmac.med.harvard.edu.

Jung, C. (1933). *Modern man in search of soul.* New York: Harcourt, Brace and World.

Kann, L., Kinchen, S. A., Williams, B. I., Ross, J. G., Lowry, R., Grunbaum, J., & Koble, L. J. (2000). Youth risk behavior surveillance—United States, 1999. *Morbidity and Mortality Weekly Report, 49,* SS-5.

Kenney, J. W., Reinholtz, C., & Angelini, P. J. (1998). Sexual abuse, sex before age 16 and high-risk behaviors of young females with sexually transmitted diseases. *Journal of Obstetric, Gynecologic and Neonatal Nursing, 27*(1), 54–63.

Klaas, D. (1998). Testing two elements of spirituality in depressed and non-depressed elders. *International Journal of Psychiatric Nursing, 4*(2), 452–462.

Klitzman, R. L., Pope, H. G., & Hudson, J. I. (2000). MDMA ("Ecstasy") abuse and high-risk sexual behaviors among 169 gay and bisexual men. *American Journal of Psychiatry, 157*(7), 1162–1164.

Klotz, L. H. (1999). Why is the rate of testicular cancer increasing? *Canadian Medical Association Journal, 160,* 213–214.

Levinson, D. J. (1978). *The seasons of a man's life.* New York: Alfred A. Knopf.

Levinson, D. J. (1986). Conception of adult development. *American Psychologist, 41,* 3–13.

Lindeman, C. A., & McAthie, M. (1999). *Fundamentals of contemporary nursing practice.* Philadelphia: W. B. Saunders.

McMurdo, M. (1999). Exercise in old age: Time to unwrap the cotton wool. *British Journal of Sport Medicine, 33,* 295–300.

Mendenhall, B. (1999). *Bridging the generation gap.* [On-line]. Available: http://lifematters.com/bridge.html.

Murray, R. B., & Zentner, J. P. (2001). *Health promotion strategies throughout the life span* (7th ed.). Upper Saddle River, NJ: Prentice-Hall.

National Diabetes Information Clearinghouse. (2001). *Diabetes in American Indians and Alaska natives.* [On-line]. Available: www.niddk.nih.gov/health/diabetes/pubs/amindian/amindian.htm.

Newman, B., & Newman, P. (1999). *Development through life: A psychosocial approach* (7th ed.). Belmont, CA: Brooks/Cole.

O'Hare, T. (1999). Risky sex and drinking context in young women and men. *Journal of Human Behavior in the Social Environment, 2*(4), 1–18.

Ostir, G. V., Markides, K. S., Black, S. A., & Goodwin, J. S. (2000). Emotional well-being predicts subsequent functional independence and survival. *Journal of American Geriatric Society, 48*(5), 473–478.

Papalia, D., & Olds, S. (1998). *Human development* (3rd ed.). Boston: McGraw-Hill.

Quigley, D. G., & Schatz, M. S. (1999). Men and women and their responses in spousal bereavement. *Hospice Journal: Physical, Psychosocial, and Pastoral Care of the Dying, 14*(2), 65–78.

Read, J., & Argyle, N. (1999). Hallucinations, delusions and thought disorders among adult psychiatric inpatients with a history of child abuse. *Psychiatric Services, 50*(11), 1467–1472.

Riegel, K. F. (1973). Dialectical operations: The final period of cognitive development. *Human Development, 16,* 346–370.

Rogers, M. A. (1970). *Theoretical basis of nursing.* Philadelphia: F. A. Davis.

Ryan, A. A., & Scullion, H. F. (2000). Nursing home placement: An exploration of the experience of family carers. *Journal of Advanced Nursing, 32*(5), 1187–1195.

Sarna, L. (1995). Cancer in the elderly. In M. Stanley & P. G. Beare (Eds.), *Gerontological nursing* (pp. 323–337). Philadelphia: F. A. Davis.

Sheehy, G. (1995). *New Passages*. New York: Random House.

Skidmore, D., & Hayter, E. (2000). Risk and sex: Ego-centricity and sexual behavior in young adults. *Health, Risk & Society, 2*(1), 23–32.

Smelzer, S. C., & Bare, B. G. (2000). *Textbook of medical surgical nursing*. Philadelphia: J. B. Lippincott.

Staton, M., Leukefeld, C., Logan, T. K., Zimmerman, R., Lynam, D., Milich, R., Martin, C., McClanahan, K., & Clayton, R. (1999). Risky sex behavior and substance use among young adults. *Health and Social Work, 24*(2), 147–154.

Stein, L. M., & Bienenfeld, D. (1992). Hearing impairment and its impact on elderly patients with cognitive, behavioral, or psychiatric disorders: A literature review. *Journal of Geriatric Psychiatry, 25,* 145–156.

Swagerty, D. L., Takahashi, P. Y., & Evans, J. M. (1999). Elder mistreatment. *American Family Physician, 59*(10), 2804–2808.

Taylor, C., Lillis, C., & LeMone, P. (2001). *Fundamentals of nursing* (4th ed.). Philadelphia: J. B. Lippincott.

Timon, M. (2001). *Caring for caregivers*. [On-line]. Available: www.workingwoman.com.

Townsend, M. C. (2000). *Psychiatric mental health nursing* (3rd ed.). Philadelphia: F. A. Davis.

U.S. Department of Health and Human Services. (2000). *Healthy people 2010: Understanding and improving health* (2nd ed.). Washington, DC: U.S. Government Printing Office. [On-line]. Available: http://www.health.gov/healthypeople.

U.S. Public Health Service. (1999). At a glance: Suicide among the elderly. *The Surgeon General's Call to Prevent Suicide*. Washington, DC: Author. [On-line]. Available: http://www.surgeongeneral.gov/library/calltoaction/fact2.htm.

Varcarolis, E. M. (2002). *Foundations of psychiatric mental health nursing* (4th ed.). Philadelphia: W. B. Saunders.

Ward, D. (2000). Adult/elderly care nursing. Ageism and the abuse of older people in health and social care. *British Journal of Nursing, 9*(9), 560–563.

Wasaha, S., & Angelopoulos, F. M. (1996). What Every Woman Should Know About Menopause. *American Journal of Nursing, 96*(1), 24–32.

Wechsler, H., Lee, J. E., Kuo, M., & Lee, H. (2000). College binge drinking in the 1990's: A continuing problem: Results of the Harvard School of Public Health 1999 college alcohol study. *Journal of American College Health, 48*(5), 199–210.

Wilkes, L., LeMiere, J., & Walker, E. (1998). Nurses in an acute care setting: Attitudes to and knowledge of older people. *Geriaction, 16*(1), 9–16.

Wingerson, N. (1992). Psychic loss in adult survivors of father-daughter incest. *Archives of Psychiatric Nursing, 6*(4), 239–244.

Zimmer, J. C., & Thurston, W. E. (1998). Attitudes, beliefs and practices of nursing students concerning HIV/AIDS: Implications for prevention in women. *Health Care for Women International, 19*(4), 327–342.

CHAPTER 24: FRAMEWORKS FOR ASSESSING FAMILIES

Aerts, E. (1993). Bringing the institution back in. In P. A. Cowan, D. Field, D. A. Hansen, A. Skolnick, & G. E. Swanson (Eds.). *Family, self, and society: Toward a new agenda for family research* (pp. 3–41). Hillsdale, NJ: Lawrence Erlbaum Associates.

Andrews, M. M. (1995). Transcultural nursing care. In M. M. Andrews & J. S. Boyle (Eds.), *Transcultural concepts in nursing care* (2nd ed., pp. 49–96). Philadelphia: J. B. Lippincott.

Associated Press. (1994, February 15). Welfare cases rise as debate over reform heats up. *Marin Independent Journal,* A7.

Auger, J. R. (1976). *Behavioral systems and nursing*. Englewood Cliffs, NJ: Prentice Hall.

Baker, D. (1996). *King's Theory and case management of high-risk senior citizens within a health maintenance organization*. Unpublished paper.

Barstow, D. G. (1999). Female genital mutilation: The penultimate gender abuse. *Child Abuse and Neglect, 23,* 501–510.

Becvar, D. S., & Becvar, R. J. (2000). *Family therapy: A systemic integration* (4th ed.). Boston: Allyn & Bacon.

Blue, C. L., Brubaker, K. M., Fine, J. M., Kirsch, M. J., Papazian, K. R., Riester, C. M., & Sobiech, M. A. (1994). Sister Callista Roy: Adaptation model. In A. Marriner-Tomey (Ed.), *Nursing theorists and their work* (3rd ed., pp. 246–268). St. Louis, MO: Mosby-Yearbook.

Brinson, S. V., & Brunk, Q. (2000). Hospice family caregivers: An experience in coping. *Hospice Journal, 15*(3), 1–12.

Bronfenbrenner, U. (1977). Toward an experimental ecology of human development. *American Psychologist, 7,* 513–531.

Carter B., & McGoldrick, M. (1989). Overview: The changing family life cycle: A framework for family therapy. In B. Carter & McGoldrick (Eds.), *The changing family life cycle,* (pp. 3–28) Boston: Allyn & Bacon.

Carter, B., & McGoldrick, M. (1999). Overview: The expanded family life cycle: Individual, family, and social perspectives. In B. Carter & M. McGoldrick (Eds.), *The expanded family life cycle: Individual, family, and social perspectives* (3rd ed., pp. 1–26). Boston: Allyn & Bacon.

Chan, R. W., Raboy, B., & Patterson, C. J. (1998). Psychosocial adjustment among children conceived via donor insemination by lesbian and heterosexual mothers. *Child Development, 69,* 443–457.

Chang, B. L. (1999). Cognitive-behavioral intervention for homebound caregivers of persons with dementia. *Nursing Research, 48,* 173–181.

Chou, K., LaMontagne, L. L., & Hepworth, J. T. (1999). Burden experienced by caregivers of relatives with dementia in Taiwan. *Nursing Research, 48,* 206–214.

Combrinck-Graham, L. (1985). A developmental model for family systems. *Family Process, 24,* 139–150.

Cuellar, I., & Glazer, M. (1996). The impact of culture on the family. In M. Harway (Ed.), *Treating the changing family: Handling normative and unusual events.* American Counseling Association. New York: John Wiley & Sons.

Duvall, E. M. (1977). *Marriage and family development*. Philadelphia: J. B. Lippincott.

Duvall, E. M., & Miller, B. C. (1985). *Marriage and family development* (6th ed.). New York: Harper and Row.

Edelberg, H. K., Lyman, K., & Wei, L. Y. (1998). Notation of previous falls in admission record of hospitalized elderly. *Aging, 10*(1), 67–70.

Edelberg, H. K. (2001). Falls and function: How to prevent falls and injuries in patients with impaired mobility. *Geriatrics, 56*(3), 41–45.

Enevold, G., & Courts, N. J. (2000). Fall prevention program for community-dwelling older adults and their caregivers. *Home Healthcare Nurse Manager, 4*(4), 22–28.

Feeley, N., & Gottlieb, L. N. (2000). Nursing approaches for working with family strengths and resources. *Journal of Family Nursing, 6,* 9–24.

Friedman, M. M. (1998). *Family nursing: Theory and practice* (4th ed.). Stamford, CT: Appleton & Lange.

Friedemann, M. (1999). The concept of family nursing. In G. D. Wegner & R. J. Alexander (Eds.), *Readings in family nursing* (2nd ed., pp. 13–22). Philadelphia: J. B. Lippincott.

Fulmer, R. (1999). Becoming an adult. In B. Carter & M. McGoldrick (Eds.), *The expanded family life cycle: Individual, family, and social perspectives* (3rd ed., pp. 215–230). Boston: Allyn & Bacon.

Geissler, E. M. (1991). Transcultural nursing and nursing diagnoses. *Nursing and Health Care, 12,* 190–203.

Giger, J. N., & Davidhizar, R. E. (1999). *Transcultural nursing: Assessment and intervention.* St. Louis, MO: Mosby.

Gilliss, C. L. (1993). Family nursing research theory and practice. In G. D. Wegner & R. J. Alexander (Eds.), *Reading in family nursing* (pp. 34–42). Philadelphia: J. B. Lippincott.

Gilliss, C. L. (1999). Family nursing research: Theory and practice. In G. D. Wegner & R. J. Alexander (Eds.), *Readings in family nursing* (2nd ed., pp. 34–42). Philadelphia: J. B. Lippincott.

Hare, J., & Richards, L. (1993). Children raised by lesbian couples: Does context of birth affect father and partner involvement? *Family Relations, 42,* 249–255.

Harway, M., & Wexler, K. (1996). Setting the stage for understanding and treating the changing family. In M. Harway (Ed.). *Treating the changing family: Handling normative and unusual events.* New York: John Wiley & Sons.

Herrick, C. A., & Goodykoontz, L. (1999). Neuman's systems model for nursing practice as a conceptual framework for a family assessment. In G. D. Wegner and R. J. Alexander (Eds.), *Readings in family nursing* (2nd ed., pp. 72–82). Philadelphia: J. B. Lippincott.

Johnson, N. E., & Climo, J. (2000). Aging and eldercare in lesser developed countries. *Journal of Family Issues, 21,* 683–691.

King, I. M. (1981). *A theory for nursing: Systems, concepts, process.* New York: John Wiley.

King, I. M. (1986). *Curriculum and instruction in nursing.* Norwalk, CT: Appleton-Century-Crofts.

King, I. M. (1994). Quality of life and goal attainment. *Nursing Science Quality, 7,* 29–32.

Lindgren, C. L. (1993). The caregiver career. *Image, 25,* 214–219.

Macklin, E. D. (1987). Nontraditional family forms. In M. B. Sussman & S. K. Stienmetz (Eds.), *Handbook of marriage and the family.* New York: Plenum.

Malone, J. A. (1998). Family themes across settings and populations: Content analysis. In B. Vaughan-Cole, M. A. Johnson, J. A. Malone, & B. L. Walker (Eds.), *Family nursing practice* (pp. 321–346). Philadelphia: W. B. Saunders.

Marciano, T. (1991). A postscript on wider families: Traditional family assumptions and cautionary notes. *Marriage and Family Review, 17,* 159–163.

Marciano, T., & Sussman, M. B. (1991). Wider families: An overview. *Marriage and Family Review, 17,* 1–7.

Martin, K. S., & Scheet, N. J. (1992). *The Omaha system: Applications for community health nursing.* Philadelphia: W. B. Saunders.

McGoldrick, M., & Carter, B. (1999). Remarried families. In B. Carter & M. McGoldrick, (Eds.), *The expanded family life cycle: Individual, family, and social perspectives* (3rd ed., pp. 417–435). Boston: Allyn & Bacon.

McGoldrick, M., Gerson, R., & Shellenberger, S. (1999). Genograms: Assessment and intervention (2nd ed.). New York: W. W. Norton.

Neuman, B. (1983). Family intervention using the Betty Neuman health care systems model. In I. W. Clements & F. B. Roberts (Eds.), *Family health: A theoretical approach to nursing care* (pp. 161–175). New York: John Wiley & Sons.

North American Nursing Diagnosis Association. (2001). *NANDA Nursing Diagnoses: Definitions and Classification 2001–2002.* Philadelphia: Author.

Otto, H. A. (1963). Criteria for assessing family strength. *Family Process, 2,* 329–338.

Pepin, J. I. (1992). Family caring and caring in nursing. *Image, 24,* 127–131.

Petze, C. F. (1991). Health promotion for the well family. In B. W. Spradley (Ed.), *Readings in community health nursing* (4th ed., pp. 355–364). New York: J. B. Lippincott.

Pinderhughes, E. B. (1983). Empowerment for our clients and for ourselves. *Social Casework: The Journal of Contemporary Social Work, 6,* 331–338.

Pittman, K. P., Wold, J. L., Wilson, A. H., Huff, C., & Williams, S. (2000). Community connections: Promoting family health. *Family and Community Health, 23,* 72–78.

Rawsky, E. (1998). Review of the literature on falls among the elderly. *Image: Journal of Nursing Scholarship, 30,* 47–52.

Resnick, B. (1999). Falls in a community of older adults: Putting research into practice. *Clinical Nursing Research, 8,* 251–266.

Rogers, M. (1990). Nursing: Science of Unitary, Irreducible, Human Beings: Update 1990. In E. A. M. Barrett (Ed.), *Visions of Rogers' science-based nursing* (pp. 5–11). New York: National League of Nursing.

Rogers, M. E. (1992). Nursing science and the space age. *Nursing Science Quarterly, 5,* 27–34.

Rosenberg, E. B. (1992). *The adoption life cycle: The children and their families through the years.* New York: The Free Press.

Roy, Sr. C. (1983). Roy adaptation model. In I. W. Clements & F. B. Roberts (Eds.), *Family health: A theoretical approach to nursing care* (pp. 255–278). New York: John Wiley & Sons.

Rubin, R. M., & Riney, B. J. (1994). *Working wives and dual-earner families,* Wesport, CT: Praeger.

Schumacher, K. I., Stewart, B. J., Archbold, P. G., Dodd, M. J., & Dibble, S. L. (2000). Family caregiving skill: Development of the concept. *Research in Nursing and Health, 23,* 191–203.

Silva, M. C. (1999). Needs of spouses of surgical patients: A conceptualization within the Roy Adaptation Model. In G. D. Wegner & R. J. Alexander (Eds.), *Readings in family nursing* (2nd ed., pp. 43–60). Philadelphia: J. B. Lippincott.

Solomon, C. M. (1992). Work/family ideas that break boundaries. *Personnel Journal, 71*(10), 112–117.

Spector, R. E. (2000). *Cultural diversity in health and illness* (5th ed.). Upper Saddle River, NJ: Prentice-Hall.

Spiegel, J. (1982). An ecological model of ethnic families. In M. McGoldrick, J. K. Pearce, & J. Giordano (Eds.), *Ethnicity and family therapy* (pp. 31–51). New York: Guilford.

Staples, R. (1989). Family life in the 21st century: An analysis of old forms, current trends, and future scenarios. In C. L. Gilliss, B. L. Highley, B. M. Roberts, & I. M. Martinson (Eds.), *Toward a science of family nursing* (pp. 156–170). Menlo Park. CA: Addison-Wesley.

Szapoeznik, J. B., Kurtines, W. M. (1993). Family psychology and cultural diversity. *American Psychologist, 18,* 400–407.

Treacher, A. (2000). Narrative and fantasy in adoption: Toward a different theoretical understanding. In A. Treacher & I. Katz (Eds.), *The dynamics of adoption: Social and personal perspectives* (pp. 11–26). Philadelphia: Jessica Kingsley.

Triseliotis, J. (2000). Identity-formation and the adopted person revisited. In A. Treacher & I. Katz (Eds.), *The dynamics of adoption: Social and personal perspectives* (pp. 81–99). Philadelphia: Jessica Kingsley.

U.S. Bureau of the Census. (1999). *Statistical Abstractal Abstracts of the US: 1999* (119 ed.). Washington, DC: U.S. Government Printing Office.

U.S. Department of Health and Human Services. (2000). *Healthy people 2010: Understanding and improving health.* Washington, DC: Author.

von Bertalanffy, L. (1950). The theory of open systems in physics and biology. *Science, 111,* 25–29.

Wallerstein, J. S. (1995). The early psychological tasks of marriage: Part 1. *American Journal of Orthopsychiatry, 65,* 640–650.

Wallerstein, J. S. (1996). The psychological tasks of marriage: Part 2. *American Journal of Orthopsychiatry, 66,* 217–227.

Wallerstein, J. S., & Blakeslee, S. (1995). *The good marriage: How and why love lasts.* New York: Houghton Mifflin.

Walsh, W. M. (1992). Twenty major issues in remarriage families. *Journal of Counseling and Development, 70,* 709–715.

Whall, A. L. (1991). Family system theory: Relationship to nursing conceptual models. In A. L. Whall & J. Fawcett (Eds.), *Family theory development in nursing: State of the science and art* (pp. 317–341). Philadelphia: F. A. Davis.

Whall, A. (1999). The family as the unit of care in nursing: A historical review. In G. D. Wegner & R. J. Alexander (Eds.), *Readings in family nursing* (2nd ed., pp. 3–12). Philadelphia: J. B. Lippincott.

Wright, L. M., & Leahey, M. (2000). *Nurses and families: A guide to family assessment and intervention* (3rd ed.), Philadelphia: F. A. Davis.

CHAPTER 25: FAMILY FUNCTIONS AND PROCESSES

Anderson, C. M. (1999). Single-parent families: Strengths, vulnerabilities, and interventions. In B. Carter & M. McGoldrick (Eds.), *The expanded family life cycle: Individual, family, and social perspectives* (3rd ed., pp. 399–416). Needham Heights, MA: Allyn & Bacon.

Arrighi, B. A., & Maume, D. J. (2000). Workplace subordination and men's avoidance of housework. *Journal of Family Issues, 21,* 464–487.

Beavers, W. R., & Hampson, R. B. (1993). Measuring family competence: The Beavers Systems Model. In F. Walsh (Ed.), *Normal family processes* (2nd ed., pp. 73–103). New York: Guilford.

Becvar, D. S., & Becvar, R. J. (2000). *Family therapy: A systematic integration* (4th ed.). Needham Heights, MA: Allyn & Bacon.

Bisagni, G. M., & Eckenrode, J. (1995). The role of work identity in women's adjustment to divorce. *American Journal of Orthopsychiatry, 65,* 574–583.

Carson, V. B., & Arnold, E. N. (1996). *Mental health nursing: The nurse–patient journey.* Philadelphia: W. B. Saunders.

Carter, B., & McGoldrick, M. (1999a). Coaching at various stages in the life cycle. In B. Carter & M. McGoldrick (Eds.), *The expanded family life cycle: Individual, family, and social perspectives* (3rd ed., pp. 436–454). Needham Heights, MA: Allyn & Bacon.

Carter, B., & McGoldrick, M. (1999b). Overview: The expanded family life cycle: Individual, family, and social perspectives. In B. Carter & M. McGoldrick (Eds.), *The expanded family life cycle: Individual, family, and social perspectives* (3rd ed., pp. 1–26). Needham Heights, MA: Allyn & Bacon.

Crosbie-Burnett, M., & Helmbrecht, I. (1993). A descriptive empirical study of gay male stepfamilies. *Family Relations, 42,* 256–262.

Curran, D. (1983). *Traits of a healthy family.* Minneapolis, MN: Winston.

Davis, R. E. (2000). The convergence of health and family in the Vietnamese culture. *Journal of Family Nursing, 6,* 136–156.

Epstein, N. B., Bishop, D., Ryan, C., Miller, I., & Keitner, G. (1993). The McMaster Model: View of healthy family functioning. In F. Walsh (Ed.), *Normal family processes* (2nd ed., pp. 138–160). New York: Guilford.

Friedman, M. M. (1998). *Family nursing theory and practice: Research* (4th ed.). Stamford, CT: Appleton & Lange.

Galvin, K. M., & Brommel, B. J. (1986). *Family communication, cohesion, and change.* Glenview, IL: Scott, Foresman.

Garbarino, J. (1993). Reinventing fatherhood. *Families in Society: The Journal of Contemporary Human Services, 74,* 51–54.

Hanson, S. M. H. (2001). *Family health care nursing: Theory, practice, and research* (2nd ed.). Philadelphia: F. A. Davis.

Heiney, S. P. (1999). Assessing and intervening with dysfunctional families. In G. D. Wegner & R. J. Alexander (Eds.), *Readings in family nursing* (pp. 392–402). Philadelphia: J. P. Lippincott.

Janosik, E. H. (1994). *Crisis Counseling* (2nd ed.). Boston: Jones & Bartlett.

Janosik, E. H., & Green, E. (1992). *Family life: Process and practice,* Boston: Jones & Bartlett.

McCubbin, M. A. (1989). Family stress and family strengths: A comparison of single- and two-parent families with handicapped children. *Research in Nursing and Health, 12,* 101–110.

McCubbin, M. A. (1993). Family stress theory and the development of nursing knowledge about family adaptation. In S. L. Feetham, S. B. Meister, J. M. Bell, & C. L. Gilliss (Eds.), *The nursing of families* (pp. 46–58). Newbury Park, CA: Sage.

McCubbin, M. A., & McCubbin, H. J. (1989). Theoretical orientation to family stress and coping. In C. R. Figley (Ed.), *Treating stress in families* (pp. 3–43). New York: Brunner/Mazel.

McCubbin, M. A., & McCubbin, H. J. (1993). Families coping with illness: The resiliency model of family stress, adjustment, and adaptation. In C. B. Danielson, B. Hamel-Bissell, & P. Winstead-Frye (Eds.), *Families, health, and illness* (pp. 21–63). St. Louis, MO: Mosby-Yearbook.

Moorehouse, M. J. (1993). Work and family dynamics. In P. A. Cowan, D. Field, D. A. Hansen, A. Skolnick, & G. E. Swanson (Eds.), *Family, self, and society: Toward a new agenda for family research* (pp. 265–386). Hillsdale, NJ: Laurence Erlbaum Associates.

Moriarty, H. J. (1990). Key issues in the family research process: Strategies for nurse researchers. *Advances in Nursing Science, 12*(3), 1–14.

Murrell, N. L., Scherzer, T., Ryan, M., Frappier, N., Abrams, A., & Roberts, C. (2000). The AfterCare Project: An intervention for homeless childbearing families. *Community Health, 23*(3), 17–27.

Olson, D. H. (1993). Circumplex model of marital and family systems: Assessing family functioning. In F. Walsh (Ed.), *Normal family processes* (2nd ed., pp. 104–137). New York: Guilford.

Petro, N. G. (1999). Transformation of the family system during adolescence. In B. Carter & M. McGoldrick (Eds.), *The expanded family life cycle: Individual, family, and social perspectives* (3rd ed., pp. 274–286). Needham Heights, MA: Allyn & Bacon.

Pratt, L., (1976). *Family structure and effective health behavior. The energized family.* Boston: Houghton-Mifflin.

Riper, M. V. (2000). Family variables associated with well-being in siblings of children with Down syndrome. *Journal of Family Nursing, 6,* 267–286.

Shapiro, A. F., Gottman, J. M., & Carrere, S. (2000). The baby and the marriage: Identifying factors that buffer against decline in marital satisfaction after the first baby arrives. *Journal of Family Psychology, 14,* 59–70.

Stevenson-Hinde, J., & Akister, J. (1996). The McMaster model of family functioning: Observer and parental ratings in a nonclinical sample. *Family Process, 34,* 337–347.

Strober, M. H. (1988). Two earner families. In M. H. Strober & S. F. Dornbusch (Eds.), *Feminism, children and the new family* (pp. 161–190), New York: Guilford.

Townsend, M. C. (2000). *Psychiatric mental health nursing: Concepts of care* (3rd ed.). Philadelphia: F. A. Davis.

U.S. Department of Health and Human Services. (1990). *Identifying successful families: An overview of constructs and selected measures.* Washington, DC: U.S. Government Printing Office.

Varcarolis, E. M. (1998). *Foundations of psychiatric mental health nursing* (3rd ed.). Philadelphia: W. B. Saunders.

Walsh, F. (1993). Conceptualization of normal family processes. In F. Walsh (Ed.), *Normal family processes* (2nd ed., pp. 3–69). New York: Guilford.

Walsh, F. (1998). *Strengthening family resilience.* New York: Guilford.

Wright, L. M., & Leahey, M. W. (2000). *Nurses and families: A guide to family assessment and intervention* (3rd ed.). Philadelphia: F. A. Davis.

Zacks, E., Green, R. J., & Marrow, J. (1988). Comparing lesbian and heterosexual couples on the circumplex model: An initial investigation. *Family Process, 27,* 471–484.

CHAPTER 26: COMMUNICABLE DISEASES

Ackers, M. L., & Herwaldt, B. L. (1997). An outbreak in 1996 of cyclosporiasis associated with imported raspberries. *New England Journal of Medicine, 336*(22), 1548–1557.

AIDS fear brings syphilis decline. (1994, November 7). *AIDS Weekly,* No. 1, p. 10.

American Nurses Association. (1997). *Position Statement on Tuberculosis and Public Health Nursing* [On-line]. Available: http://www.ana.org/readroom/position/blood/bltbhl.htm.

Bloom, A. S., Curran, J. W., Elsner, L. G., Gwinn, M., Mofenson, L. M., Moore, J. S., Moseley, R. R., Peterson, H. B., Rogers, M. F., & Simonds, R. J. (1995, July 7). U.S. Public Health Service recommendations for human immunodeficiency virus counseling and voluntary testing for pregnant women, Part I. *Morbidity and Mortality Weekly Report, 44* (RR-7: i-7).

Carpenter, C. C. J., Fischl, M. A., Hammer, S. M., Hirsch, M. S., Jacobsen, D. M., Katzenstein, D. A., Montaner, J. S. G., Richman, D. D., Saag, M. S., Schooley, R. T., Thompson, M. A., Vella, S., Yeni, P. G., & Volberding, P. A. (1997). Antiretroviral therapy for HIV infection in 1997: Updated recommendations of the International AIDS Society USA Panel. *Journal of the American Medical Association, 277*(24), 1962–1969.

Cates, W. (1999). Estimates of the incidence and prevalence of sexually transmitted diseases in the United States. *Sexually Transmitted Diseases 26*(Suppl.), S2–S7.

Centers for Disease Control and Prevention. (1991). Rabies prevention—United States. Recommendations of the immunization practices advisory committee (ACIP). *Morbidity and Mortality Weekly Report, 40*(RR-3).

Centers for Disease Control and Prevention. (1996a). Human rabies—Connecticut, 1995. *Morbidity and Mortality Weekly Report, 45,* 207–209.

Centers for Disease Control and Prevention. (1996b). *Preventing foodborne illness: Escherichia coli O157H7.* Division of Bacterial and Mycotic Diseases, National Center for Infectious Diseases. Atlanta, GA: Author.

Centers for Disease Control and Prevention. (1997a). An unusual hantavirus outbreak in southern Argentina: Person to person transmission? *Emerging Infectious Diseases, 3*(2). National Center for Infectious Diseases. Atlanta, GA: Author.

Centers for Disease Control and Prevention. (1997b). Hantavirus pulmonary syndrome—Chile, 1997. *Morbidity and Mortality Weekly Report 46*(40), 949.

Centers for Disease Control and Prevention. (1997c). Hepatitis Branch. Atlanta, GA: Author.

Centers for Disease Control and Prevention. (1997d). Hepatitis A associated with consumption of frozen strawberries—Michigan, March, 1997. *Morbidity and Mortality Weekly Report 46*(13), 288.

Centers for Disease Control and Prevention. (1998a). *Preventing emerging infectious diseases: A strategy for the 21st century.* Atlanta, GA: Public

Health Service, U.S. Department of Health and Human Services.

Centers for Disease Control and Prevention. (1998b). Guidelines for the treatment of sexually transmitted diseases. *Morbidity and Mortality Weekly Report, 46*(No. RR-1).

Centers for Disease Control and Prevention. (1998c). Universal precautions for prevention of transmission of HIV, hepatitis B virus and other bloodborne pathogens in health care settings. *Morbidity and Mortality Weekly Report, 37,* 377–382.

Centers for Disease Control and Prevention. (1999a). Division of STD/HIV Prevention, 1999. U.S. Department of Health and Human Services. Atlanta, GA.

Centers for Disease Control and Prevention. (1999a). The concept of emergence. *Morbidity and Mortality Weekly Report, 48*(RR-13), 29–31.

Centers for Disease Control and Prevention. (1999b). *Manual for the surveillance of vaccine preventable diseases.* Atlanta, GA: Author.

Centers for Disease Control and Prevention. (2000a). *AIDS information: Statistical projections and trends.* [On-line]. Available: http://www.cdc.gov/hiv/dhap.htm.

Centers for Disease Control and Prevention. (2000b). *AIDS information: Transfusions and HIV infection.* [On-line]. Available: http://www.cdc.gov/hiv/stats/exposure.htm.

Centers for Disease Control and Prevention. (2000c). *AIDS transmission to women.* [On-line]. Available: http://www.cdc.gov/hiv/graphics/women.htm.

Centers for Disease Control and Prevention. (2000d). *Food and water borne bacterial diseases.* [On-line]. Available: http://www.cdc.gov/ncidod/dbmd/diseaseinfo/foodborneinfections_t.htm.

Centers for Disease Control and Prevention. (2000d). Case definitions for infectious conditions under public health surveillance. *Morbidity and Mortality Weekly Report, 46*(RR-10, rev.).

Centers for Disease Control and Prevention. (2000e). *National immunization program: Contraindications to pediatric immunization.* [On-line]. Available: http://www.cdc.gov/nip/recs/contraindications.htm.

Centers for Disease Control and Prevention. (2000f). *Trends in STDs in the United States 2000.* [On-line]. Available: http://www.cdc.gov/nchstp/dstd/Stats_Trends/Trends2000.pdf.

Centers for Disease Control and Prevention. (2001a). *Standards for pediatric immunization practices.* [On-line]. Available: http://www.cdc.gov/od/nvpo/standar.htm.

Centers for Disease Control and Prevention. (2001a). *Infectious diseases designated as notifiable at the national level—United States.* [On-line]. Available: http://www.cdc.gov/epo/dphsi/phs/infdis.htm.

Centers for Disease Control and Prevention. (2001b). *NCHSTP program briefing 2001: Division of TB elimination.* [On-line]. Available: http://www.cdc.gov/nchstp/od/2000program.

Centers for Disease Control and Prevention. (2002, January 15). *Nationally notifiable infectious diseases: United States, 2002* [On-line]. Available: http://www.cdc.gov/epo/dphsi/phs/infdis.htm.

Chin, J. E. (2000). *Control of communicable diseases manual* (17th ed.). Washington, DC: American Public Health Association.

Coburn, T., & Pelosi, N. (1997, September 1). Should the HIV be treated like other infectious disease? *Insight on the News, 13*(32), 24.

Deasy, J. (1996). The bite of rabies: Prevention and control strategies for rabies zoonosis. *Physician Assistant, 20*(10), 49–57.

De Vincent-Hayes, N. (1995, December). Hepatitis. *Current Health, v22*(4), 20–22.

Donovan, P. (1993). *Testing positive: Sexually transmitted disease and the public health response.* New York: Alan Guttmacher Institute.

Donovan, P. (1997). Confronting a hidden epidemic: The Institute of Medicine's Report on sexually transmitted diseases. *Family Planning Perspectives, 29,* 87–90.

Edmunds, W. J., Medley, G. F., Nokes, D. J., Hall, A. J., & Whittle, H. C. (1993). The influence of age on the development of the hepatitis B carrier state. *Lancet, 337,* 197–201.

Eng, T. R., & Butler, W. T. (Eds.). (1996). *The hidden epidemic: Confronting sexually transmitted diseases.* Committee on Prevention and Control of Sexually Transmitted Diseases. Institute of Medicine, Division of Health Promotion and Disease Prevention. Washington, DC: National Academy Press.

Feikin, D. R., Lezotte, D. C., Hamman, R. F., Salmon, D. A., Chen, R. T., Hoffman, R. E. (2000). Individual and community risks of measles and pertussis associated with personal exemptions to immunization. *Journal of the American Medical Association, 284,* 3145–3150.

Getty, V. (1997, April 25). Hepatitis A in Michigan. *USDA News Release.* Washington, DC: U.S. Department of Agriculture.

Girou, E., Schortgen, F., Delclaux, C., Brun-Buisson, C., Blot, F., Lefort, Y., Lemaire, F., & Brochard, L. (2000). Association of noninvasive ventilation with nosocomial infections and survival in critically ill patients. *Journal of the American Medical Association, 284*(18), 2361–2368.

Gordis, L. (1996). *Epidemiology.* Philadelphia: W. B. Saunders.

Hanlon, J. J., & Picket, G. E. (1979). *Public health administration and practice.* St. Louis, MO: C. V. Mosby.

Hemming, V. G., Palmer, A. L., Sinnot, J. T., & Glaser, V. (1997). Bracing for the cold and flu season. *Patient Care, 31*(15), 47–54.

Henderson, C. (1997, February 10). The link between HIV and other STDs. *AIDS Weekly Plus,* p. 16.

Hutchinson, C. M., Hook, E. W., Shepherd, M., Verley, J., & Rompalo, A. M. (1994, July 15). Altered clinical presentation of early syphilis in patients with human immunodeficiency virus infection. *Annals of Internal Medicine, 121*(2), 94–100.

Kuss, T., Proulx-Girouard, L., Lovitt, S., Katz, C. B., & Kennelly, P. (1997). A public health nursing model. *Public Health Nursing, 14*(2), 81–91.

LaPook, J. (1995). Hepatitis (liver disorders, Chapter 22). In *The Columbia University College of physicians and surgeons complete home medical guide edition 3,* (3rd ed., pp. 596–597).

Leccese, C. (1997). The best news yet: AIDS in 1997. *Advance for Nurse Practitioners, 5*(12), 25–30.

Lederberg, J., & Shope, R. E. (1992). *Emerging infections: Microbial threats to health in the United States.* Washington, DC: National Academy Press.

Mandell, G. L., Bennett, J. E., & Dolin, R. (Eds.). (1995). *Principles and practices of infectious diseases* (4th ed.). New York: Churchill-Livingston.

Miller, D. M., & Brodell, R. T. (1996). Human papillomavirus infection: Treatment options for warts. *American Family Physician, 53*(1), 135–144.

NJMC National Tuberculosis Center. (2001). *A brief history of tuberculosis.* [On-line]. Available: http://www. umdnj. edu/ntbcweb/history.html. Newark, NJ: Author.

Peters, S. (1997a). The state of pediatric immunizations today. *Advance for Nurse Practitioners, 5*(2), 43–49.

Peters, S. (1997b). Influenza update: An overview of the 1996–97 flu season. *Advance for Nurse Practitioners, 5*(1), 33–38.

Plotkin, S. A. (1996, February). Varicella vaccine (commentary). *Pediatrics, 97*(2), 251(3).

Prevention and Control of Influenza. (1997). Recommendations of the Advisory Committee on Immunization Practices (ACIP). *Morbidity and Mortality Weekly Report, 46*(RR-9), 1–25.

Prevention of hepatitis A through active or passive immunization. (1996). Recommendations of the Advisory Committee on Immunization Practices (ACIP). *Morbidity and Mortality Weekly Report, 45*(RR-15), 1–30.

ProMED. (2000). *Pathogenic microbes and infectious diseases.* [On-line]. Available: http://www.fas.org/promed/about.

Rodier, G. (1997). WHO response to epidemics. *World Health, 50*(1), 7–9.

Rupprecht, C. E., & Smith, J. S. (1994). Raccoon rabies—the re-emergence of an epizootic in a densely populated area. *Seminars in Virology, 5,* 155–164.

Satchell, M., & Hedges, S. J. (1997, September 1). The next bad beef scandal; cattle feed now contains things like chicken manure and dead cats. *U.S. News & World Report, 123*(8), 22–25.

Shovein, J. T., Damazo, R. J., & Hyams, I. (2000, March). Hepatitis A: How benign is it? *American Journal of Nursing, 100*(3), 43–48.

SmithKline Beecham. (1997, February 3). *PR Newswire.*

Stein, R. (1993). The ABC's of hepatitis. *American Health, 12*(5), 65–70.

Strausbaugh, L. J. (1997, January). Emerging infectious diseases: A challenge to all. *American Family Physician, 55*(1), 111–118.

Tauxe, R. (1997). Emerging foodborne diseases: An evolving public health challenge. *Emerging Infectious Diseases, 3*(4), 425–434.

Uhaa, I. J., Dato, V. M., Sorhage, F. E., Beckly, J. W., Roscoe, D. E., Gorsky, R. D., & Fishbein, D. B. (1992). Benefits and costs of using an orally absorbed vaccine to control rabies in raccoons. *Journal of the American Veterinary Medicine Association, 201,* 1873–1882.

U.S. Department of Health and Human Services. (1992). *Lyme disease: The facts the challenges.* NIH Publication No. 92-3193.

Walker, D. H., Barbour, A. G., Oliver, J. H., Lane, R. S., Dumler, J. S., Dennis, D. T., Persing, D. H., Azad, A. F., & McSweegan, E. (1996). Emerging bacterial zoonotic and vector-borne diseases: Ecological and epidemiological factors. *Journal of the American Medical Association, 275*(6), 463–470.

World Health Organization. (1997a, March 26). *Pap cytology screening: Most of the benefits reaped?* WHO and EUROGIN Report on Cervical Cancer Control.

World Health Organization. (1997b). *Global causes of death, 1996.* [On-line]. Available: http://www.who.ch/whr/1997/fig2e.gif.

World Health Organization. (2000a). *Overcoming antimicrobial resistance: World Health Organization report on infectious diseases 2000.* Geneva, Switzerland: Author.

World Health Organization. (2000b). *The WHO golden rules for safe food preparation.* [On-line]. Available: http://www.who.int/fsf.

CHAPTER 27: CHRONIC ILLNESS

Airhihenbuwa, C., & Harrison, I. (1993). Traditional medicine in Africa: Past, present, and future. In P. Conrad & E. Gallagher (Eds.), *Health and health care in developing countries.* Philadelphia: Temple University Press.

American Cancer Society. (2002). *Cancer Facts & Figures—2000.* Atlanta: Author.

American Nurses Association. (1986). Community Health Nurse Division. *Standards of community health nursing practice* (Publication. No CH-10). Kansas City, MO: Author.

American Public Health Association. (1981). Public Health Nursing Section. *The definition and role of public health nursing in the delivery of health care.* Washington, DC: Author.

Americans with Disability Act of 1990. (1991). Public Law 101–336, 1004 Stat. 328.

Anderson, J. M. (1991). Immigrant women speak of chronic illness: The social construction of the devalued self. *Journal of Advanced Nursing, 16,* 710–717.

Baker, N. (1996). Psychological adaptation of the child, adolescent, and family with physical illness. In P. D. Barry (Ed.), *Psychosocial nursing. Care of physically ill patients and their families* (3rd ed., pp. 505–524). Philadelphia: Lippincott-Raven.

Bauer, T., & Barron, C. (1995). Nursing interventions for spiritual care: Preferences of the community based elderly. *Journal of Holistic Nursing, 13*(3), 268–279.

Benner, P., & Wrubel, J. (1989). *The primacy of caring.* Menlo Park, CA: Addison-Wesley.

Bennett, J. (2000). Empowering persons affected by acquired immunodeficiency syndrome. In J. F. Miller, (Ed.), pp. 21–53). *Coping with chronic illness* (3rd ed.). Philadelphia: F. A. Davis.

Blevins, D., Berg, J., & Dunbar-Jacob, J. (1998). Compliance. In I. M. Lubkin & P. D. Larsen (Eds.), *Chronic Illness: Impact and Interventions* (4th ed.). Boston: Jones & Bartlett.

Boland, D., & Sims, S. L. (1996). Family care giving at home as a solitary journey. *IMAGE: Journal of Nursing Scholarship, 28*(1), 55–58.

Brillhart, B. (2000). Nursing management: Patient with a stroke. In S. M. Lewis, M. M. Heitkemper, & S. R. Dirksen (Eds.), *Medical-surgical nursing: Assessment and management of clinical problems* (5th ed., pp. 1645–1652). St. Loius, MO: Mosby.

Callaghan, D. (1992). *Living with diabetes: A qualitative study.* Unpublished master's thesis, University of Manchester, Manchester.

Callaghan, D., & Williams, A. (1994). Living with diabetes: Issues for nursing practice. *Journal of Advanced Nursing, 20,* 132–139.

Canadian Charter of Rights and Freedoms. (1982). Ottawa: Government of Canada.

Canadian Public Health Association. (1990). *Community health—public health nursing in Canada.* Ottawa: Author.

Charmaz, K. (1983). Loss of self: A fundamental form of suffering in the chronically ill. *Sociology of Health and Illness, 5*(2), 168–195.

Charmaz, K. (1991). *Good days, bad days: The self in chronic illness and time.* New Brunswick, NJ: Rutgers University Press.

Coates, V., & Boore, J. (1995). Self-management of chronic illness: Implications for nursing. *International Journal of Nursing Studies, 32*(6), 628–640.

Cohen, C. A., Pushkar Gold, D., Shulman, K. I., & Zucchero, C. A. (1994). Positive aspects of caregiving: An overlooked variable in research. *Canadian Journal of Aging, 13*(3), 378–391.

Conrad, P. (1987). The experience of chronic illness: Recent and new directions. In J. A. Roth & P. Conrad (Eds.), *Research in the sociology of health care: The experiences and management of chronic illness.* Greenwich, CT: JAI Press.

Conrad, P. (1990). Qualitative research on chronic illness: A commentary on method and conceptual development. *Social Science and Medicine, 30*(11), 1257–1263.

Conrad, P., & Gallagher, E. (1993). Introduction. In P. Conrad & E. Gallagher (Eds.), *Health and health care in developing countries.* Philadelphia: Temple University Press.

Corbin, J., & Strauss, A. L. (1987). Accompaniments of chronic illness: Changes in body, self, biography, and biographical time. *Sociology of Health Care, 6,* 249–281.

Corbin, J., & Strauss, A. L. (1988). *Unending work and care: Managing chronic illness at home.* San Francisco: Jossey-Bass.

Corbin, J., & Strauss, A. L. (1992). A nursing model for chronic illness management based upon the trajectory framework. In P. Wong (Ed.), *The chronic illness trajectory framework: The Corbin and Strauss nursing model* (pp. 9–28). New York: Springer Publishing Company.

Corbin, J., & Cherry, J. (1997). Caring for the aged in the community. In E. Swanson & T. Tripp-Reimer (Eds.), *Advances in gerontological nursing: Chronic illness and the older adult* (pp. 62–81). New York: Springer Publishing Company.

Corbin, J. M. (1998). The Corbin and Strauss chronic illness trajectory model: An update. *Scholarly Inquiry*

for Nursing Practice: An International Journal, 12(1) 33–41.

Curtin, M. & Lubkin, I. M. (1998). What is chronicity. In I. M. Lubkin & P. D. Larsen (Eds.), *Chronic illness: Impact and interventions* (4th ed.). Boston: Jones & Bartlett.

Division of General Pediatric and Adolescent Health and the Regents of the University of Minnesota. (2001). *Center for Children with Chronic Illness and Disability.* [On-line]. Available: http://www.peds.umn.edu/peds-adol/cc.html.

Epp, J. (1986). *Achieving health for all: A framework for health promotion.* Ottawa, Canada: National Health and Welfare.

Fahlberg, L. L., Poulin, A. L., Girdano, D. A., & Dusek, D. E. (1991). Empowerment as an emerging approach in health education. *Journal of Health Education, 22*(3), 185–193.

Ficke, H. (1995). Being a caregiver and a bread winner, too. *BC Caregiver News, 1*(3), 1.

Funnel, M., Anderson, M. R., Arnold, M. A., Barr, P. A., Donnelly, M. Johnson, P. D., Taylor-Moon, D., & White, N. H. (1991). Empowerment: An idea whose time has come in diabetes education. *Diabetes Education, 17*(1), 37–41.

Funnel, M. M. (2000). Helping patients take charge of their chronic illnesses. *Family Practice Management, 7*(3), 47–52.

Gerhardt, U. (1990). Qualitative research on illness: The issue and the story. *Social Science and Medicine, 30*(11), 1161–1172.

Given, B. A., & Given, C. W. (1998). Health promotion for family caregivers of chronically ill elders. *Annual Review of Nursing Research, 16,* 197–217.

Harkness, G. A. (1995). *Epidemiology in nursing practice.* St. Louis, MO: Mosby.

Hartrick, G., Lindsey, A. E., & Hills, M. (1994). Family nursing assessment: Meeting the challenge of health promotion. *Journal of Advanced Nursing, 20,* 85–91.

Hymovich, D. P., & Hagopian, G. A. (1992). *Chronic illness in children and adults: A psychosocial approach.* Philadelphia: Saunders.

Joachim, G., & Acorn, S. (2000). Stigma of visible and invisible chronic conditions. *Journal of Advanced Nursing, 32*(1), 243–248.

Kozier, B., Erb, G., Berman, A., & Burke, K. (2000). *Fundamentals of nursing: Concepts, process and practice* (6th ed.). Redwood City, CA: Addison-Wesley.

Labonte, R. (1990). Empowerment: Notes on community and professional dimensions. *Canadian Research on Social Policy, 26,* 64–75.

Lazarus, R., & Folkman, S. (1984). *Stress, appraisal and coping.* New York: Springer.

Lindsey, L. (1993). *Health within illness: Experiences of the chronically ill/disabled.* Unpublished doctoral dissertation, University of Victoria, Victoria, British Columbia, Canada.

Lindsey, L. (1995). The gift of healing in chronic illness/disability. *Journal of Holistic Nursing, 13*(4), 287–305.

Lindsey, L. (1996). Health within illness: Experiences of chronically disabled people. *Journal of Advanced Nursing, 24,* 465–472.

Lindsey, L. (1997). Experiences of the chronically ill: A covert caring for the self. *Journal of Holistic Nursing, 15*(3), 227–242.

Lubkin, I. M., & Payne, M. (1998). Family caregivers. In I. M. Lubkin & P. D. Larsen (Eds.), *Chronic illness: Impact and interventions* (4th ed., pp. 258–281). Boston: Jones & Bartlett.

Meeberg, G. A. (1993). Quality of life: A concept analysis. *Journal of Advanced Nursing, 18,* 32–38.

Michael, S. R. (1996). Integrating chronic illness into one's life: A phenomenological inquiry. *Journal of Holistic Nursing, 14*(3), 251–267.

Miller, J. F. (2000a). Client power resources. In J. F. Miller (Ed.), *Coping with chronic illness* (3rd ed., pp. 3–21). Philadelphia: F. A. Davis.

Miller, J. F. (2000b). Analysis of coping with illness. In J. F. Miller (Ed.), *Coping with chronic illness* (3rd ed., pp. 21–53). Philadelphia: F. A. Davis.

Mishel, M. H. (1999) Uncertainty in chronic illness. *Annual Review of Nursing Research, 17,* 269–294.

Mishel, M. H., & Braden, C. J. (1988). Finding meaning: Antecedents of uncertainty in illness. *Nursing Research, 37*(2), 98–103, 127.

National Center for Health Statistics. (1996). DHHS release latest progress report on prevention. *1996 Fact Sheet.* Hyattsville, MD: Public Health Service.

National Center for Health Statistics. (1999). *Vital and health statistics:*

Current estimates from the national health interview survey, 1996 (Vol. 10, No. 200). Hyattsville, MD: Author.

National Center for Health Statistics. (2000). *Deaths: Final data for 1998.* (Vol. 48, No. 11). 48(11) Hyattsville, MD: Public Health Service.

Neuberger, G., & Woods, C. T. (1998). Alternative modalities. In I. M. Lubkin & P. D. Larsen (Eds.), *Chronic illness: Impact and interventions* (4th ed., pp. 407–425). Boston: Jones & Bartlett.

Peters, D. (1998). Individual and family growth and development. In I. M. Lubkin & P. D. Larsen (Eds.), *Chronic illness: Impact and interventions* (4th ed, pp. 26–51). Boston: Jones & Bartlett.

Roberson, M. H. B. (1992). The meaning of compliance: Patient perspectives. *Qualitative Health Research, 2*(1), 7–26.

Rutman, D. (1995). *Caregiving as women's work. Women's experiences of powerlessness and powerfulness.* Victoria, Canada: University of Victoria.

Saylor, C., & Yoder, M. (1998). Stigma. In I. M. Lubkin & P. D. Larsen (Eds.), *Chronic illness: Impact and interventions* (4th ed., pp. 103–120). Boston: Jones & Bartlett.

Statistics Canada. (2000a). *Age-standardized mortality rates* (Publication No. 82F0075XCB). Ottawa: Author.

Statistics Canada. (2000b). *Population predications for 2001, 2006, 2011, 2016, 2021 and 2026, July 1. CANSOM, Matrix 6900.* Ottawa: Author.

Statistics Canada. (2001). *Health Reports: How healthy are Canadians?* (Vol. 12, No. 3). Ottawa: Author.

Sterling-Fisher, C. E. (1998). Spiritual care and chronically ill clients. *Home Healthcare Nurse, 16*(4), 243–249.

Strauss, A. L. (1975). *Chronic illness and quality of life.* St. Louis: C. V. Mosby.

Subedi, J., & Subedi, S. (1993). The contribution of modern medicine in a traditional system: The case of Nepal. In P. Conrad & E. Gallagher (Eds.), *Health and health care in developing countries.* Philadelphia: Temple University Press.

Thorne, S. E. (1993). *Negotiating health care: The social context of chronic illness.* Newbury Park, CA: Sage.

Thorne, S. E., Nyhlin, K. T., & Paterson, B. L. (2000). Attitudes toward patient expertise in chronic illness. *International Journal of Nursing Studies, 37,* 303–311.

Tomm, K. (1988). Interventive interviewing: Part III. Intending to ask linear, circular, strategic, or reflexive questions? *Family Process, 27*(1), 1–15.

U.S. Bureau of the Census. (2000). *Profiles of general demographic characteristics: 2000 census of population and housing, United States.* Washington, DC: Author.

U.S. Department of Health and Human Services. (1992). *Healthy people 2000: National health promotion and disease prevention objectives.* Summary report. Boston: Jones & Bartlett.

U.S. Department of Health and Human Services. (1998). *Health, United States, 1998 with socioeconomic status and health chartbook.* Hyattsville, MD: Author.

U.S. Department of Health and Human Services. (1999a). *Vital and health statistics: Current estimates from the national health interview survey, 1996.* Hyattsville, MD: Author.

U.S. Department of Health and Human Services. (1999b). *Health, United States, 1999 with health and aging chartbook.* Hyattsville, MD: Author.

U.S. Department of Health and Human Services. (1999c). *Chronic diseases and their risk factors: The nation's leading causes of death.* Hyattsville, MD: Author.

U.S. Department of Health and Human Services. (2000a). *Healthy people 2010.* Boston: Jones & Bartlett.

U.S. Department of Health and Human Services. (2000b). *Health, United States, 2000 with adolescent health chartbook.* Hyattsville, MD: Author.

Walton, J. (1996). Spiritual relationships: A concept analysis. *Journal of Holistic Nursing, 14*(3), 237–250.

Washington Department of Health. (1993). *A progress report from the Washington state core government public health functions task force. Core public health functions.* Olympia, WA: Author.

Watson, J. (1988). *Nursing: Human science and human care: A theory of nursing.* New York: National League for Nursing.

White, N., & Lubkin, I. M. (1997). Illness trajectory. In I. M. Lubkin & P. D. Larsen (Eds.), *Chronic illness: Impact and interventions* (4th ed., pp. 53–76). Boston: Jones & Bartlett.

World Bank. (1993). *World development report: 1993 investing in health.* Executive summary. Oxford, England: Oxford University Press.

World Health Organization. (1974). *Community health nursing.* WHO Expert Committee Report No. 558. Geneva: Author.

World Health Organization. (1978). *Alma-Ata 1978: Primary health care. Report of the international conference on primary health care.* Geneva: Author.

World Health Organization. (1980). *International Classification of Impairments, Disabilities and Handicaps.* Geneva: Author.

World Health Organization. (1985). *Report of a WHO study group. Technical Report Series 727.* Geneva: Author.

World Health Organization. (1986). *Ottawa charter for health promotion.* Ottawa, Ontario, Canada: World Health Organization, Health and Welfare Canada, and Canadian Public Health Association.

Wright, L. M., & Leahey, M. (2000). *Nurses and families: A guide to family assessment and intervention* (3rd ed.). Philadelphia: F. A. Davis.

Wuest, J. (1993). Removing the shackles: A feminist critique of noncompliance. *Nursing Outlook, 41*(5), 217–224.

Zarate, A. O. (1994). *International mortality chartbook: Levels and trends, 1955–91.* Hyattsville, MD: Public Health Service.

CHAPTER 28: DEVELOPMENTAL DISORDERS

Administration of Developmental Disabilities. (1999). [On-line]. Available: www.acf.dhhs.gov/programs.

Administration of Developmental Disabilities (2000). *ADD Fact Sheet.* [On-line]. Available: http://www.acf.dhhs.gov/programs/add/Factsheet.htm.

American Academy of Pediatrics. (1996). Policy statement on sexuality education of children and adolescents with developmental disabilities (RE9603). *Pediatrics, 97*(2), 275–278.

American Association on Mental Retardation. (2000). *About AAMR, Mission Statement.* [On-line]. Available: www.aamr.org.

American Cerebral Palsy Information Center. (2001). Cerebral palsy statistics. [On-line]. Available: www.cerebralpalsy.org.

American Psychiatric Association. (2000). *Diagnostic and statistical manual of mental disorders* (DSM-IV-TR) (4th ed.). Washington, DC: Author.

Americans with Disabilities Act. (1990).

Association of Retarded Citizens (ARC). (1997, 1998, 2000). Position statements. [On-line]. Available: www. thearc.org.

Association of Retarded Citizens. (2001). *Introduction to mental retardation.* [On-line]. Available: www.thearc.org.

Batshaw, M. (1997). *Children with disabilities.* Baltimore: Paul H. Brookes Publishing Co.

Bigby, C. (1998). Parental substitutes? The role of siblings in the lives of older people with intellectual disability. *Journal of Gerontological Social Work, 29*(1), 3–21.

Black, M. and Matula, K. (2002). *Essentials of Bayley Scale of Infant Development II.* New York: Wiley & Sons, Inc.

Bogdan, R., & Taylor, S. (1999). *Building stronger communities for all: Thoughts about community participation for people with developmental disabilities. President's Committee on Mental Retardation's Forgotten Generations Conference.* [On-line]. Available: http://soeweb.syr.edu/thechp/pcmr.html.

Braddock, D., & Hemp, R. (2000). *Developmental disability services in Indiana: Assessing Progress through 2000.* [On-line]. Available: www. state. in.us/fssa/servicedisabl/olmstead/devdisabil.html.

Brown, A. (2001). *Masspsy.com,9:1.* [On-line]. Available: www.masspsy. com/columnists/brown_9910.html.

CDC (2001). *Facts.* [On-line]. Available at: http://www.cdc.gov/ncbdd/dd/default.htm.

Centers for Disease Control and Prevention. (1998). *Birth defects and pediatric genetics.* [On-line]. Available: www.cdc.gov/nceh/cddh/BD/bdpghome.htm.

Centers for Disease Control and Prevention. (2000). *Disabilities branch: Neurodevelopmental therapies & mandated benefits sunrise review.* [On-line]. Available: www.cdc.gov/nceh/cddh/ddhome.html.

Center for Fetal Diagnosis and Treatment. (2001). *About the Center.* [On-line]. Available: http://fetalsurgery. chop.edu.

Cerebral Palsy Information Central. (2001). *Watch your language.* [On-line]. Available: www.geocities.com/HotSprings/Sauna/4441.

Children and adults with attention deficit/hyperactivity disorder. (2001).

[On-line]. Available: www.chadd.org/facts/add_facts03.hrm.

Clark, M. J. (1999). *Nursing in the community* (3rd ed.). Stamford, CT: Appleton & Lange.

Clemen-Stone, S., McGuire, S. L., & Eigsti, D. G. (1998). *Comprehensive community health nursing* (5th ed.). St. Louis, MO: Mosby.

Coerver, T. (1999). *Looking for information re: dual diagnosis (mental illness and developmental disorders).* [On-line]. Available: www.nwlink.com.

Council of Regional Networks for Genetic Services.(CORN). (1998). Newborn Screening Committee. *National Newborn Screening Report — 1993.* Atlanta, GA: CORN.

Developmental Disabilities Assistance and Bill of Rights Act. (1996). Public Law 104-183, Section 102.

Doenges, M. E., Moorhouse, M. F., & Geissler, A. C. (2000). *Nursing care plans* (5th ed.). Philadelphia: F. A. Davis.

Dzienkowski, R., Smith, K., Dillow, K, & Yucha, C. (1996). Cerebral palsy: A comprehensive review. *Nurse Practitioner, 21,* 45–59.

Engel, J. (1999). Message from the President. *Epileptic Disorders, 1*(1), 5–6.

Epilepsy and Brain Mapping Program. (2000). [On-line]. Available: www. epipro.com.

Epilepsy Foundation of America. (2001). History & milestones: Seizure recognition. [On-line]. Available: www. efa.org.

Federal Register. (1999). Department of Education Rules and Regulations, Vol. 64, p. 121.

Glascoe, S. F. (1999). Using parents' concerns to detect and address developmental and behavioral problems. *Journal of the Society of Pediatric Nursing, 4,* 24–36.

Goldman, L. (1998). Diagnosis and treatment of attention-deficit/hyperactivity disorder in children and adolescents. *Journal of the American Medical Association, 279,* 1100–1107.

Hansma, M. (1997). Disaster plans for disabled students. *Public Risk, 4,* 27–28.

Healthy people 2010. (2000). [On-line]. Available: http://health.gov/healthypeople/Document/html/jih/jih_1.htm.

Heller, T., & Factor, A. (2001). Rehabilitation Research and Training Center on Aging and Developmental Disability, Institute on Disability and Human Development. University of Illinois at Chicago. *Older adults with mental*

retardation and their aging family caregivers. [On-line]. Available: www. uic.edu/org/rrtcamr/FACTS399.html.

Individuals with Disabilities Act. (1990, 1997). [On-line]. Available: www. ideapractices.org.

Individuals with Disabilities Education Act (P. L. 944-142). *Education of All Handicapped Children Act.* [On-line]. Available: http://www.scn.org/~bk269/94-142.html.

Ingram. D. (1993). Association of Retarded Citizens' Department of Research and Program Services, Family Support Services. *Parents who have mental retardation.* [On-line]. Available: www.thearc.org.

International classification of impairments, disabilities and handicaps. (2001). [On-line]. Available: www. who.int/icidh.

International Classification of Seizures. (2002). Information leaflets: Seizures. [On-line]. Available: www.epilepsynse. org.uk/pages/info/leaflets/seizures.cmf.

International Dyslexia Association. (1998). [On-line]. Available: www. interdys.org/abcsofdyslexia.

International League against Epilepsy. (2002). *ILAE Epilepsy classification and terminology overview.* [On-line]. Available: www.ilae-epilepsy.org.

Job Accommodation Network. (2001). *An overview of the American's with Disabilities Act.* [On-line]. Available: janweb.icdi.wvu.edu/kinder/overview.htm.

Kee, J. L., & Hayes, E. R. (2000). *Pharmacology* (3rd ed.). Philadelphia: W. B. Saunders.

Keith, L. G., Ozeszczuk, J. J., & Keith, D. M. (2000). Multiple gestation: Reflections on epidemiology, causes, and consequences. *International Journal of Fertility, 45/3,* 206–214.

Kewley, G., & Latham, P. (2000). Children with ADHD: How to manage an important condition. *Community Practitioner, 75*(4), 562–565.

Knoblauch, B. (1998). *An overview of the Individuals with Disabilities Education Act Amendments of 1997,* (P.L. 105-17) ERIC Digest. [On-line]. Available: www.ed.gov/databases/ERIC_Digests/ed/430325.html.

Kramer, R. A., Allen, P., & Gergen, P. J. (1995). Health and social characteristics and children's cognitive functioning: Results from a national cohort. *American Journal of Public Health, 85,* 312–318.

Lacy, B. K. (2000). Aging with cerebral palsy: A consumer's perspective. *Aging in Action, 15*(1), 1–20.

Luckmann, J. (1999). *Transcultural communication in nursing.* Clifton Park, NY: Delmar Learning.

Morse, J., & Colatarci, S. (1994). The impact of technology. In S. P. Roth & J. S. Morse (Eds.), *A life span approach to nursing care for individuals with developmental disabilities* (pp. 351–383). Baltimore: Paul H. Brookes Publishing.

Murray, R. B., & Zentner, J. P. (2001). *Health promotion strategies through the life span* (7th ed.). Upper Saddle River, NJ: Prentice-Hall.

National Information Center for Children and Youth with Disabilities. (1994). *Children with disabilities: Understanding sibling issues.* Washington, DC.

National Information Center for Children and Youth with Disabilities. (2001). *NICHCY Search for organizations.* [On-line]. Available: www. nichcy.org.

National Institute of Disability and Rehabilitation Research. (2001). *Research & Statistics.* (2001). [On-line]. Available: www.ed.gov/offices/OSERS/NIDRR.

National Institutes of Health. (1998). Consensus statements: 110. Diagnosis & treatment of attention deficit hyperactivity disorder. (2001). [On-line]. Available: odp.od.nih.gov/consensus/cons/110/110_statement.htm.

National Institute of Neurological Disorders and Strokes. *What is epilepsy?* (2001). [On-line]. Available: www. ninds.nih.gov.

Niebuhr, V. N., & Smith, L. R. (1993). The school nurse's role in attention deficit hyperactivity disorder. *Journal of School Health, 63*(2), 112–115.

Pacer (1995). *What makes a good individual education plan for your child?* [On-line]. Available: www.pacer.org/parent/iep.

Persons with Disabilities. (2001). *The UN and persons with disabilities.* [On-line]. Available: www.un.org/esa/socdev/enable.

Priaulx, E. (2000). P & A's are monitoring community placements. *Protection and Advocacy Systems News, 5*(1).

Rapp, C. E., & Torres, M. M. (2000). The adult with cerebral palsy. *Archives of Family Medicine, 9,* 466–472.

Sarasquetta, L. (1998, Spring). On Chronic Sorrow. *Hydrocephalus Association Newsletter.* [On-line]. Available: www.hydroassoc.org/newsletter/.

Schwier, K. M. (1995). *Couples with intellectual disabilities talk about living and loving.* Rockville, MD: Woodbine House.

Sheerin. (1998). Parents with learning disabilities: A review of the literature. *Journal of Advanced Nursing, 28*(1), 126–133.

Smelzer, S. C., & Bare, B. G. (2000). *Textbook of medical surgical nursing* (9th ed.). Philadelphia: J. B. Lippincott.

Spencer, E. (1960). *The light in the piazza.* New York: McGraw-Hill.

Statement by the president. (2000). [On-line]. Available: www.acf.dhhs.gov/ news.

Stewart, G. W., & Laraia, M. T. (1998). *Principles and practice of psychiatric nursing* (6th ed.). St. Louis, MO: Mosby.

Townsend, M. C. (2000). *Psychiatric mental health nursing.* Philadelphia: F. A. Davis.

United Cerebral Palsy. (2001). *Health & wellness* [On-line]. Available: www. ucp.org.

U.S. Department of Health and Human Services. (2000). *Care, rehabilitation, research, and disability prevention* [On-line]. Available: www.cdc.gov/ncipc/dacrrdp/dacrrdp.htm.

Valenti-Hein, D., & Schwartz, L. (1995). *The sexual abuse interview for those with developmental disabilities.* Santa Barbara: CA: James Stanfield Company.

Varcarolis, E. (1998). *Foundations of psychiatric mental health nursing* (3rd ed.). Philadelphia: W. B. Saunders.

WHO/ILAE/IBE global campaign against epilepsy. (1997). [On-line]. Available: www.who.int/msa/mnh/nrs/neuro3.htm.

Wittert, D. (2001). Parental reactions to having a child with disabilities. *Nursing Spectrum Career Fitness.* [On-line]. Available: http://community.nursingspectrum.com.

Wolbring, G. (2000). In focus: Risk and prevention of maltreatment of children with disabilities. [On-line]. Available: www.nccanch@calib.com.

Wolfensberger, W. (1972). *Normalization: The principle of normalization in human services.* Toronto: National Institute on Mental Retardation.

Wong, D. (1999). *Whaley and Wong's nursing care of infants and children* (6th ed.). St. Louis, MO: Mosby

World Health Organization. (1997). *International classification of functioning and disability (ICIDH-2): Beta-1 draft for field Trails,* Geneva, Switzerland: Author.

Zubal, R., & Drake, S. (2001). *Internet resources concerning people with developmental disabilities.* [On-line]. Available: htt://soeweb.syr.edu/thechp/internet.html.

CHAPTER 29: MENTAL HEALTH AND ILLNESS

American Nurses Association. (1994). *Statement on the scope and standards of psychiatric-mental health clinical nursing practice.* Washington, DC: Author.

American Psychiatric Association. (1993). *Idea and information exchange for disaster response.* Washington, DC: Author.

American Psychiatric Association. (2000). *Diagnostic and statistical manual of mental disorders* (text revision). Washington, DC: Author.

Barreira, P. J., & Cohen, B. M. (2000, November 13). Second class care for mental health? *Boston Globe,* pp. Op-Ed.

Brittingham, A. (2000). *The foreign-born population in the United States: Population characteristics.* Washington, DC: U.S. Census Bureau.

Ditton, P. M. (1999). *Mental health and treatment of inmates and probationers* (Rep. No. NCJ 174463). Washington, DC: Bureau of Justice Statistics, U.S. Department of Justice.

Dowrick, C., Dunn, G., Ayuso-Mateos, J. L., Dalgard, O. S., Page, H., Lehtinen, V., Casey, P., Wilkinson, C., Vazquez-Barquero, J. L., & Wilkinson, G. (2000). Problem solving treatment and group psychoeducation for depression: Multicentre randomised controlled trial. *British Medical Journal, 321,* 1450–1456.

Firestone, R. W. (1997). *Suicide and the inner voice: Risk assessment, treatment, and case management.* Thousand Oaks, CA: Sage.

Freud, S. (1938). In A. A. Brill (Ed. and Trans.), *The basic writings of Sigmund Freud.* New York: The Modern Library.

Frisch, N. C., & Frisch, L. E. (2002). The client who is suicidal. In N. C. Frisch & L. E. Frisch (Eds.), *Psychiatric mental health nursing* (2nd ed., pp. 303–327). Clifton Park, NY: Delmar Learning.

Golden, B. (1994). *Mental health screening.* Unpublished.

Guarnaccia, P. J., & Lopez, S. (1998). The mental health and adjustment of immigrant and refugee children.

Child and Adolescent Psychiatry Clinics of North America, 7, 537.

Guy, W. (1976). *Abnormal Involuntary Movement Scale (AIMS).* Rockville, MD: National Institute of Mental Health.

Kaminski, P., & Harty, C. (1999). From stigma to strategy. *Nursing Standard, 1*(38), 36–40.

Kaplan, H. I., Sadock, B. J., Grebb, J. A. (1998). *Synopsis of psychiatry: Behavioral sciences, clinical psychiatry.* Baltimore: Williams & Wilkins.

Kessler, R. C., McGonagle, K. A., Zhao, S., Nelson, C., Hughes, M., Eshleman, S., Wittchen, H. U., & Kendler, K. S. (1994). Lifetime and 12-month prevalence of DSM-III-R psychiatric disorders in the United States. *Archives of General Psychiatry, 51*(8), 8–19.

Kim, S. (1998). Our of darkness. *Reflections, 24,* 8–12.

Maslow, A. H. (1962). *Toward a psychology of living.* Princeton, NJ: Van Nostrand.

Martin, K. S., & Scheet, N. J. (1992). *The Omaha system: Applications for community health nursing.* Philadelphia: W. B. Saunders.

Meleis, A. L. (1997). *Theoretical nursing: Development and progress* (3rd ed.). Philadelphia: Lippincott-Raven.

Melville, H. (n.d.). In W. J. Clinton, Remarks by the president at memorial service for Al Shanker (April 9, 1997) [On-line]. Retrieved February 25, 2002: http://www.ed.gov/PressReleases/04-997/040997pa.html.

Murray, C. L. (1996). *The global burden of disease: A comprehensive assessment of mortality and disability from diseases, injuries, and risk factors in 1990 and projected.* Boston: Harvard School of Public Health.

Murray R. B., & Baier M. (1993). Use of therapeutic milieu in a community setting. *Journal of Psychosocial Nursing, 31*(10), 11–16.

National Alliance for the Mentally Ill. (2000). *History and mission of NAMI.* Arlington, VA: Author. [On-line]. Available: http://www.nami.org/history.htm.

National Institute of Mental Health. (1999). *Suicide Facts* [On-line]. Available: http://www.nimh.nih.gov/publicat/suicidefacts.cfm.

North American Nursing Diagnosis Association. (2001). *NANDA nursing diagnoses: Definitions and classifica-*

tion 2001–2002. Philadelphia: Author. Taylor, S. G., & Renpenning, K. M.

Ohlund, G. (1997). Psychiatric home care benchmarking study. Unpublished study cited in B. J. Taylor, V. B. Carson, & T. Bales, Home Healthcare Nurses Association psychiatric home care nursing position statement. *Home Healthcare Nurse, 17,* 149–152.

Orem, D. E., (2001). *Nursing concepts of practice* (6th ed.). St. Louis, MO: Mosby-Yearbook.

Peplau, H. E. (1952). *Interpersonal relations in nursing.* New York: G. P. Putnam's Sons.

Porter, R. (1989). *A social history of madness: The world through the eyes of the insane.* New York: E. P. Dutton.

Rabins, P. V., Black, B. S., Roca, R., German, P., McGuire, M., Robbins, B., Rye, R., & Brant, L. (2000). Effectiveness of a nurse-based outreach program for identifying and treating psychiatric illness in the elderly. *Journal of the American Medical Association, 283,* 2802–2809.

Saulnier, C. F. (1998). Prevalence of suicide attempts and suicidal ideation among lesbian and gay youth. In L. M. Sloan & N. S. Gustavsson (Eds.), *Violence and social injustice against lesbian, gay and bisexual people.* New York: Harrington Park Press.

Skinner, B. F. (1953). *Science and human behavior.* New York: Macmillan.

Sullivan, H. S. (1953). In H. S. Perry, and M. L. Gawel, (Eds.), *The interpersonal theory of psychiatry.* New York: W. W. Norton & Co.

Taylor, B. J., Carson, V. B., & Bales, T. (1999). Home Healthcare Nurses Association psychiatric home care nursing position statement. *Home Healthcare Nurse, 17,* 149–152.

Tye, L. (2001, June 5). Mentally ill at risk of early death, state finds. *Boston Globe,* pp. A1, A13.

U.S. Department of Health and Human Services. (1996). *Healthy people 2000: Midcourse review and 1995 revisions.* Sudbury, MA: Jones & Bartlett.

U.S. Department of Health and Human Services. (1999). *Mental health: A report of the surgeon general.* Rockville, MD: Public Health Service.

U.S. Department of Health and Human Services. (2000). *Healthy people 2010.* Washington, DC: Author.

Walker, P. F., & Jaranson, J. (1999). Refugee and immigrant health care. *Medical Clinics of North America, 83,* 1103–1120.

Weiden, P., & Havens, L. (1994). Psychotherapeutic management techniques in the treatment of outpatients with schizophrenia. *Hospital and Community Psychiatry, 45*(6), 549–555.

Whooley, M. A., & Simon, G. E. (2000). Managing depression in medical outpatients. *New England Journal of Medicine, 343,* 1942–1950.

World Health Organization. (1992). *Psychosocial consequences of disasters: Prevention and management.* Geneva: Author.

CHAPTER 30: FAMILY AND COMMUNITY VIOLENCE

Abracen, J., Looman, J., & Anderson, D. (2000). Alcohol and drug abuse in sexual and nonsexual violent offenders. *Sexual Abuse, 12*(4), 263–274.

Affara, F. A. (2000). When tradition maims. *American Journal of Nursing, 100*(8), 52–63.

Allan, M. A. (1998). Elder abuse: A challenge for home care nurses. *Home Healthcare Nurse, 16*(2), 103–110.

Bandura, A. (1973). *Aggression: A social learning analysis,* Englewood Cliffs, NJ: Prentice Hall.

Baron, R. A. (1977). *Human aggression.* New York: Plenum.

Bethea, L. (1999). Primary prevention of child abuse. *American Family Physician, 59*(6), 1577–1585.

Bogard, M. (1992). Values in conflict: Challenges to family therapists' thinking. *Journal of Marital and Family Therapy, 18*(3), 245–256.

Brody, J. E. (1999). Guns in the house endanger innocent lives. In H. H. Kim (Ed.), *Guns and violence* (pp. 152–154). San Diego: Greenhaven.

Bull, M. J., Agran, P., Laraque, D., Pollack, S. H., Smith, G. A., Spivak, H. R., Tenenbein, M., & Tully, S. B. (2000). Firearm-related injuries affecting the pediatric population. *American Academy of Pediatrics, 105*(4), 888–895.

Butler, M. J. (1995). Domestic violence—A nursing imperative. *Journal of Holistic Nursing, 13*(1), 54–69.

Campbell, J., & Humphreys, J. (1984). *Nursing care of victims of violence.* Reston, VA: Reston Publishing.

Campell, J. G. (1992). Violence against women. *Nursing and Health Care, 13,* 467–470.

Cassidy, K. (1999). How to assess and intervene in domestic violence situations. *Home Healthcare Nurse, 17*(10), 665–670.

Christensen, L. W. (1999). *Understanding the deadly minds of America's street gangs.* Boulder, CO: Paladin.

Christoffel, K. K., Spivack, H., & Witwer, M. (2000). Youth violence prevention: The physician's role. *Journal of the American Medical Association, 283*(9), 1202–1203.

Clarke, P. N., Pendry, N. C., & Kim, Y. S. (1997). Patterns of violence in homeless women. *Western Journal of Nursing Research, 19,* 490–500.

Community United Against Violence. (1998). [On-line]. Available: www.xq.com/cuav.truths.

Council on Ethical and Judicial Affairs, American Medical Association. (1992). Physicians and domestic violence: Ethical considerations. *Journal of the American Medical Association, 267,* 3190–3193.

Crowell, N. A., & Burgess, A. W. (Eds.). (1996). *Understanding violence against women.* Washington, DC: National Academy Press.

Dahlberg, L. I., & Potter, L. B. (2001). Youth violence. *American Journal of Preventive Medicine, 20*(15), 3–14.

D'Antonio, M. (1999). Ways to reduce gun violence: An overview. In H. H. Kim (Ed.), *Guns and violence* (pp. 164–169). San Diego, CA: Greenhaven.

Dobash, R. E., & Dobash, R. P. (1992). *Women, violence, and social change.* New York: Routledge.

Duhaine, A. C., Christion, C. W., Rorke, L. B., & Zimmerman, R. A. (1998). Nonaccidental head injury in infants: The shaken baby syndrome. *New England Journal of Medicine, 338,* 1822–1829.

DuRant, R. H., Krowchuk, D. P., Kreiter, S., Sinal, S. H., & Woods, C. R. (1999). Weapon carrying on school property among middle school students. *Archives of Pediatric and Adolescent Medicine, 153,* 21–26.

Eisenstat, S. A., & Zimmer, B. (1998). Providing medical care and advocacy for survivors of domestic abuse, *Journal of Clinical Outcomes Management, 5*(5), 54–64.

Erhart, J. K., and Sandler, B. R. (1985). *Myths and realities about rape.* Washington, DC: Project on the Status and Education of Women.

Eyler, A. E., & Cohen, M. (1999). Case studies in partner violence. *American Family Physician, 60*(9), 2569–2576.

Fauman, M. A. (1994). *Study guide to DSM-IV.* Washington, DC: American Psychiatric Press, Inc.

FBI Hate Crimes Statistics, (2001). [On-line]. Available: www.fbi.gov/ucr/98hate.pdf.

Fee, E. & Brown, T. M. (2001). Preemptive biopreparedness: Can we learn anything from history? *American Journal of Public Health, 91,* 721–726.

Feldhaus, K. M., & Kaminsky, R. (1999). Lifetime sexual assault prevalence rates and reporting patterns in an emergency department population, *Academic Emergency Medicine, 6*(5), 547–556.

Fingerhut, L. A., Ingram, D. D., & Feldman, J. J. (1998). Homicide rates among US teenagers and young adults: Differences by mechanism, level of urbanization, race and sex. *Journal of the American Medical Association, 28*(5), 423–427.

Fromme, E. (1977). *The anatomy of human destructiveness.* Harmondsworth, England: Penguin.

Fullilove, M. T., Heon, V., Jimenez, C., Parsons, C., Green, L. L., & Fullilove, R. E. (1998). Injury and anomie: Effects of violence on an inner-city community. *American Journal of Public Health, 88,* 924–927.

Gilgun, J. F. (1999). *Detecting the potential for violence* (pp. 174–190). Twin Cities: University of Minnesota, School of Social Work, Minnesota Center Against Violence and Abuse.

Graham-Bermann, S. A. (2001). Designing intervention evaluations for children exposed to domestic violence: Applications of research and theory. In S. A. Graham-Bermann & J. L. Edleson (Eds.), *Domestic violence in the lives of children* (pp. 237–267). Washington, DC: American Psychological Association.

Gray-Vickrey, P. (2000). Protecting the elder, *Nursing 2000, 30*(7), 34–38.

Greenwalt, B. C., Sklare, G., & Portes, P. (1998). The therapeutic treatment provided in cases involving physical child abuse: A description of current practices. *Child Abuse and Neglect, 22,* 71–78.

Hall, L. A., Sachs, B., & Rayens, M. K. (1998). Mothers' potential for child abuse: The roles of childhood abuse and social resources. *Nursing Research, 47,* 87–95.

Helpnetwork (2002). *Trigger Locks: What we know and what's needed.* [On-line]. Available: http://www.helpnetwork.org/firearms/resources trigger.html.

Henderson, H. (2000). *Gun control.* New York: Facts on File, Inc.

Hennes, H. (1998). Review of violence statistics among children and adolescents in the U.S. *Pediatric Clinics of North America, 45*(2), 269–280.

Henritig, F. (2001). Biological and chemical terrorism defense: A view from the "front lines" of public health. *American Journal of Public Health, 91,* 718–720.

Herman-Giddens, M. E., Brown, G., & Verbiest, S. (1999). Underascertainment of child abuse mortality in the United States, *Journal of the American Medical Association, 282,* 463–467.

Hernandez, A. (1998). *Peace in the streets: Breaking the cycle of gang violence.* New York: Child Welfare League of America.

Hetherton, J. (1999). The idealization of women: Its role in the minimization of child sexual abuse by females. *Child Abuse and Neglect, 23,* 161–174.

Hoffman, B. (1998). *Inside terrorism.* New York: Columbia University Press.

Horne, S. (1999). Domestic violence in Russia. *Journal of the American Psychologist Association, 54*(1), 55–61.

Humphreys, J. C. (2001). Growing up in a violent home: The lived experience of daughters of battered women. *Journal of Family Nursing, 7,* 244–260.

Hunt, G., & Joe-Laidler, K. (2001). Situations of violence in the lives of girl gang members. *Health Care for Women International, 22,* 363–384.

Jennings, J. L., & Murphy, C. M. (2000). Male-male dimensions of male-female battering: A new look at domestic violence. *Psychology of Men and Masculinity, 1*(1), 21–29.

Johnson, C. D., Fein, J. A., Campbell, C., & Ginsburg, K. R. (1999). Violence prevention in the primary care setting. *Archives of Pediatric Medicine, 153,* 531–535.

Kaplan, H. B. (1975). *Self-attitudes of deviant behavior.* Pacific Palisades, CA: Goodyear.

Kellerman, A. L. (1994). Annotation: Firearm-related violence—What we don't know is killing us. *American Journal of Public Health, 84*(4), 541–542.

Korbin, J. E., Coulton, C. J., Lindstrom-Ufuti, H., & Spilbury, J. (2000). Neighborhood view on the definition and etiology of child maltreatment. *Child Abuse and Neglect, 24*(12), 1509–1527.

Kozu, J. (1999). Domestic violence in Japan. *Journal of the American Psychologist Association, 54*(1), 50–54.

Lamberg, L. (1998a). Mental illness and violent acts: Protecting the patient and the public. *Journal of the American Medical Association, 280*(5), 407–408.

Lamberg, L. (1998b). Preventing school violence: No easy answer. *Journal of the American Medical Association, 280*(5), 404–406.

Lamberg, L. (1998c). Good news on guns but not for everyone [Medical news and perspectives]. *Journal of the American Medical Association, 280*(5), 403–404.

Lee, S. S., Gergerich, S. G., Waller, L. A., Anderson, A., & McGovern, P. (1999). Work related assault injuries among nurses. *Epidemiology, 10,* 685–691.

Lie, G., Schlitt, R., Bush, J., Montagne, M., & Reyes, L. (1991). Lesbians in currently aggressive relationships: How frequently do they report aggressive past relationships? *Violence and Victims, 6,* 121–135.

Littrell, K., & Littrell, S. (1998). Current understanding of violence and aggression: Assessment and treatment. *Journal of Psychosocial Nursing, 36*(12), 18–24.

Lewis, M. L., & Dehn, D. S. (1999). Violence against nurses in outpatient mental health settings. *Journal of Psychosocial Nursing, 37*(6), 29–33.

Loulan, J. (1987). *Lesbian passion: Loving ourselves and each other.* San Francisco: Spinsters/Aunt Lute.

Mayer, B. W., & Burns, P. (2000). Differential diagnosis of abuse injuries in infants and young children. *Nurse Practitioner, 25*(10), 15–35.

McAllister, M. (2000). Domestic violence: A lifespan approach to assessment and intervention. *Primary Care Practice, 4*(2), 174–189.

McWhirter, P. T. (1999). La violencia privada: Domestic violence in Chile. *Journal of the American Psychologist Association, 54*(1), 37–40.

Mitka, M. (2001). Watch what kids are watching. *Journal of the American Medical Association, 285*(1), 27.

Molnar, B. E., Buka, S. L., & Kessler, R. C. (2001). Child sexual abuse and subsequent psychopathology: Results from the National Comorbidity Survey. *American Journal of Public Health, 91,* 753–760.

Morris, M. R. (1998). Elder abuse: What the law requires. *RN, 61*(8), 52–53.

Mulryan, K., Cathers, P., & Fagin, A. (2000). Protecting the child. *Nursing 2000, 30*(7), 39–43.

National Center for Injury Prevention and Control, Centers for Disease Control and Prevention. (2001, January 12). [On-line]. Available: http://www.cdc.gov.

Nelson, B. S., & Wampler, K. S. (2000). Systemetic effects of trauma in clinic couples: An exploratory study of secondary trauma resulting from childhood abuse. *Journal of Marital and Family Therapy, 25,* 171–184.

Nester, C. B. (1998). Prevention of child abuse and neglect in the primary care setting. *Nurse Practitioner, 23*(9), 61–70.

Nicolette, J., & Nuovo, J. (1999). Reframing our approach to domestic violence: The cyclic batterer syndrome. *American Family Physician, 60*(9), 2498–2501.

Noel, N. L., & Yam, M. (1992). The pregnant battered woman. *Nursing Clinics of North America, 27*(4), 871–883.

Nolan, P., Dallender, J., Soares, J., Thomsen, S., & Arnetz, B. (1999). Violence in mental health care: The experiences of mental health nurses and psychiatrists. *Journal of Advanced Nursing, 30,* 934–941.

Oriel, K. A., & Fleming, M. F. (1998). Screening men for partner violence in a primary care setting. A new strategy for detecting domestic violence. *Journal of Family Practice, 46*(6), 493–498.

Perrin, K. M., Boyett, T. P., & McDermott, R. J. (2000). Continuing education about physically abusive relationships: Does education change the perceptions of health care practitioners? *Journal of Continuing Education in Nursing, 31*(6), 269–274.

Pistorello, J., & Follette, V. M. (1998). Childhood sexual abuse and couples' relationships: Female survivors' reports in therapy groups. *Journal of Marital and Family Therapy, 24,* 473–485.

Powell, T. (1999). Gun ownership is an effective means of self-disclosure. In H. H. Kim (Ed.), *Guns and violence* (pp. 144–146). San Diego, CA: Greenhaven.

Purcell, M. A. (1998). Spiritual abuse. *American Journal of Hospice & Palliative Care, 15,* 227–231.

Quina, K., and Carlson, N. I. (1989). *Rape, incest, and sexual harassment.* New York: Praeger Press.

Randall, T. (1992). Adolescents may experience home, school abuse: their future draws researchers concerns. *Journal of the American Medical Association, 267,* 3127–3131.

Rasekh, Z., Bauer, H. M., Manos, M. M., & Iocopino, V. (1998). Women's health and human rights in Afghanistan, *Journal of the American Medical Association, 280*(5), 449–455.

Romans, S. E., Poore, M. R., & Martin, J. L. (2000). The perpetrators of domestic violence. *Medical Journal of Australia, 173,* 484–488.

Rosado, C. (1999). Spiritual involvement would reduce gun violence. In H. H. Kim (Ed.), *Guns and violence* (pp. 170–178). San Diego: Greenhaven.

Rossman, B. B. R. (2001). Longer term effects of children's exposure to domestic violence. In S. A. Graham-Bermann & J. L. Edleson (Eds.), *Domestic violence in the lives of children* (pp. 35–65). Washington, DC: American Psychological Association.

Runyan C. W. (2001). Moving forward with research on the prevention of violence against workers. *American Journal of Preventive Medicine, 20,* 169–172.

Sams, D. L. (2001). First star: A new approach to the fight against child abuse and neglect. *Caring, 30*(6), 30–32.

Scales, J., Fleischer, A. B., & Sinal, S. H. (1999). Skin lesions that mimic abuse. *Contemporary Pediatrics, 16*(1), 136–147.

Schroeder, M., & Weber, J. R. (1998). Promoting domestic violence education for nurses. *Nursing Forum, 33*(4), 13–21.

Schulte, J. M., Nolt, B. J., Williams, R. L., Sprinks, C. L. & Hillstein, J. J. (1998). Violence and threats of violence experienced by public health fieldworkers. *Journal of the American Medical Association, 280,* 439–442.

Seedat, S., & Stein, D. J. (2000). Trauma and post-traumatic stress disorder in women: A review, *International Clinical Psycopharmacology, 15*(Suppl. 3), 25–33.

Siann, G. (1985). *Accounting for aggression and violence.* London: Allen & Urwin.

Siebel, B. J. (2000). The case against the gun industry. *Public Health Reports, 115,* 410–418.

Smith, D. W., Letourneau, E. J., Saunders, B. E., Kilpatrick, D. G., Resnick, H. S., & Best, C. L. (2000). Delay in disclosure of childhood rape: Results from a national survey. *Child Abuse and Neglect, 24*(2), 273–287.

Smith-DiJulio, K. (1998). Families in crisis: Family violence. In E. M. Varcarolis (Ed.), *Foundations of psychiatric mental health nursing* (3rd ed., pp. 387–418). Philadelpia: W. B. Saunders.

Snyder, H. N. (2000). *Sexual assault of young children as reported to law enforcement: victim, incident, and offender characteristics.* BJS Report, NCJ 182990. Washington, DC: National Center for Juvenile Justice.

Song, L., Singer, M. I., & Anglin, T. (1998). Violent exposure and emotional trauma as contributors to adolescent's violent behavior. *Archives of Pediatric and Adolescent Medicine, 152,* 531–536.

Stanton, B., Baldwin, R. M., & Rachuba, L. A. (1997). A quarter century of violence in the United States: An epidemiological assessment. *Psychiatric Clinics in North America, 20*(2), 269–282.

Storr, A. (1968). *Human aggression.* Harmondsworth, England: Penguin.

Straus, M. (2000). Corporal punishment and primary prevention of physical abuse. *Child Abuse and Neglect, 24*(9), 1109–1114.

Stewart, P. (1995). *Extinguishing the light.* Unpublished manuscript.

Swagerty, D. L., Takahashi, P. Y., & Evans, J. M. (1999). Elder mistreatment. *American Family Physicians, 59*(10), 2804–2808.

The Terrorist Research Center (1997). *The basics of terrorism: Part 1.* [On-line]. Available: www.terrorism.com/terrorism/bpart1.html.

The Terrorist Research Center (1997). *The future of terrorism: Part 6.* [On-line]. Available: www.terrorism.com/terrorism/bpart1.html.

Thobaben, M. (1998). Survivors of violence or abuse. In N. C. Frisch & L. F. Frisch (Eds.), *Psychiatric mental health nursing* (pp. 559–605). Clifton Park, NY: Delmar Learning.

Tjaden, P., & Thoennes, N. T. (2000). *Extent, nature, and consequences of intimate partner violence series: Research report.* Washington, DC: National Institute of Justice and the Centers for Disease Control and Prevention.

Toomey, S., & Bernstein, H. (2001). Child abuse and neglect: Prevention and intervention. *Current Opinions in Pediatric, 13,* 24–25.

Townsend, M. C. (2000). *Psychiatric mental health nursing: Concepts of care* (3rd ed.). Philadelphia: F. A. Davis.

United Nations. (2001). *Latest UN news.* [On-line]. Available: www.un.org/News/dh/latest/page2.html.

Urbancic, J. C. (2000). Survivors of family violence. In K. M. Fortinash & P. A. Holoday-Worret (Eds.), *Psychiatric mental health nursing* (2nd ed., pp. 618–651). St. Louis: Mosby.

U.S. Department of Health and Human Services. (1998). *Child Maltreatment, 1998.* Reports from the State to the National Child Abuse and Neglect. Washington, DC: U.S. Government Printing Office

U.S. Department of Justice. (1998). *Violence by intimates: Analysis of data on crimes by current or former spouses, boyfriends and girlfriends* Washington, DC: U.S. Government Printing Office.

U.S. Department of Health and Human Services Center for Disease Control and Prevention (1999). Non-fatal and fatal firearm related injuries in the U.S. 1993–1997. *MMWR Morbidity and Mortality Weekly Report, 48,* 1029–1034.

U.S. Department of Health and Human Services. (2000). *Healthy people 2010.* Washington, DC: Author.

U.S. Department of Health and Human Services, CDCP, (2002). [On-line]. Available: www.health.gov/healthypeople/document/html/volume2/15injury.html.

Walker, L. (1999). Psychology and domestic violence around the world. *Journal of the American Psychologist Association, 54*(1), 21–29.

Walker, L. E. (1979). *The battered woman.* New York: Harper & Row.

Webster, S., (2002). Violence: a hidden health epidemic. [On-line]. Available: http:/detnews.com/specialreports/2000/violence/sunlead2/sunlead2.html.

Worling, J. R., & Curwen, T. (2000). Adolescent sexual offender recidivism: Success of specialized treatment and implications for risk prediction. *Child Abuse and Neglect, 24*(7), 965–982.

Youth Violence Prevention: the physician's role. *Journal of the American Medical Association. March 1, 2000, 283,* 1202–1203.

Zoeller, L. A., Goodwin, M. I., & Foa, E. B. (2000). PTSD severity and health perceptions in female victims of sexual assault. *Journal of Trauma and Stress, 13*(4), 635–649.

CHAPTER 31: SUBSTANCE ABUSE

Abel, E., & Sokol, R. (1991). A revised conservative estimate of the incidence of FAS and its economic impact. *Alcoholism Clinical and Experimental Research, 15*(3), 514–524.

Adams, W. L. (1995). Interactions between alcohol and other drugs. *International Journal of the Addictions, 30*(13, 14), 1903–1923.

Agency for Health Care Policy and Research. (1996). Smoking cessation clinical practice guideline (consensus statement). *Journal of the American Medical Association, 275*(16), 1270–1281.

Ambrosone, C. B., Freudenheim, J. L., Graham, S., Marshall, J. R., Vena, J. E., Brasure, J. R., Michalek, A. M., Laughlin, R., Nemoto, T., Gillenwater, K. A., Harrington, A. M., & Shields, P. G. (1996). Cigarette smoking. *N*-acetyltransferase 2 genetic polymorphisms, and breast cancer risk. *Journal of the American Medical Association, 276*(18), 1494–1502.

American Geriatrics Society. (2001). *Geriatric pharmaceutical care guidelines. Clinical evaluation and review.* Philadelphia: University of the Sciences.

American Psychiatric Association. (1994). *Diagnostic and statistical manual of mental disorders* (4th ed.). Washington, DC: Author.

Amodeo, M. (1995). The therapist's role in the drinking stage. In S. Brown (Ed.), *Treating alcoholism* (pp. 95–132). San Francisco: Jossey–Bass.

Annas, G. J. (1996). Cowboys, camels and the first amendment. *New England Journal of Medicine, 335*(23), 1779–1784.

A survey of illegal drugs: High time. (2001, July 28–August 3). *Economist, 360* (8232), special section.

Bara, A. L. & Barley, E. A. (2002). Caffeine for asthma (Cochrane Review).

In: the Cochrane Library: Oxford: Update Software. [On-line]. Available: www.medscape.com/viewarticle/422087

Baum, A. S., & Burnes, D. W. (1993). *A nation in denial: The truth about homelessness*. San Francisco: Westview Press.

Bean, M. (1984). Clinical implications of models for recovery from alcoholism. *Advances in Alcohol and Substance Abuse, 3,* 91–104.

Becker, K. L. & Walton-Moss, B. (2001). Detecting and addressing alcohol abuse in women. *The Nurse Practitioner, 26*(10), 13–25.

Beebe, D. K., & Walley, E. (1995). Smokable methamphetamine ("ice"): An old drug in a different form. *American Family Physician, 51*(2), 449–454.

Beim, A. (1995). Quitting for good. *American Health, 14*(7), 88–90.

Blum, K., Cull, J. G., Braverman, E. R., & Comings, D. E. (1996). Reward deficiency syndrome. *American Scientist, 84*(2), 132–146.

Broder, J. M. (1997, March 21). Cigarette maker concedes that smoking can cause cancer. *New York Times*, p. 1.

Brown, R. L., Leonard, T., Saunders, L. A., & Papasoiliotis, O. (2001). A two-item conjoint screen for alcohol and other drug problems. *Journal of the American Board of Family Practice, 14*(2), 95–106.

Brown, S. (1995). Introduction: Treatment models. In S. Brown (Ed.), *Treating alcoholism* (p. 17). San Francisco: Jossey-Bass.

Buckley, W. F. (1996). The California marijuana vote. *National Review, 48*(24), 62–64.

Calhoun, G. (1996). Prenatal substance afflicted children: An overview and review of the literature. *Education, 117*(1), 30–39.

Centers for Disease Control and Prevention. (1995a). Increasing morbidity and mortality associated with abuse of methamphetamine. *Morbidity and Mortality Weekly Report, 44*(47), 882–887.

Centers for Disease Control and Prevention. (1995b). Symptoms of substance abuse dependence associated with use of cigarettes, alcohol, and illicit drugs—United States, 1991–1992. *Morbidity and Mortality Weekly Report, 44*(44), 830–835.

Centers for Disease Control and Prevention. (1995c). Syringe exchange programs—United States, 1994–1995.

Journal of the American Medical Association, 274(16), 1260–1262.

Centers for Disease Control and Prevention. (1996a). *HIV/AIDS surveillance report*. Washington, DC: Author.

Centers for Disease Control and Prevention. (1996b). Scopolamine poisoning among heroin users. *Morbidity and Mortality Weekly Report, 45*(22), 457–461.

Centers for Disease Control and Prevention (2000). Tobacco information and prevention source (TIPS). National Center for Chronic Disease Prevention and Health Promotion [On-line]. Available: http://www.cdc.gov/tobacco/issue.htm.

Centers for Disease Control and Prevention. (2000a). Mortality and Morbidity Reports. *Heroin overdose deaths—Multnomah County, Oregon, 1993–1999.* [On-line]. Available: http://nurses/medscape.com/govmt/CDC/MMWR/2000/07.00/mmwr4928.01/mmwr4928.01.htm.

Centers for Disease Control and Prevention. (2000b). Mortality and Morbidity Reports. *Use of FDA-approved pharmacologic treatments for tobacco dependence—United States, 1984–1998.* [On-line]. Available: http://nurses.Medscape.com.govmt/CDC/MMWR/2000/07.00/mmwr4929.04/mmwr4929.04.

Centers for Disease Control and Prevention (2001). Update: Syringe exchange programs—United States: Report, 1998. *Morbidity and Mortality Weekly Report, 50*(19), 384–387.

Centers for Disease Control and Prevention. (2001). *Morbidity and Mortality Weekly Report, 50,* 384–387.

Chaisson, R. E., Bacceheti, P., Osmond, D., Bradie, B. Sande, M. A., & Moss, A. R. (1989). Cocaine use and HIV infection in intravenous drug users in San Francisco. *Journal of the American Medical Association, 261,* 561–565.

Chapman, S. (1997). The lie of the needle: Clinton shoots down needle exchange. *New Republic, 216*(13), 11–13.

Chaudhuri, J. D. (2000). An analysis of the teratogenic effects that could possibly be due to alcohol consumption by pregnant mothers. *Indian Journal of Medical Science, 54,* 425–431.

Coombs, R. H. (1997). *Drug-impaired professionals*. Boston: Harvard University.

Coutinho, R. A. (1995). Needle exchange programs—Do they work?

American Journal of Public Health, 85(11), 490–492.

Cramer, C., & Davidhizar, R. (1999). FAS/FAE: Impact on children. *Journal of Child Health Care, 3*(3), 31–34.

Dejin-Karlsson, E., Hanson, B. S., Ostergren, P. M., Sjoberg, N., & Marsal, K. (1998). Does passive smoking in early pregnancy increase the risk of small-for-gestational-age infants? *American Journal of Public Health,* 1523–1527.

Delbanco, T. L. (1996). Patients who drink alcohol: Pain, pleasure and paradox (editorial). *Journal of the American Medical Association, 275*(10), 803–805.

Des Jarlais, D. C., Paone, D., Friedman, S. R., Peyser, N., & Newman, R. G. (1995). Regulating controversial programs for unpopular people: Methadone maintenance and syringe exchange programs. *American Journal of Public Health, 85*(11), 1577(8).

DiFranza, J. R., & Librett, J. J. (1999). State and federal revenues from tobacco consumed by minors. *American Journal of Public Health, 89,* 1106–1108.

Dority, B. (1997). The rights of Joe Camel and the Marlboro man. *Humanist, 57*(1), 34–37.

Drake, R. E., & Mueser, K. T. (1996). Alcohol-use disorder and severe mental illness. *Alcohol Health and Research World, 20*(2), 86–94.

Dumas, L. (1991). Cocaine addicted women in home care. *Home Health Care Nurse, 10*(1), 12–17.

Dumas, L. (1992a). Addicted women: Profiles from the inner city. *Nursing Clinics of North America, 27*(4), 901–915.

Dumas, L. (1992b). Lung cancer in women: Rising epidemic, preventable disease. *Nursing Clinics of North America, 27*(4), 859–869.

Dumont, M. P. (1992). *Treating the poor.* Belmont, MA: Dympha Press.

Easley-Allen, C. (1992). Families in poverty. *Nursing Clinics of North America, 27* 337–408.

Ebersole, P., & Hess, P. (1998). *Toward healthy aging human needs and nursing response* (5th ed.). St. Louis, MO: Mosby.

Ecstasy points the way to new treatments for Parkinson's disease. [On-line]. Available: http://www.drugabuse.gov/Infofax/nationtrands.html; http://nurses.medscape.com/reuters/prof/2001/02/02.15/20010214clin002.html.

Faden, V. B., & Graubard, B. I. (2000). Maternal substance use during pregnancy and developmental outcome at age three. *Journal of Substance Abuse, 12,* 329–340.

Faltz, B. G. (1998). Substance abuse disorders. In A. Boyd & M. A. Nihart (Eds.), *Psychiatric nursing: Contemporary practice.* Philadelphia: J. B. Lippincott Company.

Federal Report. (2001). *Federal report says US children's well-being is improving.* [On-line]. Available: http://nurses.medscape.com/reuters/prof/2001/07/07.20/20010719pub1001. html.

Fillmore, K. M., Golding, J. M., Kniep, S., Leino, E. V., Shoemaker, C., Ager, C. R., Ferrer, H. A., Ahlstrom, S., Allenbeck, F., Amundsen, A. (1995). Gender differences for the risk or alcohol-related problems in multiple national contexts. *Recent Developments in Alcohol, 12,* 409–439.

Fink, A., Hays, R., Moore, A., & Beck, J. (1996). Alcohol-related problems in older persons: Determinants, consequences, and screening. *Archives of Internal Medicine, 156*(11), 1150–1157.

Finkelstein, N. (1994). Treatment issues for alcohol-and-drug-dependent-pregnant and parenting women. *Health and Social Work, 19*(1), 7–16.

Fishbein, D. H., & Pease, S. E. (1996). *The dynamics of drug abuse.* Boston: Allyn and Bacon.

Flexnor, S. B., & Hauck, L. C. (Eds.). (1993). *Random House unabridged dictionary* (2nd ed.). New York: Random House.

Frisch, N. C. & Frisch, L. E. (1998). Psychiatric mental health nursing. Clifton Park, NY: Delmar Learning.

Gentilello, I. M., Rivara, F., Donovan, D. M., Villaveces, A., Daranciang, E., Dunn, C. W., & Reis, R. R. (2000). Alcohol problems in women admitted to a level I trauma center: A gender-based comparison. *Journal of Trauma 48,* 108–114.

Gierdingen, D., McGovern, P., Bekker, M., Lundberg, U. & Willemsen, T. (2000). Women's work roles and their impact on health, well-being, and career: Comparisons between the United States, Sweden, and the Netherlands. *Women and Health, 31*(4), 1–20.

Gold, M. (1991). *The good news about drugs and alcohol.* New York: Villard Press.

Goldberg, M. E. (1995). Substance-abusing women: False stereotypes and real needs. *Social Work, 40*(6), 789–799.

Goldstein, A. O., Sobel, R. A., & Newman, G. R. (1999). Tobacco and alcohol use in G-rated childrens' animated films. *Journal of the American Medical Association, 281,* 1131–1136.

Gomberg, E. S. (1995). Older women and alcohol: Use and abuse. *Recent Developments in Alcoholism, 12,* 61–79.

Goroll, A. H., May, L., & Mulley, A. G. (2000). *Primary care medicine* (4th ed.). Philadelphia: Lippincott-Raven.

Hader, S. L., Smith, D. K., Moore, J. S., & Holmberg, S. D. (2001). HIV infection in women in the United States: Status at the Millennium. *Journal of the American Medical Association, 285*(9), 1186.

Henderson, C. W. (2001). Excluding women from mecial studies hinders progress, widens gender gap. *Women's Health Weekly,* p. 3.

Hennessey, M. B. (1992). Identifying the woman with alcohol problems: The nurse's role as gatekeeper. *Nursing Clinics of North America, 27*(4), 917–924.

Herbert, J. T., Hunt, B., & Dell, G. (1994). Counseling gay men and lesbians with alcohol problems. *Journal of Rehabilitation, 60*(2), 52–58.

Hewitt, B. G. (1995). The creation of the National Institute on Alcohol Abuse and Alcoholism: Responding to America's alcohol problem. *Alcohol Health and Research World, 19*(1), 12–17.

Hughes, T. L., & Smith, L. L. (1994). Is your colleague chemically dependent? *American Journal of Nursing, 94*(9), 30–35.

Humphreys, K. (1999). Professional Interventions that facilitate 12-step, self-help group involvement. *Alcohol Research and Health 23*(2), 93.

Igoe, J. (1994). School nursing. *Nursing Clinics of North America, 29*(3), pp. 443–457.

Julien, R. M. (1985). *A primer of drug action* (4th ed.). New York: W. H. Freeman and Company.

Kinney, J. (1991). *Clinical manual of substance abuse.* St. Louis: Mosby-Yearbook.

Klatsky, A., Friedman, G., & Armstrong, M. (1990). Coffee use prior to myocardial infarction restudied: Heavier intake may increase the risk. *American Journal of Epidemiology, 132,* 479–488.

LaDuke, S. (2000). The effects of professional discipline on nurses. *American Journal of Nursing, 100*(6), 26–33.

Lamarine, R. J. (1994). Selected health and behavioral effects related to the use of caffeine. *Journal of Community Health, 19*(6), 449–477.

Landry, M., & Smith, D. E. (1987). Crack: Anatomy of an addiction. *California Nursing Review, 9*(3), 28–31, 39–46.

Lee, R. (2000). Health care problems of lesbian, gay, bisexual, and transgender patients. *Western Journal of Medicine, 177,* 403–408.

Lehne, R. A. (1995). *Pharmacology for nursing care* (2nd ed.). Philadelphia: W. B. Saunders.

Lehne, R. A. (2000). *Pharmacology for nursing care* (4th ed.). Philadelphia: Saunders.

Leo, J. (1996). The voters go to pot. *U.S. News & World Report, 121*(17), 23.

Levine, H. G. (1978). The discovery of addiction: Changing conceptions of habitual drunkenness in America. *Journal of Studies on Alcohol, 39*(1), 143–169.

Liberto, J. G., & Oslin, D. W. (1995). Early versus late onset of alcoholism in the elderly. *International Journal of the Addictions, 30*(13–14), 1799–1818.

Liftik, J. (1995). Assessment. In S. Brown, (Ed.). *Treating alcoholism* (pp. 57–94). San Francisco: Jossey-Bass.

Ling, W., & Wesson, D. R. (1990). Drugs of abuse—Opiates. *Addiction Medicine* (Special issue). *Western Journal of Medicine, 152,* 565–572.

Liu, S., Siegel, P. Z., Brewer, R. D., Mokdad, A. H., Sleet, D. A., & Serdula, M. (1997). Prevalence of alcohol impaired driving: Results from a national self-reported survey of health behaviors. *Journal of the American Medical Association, 277*(2), 122–126.

Lurie, P., & Drucker, E. (1997). An opportunity lost: HIV infections associated with lack of a national needle-exchange programme in the USA. *Lancet, 349*(9052), 604–609.

Maher, L. (1992). Punishment and welfare: Crack cocaine and the regulation of mothering. *Women and Criminal Justice, 3*(2), 35–70.

Margolin, A. (2000). Randomized controlled trial of auricular acupuncture for cocaine dependence. (2000). *Archives of Internal Medicine, 160,* 2305–2312.

Martin, S. E. (1997). Alcohol and homicide: A deadly combination of two American traditions, *Journal of Studies on Alcohol, 58*(1), 107.

McKim, W. A. (1986). *Drugs and behavior: An introduction to behavioral pharmacology.* Upper Saddle River, NJ: Prentice-Hall.

McKinlay, J. B. (1974). The case for refocusing upstream: The political economy of illness, applying behavioral science to cardiovascular risk. In *Proceedings of the American Heart Association Conference,* Seattle, WA.

McKinlay, J. B. (1993). Health promotion through healthy public policy: The contribution of complementary research methods. *Canadian Journal of Public Health, 4*(19), 109–117.

Mendelson, J. (2000). *Club drug 'Ecstasy' increases heart rate, blood pressure and cardiac output.* [On-line]. Available: http://nurses.medscape. com/reuters/prof/2000.

Meyer, R. E. (1996). The disease called addiction: Emerging evidence in a 200-year debate. *Lancet, 347*(8995), 162–167.

Miller M. P. P., Gillespie, J., Billian, A., & Davel, S. (2001). Prevention of smiling behaviors in middle school students: Student nurse interventions. *Public Health Nursing, 18*(2), 77–81.

Monroe, J. (1996). A deadly narcotic: Heroin. *Current Health 2, 23*(2), 13–16.

Morganthau, T. (1997). The war over weed. *Newsweek, 129*(5), 20–23.

Morrison, J. (1995). DSM-IV made easy: *The clinician's guide to diagnosis.* New York: Guilford.

Mosher, J. F. (1994). Alcohol advertising and public health: An urgent call for action. *American Journal of Public Health, 84*(2), 180–182.

Murin, S., & Inciardi, J. (2001). Cigarette smoking and the risk of pulmonary metastasis from breast cancer. *Chest, 119*(6), 1196.

Murin, S. (2001). *Cigarette smoking and the risk of pulmonary metastis from breast cancer.* [On-line]. Available: http://nursins.medscape.com/ACCP/chest/2001/v119n06/ch1196.01.muri/ch119b.02.mur-01.html.

Myers, M. (1988). Effects of caffeine on blood pressure. *Archives of Internal Medicine, 148,* 1189–1193.

Myers, M. (1991). Caffeine and cardiac arrhythmias. *Annals of Internal Medicine, 114,* 147–150.

National Center for Health Statistics. (1995). *Health United States.* Hyattsville, MD: Public Health Services.

National Council on Alcoholism and Drug Dependence (2000). *Alcoholism and alcohol related problems: A sobering look.* [On-line]. Available: http://www.ncadd.org/facts/problems.html.

National Institute on Drug Abuse Research Report Series. (2001). *Heroin: Abuse and addiction.* [On-line].

Available: http://165.112.78.61/ResearchReports/heroin/heroin2html.

National Highway Traffic Safety Administration impaired driving program. (2001). [On-line]. Available: http://www.nhtsa.dot.gov/people/injury/alcohol/facts.html.

Nelson, D. E., Giovino, G. A., Emont, S. L., Brackbill, R., Cameron, L. L., Peddicord, J., & Mowery, P. D. (1994). Trends in cigarette smoking among US physicians and nurses. *Journal of the American Medical Association, 271*(16), 1273–1276.

NIDA Infofax. (2001a). *Crack and cocaine (13546).* [On-line]. Available: 165.112.78.61/Infofax/cocaine.html.

NIDA Infofax. (2001b). *Heroin (13548).* [On-line]. Available: 165.112.78.61/Infofax/heroin.html.

NIDA Infofax. (2001c). *High school and youth trends (13565).* [On-line]. Available: http://165.112.78.61/Infofax/HSYouthtrends.html.

NIDA Infofax. (2001d). *MDMA (Ecstasy) (13547).* [On-line]. Available: http://www.165.112.78.61/Infofax/ecstasy.html.

NIDA Infofax. (2001e). *Methamphetamine (13552).* [On-line]. Available: 165.112.78.61/Infofax/methamphetamine.html.

NIDA Infofax. (2001f). *Marijuana (13551).* [On-line]. Available: http://165.112.78.61/Infofax/marijuana.html.

NIDA Infofax. (2001g). *Nationwide trends (13567).* [On-line]. Available: http://www.165.112.78.61/Infofax/nationtrends.html.

NIDA Notes. (2001a). *About anabolic steroid abuse.* [On-line]. Available: http://www.165.112.78.61/NIDA_Notes/NNVol15N3/tearhoff.htm.

NIDA Notes. (2001b). *Facts about prescription drug abuse and addiction.* [On-line]. Available: http:// 165.112.78.61/NIDA_Notes/NNVol16N3/tearoff.html.

O'Brien, C. P., & McLellan, A. T. (1996). Myths about the treatment of addiction. *Lancet, 347*(8996), 237–241.

Oppenheimer, E. (1991). Alcohol and drug abuse among women—An overview. *British Journal of Psychiatry, 158*(Suppl. 10), 36–44.

Palmer, C. F. (1896). *Inebriety: Its source, prevention and cure* (3rd ed.). New York: Fleming H. Revell.

Pietinen, P., Geboers, J., & Kesteloot, H. (1988). Coffee consumption and serum cholesterol: An epidemiological study in Belgium. *International*

Journal of Epidemiology, 17, 98–104.

Pope, H. G. (2001). Letter to *New England Journal of Medicine. NIDA Notes, 51*(6).

Portnoy, F., & Dumas, L. (1994). Nursing for the public good. *Nursing Clinics of North America, 29*(3), 371–376.

Prothrow-Stith, D. (1990). The epidemic of violence and its impact on the health care system. *Henry Ford Hospital Medical Journal, 38*(2,3), 175–177.

Prothrow-Stith, D. (1996). *Violence prevention curriculum for Massachusetts.* Teen Age Health Teaching Modules. Newton, MA: Education Development Center.

Ray, O. (1983). *Drugs, society, and human behavior.* St. Louis, MO: C. V. Mosby.

Reichman, M. E. (1994). Alcohol and breast cancer. *Alcohol, Health and Research World, 18*(3), 182–185.

Reuters ABC news. (2001). [On-line]. Available: http://dailynews.yahoo.com.h.nm.20010703/hl/pot_offenders_ 1.html.

Rodriguez, M. A., & Brindis, C. D. (1995). Violence and Latino youth: Prevention and methodological issues. *Public Health Reports, 110*(3), 260–268.

Rogers, A. (1997). Seeing through the haze: Can marijuana ever be good medicine? *Newsweek, 129*(2), 60.

Rosenberg, L. (1990). Coffee and tea consumption in relation to the risk of large bowel cancer: A review of epidemiological studies. *Cancer Letters, 52,* 163–171.

Rosenberg, L., Metzger, L. S., & Palmer, J. R. (1993). Alcohol consumption and risk of breast cancer: A review of the epidemiologic evidence. *Epidemiological Review, 15,* 133–144.

Schiff, L. (2001). Canada becomes the first to allow medical marijuana. *RN, 64*(10), 16.

Schuckit, M. A. (1983). Alcoholism and other psychiatric disorders. *Hospital and Community Psychiatry, 34*(11), 1022–1027.

Schuckit, M. A., & Monteiro, M. G. (1988). Alcoholism, anxiety and depression. *British Journal of Addictions 83*(12), 1373–1380.

Schwenk, T. (2000). Alcohol use in adolescents. The scope of the problem and strategies for intervention. *Physician and Sportsmedicine, 28*(6), 71.

Sluder, L. C., Kinnison, L. R., & Cates, D. (1996). Prenatal drug exposure:

Meeting the challenge. *Childhood Education, 73*(2), 66–70.

Steroid abusers may go on to abuse opioids, too. Study reported in a letter to *New England Journal of Medicine. NIDA Notes, 15* (6).

Strain, E. C., Mumiford, G. K., Silverman, K., & Griffiths, R. R. (1994). Caffeine dependence syndrome: Evidence from case histories and experimental examinations. *Journal of the American Medical Association, 272*(13), 1043–1049.

Streissguth, A. (1997). *Fetal alcohol syndrome: A guide for families and communities.* Baltimore: Brooks.

Stocker, S. (2001). *NIDA Notes: Cocaine abuse may lead to strokes and mental deficits.* [On-line]. Available: http://www.165.112.78.61/NIDA_Notes/NNVol13/Cocaine.html.

Substance Abuse and Mental Health Service Administration. (2001b). *HSS report shows drug use rates stable, youth tobacco use declines.* [On-line]. Available: http://www.samhas.gov/oas/nhsda/2khhspress.html.

Sullivan, E. J., Handley, S. M., & Connors, H. (1994). The role of nurses in primary care: Managing alcohol abusing patients. *Alcohol, Health and Research World, 18*(2), 158–162.

Talashek, M. L., Laina, C. S., Gerace, M., & Starr, K. L. (1994). The substance abuse pandemic: Determinants to guide interventions. *Public Health Nursing 11*(2), 131–139.

Teinowitz, I. (1997). Justice Department backs FDA, sees cig ad/kids linkage. *Advertising Age, 68*(3), 39.

Thompson, H. R. (1995). Gender differences in alcohol metabolism. Physiological responses to ethanol. *Recent Developments in Alcohol, 1005,* 163–179.

Tierney, L. A., McPhee, S. J., & Papadakis, M. A. (2001). Eds. (2000). *Current medical diagnosis and treatment.* New York: Lange Books McGraw-Hill.

Trevisan, L. A., Boutros, N., Petrakis, I. L., & Krysta, J. H. (1998). Complications of alcohol withdrawal: pathophysiological insights. *Alcohol Health & Research World, 22*(1), 61–66.

University of California. (1994, April). *Berkeley Wellness Letter, 10*(4), 7.

U.S. Department of Health and Human Services. (1990a). *Alcohol and Health.* DHHS Publication No. (ADM) 90–1656. Washington, DC: U.S. Government Printing Office.

U.S. Department of Health and Human Services. (1990b). *Healthy people 2000: National health promotion and disease prevention objectives.* DHHS Publication No. PHS 91–50212. Washington, DC: U.S. Government Printing Office.

U.S. Department of Health and Human Services. (1992). Alcohol related injuries and violence. *Prevention Pipeline, 5*(3), 3–10.

U.S. Department of Health and Human Services. (1994a). *National household survey on drug abuse: Population estimates 1993.* DHHS Publication No. (SMA) 94–3017. Washington, DC: U.S. Government Printing Office.

U.S. Department of Health and Human Services. (1994b). *National survey results on drug use from the monitoring the future study, 1975–1993.* Vol. 1: *Secondary school students.* NIH Publication No. 94–3809. Washington, DC: U.S. Government Printing Office.

U.S. Department of Health and Human Services. (1996). *Healthy People 2000: Midcourse review and 1995 revisions.* Sudbury, MA: Jones & Bartlett.

U.S. Department of Health and Human Services. (2000a). *Healthy People 2010: Understanding and Improving Health.* 2nd. ed. Washington, DC: U.S. Government Printing Office.

U.S. Department of Health and Human Services. (2000b). Tenth Special Report to the U.S. Congress on Alcohol and Health. [On-line]. Available: http://www.niaaa.nih.gov/publications/10report/chap07a.pdf

U.S. Department of Health and Human Services. National Institutes of Health. National Institute on Drug Abuse (2000c). Research Report Series: Heroin. Washington, DC: U.S. Government Printing Office.

Varitiainen, E., Paavola, M., McAlister, A., & Puska, P. (1998). Fifteen-year follow-up of smoking prevention effects in the North Karelia Youth Project. *American Journal of Public Health, 58,* 81–85.

Volkow, N. D., Chang, L., Wang, G. J., Fowler, J. S., Leonido-Yee, M., Franceschi, M., Sedler, M. J., Gatley, S. J., Hitzemann, R., Ding, Y. S., Logan, J., Wong, Christopher and Miller, E. N. (2001). Association of dopamine transporter reduction with psychomotor impairment in methamphetamine abusers. *American Journal of Psychiatry 158* (3)377.

Wallace, J. (1977). Alcoholism from the inside out: A phenomenological analysis. In N. J. Estes & M. E. Heine-mann (Eds.), *Alcoholism* (pp. 3–14). St. Louis, MO: C. V. Mosby.

Warren, T., Rowlingson, K. & Whyly, E. (2001). Female finances: Gender wage gaps and gender assets gaps. *Work, Employment, and Society: 15,* 465–488.

Watters, J. K., Estilo, M. J., Clark, G. L., & Lorvick, J. (1994). Syringe and needle exchange as HIV/AIDS prevention for injection drug users. *Journal of the American Medical Association, 271*(2), 115–121.

Webber, R. (2001). *Marijuana addictive? Study "clear" but opinions differ.* [On-line]. Available: http://www.Cbshealthwatch.com/cx/viewarticle/234198.

Weiner, L., & Larsson, G. (1987, Summer). Clinical prevention of fetal alcohol effects, a reality: Evidence for the effectiveness of intervention. *Alcohol Health and Research World,* 60–65.

Weiner, L., Morse, B., & Garrido, P. (1989). FAS/FAE focusing prevention on women at risk. *International Journal of the Addictions, 24*(5), 385–395.

Weiner, L., Rosett, H. L., & Mason, E. A. (1985). Training professionals to identify and treat pregnant women who drink heavily. *Alcohol, Health and Research World, 1,* 32–36.

Wilsnack, S., & Wilsnack, R. (1991). Prevalence and magnitude of perinatal substance abuse exposures in California. *New England Journal of Medicine, 325,* 775–782.

Wilson, E. (2000). *The First International conference on Women, Health Disease, and Stroke: Science and policy in action. Women's Health Conference Summaries* [On-line] Available: http://nurses.Medscape.com/medscapte./CNO/2000/FICWHDS?FICWHDS-1.html.

Witters, W. L., & Venturelli, P. J. (1988). *Drugs and society* (2nd ed.). Boston: Jones & Bartlett.

Woody, G. (1996) The challenge of dual diagnosis (alcoholism and psychiatric disorder). *Alcohol, Health and Research World, 20*(2), 76–81.

Yost, D. A. (1996). Alcohol withdrawal syndrome. *American Family Physician, 54*(2), 657–666.

CHAPTER 32: POVERTY

Amarasingham, R., Spalding, S. H., & Anderson, R. J. (2001). Disease conditions most frequently evaluated among the homeless in Dallas. *Journal of Healthcare for the Poor and Underserved, 12*(2), 162–176.

Basch, P. (1999). *Textbook of international health* (2nd ed.). Oxford, England: Oxford University Press.

Beeghley, L. (2000). *The structure of social stratification in the United States* (3rd ed.). Boston: Allyn and Bacon.

Broyles, R. W., McAuley, W. J., & Baird-Holmes, D. (1999). The medically vulnerable: Their health risks, health status, and use of physician care. *Journal of Health Care for the Poor and Underserved, 10*(2), 186–200.

Chandra, N. C., Ziegelstein, R. C., & Rogers, W. J. (1998). Observations of the treatment of women in the United States with myocardial infarction: A report from the National Registry of Myocardial Infarction—I. *Archives of Internal Medicine, 158,* 981–988.

Chaturvedi, N., Jarrett, J., Shipley, M. J., & Fuller, J. H. (1998). Socioeconomic gradient in morbidity and mortality in people with diabetes: Cohort study findings from the Whitehall study and the WHO multinational study of vascular disease in diabetes. *British Medical Journal, 316,* 100–106.

Collins, R. (1974). *Conflict sociology: Toward an explanatory science.* New York: Academic Press.

Dahrendorf, R. (1959). *Class and class conflict in industrial society.* Palo Alto, CA: Stanford University Press.

Davidson, L., & Krackhardt, D. (1975). *Structural change and the disadvantaged: An empirical test of culture of poverty/situational theories of hard core work behavior.* Paper presented to annual meeting of the American Sociological Association, San Francisco.

Davis, K., Moore, W. E. (1945). Some principles of stratification. *American Sociological Review, 10,* 242–249.

Domhoff, G. W. (1999). *Who rules America? Power and politics in the year 2000* (3rd ed.). Mountain View, CA: Mayfield Publishing.

Galbraith, J. K. (1979). *The nature of mass poverty.* Cambridge MA: Harvard University Press.

Gans, H. J. (1972). The positive functions of poverty. *American Journal of Sociology, 78,* 275–289.

Harrington, M. (1962). *The other America: Poverty in the United States.* New York: Macmillan.

Haub, C., & Cornelius, D. (1999). *World population data sheet.* Washington, DC: Population Reference Bureau.

Henslin, J. M. (2000). *Social problems* (5th ed.). Upper Saddle River, NJ: Prentice-Hall.

Higgs, R. Z., & Kinzel, D. (2001). Personal communication.

Hingson, R., Heeren, T., & Zakocs, R. (2001). Age of drinking onset and involvement in physical fights after drinking. *Pediarics, 108,* 872.

Huggins, M. K. (1993). *Lost childhoods: Assassinations of youth in democratizing Brazil.* Paper presented at the annual meeting of the American Sociological Association.

Kaguskar, S., Bradshaw, H., & Rayner, M. (1997). *Coronary heart disease statistics.* London: British Heart Foundation.

Lewis, O. (1966a). The culture of poverty. *Scientific American, 115,* 19–25.

Lewis, O. (1966b). *La Vida.* New York: Random House.

Makuc, D. M., Breen, N., & Freid, V. (1999). Low income, race, and the use of mammography. *Health Services Research, 34*(1), 229–239.

Manson-Siddle, C. J., & Robinson, M. B. (1998). Super profile analysis of socioeconomic variations in coronary investigation and revascularization rates. *Journal of Epidemiology and Community Health, 52,* 507–512.

McNeil, D. G. (1999, January 15). In Angola's capital, life does not yet imitate art. *New York Times.* p. 4.

Mills, C. W. (1956). *The power elite.* New York: Oxford University Press.

Muraskin, W. (1998). *The politics of international health.* Albany, NY: State University of New York Press.

National Coalition for the Homeless. (2000). *Report on Homelessness for the Year 2000.* New York: Author.

Rathore, S. S., Berger, A. K., Weinfert, K. P., Feinleib, M., Oetgen, W. J., Gersh, B. J., & Schulman, K. A. (2000). Race, sex, poverty, and the medical treatment of acute myocardial infarction in the elderly. *Circulation, 102*(6), 642–648.

Robinson, N., Lloyd, C. E., & Stevens, L. K. (1998). Social deprivation and mortality in adults with diabetes mellitus. *Diabetic Medicine, 15,* 205–212.

Rodman, H. (1963). The lower class values stretch. *Social Forces, 42,* 205–215.

Rossi, P. H. (1989). *Down and out in America: The origins of homelessness.* Chicago: University of Chicago Press.

Schellenberg, J. A. (1996). *Conflict resolution: Theory, research, and practice.* Albany: New York University Press.

Schulman, K. A., Berlin, J. A., & Harless, W. (1999). The effect of race and sex on physicians' recommendations for cardiac catheterization. *New England Journal of Medicine, 340,* 618–626.

Szaz, T. S. (1998). *Cruel compassion: Psychiatric control of society's unwanted.* Syracuse: Syracuse University Press.

U.S. Bureau of the Census. (2000). *Statistical Abstract of the United States: The national data book.* Washington, DC: US Government Printing Office.

Valentine, C. A. (1968). *Culture and poverty: Critique and counter proposals.* Chicago: University of Chicago Press.

Walton, M. A. (2001). Diversity in relapse prevention needs: Gender and race comparisons among substance abuse treatment patients. *American Journal of Drug and Alcohol Abuse. 27,* 225–240.

World Health Organization. (1999b). *International classification of impairments, disabilities and handicaps: A manual of classification relating to the consequences of disease.* Geneva, Switzerland: Author.

Zerwekh, J. V. (2000). Caring on the ragged edge: Nursing persons who are disenfranchised. *Advances in Nursing Science, 22*(4), 47–61.

CHAPTER 33: HOMELESSNESS

Ayerst, S. L. (1999). Depression and stress in street youth. *Adolescence, 34*(135), 567–575.

Bassuk, E. L., Weinreb, L. F., Buckner, J. C., Browne, A., Salomon, A., & Bassuk, S. S. (1996). The characteristics and needs of sheltered homeless and low-income housed mothers. *Journal of the American Medical Association, 276*(8), 640–646.

Baum, A. S., & Burnes, D. W. (1993). *A nation in denial: The truth about homelessness.* San Francisco: Westview Press.

Bogue, D. J. (1963). *Skid row in American cities.* Chicago, IL: University of Chicago, Community and Family Study Center.

Buhrich, N., Hodder, T., & Teesson, M. (2000). Lifetime prevalence of trauma among homeless people in Sydney.

Australia and New Zealand Journal of Psychiatry, 34(6), 963–966.

Burt, M. R. (1992). *Over the edge: The growth of homelessness in the 1980s.* New York: Russell Sage Foundation (The Urban Institute Press, Washington, DC).

Centers for Disease Control and Prevention. (1992). Prevention and control of tuberculosis among homeless persons. *Morbidity and Mortality Weekly Report, 41*(RR-5), 13–23.

Centers for Disease Control and Prevention. (1993). *TB-HIV: The connection: What health care workers should know.* Washington, DC: U.S. Government Printing Office.

Centers for Disease Control and Prevention. (1994). *Core curriculum on tuberculosis: What the clinician should know* (3rd ed.). Washington, DC: U.S. Government Printing Office.

Centers for Disease Control and Prevention. (2000a). Division of tuberculosis Elimination, Surveillance Reports, *Reported tuberculosis in the United States.* [On-line]. Available: http://www.cdc.gov/nchstp/tb/surv/surv2000/pdfs/tl.pdf.

Centers for Disease Control and Prevention. (2000b). Hypothermia-related deaths—Suffolk County, New York, January 1999–March 2000, and United States, 1979–1998. *Morbidity and Mortality Weekly Report, 50*(4), 53–57.

Centers for Disease Control and Prevention. (2001). *Tuberculosis cases and case rates per 100,000 population deaths and death rates per 100,000 population: United States 1953–2000.* [On-line]. Available: http://www.cdc.gov/nchstp/tb/surv/surv2000/pdfs/tl.pdf.

Chinman, M. J., Rosenheck, R., & Lam, J. A. (2000). The case management relationship and outcomes of homeless persons with serious mental illness. *Psychiatric Services, 51*(9), 1142–1147.

Chosidow, O. (2000). Scabies and pediculosis. *Lancet, 355*(9), 206, 819–826.

Council of State Governments. (2000). Welfare reform—four years later. *Spectrum: Journal of State Government, 73*(4), 20.

Dail, P. W. (2000). Introduction to the symposium on homelessness. *Policy Studies Journal, 28*(2), 331.

DeMatteo, D., Major, C., Block, B., Coates, R., Fearon, M., Goldberg, E., King, S. M., Millson, M., O'Shaugh-nessy, M., & Read, S. E. (1999). Toronto street youth and HIV/AIDS: Prevalence, demographics, and risks. *Journal of Adolescent Health, 25*(5), 358–366.

Dennis, D. L., Cocozza, J. J., & Steadman, H. J. (1999). What do we know about systems integration and homelessness? In L. B. Fosburg & D. L. Dennis (Eds.), *Practical lessons: The 1998 Symposium on Homelessness Research.* Washington, DC: U.S. Department of Housing and Urban Development.

DiBlasio, F. A., & Belcher, J. R. (1993). Social work outreach to homeless people and the need to address self esteem. *Health and Social Work, 8*(4), 201.

Eighner, L. (1993). *Travels with Lisbeth.* New York: St. Martin's Press.

Fergusen, M. A., & Ragosta, C. W. (1998). Homeless at risk of mortality: A proactive approach to vulnerable "repeaters." *Journal of Emergency Nursing, 24*(6), 546–550.

Finland: National strategy delivers positive results. (1998). [On-line]. Available: http://www.feantsa.org.

Fisher, B., Hovell, M., Hofstetter, C. R., & Hough, R. (1995). Risks associated with long-term homelessness among women: Battery, rape and HIV infection. *International Journal of Health Services, 25*(2), 351–369.

From welfare to worsefare. (2000). *Business Week, 3702,* 103.

Goldsmith, J. (1995). Breaking the barrier of not caring: Urban nursing. *Reflections, 21*(2), 8–10.

Gorzka, P. A. (1999). Homeless parents' perception of parenting stress. *Journal of Child and Adolescent Psychiatric Nursing, 12*(1), 7–15.

Harrington, M. (1962). *The other America: Poverty in the United States.* Baltimore: Penguin Books.

Health Care for the Homeless Mobilizer. (2001), Vol. 5, Issue 2. [On-line]. Available: http://www.nhchc.org.

Henderson, V. (1966). *The nature of nursing.* New York: MacMillan Company.

Herlihy-Starr, C. (1982). They are their brother's keepers. *Boston College Magazine, VLV* (2), 16–19.

Jones, R. E. (1983). Street people and psychiatry: An introduction. *Hospital and Community Psychiatry, 34*(9), 807–811.

Kakuchi, S. (1996). Japan's painful changes. *MacLean's, 109*(2), 18–21.

Katz, J. L. (1996). Welfare overhaul law (provisions of the personal responsibility and work opportunity reconcil-iation act of 1996). *Congressional Quarterly Weekly Report, 54*(38), 2696–2706.

Koegel, P., Burnham, M. A., & Baumohl, J. (1996). In J. Baumoh (Ed.), *The causes of homelessness in America.* New York: Oryx Press.

Kozol, J. (1988). *Rachel and her children: Homeless families in America.* New York: Crown Publishers.

Lebow, J. M., Bierer, M. F., O'Connell, J. J., Orav, E. J., & Brennan, T. A. (1998). Risk factors for death in homeless adults in Boston. *Archives of Internal Medicine, 158*(13), 1454–1460.

Lebow, J. M., O'Connell, J. J., Oddleifson, S., Gallagher, K. M., Seage, G. R., & Freedberg, K. A. (1995). AIDS among the homeless of Boston: A cohort study. *Journal of Acquired Immune Deficiency Syndromes and Human Retrovirology, 8*(3), 292–296.

Lenehan, G., McInnis, B. N., O'Donnell, D., & Hennessey, M. (1985). A nurses' clinic for the homeless. *American Journal of Nursing, 85,* 1237–1240.

MacDonald, N. E., Fisher, W. A., Wells, G. A., Doherty, J. A., & Bowie, W. R. (1994). Canadian street youth: Correlates of sexual risk-taking activity. *Pediatric Infectious Disease Journal, 13*(8), 690–697.

Mauch, D., & Mulkern, V. (1992). The McKinney Act. In P. O'Malley (Ed.), *Homelessness: New England and beyond* (pp. 419–430). Boston: University of Massachusetts Press.

McGinnis, B. (1995). Tuberculosis among the homeless: The Pine Street Inn experience. In F. L. Cohen & J. Durham (Eds.), *Tuberculosis: A source book for nursing practice* (pp. 229–240). New York: Springer Publishing Company.

McMurray, D. (1990). Family breakdown causes homelessness. In L. Orr (Ed.), *The homeless: Opposing viewpoints* (pp. 71–74). San Diego, CA: Greenhaven Press.

McMurray-Avila, M. (1998). *Organizing health services for homeless people: A practical guide.* Nashville: National Health Care for the Homeless Council.

McMurray-Avila, M., Gelberg, L., & Breakey, W. R. (1999). Balancing act: Clinical practices that respond to the needs of homeless people. In L. B. Fosburg & D. L. Dennis (Eds.), *Practical lessons: The 1998 Symposium on Homelessness Research.*

Washington, DC: U.S. Department of Housing and Urban Development.

Millions still face homelessness in a booming economy. (2000). Washington, DC: The Urban Institute. [On-line]. Available: http://www/urban. org.

National Coalition for the Homeless. (1999a). *NCH Fact Sheet #1: Why are people homeless?* Washington, DC: Author.

National Coalition for the Homeless. (1999b). *NCH Fact Sheet #2: How many people experience homelessness?* Washington, DC: Author.

National Coalition for the Homeless. (1999c). *NCH Fact Sheet #6: Addiction disorders and homelessness?* Washington, DC: Author.

National Coalition for the Homeless. (1999d). *NCH Fact Sheet #7: Homeless families with children.* Washington, DC: Author.

National Coalition for the Homeless. (1999e). *NCH Fact Sheet #8: Health care and homelessness.* Washington, DC: Author.

National Coalition for the Homeless. (1999f). *NCH Fact Sheet #9: Homeless veterans.* Washington, DC: Author.

National Coalition for the Homeless. (1999g). *NCH Fact Sheet #15: Homelessness among elderly persons.* Washington, DC: Author.

O'Connell, J. J. (1999). *Utilization and costs of medical services by homeless persons: A review of the literature and implications for the future.* Nashville: National Health Care for the Homeless Council.

Parmentier, C. (Ed.). (1998). *Europe against exclusion: Housing for all.* Brussels: FEANTSA (European Federation of National Organisations Working with the Homeless). [On-line]. Available: www.feantsa.org.

Polikow, V. (1998) Homeless children and their families: The discards of the postmodern 1990s. In S. Books (Ed.). *Invisible children in the society and its schools* (pp. 3–22). Mahwah, NJ: Lawrence Erlbaum Associates.

Poverty amidst plenty 2001: Unspent TANF funds and persistent poverty. (2001). National Campaign for Jobs and Income Support. [On-line]. Available: www.nationalcampaign.org.

Redburn, F. S., & Buss T. F. (1986). *Responding to America's homeless: Public policy alternatives.* New York: Praeger.

Redlener, I., & Johnson, D. (1999) *Still in crisis: The health status of New York's homeless children.* The Children's Health Fund. [On-line]. Available: http://www.childrenshealthfund. org/hshc4.html.

Ringwalt, C. L., Greene, J. M., Robertson, M., & McPheeters, M. (1998). The prevalence of homelessness among adolescents in the United States. *American Journal of Public Health, 88*(9), 1325–1330.

Rosenheck, R., Bassuk, E., & Salomon, A. (1999). Special populations of homeless Americans. In L. B. Fosburg & D. L. Dennis (Eds.), *Practical lessons: The 1998 Symposium on Homelessness Research.* Washington, DC: U.S. Department of Housing and Urban Development.

Silliman, K., Yamanoha, M. M., & Morrissey, A. E. (1998). Evidence of nutritional risk in a population of homeless adults in rural northern California. *Journal of the American Dietetic Association, 98*(8), 908–910.

Sleegers, J. (2000). Similarities and differences in homelessness in Amsterdam and New York City. *Psychiatric Services, 51*(1), 100–104.

Smereck, G. A., & Hockman, E. M. (1998). Prevalence of HIV infection and HIV risk behaviors associated with living place: On-the-street homeless drug users as a special target population for public health intervention. *Americal Journal of Drug and Alcohol Abuse, 24*(2), 299–319.

Somers, S. A., Rimel, R. W., Shmavonian, N., Waxman, L. D., Reyes, L. M., Wobido, S. L., & Brickner, P. W. (1990). Creation and evolution of a national health care for the homeless program. In P. W. Brickner, L. K. Scharer, B. Conanan, M. Savarese, & B. C. Scanlan (Eds.), *Under the safety net* (pp. 56–66). New York: W. W. Norton Company.

Song, J. Y. (1999) *HIV/AIDS and homelessness: Recommendations for clinical practice and public policy.* National Health Care for the Homeless Council. Mahwah, NJ: HCH Clinicians Network.

SSI and SSD Benefits termination as seen in HCH projects. (1999). National Health Care for the Homeless Council. [On-line]. Available: http:// www.nhchc.org/SSI.html.

State income inequality continued to grow in most states in the 1990s, despite economic growth and tight labor markets. (2000). Center on Budget and Policy Priorities, Washington, DC. [On-line]. Available: http:// www.cbpp.org/1-18-00sfp.htm.

St. Lawrence, J. S., & Brasfield, T. L. (1995). HIV risk behavior among homeless adults. *AIDS Intervention and Prevention, 7*(1), 22–31.

Strasser, J. A., Damrosch, S., & Gaines, J. (1991). Nutrition and the homeless person. *Journal of Community Health Nursing, 8*(2), 65–73; *American Journal of Diseases of Children, 145*(4), 431–436.

Torrey, E. F. (1998). *Out of the shadows, confronting America's mental illness crisis.* New York: John Wiley and Sons.

U.S. Bureau of the Census. (2001). *Poverty in the United States, 1999.* [On-line]. Available: http://www. census.gov/hhes/poverty/poverty99/ pov99.html.

U.S. Bureau of the Census (2001). Poverty 1999 Graph [On-line]. Available: http://www.census.gov/hhes/ poverty/poverty99/povfam99.html.

U.S. Conference of Mayors. (2000). *A status report on hunger and homelessness in America's cities.* Washington, DC: Author.

U.S. Department of Health and Human Services. (1990). *Healthy people 2000: National health promotion and disease prevention objectives.* DHHS Publication No. PHS 91-50212. Washington, DC: U.S. Government Printing Office.

U.S. Department of Health and Human Services. (2000). *Healthy people 2010: National health promotion and disease prevention objectives.* Washington, DC: U.S. Government Printing Office.

Wagner, J., & Menke, E. M. (1991). Stressors and coping behaviors of homeless, poor, and low-income mothers. *Journal of Community Health Nursing, 8*(2), 75–84.

Walters, A. S. (1999). HIV prevention in street youth. *Journal of Adolescent Health, 25*(3), 187–198.

Watson, J. (1985). *Nursing: Human science and human care.* Norwalk, CT Appleton Century Crofts.

Whitbeck, L. B., & Hoyt, D. R. (1999). *Nowhere to grow: Homeless and runaway adolescents and their families.* New York: Aldine De Gruyter.

Wright, J. D. (1990). The health of homeless people: Evidence from the National Health Care for the Homeless Program. In P. W. Brickner, L. K. Scharer, B. Conanan, M. Savarese, & B. C. Scanlan (Eds.), *Under the safety net* (pp. 15–31). New York: W. W. Norton Company.

Wright, J. D., Rubin, B. A., & Devine, J. A. (1998). *Beside the golden door: Policy, politics, and the homeless.* New York: Aldine De Gruyter.

Zuckerman, D. M. (2000a). The evolution of welfare reform: Policy changes and current knowledge. *Journal of Social Studies, 56*(4), 811.

Zuckerman, D. M. (2000b). Welfare reform in America: A clash of politics and research. *Journal of Social Studies, 56*(4), 587.

CHAPTER 34: RURAL HEALTH

Alcott, L. M. (1863). *Hospital sketches.* New York: Hurst & Company.

American Nurses Association, Rural/Frontier Health Care Task Force. (1996). *Rural/frontier nursing. The challenge to grow.* Washington, DC: Author.

American Psychological Association. (2001, June 14). *The behavioral health care needs of rural women.* [On-line]. Available: http://www.apa.org/rural/ruralwomenexec.pdf.

Austin, B. (1999). Time to build clinical linkages with your home health provider 7 "S" model for home health: A tool for discharge planning. *The New Definition, 14*(2). Retrieved January 25, 2001. [On-line]. Available: http://www.cfcm.com/newdefinition14 2.htm.

Bigbee, J. L. (1993, March). The uniqueness of rural nursing. *Nursing Clinics of North America, 28*(1), 131–144.

Bugarin, A., & Elias, L. (1998). *Farmworkers in California.* California Research Bureau. California State Library. CRB-98-00. Retrieved June 18, 2001. [On-line]. Available: http://www. library.ca.gov/crb/98/07/98007apdf.

Bushy, A. (1991). *Rural nursing,* (Vol. 1) Newbury Park, CA: Sage.

Bushy, A. (2000). *Meeting the special needs of the rural community.* Retrieved January 24, 2001. [On-line]. Available: http://www.nursece.com/RuralHealth.htm.

Center for Health Policy. (1997). *Factors affecting children's health: A rural profile, 1*(2). [On-line]. Available: www/gmu.edu/departments/chp/rhr/brief2.

Centers for Disease Control and Prevention. (1992, June 6). Prevention and control of tuberculosis in migrant farm workers: Recommendations of the advisory council for the elimination of tuberculosis. *Morbidity and Mortality Weekly Report.*

Colorado AHEC Program, University of Colorado Health Sciences Center. (1997). *Interdisciplinary rural team training.* Retrieved June 18, 2001. [On-line]. Available: http://www.uchsc.edu/ahec/finaid/manual/mod2.htm.

Colorado Migrant Health Program. (1998). Internet page.

Community Oriented Primary Care. (1998). *Practical illustrations of COPC.* The George Washington University Medical Center, School of Public Health and Health Services. Retrieved January 28, 2001. [On-line]. Available: http://learn.gwumc.edu/sphhs/pubh280/copcbib.htm#principles.

D'Arrigo, T., & Keegan, A. (2000). *Diabetes & Latinos: Community at risk. Diabetes Forecast.* American Diabetes Association. Retrieved June 18, 2001. [On-line]. Available: http://www. diabetes.org/diabetesforcast. 00June.

Davis, R., & Magilvy, J. (2000). Quiet pride: The experience of chronic illness by rural older adults. *Journal of Nursing Scholarship, 32*(4), 385–390.

Dougherty, S. (1996). *Half of all US farmworkers may be infected with TB, and as many as 4 to 5 percent are infected with HIV. 1996 National Farmworker Health Conference.* Retrieved June 18, 2001. [On-line]. Available: http://www.thebody.com/iapac/farmwork.html.

Grun, B. (1991). *The timetables of history* (3rd ed.). New York: Simon & Schuster.

Gwyther, M., & Jenkins, M. (1998). Migrant farmworker children: Health status, barriers to care, and nursing innovations in health care delivery. *Journal of Pediatric Health Care, 12*(2), 60–66.

Hagopian, A. & Hart, L. G. (2001). *Rural hospital flexibility program tracing project.* Rural Policy Research Institute. [On-line]. Available: http://www.rapri.org.

Health Resources and Services Administration. (1998, February 11). *The migrant health program.* [On-line]. Available: http://www.access.gpo.gov/usbudget.

Health Resources and Service Administration, Office of Rural Health Policy. (2000). *Capital area rural health roundtable: Selected federal programs meeting the health care needs of rural Americans.* Retrieved January 28, 2001. [On-line]. Available: http://www.gmu.edu/departments/chp/rhr/federalprgms oo.pdf.

Henderson, T., & Coopey, J. (2000). *Ensuring the survival of critical access hospitals: The new Medicare rural hospital flexibility program and the important role for states.* Retrieved January 25, 2001. [On-line]. Available: http://www.ruralhealth.hrsa.gov/IssueBriefl.htm.

Herek, G. M. & Berrill, K. T. (1992). *Hate crimes: Confronting violence against lesbians and gay men.* Newbury Park: Sage.

Lee, B.C., Jenkins, L. S., Westaby, J. D. (1997). Factors influencing exposure of children to major hazards on family farms. *Journal of Rural Health, 13*(3), 206–215.

Lee, H. J. (1993). Health perceptions of middle, "new middle," and older rural adults. *Family Community Health, 16*(1), 19–27.

Migrant Clinician Network. (2001, January 29). *The farmworker population: Background.* [On-line]. Available: http://www.migrantclinician.org/about/migback.html.

National Agricultural Statistics Service (NASS). (1999). *1998 Childhood agricultural injuries.* [On-line]. Available: http://msda.manlib.cornell.edu/reports.

National Center for Farmworkers Health. (2001a, January 29). *Facts about farmworkers.* [On-line]. Available: http://www.ncfh.org/aboutfds. htm.

National Center for Farmworker Health. (2001b). *About America's farmworkers: Population demographics.* [On-line]. Available: http://www.ncfh.org/aboutfws.htm#intro.

National Institute of Mental Health. (2000). *Research on mental disorders in rural and frontier populations.* Retrieved January 28, 2001. [On-line]. Available: http://grants.nih.gov/ grants/guide/pa-files/PA-00-082.html.

National Rural Development Partnership. (2001, January 28). *Health Care Task Force.* [On-line]. Available: http://www.rurdev.usda.gov/nrdp/healthcare.html.

National Rural Health Association. (1998, February). *Rural health services, rural communities and reform: A vision for health reform models for America's rural communities.* [On-line]. Available: http://www.nrharural.org.

National Rural Health Association. (1999a). *Access to health care for the uninsured in rural and frontier America.* Retrieved January 24, 2001. [On-line]. Available: http://www.nrharural.org/dc/issuepapers/ipaper15.html.

National Rural Health Association: (1999b). *Mental health in rural America.* Retrieved January 24, 2001. [On-line]. Available: http://www.nrharural.org/dc/issuepaper/ipaper14.html.

National Rural Health Association. (2000, January 28). *Rural and frontier emergency medical services toward the year 2000.* [On-line]. Available: www.nrharural.org/pagefile/issuepaper/paper9.html.

National Rural Recruitment and Retention Network (3R Net). (2001, January 28). *The rural recruitment and retention network.* [On-line]. Available: http://www.3rnet.org/index.asp.

Patton, S. (1995). Empowering women: Improving a community's health. *Nursing Management, 26*(3), 36–38.

Reeves, M., Schafer, K., Hallward, K., & Katten, A. (1999). *Fields of poison: California farmworkers and pesticides.* Pesticide Action Network North America (PANNA). Retrieved June 18, 2001. [On-line]. Available: http://www.globalexchange.org/farmworkers/fieldsOfPoison.html.

Ricketts, T. C., Johnson-Webb, K. D., & Taylor, P. (1998). *Definitions of rural: A handbook for health policy makers and researchers.* Contract Number HRSA 93-857(P). Washington, DC: U.S. Department of Health and Human Services, Federal Office of Rural Health Policy.

Robinson, J. W., & Savage, G. T. (2000). Small, rural hospitals: A fight for survival. *Online Journal of Rural Nursing and Health Care, 1*(1). Retrieved January 27, 2001. [On-line]. Available: http://www.rno.org/journal.

Rogers, C. (1999). Growth of the oldest old population and future implications for rural areas. *Rural Development Perspectives 4(3).* [On-line]. Available: http://www.ers.usda.gov/publications/rdp/rdpoct99/rdpoct99d.pdf.

Rural Policy Research Institute. (2000). *The economic importance of the health care sector.* Retrieved January

27, 2001. [On-line]. Available: http://www.rupri.org/pubs/archive/old/health/orhw/orhw11/index.html.

Runyan, J. L. (1998). *Injuries and fatalities on U.S. farms.* Economic Research Service, U.S. Department of Agriculture. Retrieved January 29, 2001. [On-line]. Available: http://www.ers.usda.gov/publications/summaries/aib739.htm.

Runyan, J. L. (2000). *Summary of federal laws and regulations affecting agricultural employers, 2000.* Economic Research Service, U.S. Department of Agriculture. Agricultural Handbook No. 719. July 2000. Retrieved January 29, 2001. [On-line]. Available: http://www.ers.usda.gov/Publications/ah719/index.htm.

Shupe, W. D. (1980). Introduction. In A. Sovotny & C. Smith (Eds.), *Images of healing* (pp. 8–11). New York: Macmillan.

Smith, L., & Weinert, C. (2000). Telecommunication support for rural women with Diabetes. *Diabetes Educator, 26*(4), 645–655.

Sternas, K. A., O'Hare, P., Lehman, K., & Milligan, R. (1999). Nursing and medical student teaming for service learning in partnership with the community: An emerging holistic model for interdisciplinary education and practice. *Holist Nursing Practice, 13*(2), 66–77.

The Association of State and Territorial Health Officials (ASTHO). (Aug., 1999). *Telehealth* [On-line]. Available: http://www.astho.org/access/documents/abriefs/abriefs99/abrief0899.html.

U.S. Bureau of the Census. (2000). *Metropolitan area population estimates for July 1, 1999 and population change for April 1, 1990 to July 1, 1999 (includes April 1, 1990 population estimates base).* Retrieved January 24, 2001. [On-line]. Available: http://www.census.gov/population/estimates/metro-city/ma99-01.txt.

U.S. Bureau of the Census. (2001a, January 24). *About metropolitan areas.* [On-line]. Available: http://www.census.gov/population/www/estimates/aboutmetro.html.

U.S. Bureau of the Census. (2001b, January 24). *Census 2000 geographic definitions.* [On-line]. Available: http://www.census.gov/geo/www/UR.

U.S. Bureau of the Census. (2001c, June 17). *Profile of general demographic characteristics: 2000 census of population and housing United States.*

[On-line]. Available: http://blue.census.gov/Press-Release/www/2001/2khus.pdf.

U.S. Department of Agriculture. (1999). National Agricultural Statistics Service. *1998 childhood agricultural injuries.* Retrieved January 29, 2001. [On-line]. Available: http://usda.mannlib.cornell.edu.

U.S. Department of Agriculture. (2000a). Economic Research Service. *Farm labor: farm safety.* Retrieved January 29, 2001. [On-line]. Available: http://www.ers.usda.gov/Briefing/farmlabor/farmsafety.

U.S. Department of Agriculture. (2000b). Economic Research Service. *Measuring rurality: County typology codes.* Retrieved January 24, 2001. [On-line]. Available: http://www.ers.usda.gov/Briefing/Rurality/Typology/index.htm.

U.S. Department of Agriculture. (2000c). Economic Research Service (ERS). *Measuring rurality: What is rural? Retrieved January 24, 2001.* [On-line]. Available: http://www.ers.usda.gov/Briefing/Rurality/whatisrural.

U.S. Department of Agriculture. (2000d). Economic Research Service. *Rural population and migration: Rural population change.* Retrieved June 14, 2001. [On-line]. Available: http://www.ers.usda.gov/briefing/Population/popchange.

U.S. Department of Agriculture. (2001, January 27). *Migrant and Seasonal Agricultural Worker Protection Act.* [On-line]. Available: http://www.usda.gov/oce/oce/labor-affairs/mspasumm.htm#Requirements.

U.S. Department of Health And Human Services. (1999a). The National Institute For Occupational Safety And Health. *NIOSH childhood agricultural injury prevention initiative.* Retrieved January 29, 2001. [On-line]. Available: http://www.cdc.gov/niosh/childagz.html.

U.S. Department of Health and Human Services. (1999b). Health Care Financing Administration. *Medicare managed care operational policy letter #46.* Retrieved January 28, 2001. [On-line]. Available: http://www.hcfa.gov/medicare/op1046.htm.

U.S. Department of Health and Human Services. (2000a). Health Care Financing Administration. *1999 Medicaid managed care enrollment report glossary.* Retrieved January 28, 2001. [On-line]. Available: http://www.hcfa.gov/medicaid/mcgloss9.htm.

U.S. Department of Health and Human Services. (2000b). *Healthy people 2010: Understanding and improving health (HP 2010)* (2nd ed.). Washington, DC: U.S. Government Printing Office.

U.S. Department of Health and Human Services. (2001a, January 29). Indian Health Service. *Indian Health Service.* [On-line]. Available: http://www.ihs.gov.

U.S. Department of Health and Human Services. (2001b, January 29). Indian Health Service. *Indian health service medical programs.* [On-line]. Available: http://www.ihs.gov/MedicalPrograms/index.asp.

U.S. Department of Health and Human Services. (2001c, January 27). The National Institute for Occupational Safety and Health. *About NIOSH research and services.* [On-line]. Available: http://www.cdc.gov/niosh/training.html#erc.

U.S. Department of Labor. (2000). *Findings from the National Agricultural Workers Survey (NAWS) 1997–1998. A demographic and employment profile of United States farmworkers. (NAWS).* Retrieved June 18, 2001. [On-line]. Available: http://www.dol.gov/dol/asp/public/programs/agworker/report_8.pdf.

U.S. Department of Labor. (2001, January 27). Occupational Safety and Health Administration. *The OSH Act. Public Law 91-596, 91st Congress, S.2193, December 29, 1970.* [On-line]. Available: http://www.oshaslc.gov/OshAct data/OSHACT. html.

U.S. Executive Office of the President. (1998). *Budget of the United States government fiscal year 1999.* [On-line]. Available: http://www.whitehouse.gov/omb.

Weinert, C., & Burman, M. (1999). The sampler quilt. In A. S. Hinshaw, S. L. Feetham, & J. L. Shaver (Eds.), *Handbook of clinical nursing research* (pp. 75–86). Thousand Oaks, CA: Sage.

Zelarney, P. T., & Ciarlo, J. A. (2000). *Defining and describing frontier areas in the United States: An update: Letter to the field no. 22.* Frontier Mental Health Resource Network. Retrieved January 24, 2001. [On-line]. Available: http://www.wiche.edu/MentalHealth/Frontier/index.htm.

INDEX

Student Tutorial CD-ROM to Accompany Community Health Nursing, 2nd Edition

Standard Flash!
System Requirements

- 100 MHz Pentium w/24 MB of RAM
- Windows™ 95 or newer
- Sound card and speakers
- SVGA 24-bit color display
- 8 megabytes of free disk space

Microsoft® is a registered trademark and Windows™ and NT™ are trademarks of Microsoft Corporation. Netware™ is a trademark of Novell, Inc.

[**Note:** Sound card and speaker are ONLY required for products that include sound.]
Set Up Instructions

1. Double click My Computer
2. Double click the Control Panel icon
3. Double click Add/Remove Programs
4. Click the Install button and follow the on screen prompts from there.

License Agreement for Delmar Learning, a division of Thomson Learning, Inc.
Educational Software/Data

You the customer, and Delmar Learning, a division of Thomson Learning, Inc. incur certain benefits, rights, and obligations to each other when you open this package and use the software/data it contains. BE SURE YOU READ THE LICENSE AGREEMENT CARE-FULLY, SINCE BY USING THE SOFT-WARE/DATA YOU INDICATE YOU HAVE READ, UNDER-STOOD, AND ACCEPTED THE TERMS OF THIS AGREE-MENT.

Your rights:

1. You enjoy a non-exclusive license to use the software/data on a single microcomputer in consideration for payment of the required license fee, (which may be included in the purchase price of an accompanying print component), or receipt of this software/data, and your acceptance of the terms and conditions of this agreement.
2. You acknowledge that you do not own the aforesaid software/data. You also acknowledge that the software/data is furnished "as is," and contains copyrighted and/or proprietary and confidential infor-mation of Delmar Learning, a division of Thomson Learning, Inc. or its licensors.

There are limitations on your rights:

1. You may not copy or print the software/data for any reason whatsoever, except to install it on a hard drive on a single microcomputer and to make one archival copy, unless copying or printing is expressly permitted in writing or statements recorded on the diskette(s).
2. You may not revise, translate, convert, disassemble or otherwise reverse engineer the software/data except that you may add to or rearrange any data recorded on the media as part of the normal use of the software/data.
3. You may not sell, license, lease, rent, loan or other-wise distribute or network the software/data except that you may give the software/data to a student or and instructor for use at school or, temporarily at home.

Should you fail to abide by the Copyright Law of the United States as it applies to this software/data your license to use it will become invalid. You agree to erase or otherwise destroy the software/data immediately after receiving note of termination of this agreement for violation of its provisions from Delmar Learning.

Delmar Learning, a division of Thomson Learning, Inc gives you a LIMITED WARRANTY covering the enclosed software/data. The LIMITED WARRANTY follows this License.

This license is the entire agreement between you and Delmar Learning, a division of Thomson Learning, Inc. interpreted and enforced under New York law.

LIMITED WARRANTY

Delmar Learning, a division of Thomson Learning, Inc. warrants to the original licensee/purchaser of this copy of microcomputer software/data and the media on which it is recorded that the media will be free from defects in material and workmanship for ninety (90) days from the date of original purchase. All implied warranties are limited in duration to this ninety (90) day period. THEREAFTER, ANY IMPLIED WARRANTIES, INCLUDING IMPLIED WARRANTIES OF MERCHANTABILITY AND FITNESS FOR A PARTICULAR PURPOSE, ARE EXCLUDED. THIS WARRANTY IS IN LIEU OF ALL OTHER WARRANTIES, WHETHER ORAL OR WRITTEN, EXPRESS OR IMPLIED.

If you believe the media is defective please return it during the ninety day period to the address shown below. Defective media will be replaced without charge provided that it has not been subjected to misuse or damage.

This warranty does not extend to the software or information recorded on the media. The software and information are provided "AS IS." Any statements made about the utility of the software or information are not to be considered as express or implied warranties.

Limitation of liability: Our liability to you for any losses shall be limited to direct damages, and shall not exceed the amount you paid for the software. In no event will we be liable to you for any indirect, special, incidental, or consequential damages (including loss of profits) even if we have been advised of the possibility of such damages.

Some states do not allow the exclusion or limitation of incidental or consequential damages, or limitations on the duration of implied warranties, so the above limitation or exclusion may not apply to you. This warranty gives you specific legal rights, and you may also have other rights which vary from state to state. Address all correspondence to: Delmar Learning, a division of Thomson Learning, Inc., 5 Maxwell Drive, P.O. Box 8007, Clifton Park, NY 12065-8007. Attention: Technology Department